W9-CHP-521

The Adult Hip

SECOND EDITION

The Adult Hip

SECOND EDITION

Volume I

EDITORS

■ JOHN J. CALLAGHAN, MD

The Lawrence and Marilyn Dorr Chair
Professor of Orthopaedics & Rehabilitation and Bioengineering
University of Iowa
Veterans Administration Hospital
Iowa City, Iowa

■ AARON G. ROSENBERG, MD

Professor of Orthopaedic Surgery
Department of Orthopaedic Surgery
Rush University Medical Center
Chicago, Illinois

■ HARRY E. RUBASH, MD

Chief of Orthopaedic Surgery
Massachusetts General Hospital
Edith M. Ashley Professor
Harvard Medical School
Boston, Massachusetts

● Lippincott Williams & Wilkins
a Wolters Kluwer business
Philadelphia · Baltimore · New York · London
Buenos Aires · Hong Kong · Sydney · Tokyo

Acquisitions Editor: Robert Hurley
Managing Editor: Michelle LaPlante
Marketing Director: Sharon Zinner
Project Manager: Fran Gunning
Manufacturing Manager: Benjamin Rivera
Designer Coordinator: Holly Reid McLaughlin
Compositor: TechBooks
Printer: Edwards Brothers

© 2007 by LIPPINCOTT WILLIAMS & WILKINS
530 Walnut Street
Philadelphia, PA 19106 USA
LWW.com

All rights reserved. This book is protected by copyright. No part of this book may
be reproduced in any form or by any means, including photocopying, or utilized
by any information storage and retrieval system without written permission from
the copyright owner, except for brief quotations embodied in critical articles and
reviews. Materials appearing in this book prepared by individuals as part of their
official duties as U.S. government employees are not covered by the above-
mentioned copyright.

Printed in the USA

Library of Congress Cataloging-in-Publication Data

The adult hip / editors, John J. Callaghan, Aaron G. Rosenberg, Harry
    E. Rubash. — 2nd ed.
      p. ; cm.
    Includes bibliographical references and index.
    ISBN 13: 978-0-7817-5092-9
    ISBN 10: 0-7817-5092-X (alk. paper)
    1. Hip joint—Surgery.   2. Hip joint—Diseases.   3. Artificial hip joint.
I. Callaghan, John J.   II. Rosenberg, Aaron G.   III. Rubash, Harry E.
    [DNLM: 1. Hip Joint—surgery.   2. Biocompatible Materials.
3. Bone Diseases—surgery.   4. Hip Prosthesis.   5. Hip.   6. Joint
Diseases—surgery.   WE 860 A2435 2007]
    RD549.A36 2007
    617.5′81—dc22

                                                                    2006024802

Care has been taken to confirm the accuracy of the information presented and to
describe generally accepted practices. However, the authors, editors, and publisher
are not responsible for errors or omissions or for any consequences from application of the information in this book and make no warranty, expressed or implied,
with respect to the currency, completeness, or accuracy of the contents of the publication. Application of this information in a particular situation remains the professional responsibility of the practitioner.

The authors, editors, and publisher have exerted every effort to ensure that drug
selection and dosage set forth in this text are in accordance with current recommendations and practice at the time of publication. However, in view of ongoing
research, changes in government regulations, and the constant flow of information
relating to drug therapy and drug reactions, the reader is urged to check the package insert for each drug for any change in indications and dosage and for added
warnings and precautions. This is particularly important when the recommended
agent is a new or infrequently employed drug.

Some drugs and medical devices presented in this publication have Food and
Drug Administration (FDA) clearance for limited use in restricted research settings.
It is the responsibility of the health care provider to ascertain the FDA status of
each drug or device planned for use in their clinical practice.

To purchase additional copies of this book, call our customer service department at (800) 638-3030 or fax orders to (301) 824-7390. International customers
should call (301)714-2324.

Visit Lippincott Williams & Wilkins on the Internet: at LWW.com. Lippincott
Williams & Wilkins customer service representatives are available from 8:30 am to
6 pm, EST.

                    10 9 8 7 6 5 4 3 2 1

To my wife, Kim,
and our children, Patrick and Katie,
for their love, friendship, and never-ending support,
as well as for their uncanny ability to keep me balanced and grounded
J.J.C.

To my wife, Iris,
whose love, support, and example fill my life and world,
and to our wonderful children, AJ, Jess, Becca, and Cody,
who put everything into perspective
A.G.R.

To my wife, Kimberly, for her
love, support, and friendship for over 3 decades
H.E.R.

Contents

Preface

As students of hip surgery, we are acutely aware of the giants in our field who have paved the way for our contemporary ability to diagnose and treat hip diseases. We are fortunate to live in a time when access to information is more readily obtained than it was in the past. This second edition of *The Adult Hip* represents our contribution to this reality.

We developed this second edition of *The Adult Hip* to provide a comprehensive, organized text on adult hip pathology and treatment. The enormous amount of investigative work that has been performed and reported on the normal hip, the disease processes affecting it, and treatment of these diseases are provided by this one complete and convenient source. We were fortunate to attract the most respected world authorities in this field, and the book reflects the depth of their various knowledge and expertise.

The 112 chapters in this edition of *The Adult Hip* are organized as two volumes with seven major sections. The *"Basic Science"* section provides the necessary underpinnings for sound clinical judgment. It includes pertinent information concerning anatomy, biomaterial, wear, the biology of grafts, and osteolysis, as well as issues related to bearing surface options. Distinctive features of the clinical sections include beautifully illustrated chapters on surgical anatomy and minimally invasive and standard approaches, as well as in-depth coverage of alternatives to arthroplasty. In addition, eminent authorities provide detailed analyses on evaluation and imaging of the hip, the various disorders that affect the adult hip, and important details of perioperative management from anesthesia and nursing standpoints.

Because it remains the most performed hip operation, total hip arthroplasty receives exhaustive attention, including indications, contraindications, technical details, complications, and outcomes, as well as the economic impact of both primary and revision procedures. The inclusion of multiple authors, representing varying and sometimes opposing points of view, accurately represents the profusion of surgical techniques and approaches to the problem of contemporary hip arthroplasty. In addition, multiple authors have represented the various implant options in primary and revision surgery. Some of these approaches are so new that their utility is not yet clear; but they represent potential solutions to problems that have not yet been adequately addressed.

This text can serve as a comprehensive review for medical students, researchers, and students in the basic sciences related to hip reconstruction, orthopaedic residents, and fellows in adult reconstructive hip surgery. At the same time, it is a valuable resource for those seeking practical advice and expertise concerning the details of hip reconstruction, including general orthopaedic surgeons, experienced hip surgeons, and others who care for patients with hip problems. All of these groups will find information to broaden their scope of knowledge and clinical performance.

Our goal for this edition of *The Adult Hip* is to set a new standard for a text on adult hip surgery. We hope that we have captured the extensive advances in the field of hip surgery, especially since the development of total hip arthroplasty, and that all readers will better understand the disorders of the adult hip and their treatments.

Acknowledgments

Many people have helped to make the second edition of *The Adult Hip* even more comprehensive than the first: my father Don who is recently deceased, and my ever inspiring mother Jeanne, who promoted intellectual curiosity and the search for truth; my teachers, from whose inspiration came my devotion to the profession; Emil T. Hofman and the faculty at the University of Notre Dame; Wilton H. Bunch and the faculty at Loyola Stritch School of Medicine; Richard C. Johnston, my father in hip surgery, and the faculty at the University of Iowa; Eduardo A. Salvati, my mentor in hip surgery, and the faculty at the Hospital for Special Surgery; my friends and colleagues in the Hip Society; my students who have endured my passion for the understanding of the hip and the dissemination of that understanding; Lori Yoder, my secretary, who handled all of the issues of a complex practice during the preparation of this book; Steve Liu, my devoted research associate and friend who handled all the coordination of faxes, messages, and manuscripts crucial to the timely completion of this book; Robert Hurley and the publishers at Lippincott Williams & Wilkins, who handled every detail of the editing process and assured the timely submission of manuscripts, which is indeed a huge task for such a production as this book; and finally, most importantly, the authors, who have sacrificed their time and energy in the preparation of this text.

—J. J. C.

My contributions would not be possible without my mentors: Henry J. Mankin, MD and Jorge O. Galante, MD, who guided my development as a surgeon, educator, and investigator. I am abundantly grateful for my partners, especially Joshua Jacobs, MD and Wayne Paprosky, MD, who have provided wise counsel and strong support through the years, and for the dedicated work of Regina Barden, RN, whose attention to detail, comprehensive patient care, and search for truth and excellence in research have been an inspiration both for me and for my patients for 20 years.

—A. G. R.

Many people have been instrumental in the completion of the second edition of *The Adult Hip*: my eighty-three-year-old, mother, whose work ethic and dedication to her family continues to inspire me; Dr. William H. Harris, whose compassion and genius have guided the field of arthroplasty for more than three decades and who continues to teach me what it means to be an educator, investigator, gentleman, and leader; Dr. James H. Herndon, whose wisdom, insight, leadership, and mentoring have contributed to the success of so many academic orthopaedists; my Residents and Fellows, who have tolerantly endured my determination to pursue this important project; Karen Bernstein, Clinical Research Editor, who works hard and has an amazing ability to multitask so many important projects in our offices at the MGH; and the many authors and co-authors who have contributed to the success of this most up-to-date version of primary and hip arthroplasty.

—H. E. R.

Foreword

Advances in the field of total hip replacement surgery are occurring at an accelerating rate. Simply consider the recent remarkable advances in the concepts, techniques, and materials of total hip replacement. For example, the number one long term problem in total hip replacement for the first forty years was periprosthetic osteolysis. Our present understanding of this problem is dramatically better than it was with the last edition of *The Adult Hip*. With the improvement in the conceptual features of periprosthetic osteolysis have come improvements in implant design, materials, and surgical techniques. This second edition of *The Adult Hip* consolidates and integrates this rapidly increasing information.

This two-volume set is much more than just a text on total hip surgery; it provides succinct presentations of the most up to date primary and revision hip surgery, development, anatomy, and biomechanics, as well as an especially strong section on biomechanics, wear and bearing surface options. In addition to a detailed presentation of perioperative considerations, the text provides important information on the alternatives to total hip arthroplasty.

It is a substantial achievement to bring all of these advances into one beautifully integrated text that comprehensively assesses the current state-of-the-art advances in adult hip surgery. The editors are vigorous, thoughtful, and critical. They have selected outstanding contributors and have ensured that the presentations are balanced, inclusive, and lucid. The authors draw deeply from the wellsprings of creative innovation and evaluation of all aspects of total hip replacement, enabling the reader to benefit from their skills and knowledge.

Finally, this text deals admirably with the three important "hows" of adult hip surgery: how to assess problems, how to interpret concepts, and how to manage patients.

The editors and contributors to this second edition are to be congratulated. We, as surgeons, gain immeasurably from this compilation of timely advances, enabling us to better serve our patients.

—William H. Harris, MD

Contributors

ROY K. AARON, MD
Professor
Department of Orthopaedic Surgery
Brown Medical School
Providence, Rhode Island

MICHAELENE ABRAN, RN, BSN
Clinical Nurse Coordinator
Medical Surgical Nursing
Rush University Medical Center
Chicago, Illinois

SANJEEV AGARWAL, FRCS
Specialist Registrar
Department of Orthopaedics
Leeds Orthopaedic Program
Leeds, United Kingdom

AJAY AGGARWAL
Department of Orthopaedics Surgery
University of Iowa Hospitals
      and Clinics
Iowa City, Iowa

MAURICE ALBRIGHT, MD
Instructor
Department of Orthopaedic Surgery
Harvard Medical School
Assistant in Orthopaedics
Department of Orthopaedic Surgery
Massachusetts General Hospital
Boston, Massachusetts

THOMAS P. ANDRIACCHI, PhD
Professor
Department of Mechanical Engineering and
Department of Orthopaedic Surgery
Stanford University
Stanford, California

MICHAEL J. ARCHIBECK, MD
Joint Replacement Surgeon
New Mexico Center for Joint
      Replacement Surgery
New Mexico Orthopaedics
Albuquerque, New Mexico

DEREK R. ARMFIELD, MD
Assistant Professor
Department of Radiology
University of Pittsburgh School of Medicine
University of Pittsburgh Medical Center
Pittsburgh, Pennsylvania

MIGUEL A. AYERZA, MD
Department of Orthopaedic Surgery
Italian Hospital of Buenos Aires
Buenos Aires
Argentina

W. TIMOTHY BALLARD, MD
Chattanooga, Tennessee

REGINA M. BARDEN, RN, BSN, ONC
Orhopaedic Nurse Clinician
Department of Orthopaedics
Rush University Medical Center
Chicago, Illinois

WILLIAM L. BARGAR, MD
Assistant Clinical Professor
Department of Orthopaedic Surgery
University of California Davis School of Medicine
Sutter General Hospital
Sacramento, California

ROBERT L. BARRACK, MD
Charles and Joanne Knight Distinguished Professor of
      Orthopaedic Surgery
Department of Orthopaedic Surgery
Washington University School of Medicine
Director, Adult Reconstructive Surgery
Chief of Staff
Department of Orthopaedic Surgery
Barnes-Jewish Hospital
St. Louis, Missouri

SUSAN E. BARRETT, MD, MPH
Mulroy Orthopaedics in Sports Medicine
Milford, Massachusetts

JOHN W. BARRINGTON, MD
Surgeon
Texas Center for Joint Replacement
Plano, Texas

ANUJ BELLARE, PhD
Assistant Professor
Department of Orthopedic Surgery
Harvard Medical School
Director, Orthopedic Nanotechnology Laboratory
Department of Orthopedic Surgery
Brigham and Women's Hospital
Boston, Massachusetts

RICHARD A. BERGER, MD
Assistant Professor of Orthopaedics
Department of Orthopedic Surgery
Rush Medical College
Chicago, Illinois

ARNOLD T. BERMAN
Department of Orthopaedic Surgery
Allegheny University Hospitals
Philadelphia, Pennsylvania

DANIEL J. BERRY, MD
Professor and Chair
Department of Orthopedic Surgery
Mayo Clinic
Rochester, Minnesota

HARI P. BEZWADA, MD
Assistant Clinical Professor
Department of Orthopaedic Surgery
University of Pennsylvania School of Medicine
Orthopaedic Surgeon
Pennsylvania Orthopaedics
Pennsylvania Hospital
Philadelphia, Pennsylvania

RUDI G. BITSCH, MD

JONATHAN BLACK, PhD, FBSE
Hunter Professor Emeritus of Bioengineering
Clemson University
Clemson, South Carolina

J. DAVID BLAHA, MD
Professor of Adult Joint Reconstruction
Department of Orthopaedic Surgery
University of Michigan
Ann Arbor, Michigan

SORIN BLENDEA, MD
Clinical Research Fellow
The Western Pennsylvania Hospital
Institute for Computer-Assisted Orthopaedic Surgery
Pittsburgh, Pennsylvaina
Orthopaedic Surgery Resident
Centre Hospitalier Universitaire Grenoble
Grenoble, France

PAUL M. BOEHM, MD
Associate Professor
Department of Orthopaedic Surgery
University Tuebingen
Tuebingen, Germany
Head
Department of Orthopaedic Surgery
High-Tech-Clinic
Nuremberg, Germany

PATRICK BOLAND, MD
Preceptor, Weill Medical College
Cornell University
Clinical Member and Attending Orthopaedic Surgery
Memorial Sloan Kettering Cancer Center
New York, New York

LIEUTENANT COMMANDER ERIC G. BONENBERGER, MD
Arthroplasty Section Head
Department of Orthopaedic Surgery
Naval Hospital Jacksonville
Staff Orthopaedic Sugeon
Department of Orthopaedic Sugery
University of Florida and Shands
Jacksonville, Florida

TODD A. BORUS, MD
Fellow
Department of Orthopaedic Surgery
Brigham and Women's Hospital
Boston, Massachusetts

TOREY P. BOTTI, MD
Resident in Orthopaedic Surgery
Division of Orthopaedics
The University of Chicago Hospitals and Clinics
Chicago, Illinois

F. BOTTNER

ROBERT B. BOURNE, MD, FRCSC
Professor
Department of Surgery
University of Western Ontario
Chair and Chief
Division of Orthopaedic Surgery
London Health Sciences Centre
London, Ontario
Canada

KEVIN J. BOZIC, MD, MBA
Assistant Professor in Residence
Department of Orthopaedic Surgery
University of California, San Francisco
San Francisco, California

BARRY D. BRAUSE, MD
New York, New York

MARTHA F. BRINSON, MSN
Staff
Southern Joint Replacement Institute
Nashville, Tennessee

BARRETT S. BROWN, MD
Department of Orthopedic Surgery
University of Kansas Medical Center
Kansas City, Kansas

CALVIN R. BROWN, JR., MD
Associate Professor of Medicine
Section of Rheumatology
Rush Medical College
Chicago, Illinois

THOMAS D. BROWN, PhD
Richard and Janice Johnston Chair of Orthopaedic
    Biomechanics
Department of Orthopaedics and Rehabilitation
University of Iowa
Iowa City, Iowa

WILLIAM D. BUGBEE, MD
Associate Professor
Department of Orthopaedics
University of California at San Diego
La Jolla, California

PIETER BUMA, PhD
Department of Orthopaedics
Radboud University Nijmegen Medical Centre
Nijmegen, The Netherlands

DENNIS W. BURKE, MD
Department of Orthopaedic Surgery
Massachusetts General Hospital
Harvard Medical School
Boston, Massachusetts

R. STEPHEN J. BURNETT, MD, FRCS(C)
Assistant Professor
Department of Orthopedic Surgery
Washington University School of Medicine
Staff Physician
Barnes-Jewish Hospital
Barnes-Jewish West County Hospital
St. Louis, Missouri

CONSTANT A. BUSCH, MB BS, BSC (HONS), FRCS (ENG), FRCS (TR AND ORTH)
Consultant Orthopaedic Surgeon
Rowley Bristow Orthopaedic Unit
Ashford and St. Peter's NHS Trust
Chertsey, Surrey
United Kingdom

MIGUEL E. CABANELA, MD
Professor
Department of Orthopedic Surgery
Mayo Clinic College of Medicine
Consultant
Department of Orthopedic Surgery
Mayo Clinic
Rochester, Minnesota

JOHN J. CALLAGHAN, MD
The Lawrence and Marilyn Darr Chair
Professor of Orthopaedics and Bioengineering
University of Iowa
Professor
Department of Orthopaedics
    and Rehabilitation
University of Iowa Health Care
Iowa City, Iowa

WILLIAM N. CAPELLO, MD
Professor
Department of Orthopaedics
Indiana University
Surgeon
Department of Orthopaedics
Clarian Health
Indianapolis, Indiana

JOHN A. F. CHARITY, MD
Research Fellow
Princess Elizabeth Orthopaedic Centre
Royal Devon and Exeter NHS Trust
Exeter, Devon, England
United Kingdom

PETER P. CHIANG, MD
Orthopaedic Surgeon, Adult Reconstruction
Department of Orthopaedic Surgery
Exempla Good Samaritan Hospital
Layfayette, Colorado

E. S. CHOI, MD

MICHAEL J. CHRISTIE, MD
Associate Clinical Professor
Department of Orthopaedics and Rehabilitation
Vanderbilt University Medical Center
Director
Southern Joint Replacement Institute
Nashville, Tennessee

JOHN C. CLOHISY, MD
Associate Professor
Department of Orthopaedic Surgery
Washington University School of Medicine
Co-Chief, Adult Reconstructive Surgery
Department of Orthopaedic Surgery
Barnes-Jewish Hospital
St. Louis, Missouri

DENNIS K. COLLIS, MD
Associate Clinical Professor
Department of Orthopaedics
Oregon Health Sciences University
Portland, Oregon
Orthopedic Surgeon
Sacred Heart Medical Center
Eugene, Oregon

ROY D. CROWNINSHIELD, PhD
Professor
Department of Orthopaedic Surgery
Rush Medical College
Chicago, Illinois

FRANCIS P. CYRAN, MD
Assistant Professor
Department of Orthopaedic Surgery
University of Californa, Los Angeles
Attending Staff Surgeon
Department of Orthopaedic Surgery
UCLA Healthcare Westwood and Santa Monica
Santa Monica, California

JAMES A. D'ANTONIO, MD
Greater Pittsburgh Orthopedic Associates
Moon Township, Pennsylvania

LAWRENCE P. DAVIS, MD
Associate Professor
Department of Radiology
Wayne State University
Detroit, Michigan

DAVID K. DEBOER, MD
Assistant Clinical Professor
Department of Orthopaedics and Rehabilitation
Vanderbilt University Medical Center
Director
Southern Joint Replacement Institute
Nashville, Tennessee

CRAIG J. DELLA VALLE, MD
Assistant Professor
Department of Orthopaedic Surgery
Rush University Medical Center
Chicago, Illinois

DOUGLAS A. DENNIS, MD
Adjunct Professor
Department of Biomedical Engineering
University of Tennessee
Knoxville, Tennessee
Co-Director, Porter Center for Joint Replacement
Department of Orthopaedic Surgery
Porter Adventist Hospital
Denver, Colorado

PAUL E. DICESARE, MD
Professor of Orthopaedic Surgery
    and Cell Biology
New York University School of Medicine
Director
Musculoskeletal Research Center
Chief, Adult Recontructive Service
New York University Hospital
    for Joint Diseases
New York, New York

ANTHONY M. DIGIOIA III, MD
Clinical Associate Professor
Department of Orthopaedic Surgery
University of Pittsburgh School of Medicine
Orthopaedic Surgeon
Renaissance Orthopaedics
Magee-Women's Hospital
Pittsburgh, Pennsylvania

LAWRENCE D. DORR, MD
Director
Arthritis Institute
Centinela Freeman Regional Medical Center
Inglewood, California

PATRICK J. DUFFY, MBCHB, FRCS
Former Clinical and Research Fellow
Department of Orthopaedics
University of British Columbia
Former Clinical and Research Fellow
Division of Lower Limb Reconstruction and
    Oncology
Department of Orthopaedics
Vancouver General Hospital
Vancouver, British Columbia

CLIVE P. DUNCAN, MD, MSc, FRCSC
Professor and Chairman
Department of Orthopaedics
University of British Columbia
Head
Department of Orthopaedics
Vancouver General Hospital
Vancouver, British Columbia

SRIDHAR M. DURBHAKULA, MD
Clinical Instructor
Department of Orthopaedic Surgery
Johns Hopkins Hospital
Baltimore, Maryland

JEFFREY J. ECKARDT, MD
Professor
Helga and Walter Oppenheimer Chair of Musculoskeletal
    Oncology
Department of Orthopaedic Surgery
University of California, Los Angeles
Vice Chair
Department of Orthopaedic Surgery
UCLA Medical Center
Santa Monica, California

THOMAS A. EINHORN, MD
Professor and Chairman
Department of Orthopaedic Surgery
Boston University Medical Center
Boston, Massachusetts

ROGER H. EMERSON, JR., MD
Associate Clinical Professor
Department of Orthopaedic Surgery
University of Texas Southwestern
    Medical School
Dallas, Texas
Active Staff
Department of Orthopaedic Surgery
Presbyterian Hospital of Plano
Plano, Texas

CHARLES A. ENGH, MD
Anderson Orthopaedic Research Institute
Anderson Orthopaedic Clinic
Alexandria, Virginia

BRIAN G. EVANS, MD
Department of Orthopaedic Surgery
Georgetown University Medical Center
Washington, D.C.

BRIAN T. FEELEY, MD
University of California School of Medicine
Los Angeles, California

JUDY R. FEINBERG, PhD
Indiana University School of Medicine
Department of Orthopaedic Surgery
541 Clinical Drive – CL600
Indianapolis, Indiana

ANTHONY B. FIORILLO, MD
Francis X. Solano, Jr.
Department of Medicine
University of Pittsburgh Medical Center
Pittsburgh, Pennsylvania

ALFONS FISCHER, PROF. DR.-ING.
Professor
Department of Material Science and Engineering
University of Duisburg-Essen
Duisburg, Germany

ROBERT H. FITZGERALD, JR., MS, MD
Professor and Chairman
Department of Orthopaedic Surgery
Hospital of the University of Pennsylvania
Philadelphia, Pennsylvania

VINCENT A. FOWBLE, MD
Palm Beach Orthopaedic Institute
Palm Beach Gardens, Florida

ANDREW A. FREIBERG, MD
Assistant Professor
Department of Orthopedic Surgery
Harvard Medical School
Chief
Adult Reconstructive Service
Massachusetts General Hospital
Boston, Massachusetts

ANIL K. GAMBHIR, FRCS
Consultant Orthopaedic Surgeon
Centre for Hip Surgery
Wrightington Hospital
Wigan, Lancashire, England
United Kingdom

JEAN W. M. GARDENIERS, MD, PhD
Department of Orthopaedics
Radboud University Nijmegen Medical Centre
Nijmegen, The Netherlands

TIMOTHY M. GANEY, PhD
Orthopaedic Research Director
Georgia Baptist Medical Center
Atlanta, Georgia

KEVIN L. GARVIN, MD
Professor and Chair
Department of Orthopaedic Surgery
University of Nebraska Medical Center
Omaha, Nebraska

RUDOLPH G. T. GEESINK, MD, PhD
Professor
Department of Orthopaedic Surgery
University of Maastricht, the Netherlands
Head
Department of Orthopaedic Surgery
University Hospital Maastricht
Maastricht, The Netherlands

GRAHAM A. GIE, FRCSEd
Honorary Research Fellow
Department of Engineering Science
University of Exeter
Consultant Orthopaedic Surgeon
Princess Elizabeth Orthopaedic Centre
Royal Devon and Exeter NHS Hospital Trust
Exeter, Devon
England

JEREMY L. GILBERT, PhD
Professor of Biomaterials and Associate Dean for
    Research and Doctoral Programs
Department of Biomedical and Chemical Engineering
College of Engineering and Computer Science
Syracuse University
Syracuse, New York

ANDREW H. GLASSMAN, MD, MS
Associate Professor
Department of Orthopaedics Surgery
Ohio State University College of Medicine
Director, Total Joint Replacement Service
Department of Orthopaedic Surgery
Ohio State University Hospitals
Columbus, Ohio

VICTOR M. GOLDBERG, MD
Professor
Department of Orthopaedics
Case Western Reserve University
Attending
Department of Orthopaedics
University Hospital of Cleveland
Cleveland, Ohio

STUART GOODMAN, MD, PhD, FRCSC, FACS, FBSE
Professor
Department of Orthopaedic Surgery
Stanford University
Stanford University Medical Center
Stanford, California

ROBERT R. L. GRAY, MD
Resident
Department of Orthopedic Surgery
Rush University Medical Center
Chicago, Illinois

PETER GRISS
der Philipps Universitat
Marburg, Germany

ALLAN E. GROSS, MD, FRCSC, O. ONT.
Full Professor
Department of Surgery
Faculty of Medicine
University of Toronto
Staff Orthopaedic Surgeon
Department of Surgery
Division of Orthopaedics
Mount Sinai Hospital
Toronto, Ontario
Canada

WILLIAM G. HAMILTON, MD
Clinical Instructor
Anderson Orthopaedic Research Institute
Orthopaedic Surgeon
Department of Orthopaedic Surgery
Inova Mount Vernon Hospital
Alexandria, Virginia

BRETT J. HAMPTON, MD
Director, Adult Reconstruction
Department of Orthopaedics and Rehabilitation
Walter Reed Army Medical Center
Washington, DC

ARLEN D. HANSSEN, MD
Professor
Department of Orthopedic Surgery
Mayo Clinic
Rochester, Minnesota

WILLIAM H. HARRIS, MD
Chief Hip and Implant Unit
Director
Orthopaedic Bromechanics Laboratory
Clinical Professor
Department of Orthopaedic Surgery
Massachusetts General Hospital
Boston, Massachusetts

JAMES M. HARTFORD, MD
Staff Physician
Department of Orthopedic Surgery
Palo Alto Medical Foundation
Palo Alto, California

MICHAEL HAWKINS

WILLIAM L. HEALY, MD
Professor
Department of Orthopaedic Surgery
Boston University Medical Center
Boston, Massachusetts
Chairman
Department of Orthopaedic Surgery
Lahey Clinic
Burlington, Massachusetts

DAVID A. HECK, MD
Dallas, Texas

CHRISTIAN HEISEL, MD
Heidelberg, Germany

KELLY J. HENDRICKS, MD
Assistant Professor
Department of Orthopaedic Surgery
Adult Reconstruction
University of Kansas Medical Center
Kansas City, Kansas

NICOLETTE H.M. HOEFNAGELS, MSc
Department of Orthopaedic Surgery
University Hospital Maastricht
Maastricht, The Netherlands

DONALD W. HOWIE, PhD, FRACS, MBBS
Professor and Head
Department of Orthopaedics and Trauma
Univesity of Adelaide
Clinical Director
Orthopaedic and Trauma Service
Royal Adelaide Hospital
Adelaide, South Australia

WILLIAM J. HOZACK, MD
Professor
Department of Orthopedic Surgery
Rothman Institute Orthopedics
Chief
Hip and Knee Replacement Service
Thomas Jefferson University Medical School
Philadelphia, Pennsylvania

WELLINGTON K. HSU, MD
Resident Surgeon
Department of Orthopaedic Surgery
University of California, Los Angeles Medical Center
Los Angles, California

RIK HUISKES, PhD
Professor of Orthopaedic Biomechanics
Department of Biomedical Engineering
Eindhoven University of Technology
Eindhoven, The Netherlands

DAVID S. HUNGERFORD, MD
Professor
Department of Orthopaedic Surgery
Johns Hopkins University
Attending
Department of Orthopaedics
Good Samaritan Hospital
Baltimore, Maryland

MARC W. HUNGERFORD, MD
Assistant Professor
Department of Orthopedic Surgery
Johns Hopkins University
Baltimore, Maryland

MICHAEL H. HUO, MD
Associate Professor
Department of Orthopedic Surgery
University of Texas Southwestern Medical Center
Dallas, Texas

DEBRA E. HURWITZ, PhD
Associate Professor
Department of Orthopedic Surgery
Rush University Medical Center
Chicago, Illinois

RICHARD IORIO, MD
Associate Professor
Department of Orthopaedic Surgery
Boston University Medical Center
Boston, MA
Senior Attending Orthopaedic Surgeon
Lahey Clinic Medical Center
Burlington, Massachusetts

JOSHUA J. JACOBS, MD
Crown Family Professor of Orthopaedic Surgery
Department of Orthopaedics
Rush University Medical Center
Chicago, Illinois

VICTOR T. JANDO, MD CM, FRCSC
Former Clinical and Research Fellow
Department of Orthopaedics
University of British Columbia
Former Clinical and Research Fellow
Division of Lower Limb Reconstruction and
    Oncology
Department of Orthopaedics
Vancouver, British Columbia

BRANISLAV JARAMAZ, PhD
Scientific Director
Institute for Computer-Assisted Orthopaedic Surgery
The Western Pennsylvania Hospital
Pittsburgh, Pennsylvania

MURALI JASTY, MD
Associate Clinical Professor
Department of Orthopaedic Surgery
Massachusetts General Hospital
Boston, Massachusetts

WILLIAM A. JIRANEK, MD
Associate Professor
Department of Orthopaedic Surgery
Medical College of Virginia
Virginia Commonwealth University
Chief, Adult Reconstruction Section
Department of Orthopaedic Surgery
Virginia Commonwealth University Health System
Richmond, Virginia

JAMES D. JOHNSTON
Division of Orthopaedic Engineering Research
University of British Columbia
Vancouver, British Columbia
Canada

RICHARD C. JOHNSTON, MD
Department of Orthopaedics
University of Iowa
Iowa City, Iowa

MICHAEL N. KANG, MD
Arthritis Service Clinical Fellow
Department of Orthopaedic Surgery
Stanford University Medical Center
Postdoctoral Clinical Fellow
Department of Orthopaedic Surgery
Stanford Hospital and Clinics
Stanford, California

PETER R. KAY, FRCS
Senior Lecturer
Department of Orthopaedics
Manchester University
Manchester, England
Chairman
Wrightington Hospital
Lancashire, England
United Kingdom

BRYAN T. KELLY, MD
Hospital for Special Surgery
New York, New York

JAMES A. KEENEY, MD
Orthopaedic Surgery Clinic
Wilford Hall Medical Center
San Antonio, Texas

HEINO KIENAPFEL, MD, PhD
der Philipps Universitat
Marburg, Germany

SHIN-YOON KIM, MD, PhD
Professor
Department of Orthopedic Surgery
Kyungpook National University, School of Medicine
Chairman
Department of Orthopedic Surgery
Kyungpook University Hospital
Daegu, Korea

RICHARD D. KOMISTEK, PhD
Professor
Department of Biomedical Engineering
University of Tennessee
Knoxville, Tennessee

PAUL F. LACHIEWICZ, MD
Professor
Department of Orthopaedics
University of North Carolina at Chapel Hill
Attending Surgeon, Department of Orthopaedics
University of North Carolina Hospitals
Chapel Hill, North Carolina

TONY D. LAMBERTON, FRACS
Consultant Orthopaedic Surgeon
Department of Orthopaedic Surgery
Tauranga Hospital
Tauranga, New Zealand

CARLOS J. LAVERNIA, MD
Adjunct Clinical Professor
Department of Othopaedics
University of Miama
Medical Director
Department of Orthopaedics
Mercy Hospital
Miami, Florida

JO-ANNE E. LEE, MS
Nurse Practitioner
Department of Orthopedics
New England Baptist Hospital
Boston, Massachusetts

JACK E. LEMONS, MS, PhD
Professor
Department of Prosthodontics and Biomaterials
University of Alabama at Birmingham
Birmingham, Alabama

SETH S. LEOPOLD, MD
Associate Professor
Department of Orthopaedics and Sports Medicine
University of Washington Medical Center
Seattle, Washington

BRETT R. LEVINE, MD, MS
Adult Reconstruction Fellow
Department of Orthopaedics
Rush University Medical Center
Chicago, Illinois

HARLAN B. LEVINE, MD
Hartzband Joint Replacement Institute
Paramus, New Jersey

DAVID G. LEWALLEN, MD
Professor
Mayo Clinic College of Medicine
Chair, Division of Adult Recontruction
Department of Orthopaedic Surgery
Mayo Clinic
Rochester, Minnesota

JAY R. LIEBERMAN, MD
Professor
Department of Orthopaedic Surgery
David Geffen School of Medicine at UCLA
Physician
Departments of Joint Replacement and Orthopaedic Trauma
UCLA Medical Center
Santa Monica, California

CHRISTOPHER B. LYNCH

ANDREW D. MACDOWELL, MA, FRCS
Lecturer
Department of Orthopaedics and Trauma
University of Adelaide
Joint Replacement Fellow
Orthopaedic and Trauma Service
Royal Adelaide Hospital
Adelaide, South Australia

R. MAHFOUZ

CRAIG R. MAHONEY, MD
Des Moines, Iowa

DAVID R. MAISH

CYNTHIA W. MAJERSKE, MD
Department of Physical Medicine
　and Rehabilitation
University of Pittsburgh Medical Center
Pittsburgh, Pennsylvania

WILLIAM J. MALONEY, MD
Professor and Chairman
Department of Orthopaedic Surgery
Stanford University Medical Center
Chairman
Department of Orthopaedic Surgery
Stanford Hospital and Clinics
Stanford, California

MICHAEL T. MANLEY, PhD
Consultant Biomedical Engineer
Ridgewood, New Jersey

DAVID W. MANNING, MD
Assistant Professor
Department of Surgery
Section of Orthopaedics
University of Chicago
Assistant Professor of Surgery and
　Adult Reconstruction
Department of Surgery
Section of Orthopaedics
University of Chicago Hospitals
Chicago, Illinois

JOHN M. MARTELL, MD
Associate Professor of Surgery
Department of Orthopaedic Surgery
University of Chicago
Chicago, Illinois

BASSAM A. MASRI MD, FRCSC
Associate Professor
Department of Orthopaedics
University of British Columbia
Head
Division of Lower Limb Reconstruction
　& Oncology
Department of Orthopaedics
Vancouver General Hospital
Vancouver, British Columbia

JAMES P. MCAULEY, MD, FRCSC
Associate Clinical Professor
Department of Orthopaedic Surgery
University of Maryland
College Park, MD
Consultant
Anderson Orthopaedic Institute and
Anderson Orthopaedic Research Institute
Inova Mount Vernon Hospital
Alexandria, Virginia

JOSEPH C. MCCARTHY, MD
Clinical Professor
Department of Orthopaedic Surgery
Tufts University School of Medicine
Clinical Professor of Orthopedic Surgery
Department of Orthopedics
New England Baptist Hospital
Boston, Massachusetts

THOMAS A. MCDONALD, MD
Foot and Ankle Surgery
New England Orthopaedic Surgeons
Springfield, Massachusetts

WILLIAM A. McGANN, MD
St. Mary's Medical Center
Orthopaedic Education
San Francisco, California

HARRY A. McKELLOP, PhD
Associate Professor
Department of Orthopaedics and Biomedical Engineering
The Vermont Luck Orthopaedic
Research Center
University of Southern California
Los Angeles, California

PATRICK A. MEERE, MD
Clinical Assistant Professor
Department of Orthopaedic Surgery
Chief, Ortho A Service
Department of Orthopaedic Surgery
New York University Hospital for Joint Diseases
New York, New York

R. MICHAEL MENEGHINI, MD
Orthopaedic Surgeon
Joint Replacement Surgeons of Indiana
St. Vincent Center for Joint Replacement
Indianapolis, Indiana

MICHAEL D. MILLER, MD
Associate Professor Department of Orthopedic Surgery
University of Arizona
Department of Orthopedic Surgery
University Medical Center
Tucson, Arizona

MICHAEL B. MILLIS, MD
Associate Professor
Clinical Orthopaedic Surgery
Harvard Medical School
Director, Adolescent and Young Adult Hip Unit
Children's Hospital
Boston, Massachusetts

STEPHEN B. MURPHY, MD
Center for Computer Assisted and Reconstructive Surgery
New England Baptist Hospital
Boston, Massachusetts

CRAIG G. MOHLER, MD
Othro Healthcare
Eugene, Oregon

MICHAEL A. MONT, MD
Reuben Institute for Advanced Orthopaedics
Baltimore, Maryland

J. CRAIG MORRISON, MD
Director
Southern Joint Replacement Institute
Nashville, Tennessee

MICHAEL C. MUNIN, MD
Department of Physical Medicine and Rehabilitation
University of Pittsburgh Medical Center
Pittsburgh, Pennsylvania

ORHUN K. MURATOGLU, PhD
Associate Professor
Department of Orthopaedic Surgery
Harvard Medical School
Co-director
Alan Gerry Scholar and Deputy Director
Harris Orthopaedic Biomechanics and Biomaterials
    Laboratory
Massachusetts General Hospital
Boston, Massachusetts

STEPHEN B. MURPHY, MD
Assistant Professor
Department of Orthopedic Surgery
Tufts University School of Medicine
Associate Orthopedic Surgeon
Center for Computer Assisted and Reconstructive Surgery
Department of Orthopedic Surgery
New England Baptist Hospital
Boston, Massachusetts

D. LUIS MUSCOLO, MD
Director
Research Laboratory
Vice-Chairman
Department of Orthopaedic Surgery
Italian Hospital of Buenos Aires
Buenos Aires, Argentina

TAKASHI NISHII, PhD
Assistant Professor
Department of Orthopaedic Surgery
Osaka University Medical School
Suita, Osaka
Japan

PHILIP C. NOBLE, PhD
Barnhart Professor
Department of Orthopedic Surgery
Baylor College of Medicine
John S. Dunn Professor
Department of Orthopedic Research
The Methodist Hospital
Houston, Texas

JOHN A. OGDEN, MD
Clinical Professor
Director of Orthopaedics
Georgia Baptist Medical Center
Atlanta, Georgia

MICHAEL R. O'ROURKE, MD
Assistant Professor
Department of Orthopaedics and Rehabilitation
University of Iowa
Iowa City, Iowa

WAYNE G. PAPROSKY, MD, FACS
Rush Presbyterian St. Luke's Medical Center
Chicago, Illinois
Central Dupage Hospital
Winfield, Illinois

JAVAD PARVIZI, MD, FRCS
Associate Professor
Department of Orthopedics
Rothman Institute at Thomas Jefferson University
Philadelphia, Pennsylvania

LEONARD F. PELTIER,* MD, PhD
Professor Emeritus
Section of Orthopaedics
The University of Arizona
College of Medicine
Tucson, Arizona

CHRISTOPHER L. PETERS, MD
Associate Professor
Department of Orthopaedics
University of Utah
Salt Lake City, Utah

*(Deceased)

MARC J. PHILLIPON, MD
Clinical Research
Steadman Hawkins Research Foundation
Orthopaedic Surgeon
Steadman Hawkins Clinic
Vail, Colorado

HOLLIS G. POTTER, MD
Professor
Department of Radiology
Weill Medical College of Cornell University
Chief, Division of MRI
Department of Radiology and Imaging
Hospital for Special Surgery
New York, New York

STEVEN A. PURVIS, DO

LOUIS QUARTARARO, MD
Department of Orthopaedic Surgery
Allegheny University Hospitals
Philadelphia, Pennsylvania

DHEERAJ K. RAJAN, MD
Department of Radiology
Wayne State University
Detroit, Michigan

AMAR S. RANAWAT, MD
Assistant Attending Surgeon
The Department of Orthopaedic Surgery
Lenox Hill Hospital
New York, New York

CHITRANJAN S. RANAWAT, MD
James A. Nicholas Chairman
Department of Orthopaedic Surgery
Lenox Hill Hospital
New York, New York

AARON G. ROSENBERG, MD
Professor of Orthopaedic Surgery
Rush University Medical Center
Department of Orthopaedic Surgery
Chicago, Illinois

HARRY E. RUBASH, MD
Edith M. Ashley Professor of Orthopedic Surgery
Harvard Medical School,
Chief, Orthopaedic Surgery
Massachusetts General Hospital,
Boston, Massachusetts

KHALED J. SALEH, MD, MSc, FRCS, FACS
Associate Professor
Division Head, Adult Reconstruction
Department of Orthopedic Surgery
University of Virginia
Charlottesville, Virginia

EDUARDO A. SALVATI, MD
Professor of Clinical Orthopaedic Surgery
Director Hip and Knee Services
The Hospital for Special Surgery and New York Hospital
Weill Medical College of Cornell University
New York, New York

THOMAS P. SCHMALZRIED, MD
Associate Director
Joint Replacement Institute
Orthopaedic Hospital
Los Angeles, California

PERRY L. SCHOENECKER, MD
Professor
Department of Orthopedic Surgery
Washington University School of Medicine
Chief of Staff
Shriner's Hospital for Children
St. Louis, Missouri

B. WILLEM SCHREURS MD, PhD
Orthopaedic Surgeon
Department of Orthopaedics
Radboud University Nijmegen Medical Centre
Nijmegen, The Netherlands

STEVEN F. SCHUTZER, MD
Clinical Associate Professor
Department of Orthopedic Sugery
University of Connecticut
John Dempsey Hospital
Farmington, Connecticut
Senior Staff and Co-director of Adult Reconstruction Service
Hartford Hospital
Hartford, Connecticut

JOSEPH H. SCHWAB, MD

THOMAS P. SCULCO, MD
Professor and Chair
Department of Orthopedic Surgery
Weill Cornell Medical College
Surgeon-in-Chief
Hospital for Special Surgery
New York, New York

CHRISTOPHER E. SELGRATH, DO
Associate Professor
Department of Surgery
Philadelphia College of Osteopathic Medicine
Philadelphia, PA
Staff
Department of Surgery
Center for Advanced Orthopaedics
East Norriton, Pennsylvania

MANISH K. SETHI, MD
Resident
Department of Orthopedic Surgery
Massachusetts General Hospital
Boston, Massachusetts

CAMBIZE SHAHRDAR
Shreveport, Louisianna

ARUN S. SHANBHAG, PhD, MBA
Assistant Professor
Department of Orthopaedic Surgery
Harvard Medical School
Massachusetts General Hospital
Boston, Massachusetts

NIGEL E. SHARROCK, MB, ChB
Clinical Professor
Department of Anesthesiology
Weill Medical College of Cornell University
Attending Anesthesiologist
Department of Anesthesiology
Hospital for Special Surgery
New York, New York

RAFAEL J. SIERRA, MD
Assistant Professor
Senior Associate Consultant
Department of Orthopedic Surgery
Mayo Clinic
Rochester, Minnesota

MAURICIO SILVA, MD

CRAIG D. SILVERTON, MD
Chief-Adult Reconstructive Surgery
Department of Orthopaedic Surgery
Henry Ford Hospital
Detroit, Michigan

RAJ K. SINHA
Department of Orthopaedic Surgery
University of Pittsburgh Medical Center
Pittsburgh, Pennsylvania

TOM J. J. H. SLOOFF, MD, PhD
Emeritus Professor
Department of Orthopaedics
Radboud University Nijmegen Medical Centre
Nijmegen, The Netherlands

FRANCIS X. SOLANO, JR., MD
Clinical Associate Professor of Medicine
Department of Medicine
University of Pittsburgh
Medical Center
Pittsburgh, Pennsylvania

SCOTT M. SPORER, MD, MS
Assistant Professor
Department of Orthopaedic Surgery
Rush University Medical Center
Chicago, Illinois
Attending
Department of Orthopaedic Surgery
Central Dupage Hospital
Winfield, Illinois

BERNARD N. STULBERG, MD
Director
Center for Joint Reconstruction
Cleveland Orthopaedic and Spine Hospital
Cleveland, Ohio

PETER G. SULTAN

NOBUHIKO SUGANO, MD, PhD
Assistant Professor
Department of Orthopaedic Surgery
Osaka Kosei-Nenkin Hospital
Suita, Osaka
Japan

CHRISTI J. SYCHTERZ
Anderson Orthopaedic Research Institute
Anderson Orthopaedic Clinic
Alexandria, Virginia

MASAKI TAKAO
Department of Orthopaedic Surgery
Osaka University Graduate School of Medicine
Osaka, Japan

JOSEPH J. THOMAS, RN, BSN
Coordinator
Center for Advanced Bloodless Medicine and Surgery
Fairview Hospital
Cleveland, Ohio

JOHN F. TILZEY, MD, PhD
Clinical Instructor
Department of Orthopaedic Surgery
Boston University Medical Center
Boston, Massachusetts
Attending Surgeon
Department of Orthopaedic Surgery
Lahey Clinic
Burlington, Massachusetts

JOHN TIMPERLEY, FRCS
Honorary Research Fellow
Department of Engineering Science
University of Exeter
Consultant Orthopaedic Surgeon
Princess Elizabeth Orthopaedic Centre
Royal Devon and Exeter NHS Hospital Trust
Exeter, Devon, England
United Kingdom

ANDREW D. TOMS, MB, ChB, FRCS, MSc, FRCS
Former Clinical and Research Fellow
Department of Orthopaedics
University of British Columbia
Former Clinical and Research Fellow
Division of Lower Limb Reconstruction and Oncology
Department of Orthopaedics
Vancouver General Hospital
Vancouver, British Columbia
Canada

JEFFREY D. TOWERS, MD
Associate Professor
Department of Radiology
University of Pittsburgh School of Medicine
University of Pittsburgh Medical Center
Pittsburgh, Pennsylvania

ROBERT T. TROUSDALE, MD
Mayo Clinic
Rochester, Minnesota

IAN Y. Y. TSOU, FRCR (UK)
MRI Research Fellow
Department of Radiology and Imaging
Hospital for Special Surgery
New York, New York

THOMAS P. VAIL, MD
Professor
Division of Orthopaedic Surgery
Department of Surgery
Duke University Medical Center
Durham, North Carolina

NICO J. J. VERDONSCHOT, PHD
Assistant Professor
Department of Orthopaedics
Director, Biomechanics Section
Orthopaedic Research Lab
Radboud University Nijmegen Medical Centre
Nijmegen, The Netherlands

FRAZER A. WADE

RAY C. WASIELEWSKI, MS, MD
Clinical Associate Professor
Department of Orthopaedics
Ohio State University
Director of Orthopaedic Research
Department of Orthopaedics
Grant Medical Center
Columbus, Ohio

STUART L. WEINSTEIN, MD
Ignacio V. Ponseti Chair and Professor of Orthopaedic Surgery
Department of Orthopaedic Surgery
University of Iowa
Iowa City, Iowa

JEAN WELTER

DENNIS R. WENGER, MD
Pediatric Orthopedic and Scoliosis Center
San Diego, California

RICHARD E. WHITE, JR., MD
Clinical Assistant Professor
Department of Orthopaedic Surgery and Rehabilitation
University of New Mexico School of Medicine
Albuquerque, New Mexico

MARKUS A. WIMMER, PhD
Assistant Professor
Department of Orthopedic Surgery
Rush University Medical Center
Director, Section of Tribology
Department of Orthopedic Surgery
Rush University Medical Center
Chicago, Illinois

PHILIP Z. WIRGANOWICZ, MD
Kaiser Permanente
Oakland Medical Center
Hospital Building, 1st Floor
280 W. MacArthur Blvd.
Oakland California

JEFFREY D. YERGLER, MD
South Bend Orthopaedic Associates
South Bend, Indiana

ERIK N. ZEEGEN, MD
Assistant Clinical Professor
Department of Orthopaedic Surgery
University of California, Los Angeles
Santa Monica, California
Attending Surgeon
Department of Orthopaedic Surgery
Encino-Tarzana Regional Medical Center
Encino, California

JOSEPH D. ZUCKERMAN, MD
Professor and Chairman
Orthopaedic Surgery
New York University School of Medicine
Surgeon-in-Chief
New York Hospital for Joint Diseases
New York, New York

History of Hip Surgery

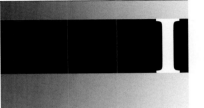

A History

of Hip Surgery

*Leonard F. Peltier**

In the beginning, the prospect of operating on the hip deterred even the most aggressive surgeons. Prior to the introduction of anesthesia and antiseptic/aseptic precautions, the success rate of any operation on the hip was so low that such procedures were limited to those cases of trauma or infection for which it was a last resort. The introduction of anesthesia in 1847 permitted more care and deliberation in the carrying out of an operation, but surgeons still watched in frustration and despair as their patients regularly died of wound infection. The introduction by Lister (1865) of the antiseptic method of preventing such infections began the development of an operating room ritual, replacing antisepsis with asepsis. Although surgeons did not rush to adopt Lister's methods, there was a slow but continuous decrease in the incidence of postoperative wound infections as technical improvements in sterilization were made. Landmarks along the way were the introduction of rubber gloves by William S. Halsted in 1890 and the development of the "no-touch technique" and other innovations by W. Arbuthnot Lane in 1902 (48,132). The evolution of the operating room ritual was still continuing when Charnley (Fig. 1-1) introduced his "Clean Air Operating Enclosure" in 1964 in an effort to control bacteriologic contamination through the air (24). The result of the improvements in anesthesia, preoperative and postoperative care, and especially the aseptic operating room ritual has been to make the risk of an operation on the hip very low, encouraging the widespread acceptance of elective surgery.

The development of hip surgery was closely associated with the treatment of tuberculosis. With the exception of trauma and an occasional case of acute hematogenous arthritis, tuberculous joint disease was the most common indication for operative intervention until the introduction of effective antibiotic treatment for tuberculosis in the years following World War II. The presence of systemic tuberculosis greatly influenced the operative mortality, postoperative morbidity, and long-term survival associated with any operations on the tuberculous hip.

In children, open reduction of congenital dislocations of the hip and operations to improve function in patients with unreduced congenital dislocations of the hip developed along with the treatment of tuberculosis. The operative treatment of acute fractures and for ununited fractures of the femoral neck depended to a large extent on the development of the x-ray and of metallic internal fixation devices.

The slowly increasing life expectancy following World War I was associated with an increasing population of patients with chronic joint disease. The demand for the relief of pain and disability due to such arthritides led to the development of operations such as osteotomy and arthroplasty to remedy these problems.

Although hip surgery had its roots in the 19th century, its greatest period of growth and development has occurred in the 20th century, and many of those who contributed to its amazing success are among our contemporaries.

AMPUTATION AT THE HIP JOINT

For the surgeons of the 18th and 19th centuries amputation of the lower extremity through the hip joint was the simplest operation in concept and the most difficult in execution.

---

* Deceased

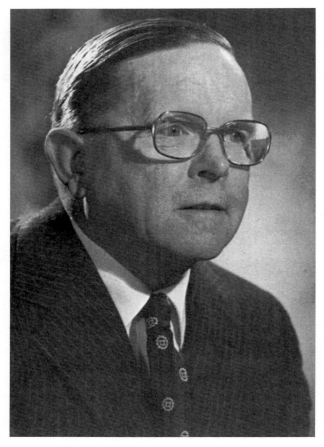

Figure 1-1 John Charnley (1911–1982).

Sauveur Francois Morand, a student of Cheselden and a surgeon at La Charite in Paris, in 1729 was the first to seriously consider the possibility of carrying out such an amputation (100). Following his gambit, there appeared a large literature regarding the possibility of performing such an operation with patient survival, as well as extensive discussions regarding the ethics of attempting such a mutilating and dangerous procedure. Subsequently, anecdotal reports of hip disarticulation for wounds and for infection, particularly tuberculosis, accumulated. In 1812, for example, Larrey described a successful amputation through the hip joint in an officer of the dragoons wounded by a missile in a battle before Moscow (70). Astley Cooper successfully carried out an elective disarticulation of the hip in 1824 in a 40-year-old patient with a chronic infection involving the whole upper end of the femur (20). By 1867 there had been reported 111 such operations with 46 survivors, a mortality rate of 57% (102). During the Civil War (1861–1865) there were 19 primary disarticulations of the hip for missile wounds with a mortality rate of 95%; 9 secondary disarticulations with a mortality rate of 78%; and 7 cases of reamputation with a mortality rate of 43% (101). During the next century the operative mortality for all types of hip disarticulation continued to drop, reaching an acceptable level after World War II. Hip disarticulation has remained in the surgical armamentarium primarily as tool for the control of malignant tumors of the bone and soft tissue, rarely for

trauma. The basic technique of the operation was well described by Boyd (17).

HIP JOINT RESECTION

Although amputations through the hip joint were unusual, other amputations for trauma and infection, usually tuberculous, were carried out frequently during the 18th century. Sentient surgeons, however, began to consider the possibility of limb-sparing operations. On February 9, 1769, at a meeting of the Royal Society, Charles White described the case of a 14-year-old boy with a large abscess, probably tuberculous, in his left shoulder (149). He had treated the patient by drainage of the abscess and resection of the necrotic portion of the upper end of the humerus. The result was as favorable as it was surprising, with preservation of the arm and a high level of function. While White never carried out a hip joint resection on a living patient, he did carry out such an operation on a cadaver and proved to his satisfaction that it was feasible. The substitution of joint resection for amputation was popularized by Park and Moreau (102). James Syme was an ardent advocate of joint resection but believed that it was not a feasible operation at the hip (131). It was not until 1822 that a hip joint resection was carried out in a patient with a chronic abscess of the joint with dislocation of the head of the femur by Anthony White at Westminster Hospital, London (148). Postoperatively the deformity was corrected and the patient was treated as for an open fracture using a long splint. Twelve months later the wound had healed and the patient had regained a remarkable level of function.

Joint resection was the first orthopedic operation for which special instrumentation was developed. Moreau had a flexible saw, "with joints like the chain of a watch," constructed by an instrument maker in London in 1790 (102). This was passed around the bone by means of a large needle. Bernhard Heine of Wurzburg took this idea a step farther when in 1832 he developed his "chain osteotome" (119). This progenitor of the present ubiquitous chain saw was considered a real advance because it allowed division of the bone quickly through a small incision. Heine received the important Monthyon Prize in Paris for this invention in 1835. Heine also carried out extensive animal experiments studying the process of regeneration of bony tissue following resection (142). Louis Ollier of Lyon also used the operation of resection as a means of studying bone regeneration and the function of the periosteum, both in his patients and in experimental animals. In his two-volume work on these subjects he gives a good description of the operation of hip resection in a patient (99).

By the middle of the 19th century resection of the hip joint was well accepted, being described by Erichsen as "not difficult in performance" (34). Postoperatively the patients were managed by being placed in a long splint.

In the United States, Lewis Sayre became the great exponent of hip joint resection for chronic infections. His first such procedure, carried out in 1854, was on a 9-year-old girl with "morbus coxarius," probably tuberculosis. The case was thoroughly discussed in his lectures (113). Accompanying this report is an analysis of 59 of his hip resections with 39 survivors. Eight patients died during the immediate postoperative period. The remainder died of late complications, usually of the lesser trochanter depending on the site of the disease. Postoperatively the patients were treated in traction on a frame. The control of tuberculosis by the use of antibiotic drugs has almost left this operation without an indication except as a salvage operation in cases of infected prostheses.

In addition to applying this operation to tuberculous and other infected cases, Girdlestone also used it in some cases of severe bilateral osteoarthritis of the hips, simply resecting the head and neck of the femur to gain mobility (43).

ARTHRODESIS

The concept of stiffening a joint in order to improve function by providing stability had been introduced by Eduard Albert (Fig. 1-3) in 1882 when he carried out an ankle fusion in a patient with postpoliomyelitis paralysis (5). The concept was taken up quickly by other surgeons. Heusner and Lampugnani soon reported cases of fusion of the hip for old congenital dislocations of the hip (54,67).

While arthrodesis was used also for paralytic deformities, it found its greatest use in the treatment of tuberculous joint disease. Over a long period of time, clinicians had observed that an occasional case of tuberculous joint disease ceased to

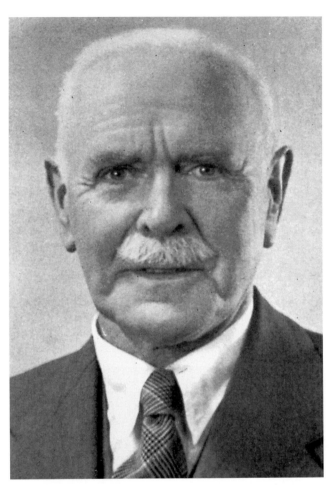

Figure 1-2   Gathorne Robert Girdlestone (1881–1950).

tuberculosis. Sayre toured Europe discussing hip resection and was decorated by the Norwegian Crown for his work. In 1876, at the International Medical Congress in Philadelphia, Sayre demonstrated the operation before a group of surgeons including Lister (62). Gibney, in New York, supported Sayre and recognized the value of the operation in preventing and even reversing the progress of "lardaceous degeneration" or secondary amyloidosis, a common cause of death in bone and joint tuberculosis (39). Volkmann, in Leipzig, was more conservative and believed that hip resection should be done only as a life-saving procedure (143). The French surgeons also maintained a very conservative attitude toward hip joint resection for tuberculosis, Calot believing it to be a bad operation (21).

More recently, the surgeon most closely identified with the procedure known as hip joint resection was Gathorne Robert Girdlestone in Oxford (Fig. 1-2). In his book on bone and joint tuberculosis published in 1940, Girdlestone outlined the essential steps of the operation (44). They were (a) a complete exposure of the anterior and upper aspect of the joint, (b) excision of the capsule and synovia, (c) division of all structures inserted into the greater trochanter, (d) dislocation of the remains of the head of the femur and cleaning out the acetabulum, and (e) a transverse osteotomy usually just above

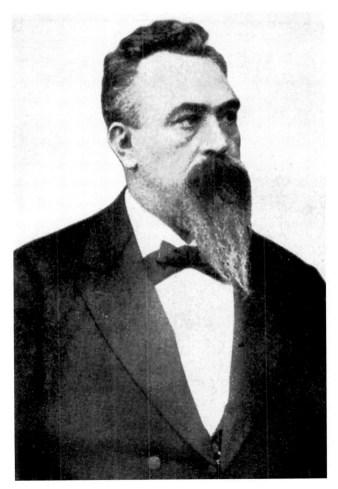

Figure 1-3   Eduard Albert.

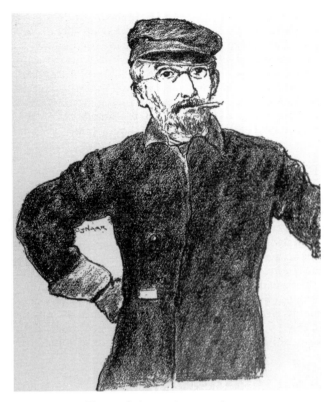

Figure 1-4   Hugh Owen Thomas.

progress or became "arrested" when the affected joint became stiff. Indeed, a good deal of conservative treatment with splints and frames was directed to producing just such a spontaneous ankylosis. Hugh Owen Thomas (Fig. 1-4), whose treatment of hip disease was based on the dictum "rest, absolute, uninterrupted, and prolonged," considered that a good end result of his treatment was an ankylosed hip in the best functional position (133). It is surprising, then, that surgical arthrodesis of a tuberculous joint was not carried out until 1911 when Russell Hibbs of New York (Fig. 1-5) first reported such an operation in a patient with tuberculosis of the knee.

While in knee fusion it was possible to resect the articular cartilage of the joint and to oppose two relatively large flat cancellous bone surfaces, after removing the articular cartilage from the femoral head and the acetabulum, the surgeon was left with a cup and saucer configuration that severely limited the area of cancellous bone apposition. In cases of tuberculosis, in addition, it was deemed advisable to avoid entering the joint. For this reason a large number of methods of extra-articular hip fusion have been described. In 1926, Hibbs reported preliminary results after an extracapsular hip fusion for tuberculosis in which he advanced the greater trochanter upward to impinge on the pelvis (58). Variations of this method of bridging the space between the greater trochanter and the wing of the ilium with a graft either from the trochanter or the ilium were reported by many surgeons (38,53,153). Biomechanically, all of these grafts were placed under tension. Other operations were quickly designed for extra-articular hip fusion where the grafts were under compression. Although others had tried, Trumble was the first surgeon to design such

a satisfactory ischiofemoral fusion (140). This was further improved by Brittain who incorporated a femoral osteotomy in the operation, which allowed for better correction of the deformity (19). Immobilization during the healing period was provided by plaster of paris spicas.

Hip fusions were carried out for indications other than tuberculosis, such as advanced osteoarthritis and old congenital deformities. In the absence of sepsis, intra-articular fusions could be performed. One of the simplest techniques was that of Watson-Jones who simply drove a long triflanged nail up the femoral neck and across the joint into the acetabulum (146). This was useful only in patients with a minimal amount of motion and deformity. Charnley improved on this technique by shaping the head of the femur and dislocating it centrally into a hole in the acetabulum (25). This allowed correction of the deformity and provided a better environment for producing solid union. These techniques did not entirely eliminate the need for additional fixation in all cases. With advances in the internal fixation of fractures and the introduction of very large plates, hip fusion techniques were devised using the Cobra plate, which extended from the ilium to the upper femoral shaft (94). This provided excellent fixation.

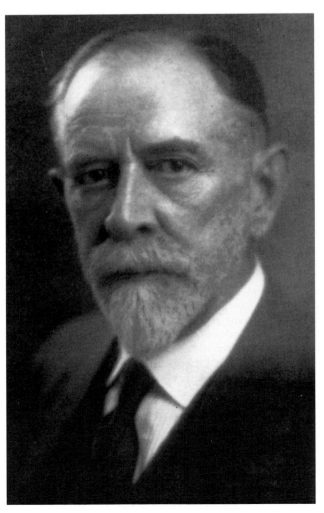

Figure 1-5   Russell A. Hibbs.

OSTEOTOMY

There were indications for operation on the hip other than infection and trauma. As surgeons became more experienced, the presence of deformity and/or functional impairment due to conditions involving the hip joint stimulated them to devise new operations. In the evolution of the various indications and techniques for osteotomy, there was a subtle interplay between operations to correct deformity and operations to produce deformity to increase function. In contrast to amputations and resections, osteotomies of the hip were useful in many conditions and were helpful in solving many problems. This explains the large number and variety of such procedures.

John Rhea Barton of Philadelphia (Fig. 1-6) performed the first osteotomy of the hip on November 22, 1826 (10). His patient, a 21-year-old sailor, had been injured in a fall at sea 20 months previously, suffering an injury variously diagnosed as a contusion of the hip, a dislocation, or a fracture. At the time he was seen by Barton, the hip was ankylosed in severe flexion and adduction and there was considerable swelling about the hip joint. After observing him in the hospital for almost a year, Barton carried out his carefully planned operation. Having had a strong narrow saw manufactured for the purpose, Barton made a short muscle-splitting incision over the upper end of the femur and divided the bone at the level of the base of the neck of the femur. Postoperatively the wound healed by secondary intention with only one bout of erysipelas. The deformity was corrected and a deliberate effort was made to keep the osteotomy from healing so as to produce a pseudoarthrosis. Four months after the operation the patient was able to walk and had a useful range of motion in his hip.

Bernard Langenbeck, the leading German surgeon of his generation, was aware of Barton's work and, based on this knowledge and the experience with bone surgery gained during a war in 1848, developed his method of subcutaneous osteotomy (68). Through a small incision, a drill was used to perforate the bone. A sharp-pointed narrow saw was inserted into the drill hole and used to partially divide the bone. When the bone was weakened sufficiently, the remainder was broken through by manipulation. Langenbeck applied his method to old ricketic deformities of the tibia. Mayer published a major paper on osteotomy in 1856 (79). He reported his experience in his clinic in Wurzburg with 17 patients including an 8-year-old girl in whom he carried out a high femoral osteotomy for an ankylosed hip. He derived the operation from other subcutaneous operations introduced by Delpech and Stromeyer and reviewed the experience of European and American surgeons. Lewis Sayre reported two cases of osteotomy through the trochanteric region with the aim of producing an "artful pseudarthrosis" in 1863 (112).

Richard Volkmann, a friend and admirer of Lister, was the first surgeon to carry out osteotomies using antiseptic precautions (144). In 1879, William Adams reviewed the subject of osteotomy as it was carried out in England (2). He adopted Lister's antiseptic technique only after Ogston in Aberdeen had done the first such case in Britain in 1876. The London surgeon Gant was an early proponent of osteotomy of the femur just below the lesser trochanter for fixed deformities of the hip (37). As a result of his experience with the treatment of congenital dislocations of the hip and the treatment of old wounds of the hip during World War I, Lorenz (Fig. 1-7) devised his bifurca-

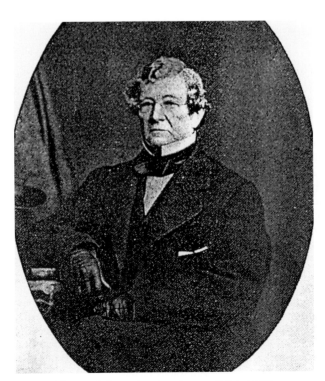

Figure 1-6 John Rhea Barton (1796–1878).

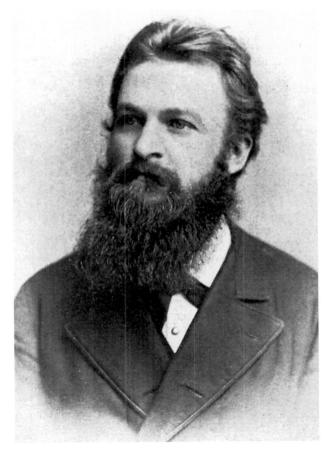

Figure 1-7 Adolf Lorenz.

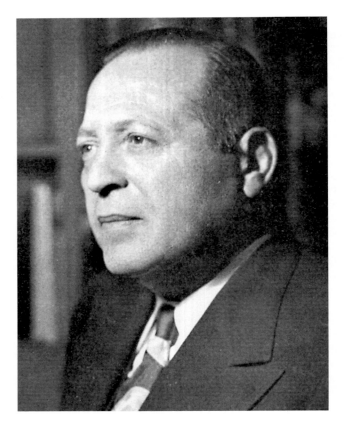

Figure 1-8   Henry Milch (1895–1964).

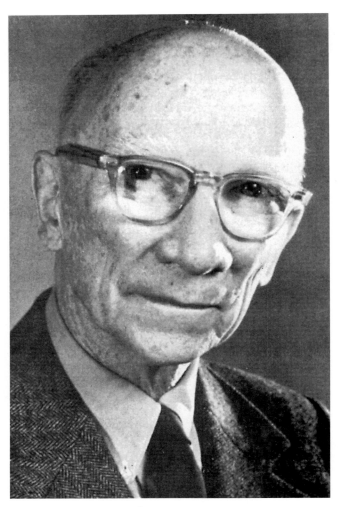

Figure 1-9   Alfred Rives Schanz.

tion osteotomy to correct deformity and to restore stability during weight bearing (74). Henry Milch of New York (Fig. 1-8) became interested in Lorenz's osteotomy and did a great deal to explain the biomechanics of its success. In 1943, Milch reported two patients with ankylosis of the hip in whom, to regain useful motion, he had resected the femoral head and neck and performed a high femoral "pelvic support" osteotomy (87). This operation has also been performed by other surgeons with success (28). Through his work, the procedure became a staple of the orthopedic armamentarium (88,89). This osteotomy had wide application and became the prototype of the high femoral pelvic support osteotomies.

Postoperatively, following all of the osteotomies, the patients were immobilized in splints, in traction, or in plaster of paris dressings. Skeletal fixation of the osteotomy fragments was a relatively late development. It was not until 1924 that Schanz (Fig. 1-9) described the use of external skeletal fixation to control and immobilize the components of his osteotomy (115). Two large screws were placed, one above and one below the line of the osteotomy prior to dividing the bone. After the osteotomy, the ends of the screws were brought out through the wound and held in place by a special clamp. This form of external skeletal fixation gave good control of the fragments and introduced more precision into the operation, but still relied on the use of a plaster of paris spica. Originally designed for the treatment of congenital dislocations of the hip, Schanz soon adapted his operation to the treatment of old ununited fractures of the neck of the femur (114). The level of the femoral osteotomy as carried out by Schanz varied with each case but was almost always below the lesser trochanter.

It was Blount of Milwaukee (Fig. 1-10) who described the first effective system of internal fixation for high femoral osteotomies in 1943 (12). Using his blade plate in many configurations, Blount was able to precisely plan and carry out a wide variety of osteotomies and fix them well enough that no additional splints or spicas were required. The patients could be allowed out of bed and became ambulatory with aides shortly after the operation. As techniques of internal fixation improved, the internal fixation of the osteotomy fragments became even more secure (93). Such internal fixation permitted exact planning for the final angulation and/or displacement of the bony fragments and insured against any change in the desired configuration during the healing process, while at the same time permitting the patient to be active.

Osteotomies of the femur and pelvis have become important procedures in the management of patients with congenital dislocations of the hip. The reduction of an old congenital dislocation of the hip by means of an operation was first described by Alfonso Poggi of Bologna in 1880 (107). The open reduction of congenital dislocations of the hip was popularized by Albert Hoffa who believed that it should be carried out early, in young children, rather than be delayed (59,60).

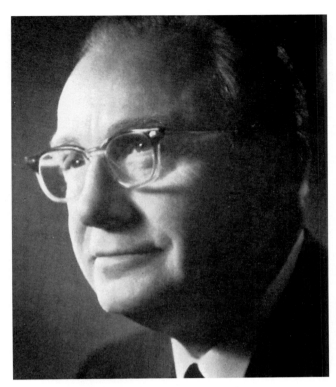

Figure 1-10   Walter Putnam Blount.

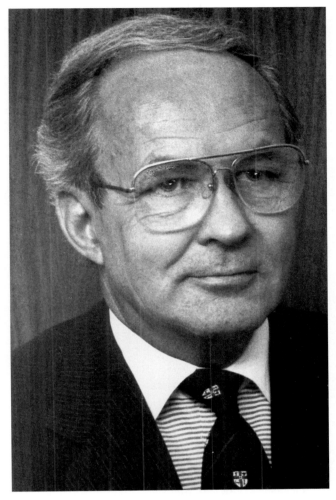

Figure 1-11   Robert B. Salter.

The anterior approach as described by Salter (Fig. 1-11) became the most commonly used avenue through which open reduction was accomplished (111). An alternative medial approach was developed by Ludloff (76). This has remained a very viable option (35). As an aid to the reduction, Swett described an osteotomy of the shaft of the femur that short-ened it (130). Osteotomies were also carried out to correct rotation deformities of the upper end of the femur after a reduction had been obtained (125).

In the early years of the 20th century, few children with con-genital dislocations of the hip had open reductions because the diagnosis was usually made late and the results of open reduc-tion in late cases were not satisfactory. With the introduction of the x-ray and with increasing emphasis on early diagnosis, open reduction during the first year of life became the usual treatment if closed reduction could not be accomplished.

The bifurcation osteotomy of Adolf Lorenz was widely used in older patients whose hips could not be reduced (74). In this operation, the position of the dislocated head of the femur remained unchanged; the oblique osteotomy took place at the level of the acetabulum, and the proximal end of the distal fragment was placed in the acetabulum (129). As the osteotomy healed, the bone spike placed in the acetabu-lum atrophied, and the end result was a high pelvic support osteotomy. Schanz carried out his osteotomy through the shaft of the femur more distally, at the level of the ischial tuberosity (115).

Operations for the treatment of congenital dislocations of the hip were also carried out on the acetabular side. The first of these were designed to cover the head by extending the acetabular roof laterally by means of the "shelf operation." In 1915, Albee (Fig. 1-12) described an operation to stabilize

paralytic and congenital dislocations of the hip that consisted of turning down the lateral roof of the acetabulum and main-taining its position by means of a bone graft (4). Among the surgeons who modified and popularized the shelf operation, Gill of the University of Pennsylvania was the most prominent (40–42). In spite of its apparent inadequacy, the long-term results of such operations were surprisingly good (57). The operations of Pemberton, Steele, Chiari, and Salter were all directed to providing better coverage of the femoral head by means of turning down the roof of the acetabulum, displacing the acetabulum medially, or reorienting the entire acetabulum (27,105,111,128).

Osteotomies of the upper end of the femur, in addition to being useful in the management of hip problems in infants and children, proved to be of great value in the management of osteoarthritis of the hip in adults. In Vienna, Hass, an asso-ciate of Lorenz, applied the bifurcation osteotomy to the treat-ment of osteoarthritis of the hip with some success (46). In Great Britain both Malkin and McMurray had similar results (78,83).

McMurray of Liverpool (Fig. 1-13) is generally credited with popularizing high femoral osteotomy for this purpose (84). In 1939 he reported on a series of 42 patients on whom he had

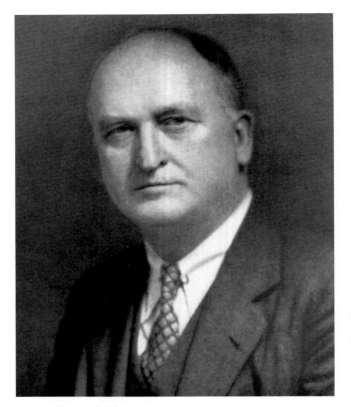

Figure 1-12 Fred Houdlett Albee (1876–1945).

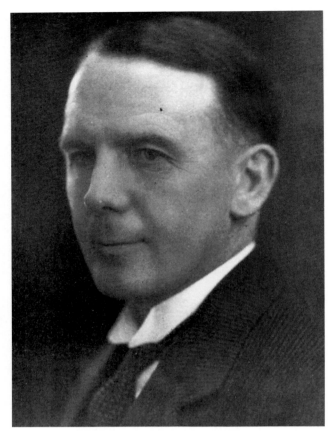

Figure 1-13 T. P. McMurray.

carried out an oblique osteotomy through the intertrochanteric region with displacement of the distal fragment medially. He believed that the operation favorably affected the weight-bearing line, relieving the hip from stress, and exposed a new portion of the articular surface of the head of the femur to the articular surface of the acetabulum. The patients were immobilized in a plaster of paris spica postoperatively. The introduction of effective internal fixation quickly made it possible to discard the spica and improved the convalescence. Many types and techniques of high femoral osteotomies were used in the treatment of osteoarthritis of the hip (72).

The relief of pain gained by these operations was generally satisfactory and lasting. Interestingly enough, the success of the operation did not depend on the degree of displacement of the osteotomy. The important factor appeared to be the complete division of the femur (1,97). This, coupled with the immediate relief of hip pain following the operation, pointed to circulatory changes in the proximal fragment, rather than mechanical factors, as the cause of the improvement. There was good evidence to indicate that repair of the articular cartilage of the head of the femur occurred months and years following the osteotomy (50).

The value of high femoral osteotomy for the treatment of osteoarthritis of the hip can be assessed by this statement of the well-known total joint surgeon William H. Harris of Boston, writing in 1995: "On the basis of its clinical results, and because of the well known adverse effects of hip replacements in young patients, osteotomy remains the preferred operative procedure in patients who are suitable candidates and who are less than forty-five to fifty years old" (50).

The usefulness of the high femoral osteotomies extended to yet another problem, as we shall see when we discuss the treatment of fractures of the neck of the femur.

FRACTURES OF THE HIP

The treatment of fractures about the hip has presented problems for surgeons since the time of Hippocrates. In 1822, Astley Cooper classified these fractures as intracapsular and extracapsular on the basis of their blood supply and stated that he had never seen a healed intracapsular fracture (31). In 1857, the American surgeon Frank Hastings Hamilton reviewed the results of the treatment of 39 cases of fractured hips, both intra- and extracapsular, and found all to be "imperfect" (49). The failure of nonoperative methods of treatment encouraged surgeons to seek other solutions.

At a meeting of the Deutsche Gesellschaft für Chirurgie in April 1878, Bernard Langenbeck described the open reduction and internal fixation of an ununited extracapsular hip fracture with a silver-plated metal screw (69). At the same meeting, Friedrich Trendelenberg presented his case of a man with a fresh extracapsular fracture of the hip that he had openly reduced and fixed with an ivory peg (138). Although there are other anecdotal reports of this type, it was Nicolas Senn of Chicago who demonstrated that (a) intracapsular fractures of the hip sometimes healed and (b) internal fixation of such fractures in cats could result in healing (117,118). On this basis, in 1883, he urged open reduction and internal fixation in such cases. However, in view of the strenuous opposition of all of his surgical colleagues, he abandoned his proposal. Twenty years later, Royal Whitman of New York demonstrated that the reduction and immobilization of intracapsular hip fractures by means of a hip spica could lead to healing in a substantial number of patients (150).

Dissatisfaction with the cumbersome plaster immobilization spurred surgeons to explore better methods. In 1912, Fred Albee of New York began to carry out open reduction and internal fixation of intracapsular fractures using anterior and lateral incisions (3). The fracture was fixed with a bone graft taken from the patient's tibia. Hey-Groves of Bristol carried out similar operations using pegs of ivory and beef bone as well as autogenous grafts for fixation (56). With the introduction by Sherman of stainless steel surgical appliances in 1912, the use of other materials for fixation was gradually phased out (120).

In 1917, Smith-Petersen of Boston (Fig. 1-14) combined the anterior and lateral incisions into one larger incision that gave exposure to the entire upper end of the femur (123). Through this incision he was able to open the capsule of the hip joint, reduce the fracture, and insert a nail through the lateral cortex of the trochanter. To fix the fracture, Smith-Petersen

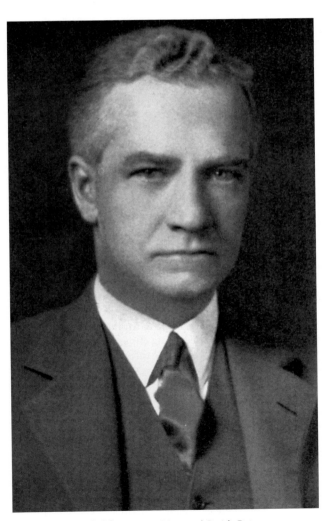

Figure 1-14 Marius Nygaard Smith-Petersen.

designed a triflanged nail which more effectively prevented rotation of the fragments (124). Hand in hand with the new nail design came improvements in the fracture table and the equipment for intraoperative x-rays to determine the position of the fracture fragments (52). The addition of a central hole to the original Smith-Petersen nail by Sven Johansson greatly improved the ease of placing the nail because it could be inserted over a guide pin through a small lateral incision (63). The result of this evolution was to make closed reduction and internal fixation of fractures of the neck of the femur the standard method of treatment (106).

Friedrich Pauwels, a student of Schanz, was one of the first to thoroughly study the biomechanics of intracapsular hip fractures and to describe a classification that had a predictive value for the prognosis (103). This was based on his knowledge of the effects of forces of compression, tension, and shear on fracture healing. He applied this knowledge specifically to the configuration of fractures of the neck of the femur before and after reduction, and concluded that those in a compression mode had a more favorable prognosis than those in which shear and tension predominated. In addition to emphasizing the importance of achieving a primary reduction in a compression mode, when this failed or in cases of ununited fractures, he advocated carrying out a high femoral osteotomy to produce a compression mode.

In spite of the progress that had been made, the results were far from satisfactory due to the complications of nonunion and aseptic necrosis. This was especially true in cases of fractures of the neck of the femur in children (6,61). In 1934, Kellogg Speed, in his Fracture Oration before the Clinical Congress of the American College of Surgeons, spoke of the intracapsular hip fracture as the "unsolved fracture" (127). Nineteen years later, in 1953, in his presidential address to the American Orthopedic Association, James A. Dickson again spoke of this fracture as the "unsolved fracture" (32).

For the management of ununited fractures of the neck of the femur there were several surgical options depending on the presence of a viable head of the femur, of aseptic necrosis, and of resorption of the neck. In an ideal case, the fracture could be reduced into an optimum position and renailed, sometimes with an accompanying autogenous bone graft (126). If the head of the femur was viable but the neck resorbed, the Brackett operation could be performed (18). In this operation, the hip joint was exposed, the fibrous scar tissue excised, and the base of the head curetted down to bleeding bone, forming a slight cup. The remnant of the neck was removed, and the greater trochanter was resected. The stump of the trochanter was then opposed to the head and immobilized. Vernon Luck improved the Brackett operation by transplanting the greater trochanter distally after the resection in order to preserve abduction (75). When the head was not viable it could be removed, and after transferring the greater trochanter distally, the stump of the end of the femur was placed in the acetabulum, in other words, the Whitman reconstruction operation (151).

The osteotomies devised by McMurray and by Schanz were effectively used for the treatment of ununited fractures of the neck of the femur when the head of the femur was viable (85,114). When the head of the femur was not viable and had to be resected, various methods of arthroplasty were employed.

The problem of avascular necrosis was particularly complicated because of the problem of establishing an early diagnosis and the difficulty of reestablishing circulation to the necrotic area of bone. To accomplish the latter, Bonfiglio and Voke proposed an operation consisting of introducing an autogenous bone graft up the neck of the femur into the necrotic area of the head (15,16). Others advocated the use of bone grafts on a muscle pedicle in order to promote union and treat aseptic necrosis (65,86).

As early as 1927, Hey-Groves had replaced the head of the femur of a patient using a prosthesis made of ivory (55). Moore and Bohlman replaced the head and upper end of the femur with a metal prosthesis after resecting a giant cell tumor in 1940 (92). In 1949 the Judet brothers in France reported their experience with the use of an acrylic-stemmed prosthesis in 76 patients undergoing arthroplasty (64). The acrylic prosthesis was quickly introduced in the treatment of fresh intracapsular hip fractures. Metallic-stemmed femoral head prostheses were designed by McBride and Thomson (80,135). It became apparent that such designs were not sufficiently stable, and after a period of trial and error, the stemmed prostheses developed by Austin Moore and Frederick Thompson became the devices of choice for the treatment of fresh fractures of the femoral neck (91,134). As we shall see, the experience gained with these prosthetic devices gave strong impetus to the subsequent development of total hip replacement arthroplasty.

While extracapsular fractures could be healed in most cases by treatment in traction, prolonged bed rest in elderly patients had a high morbidity. It was recognized very early that the use of a peg or a nail for the internal fixation of extracapsular hip fractures did not provide adequate fixation. In 1914, M. E. Preston devised a screw with a side plate to be used for these fractures (108). The number and variety of internal fixation devices used to internally fix extracapsular fractures of the hip rapidly grew in number. They all incorporated a nail or screw for the proximal fragment and a side plate or intramedullary device for fixation of the femoral shaft. In the exhibit prepared by the Committee on the History of Orthopedic Surgery of the American Academy of Orthopedic Surgeons (AAOS) in 1988, over 80 devices of various designs were collected, and the exhibit was far from complete (see the exhibits at the end of this chapter) (30). Others have described similar assemblies of orthopedic appliances, each with its champion (103,137,139,154). Because of their natural tendency to heal, almost any type of internal fixation device can be used in the treatment of extracapsular fractures of the hip, if it is used properly.

ARTHROPLASTY

The original intent of the operation called arthroplasty was to restore motion to an ankylosed joint. This concept has been expanded to include the restoration, as far as possible, of the integrity and functional power of a diseased joint. As the MacAuslands pointed out, while a resection restores motion, an arthroplasty, to be successful, must not only restore motion but also provide stability of the joint—a crucial difference (99).

Although John Rhea Barton performed an osteotomy of the hip rather than an arthroplasty in 1826, his statement regarding the indications for this procedure could be applied to the operation of hip arthroplasty today.

> I hope I will not be understood as entertaining the belief, that this treatment will be applicable to, and judicious in, every case of anchylosis. I believe the operation would be justifiable only under the following circumstances, viz. where the patient's general health is good, and his constitution is sufficiently strong; where the rigidity is not confined to the soft parts, but is actually occasioned by a consolidation of the joint; where all the muscles and tendons that were essential to the ordinary movements of the former joint are sound, and not incorporated by firm adhesions with the adjacent structure; where the disease causing the deformity has entirely subsided; where the operation can be performed through the original point of motion, or so near to it, that the use of most of the tendons and muscles will not be lost; and, finally, where the deformity, or inconvenience, is such as will induce the patient to endure the pain, and incur the risks of an operation (10).

While in an arthrodesis the purpose of the operation was to create raw cancellous bone surfaces on each side of the joint and to hold them in rigid apposition, in an arthroplasty the purpose of the operation was to shape the ends of the bones and to hold the surfaces apart, almost always using some material interposed between the fragments. A wide variety of materials was used by different surgeons. In Chicago, J. B. Murphy developed procedures for arthroplasty for all of the major joints using a flap of fascia and fat interposed between the remodeled joint surfaces (96). The reamers that he designed for shaping the head of the femur and acetabulum were used for this purpose by orthopedic surgeons for many years. In 1917, William S. Baer (Fig. 1-15), the founder of the Department of Orthopedics at the Johns Hopkins Medical School, reported on a series of 100 arthroplasties in which he had used chromicized sheets of pig bladder as the interposing membrane (9). For a short time, "Baer's membrane" was widely used for arthroplasty. Fascia lata removed from the patient was also used as an interposing membrane in hip arthroplasty (22,96,109). For the treatment of older children with congenital dislocations of the hip, Colonna carried out a procedure in which the capsule of the hip joint was used as an interposing membrane as well as a means to retain the hip in the acetabulum (29). Kallio, in Helsinki, had success using the dermal layer of the skin taken from the patient as an interposing membrane in hip arthroplasty (66). Dermal arthroplasty is still used occasionally in smaller joints.

Marius Nygaard Smith-Petersen of Boston began working on other materials to use for arthroplasties of the hip in 1923 (122). At first he tried using cups made of glass, which broke; then cups of Bakelite, an early plastic material that also failed. He achieved success 15 years later with the adoption of cups made of vitallium, the first nonreactive metal alloy to be used in orthopedic surgery (124). "Mold arthroplasty," as Smith-Petersen called his operation, was carried out through his anterior lateral incision and consisted of a revision of both the head of the femur and the rim of the acetabulum. Vitallium cups of varying diameter and depth were used. The operation was followed by a prolonged hospital stay for physical therapy and rehabilitation. The results were impressive; 82% good or satisfactory results in 1000 cases (8). Smith-Petersen's mold arthroplasty became the method of choice for hip arthroplasty. John Schwartzmann

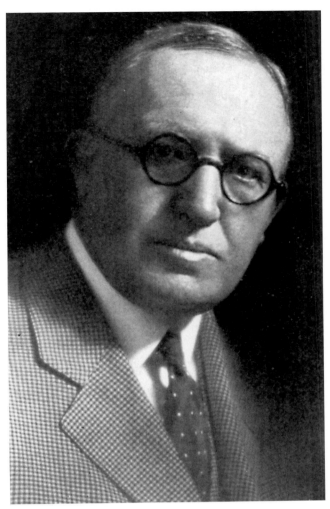

Figure 1-15 William S. Baer.

showed that this operation was particularly useful in patients with rheumatoid arthritis (116).

The most sophisticated interposition arthroplasty procedure was devised by Bateman, who developed the bipolar prosthesis (11). Like the mold arthroplasty, the bipolar prosthesis provided two planes of motion: the first between a large cup and the acetabulum, the second between a femoral component and a high-density polyethylene surface inside of the cup. This device has been used in a large variety of primary and secondary operations on the hip.

TOTAL HIP ARTHROPLASTY

The hemiarthroplasty of the Judet brothers and the interposition mold arthroplasty of Smith-Petersen gave surgeons experience with reconstructive hip surgery and stimulated new ideas and directions for improving the technique and the results. Themistocles Gluck, working in Berlin during the last decade of the 19th century, had demonstrated that the human body could tolerate large foreign bodies and had designed total knee joints made of ivory, which he fixed in place with a cement consisting of a mixture of resin and pumice or plaster of paris (45). Gluck's work was based on a long series of animal experiments. His clinical cases were all in patients with joints destroyed by tuberculosis or other serious disease. It was not until 1938 that Philip Wiles of London implanted matched acetabular and femoral components made of stainless steel as hip replacements in six patients with Still disease (152). The acetabulum was stabilized with screws and the head component with a stem, sideplate, and screws. World War II intervened and after the war Wiles did not pursue his ideas any farther.

With hemiarthroplasties becoming popular for the treatment of intracapsular hip fractures, it was logical to expand the operation to include an acetabular component. All-metal combinations were introduced by McKee and Farrar and Ring in England and by Haboush, Urist, and McBride in the United States (47,81,82,110,141). While the use of these prostheses gave surgeons further experience with what had become known as total hip arthroplasty, the results were not entirely satisfactory because of problems with loosening of the components and wear between the opposing metal surfaces.

It was John Charnley who led the way in establishing total hip replacement as a useful procedure—one that could be performed by any well-trained orthopedic surgeon, anywhere in the world. Charnley's method was the culmination of many years of hard work in the laboratory and in the clinic. Success did not come easily. His life and work are well presented in the biography by William Waugh (147). His most important intellectual breakthrough was his concept of the low-friction arthroplasty (26). Previously, all surgeons had substituted prostheses that were the same size and configuration as normal human anatomy. Charnley greatly reduced the diameter of the head on the femoral stem to a diameter of 22 mm to improve the frictional torque. Muller followed suit by introducing a design with a femoral head diameter of 32 mm (95). Charnley's attention was called to the possibilities of using methyl methacrylate cement by Leon Wiltsie of Los Angeles, and Charnley quickly adopted it (23). After an initial failure with the use of polytetrafluoroethylene (Teflon) as a bearing surface, he adopted high molecular weight polyethylene, which was satisfactory. With his design, the materials, and the technique of the operation in place, the use of the procedure spread quickly everywhere except the United States, where there was some delay awaiting the approval of the acrylic cement by the Food and Drug Administration.

Initially, total hip replacement using methyl methacrylate as a bone cement was thought to be a very forgiving operation. Errors in resecting bone and reaming could be made up by the addition of more cement. Unfortunately, this led to increased loosening. The operative technique has become more and more exact, and cementing technique more crucial. Robin Ling pointed out the importance of careful preparation of the bone surfaces and of forcing the cement into the bone by pressure (71). Jo Miller expanded this idea and introduced low-viscosity cement (90). William Harris studied and popularized the use of improved cementing techniques (51,98).

In a reaction to problems incident to the use of the acrylic cement, efforts were made to promote a more biological fixation by eliminating the cement altogether and providing a stem with a porous surface allowing for bone ingrowth. Pillar and Galante's research groups were pioneers in the study of this approach (13,14,36). The introduction of femoral components made of titanium also allowed fixation without the use of bone cement and without porous coating (73). The use of uncemented implants, both for the stem and for the acetabular components, has placed a high premium on technical skill and has made the procedures much more precise.

Was it necessary to resect so much of the proximal femur to provide a satisfactory arthroplasty? Answering in the negative were those surgeons who developed a resurfacing procedure called the "double-cup arthroplasty." Charnley tried this approach early in his work but abandoned it because of unsatisfactory results (26). In the United States, Haboush and Townley developed procedures of this type that saved most of the neck of the femur (47,136). In Europe, Wagner, among others, worked on this approach (145). The procedure of double-cup arthroplasty has not been widely adopted, but in the hands of enthusiasts such as Amstutz it has yielded good results (7).

CONCLUSIONS

The rapid development of hip surgery in the 20th century, with continuing biomechanical and technical innovations, has led to an explosion of information that has often been difficult for the orthopedic surgeon to absorb. Rapid communication among surgeons and surgical groups has become even more necessary. The general orthopedic societies and journals have been unable to keep up with the flood of papers and symposia coming from clinics and laboratories throughout the world. For this reason, the Hip Society was founded in 1968. Through its annual meetings, this society has provided the forum needed for this increasingly important area of orthopedic endeavor.

The following exhibits are reproduced from the outstanding collection of hip arthroplasty devices collected by the AAOS and currently on display at the Academy Building in Rosemont, Illinois. Permission has been granted by the AAOS to reproduce this collection, which allows the contemporary surgeon an appreciation of the large number of surgeons who have contributed to the current design philosophies underlying the modern total hip replacement. We would particularly like to thank the Academy Committee on the History of Orthopaedic Surgery: Rocca A. Calandruccio, M.D.; Robert J. Graham, M.D.; Leonard F. Peltier, M.D.; Marshall R. Urist, M.D.; and Sidney Weisman, M.S. (consultant).

REFERENCES

1. Adam A, Spence AJ. Intertrochanteric osteotomy for osteoarthritis of the hip. *J Bone Joint Surg.* 1958;40B:219–226.
2. Adams W. On subcutaneous osteotomy. *BMJ.* 1879;2:604–606.
3. Albee F. *Bone graft surgery.* Philadelphia: WB Saunders; 1917.
4. Albee FH. The bone graft wedge: its use in the treatment of relapsing, acquired, and congenital dislocation of the hip. *N Y Med J.* 1915;52:433–435.
5. Albert E. Einige Falle von kustlicher Ankylosebildung an paralytischen Gliedmassen. *Wien Med Press.* 1882;23:725–728.
6. Allende C, Lezama LG. Fractures of the neck of the femur in children. *J Bone Joint Surg.* 1951;33A:387–395.
7. Amstutz HC, Graff-Radford A, Mai LL, et al. Surface replacement of the hip with the Tharies system. *J Bone Joint Surg.* 1981;63A:1069–1077.
8. Aufranc OE. Constructive hip surgery with a vitallium mold: a report of 1000 cases of arthroplasty of the hip over a 15 year period. *J Bone Joint Surg.* 1957;39A:237–248.
9. Baer WS. Arthroplasty with the aid of animal membrane. *Am J Orthop Surg.* 1918:16:1–29, 94–115, 171–199.
10. Barton JR. On the treatment of anchylosis, by the formation of artificial joints. *Am Med Surg J.* 1827;3:279–292.
11. Bateman JE, ed. Symposium: bipolar femoral prosthesis. *Clin Orthop.* 1990;251:2–133.
12. Blount WP. Blade-plate fixation for high femoral osteotomies. *J Bone Joint Surg.* 1943;25:310–339.
13. Bobyn JD, Pilliar RM, Cameron HU, et al. Porous surfaced layered prosthetic devices. *J Biomed Eng.* 1975;10:126–131.
14. Bobyn JD, Pilliar RM, Cameron HU, et al. The optimum pore size for the fixation of porous surfaced metal implants by the ingrowth of bone. *Clin Orthop.* 1980;150:126–131.
15. Bonfiglio M. Aseptic necrosis of the femoral head in dogs: effect of drilling and bone grafting. *Surg Gynecol Obstet.* 1954;98:591–599.
16. Bonfiglio M, Voke EM. Aseptic necrosis of the femoral head and non-union of the femoral neck. *J Bone Joint Surg.* 1968;50A:48–66.
17. Boyd HB. Anatomic disarticulation of the hip. *Surg Gynecol Obstet.* 1947;84:346–349.
18. Brackett EG. Fractured neck of the femur; operation of transplantation of femoral head to trochanter. *Boston Med Surg J.* 1925;192:1118–1120.
19. Brittain HA. Ischiofemoral arthrodesis. *Br J Surg.* 1941;29:93–104.
20. Brock RC. *The life and work of Astley Cooper.* Edinburgh: Livingstone; 1952:66–71.
21. Calot F. *Indispensable orthopaedics.* London: Bailliere, Tindall and Cox; 1914:381.
22. Campbell WC. Arthroplasty of the hip: an analysis of 48 cases. *Surg Gynecol Obstet.* 1926;43:9–17.
23. Charnley J. Anchorage of the femoral head prosthesis to the shaft of the femur. *J Bone Joint Surg.* 1960;42B:28–30.
24. Charnley JA. Clean-air operating enclosure. *Br J Surg.* 1964;51:202–205.
25. Charnley JA. *Compression arthrodesis.* Edinburgh: Churchill and Livingstone; 1953.
26. Charnley J. *Low friction arthroplasty of the hip.* New York: Springer-Verlag; 1970.
27. Chiari K. Ergebnisse mit der Beckenosteotomie als Pfannendachplastik. *Z Orthop.* 1955;87:14–26.
28. Chicote-Campos F, Schlegel KF. Resection of the femoral head with or without angulation osteotomy. In: Rutt A, ed. *Coxarthrosis.* Stuttgart: Thieme; 1976:51–65.
29. Colonna PC. An arthroplastic procedure for congenital dislocation of the hip. *Surg Gynecol Obstet.* 1936;63:771–778.
30. Committee on the History of Orthopaedic Surgery, American Academy of Orthopaedic Surgeons, unpublished data, 1988.
31. Cooper A. *A Treatise on dislocations and on fractures of the joints.* London: Longman, Hurst, Rees, Orme and Brown; 1822:114–175.
32. Dickson JA. The "unsolved" fracture, a protest against defeatism. *J Bone Joint Surg.* 1953;35A:805–822.
33. Erichsen J. *The science and art of surgery, an American edition.* Philadelphia: Henry C Lea; 1866:657.
34. Ferguson AB. Primary open reduction of congenital dislocations of the hip using a median adductor approach. *J Bone Joint Surg.* 1973;55A:671–689.
35. Galante J, ed. Symposium: total joint arthroplasty without cement. *Clin Orthop.* 1983;176:7–114.
36. Gant FJ. Subcutaneous osteotomy below the trochanters. *BMJ.* 1879;2:606–607.
37. Ghormley RD. Use of the anterior superior spine and crest of the ilium in surgery of the hip joint. *J Bone Joint Surg.* 1931;13:784–798.
38. Gibney VP. *The hip and its diseases.* New York: Bermingham and Co.; 1884:391.
39. Gill B. Operation for old congenital dislocation of the hip. *Surg Clin N Am.* 1926;6:147–153.
40. Gill B. Operation for old or irreducible congenital dislocations of the hip. *J Bone Joint Surg.* 1928;10:698–707.
41. Gill B. Plastic reconstruction of an acetabulum in congenital dislocation of the hip: the shelf operation. *J Bone Joint Surg.* 1935;17:48–59.

42. Girdlestone GR. Discussion on treatment of unilateral osteoarthritis of the hip-joint. *Proc R Soc Med.* 1945;38:323.
43. Girdlestone GR. *Tuberculosis of bone and joints.* Oxford: Oxford University Press; 1940:81–83.
44. Gluck T. Die Invaginationsmethode der Osteo- und Arthroplastik. *Berl Klin Wochenschr.* 1890;28:732–736, 752–757.
45. Haas J. Neue Anwendungsgebiete der Lorenz'schen Bifurkation (Gabelung des oberen Femurendes). *Zentralbl Chir.* 1927;54:783–785.
46. Haboush EJ. A new operation for arthroplasty of the hip based on biomechanics, photoelasticity, fast setting dental acrylic, and other considerations. *Bull Hosp Joint Dis.* 1953;14:242–247.
47. Halsted WS. *The employment of fine silk in preference to cat-gut: the advantages of transfixing tissues and vessels in controlling haemorrhage. Also, an account of the introduction of gloves, gutta-percha tissue and silver foil.* Boston: Welch Bibliophilic Society; 1939.
48. Hamilton FH. *Deformities after fracture, part III.* Philadelphia: TK & PG Collins; 1857:63–54.
49. Harris WH, Enneking WF. Characteristics of the articular cartilage formed after intertrochateric osteotomy. *J Bone Joint Surg.* 1995;77A:602–607.
50. Harris WH, McCarthy JC, O'Neill OA. Femoral component loosening using contemporary techniques of femoral cement fixation. *J Bone Joint Surg.* 1982;64A:1063–1067.
51. Hawley GW. A new fracture, X-ray and orthopedic table. *Am J Surg.* 1932;18:19–25.
52. Henderson MS. Combined intra-articular and extra-articular arthrodesis for tuberculosis of the hip joint. *J Bone Joint Surg.* 1933;15:51–57.
53. Heusner L. Uber Ursachen, Geschichte, und Behandlung der angeborener Huftluxation. *Z Orthop Chir.* 1885;5:16.
54. Hey-Groves E. Some contributions to reconstructive surgery. *Br J Surg.* 1927;14:486–517.
55. Hey-Groves E. Treatment of fractured neck of the femur with especial regard to results. *J Bone Joint Surg.* 1930;12:1–11.
56. Heyman CH. Long-term results following a bone shelf operation for congenital and some other dislocations of the hip in children. *J Bone Joint Surg.* 1963;45A:1113–1146.
57. Hibbs RA. A preliminary report of twenty cases of hip joint tuberculosis treated by an operation devised to eliminate motion by fusing the joint. *J Bone Joint Surg.* 1926;8:522–533.
58. Hoffa A. Luxations congenitales de la hanche. *Rev Orthop.* 1890:24–41.
59. Hoffa A. Zur operativen Behandlung der angeborenen Huftgelenkverrenkung. *Zentralbl Chir.* 1892;19:921–924.
60. Ingram AJ, Bachynski B. Fractures of the hip in children. *J Bone Joint Surg.* 1953;35A:867–886.
61. Kelly HA, Burrasge WL. *Dictionary of American medical biography.* New York: Appleton; 1928:1079–1080.
62. Johansson S. On the operative treatment of medial fractures of the neck of the femur. *Acta Orthop Scand.* 1932;3:362–392.
63. Judet R, Judet J. Essais de reconstruction prothetique de la. hanche apres resection de la tete femorale. *J Chir.* 1949;65:17–24.
64. Judet R, Judet J. Treatment of fractures of the femoral neck by pedicled graft. *Presse Med.* 1961;2:452–453.
65. Kallio KE. Skin arthroplasty of the hip joint. *Acta Orthop Scand.* 1957;26:327–328.
66. Lampugnani L. La decapitazione del femore nella lussazione congenita dell'anca. *Giorn R Acad Med Torino.* 1885;33: 538–551.
67. Langenbeck B. Die subcutane Osteotomie. *Dtsch Klinik.* 1854;6:327–330.
68. Langenbeck B. Protokolle, Discussionen, kleinere Mittheilungen. *Verh Dtsch Ges Chir.* 1878(suppl):92–93.
69. Larrey DJ. *Memoires de chirurgie militaire, et campagnes.* Vol 4. Paris: J. Smith; 1817:50–51.
70. Lee AC, Ling RSM, Vangala SS, et al. Some clinically relevant variables affecting the mechanical behavior of bone cement. *J Bone Joint Surg.* 1978;60B:137.
71. Leger W. Proximal osteotomies of the femur without effect on the position of the head. In: Rutt A, ed. *Coxarthrosis: surgical and conservative treatment.* Stuttgart: Thieme; 1976:33–42.
72. Lintner F, Zweymuller K, Brand G. Tissue reactions of surrounding tissue to the cementless hip implant Ti-6AI.40 after implantation period of seven years. *Arch Orthop Trauma Surg.* 1988;107; 357–366.
73. Lorenz A. Ueber die Behandlung der irreponiblen angeborenen Huftluxationen und der Schenkelhalspseudarthrosen mittles Gabelung (Bifurkation desoberen Femurendes). *Wien Med Wochenschr.* 1919;32:997–999.
74. Luck VJ. Reconstruction operation for pseudoarthrosis and resorption of the neck of the femur. *J Iowa Med Soc.* 1938;28:620–622.
75. Ludloff K. Zur blutingen Einrenkung der angeborenen Huftluxation. *Z Orthop Chir.* 1908;22:272–276.
76. Malkin SAS. Femoral osteotomy in treatment of osteoarthritis of the hip. *BMJ.* 1936;1:304–305.
77. Mayer A. Historische und statistiche Notizen. Die von Dr. Mayer verrichtet Osteotomien. *Dtsch Klinik.* 1856;8:119–121, 140–141, 169–170, 178–180, 187–188, 200–202.
78. McBride ED. A femoral head prosthesis for the hip-joint. *J Bone Joint Surg.* 1952;34A:989–996.
79. McBride ED. The flanged acetabular replacement prosthesis. *Arch Surg.* 1961;83:721–728.
80. McKee GK, Watson-Farrar J. Replacement of arthritic hips by the McKee-Farrar prosthesis. *J Bone Joint Surg.* 1966;48B:245–259.
81. McMurray TP. Osteoarthritis of the hip joint. *Br J Surg.* 1938;22:718–727.
82. McMurray TP. Osteo-arthritis of the hip joint. *J Bone Joint Surg.* 1939;21:1–11.
83. McMurray TP. Ununited fractures of the neck of the femur. *J Bone Joint Surg.* 1936;18:319–327.
84. Meyers MH, Harvey JP, Moore TM. The muscle pedicle bone graft in the treatment of displaced fractues of the femoral neck. *Orthop Clin N Am.* 1974;5:779–792.
85. Milch H. Resection of the femoral neck with pelvic support osteotomy for ankylosis of the hip. *Surgery.* 1943;13:55–61.
86. Milch H. The bifurcation operation. *Surgery.* 1940;8:686–698.
87. Milch H. The "pelvic support" osteotomy. *J Bone Joint Surg.* 1941;23:581–595.
88. Miller J. Pressure penetration of low viscosity acrylic cement for improved fixation of arthroplasty components. *J Bone Joint Surg.* 1982;64B:619.
89. Moore AT. The self-locking metal hip prosthesis. *J Bone Joint Surg.* 1957;39A:811–827.
90. Moore AT, Bohlman HR. Metal hip joint: a case report. *J Bone Joint Surg.* 1943;25:688–692.
91. Muller HK. Intertrochanteric angulation osteotomy in the treatment of coxarthrosis. In: Rutt A, ed. *Coxarthosis: surgical and conservative treatment.* Stuttgart: Thieme; 1976:23–32.
92. Muller ME, Allkgower M, Schneider RT, et al. *Manual of internal fixation.* 2nd ed. New York: Springer-Verlag; 1979.
93. Muller ME, Boltzy X. Artificial hip joints made from Protosol. *Bull Assoc Study Problems Intern Fixation.* 1968:1–5.
94. Murphy JB. Arthroplasty of ankylosed joints. *Trans Am Surg Assoc.* 1913;31:67–137.
95. Nicoll EA, Holden NT. Displacement osteotomy in the treatment of osteoarthritis of the hip. *J Bone Joint Surg.* 1961;43B:50–60.
96. Oh I, Carlson C, Tomford W, et al. Improved fixation of the femoral component after total hip replacement using a methacrylate intramedullary plug. *J Bone Joint Surg.* 1978;60A:608–613.
97. Ollier L. *Traite experimental et clinique de la regeneration des os et de la production artificielle du tissu osseux.* Vol 2. Paris: Masson et Fils; 1867:385–386.
98. Otis GA. *A report of amputations at the hip-joint in military surgery.* Washington, DC: Government Printing Office; 1867.
99. Otis GA. *A report on excisions of the head of the femur for gunshot injury.* Washington, DC: Government Printing Office; 1869.
100. Park H, Moreau PF. *Cases of the excision of carious joints.* Glasgow: Brash and Reed; 1806.
101. Pauwels F. *Der Schenkelhalsbruch, Ein Mechanisches Problem, Grundlagen des Heilungsvorganges Prognose und kausale Therapie.* Stuttgart: Ferdinand Enke Verlage; 1935.
102. Pemberton PA. Pericapsular osteotomy of the ilium for treatment of congenital subluxation and dislocation of the hip. *J Bone Joint Surg.* 1965;47A:65–86.
103. Plummer WW. Comments on lateral fixation in fresh fractures of the neck of the femur. *J Bone Joint Surg.* 1938;20:97–107.
104. Poggi A. Contributio alla cura creenta della luzzazione congenita coxofemorale unilaterale. *Arch Orthop.* 1880;7:105.

105. Preston ME. New appliance for the internal fixation of fractures of the femoral neck. *Surg Gynecol Obstet.* 1914;18:260–261.
106. Putti V. Arthroplasty. *J Orthop Surg.* 1921;3:421–430.
107. Ring PA. Complete replacement arthroplasty of the hip by the Ring prosthesis. *J Bone Joint Surg.* 1968;50B:720–731.
108. Salter RB. Innominate osteotomy in the treatment of congenital dislocation and subluxation of the hip joint. *J Bone Joint Surg.* 1961;43B;3:518–539.
109. Sayre LW. A new operation for artificial hip joint in bony anchylosis. Illustrated by two cases. *Trans Med Soc N Y.* 1863:111–127.
110. Sayre LW. *Lectures on orthopedic surgery and diseases of the joints.* New York: Appleton; 1876:297–327.
111. Schanz A. Ueber die nach Schenkelhalsbruchen zuruckbleibenden Gehstorungen. *Munch Med Wochenschr.* 1925;51:730–732.
112. Schanz A. Zur Behandlung der veralteten angeborenen Huftverrenkung. *Munch Med Wschr.* 1922;69:930–931.
113. Schwartzmann JR. Arthroplasty of the hip in rheumatoid arthritis. *J Bone Joint Surg.* 1959;41A:705–721.
114. Senn N. A case of bony union after impacted intracapsular fracture of the neck of the femur. *Trans Am Surg Assoc.* 1883;1:167–170.
115. Senn N. Fractures of the neck of the femur. *Trans Am Surg Assoc.* 1883;1:333–352.
116. Seufert WD. The chain osteotome by Heine. *J Hist Med Allied Sci.* 1980;35:454–459.
117. Sherman WO. Vanadium steel bone plates and screws. *Surg Gynecol Obstet.* 1912;14:629–634.
118. Smith-Petersen MN. Evolution of mold arthroplasty of the hip. *J Bone Joint Surg.* 1949;30B:59–75.
119. Smith-Petersen MN. New supra-articular subperiosteal approach to the hip joint. *Am J Orthop.* 1917;15:592–595.
120. Smith-Petersen MN, Cave EF, VanGorder GW. Intracapsular fractures of the neck of the femur. *Arch Surg.* 1931;715–759.
121. Sommerville EW. The direct approach to congenital dislocation of the hip. *J Bone Joint Surg.* 1957;39B:623–640.
122. Speed JS, ed. *Campbell's operative orthopedics.* 2nd ed. St. Louis: CV Mosby; 1949:654–659.
123. Speed K. The unsolved fracture. *Surg Gynecol Obstet.* 1935;60:341–352.
124. Steele HH. Triple osteotomy of the innominate bone. *Clin Orthop.* 1977;122:116–127.
125. Steindler A. *Orthopedic operations.* Oxford: Blackwell Ltd; 1947:203.
126. Swett PP. An operation for reduction of certain types of congenital dislocations of the hip. *J Bone Joint Surg.* 1928;10:675–686.
127. Syme J. *The principles of surgery.* Philadelphia: Carey and Lea; 1832:352–353.
128. Tanner WE. *Sir W. Arbuthnot Lane, Bart. His life and work.* Baltimore: Williams & Wilkins; 1946:105.
129. Thomas HO. *Diseases of the hip, knee, and ankle joints with their deformities, treated by a new and efficient method.* 2nd ed. Liverpool: Dobb; 1876:27–86.
130. Thompson FR. Two and a half years' experience with a vitallium intramedullary prosthesis. *J Bone Joint Surg.* 1954;36A:489–500.
131. Thomson JEM. A prosthesis for the femoral head. *J Bone Joint Surg.* 1952;34A:175–182.
132. Townley CO. Hemi and total articular replacement arthroplasty of the hip with fixed femoral cup. *Orthop Clin N Am.* 1982;13:869–894.
133. Treharne RW. The compresson hip screw: the 25th aniversary of its development. *Orthop Rev.* 1982;11:45–52.
134. Trendelenberg F. Protokolle, Discussionen, kleinere Mittheilungen. *Verh Dtsch Ges Chir Suppl 1.* 1878:90–92
135. Tronzo RG. Hip nails for all occasions. *Orthop Clin N Am.* 1974;5:479–491.
136. Trumble HC. A method of fixation of the hip joint by means of an extra-articular bone graft. *Aust N Z J Surg.* 1932;1:413–420.
137. Urist M. The principles of hip-socket arthroplasty. *J Bone Joint Surg.* 1957;39A:786–810.
138. Vogler K, Redenz E, Walter H, et al. *Bernhard Heine's Versuche uber Knochenregeneration, Sein Leben und seine Zeit.* Berlin: Springer-Verlag; 1926.
139. Volkmann R. Die Krankheiten der Bewegungsorgane. In: Pitha F, Billroth T, eds. *Handbuch der algemeinen und speciellen Chirurgie.* Vol 2. Erlangen: Enke; 1865:554.
140. Volkmann R. Professor Volkmann on antiseptic osteotomy. *Edinburgh Med Surg J.* 1875;10:740–745.
141. Wagner H. Surface replacement arthroplasty of the hip. *Clin Orthop* 1978;134:102–136.
142. Watson-Jones R. Arthrodesis of the osteoarthritic hip. *JAMA.* 1938;110:278–280.
143. Waugh W. *John Charnley: the man and the hip.* London: Springer-Verlag; 1990.
144. White A. Letter from Lionel Beale. *Lond Med Gazette.* 1832;9:853.
145. White C. *Cases in surgery with remarks.* Part 1. London: Johnston; 1770:51–67.
146. Whitman R. A new treatment for fractures of the neck of the femur. *Med Record (N Y).* 1904;65:441–447.
147. Whitman R. Reconstruction operation for ununited fracture of the neck of the femur. *Surg Gynecol Obstet.* 1921;32:479–486.
148. Wiles P. The surgery of the osteoarthritic hip. *Br J Surg.* 1958;45:488–497.
149. Wilson JC. Extra-articular fusion of tuberculous hip joint. *Calif West Med.* 1927;27:774–776.
150. Zuckerman JD. The internal fixation of intracapsular hip fractures: a review of the first one hundred years. *Orthop Rev.* 1982;11:85–95.

Exhibit Figure 1-1   Cup Arthroplasty. While not the first arthroplasty performed in the United States, the Smith-Peterson cup arthroplasty was the first popular attempt to resurface the hip. **a:** An original plaster model of the Smith-Peterson cup from 1923. Wax was used as a template, and glass molds were made from the plaster cast. Glass blower Macallister Bicknell of Cambridge, Massachusetts, contributed to the technical aspects of this manufacturing technique. **b, c:** Originally made of a celluloid material (Viscaloid), these cups proved experimentally and clinically to produce a severe foreign body reaction. They were abandoned and 8 years passed before success was achieved. **d–f:** The years 1933–1936 represented a return to glass, now called by the trade name Pyrex. **d** is an imperfect mold, **e** an unstressed mold, and **f** a retrieval after 25 months of service in an active waitress. The cup was removed for revision to a vitallium replacement, necessitated by the fact that of the 17 other glass cups inserted this was the only one that did not break. **g, h:** An unused and a retrieved Bakelite cup. The only one of its kind inserted, the squeaking of this hip joint was used by the gas station attendant in whom it was implanted to remind his customers that they might need a lube job. **i–k:** Dr. Smith-Petersen's dentist, Dr. John Cooke, recommended the use of vitallium as a suitable material for the mold arthroplasty. **i** is an original, unsatisfactory mold; **j** is a never implanted model with a peripheral rim to prevent protrusion, and **k** is the final model used from 1938 through 1952. **l–o: l** is an unused vitallium mold, which can be compared in terms of surface polish to **m**, which is a 28-year successful retrieval specimen. **n** and **o** are 19-year retrievals. **p–t: p** is a lost wax casting model used to create **q**, the unpolished vitallium casting. The finished product, **r**, represents 8 hours of machine polishing. **s** and **t** represent 11 and 20 years of service, respectively. Note the high degree of polishing present from service. **u–x:** Similar cup arthroplasty specimens from the decades prior to total hip replacement. **y:** Laing developed the same mold design in titanium in 1960. **z, aa: z** and **aa** are later models of similar design. **bb, cc:** Albee and Pearson designed and implanted a socket in vitallium in 1940–1944 **(bb)**, whereas Urist's design is from 1951 **(cc)**.

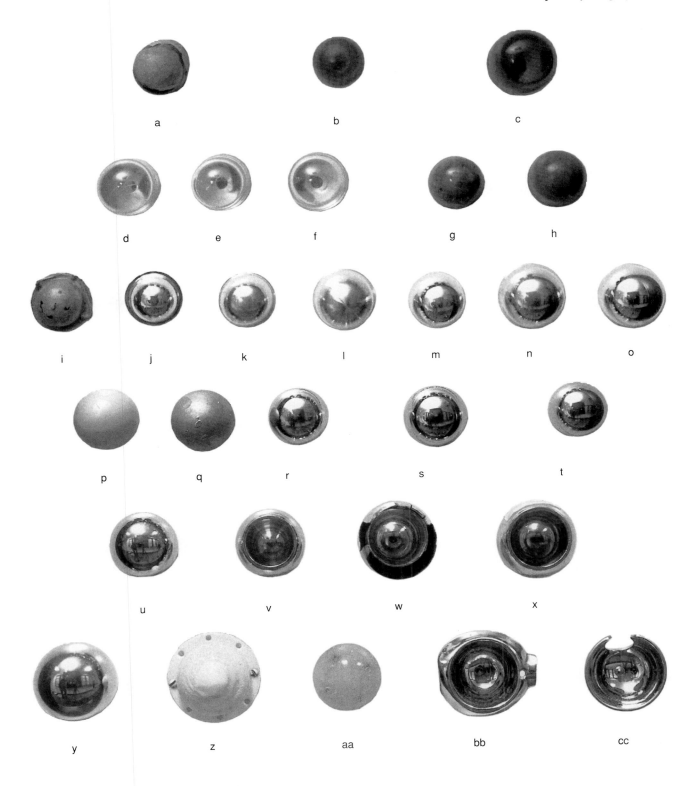

a

b

c

d   e   f   g   h

i   j   k   l   m   n   o

p   q   r   s   t

u   v   w   x

y   z   aa   bb   cc

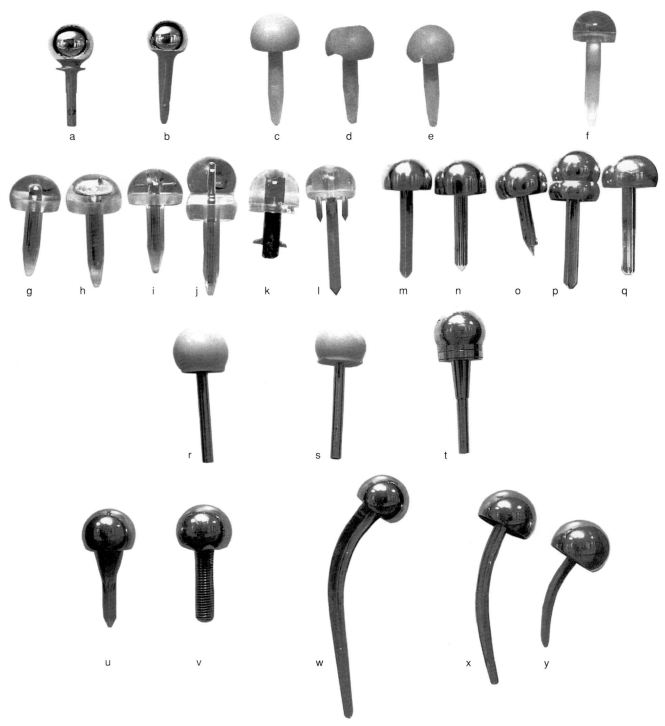

Exhibit Figure 1-2   Short-Stem Femoral Head Prosthesis. Short-stem femoral head prostheses were an important contribution to total hip arthroplasty. They had, as Charnley noted, a defective load bearing capacity. **a, b:** Initially made by Hohlman in 1939 and 1940, these vitallium femoral head prostheses represent the original **(a)** and improved **(b)** versions. **c–f:** About 1946, Judet reproduced the short-stem design in acrylic-polymethyl methacrylate. Molded at room temperature and pressure, the acrylic is opaque, as seen in **c**. Head erosion was produced by shear stress and produced typical defects in the overhanging lip. **d** and **e** represent 2-year retrievals. **f** represents the clear material acrylic yields when moulded at higher temperatures and pressures. **g–l:** These stems represent modifications to the original acrylic design and include metal reinforcing stems and supplemental fixation flanges. **m–q:** These stems are unidentified as to the designer but were developed in the same era and are examples of Smith-Petersen nails welded onto a solid or hollow-headed cup. The addition of flanges for fixation and cannulation for the insertion over guidewires can be noted. **r–t:** These stems represent a materials modification. Roger Anderson designed this nylon headed implant. Unfortunately, the nylon was susceptible to in vivo loss of tensile strength and resulted in material loss, dimensional change, and severe accompanying tissue reaction. **u, v:** These implants designed in 1950 by J. E. Thompson are called lightbulb prostheses due to their shape. Note solid heads with truncated smooth **(u)** and threaded **(v)** stem designs. **w–y:** Charles Townley of Pt. Huron, Michigan, redesigned the basic short-stem femoral head replacement to achieve increased intramedullary fixation. Initial stem length was considerably shortened in newer designs, and eventually the stem was combined with an acetabular component to create a total hip arthroplasty.

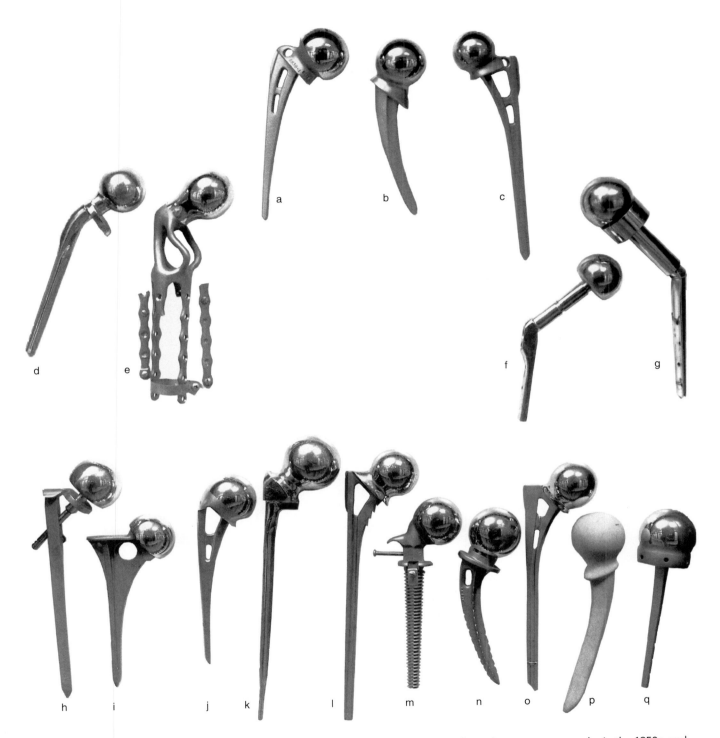

Exhibit Figure 1-3   Long-Stem Femoral Head Prosthesis. Long-stem femoral head prostheses became more popular in the 1950s, and multiple design modifications were the rule rather than the exception. **a–c:** Moore, based on experience with Bohlman, fenestrated the prosthetic stem to reduce its weight in 1950 **(a)**. A similar nonfenestrated design by F. R. Thompson in 1951 **(b)**, and the 1961 modification of the Moore design **(c)**. Called self-locking by virtue of its long, straight I-beam stem implanted in the curved intramedullary canal, bone chips were placed in the fenestrations to get bone growth across them as an afterthought. **d:** Intramedullary stem prosthesis designed by Eicher in 1951. **e:** In 1940 Moore created an upper third femur replacement for management of a giant cell tumor. Bohlman supervised the design to reduce its overall weight. This replica was inserted by Walter G. Stuck, M.D., of San Antonio, Texas for a similar case. It survived 20 years of use before the femur fractured at the lower end of the device. **f, g:** Well-known instrument makers Jaenichen and Collison developed these multisegment trunnion designs with side plates. **h–o:** These stems represent additional design modifications based on the original concepts. Lippman prosthesis 1952 **(h)**, Jergensen prosthesis 1960 **(i)**, Michele medial displacement prosthesis 1947 **(j)**, Leinbach prosthesis 1947 **(k)**, Townley prosthesis **(l)**, McBride screw-in prosthesis 1948 **(m)**, Scuderi trunnion prosthesis **(n)**, Cathcart ellipsoid-head prosthesis **(o)**. **p, q:** Smith-Brown experimental ceramic **(p)** prosthesis and Aufranc shaft prosthesis for special cases, 1973 **(q)**.

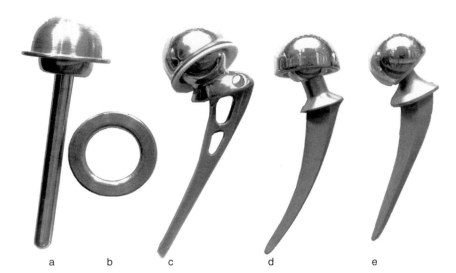

a   b   c   d   e

Exhibit Figure 1-4 Bipolar Replacement. Bipolar cups were introduced as early as 1950. While initially lined with Teflon, the inferior mechanical characteristics and subsequent biological reaction caused a search for a better bearing material. High molecular weight polyethylene was identified by Charnley in the 1960s and was subsequently used in many articulation designs. **a–c:** A McKeever-Collison collaboration from about 1950. The bearing **(b)** is Teflon. Trease designed this Teflon-lined cup **(c)** to mate with the Moore stem in 1960. **d, e:** Gilbert and Bateman designed polyethylene bipolar cups. These designs are from 1973.

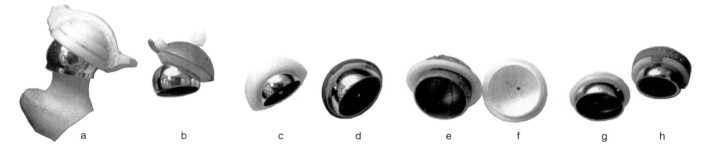

a   b   c   d   e   f   g   h

Exhibit Figure 1-5 Resurfacing Arthroplasty. Resurfacing arthroplasty, replacement of both the femoral and acetabular sides of the joint without violating the femoral canal, was investigated in the 1970s. Problems with maintaining the viability of the bone under the resurfaced femoral head, eventual loosening of the socket with substantial acetabular bone loss due to the large size of the component, and femoral neck fracture were all problematic in most series. Note that methacrylate fixation was popular on both sides of the articulation until porous ingrowth became available. **a:** 1971 Italian design of Paltrinieri-Tretani. **b:** M. A. R. Freeman design from 1979. Note the use of flanged polyethylene pegs instead of cement for fixation of the cup. **c, d:** The Indiana Conservative Cup designed in Indianapolis by Eicher in the late 1960s and early 1970s, redesigned by William Capello, his student in the late 1970s. Note metal backing of acetabular liner. **e, f:** The original Wagner design with metal head, metal-backed polyethylene socket with low-profile metal backing. **g, h:** Harlan Amstutz of UCLA continued to modify his THARIES resurfacing arthroplasty from the cemented all polyethylene cup **(g)** of the late 1970s through the era of porous ingrowth in the early 1990s, as seen in the fixation surface of the cup on **h.**

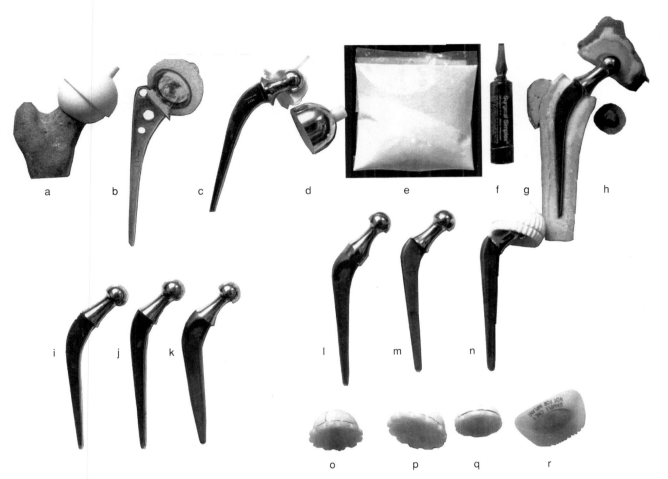

Exhibit Figure 1-6 Charnley Total Hip Arthroplasty. Myriad aspects of hip replacements were investigated, popularized, and some would say perfected by Sir John Charnley. He made many original contributions to the science and art of hip surgery, including the materials used and the methods of the fixation of the implants, as well as the design of the implants. He worked hard to reduce operative complications and postoperative morbidity. His development of the low-friction arthroplasty concept led to his being called the father of the total hip arthroplasty. **a–c:** Initially incorporating Teflon, this polymer was brittle and unsuitable. It generated wear debris rapidly, and this debris produced a significant tissue response. **a** represents original Charnley resurfacing components from 1958, which were press-fit. **b** has a large head and press-fit stem, which were mated with a Teflon cup (1958–1960). **c** represents the adoption of a smaller (22-mm) head diameter, which produced lower frictional torque and was developed in 1960–1962,one of many pioneering developments by Charnley. This retrieval demonstrates extensive wear in the bisected Teflon cup. Polyethylene as a bearing surface **(d)** was another significant contribution of Charnley's still utilized in today's total hip replacement. In 1963 a press-fit metal-backed polyethylene shell was utilized. **e, f:** The original methyl methacrylate powder and monomer still in use today. **g:** Cross section of a cemented Charnley stem and polyethylene cup. **h:** The wire mesh Mexican hat designed to plug the centering hole created in the medial wall of the acetabulum to center the acetabular cartilage reamers. This device was utilized to prevent cement from extruding into the pelvis. **i–k:** Modifications of the original Charnley stem. **i** represents the standard round-back stem, **j** a straight stem, and **k** the Cobra stem with anterior and posterior flanges on the lateral shoulder to aid in cement pressurization during insertion. **l–n:** Additional modifications of the original Charnley system. **o–r:** Modifications of cup design included addition of a radiographic marking wire in the cup **(o)**, an extended posterior wall to minimize dislocation **(p)**, an eccentric socket in the smaller sizes to maximize material where wear is expected **(q)**, and the Ogee cup designed with peripheral flanges to contain and pressurize cement during implantation **(r)**.

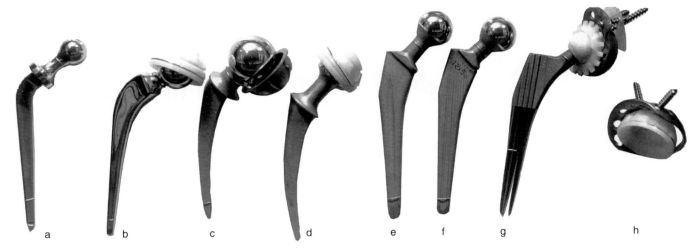

a   b   c   d   e   f   g   h

Exhibit Figure 1-7   Muller Total Hip Arthroplasty. Maurice E. Muller made substantial design modifications during the 1960s. **a:** In 1961 a thin curved-stem implant with Teflon socket and small head was press-fit. **b:** In 1963 polyethylene was adapted as the bearing surface. The implant was cemented. Note the hole in the inferior aspect of the head to trap wear debris. **c:** Metal on metal articulation allowed for a polyethylene liner that could be interposed between the standard head and cup bearings. **d:** The Charnley-Muller stem with curved banana-shaped stem and poly cup; a popular implant in the 1970s. **e, f:** Two modifications of the Muller straight-stem design introduced in 1977. These stems had longitudinal ridges. **g:** In 1988 the cementless self-locking system was produced. This system incorporated the longitudinal ridges seen in the previous design but added a distal clothes pin for press-fitting, modular collar, and modular heads in cobalt-chrome or ceramic, as well as a metal-backed porous-surfaced cup fixed with titanium screws. **h:** Developed in 1977, this acetabular roof-reinforcing ring was developed for screw fixation into iliac and remaining acetabular bone in cases where acetabular bone stock was thought to be insufficient to hold the cemented socket. The polyethylene cup was cemented into the ring.

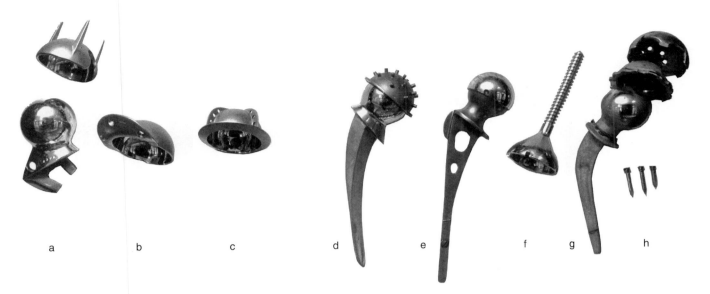

a   b   c   d   e   f   g   h

Exhibit Figure 1-8   Metal-on-Metal Total Hip Arthroplasty. Metal on metal as an articulation was attempted in the 1950s and further modified during the 1960s. More recent concerns about poly-ethylene wear debris have sparked a renewal of interest in this articulation in the 1990s. **a–c:** These sockets were mechanically fixed to the pelvis and were initially designed for acetabular arthroplasty. However, they were also used with the nonpolar Moore and Thompson prostheses for metal-on-metal total hip replacements: Urist, 1951 **(a)**, Gaenslen, 1953 **(b)**, and McBride, 1961 **(c)**. **d:** The first popular metal-on-metal total hip was the McKee-Farar. **e, f:** Ring designed an acetabular component with a massive threaded stem that obtained purchase in the ilium and occasionally traversed the sacroiliac joint. **g, h:** The Stanmore hip designed by Duff, Barclay, and Scales employed a two-piece acetabular shell, which was assembled at the time of surgery.

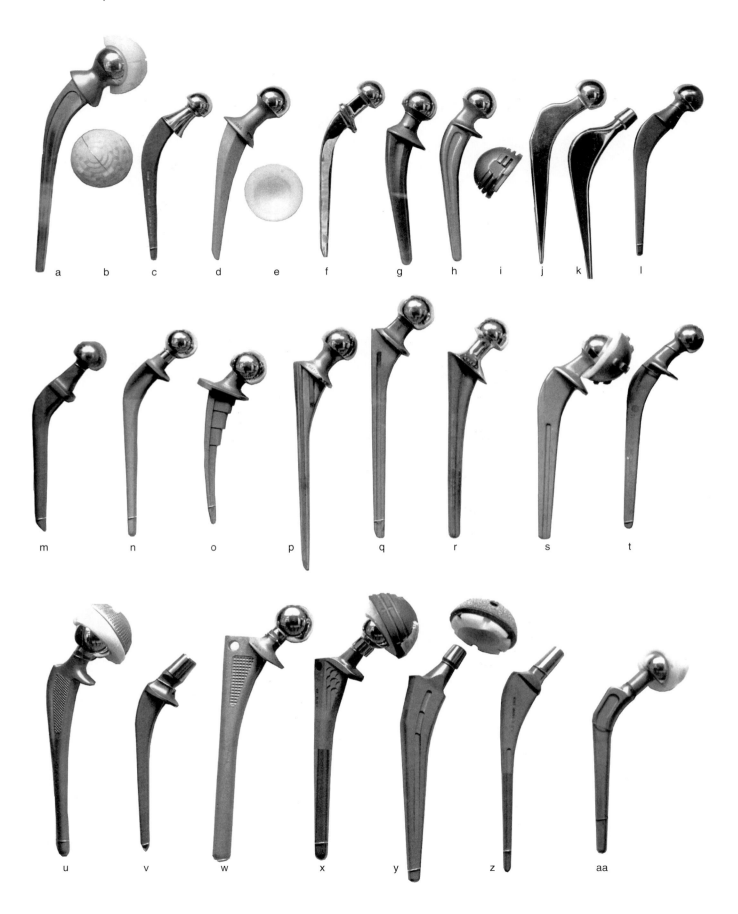

a   b   c   d   e   f   g   h   i   j   k   l

m   n   o   p   q   r   s   t

u   v   w   x   y   z   aa

◄─────────────────────────────────

Exhibit Figure 1-9   Cemented Total Hip Arthroplasty. Literally hundreds of cemented total hip designs followed on these pioneering efforts. During the late 1970s it seemed that every engineering finding led to new stem design modifications. **a:** Bucholz from Germany designed this 38-mm head, I-beam stem with rather sharp internal radii. The socket was 1.5 mm in diameter larger than the head, with an elliptic recess in the anterior aspect of the cup. **b:** An additional socket design by Bucholz. **c:** Bechtol of California produced the first Charnley-type stem in the United States. Head size was 25 mm. **d:** Otto Aufranc and Roderick Turner in Boston developed the Aufranc-Turner stem featuring a 32-mm head, oval neck cross section, and sharp edges at the corners of the stem. **e:** A polyethylene cup designed for the stem seen in **d**. **f:** Harlan Amstutz of California developed the Trapezoidal 28, which featured a trapezoidal cross section at the head and neck. Later models adopted a square cross section. **g:** The CAD hip (computer-assisted design) was cast and featured a 32-mm head and a broad short stem with more gentle radii at the stem margins. **h, i:** The HD-2 stem designed and popularized by William Harris, M.D., of Boston. This stem was forged and featured a larger collar and smaller stem configuration. The metal shell allowed for polyethylene liner exchange. **j, k:** Robin Ling of Exeter, U.K., designed with a collarless stem **(j)**, which featured tapered surfaces in both planes. This was designed to allow for stem subsidence within the cement mantle. Later design **(k)** featured polished surfaces. **l:** The STH hip designed by Augusto Sarmiento, M.D., appeared to mimic the design of Charnley but was produced in titanium, representing the first use of titanium for a total hip stem in the United States. **m:** Phillip Wilson, M.D., and Al Burstein, Ph.D., of New York designed the DF-80, which was intended to fill 80% of the intramedullary canal diameter. **n:** The IOWA Hip, developed in conjunction with University of Iowa engineers, was popularized by surgeon/implant designer Richard Johnston. It features a cylindrical stem distally and rounded borders to minimize cement strain concentrations. **o:** Charles Townley, M.D., of Michigan developed this stem with an exceptionally broad proximal platform and collar and step-graduated stem taper. **p–r:** Fatigue failure of stems led to attempts to strengthen the stem with I-beam construction. Additional modifications to minimize cement strains were added, as noted in this Mitchetti-Brown **(p)** stem. Mack Clayton of Denver, Colorado, designed a stem that featured a distal taper plus I-beam **(q)**, whereas Rocco Callundrucio, M.D., designed the Titan stem, which featured a compressed oval cross section. **s:** Indong Oh designed this stem to provide compressive stresses on the cement. **t:** This stem was similar to the Charnley in stem geometry but featured a collar. **u–x:** In the 1980s design modifications appeared that textured the stem to improve interlocking OC stem and cement. Centralization of the stem was accomplished by the addition of distal centralizers to allow for a more uniform cement mantle. In addition, head and neck modularity was introduced. This modification is seen on most implants dating from this period forward. While providing several advantages for the operating surgeon, as in any design choice, multiple disadvantages were eventually noted as well. These are well described in multiple sections of the text. The precision hip featured both proximal and distal centralizers as well as proximal stem macrotexturing **(u)**. **v** shows a stem that was similar to the Charnley in stem geometry but featured a collar. The cemented medullary locking stem (CML) **(w)** utilized a preformed polymethyl methacrylate centralizer in addition to proximal macrotexturing as did the Proforma stem **(x)**. **y:** This stem featured a straight bluntly tapered geometry with longitudinal grooves to resist rotational forces. Note the absence of a collar. **z:** Proximal stem grit blasting to improve cement stem bonding was a feature of this Mallory-Head implant designed by William Head, M.D., and Thomas Mallory, M.D.. **aa:** Nas Eftekhar, M.D., of New York modified the neck angle and proximal stem of the Charnley-type design.

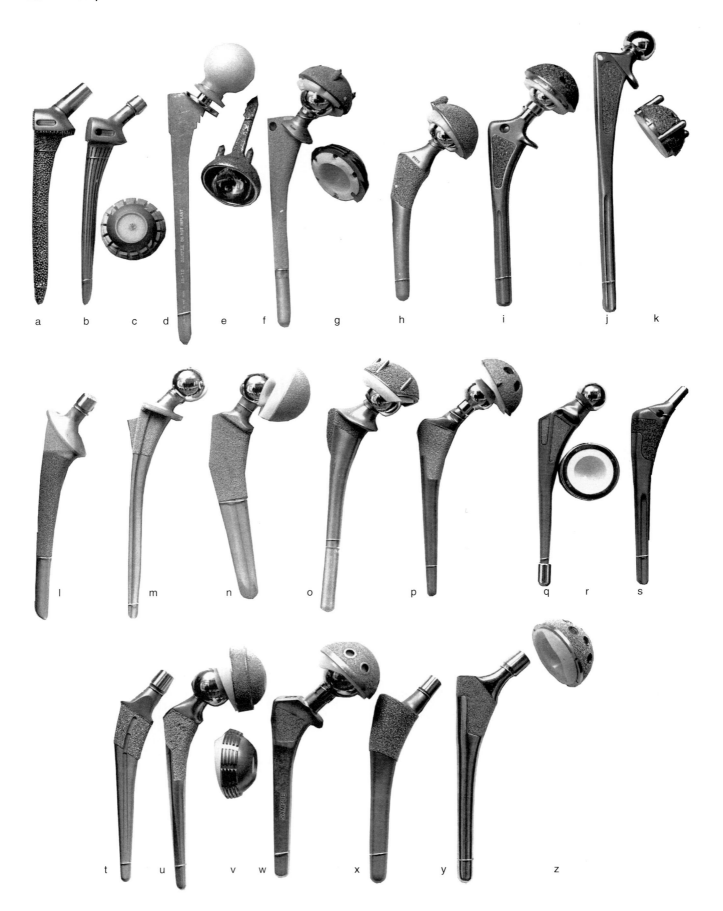

←

Exhibit Figure 1-10   Metal-Coated Total Hip Arthroplasty. Beginning in the 1970s and continuing through the end of the century, ortho-pedic surgeons have attempted to eliminate bone cement as a secondary fixation substance and obtain direct fixation of bone to the implant. Because of the mechanical requirements of stem stability, bone implant apposition, and the biological nature of the interface, mul-tiple design modifications at regular intervals have marked the development of this path toward improving implant longevity. **a–c:** Gerald Lord of France developed the Madreporique implant **(a)**, which had a macroscopic beaded surface and was coated throughout its length. Extraction of a well-ingrown stem was a daunting task. The later version incorporated a roughened surface and longitudinal flutes to pro-vide for rotational stability **(b)**. A mainstay of European design through the 1970s, 1980s, and 1990s has been the threaded screw ring cup **(c)** for acetabular fixation. Results of this cup in the hands of many American surgeons show high migration and loosening rates. **d, e:** Tronzo of Florida designed this stainless steel implant in the 1970s. A trunnion on the stem accepted a polyethylene head, and the long spiked acetabular component, which had a porous surface, accepted a polyethylene liner. **f–s:** First-generation modern cementless stems employed a multitude of different and, in many cases, contrary design features. A pioneer in the use of porous-surfaced stems was Emmet Lunceford, M.D., who along with Pillar and Engh designed the Anatomic Medullary Locking Stem **(f)**. It featured varying lengths of porous coating (proximal, 5/8th seen here, and fully coated). It was matched to a porous cup impacted in place, with rotational stability augmented by small spikes. One of the most commercially successful of the earlier cementless designs, the porous-coated anatomic (PCA) was designed by David Hungerford and Robert Kenna **(g)**. The implant was anatomic in shape and employed a circumferentially beaded surface over the proximal third of the implant. The cup had two small porous pegs at the superolateral surface, which augmented rotational sta-bility. **h** represents an alternate screw-in threaded socket design available with this component. The straight-stem prosthesis (designed by William H. Harris, M.D., of Boston and Jorge O. Galante, M.D., of Chicago: the H-G hip) utilized fiber metal as the porous substrate **(i)**. The pad surface was not circumferential. This was seen over time to allow for the movement of joint wear debris along the intramedullary canal. The socket was also designed with a fiber metal ingrowth surface. Note the hole anteriorly for placement of a screw. The feature of screw augmentation to improve cup stability was an innovation that was eventually copied in most cups and proved particularly useful in acetab-ular component revision. Ramon Gustillo, M.D., and Richard Kyle, M.D., of Minneapolis, Minnesota, designed the Bias stem **(j, k)**, which also employed patch fiber metal ingrowth surface proximally. Stem length was substantially longer than in most other first-generation cementless implant designs, and the stem was curved to fit the isthmic region of the canal, based on the concept of intramedullary rod fix-ation. Smooth pegs and supplemental screw fixation were a feature of the cup. Roy-Camille of France designed the mini-Madreporique stem **(l)** with smaller bead diameter and less extensive coating than the Lord stem seen in Exhibit Figure 1-10a. Charles Townley, M.D., of Port Huron, Michigan, added a lateral fin to improve rotational stability to a proximally beaded implant **(m)**. The stem in **n** is very broad in the medial-lateral direction and is without a collar, similar to the designs of Muller. Leo Whitesides of St. Louis, Missouri, designed a very proximally coated stem with a lateral fin **(o)**, as seen in Exhibit Figure 1-10m. Additional innovations included a machined methyl methacry-late sleeve, which could be placed distally on the stem to improve canal fill in patients in whom the metaphyseal segment of the femur was disproportionately large in comparison to the diaphysis. Note also the cut-out segment of the inferomedial aspect of the acetabulum. This was thought to improve range of motion and minimize impingement. The Perfecta stem **(p)** had plasma-sprayed titanium as the proximal ingrowth surface and employed small fins on the periphery of the acetabulum to augment stability. The Omniflex stem **(q)** incorporated a distal bullet tip that was modular and allowed for improved diaphyseal fill and with less stem stiffness and is similar in concept to the stem in **o**. Polar view **(r)** of a cementless socket with modular polyethylene insert. The anatomic stem **(s)** was designed to match the double bow of the proximal femur for improved metaphyseal fill and greater rotational stability. Porous titanium fiber metal coating was limited to the upper third but was circumferential. **t:** The Roy-Camille mini-Madreporique cementless universal stem and cup. **u:** The Omnifit stem employed a proximally porous-coated stem and a new design of socket. Note the differing geometries of the central versus the peripheral portions of the cup. No screw holes or other stability augmentation features are present. The cup was designed to press-fit by impaction of the peripheral rim. **v:** A threaded chamfered screw-in socket. **w:** The collarless Anatomic Proximal Replacement (APR) was designed by Larry Dorr, M.D., of Los Angeles, California. The stem featured a collar and proximal patch coating. **x:** The Profile hip stem geometry was based on the compiled intramedullary canal dimensions of a large cohort of cadaver femora. **y, z:** The Optifix was a collarless stem that employed a titanium bead coating.

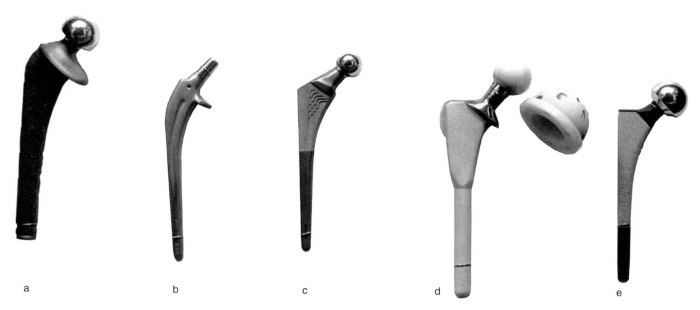

a   b   c   d   e

Exhibit Figure 1-11   Nonmetallic-Coated Total Hip Arthroplasty. Multiple attempts have been made to coat the metal stem substrate to achieve improved integration of the stem with bone and or cement or to alter the mechanical features of the stem. **a:** The Poplast stem implanted in 1966 utilized a metal substrate coated with polytetrafluoroethylene, designed by King, Homsy, and Hugh Tullos, M.D. **b:** William H. Harris, M.D., applied a layer of methyl methacrylate to the upper third of this cobalt-chrome stem to chemically bond the cement implanted at surgery to the cement applied to the stem at the time of manufacture. This was thought to help prevent stem debonding. **c:** Hydroxyapatite coating over the proximal half of the stem with normalization ridges cut into the metaphyseal region. These ridges were thought to convert shear stresses in part to compressive stresses. **d:** The Fulrong hydroxyapatite-coated stem incorporating a collar and ceramic head, as well as a hydroxyapatite-coated socket. **e:** This stem featured a titanium substrate with fused particles of engineering grade polysulfone, and solid polysulfone distally.

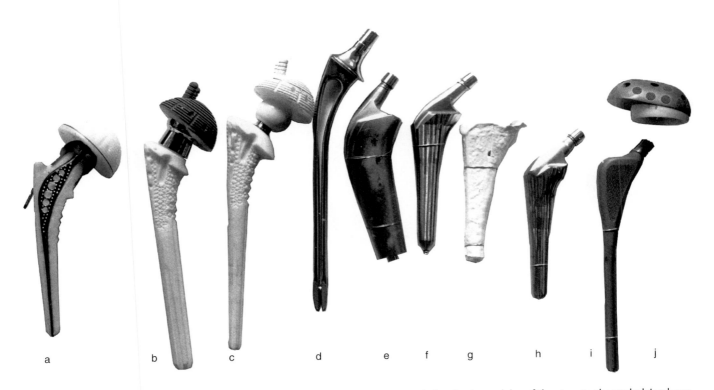

a   b   c   d   e   f   g   h   i   j

Exhibit Figure 1-12   Isoelastic and Custom-Made Prostheses. Attempts to match the elastic modulus of the stem to the underlying bone were popular throughout the 1980s. **a–c:** Bombelli, Moscher, and Mathys designed a low-modulus stem that incorporated a steel (and later a titanium) core under polyacetate resin. Cutaway view **(a)** of the stem with a cementless all-polyethylene cup. Porous metal threaded cup **(b)** and hydroxyapatite-coated polyethylene cup **(c)**. **d:** One-piece forged steel stem with four rods connected distally. **e–j:** Customization has been attempted in two major fashions. Intraoperative customization is seen in **e–h**. **e** represents a partially machined titanium blank. **f** represents the precut model, and **g** represents a Silastic mold taken intraoperatively from the intramedullary canal. An on-site facility machines the final implantable stem **(h)** according to the dimensions of the Silastic mold. **i, j:** William Bargar, M.D., of Sacramento, California, and S. David Stulberg, M.D., of Chicago, Illinois, developed custom stems and sockets (here designed for a bone-deficient acetabulum based on CT scan dimensional measurements).

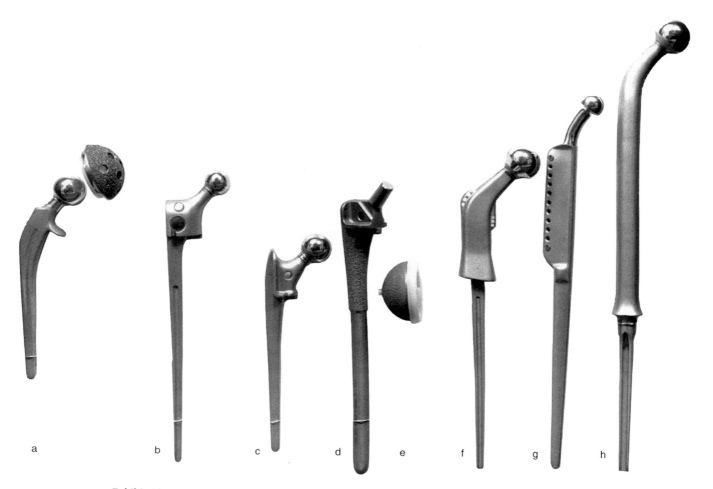

a   b   c   d   e   f   g   h

Exhibit Figure 1-13   Hybrid Hip and Replacement Prostheses. Multiple designs have incorporated substantial segmental replacement capabilities. **a:** A standard stem in terms of overall length as well as neck length for comparison purposes. **b, c:** Cemented calcar replacement stems. **d:** Stem designed for proximal porous ingrowth. **f–g:** Cemented stems designed for massive bone loss, most commonly after tumor resection.

Exhibit Figure 1-14   Press-Fit and Total Hip Arthroplasty. Multiple stems have been designed to provide an interference or press-fit. Principles of such stem design can be found in Chapter 68. **a:** The Austin-Moore, one of the original press-fit stems. **b:** The Judet prosthesis featured a large trochanteric fin and a cast, rough-textured surface. Note the cylindrical shape of the acetabulum. **c:** This stem, the Itami, featured pagoda-shaped spaces on the acetabulum and a cross-hatched surface finish on the femur. **d:** The Mittelmeir prosthesis, developed in Germany, was used in the United States for a short period of time. It featured a macrotextured stem with ceramic head and ceramic screw-in threaded cup. **e:** The Biofit stem developed by Indong Oh featured a macrotextured stem with scallops and a lateral trochanteric fin to maximize proximal fixation. **f:** The Norwich smooth stem has holes for attachment of the abductors. The porous coating is on the undersurface of the collar. **g,h:** The McCutcheon **(g)** featured a trapezoidal cross-sectional geometry and longitudinal grooves for macroscopic fixation. The Macrofit stem **(h)** oriented grooves in a curved fashion. **i, j:** These stems featured steplike normalizations designed to convert stresses from shear to compression, ostensibly better for the interface of stem and bone **(i)** or stem and cement **(j)**. **k:** The anatomically shaped stem was called the Anthropometric Total Hip and was designed by Harlan Amstutz of Los Angeles, California. **l, m:** This Russian design, the Sivash **(l)**, was designed with a one-piece articulated constrained socket. **m** represents a modification designed to improve cement fixation. **n, o:** Hugh Cameron of Canada designed this modular stem, which incorporated a porous sleeve that could be placed in the metaphysis, which could be machined to accept the part. A modular stem inserted into the sleeve could be adjusted to accommodate anteversion requirements with distal modifications such as cutting flutes or cutouts to reduce stiffness. **p, q: p** represents an attempt at a stem filling design, as seen in Exhibit Figure 1-9y, whereas **q** attempts to achieve canal fill by a modular sleeve. **r–t:** Press-fit and total hip arthroplasty. The stem designed by Deyerle in 1974 **(r, s)** employed interlocking bolts to prevent subsidence and rotation. These interlocking nail concepts were applied to revision stems in the 1980s but met with little success. These concepts were more successfully employed in the interlocking femoral fracture nails designed in the 1980s. The acetabular component **t** offered both peripheral fins and peripheral screw fixation capabilities. **u–w:** M. A. R. Freeman of London, England, designed this stem to minimize neck resection and take advantage of the potential that the remaining neck had to resist rotational forces around the stem **(u)**. The stem was inserted into a slot cut into the superior aspect of the neck and greater trochanter **(v)**. The stem was designed with hydroxyapatite coating for press-fit Press fit **(v)** and was also designed for use with cement **(w)**.

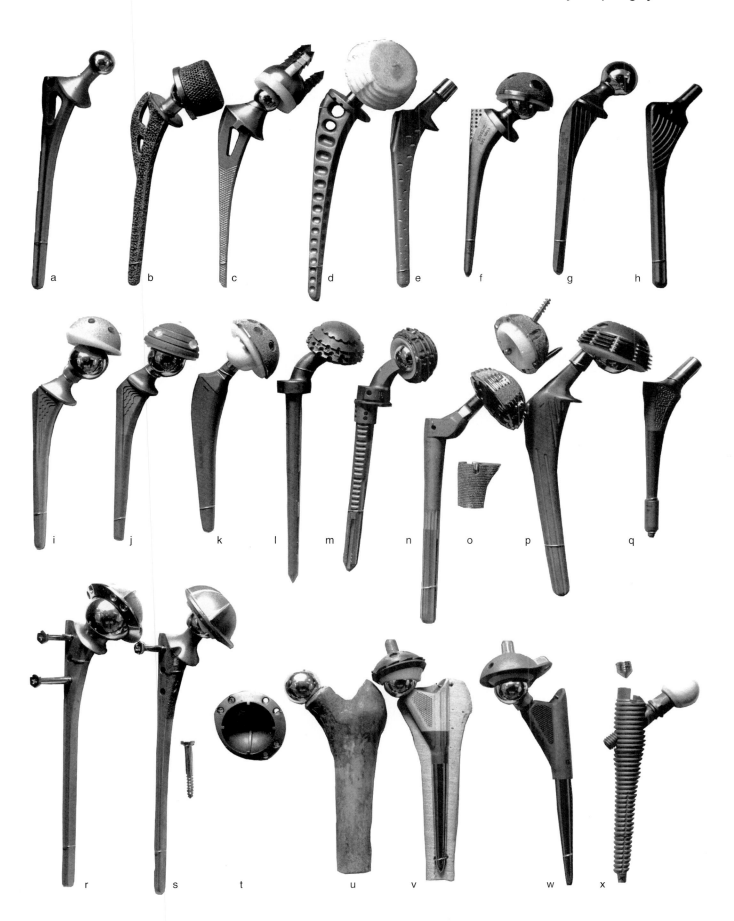

Basic Science

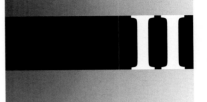

Pre- and Postnatal Development of the Hip

2

Timothy M. Ganey   *John A. Ogden*

In joining the lower extremities to the trunk, the hip joints provide an anatomic basis for upright posture and balanced locomotion. The hip joints are designed for both strength and mobility, effectively embracing walking, running, jumping, climbing, and myriad modifications and amplifications of these fundamental movements. Hence, the anatomy reflects the need for strong, heavy bones that are secured in articulation and constrained in range of motion by numerous ligaments and surrounding muscles. The adult hip emerges over the course of coaptive development as an articulation between the head of the femur and the acetabulum, ultimately reflecting the individual interpretation of and response to biological demands that are initiated intrinsically in the embryo, and functionally adapted to during progressive skeletal maturation.

Although the word *pelvis* is often used interchangeably to describe the articulated bony ring formed by the sacrum and the two hip bones, the hip joint will be considered as the femoral articulation of the lower extremity with the hip bone. This is not to discount the postural interrelationship of the spine via the sacrum, nor the potential for imbalanced loading imposed by leg-length inequality, but more to delimit the anatomy of the acetabular–femoral articulation as a regional entity of consideration. Developmental changes in either component affect the responsive growth of its companion,

and it is the maintenance of balance between the two that extends a mechanically stable range of motion through a course of skeletal maturation.

In considering the development of the hip, it is important to remember the significance of changing anatomical differences between a child and an adult, particularly with respect to potential complications. Areas of major importance include (a) the complex cartilaginous components of the acetabulum; (b) the progressive development of the proximal femur into the functionally separate lesser trochanter, greater trochanter, and capital femoral epiphyses; and (c) the susceptibilities to vascular compromise that are associated with age and anatomy. While these issues underscore the dynamics of enchondral bone formation and skeletal maturation at an individual level, they must be considered with respect to their performance selection over the long evolution of the hip.

Growth as a permanent increase in size, and morphogenesis as a change in shape, retains a basic dependency on the differentiation and emergence of specialized, functional cell lines. Ultimately, the proliferation of the cells with respect to their surrounding cell environment defines the limits of size; the larger the initial deposit of cells, the greater potential for growth. Such represents an inherent capacity for genetic or ontogenetic variation amongst members of a population. For the structures to be elucidated shortly, other variables of individual development merit consideration. The adult acetabulum is formed by the coalescence of three separate osseous components, namely, the ischium, the ilium, and the pubic bone. Although these individual components emerge from developmental fields that are separately maintained genetically, their successful functional maturation requires a coordinated response between the individual ossification centers, as well as with the head of the femur. If evolutionary pressures effectively sieve the most efficient structure over a long course of time, the genetic disposition of the tissues reflecting a best adult trait may not necessarily be in total accord with phenotypic requirements during transitional stages of development.

Considering the sudden transition of the hip at birth from flexion to nearly an extended position, a case might be made that the cartilaginous neonate articulation may be subject to subtleties of mechanical imbalance that are more apparent in some individuals.

As growth and development of the acetabulum and the proximal femur are both dependent upon cell and tissue mechanisms of endochondral ossification, small differences in structures that are present initially may lead to large-scale divergence over a course of progressive development. Understanding normal morphology of the developing hip brings a certain prognostic value to clinical assessment by extending a basis for recognizing how aberrant immature structures might potentiate compromised adult tissue biomechanical performance.

DEVELOPMENT OF THE HIP JOINT

Successful development of the vertebrate limb requires a complex set of interactions between the ectoderm and the underlying mesoderm (3,25,51). The onset of limb development, initiated by mesodermal condensation in the lateral plate mesoderm, is dependent upon inductive influences of both adjacent somite tissue (49) and the mesonephros (24). Four weeks after fertilization, the lower limb buds become evident on the anterior lateral body wall at the level of the lumbar and first sacral somites (52). Once the initial bud has formed, through as yet still incompletely understood mesenchymal–ectodermal interactions, the epithelium at the leading margin of the bud thickens and assumes a pseudostratified appearance known as the apical ectodermal ridge (AER). Further limb bud elongation occurs rapidly under the influence of the AER, and within a few days, differentiation of an intricate pattern of cartilage, bone, muscles, and other support tissues occurs.

The remarkable degree of homology between different species of vertebrates has led to several insights into pattern imprinting (5,6,20). From the available literature, much of it derived from chick limb bud studies, a few basic tenets have evolved, perhaps the foremost being that the basic recognizable components of limb outgrowth potentiate from most proximal to distal. This suggests that as cells divide in response to positional disparities, certain cells progressively adopt a more distal identity (7). As the femur and the acetabulum emerge from this mesenchymal blastema as the most proximal aspect of the limb buds, they constitute the basis for further differentiation of more distal limb structures. As proximal to distal differentiation progresses, groups of cells become committed to certain zones or regions, while other groups continue to migrate and commit more distally.

Additional studies support a genetic basis for segmentation on the anterior–posterior axis. Based on the 1978 work by Lewis in *Drosophila* (40), the vertebrate *HOX* genes have been elicited as candidates for pattern formation during morphogenesis in not only the body axis but in the limb as well (14,15). In the context of the hip articulation, the proximal extent of the fibular developmental field involves the pubic portion of the pelvis and the proximal femur, while ischial and iliac portions of the hip bones and the distal femur are associated with the tibial developmental field (39). Thus, while it would be fair to say that the acetabulum and the proximal femur evolve from a common mesenchymal mass, it is important to realize that ontogenetic separateness extends not only to the skeleton, but to the synovia, the ligaments of the joint, and the muscles and their intermuscular septa and tendons. These field patterns thus explain interrelationships of deficiency syndromes, such as the association of fibular deficiency or absence with a hypoplastic femur or proximal femoral focal deficiency.

ACETABULUM

The acetabulum is the convergence point of the three primary ossification centers: the ischium, pubis, and ilium. The acetabulum is first apparent in the 14- to 15-mm embryo as a cellular depression proximal to the developing femur, the concavity shallow and composing an arc of only 65° to 70° (52). Still essentially a skeletal blastema, further differentiation of the cartilaginous anlagen of the hip bone lags behind

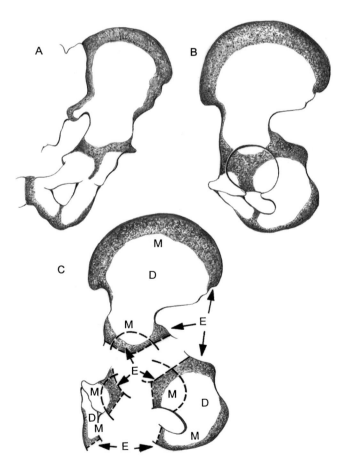

Figure 2-1 This illustration depicts the separate osseous entities from which the hip bone is composed. **A:** An anterior view does not permit a full appreciation of the acetabulum. **B:** In a true lateral view, a better grasp of the union of the separate components is apparent. **C:** An exploded view depicts the morphologic identity that each of the three component bones—ilium, ischium, and pubis—brings to the triradiate cartilage. E, epiphysis; M, metaphysis; D, diaphysis.

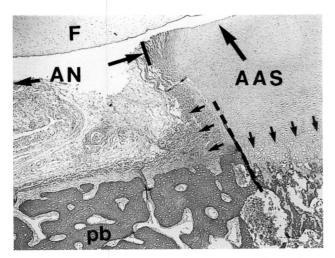

Figure 2-2 A transverse section of the prenatal acetabulum demonstrates the floor of the acetabular notch (*AN*). Note the discontinuity of the acetabular articular surface (*AAS*), and the orientation of the periosteal bone (*pb*) within the fovea. A broken line delineates areas of endochondral bone formation from a physeal-type mechanism from periosteal differentiation and membranous-type bone formation. Such morphology permits acetabular expansion that is balanced between tension-regulated periosteal proliferation within the notch, and enchondral transition at the triradiate metaphysis. F, femur.

the shaft and the femoral head at all stages. Chondrification radiates from the conjunction of the three primordia, establishing an antecedent for the triradiate cartilage, which will subsequently serve as a composite epiphysis for the acetablum. The iliac and the ishial anlagen coalesce posteri-

orly, followed shortly thereafter by fusion of the ilium with the pubic component. Finally, the ischium and the pubis fuse from their inner margins outward until all that remains of the blastemal junction is the acetabular fossa. In a manner that is similar to all growth cartilage, further enlargement of the acetabulum occurs by appositional and interstitial cell multiplication, and matrix elaboration.

Primary ossification centers for the three anlagen of the hip joint appear in the ilium at 38 to 39 mm, in the ischium variably between 105 and 124 mm, and in the pubis at 161 mm (23). Each of the three ossification centers expands centrally, converging within the acetabulum until separated only by the triradiate cartilage (Fig. 2-1). The triradiate cartilage may be considered as a composite epiphysis of the three contributing centers of the hip bone, allowing integrated growth of the acetabulum commensurate with spherical growth of the capital femur.

The acetabulum develops through four types of cartilage. The first type, the articular cartilage, is variably thick and merges imperceptibly with the second type, the undifferentiated hyaline cartilage. The hyaline cartilage, like the epiphyseal cartilage of a tubular bone, has a discrete system of cartilage canals and contributes cells to the third type, the physeal cartilage. The fourth type, the fibrocartilage of the labrum is grossly and histologically well demarcated from the adjacent hyaline and articular cartilage types. The three growth sectors—iliac, pubic, and ischial—are confluent with the respective physeal regions of the acetabulum, opposing each other through a common epiphysis: the triradiate hyaline cartilage.

Although the separate cartilages of the acetabulum imperceptibly blend in appearance, they maintain functionally separate identities. The lateral cup-shaped articular cartilage forms the articular surface with the head of the femur, while

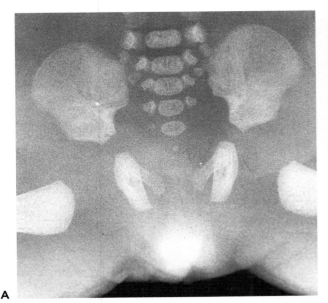
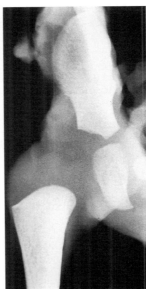
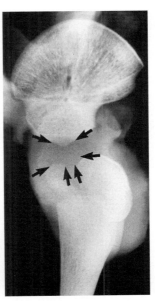

A   **B,C**

Figure 2-3 **A:** The three separate primary ossification centers of the hip bone are apparent in this third-trimester fetus. **B:** An anterior view of the dissected hip articulation does not permit the same appreciation of the separation between the joints as seen in a lateral radiograph. **C:** As the secondary center of ossification is not yet present in the proximal femur, a clear view of the contributing structures can be seen. *Arrows* are used to delineate the bipolar physes between the separate bones.

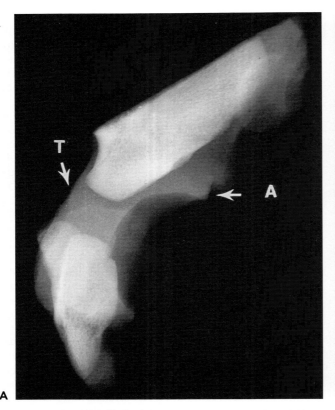

A

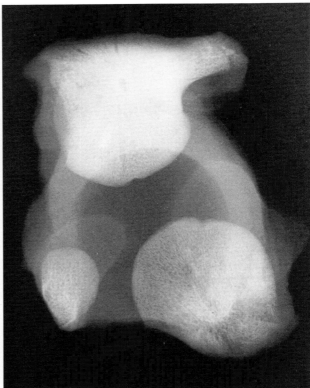

B

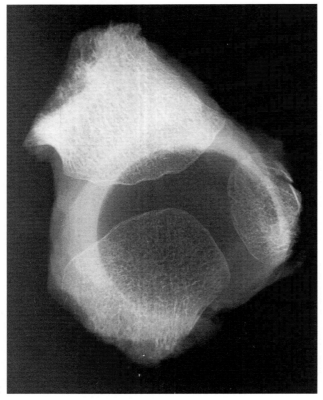

C

Figure 2-4   Direct radiographic views of the acetabulum permit a clear assessment of the developmental patterns. **A:** Duplication of a standard anterior view does not allow a full appreciation of the acetabulum from this stillborn neonate. In this radiograph, both the acetabular (*A*), and triradiate (*T*) cartilages are apparent. **B:** A radiograph perpendicular to the acetabular fossa provides an appreciation for the cartilaginous component and growth potential of the acetabulum. Note the shadow of the femoral articular circumference defined as well. **C:** As the skeleton matures, the bipolar areas of growth cartilage separating the pelvic bones narrow. Appearance of the triradiate cartilage at 4 years.

the medial triradiate component forms a continuous buttress that separates the ilium, ischium, and pubis in the region of the acetabulum (50). The triradiate cartilage assumes a Y shape, with an anterior, slightly superiorly slanted component dividing the ilium and the pubis, a posterior horizontal strip of cartilage separating the ilium and the ischium, and an inferior, near vertical one located between the ischium and the pubis.

Although all three arms of the triradiate cartilage meld peripherally with the articular cartilage of the acetabulum, a central, inferior, nonarticulating acetabular fossa exists within the medial wall of the acetabulum that is filled with a haversian fat pad known as the pulvinar. The base of this fossa consists of the ilium above the posterior horizontal flange of the triradiate cartilage, the ishium below it, and the inferior arm of the triradiate cartilage. During prenatal development, the nonarticular wall of the acetabular fossa reflects subperiosteal membranous-type modeling in accord with growth and pressure from the expanding femoral head (Fig. 2-2). The central nonarticular fossa is separated from the articular cartilage of the acetabulum by a raised bony crest known as the acetabular ridge that is highest on its inferior and posterior surfaces (10). Inferiorly, the notch in the articular surface is the site of attachment of the transverse acetabular ligament. Together with the fibrocartilaginous labrum, this ligament completes a ring around the acetabulum and adds depth to the socket.

Within the triradiate cartilage, the physis is bipolar. The germinal zone runs along the center of each arm. Small blood vessels, known as cartilage canals, permeate the central regions of the hyaline cartilage in a manner analogous to the epiphyseal centers of long bones. Extending from the central germinal zone toward each metaphysis are the dividing and the hypertrophic zones. These zones are not as wide as they are in longitudinal bones, reflecting the less rapid rates of endochondral ossification occurring in the triradiate physes (47).

The bone adjacent to each physis is analogous to the metaphysis and thus represents bone capable of considerable remodeling. This metaphyseal bone does not elaborate a subchondral plate until late in development. Therefore, the interstitial expansion of the physis and epiphysis may continue unimpeded. The intricate interrelationship between the acetabular, articular, and triradiate cartilage appears functionally necessary to accommodate progressive expansion of the acetabular concavity in response to proximal femoral growth. Thus the major function of the triradiate–acetabular cartilage is to facilitate a radial increase in absolute size of the acetabulum while maintaining a spherical congruency with the femoral head.

The triradiate cartilage in the newborn is wide relative to the size of the hip bones (Fig. 2-3). As the hip develops, the widths of the arms progressively narrow until they are approximately 5 to 6 mm wide throughout most of childhood and adolescence. Standard anteroposterior radiographs restrict interpretation of the triradiate cartilage to the composite radiolucency of the superior arms and are difficult to obtain due to the obliquity of the acetabulum and the superimposition of the capital femoral ossification center. Direct views of the acetabulum permit a fuller appreciation of its true appearance (Fig. 2-4).

As the child reaches adolescence, secondary ossification centers analogous to those seen in long bones develop within

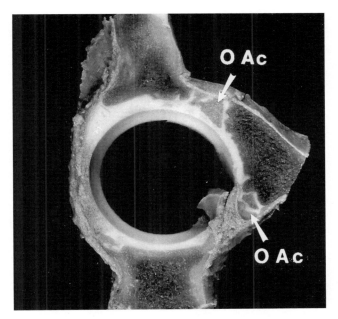

Figure 2-5 Adolescent development of the triradiate cartilage is depicted. Individual margins of the separate pelvic bones can be clearly seen. The os acetabuli (*O Ac*) are distinguished by a marrow similar in appearance to epiphyses of long bones.

the arms of the triradiate cartilage (45) (Fig. 2-5). These epiphyses expand toward the periphery of the acetabulum, in function contributing to a greater depth and surface area for femoral articulation. Radiographically interpreted as os acetabuli in the adolescent, they represent sites of coalescence between the secondary centers of ossification, and transform each bipolar growth plate of the triradiate cartilage into two separate growth plates of mirroring morphology and antipodal growth potential (47,62). They fuse at about the age of 18 years (50). The inferior ramus of the pubis and ischium also has interposed cartilage that normally fuses between the ages of 4 and 7 years. Enlargement of the ischiopubic junction is often evident radiographically and should not be misinterpreted as an osteochondrosis or healing stress fracture. Although speculative, fusion of the inferior ischial–pubic interface prior to the establishment of the secondary centers of ossification in the triradiate cartilage might serve to stabilize and couple the growth of the head of the femur with the triradiate cartilage during accelerated adolescent growth.

PROXIMAL FEMUR

Development of the proximal femoral chondro-osseous epiphysis and physis represents probably the most complex of all growth regions. Several anatomical features contribute to the uniqueness of its structure and intricacy of its maturation. These include the emergence of three ossification centers from a composite chondroepiphysis, a ligamentous attachment to the acetabulum that emanates from the center of the proximal articular surface, and the intracapsular course of the limited capital femoral blood vessels. Coupled with the continuum of the articular cartilage with the hyaline growth cartilage, an inelastic capsular girding, and muscular action rotating the femur on an axis separate from the medullary cortex, both the biomechanics and structural dynamics of the proximal femur are complex.

As alluded to in the discussion of the acetabulum, the femoral blastema is apparent during the fourth week of embryonic life in the 15-mm embryo. Shortly thereafter, the appearance of the chondrocyte phenotype initiates matrix elaboratation centrally and at both ends of the anlage. When fibroblast cellularity of the periosteum is contrasted with the abundant matrix surrounding the chondrocytes of the anlage, a silhouette of the fetal femur emerges. At the upper end of the femur, the separate morphologies of the greater and lesser trochanter also differentiate from the primitive mesenchymal blastema. Primary ossification of the anlage is initiated centrally in the anlage and proceeds both proximally and distally along the shaft of the femur. Although circumferential ossification characterizes the central diaphysis of the femur, primary ossification of the diaphyseal shaft initially remains incomplete medially and posterior at the site of the lesser trochanter, essentially notching the top of the diaphyseal cylinder (Fig. 2-6).

At birth the proximal femur is a composite chondroepiphysis with the greater trochanter, the lesser trochanter, and the capital femur forming a continuous mass of cartilage (Fig. 2-7). Within this synchondrous epiphysis, numerous cartilage canals are present that initially provide a basis for nutrition of the cartilage and later establish a conduit for cell lineages that support the differentiation of bone. Cartilage canals are actually vascular plexi, consisting of arterial, venous, and capillary components within a connective tissue support matrix. These vessels penetrate the chondroepiphysis of the proximal femur

in the 39-mm embryo and elaborate in complexity and volume with continued development of the chondroepiphysis (21,43).

Grossly, the proximal femur is structured with a spherical femoral head, variable anteversion, virtually no neck, and with a trochanteric height at a level similar to the femoral articulating surface. The normal morphology is initially characterized by a neutral articulotrochanteric distance. During ensuing developmental periods, this distance becomes increasingly positive, commensurate with the elongation of the femoral neck.

The hip capsule attaches along the intertrochanteric region superiorly, anteriorly, and posteriorly and just above the lesser trochanter inferiorly. Proximally, the capsule attaches at the interface of bone and hyaline cartilage just beyond the fibrocartilaginous labrum on the acetabular side, making the rim and its transverse acetabular ligament intracapsular structures. The greater and lesser trochanters, although differentiating as indivisible regions of the chondroepiphysis, during development assume extracapsular, apophyseal function, similar in many respects to the tibial tuberosity.

Ossification usually begins in the capital femur by 4 to 6 months postnatally, although a range of 2 to 10 months should be within normal limits (Fig. 2-8). The central nidus of ossification expands centrifugally, eventually conforming to the hemispheric shape of the articular contour. Ossification of the secondary center is coordinate with enhanced growth of the medial aspect of the metaphysis. The hip continues to exhibit a significant degree of capsular laxity, with the medial aspect becoming increasingly intracapsular. Over the 4- to 6-month period of postnatal development, the acetabular

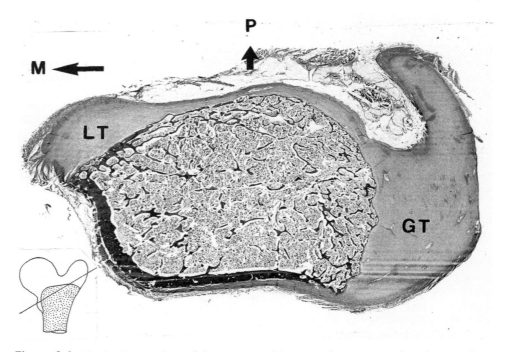

Figure 2-6   The hyaline cartilage of the greater and lesser trochanters, as well as the capital epiphysis are initially of a common mass. The lesser trochanter (*LT*) in this stillborn, full-term infant is continuous with the hyaline cartilage of the greater trochanter (*GT*). Medial (*M*) and posterior (*P*) aspects, as well as plane of section are indicated.

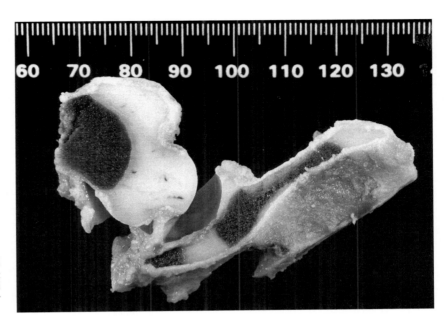

Figure 2-7 At birth, the entire proximal aspect of the femur is composed of cartilage. It is not possible to separately distinguish regional morphologies such as the greater trochanter from the capital femoral epiphysis.

labrum becomes a more evident structure and assumes an increasing role as a hip stabilizer. As this development is coincident with the appearance of the secondary center of ossification, which depends on an adequate blood supply derived from the posteriosuperior vessels, occlusion resulting in any temporary or permanent decrease in blood flow can seriously impair this stage of chondro-osseous transformation and potentially affect the ability of the capital femoral ossification center to continue maturing.

The femoral neck continues to elongate over the 6- to 12-month period and establishes a discrete capital femoral epiph-

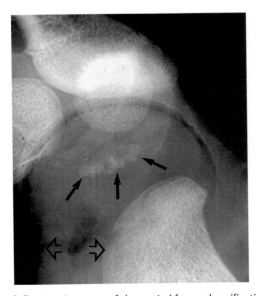

Figure 2-8 Development of the capital femoral ossification center occurs from either a central nidus, or focal centers (*short, straight arrows*) that quickly coalesce. Progressive diaphyseal maturation reduces the continuity between the greater trochanter and the capital epiphysis, in the process narrowing the cartilage of the intertrochanteric region (*open arrows*) and promoting femoral neck development.

ysis. Although a significant amount of hyaline cartilage initially bridges the greater trochanter and the capital femoral intraepiphyseal centers, elongation of the neck results in their increasing separation despite the sustained continuity. As the neck develops, the superior articular surface of the capital femur gradually becomes more proximal than the still cartilaginous greater trochanter, firmly establishing a positive articulotrochanteric distance.

Between the ages of 1 and 2 years, progressive and continuous elongation leads to a narrowing of the intraepiphyseal hyaline cartilage zone with the retention of cells typical of compressive–responsive physeal cytoarchitecture. Increased growth of the medial physis leads to a more specific definition of the capital femoral physis. Continued expansion of the secondary ossification center results in its flattening at the juxtaposition with the physis, transforming the original round shape into a hemisperical one, and establishing a bipolar growth zone between the capital femur ossification center and the metaphysis (Fig. 2-9). The hip capsule exhibits decreased laxity, and the medial physis, in response to normal hip joint mechanics, begins to angulate and also to develop mammillary processes. Akin to interlocking bone and cartilage pegs, they give the physis an undulated appearance, reaching their maximum height between the ages of 6 and 13 years. While the shear strength of the capital epiphyseal plate is greatly dependent upon the perichondrial zone of Ranvier during infancy, after 3 years of age much of the support for resisting shear is shifted to the interdigitating mammillary morphology (10,12,43).

One would suspect that the development and maintenance of secondary centers would alter the dependency of the physis to new and consistent strains, which in turn would also enable compression–tension dynamics to fulfill the Pauwel hypothesis for modeling, in that predictable patterns of response of bone growth will be mediated through biomechanical transduction. The idea of compression enhancing bone formation, and the dynamics of focal pressure imparted by an ossicle in the middle of a volume of cartilage have been explored as a

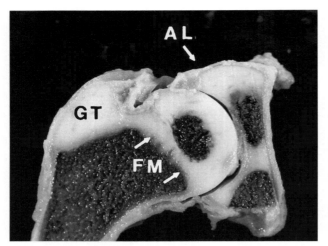

Figure 2-9 By 1 year, continued centrifugal expansion of the capital femoral ossification center results in its flattening at the interface with the femoral shaft metaphysis (*FM*). Such development establishes a growth plate that facilitates directional extension perpendicular to the new physis (*white arrows*). Continuity between the capital femur and the greater trochanter (*GT*) is maintained on the superior aspect of the femoral neck. The acetabular labrum (*AL*) plays an important role as a hip stabilizer.

remainder of the trochanteric chondroepiphysis, establishing a growth plate that develops an undulated appearance similar to that of the capital femoral epiphysis. The evolving complexity of the undulations seems related to the thinning of the intraepiphyseal cartilage and may represent a response to changing biomechanical function. During this period, the metaphysis demonstrates enhanced medial trabecular patterning along its superior neck in conjunction with an increasing intertrochanteric distance, reflecting the faster growth rate of the capital physis compared to that of the greater trochanter. In the context of Ward's treatise on the developing femur (58), the balance of compressive forces on the capital physis must be met and balanced with tensile forces tethered from the superior aspect of the femoral neck (Fig. 2-11). As tensile forces have been shown to accommodate bone differentiation without antecedent hyaline cartilage (32,33), distraction osteosynthesis of the femoral neck potentiates bone differentiation with sustained vascular supply and integrates formative modeling as a mechanistic continuum for bone growth (22).

Expansion of the greater trochanter and enlargement of the ossification center of the capital epiphysis continue over the period of 5 to 8 years. The greater trochanter often develops an additional ossification center near the proximal end of the trochanter, which rapidly fuses with the main center. The area

model for site specificity of secondary center formation (9). An issue germane to the concept of secondary center development is based on stress transduction through dissimilar mediums. Cartilage (articular–epiphyseal) to bone (metaphysis) conduction will differ from cartilage (articular) to bone (secondary center) to cartilage (physis) to bone (metaphysis) in not only signal, but in stress and strain profiles, particularly in shear. Mammillary process development, to a great extent, probably relies on restitution of neutral strain and stress abatement. The morphology of biologic tissue modeling reflects such an effort in the retention and exaggeration of the reserve zone matrix. Such production heightens the quiescent state of the physeal chondrocyte, suppresses the transition of the metaphyseal morphotype, and extends the regional growth potential. Maximum height may be an extrusion of the biological potential to react to stress in such a condition, and reflect organismal variation. Animals that attain the distinction of height have a larger and more complex mammillary process inherent to their physes, and the question must be posed whether matrix structuring to relieve stress also focally suppresses vascularization. Conceptually, the binding potential of growth plate for inhibitors of metalloproteinases (TIMP), or for decorin distribution as a mechanistic inhibitor of TGF-β would be assayable, and ongoing work may demonstrate regional distribution mirroring the morphology of the growth plate.

Continued longitudinal and interstitial growth of the femoral neck results in elongation and thinning of the intraepiphyseal area at 3 to 4 years of age, although a posterosuperior region remains as a definite mass of cartilage between the greater trochanter and the femoral head (Fig. 2-10). During this time, the greater trochanter develops a secondary center of ossification directly above the lateral metaphysis that is initiated from a single center or rapidly coalesces from multiple, small ossific foci. Ossification then extends through the

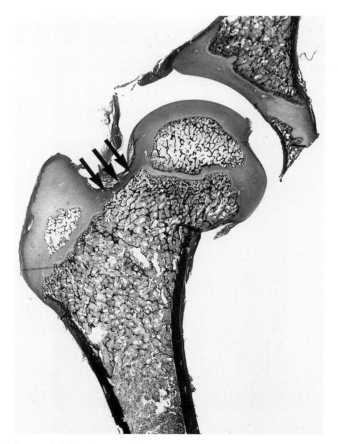

Figure 2-10 Thinning of the superior aspect of the femoral neck (*bold arrows*) characterizes the period of development between 3 and 4 years. By this time, the capital femoral epiphysis has attained a nearly hemispherical profile, domed to a subchondral articular margin, and flattened at its physeal interface.

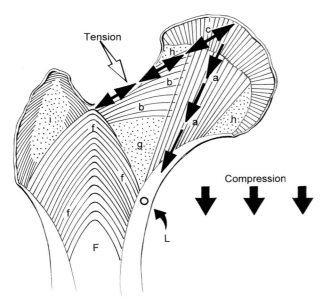

Figure 2-11 Based on Ward's model of bone formation and modeling, trabecular pattern develops in accordance with loading history. Tensile and compressive forces account for neck development, where the balance between the two determines the efficiency of proximal femur morphology. Transition of the superior, intertrochanteric region of the proximal femur from hyaline to fibrocartilage aligns the vector of growth in counterbalance to muscle forces that establish range of motion. Were the cortical shaft of the femur a fixed cylinder (*F*) with no neck, compressive force would be directed down the shaft. However, as the neck develops, increasing force is carried medially beyond the diameter of the shaft, transforming the medial aspect of the shaft into a lever arm (*L*), and establishing tensile force along the superior aspect of the femoral neck that is stimulatory to bone differentiation. Increasing length on the superior side stimulates incremental modeling along the inferior aspect associated with changing compressive force. Balance between the two modeling forces sustains the direction of the capital femur in check with optimal support through maximum range of joint articulation.

juxtaposed to the fovea capitis develops a distinct indentation in the ossification center (Fig. 2-12). By the end of this stage of development, the proximal femur has formed the final anatomic contours of anteversion, the functionally separate femoral head and trochanter, and the neck-shaft angle.

The average neck angle of the femur at birth is 138°, increasing to 145° at 1 year. After the infant begins to walk, it gradually thereafter declines until reaching the average adult angle of 120° (30). Most of the subsequent growth through adolescence will comprise the remodeling of trabecular patterns and the integrated enlargement of the capital femur and the trochanters.

Femoral torsion angle, from which anteversion is determined, is formed by the intersecting planes of the femoral condyles with a line drawn through the femoral neck and femoral head centers. If the plane of the head–neck axis passes anterior to the condylar plane, it is termed anteversion, while if passing posteriorly, it is called femoral retroversion. Femoral anteversion at birth ranges from −15° to −53°, gradually decreasing until the adult values of −14° are attained (11,57,59).

No dramatic gross morphological changes occur from 9 to 12 years. However, continued growth of the ossification cen-

ters of the trochanter and the capital femur is accompanied by widening and maturation of the femoral neck. Interdigitation of the mammillary processes into the metaphysis becomes increasingly complex. The capital femoral epiphysis, extending over and around the metaphysis anteriorly, medially, and posteriorly, might conceptually be envisaged as analogous to equatorial tipping. In gross specimens this extension creates the impression that the articular surface covers the epiphysis and the metaphysis, especially medially. In slab sections, one can see clearly that both the epiphysis and the articular surface extend over the metaphysis, a process termed lappet formation.

The intraepiphyseal fibrous growth plate that emerged at 3 to 4 years of age maintains a significant fibrocartilaginous component and, as alluded to earlier, continues to form bone by a membranous rather than an endochondral mechanism. A fairly abrupt histologic change, sometimes associated with an osseous extension analogous to the osseous ring of the zone of Ranvier, demarcates the lateral portion of the capital femoral physis from the intraepiphyseal physis. The cell columns are obliquely oriented away from the center of the intraepiphyseal region and appear to follow tensile stress patterns. As its major function, the intraepiphyseal region provides a basis for widening of the neck together with elongation and modeling. Following femoral neck fracture, reduced

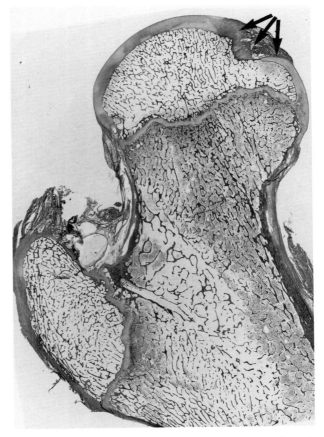

Figure 2-12 The capital femur develops a normal indentation (*arrows*) where ligamentum capitum femoris attaches, known as the fovea capitis. The superior neck region remains thin and responsive to bone differentiation in accord with tensile force.

normal cellular function could lead to a narrow, deformed femoral neck.

Whereas the period from 13 to 16 years of age characteristically is one of rapid growth, which may account for an increased susceptibility to slipped capital femoral epiphysis, it is also marked by the physiologic closure of the physis. Of the three active growth regions of the proximal femur, the capital femoral physis is the first to close. The process begins centrally with an increasing thickness of the subchondral epiphyseal plate followed by a similar thickening of the trabecular bone of the metaphysis. As a result of chondrocytes of the growth plate forming occasional clones rather than cell columns, a general attenuation of plate dynamics occurs, resulting in a thinning of the growth plate. The dense osseous plates on either side of the physis begin to join together by small bridges that gradually become larger. The fusion progresses centrifugally, eventually incorporating the entire capital femoral epiphysis. As coalition nears completion in the capital femur, a similar process begins in the greater trochanteric physis. Following the union of the metaphyseal bone with the separate epiphyses, final modeling of the remaining hyaline matrix of the capital physis establishes a subarticular, subchondral bone interface with only articular cartilage remaining.

VASCULAR SUPPLY

As seen in most biological structures, vascular distribution in the hip varies considerably. The proximal femur seems especially predisposed to vascular variation and remains uniquely susceptible to vascular disorders at any and all stages of postnatal development and growth. It is essential to understand the changing patterns of macroscopic and microscopic circulation in the context of proximal femoral development to adequately appreciate the role of the vascular supply in normal physiological development, and the consequence of ischemic changes encountered in slipped femoral capital epiphysis, femoral neck fracture, traumatic hip dislocation, developmental hip dysplasia, and Legg–Calvé–Perthes disease. The predisposition to variation may be ascribed primarily to the development of an intracapsular course for the increasingly limited blood vessels that supply the femoral head.

The extracapsular blood supply to the proximal femur is derived principally from the medial and lateral circumflex arteries. Anastomoses of the vessels are present around the hip joint, particularly over the capsule and along anterior and posterior peritrochanteric regions. With such anastomotic connections, compromise of one or more major extracapsular vessels at specific areas has potential to jeopardize functional flow in adjacent regions by a process akin to siphoning. Development and branching patterns of vessels to a great extent reflect biological demand. Vascular beds in the proximal femur encircle, anastomose, and balance separate arterial sources and venous returns that are necessary to support the metabolic demands of the developing femur. Should an element of the supply side be affected, arterial imbalance may initiate arterial flow dynamics that change not only the pattern, but the direction of flow. Such marked arterial imbalance has potential for contributing to venous stasis with regional distribution.

In the 2-month-old embryo, both extracapsular circumflex arteries to the proximal femur, the acetabular artery as a branch from the obturator to the acetabular fossa, and the artery to the ligamentum teres are present (56) (Fig. 2-13). The medial and lateral circumflex arteries anastomose to form a ring around the femoral neck base, from which a significant periosteal capillary network embraces the inferior aspect of the neck region as well as the diaphyseal portion of the proximal femur. The medial, posterior, and lateral aspects of the ring are a continuation of medial femoral circumflex artery, whereas the anterior aspect of the ring is formed by the lateral circumflex artery.

The predominant blood supply of the proximal femur, regardless of the stage of postnatal development, is derived from the deep (profunda) femoral artery. The lateral circumflex artery displays little variation, arising from the profunda artery 90% of the time, while the medial circumflex artery, although emanating from the profunda in 30% of specimens, more often arises as an independent vessel directly from the main femoral trunk (10).

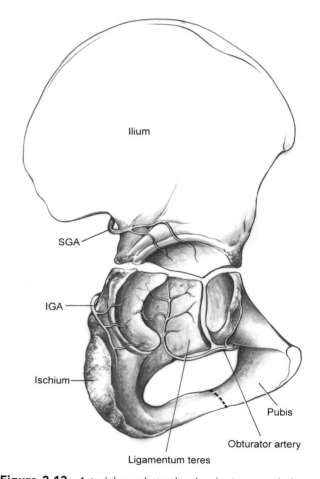

Figure 2-13 Arterial supply to the developing acetabulum is derived from branches from the internal iliac artery. The superior aspect is supported by branches from the superior gluteal artery (*SGA*), while the posterior aspect receives its vascular supply from the inferior gluteal artery (*IGA*). The floor of the acetabulum, the artery to the ligamentum teres, and the pubic portion of the acetabulum are nourished by branches of the obturator artery. Figure is a composite based on previous work by Ulloa (56) and Grant (27).

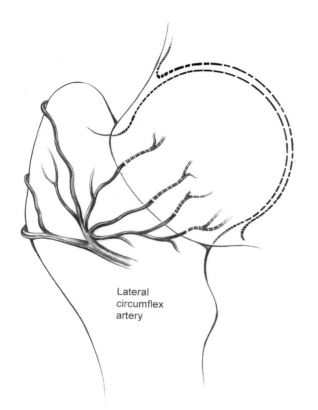

Figure 2-14 The lateral circumflex artery primarily supplies the greater trochanter but does send anterior, intracapsular branches as well to the femoral head.

During the first year of life the lateral circumflex branches supply a considerable portion of the anterior chondroepiphysis. After passing laterally and anterior to the iliospoas, the lateral femoral circumflex artery divides into several terminal branches that ascend as lateral and anterior cervical branches to the femoral head and neck. With the development and elongation of the neck, however, the lateral circumflex artery increasingly supplies the greater trochanter, the anterior femoral neck and metaphysis and decreasingly contributes to the intracapsular capital femoral circulation (Fig. 2-14).

The medial femoral circumflex artery passes posteriorly between the iliopsoas and pectineus muscles and then between the medial capsule and the obturator externus muscles. Branches provide vascular support for the medial inferior aspect of the neck between the inferomedial capsular insertion and the lesser trochanter. A small branch courses along the anterior capsular insertion, while the major portion of the medial circumflex artery traverses the posterior intertrochanteric notch as the intraepiphyseal artery and eventually crosses over to the anterosuperior aspect of the intertrochanteric groove where it anastomoses with the terminal ramifications of the lateral circumflex artery (Fig. 2-15).

At birth the two circumflex arteries supply approximately equal portions of the greater trochanter, the capital femoral hyaline cartilage, and physis, with the medial supplying the posterior aspect, and the lateral supplying the anterior half. Attachment of the hip capsule remains relatively constant, resulting in a relatively medial displacement of the capital

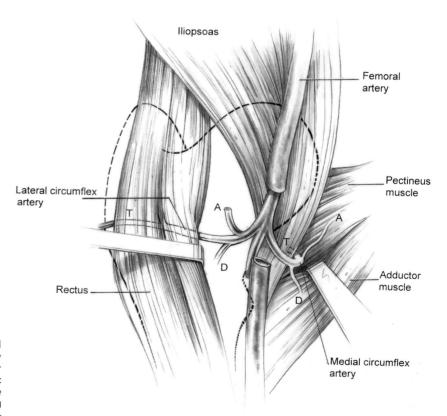

Figure 2-15 The main branch of the medial femoral circumflex artery courses posteriorly between the capsular insertion and the lesser trochanter, and along the intertrochanteric notch, where it passes anteriorly over the intertrochanteric groove before anastomosing with terminal branches of the lateral femoral circumflex artery.

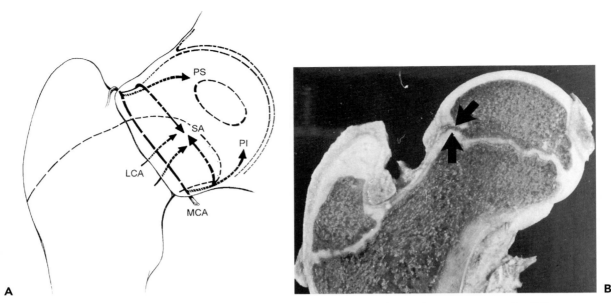

Figure 2-16 A: A subsynovial intracapsular anastomosis (*SA*) is derived from posterosuperior (*PS*) and posteroinferior (*PI*) branches of the medial circumflex artery (*MCA*). The lateral circumflex artery (*LCA*) contributes little anteriorly to this anastomosis. **B:** Several large vessels directly enter the capital femoral epiphysis from the posterior superior aspect of the femoral neck. *Arrows* depict one such vessel in this cut section of bone.

femoral epiphysis and necessitating changing circulation patterns. The lateral circumflex artery increasingly becomes the predominate blood supply to the developing intracapsular metaphysis. As the articular surface and the underlying epiphysis gradually overlap the anterior and the inferior metaphysis, fewer areas remain where the anterior vessels can penetrate. By 3 to 5 years of age, the anterior branches supply only the metaphysis, while the posteriorly located medial circumflex branches assume the primary role for vascular support of the capital femoral epiphysis throughout its development.

The medial artery establishes two important posterior circulations. Sometimes referred to as ascending cervical arteries (10), the posterior inferior artery arises from the medial circumflex artery near the lesser trochanter, penetrates the hip capsule, and courses along the inferior femoral neck. The more important system, the posterosuperior arterial system, penetrates the hip capsule and courses along the superior region of the femoral neck, often comprised of two or more arteries. The ascending arteries anastomose to form a subsynovial ring on the femoral neck surface at the articular cartilage margin. Even during the perinatal period, the superior region is characterized by several large vessels entering the chondroepiphysis (Fig. 2-16). The posteroinferior artery—which, unlike the posterosuperior system, is usually a single vessel system—courses in a much more mobile retinacular reflection, sending off minimal branches to the underlying epiphysis and metaphysis, but never directly crosses the growth plate.

ARTICULATION: CAPSULAR AND LIGAMENTOUS CONSTRAINMENT

The articulation of the proximal femur with the acetabulum is classified as an enarthrosis, or ball and socket joint. Such con-

formation permits extensive mobility through a wide range of functional motion. Although it is conceptually useful to consider the articulation as a spherical mechanical bearing, mammalian joints develop incongruities inherent to an adaptive loading history as well as to the relative position of the joints (8,26). During early development, when substantial portions of both the femur and acetabulum are composed of cartilage, precision of fit between the separate components is less critical to the dynamics of articulation than when a more static conformation is acquired. Were joint surfaces to remain incongruent during large stresses of weight, the articular surfaces would rapidly deteriorate. Fortunately, the compliance of the cartilaginous surfaces of the separate joint components coupled with synovial fluid accommodates the necessary apposition during the load phase of articulation. As many of the properties of synovial lubrication depend upon contact with articular surfaces, incongruences may bear some functional role in distribution of synovial fluid (28).

During the early condensation of the limb axis, an investment of mesodermal cells surrounds the bones as periosteum and the joints as capsule. Essentially continuous along the contour of the skeletal axis, the morphology is clearly demarcated at the transition of capsule and periosteum. While the periosteum is strongly adherent to the diaphyseal and metaphyseal aspect of the developing bone, the capsule is inadherent and inelastic, spanning and sustaining the joint as an articulation of two separate entities. Attachment occurs at the separate metaphyses of the femur and the acetabulum, within which is supported a vascular synovium. Although the collagenous capsule is inelastic, its sites of attachment are morphologically dynamic enough to permit growth and continued expansion of the articular surfaces without restricting motion. The hip joint capsule is reinforced by the iliofemoral, pubofemoral, and ischiofemoral ligaments, yet remains sensitive to stretch and serves as a mechanism for muscular feedback and pain.

The iliofemoral ligament (ligament of Bigelow) resembles an inverted Y. The apex of the ligament originates from the anterior inferior iliac spine and traverses the anterior aspect of the hip joint before dividing as a broad thickened longitudinal band that attaches along the anterior intertrochanteric line. The iliofemoral ligament limits hyperextension and lateral rotation of the hip joint and is taut in full extension. Full extension of the hip exposes the capsule and ligaments to a twisting and shortening effect that forces the head onto the acetabulum and may increase intracapsular pressure, especially when a hemarthrosis is present (46). The dynamics of such action may warrant consideration of the biomechanical imposition that an emergence of postnatal hip extension brings to a structure that has developed under the protracted mechanical bias of flexion. Little information is available detailing the relative set point of capsular fibroblast matrix elaboration with respect to chondrocyte matrix synthesis. In this regard, taking into account the inelastic nature of ligament with respect to the moldable cartilage matrix, a postero-superior compressive force may develop due to ligamentous tethering. Anatomically, this restrictive force would be most pronounced during a transition from flexion to extension, suggesting that inherent genetic competence may be one factor that determines the capacity for balance between the two tissue phenotypes, especially during developmental periods of shallow acetabular depth.

DEVELOPMENTAL DYSPLASIA OF THE HIP

A basic understanding of hip development makes it possible to conceptually envisage how inherent or acquired error in structure might manifest itself as aberrant functional morphology. Developmental dysplasia of the hip, often referred to by its acronym DDH, has been extensively used to include a broad spectrum of problems, including hips that are unstable, malformed, subluxated, or dislocated (41). Use of the original term CDH stems from its use by Ortolani in his treatise on congenital dislocation (48), although a century prior, Guillaume Dupuytren distinguished acetabular dysplasia from tuberculosis and pyoarthritic disease of hip joints that were prevalent in Europe at the time (18). Recently, DDH has been accepted as a more appropriate descriptive term that embraces the entire spectrum of skeletal development without delimiting potential onset to a prenatal timeline (1).

Because of presentation variation, much of the pathologic anatomy is dependent on type, grade, and duration of the displacement. From an anatomic standpoint, displaced hips fall into three basic classifications (44). The first is represented by those hips that are basically unstable and at risk of subluxation. Pathologic changes are minimal and severe dislocation is not present. Left untreated, they may, however, progress from subluxation to complete dislocation during growth and develop secondary changes that aggravate articular congruence. A second classification consists of those hips in which the acetabular rims show moderate changes yet remain open enough to permit anatomical reduction. Category three hips feature marked eversion of the acetabular labrum and carti-

lage as well as diminished depth of the acetabular aperture, both of which are impediments to spontaneous reduction regardless of the position of the femoral head. Once articular contact and suction from apposed surfaces are lost, joint capsule distortion from superoposterior traction of the femoral head stretches periarticular connective tissue and deforms the fibrocartilaginous rim, in the process fashioning a false acetabulum (Fig. 2-17). In addition to distracting and flattening the femoral ligament, such forces also reshape the morphology of the capital femur from one primarily spherical, to one eccentrically flattened on its medial aspect. The interplay between appositional growth of cartilage of the femoral head and the acetabulum represents one of balanced inhibition. Dislocation of the femoral head permits matrix elaboration and proliferation of hyaline matrix. Such changes in articular cartilage morphology of the acetabulum result in decreased depth of the acetabular cavity and are permissive to thickening of the articular surface of the capital femur as well. In time, the developmental trajectory resolved by separate rather than coaptive environments ceases to reflect congruent surface morphology.

The etiology of DDH is incompletely understood, although ligamentous and capsular laxity (especially due to

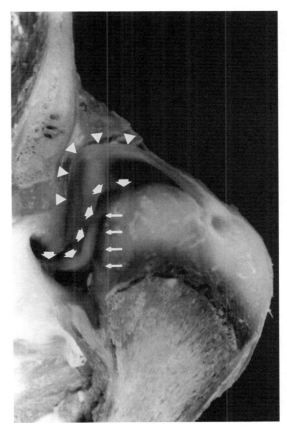

Figure 2-17 Dislocation in utero results in lateral superior displacement of the proximal femur and development of a false acetabulum (*white arrow heads*). Periarticular capsular and connective tissue proliferation in response to sustained muscular traction of the femur lengthens and flattens the femoral ligament (*short, broad arrows*), in the process reshaping the capital femoral epiphysis from a morphology normally spherical to one eccentrically flattened medially (*thin, white arrows*). Separation of the chondroepiphysis from the metaphyseal bone occurred during dissection.

hormonal changes in the last trimester), mechanical forces resulting from anatomical instability and intrauterine posture, genetic inheritance, and postnatal environmental influence are conditions that have been proposed as intrauterine contributing factors (55). It has been suggested that the hip is at increased risk for dislocation during separate periods of prenatal development that correspond to temporal as well as to maturational transitions. The first occurs during the differentiation of the hip from the mesenchymal blastema and takes into account the embryonic torsional rotation at 12 weeks responsible for midline alignment of the lower extremities (29). The suggestion is that dislocation at this stage leads to abnormal changes of all elements of the hip joint. A second period is potentiated at 18 weeks by inadequate development of the hip musculature and can result in paralytic dislocation. However, even with adequate diagnostic recognition prior to 20 weeks gestation, treatment may be obfuscated by a lack of options (42).

A final prenatal influence predisposing the hip to DDH is imparted during the final 4 weeks of gestation by abnormal mechanical forces such as breech presentation or oligohydramnios. Dunn contrasted breech presentation in 32% of abnormal infants with a 5% incidence in normal infants, suggesting that the breech birthing position, with straightened knee and hyperflexed hips, effects loss of containment of the femur within the acetabulum, and suppresses the potential of fetal kicking to alter and vary the forces (16). More recently, dynamic ultrasound has validated Dunn' theory, demonstrating that tension of the hamstrings produced by knee extension pulls the femoral head posterior when the hip is held in flexed position (54). First pregnancy is itself a factor, in that containment by the primigravid uterus and unstretched abdominal wall influence the shape of the uterine cavity during the final weeks of pregnancy.

Evidence for a genetic component to DDH suggests that prevalence follows geographic, racial, familial, and also gender parameters. In a widely cited report, Edelstein reported the incidence of hip dysplasia in the African Bantu as practically unknown, despite the fact that 897 of the 16,678 births that he examined had breech presentation (19). While it is rare in the Chinese population as well, it is more common in Native Americans and Laplanders, aside from correlations with postnatal environmental factors such as swaddling, which impose additional risk to the hip due to postural adduction and extension (38,41). A lower incidence exists in populations where children are positioned with their hips in an attitude of flexion and abduction, perhaps the most stable position for developing hips (1). As treatments are in intent designed to duplicate this posture, one might suspect that any inherent prevalence for DDH would be masked by postnatal experience within these groups.

Siblings and close relatives show an increased predilection for DDH as well. Wynne-Davies placed the risk as incremental, ultimately suggesting that a child born of an affected parent with an affected child had a 37% possibility of DDH (60). A twin study, comparing a 41% prevalence of DDH in monozygotic twins to only 2.8% in dizygotic twins, is cited to further corroborate genetic predisposition (61). Despite the apparent link, it remains unclear which traits are actually inherited, although joint laxity and shallow acetabulum would be suspected characteristics.

The maternal hormone relaxin, which contributes to remodeling of the symphysis pubis prior to childbirth, has in particular been suspected of contributing to the higher incidence of females with DDH than males (16). As the pelvic ligaments of females are more responsive to relaxin than are the males, their hips are susceptible to a lesser threshold of dislocating force.

The left side, involved two to three times as often as the right side, according to one theory results from the fetus lying more often on its left side in utero, predisposing the left leg to adduction, and the hip to dislocation due to protracted contact with the mother's sacral promontory (17). DDH has also been associated with congenital muscular torticollis (31,34) and metatarsus adductus (35,37), although these reports vary significantly with regard to incidence.

Further mechanistic support for flexion and adduction as primary effectors to posterior dislocation comes from a report of hip dislocation resulting from infantile myofibromatosis of the adductors (2). Hard, white-gray connective tissue replaced longus and brevis from origin to insertion while sparing the adductor magnus. After removing the abnormal tissue, the hip was relocated into the acetabulum. Although it was impossible to determine over what developmental interval muscle tissue had been replaced by fibrous tissue, a common final effect of the tissue aberrance was akin to inelastic tethering. Adductor attachment below and medial to the level of the femoral physis served to redirect the vector of proximal growth both away from and beyond the articular domain of the acetabulum.

Stability at birth does not imply that subsequent development will be normal, nor does instability at birth obviate the potential for full recovery. Given Barlow's finding that the incidence of spontaneous recovery approximates 58% without treatment, making an assumption that all hips will become normal is probably errant given the incidence of late-discovered subluxations (4). The possibility exists as well that clinically stable hips at birth may at some future time be subject to dysplasia, subluxation, or dislocation in accord with other risk factors (13).

CONCLUSION

Successful development and maturation of the hip require progressive integration of varying congenital, environmental, and morphological stimuli over an extensive span of time to ensure that the physiology of the adult joint will accurately reflect the paired function of the separate components. Development remains a continuum of proactive and reactive biological events that sustain capacity to render mechanical competence to the hip in static posture or ambulation, withstanding changing loads through adaptive modeling. It is this dynamic component of the developing hip that confers mobility to a spectrum of human and nonhuman morphotypes.

Although the hip is subject to some risk of developmental dysplasia, it is fortunate that most cases represent deforming rather than malforming circumstance. As such, the prognosis for recovery is based on expedient recognition of compromised anatomy and timely intervention. Recognition has been greatly enhanced by the advent first of ultrasound (53), and more recently by magnetic resonance imaging (36). With early diagnosis and treatment, many of the deforming consequences of unattended, unfocused growth can be forestalled, and corrective reduction and bracing can be used to restore the anatomy of the hip. The prognosis for recovery after re-establishment of appropriate femoral–acetabular articulation is based on a precept of developmental plasticity, by which functional anatomy and biomechanical focus retain the capacity to override discordant morphology. If the hip can be aligned to its functional optimum, congruency of the joint will develop in accordance with provisional and individual patterns of posture and gaiting.

REFERENCES

1. Aronsson DD, Goldberg MJ, Kling TF, et al. Developmental dysplasia of the hip. *Pediatrics.* 1994;94:201–208.
2. Atar D, Tenenbaum Y, Lehman WB, et al. Hip dislocation caused by infantile myofibromatosis. *Am J Orthop.* 1995;24:774–776.
3. Bardeen CR, Lewis WH. The development of the limbs, body-wall and back in man. *Am. J Anat.* 1901;1:1–36.
4. Barlow TG. Early diagnosis and treatment of congenital dislocation of the hip. *J Bone Joint Surg.* 1962;44B:292–301.
5. Brickell PM, Tickle C. Morphogens in chick limb development. *Bioessays.* 1989;11:145–149.
6. Brockes JP. Retinoids, homeobox genes, and limb morphogenesis. *Neuron.* 1989;2:1285–1294.
7. Bryant SV, Gardiner DM. Retinoic acid, local cell-cell interactions, and pattern formation in vertebrate limbs. *Develop Biol.* 1992;152:1–25.
8. Bullough PG, Goodfellow JW, Greenwald AS, et al. Incongruent surfaces in the human hip joint. *Nature.* 1968;217:1290–1292.
9. Carter DR, Wong M. Mechanical stresses and endochondral ossification in the chondroepiphysis. *J Orthop Res.* 1988;6:148–154.
10. Chung SMK. Embryology, growth, and development. In: Steinberg ME, ed. *The Hip and Its Disorders.* Philadlphia: WB Saunders; 1991.
11. Chung SMK. *Hip Disorders in Infants and Children.* Philadelphia: Lea & Feiberger; 1981.
12. Chung SMK, Batterman SC, Brighton CT. Shear strength of the human femoral capital epiphyseal growth plate. *J Bone Joint Surg.* 1976;58:94–103.
13. Davies SJM, Walker G. Problems in the early recognition of hip dysplasia. *J Bone Joint Surg.* 1984;66B:479–484.
14. Dolle P, Izpisua-Belmonte JC, Falkenstein H, et al. Coordinate expression of the murine *HOX-5* complex homeobox containing genes during limb pattern formation. *Nature.* 1989;342:767–772.
15. Duboule D, Dollle P. The structural and functional organization of the murine *HOX* gene family resembles that of *Drosophila* homeotic genes. *EMBO J.* 1989;8:1497–1505.
16. Dunn PM. The anatomy and pathology of congenital dislocation of the hip. *Clin Orthop.* 1976;119:23–27.
17. Dunn PM. *The Influence of the Intrauterine Environment in the Causation of Congenital Postural Deformities with Special Reference to Congenital Dislocation of the Hip* [M.D. thesis]. Cambridge: Cambridge University; 1969.
18. Dupuytren G. *Lecons orales de clinique chirurgicale faites a l hotel Dieu de Paris. Germer-Bailliere, 1832–34.* Le Gros Clark F, trans-ed. London: Sydenham Society; 1849:169–173.
19. Edelstein J. Congenital dislocation of the hip in the Bantu. *J Bone Joint Surg.* 1966;48B:397.
20. Eichele G. Pattern formation in vertebrate limb. *Curr Opin Cell Biol.* 1990;2:975–980.
21. Ganey TM, Love SM, Ogden JA. Development of vascularization in the chondroepiphysis of the rabbit. *J Orthop Res.* 1992;10:496–510.
22. Ganey TM, Ogden JA, Sasse J, et al. Basement membrane composition of cartilage canals during development and ossification of the epiphysis. *Anat Rec.* 1995;241:425–437.
23. Gardner E, Gray DM. Prenatal development of the human hip joint. *Am J Anat.* 1950;87:163–212.
24. Geduspan JS, Solursh M. A growth-promoting influence from the mesonephros during limb outgrowth. *Dev Biol.* 1992;151:242–250.
25. Goetnick PF. Genetic aspects of skin and limb development. In: Monroy A, Moscanna AA, eds. *Current Topics in Developmental Biology.* New York: Academic Press; 1966:253–283.
26. Goodfellow JW, Bullough PG. Studies on age changes in the human hip joint. *J Bone Joint Surg.* 1968;50B:222.
27. Grant JCB. *An Atlas of Anatomy.* Baltimore: Williams & Wilkins; 1972.
28. Greenwald AS. Biomechanics of the hip. In: Steinberg ME, ed. *The Hip and Its Disorders.* Philadelphia: WB Saunders; 1991.
29. Guidera KJ, Ganey TM, Keneally CR, et al. The embryology of tibial torsion. *Clin Orthop.* 1994;302:17–21.
30. Hensinger RN. *Standards in Pediatric Orthopedics.* New York: Raven Press; 1986:49.
31. Hummer CD, MacEwen GD. The coexistence of torticollis and congenital dysplasia of the hip. *J Bone Joint Surg.* 1972;54A:1255–1256.
32. Ilizarov GA. Basic principles of transosseous compression and distraction osteosynthesis. *Ortop Travmatol Protez.* 1971;32:7–9.
33. Ilizarov GA. The tension-stress effect on the genesis and growth of tissues. Part I. The influence of the rate and frequency of distraction. *Clin Orthop.* 1989;238:249–281.
34. Iwahara T, Ikeda A. The ipsilateral involvement of congenital muscular torticollis and congenital dysplasia of the hip. *J Jpn Orthop Assoc.* 1962;35:1221–1226.
35. Jacobs JE. Metatarsus varus and hip dysplasia. *Clin Orthop.* 1960;16:203–213.
36. Kashiwagi N, Suzuki S, Kasahara Y, et al. Prediction of reduction in developmental dysplasia of the hip by magnetic resonance imaging. *J Pediatr Orthop.* 1996;16:254–258.
37. Kollmer CE, Betz RR, Clancy M, et al. Relationship of congenital hip and foot deformities: a national Shriners Hospital survey. *Orthop Trans.* 1991;15:770.
38. Kutlu A, Memik R, Mutlu M, et al. Congenital dislocation of the hip and its realtionship to swaddling used in Turkey. *J Pediatr Orthop.* 1992;12:598–602.
39. Lewin SO, Opitz JM. Fibular a/hypoplasia: review and documentation of the fibular developmental field. *Am J Med Genet.* 1986;2:215–238.
40. Lewis EB. A gene complex controlling segmentation in *Drosophila. Nature.* 1978;276:565–570.
41. Morrissy RT. Congenital dislocation of the hip. In: Steinberg ME, ed. *The Hip and Its Disorders.* Philadelphia: WB Saunders; 1991.
42. Nishimura H. Incidence of malformations in abortions. In: Fraser FC, McKusick VA, eds. *Congenital Malformations.* Amsterdam: Excerta Medica; 1970:275.
43. Ogden JA. Changing patterns of proximal femoral vascularity. *J Bone Joint Surg.* 1974;56A:941–950.
44. Ogden JA. Dynamic pathobiology of congenital hip dysplasia. In: Tachdjian MO, ed. *Congenital Dislocation of the Hip.* New York: Churchill Livingston; 1982:93–144.
45. Ogden JA. Hip development and vascularity: relationship to chondroosseous trauma in the growing child. In: *The Hip.* Vol 9. St. Louis: CV Mosby; 1981.
46. Ogden JA. Injury to growth mechanisms of the immature skeleton. *Skel Radiol.* 1981;6:237–253.
47. Ogden JA. *Skeletal Injury in the Child.* 2nd ed. Philadelphia: WB Saunders; 1990.
48. Ortolani M. Un segno poco noto e sua importanza per la diagnosi prococe de prelussazione congenita dell anca. *Pediatria.* 1937;45:129–134.
49. Pinot M. Le role du mesoderme somitique dans la morphogenese precoce des membres de l embryon de Poulet. *J Embryol Exp Morphol.* 1970;23:109–151.
50. Ponseti IV. Growth and development of the acetabulum in the normal child. *J Bone Joint Surg.* 1978;60:575–585.
51. Saunders JW, Gasseling MT. Ectodermal–mesenchymal interactions in the origin of limb symmetry. In: Fleischmajer R, Billingham RA, eds. *Epithelial–Mesenchymal Interactions.* Baltimore: Williams & Wilkins; 1968:78–97.
52. Strayer LM Jr. Embryology of the human hip joint. *Clin Orthop.* 1971;74:221–240.
53. Suzuki S. Ultrasound and the Pavlik harness in CDH. *J Bone Joint Surg.* 1993;75B:483–487.

54. Suzuki S, Yamamuro T. The mechanical cause of congenital dislocation of the hip joint. Dynamic ultrasound study of 5 cases. *Acta Orthop Scand.* 1993;64:303–304.

55. Tachdjian MO. Congenital dysplasia of the hip. In: Tachdjian MO, ed. *Pediatric Orthopedics.* Philadelphia: WB Saunders; 1990:96–312.

56. Ulloa I. Embryonic and fetal development of the vascular system of the proximal end of the femur and acetabulum in man [in German]. *Z Orthop.* 1962;96:306–318.

57. Walker JM. Comparison of normal and abnormal human fetal hip joints: a quantitative study with significance to congenital hip disease. *J Pediatr Orthop.* 1983;3:173–183.

58. Ward FO. *Outlines of Human Osteology.* London: Renshaw; 1838.

59. Watanabe RS. Embryology of the human hip. *Clin Orthop.* 1974;98:8–26.

60. Wynne-Davies R. Heritable disorders and familial joint laxity: two etiological factors in congenital dislocation of the hip. *J Bone Joint Surg.* 1970;52B:704–716.

61. Wynne-Davies R. *Heritable Disorders in Orthopaedic Practice.* Edinburgh: Blackwell Scientific Publications; 1973.

62. Zander G. Os acetabuli and other bony periarticular calcifications at the hip joint. *Acta Radiol [Diagn] Stockh.* 1943;24:317.

The Hip

Ray C. Wasielewski

The os coxae is formed from three separate ossification centers: the ilium, the ischium, and the pubis. The innominate bone is ossified from these three primary centers as well as from secondary centers contributed by the iliac crest, the anterior inferior spine, the ischial tuberosity, the pubic symphysis, and the triradiate cartilage at the center of the acetabulum. At age 13 to 14, the mostly ossified bones of the ilium, ischium, and pubis unite in the acetabulum, forming a Y-shaped triradiate cartilage that proceeds to fusion by age 15 to 16. The other secondary centers unite and fuse between the ages of 20 and 22.

The acetabular surface is orientated approximately 45° caudally and 15° anteriorly (4,97). The acetabulum has a mostly circular contour in its superior margin, but it has only enough hemispherical depth to allow for 170° coverage of the femoral head. Femoral head coverage within the acetabulum is augmented by the labrum, which runs circumferentially around its perimeter to the base of the fovea, where it becomes the transverse acetabular ligament. Two strong osseous columns of bone surround the acetabulum, transmitting the stresses between the trunk and lower extremities (Fig. 3-1). The columns vary in thickness as they pass around the acetabulum. In general, expanding the acetabulum more than one third beyond the acetabular diameter (i.e., reaming a size 54 acetabulum beyond a size 72) will risk creating a pelvic discontinuity, rendering the columns incompetent (131). Overreaming the acetabulum during total hip arthroplasty (THA) may also prevent adequate circumferential hoop stresses when press-fitting the acetabular component into an undersized acetabulum. Excessive reaming of the columns

will also decrease the available bone depth, limiting the screw purchase needed for peripheral and transacetabular screws to augment acetabular component fixation. Reaming one quarter of the acetabular diameter is likely safe (i.e., reaming a size 56 acetabulum to a size 70), preserving approximately 75% of the cross-sectional bone of the anterior and posterior columns (131).

For arthroplasty, important surgical landmarks within the acetabulum include the anterior and posterior brim, the base of the fovea, and the transverse acetabular ligament. The anterior and posterior brim can help determine if appropriate acetabular component anteversion and flexion are present. The base of the fovea serves as a guide to the extent to which the acetabulum can be medially reamed. It is especially important to locate the fovea when a large medial osteophyte obscures the inferior aspect of the acetabulum. Failure to remove this osteophyte with adequate medial reaming may result in a lateralized acetabular component. However, medialization may be contraindicated in the patient with an inflammatory arthropathy, where protrusion of the hip may have occurred, often resulting in obliteration of the fovea. In such a case, only acetabular expansion is required along with morselized bone grafting of the medial wall defect. The transverse acetabular ligament provides a landmark to identify the inferior-most aspect of the acetabulum. It is particularly helpful when the acetabulum is dysplastic because it allows the inferior-most aspect of the acetabulum to be identified even in the congenitally dislocated hip (CDH) where the femoral head has never been within the acetabulum. This ligament also provides a restraint to inferior drifting of the acetabular reamer in cases where the superior acetabular bone is sclerotic. However, it can be a detriment when ossified, tending to force reamers superiorly, particularly in cases where the superior acetabular bone is osteopenic (e.g., in transplant patients and other patients on steroids).

The anterior superior iliac spine (ASIS) is an extra-acetabular landmark that is very helpful for identifying the location of competent acetabular bone on which to anchor the acetabulum, as well as a guide for the placement of transacetabular screws. It should be noted that as the acetabulum is moved superiorly between the columns, bone stock for screw placement decreases,

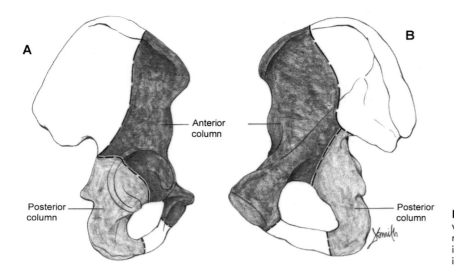

Figure 3-1 **A:** Schematic of the extrapelvic view of the pelvic bone, demonstrating the anterior and posterior columns. **B:** Schematic of the intrapelvic view of the pelvic bone, demonstrating the anterior and posterior columns.

as do the areas for safe transacetabular screw placement. The quadrant systems, as described by Wasielewski et al. (132), are useful in avoiding injury to neural and vascular structures and will be discussed in greater detail later in this chapter.

THE FEMUR

The femur is the longest and strongest bone in the human body. Its length is necessary to accomplish the biomechanical needs of gait. Its strength is necessary to transmit the muscular and weight-bearing forces. It is mostly cylindrical throughout it length, and it is anteriorly and laterally bowed in its midportion. The extent of bowing is clinically relevant because if excessive, it may not be possible to utilize long straight implants without considerable undersizing. The proximal metaphysis and neck are anteverted in relationship to the posterior aspect of the femoral condyles by approximately 15° (35,60,97). Excessive anteversion may make it difficult to utilize fixed stems (i.e., anteversion not adjustable) without considerable undersizing or osteotomy to correct the anteversion. To quantitate abnormal anteversion, a CT scan should be done to evaluate the anteversion prior to THA. It will be easier to approach and dislocate the excessively anteverted hip (as in CDH) through an anterolateral surgical approach. The retroverted hip may be more easily accessed from a posterolateral surgical approach (the old slipped capital femoral epiphysis).

The angle between the femoral shaft and the neck is approximately 125°. In most hips, the center of the femoral head is at the level of the tip of the greater trochanter. As the neck-shaft angle increases, the center of the head comes to lie above the level of the trochanter (resulting in coxa valga). A decreased neck-shaft angle results in coxa vara. Also, the distance between the center of the femoral head and the lateral aspect of the trochanter can vary independent of the neck-shaft angle (although patients with increased valgus tend to have less offset, whereas patients with increased varus have more offset). These variants are important because if they are anatomically normal, they need to be reconstructed with the use of femoral components with

similar offset and neck-shaft angulation. If the variant is pathologic, it is necessary to re-establish normal hip joint kinematics and leg length.

The proximal femoral metaphyseal orientation and shape have great variability (21,25,45,81,130). Although internal dimensions tend to correlate with one another, it is impossible to predict which configuration is present unless CT scans of the proximal femur are obtained prior to surgery. It is not until the neck cut is made during femoral arthroplasty that this geometry is best appreciated and assessed. The canal configuration may create problems for a cementless stem with fixed proximal geometries. Not only must cementless stems fit the anterior–posterior and medial–lateral dimensions of the canal, they also need to maximize the endosteal contact down the length of their porous coating. The proximal endosteal femoral geometry is demonstrated adequately for surgical planning on preoperative radiographs. Endosteal expansion of the isthmus with age results in the stovepipe femoral configuration (102,114). The proximal femur of younger patients tends to have a trumpetlike or champagne-fluted configuration. Because these different configurations affect the ability of the porous coating of a particular implant to be adequately apposed to subchondral bone, Dorr (29) and Spotorno (118) have developed indexes to characterize proximal femoral configuration. The Dorr index is a ratio of the canal diameter at the level of the lesser trochanter to the canal diameter at a point 10 cm distal (Fig. 3-2). As the canal calcar isthmus ratio (the Dorr index) approaches 1, prosthesis fill proximally and distally is compromised. Patients with stovepipe configurations may require more porous surface on their femoral implants to adequately contact the endosteal femoral surface, or a cemented implant should be considered. The ability of these indexes to predict the success of cementless femoral implants is still being elucidated. Singh et al. (113) have created an index to grade the loss of trabeculae that occurs with osteopenia. Because many of these trabeculae are removed with the required neck resection for removal of the femoral head at arthroplasty, this osteopenia measurement is likely less important than the quality of bone against the ingrowth

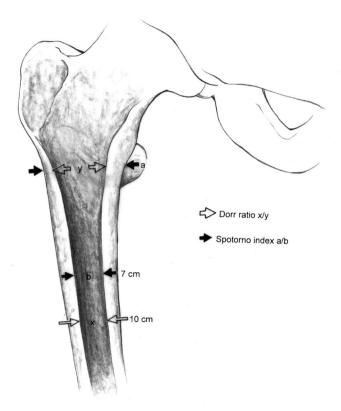

The iliofemoral ligament—often referred to as the Y liga-ment of Bigelow—is a fan-shaped ligament that resembles an inverted letter Y (Fig. 3-3A,B). The apex of the ligament is attached to the lower portion of the anterior inferior iliac spine, and the diverging fibers of the Y fan out to attach along the intertrochanteric line. The fibers of the iliofemoral liga-ment become taut in full extension, providing a check to hip extension beyond neutral. The superior portion may resist excessive external rotation. When this ligament is contracted, a flexion/internal rotation contracture may result, requiring release at total hip arthroplasty. It is particularly important to correct this internal rotation contracture if a posterior approach to the hip is done (otherwise a tendency toward hip internal rotation will result). An anterolateral approach may be preferred as it will perforce release this contracture.

The pubofemoral ligament (Fig. 3-3A) is applied to the infe-rior and medial part of the anterior capsule. It arises from the pubic portion of the acetabular rim and the obturator aspect of the superior pubic ramus, passing below to the neck of the femur to blend with the inferior-most fibers of the iliofemoral ligament. The fibers of the pubofemoral ligament become taut in hip extension and abduction. In trying to correct a hip adduction contracture at arthroplasty, these fibers may need to be released to provide for adequate hip abduction.

The ischiofemoral ligament reinforces the posterior surface of the capsule. It arises from the ischial portion of the acetab-ular rim. Its fibers spiral laterally and upward, arching across the femoral neck to blend with the fibers of the zona orbicu-laris. The spiral fibers tighten during extension but loosen or unwind during hip flexion. Other fibers traverse horizontally and attach to the inner surface of the greater trochanter, pro-viding a check to internal hip rotation (137).

The twisted orientation of the capsular ligaments sur-rounding the hip joint provides for a screw home effect in full extension. Hip extension coils and tightens these ligaments, making extension the close-packed position of the joint and the position of maximum stability (137). Interestingly, in full extension the articular surfaces of the joint are not in optimal contact. The position of optimal articular contact (flexion, abduction, and external rotation) is the loose-packed position because flexion and lateral rotation tend to uncoil the liga-ments. Because the joint surfaces are neither maximally con-gruent nor close packed, the hip joint is at greatest risk for traumatic dislocation when flexed and adducted (26,56).

HIP JOINT MUSCULATURE

The muscles of the hip joint operate as part of a closed kine-matic chain-link system. The muscles are unique in their large areas of origin and insertion (Fig. 3-4), their length, and their large cross section. These characteristics, in combination with the large range of motion available at the hip joint, result in muscle function that is dependent on limb position (Table 3-1). The range of motion accommodated at the hip is flexion 120°, extension 30°, abduction 45° to 50°, adduction 20° to 30°, inter-nal rotation 35°, and external rotation 45° (43,82). Normal gait on level ground requires at least the following hip joint ranges of motion: 30° flexion, 10° hyperextension, 5° of both abduc-tion and adduction, and 5° of both internal and external rota-tion (51). Walking on uneven terrain or stairs will increase the

Figure 3-2 Schematic diagram of the proximal femur, demon-strating the Dorr and Spotorno indexes for evaluating bone con-figuration. (From Dorr LD. Structural and cellular assessment of bone quality of proximal femur. *Bone.* 1993;14:231–242. Spotorno L, Schenk RK, Dietschi C. Personal experiences with uncemented prosthesis. *Orthopade.* 1987;16:225–238, with permission.)

surface. The influence of bone quality on successful hip replacement is presently being determined (70,99).

HIP JOINT CAPSULE AND LIGAMENTS

The articular capsule of the hip is strong and dense, contributing substantially to joint stability (Fig. 3-3). The capsule is attached along the anterior and posterior periphery of the acetabulum just outside the acetabular labrum. Making anterior and poste-rior incisions between the capsule and labrum allow retractors to be placed safely over the anterior and posterior columns. Inferiorly, the capsule is attached to the transverse acetabular lig-ament. The capsule is attached to the femur anteriorly along the intertrochanteric line, but posteriorly it has an arched free bor-der that results in only partial covering of the femoral neck (Fig. 3-3B). The femoral neck is intracapsular anteriorly, but pos-teriorly the basicervical portion and intertrochanteric crest are extracapsular. Most of the fibers of the capsule are longitudinally orientated as they traverse from the pelvis to the femur, except for the circular fibers of the zona orbicularis located posteriorly and inferiorly (Fig. 3-3B,C). Two strong accessory ligaments, the iliofemoral and the pubofemoral ligaments, reinforce the ante-rior portion of the capsule. The ischiofemoral ligament rein-forces the posterior capsule.

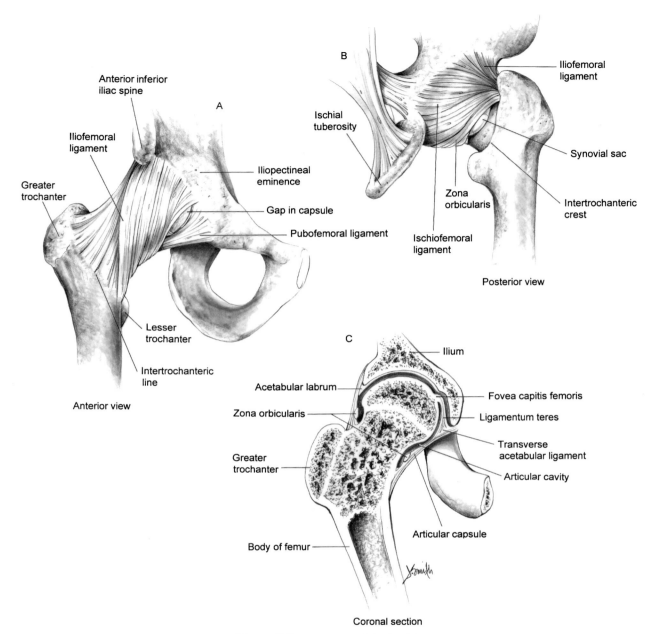

Figure 3-3   Ligaments of the hip joint.

need for joint range beyond that required for level ground, as will activities such as sitting in a chair or sitting cross-legged. Pain relief is the predominant reason for joint replacement surgery, but an understanding of the surrounding muscles can help the surgeon restore their function (15,18,73,87,94).

Flexors

The primary hip flexors are the iliopsoas, rectus femoris, and sartorius. The iliopsoas muscle consists of two separate muscles, the iliacus muscle and the psoas major muscle, which converge together into a common tendon to insert onto the lesser trochanter of the femur. The iliopsoas muscle has a broad origin including the iliac crest and fossa, sacral ala, and iliolumbar

and sacroiliac ligaments (the iliac contribution); and the sides of the bodies of the 12th thoracic through fourth lumbar vertebrae, transverse processes of the first through the fifth lumbar vertebrae, and the intervertebral disks (the psoas contribution). Its tendon is often seen traversing across the inferior aspect of the hip joint just outside the hip capsule. When an inferior capsular resection is required, it serves as an important landmark for the depth to which dissection can be carried. If this tendon is excessively taut (prearthroplasty secondary to a hip flexion contracture or after hip lengthening), the tendinous portion can be tenotomized just distal to the point it crosses over the pelvic brim, leaving the muscular portion intact.

The rectus femoris muscle crosses both the hip joint and the knee joint. It has a straight head that originates from the

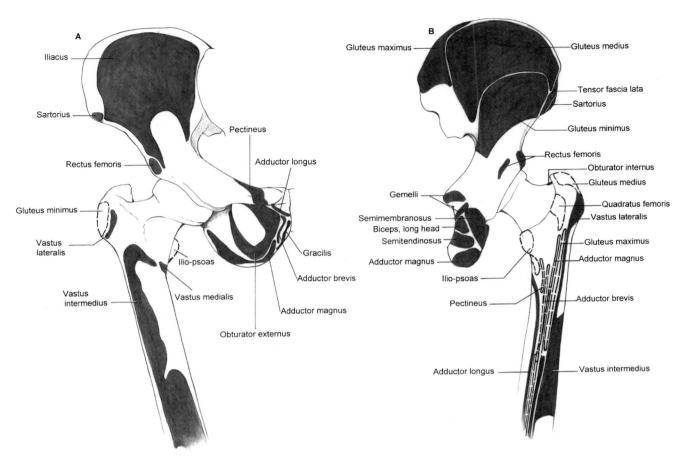

Figure 3-4 **A:** Schematic diagram of the intrapelvic view of the pelvic bone and proximal femur, demonstrating the muscle origins and insertions. **B:** Schematic diagram of the extrapelvic view of the pelvic bone and proximal femur, demonstrating the muscle origins and insertions.

anterior inferior spine of the ilium, and its reflected head originates from just above the anterior inferior rim of the acetabulum. These heads combine into a central aponeurosis and continue down the thigh to insert as a common tendon into Gerdy's tibial tuberosity. The rectus femoris flexes the hip joint and extends the knee joint. The position of the knee during hip flexion does affect its ability to generate force at the hip. The rectus femoris provides its strongest contribution to hip flexion when the knee is flexed. Knee flexion preloads the quadriceps muscles, strengthening its force across the hip joint. On the other hand, simultaneous hip flexion and knee extension considerably shorten this muscle across both joints, minimizing preload and decreasing its ability to generate a hip flexion moment. When a hip flexion contracture exists (or when the contracted hip has been lengthened by arthroplasty), release of the reflected head and transverse release of the fascia along the undersurface of the rectus may help improve knee flexion with the hip extended. After adequate release, the knee should be able to be bent to 90° with the hip in the fully extended position.

The sartorius muscle arises from the anterior superior iliac spine. It crosses the hip and knee joints to insert on the medial aspect of the proximal tibia in association with the other pes anserinus muscles. The sartorius flexes and abducts the hip, and it also flexes the knee. Although it crosses the knee, it is not substantially affected by the position of the knee because only a relatively small change in length occurs with knee motion.

The tensor fascia lata muscle originates more laterally than the sartorius on the anterolateral lip of the iliac crest. The muscle fibers are enclosed between the layers of the fascia lata, blending together to form the iliotibial band. The tensor fascia flexes, abducts, and medially rotates (weakly) the hip, although the tensor's contribution to hip abduction may be dependent on simultaneous hip flexion (57,86). The most important contribution of the tensor fascia lata may be in maintaining tension in the iliotibial band to maintain the knee in extension during stance.

Other secondary flexors are the pectineus; the adductor longus, brevis, and magnus; and the gracilis muscles; as well as the anterior portions of the gluteus minimus and medius muscles. Each is capable of contributing to hip joint flexion depending on the position of the hip. The gracilis crosses both the hip and knee joints and acts as a hip flexor when the knee is extended but not when the knee is flexed (6,13).

Extensors

The gluteus maximus and hamstring muscles are the primary hip joint extensors. These muscles receive extension assistance from the ischiocondylar fibers of the adductor magnus. The gluteus maximus is a large quadrangular muscle that originates

TABLE 3-1		
NERVE ROOT INNERVATION AND FUNCTION MUSCLE ACTION: MUSCLES OF THE HIP JOINT		
Flexors	**Iliopsoas**	N. to iliopsoas (L2, L3, L4)[a]
	Pectineus	Femoral (L2, L3, L4)[b]
	Rectus femoris	Femoral (L2, L3, L4)[b]
	Sartorius	Femoral (L2, L3, L4)[b]
	Adductors	
	Ant. portion gluteus maximus and minimus	
	Tensor fascia lata	
Extensors	**Gluteus maximus**	Inferior gluteal (L5, S1, S2)[b]
	Semimembranosus	Tibial (L4, L5, S1)[a]
	Semitendinosus	Tibial (L4, L5, S1)[a]
	Biceps femoris (long head)	Tibial (S1, S2, S3)[a]
	Adductor magnus (ischiocondyle part)	Tibial (L4, L5, S1)[a]
Abductors	**Gluteus medius**	Superior gluteal (L4, L5, S1)[b]
	Gluteus minimus	Superior gluteal (L4, L5, S1)[b]
	Tensor fascia lata	Superior gluteal (L4, L5)[b]
	Sartorius	
Adductors	**Adductor brevis**	Obturator (L2, L3)[a]
	Adductor longus	Obturator (L2, L3)[a]
	Adductor magnus (ant. part)	Obturator (L3, L4)[a]
	Gracilis	Obturator (L2, L3)[a]
	Obturator externus	Obturator (L2, L3, L4)[a]
	Pectineus	
	Hamstrings	
External rotators	**Piriformis**	N. to piriformis (S1, S2)[b]
	Quadratus femoris	N. to quad. femoris and inf. gemellus (L4, L5, S1)[a]
	Inferior gemellus	δ
	Superior gemellus	N. to sup. gemellus and obtur. internus (L4, L5, S1)[a]
	Obturator internus	δ
	Adductor muscles	
	Iliopsoas	
Internal rotators	Gluteus medius	Superior gluteal (L4, L5, S1)[b]
	Gluteus minimus	Superior gluteal (L4, L5, S1)[b]
	Tensor fascia lata	Superior gluteal (L4, L5)[b]
	Semimembranosus	Tibial (L4, L5, S1)[a]
	Semitendinosus	Tibial (L4, L5, S1)[a]
	Pectineus	
	Adductor magnus (post. part)	

N., nerve; ant., anterior; inf., inferior; sup., superior; post., posterior; quad., quadratus; obtur., obturator.
Bold type signifies major contribution to muscle action.
[a]Anterior nerve root division.
[b]Posterior nerve root division.

from the sacrum, the coccyx, the sacrotuberous ligament, and the gluteal aponeurosis overlying the gluteus medius. The uppermost fibers insert into the iliotibial band. The inferior fibers insert into the gluteal tuberosity and the lateral intermuscular septum (Fig. 3-5). The gluteus maximus is a strong hip extensor whose moment arm generates the maximum hip extension strength (to resist trunk flexion) when the hip joint is in neutral position (79). The maximus also laterally rotates the femur and stabilizes the knee through its insertion in the iliotibial tract.

The hamstrings also contribute to hip extension. These muscles are the long head of the biceps femoris, the semitendinosus,

and the semimembranosus muscles. The origin of these muscles is the ischial tuberosity. All three muscles extend the hip and flex the knee. However, their combined strength is less than that of the gluteus maximus. Hamstring strength increases with hip flexion, whereas maximus strength is decreased as the hip flexes beyond neutral (79).

Abductors

Abduction of the hip is brought about predominantly by the gluteus medius and the gluteus minimus muscles. The tensor

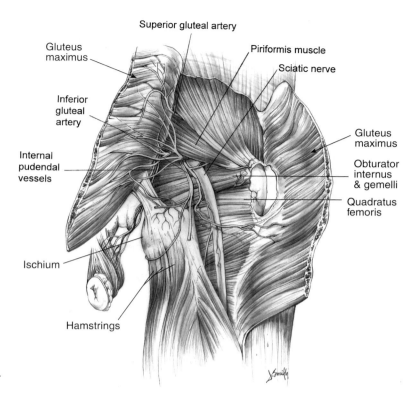

Superior gluteal artery

Gluteus maximus

Piriformis muscle

Sciatic nerve

Inferior gluteal artery

Gluteus maximus

Internal pudendal vessels

Obturator internus & gemelli

Quadratus femoris

Ischium

Hamstrings

Figure 3-5 Vascular and neural structures of the posterior aspect of the pelvis.

fascia lata may significantly contribute to abduction but only during concomitant hip flexion. The gluteus medius has anterior, middle, and posterior parts that function asynchronously during movement at the hip (116). The anterior fibers of the gluteus medius are active in hip flexion and medial rotation, whereas the posterior fibers function during extension and lateral rotation. All fibers contribute significantly to hip abduction. The gluteus minimus muscle lies deep to the gluteus medius, arising from the outer surface of the ilium, and inserting on the anterosuperior angle of the greater trochanter.

The gluteus minimus and medius muscles function together to abduct the femur during the stance phase of gait to counter the effects of the adduction moment created by the patient's weight. Using the free-body formula (74), the force required by the abductor musculature (F_{AB}) to maintain hip equilibrium during gait is $b/a \times 5W/6$, where a is the abductor moment arm, b is the distance from the center of gravity to the hip center, and W is body weight. Thus, $F_{AB} \approx 2.5W$. After total hip arthroplasty, until the abductor musculature can generate this force, the patient will have Trendelenburg sign on attempted single limb stance or have a Trendelenburg lurch with ambulation (54). The Trendelenburg lurch is the body's attempt to compensate for abductor weakness by bringing the center of gravity closer to the hip center (i.e., the patient leans toward the operative side with weight bearing decreasing the moment arm). The distance the patient with abductor weakness must shift his weight over the affected limb will be proportional to the magnitude of abductor weakness. Interestingly, the particular approach utilized for THA (e.g., Kocker, Hardinge, transtrochanteric) does not seem to influence the rate of postoperative Trendelenburg gait (84,109).

THA may also cause the gluteus minimus muscle to be tight—resulting in an internal rotation contracture—when the hip is lengthened from a shortened contracted position. It may be necessary to release the undersurface of the gluteus minimus from caudad to cephalad to allow for appropriate hip external rotation and prevent a tendency toward internal rotation that can lead to posterior hip dislocation.

Adductors

Adductor muscles of the hip include the adductor brevis, adductor longus, adductor magnus, pectineus, and gracilis. The adductor longus, brevis, and magnus muscles arise from the external surfaces of the inferior pubic ramus and the ischial ramus fanning out laterally to insert along the linea aspera. The gracilis muscle originates on the inferior pubic ramus and the edge of the symphysis pubis, inserting on the medial surface of the proximal tibia as part of the pes anserinus. The combined strength (isometric torque of adduction) of this muscle group is greater than that of abduction (76). Adduction contractures are frequently found in pathologic conditions of the hip joint. Because adduction contractures left uncorrected may result in a dislocation diathesis, an adductor tenotomy through a separate medial incision should be considered at the start of joint replacement arthroplasty to address this problem. To complete the release of a severe adduction contracture, release of the pubofemoral ligament and inferior capsule should be done when the hip joint is exposed.

External Rotators

The short muscles of external rotation include the obturator internus and externus, the superior and inferior gemellus, the quadratus femoris, and the piriformis muscles. The anterior convexity of the neck, together with the backward projection of the intertrochanteric crest, gives these muscles excellent mechanical advantage in externally rotating the hip joint (45). The obturator internus muscle originates from the inner perimeter of the obturator foramen and emerges through the lesser sciatic foramen to insert on the medial surface of the greater trochanter. The two gemelli muscles are closely associated with the obturator internus muscle, blending together as they insert into the greater trochanter. The piriformis muscle emerges from the greater sciatic foramen, inserting into the upper border of the greater trochanter. The surrounding structures are referenced relative to this tendon, prefaced by inferior and superior based on whether they exit above or below the piriformis. It is important to note that the common peroneal division of the sciatic nerve can pass through separate divisions of the piriformis in 10% of cases. Usually, the sciatic nerve passes below the piriformis to lie on top of the short external rotators (Fig. 3-5). If the surgeon tags the rotators with suture and reflects them posteriorly, the nerve is protected. The obturator externus muscle originates on the external perimeter of the obturator foramen, crossing posterior to the hip joint to insert into the trochanteric fossa. Its tendon lies just outside the posterior inferior joint capsule and can be used to reinforce the inferior closure of the posterior tissues. The quadratus femoris muscle is a thick quadrangular muscle that originates on the ischial tuberosity and inserts on the quadrate line of the femur that runs caudad from the intertrochanteric crest. Removal of this muscle is often necessary to adequately expose the lesser trochanter for neck resection level determination.

Internal Rotators

The muscles producing internal rotation of the hip joint do so secondarily, as they all have other primary functions. These muscles all have lines of pull anterior to the hip joint—directed from lateral to medial at some point through the normal hip range of motion—contributing to internal rotation. The more consistent medial rotators are the anterior fibers of the gluteus medius and minimus and the tensor fascia lata muscles. Other muscles that contribute to internal rotation are listed in Table 3-1.

EXTRAPELVIC VASCULATURE

Common Femoral Vessels

The common femoral artery is an extension of the external iliac artery as it passes under the inguinal ligament. It courses directly anterior and medial to the hip capsule, from which it is separated by only the iliopsoas tendon (Fig. 3-6). The common femoral vein becomes the external iliac vein as it passes under the inguinal ligament after receiving contributions from the profundus femoris and greater saphenous vessels. The artery is lateral to the vein at the level of the inferomedial capsule and is more susceptible to injury.

The common femoral vessels have been the most commonly reported extrapelvic vascular structures injured in association with THA. The most commonly cited mechanism of injury to the femoral vessels has been aberrant retractor placement during the surgical approach (Fig. 3-6)

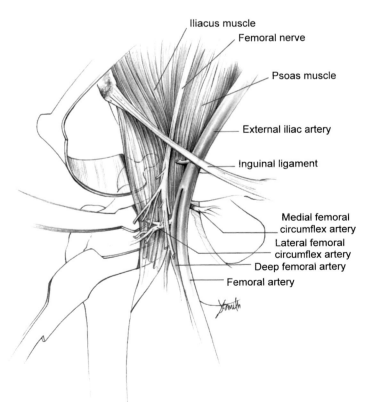

Iliacus muscle

Femoral nerve

Psoas muscle

External iliac artery

Inguinal ligament

Medial femoral
circumflex artery
Lateral femoral
circumflex artery
Deep femoral artery
Femoral artery

Figure 3-6 The femoral triangle and the position of commonly used acetabular retractors. Injury to contiguous nerves and vessels can result from aberrant retractor placement.

(7,64,77,105). This can occur during the anterior lateral approach when a retractor is placed too far medially over the anterior inferior acetabular margin. Bulk allograft placement for acetabular reconstruction (16), osteophyte resection, and resection of scar tissue from the anterior inferior acetabulum have also resulted in femoral artery injury (36,77). During cemented acetabular component fixation, extrusion of excess cement anteromedially has resulted in pseudoaneurysm formation, thrombus formation (47), and peripheral femoral arterial embolization (78). Intimal damage from the heat of polymerization is the likely cause. Prolonged cement spicule pressure has resulted in postoperative vessel erosion and pseudoaneurysm formation (28,39,46,78) and the formation of an arteriovenous fistula (77). These injuries can be avoided by placing a lap pad in this region during cementing or by removing the anterior extra-acetabular cement before polymerization.

Ischemia can present after THA without intraoperative hemorrhage in patients with severely atherosclerotic vessels. When significant vessel disease is suspected, traction on the extremity should be minimized during THA. Dislocation and reduction maneuvers (47,69,77,110,119) and complete restoration of length (69) or correction of flexion contractures must also be done with care. Intraoperative plethysmographic monitoring should be considered in high-risk patients (with calcification on x-ray). Vascular consultation should be obtained prior to hip arthroplasty if the Doppler pressure at the ankle is less than 50 mm Hg (69,110) or if there is clinical evidence of ischemia preoperatively.

Profundus Femoris Vessels

The profundus (deep) femoris artery arises from the lateral side of the femoral artery approximately 3.5 cm below the inguinal ligament. It passes posterior to the femoral artery to travel between the pectineus and adductor longus and then between the latter and the adductor brevis. The lateral circumflex artery arises from the lateral side of the proximal profundus femoris artery. It passes laterally beneath the sartorius and rectus femoris muscles on to the top of the vastus lateralis, where it divides into ascending and descending branches. The medial circumflex artery usually arises from the posteromedial profundus artery but may also arise from the femoral artery. It winds medially around the femur between the pectineus and psoas muscles and posteriorly along the intertrochanteric line to appear at the upper border of the quadratus femoris (38).

The profundus femoris vessels have been injured, although rarely, during THA. Retractor placement too far medially over the anterior inferior quadrant can result in a false aneurysm of the medial circumflex artery (Fig. 3-6) (7). Extruded cement in this region may also cause injury to the medial circumflex vessel (7). When this vessel is encountered at the superior border of the quadratus femoris muscle, it seldom causes significant hemorrhage unless injured closer to its origin. Hohmann retractor placement over the anterior hip capsule and gluteus medius has resulted in severe arterial hemorrhage from profundus femoral and lateral circumflex artery laceration (77). Osteotome use during the removal of scar and capsule during revision surgery has also resulted in injury to the lateral circumflex artery (77).

Superior Gluteal Vessels

The superior gluteal vessels are branches of the posterior division of the internal iliac artery, usually passing between the lumbosacral trunk and the first sacral nerve. The gluteal nerve travels with the artery and vein. These structures are closest to the posterior column as they exit through the superior aspect of the sciatic notch. They are relatively fixed as they pass out of the pelvis above the piriformis muscle (Fig. 3-5). Surrounding fat and extraperitoneal tissue provide 2 to 10 mm of tissue interposition between these structures and the posterior acetabular column (132). Terminal branches of these structures come to lie between the minimus and medius muscles.

Laceration of the superior gluteal artery has occurred with a fixation screw in the area of the sciatic notch (95). Injury has also occurred when a pin retractor was inserted in the direction of the notch (66). The superior gluteal vessels are as close as 2 mm from bone at this point. To minimize the risk to the superior gluteal vessels during transacetabular screw placement, the notch should be gently palpated to avoid instrument protrusion into this region.

Inferior Gluteal and Internal Pudendal Vessels

The inferior gluteal and internal pudendal vessels are the terminal branches of the anterior division of the internal iliac artery. These vessels exit the pelvis between the piriformis and coccygeus muscles to enter the gluteal region (Fig. 3-5). They are closest to the posterior column at the level of the ischial spine. The internal pudendal vessel is closer to the posterior column as it curves around the ischial spine to re-enter the pelvis through the lesser sciatic notch (Fig. 3-7). The gluteal vessels pass under the piriformis in the lower part of the greater sciatic foramen. Injury to these vessels can occur if excessively long transacetabular screws are used for acetabular component fixation. These screws would need to exit the posterior column by at least 5 mm because these structures are located at least this distance from bone (132).

INTRAPELVIC VASCULATURE

External Iliac Artery and Vein

The external iliac artery is the anterior division of the common iliac artery after its bifurcation at the level of the L5-S1 vertebral disc. It runs obliquely down the medial border of the psoas major muscle and anterior and lateral to the external iliac vein, with a portion of the muscle interposed between itself and the intrapelvic surface of the anterior column. The amount of interposed psoas muscle decreases from proximal along the arcuate line to distal at the iliopubic eminence, as the muscle becomes tendinous opposite the anterior superior quadrant (5,22,34,62,132,138). The external iliac vein accompanies the artery. Proximally, the vein runs medial and posterior to the artery. More distal, opposite the anterior superior quadrant, the vein runs medial and inferior to the artery along the medial border of the psoas with only minimal muscular and fascial interposition between itself and the pelvic brim (34,62,132,138). It is relatively immobile along the pelvic brim, being interposed between the anterior column and the parietal peritoneum (5,22,62,137,138).

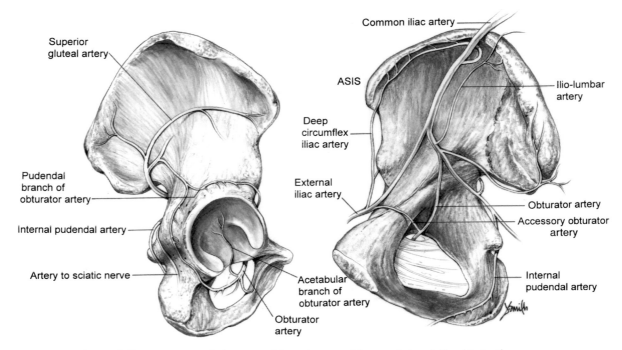

Figure 3-7 The course of the intrapelvic and extrapelvic vessels in relationship to the osseous pelvis.

Injury to the external iliac artery and vein has been reported during all phases of total hip replacement (2,7,12,17,24,46,48,49,61,63,67,69,72,77,83,98,103,108,110, 121,126,127). Reported injury to the external iliac vein is uncommon compared to external iliac artery injury (61,67,72,98,103,110). Positioning the patient with pre-existing atherosclerotic disease may result in limb ischemia from thrombosis formation or distal limb infarction from a plaque embolism (69). During the surgical approach, the vessels lie within the pelvis, but they can be injured during acetabular exposure by retractors placed too far medially over the anterior column (Fig. 3-6) (77,83,127). This risk is decreased by proximal retractor placement along the anterior column, where the interposed psoas muscle protects the vessels (75,77). Injury can also occur during preparation for placement of a cemented acetabular component from excessive medial reaming (67), excess extra-articular cement, or cement extrusion into the pelvis through an aberrant anchoring hole (72). The heat of polymerization (7,24,46,48,75,77,110,126) or direct compression (7,12,33) results in vessel thrombosis that may necessitate vessel thrombectomy (48), bypass (7), ligation (49), or repair (128). A pelvic cement restrictor or bone graft has been recommended to avoid excessive cement extrusion during acetabular component insertion (95).

Cementless acetabular component fixation often requires the use of transacetabular screws for component fixation. The external iliac vein has been lacerated during screw placement, resulting in a large retroperitoneal hematoma that necessitates evacuation and vessel repair (61). Injury can be best avoided by utilizing the posterior quadrants for screw placement (132).

Delayed injury to the external iliac vessels occurs due to socket migration (12,59,125,127), cement spicules that can result in compressive occlusion (12,46,98,103), aneurysm formation (46,49), pseudoaneurysm formation (12,63,103, 108,126), and vessel erosions (12,17). Removal of a cemented acetabular component, with cement extruded toward the iliac vessels through perforations in the anterior superior quadrant of the acetabulum, can tear the external iliac vessels (12,46,77,98). Preoperative evaluation prior to revision surgery, utilizing standard and oblique radiographs (133), arteriography (110), or contrast-enhanced CT scanning, is indicated to assess the likelihood that vessel damage will occur during acetabular component removal. An orthopedic or vascular surgeon familiar with the ilioinguinal approach can then be utilized for preliminary retroperitoneal exposure (91,104) of the external iliac vasculature before extraction of the acetabular component (72,110).

Obturator Vessels

The obturator nerve, artery, and vein most frequently traverse the lateral wall (quadrilateral surface) of the pelvis together, covered by parietal peritoneum, with the nerve located most superior and the vein most inferior (5,22,34,62,85,92,137,138). The obturator internus muscle and fascia lie lateral to these structures, separating them from the quadrilateral surface opposite the anterior inferior quadrant of the acetabulum. The obturator nerve, artery, and vein lie in contiguity at the superior and lateral aspects of the obturator foramen, where they exit the true pelvis via the obturator canal. This latter relationship is virtually a constant (22,137,138). These structures are relatively fixed at this point by the obturator membrane and surrounding peritoneum, and they are relatively nonmobile. An aberrant (accessory) artery and vein may also descend across the pelvic brim from the external iliac vessels to the obturator foramen (Fig. 3-7) (97,132).

A reported case of obturator artery injury occurred as a result of an osteophyte or cement spicule lacerating the vessel during mobilization of the head of a prosthesis during revision surgery (77). Hypothetically, injury could occur if the anterior inferior quadrant is violated or if a retractor is placed under the transverse acetabular ligament into the superolateral aspect of the obturator foramen.

Sciatic Nerve

The sciatic nerve is the continuation of the upper sacral plexus roots from the anterior and posterior divisions of L4, L5, S1, S2, and S3. The sciatic nerve consists of two peripheral nerves contained within the same connective tissue sheath: the tibial (anterior divisions) and common peroneal (posterior divisions) nerves (5) (Fig. 3-8). Most often, the sciatic nerve is one structure lying anterior and medial to the piriformis muscle just proximal to its exit from the pelvis through the greater sciatic notch. It exits below the piriformis muscle (infrapiriformis fossa), passing over the posterior lateral surface of the

posterior acetabular column. It then descends between the greater trochanter of the femur and the ischial tuberosity, crossing over the obturator internus, gemelli, and quadratus femoris muscles (Fig. 3-5).

As the sciatic nerve emerges from the sciatic notch, the fibers of the nerve are already spatially oriented with the common peroneal nerve located more laterally (53). In up to 10% of cases, the two divisions (tibial and peroneal) are distinct as they emerge from the sacral plexus, being separated by the piriformis muscle at the level of the greater sciatic foramen (9,53). The course of the common peroneal nerve descends more obliquely than that of the tibial nerve, leaving the fibers of the common peroneal nerve more superficial and more susceptible to injury (30). The peroneal division has two relatively fixed points, the sciatic notch and the head of the fibula. Also, the peroneal nerve contains large funiculi surrounded by sparse connective tissue, whereas the tibial nerve has smaller funiculi with more connective tissue. This allows the tibial division of the sciatic nerve to sustain a larger percent elongation before exhibiting evidence of neural compromise (30). A peroneal nerve palsy is differentiated

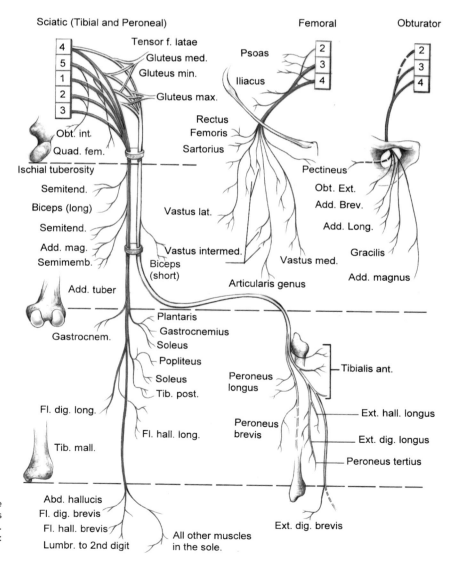

Figure 3-8 Schematic diagram of the motor distribution of the nerves of the pelvis and lower extremity. (From Anderson JE. *Grant's Atlas of Anatomy.* 4th ed. Baltimore: Williams & Wilkins; 1978, with permission.)

from a sciatic nerve palsy by electromyography (EMG) and nerve conduction velocity (NCV) findings of abnormal fibrillation potentials in the short head of the biceps, which receives innervation from two branches of the common peroneal nerve (260 mm and 150 mm above the level of the knee joint). Normal function of the gastrocnemius muscle confirms that the neural injury occurred within the peroneal division of the sciatic nerve.

Sciatic and peroneal nerve palsies are the most common forms of peripheral nerve injuries following THA (8,20,23, 27,32,96,100,106,107), with reported incidences ranging from 0.5% to 2.0% (30). The anatomic course of the sciatic nerve creates a vulnerability to injury by posterior acetabular retractors and power reamers during reconstructive surgery of the hip. This may be even more likely as incision lengths are decreased as part of minimal incision hip surgery (10,135). Revision hip surgery (30,107), increased surgical time, increased blood loss, congenital dislocation (30), and lengthening and/or lateral displacement of the extremity (30,53,134) have been associated with sciatic nerve palsies (30,53,106). Edwards et al. (30) reported that patients with peroneal nerve palsies were associated with an average lengthening of 2.7 cm (range, 1.9 to 3.7 cm), and sciatic nerve palsies were associated with an average lengthening of 4.4 cm (range, 4.0 to 5.1 cm). Isolated case reports have identified sciatic nerve injury caused by entrapment by trochanteric wiring (44,68), compression of the nerve over a spur of polymethylmethacrylate (PMMA) (19,31), and migration of broken trochanteric wires (6). Acetabular screw placement in the posterior quadrants is relatively safe, but digital palpation of the sciatic notch is prudent during drilling and screw placement. Obesity, age, surgical approach (30,53), and preoperative range of motion (140) have not been established as risk factors for the occurrence of sciatic and peroneal nerve palsies.

Nerve recovery in patients with sciatic and peroneal nerve palsies after THA has been reviewed (1,30,32,37,53,106, 107,117,134). The peroneal nerve injury fares much better than the sciatic palsy. Stretch injuries do not fair as well as direct injury (retractor, electrocautery burn, suture, and intraoperative femur fracture). Prognosis is also related to the extent of neural damage (107,122). Patients who retain some motor function after surgery or who recover some function while in the hospital are more likely to have a good recovery.

Femoral Nerve

The femoral nerve is formed from the posterior branches of the second, third, and fourth lumbar nerve roots. Within the pelvis, it overlies the iliopsoas muscle and passes into the thigh through the femoral triangle. The triangle (Fig. 3-6) lies directly anterior and medial to the hip joint, and within this space, the femoral nerve is vulnerable to injury. This triangle is defined by the inguinal ligament proximally, the sartorius muscle laterally, and the adductor longus muscle medially. The floor of the triangle is made up of the iliopsoas and pectineus muscles, and the roof, by the overlying anterior fascia. The femoral nerve, artery, and vein traverse this area in close proximity to each other. This space is relatively unyielding and offers little room for decompression of hematoma or edema (112). It supplies motor innervation to the iliacus, pectineus, sartorius, and quadriceps muscle groups. Its sensory function includes the anterior medial aspect of the thigh and the medial aspect of the leg.

The incidence of femoral nerve palsy after THA has been less well defined in comparison to sciatic and peroneal nerve palsies (8,122). In a published series of femoral palsies after THA, Simmons et al. (112) reported an incidence of 2.3% in 440 consecutive THAs. Femoral nerve palsies may occur in combination with sciatic palsies. However, the clinical manifestations (and true frequency) may be masked by the use of postoperative assistive walking devices (112). Additionally, use of the anterior approach for minimally invasive surgery places the femoral nerve in jeopardy if the surgeon strays too far medially (129).

The mechanisms of femoral nerve damage include cement extravasation (23,52,83,90,117,124,134,139), lengthening or stretch (134), hematoma (112,117,139), pseudoaneurysm, and—most commonly—retractor placement (83,112). A slightly flexed position of the patient's hip after THA may protect the femoral nerve from a postoperative traction injury. Goodfellow et al. (42) documented good results in treating femoral neuropathies in hemophiliacs by immobilization, whereas Kettlekamp and Powers (59) advocated surgical decompression in these patients. After THA, femoral nerve palsies have recovered with conservative care (139) and surgical decompression (124). Given the tight confines within the femoral triangle, when there is a progressive nerve lesion, surgical decompression may be indicated if hemorrhage is suspected as the cause of the femoral nerve palsy.

The prognosis of femoral nerve lesions after THA is similar to those of sciatic and peroneal nerve lesions, suggesting similar mechanisms. Complete entrapment of the femoral nerve by cement has a bad prognosis (134), whereas lesions secondary to impingement by spurs of PMMA may be improved by surgical removal of the spurs and neurolysis (90,134). Stretch-induced femoral neuropathy does not appear to do well (134), but quantitative analysis regarding the amount of lengthening has not been performed to the extent that it has in sciatic and peroneal palsies. In contrast to sciatic and peroneal injuries, hematoma-related femoral neuropathies fare well. Solheim and Hagen (117) and Wooten and McLaughlin (139) report good recovery of femoral nerve function after nonoperative treatment. However, surgical decompression of hematomas involving the femoral triangle may be recommended to prevent further nerve compression and irreversible damage. As with sciatic and peroneal palsies, direct neural injury caused by retractors appears to have the best prognosis for recovery of femoral nerve function (83,112).

Lateral Femoral Cutaneous Nerve

The lateral femoral cutaneous nerve is a direct branch of the lumbar plexus, arising from the posterior branches of the second and third lumbar nerves. Emerging from the psoas muscle at its lateral border, it crosses the iliac muscle deep to its fascia. Then passing distally toward the ASIS, it passes under the inguinal ligament—either superficial or deep to the sartorius muscle. It typically descends under the fascia lata on the lateral border of the sartorius. In doing such, it is close to the intermuscular interval between the tensor fasciae lata and the sartorius, descending along its medial aspect.

Injury to the lateral femoral cutaneous nerve has been uncommon in THA (13) as most surgeons use the posterior or anterolateral approaches, which do not put them in close proximity to the nerve. However, more recent use of the Smith Peterson (115) incision for cup placement in the two incision minimally invasive technique may place this nerve at increased risk (11,13). The nerve can be protected by not straying medial of the interval (101) and leaving a cuff of muscle medially for protection (65).

Obturator Nerve

The obturator nerve (anterior divisions of L2, L3, L4) crosses the quadrilateral surface of the acetabulum together with the artery and vein. The obturator internus muscle lies lateral to these structures, separating them from the bony surface. They exit the pelvis through the obturator canal at the superior lateral aspect of the obturator foramen. The nerve and vascular structures are well fixed at this point.

Obturator neuropathy appears to be a rare complication of THA (8,88,111,134). Persistent groin pain after THA, evidence of cement extrusion (88) on pelvic radiographs, clinical exam of obturator muscle strength, and positive EMG findings are needed to confirm this diagnosis. Most reports of obturator neuropathy have been secondary to intrapelvic violation by drills and/or cement (32). Violation of the medial acetabular wall as well as defects in the pubic ramus have been noted. Wire mesh used to protect the intrapelvic structures from cement penetration has been noted to be inadequate (111).

Bone grafting of all suspected defects is indicated. Screw placement as a cause of obturator nerve injury has not been reported, but given the close proximity of the obturator nerve to the quadrilateral surface of the acetabulum, avoidance of the anterior inferior acetabular quadrant for screw placement or cement penetration is necessary to prevent this complication.

Somatosensory Evoked Potentials and Electromyography

The use of somatosensory evoked potentials (SSEPs) during spinal surgery is well established (14,40,41,50,55,80,89,136). The technical aspects of the monitoring process during THA were first described by Stone et al. (120). The peroneal nerve is the most commonly injured peripheral nerve during THA (27) and is easily stimulated during surgery. Black et al. (14) reported on 100 consecutive THAs using SSEP, and Nercession et al. (80) studied 60 patients having revision or reoperation for THA. Pereles et al. (89) demonstrated that evoked potential changes were detected in 8 of 52 patients, mostly during anterior or lateral retraction of the proximal femur during primary THA. Candidates for SSEP monitoring may include high-risk patients such as those with congenital dislocation of the hip, those having revision surgery with expected limb lengthening, and possibly those with spinal stenosis or spinal dysplasias who may have highly sensitized peripheral nerves.

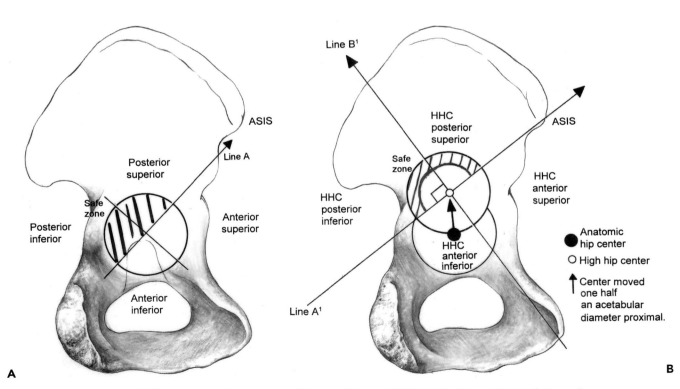

Figure 3-9   A: The quadrant system at the normal (anatomic) hip center. The posterior inferior and posterior superior quadrants are recommended for transacetabular fixation of screws in total hip arthroplasty. **B:** Schematic diagram illustrating the HHC quadrant system, which is superimposed one half of an acetabular diameter proximally over the original anatomic acetabular quadrant system. The HHC anterior quadrants (unsafe) are located in regions previously occupied by the posterior superior and posterior inferior quadrants (safe) of the original quadrant system. These formerly safe regions are no longer safe at the HHC.

Recently, spontaneous EMG has also been evaluated for its efficacy in avoiding nerve injury during revision and complex THA (93,123). This alternative real-time nerve monitoring technique detected sustained EMG activity that subsided with retractor removal and extremity repositioning but might otherwise have threatened the sciatic nerve.

THE ANATOMIC AND HIGH HIP CENTER QUADRANT SYSTEMS

The nerves and vessels that course around the acetabulum and proximal femur are demonstrated in this and many other anatomy and surgery texts (5,22,34,58,61,62,71,85,132, 137,138). The acetabular anatomy and surrounding nerves and vessels can be easily understood by using the acetabular quadrant system (132). Use of this system allows the surgeon to know the location of intrapelvic structures with respect to fixed points of reference within the acetabulum. For primary or revision acetabular arthroplasty, a line drawn from the anterior superior iliac spine through the center of the acetabulum defines anterior and posterior quadrant locations. If this line is then bisected with a perpendicular at its midpoint, four quadrants are formed. The anatomic and high hip center (HHC) quadrant systems (Fig. 3-9) can be used to locate the safe and dangerous zones for the transacetabular placement of screws; but they also can be used as a guide for retractor placement, for drilling acetabular anchoring holes for graft fixation, or to estimate bone depth in a specific acetabular zone.

The use of the anterior quadrants for the placement of screws or anchoring holes, or to help secure retractors may endanger the external iliac artery and vein and the obturator nerve, artery, and vein. The external iliac vessels lie opposite the anterior superior quadrant, and the obturator neural and vascular structures lie opposite the anterior inferior quadrant. These structures lie close to the pelvic bone, with little protective interposition of soft tissue or muscle. The risk of injury is further exacerbated by the lack of bone in the anterior quadrants (Fig. 3-10A). Violation of the inner acetabular bone opposite the anterior quadrants, with cement or transacetabular screws, should be avoided whenever possible (3). Retractor placement over the anterior column should be done with care.

The polar zone of the acetabulum is often violated during excessive reaming, placement of a cement anchoring hole, or transacetabular screw placement. Occasionally, medial migration of the acetabular component can occur with implant failure. This medial acetabular zone is opposite the external iliac vein and the obturator nerve, artery, and vein that course along the superior quadrilateral surface. The risk to these structures is increased during aging by the relatively small obturator internus muscle and the shallow acetabular bone depth opposite the structures.

The sciatic nerve and the superior gluteal nerve and vessels course opposite the posterior superior quadrant, and the inferior gluteal and internal pudendal structures are opposite the posterior inferior quadrant. In contrast to the shallow bone in the anterior quadrants, the bone depth in the posterior quadrants is 25 mm or greater in the central regions (Fig. 3-10A). Screws and anchoring holes can be placed relatively safely in these zones. In addition, the sciatic nerve can be gently displaced during retractor and screw placement, reducing the

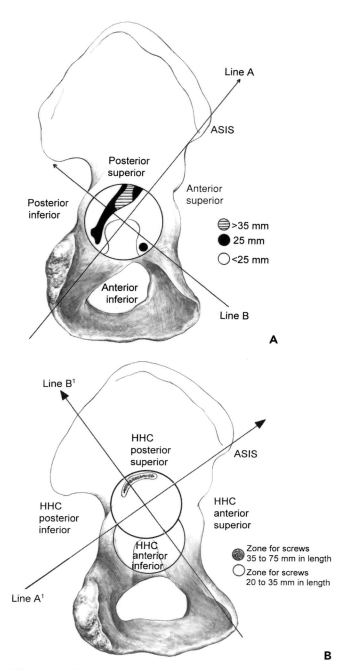

Figure 3-10   **A:** Bone depth within the quadrants. The central regions of the posterior inferior and posterior superior quadrants provide the best bone stock for screw purchase. **B:** Topographic map of the acetabular bone depth, showing a zone in the peripheral HHC posterior quadrants where screws 25 mm to greater than 35 mm can be placed up into the ilium.

likelihood of injury. The sciatic notch is easily palpable, and the superior gluteal nerve and vessels can be protected. The inferior gluteal and internal pudendal neural and vascular structures are not palpable at the level of the ischial spine. They are relatively mobile and can be protected if retractors are placed directly against the bone of the posterior column.

The quadrants for an HHC acetabulum—although constructed similarly—are different from those formed at the normal anatomic acetabulum. HHC quadrants are formed by drawing a line from the anterior superior iliac spine through the center of the newly positioned acetabulum. A second line drawn perpendicular to the first at the acetabular midpoint forms four clinically useful HHC acetabular quadrants (Fig. 3-9B).

The peripheral halves of the posterior superior and posterior inferior HHC quadrants contain the best available bone stock (Fig. 3-10B) and are relatively safe for transacetabular screw placement (Fig. 3-9B). The entire anterior superior and anterior inferior HHC quadrants, as well as the central half of the posterior superior and posterior inferior quadrants, should be avoided because of the close proximity of intrapelvic structures and the paucity of protective musculature on the inner wall of the pelvis opposite these zones.

The modified HHC and anatomic acetabular quadrant systems provide the surgeon with a reproducible intraoperative guide to the location of periacetabular neural and vascular structures. Knowledge of the mechanisms by which the nerves and vessels are injured, along with the ability to locate structures with respect to surgical landmarks, will allow the surgeon to minimize injuries during THA.

REFERENCES

1. Ahlgren S, Elmqvist D, Ljung P. Nerve lesions after total hip replacement. *Acta Orthop Scand.* 1984;55:152–155.
2. Akizuki S, Terayama K, Kobayashi S. False aneurysm of the external iliac artery during total hip replacement. *Arch Orthop Trauma Surg.* 1984;102:210–211.
3. Amstutz HC. Complications of total hip replacement. *Clin Orthop.* 1970;72:123–137.
4. Anda S, Svenningsen S, Dale LG, et al. The acetabular sector angle of the adult hip determined by computed tomography. *Acta Radiol Diagn.* 1986;27:443–447.
5. Anderson JE. *Grant's Atlas of Anatomy.* 7th ed. Baltimore: Williams & Wilkins; 1978.
6. Asnis SE, Hanley S, Shelton PD. Sciatic neuropathy secondary to migration of trochanteric wire following total hip arthroplasty. *Clin Orthop.* 1985;196:226–228.
7. Aust JC, Bredenburg CE, Murray DG. Mechanisms of arterial injuries associated with total hip replacement. *Arch Surg.* 1981;116:345–349.
8. Barrack RL, Butler RA. Avoidance and management of neurovascular injuries in total hip arthroplasty. *Instr Course Lect.* 2003;52:267–274.
9. Beaton LE, Anson BJ. The relationship of the sciatic nerve to the piriformis muscle. *Anat Rec.* 1937;70:1.
10. Belsky MR. What's new in Orthopaedic surgery. *J Am Coll Surg.* 2003;197(6):985–989.
11. Berger RA. Total hip arthroplasty using the minimally invasive two-incision approach. *Clin Orthop.* 2003;417:232–241.
12. Bergqvist D, Carlsson AS, Ericsson BF. Vascular complications after total hip arthroplasty. *Acta Orthop Scand.* 1983;54:157–163.
13. Berry DJ, Berger RA, Callaghan JJ, et al. Minimally invasive total hip arthroplasty: development, early results, and a critical analysis. *J Bone Joint Surg Am.* 2003;85A(11):2235–2246.
14. Black LL, Reckling FW, Porter SS. Somatosensory evoked potential monitored during total hip arthroplasty. *Clin Orthop.* 1991;262:170–177.
15. Bombelli R, Santore RF, Poss R. Mechanics of the normal and osteoarthritic hip: a new perspective. *Clin Orthop.* 1984;182:69–78.
16. Bose WJ, Petty W. Femoral artery and nerve compression by bulk allograft used for acetabular reconstruction. *J Arthroplasty.* 1996;11(3):348–350.
17. Brentlinger A, Hunter JR. Perforation of the external iliac artery and ureter presenting an acute hemorrhagic cystitis after total hip replacement. *J Bone Joint Surg.* 1987;69A:620–622.
18. Bullough P, Goodfellow J, O'Connor J. The relationship between degenerative changes and load-bearing in the human hip. *J Bone Joint Surg.* 1973;55B:746–758.
19. Casagrande PA, Danahy PR. Delayed sciatic-nerve entrapment following the use of self-curing acrylic. *J Bone Joint Surg.* 1971;53A:167–169.
20. Charnley J, Cupic Z. The nine and ten year results of the low-friction arthroplasty of the hip. *Clin Orthop.* 1973;95:9–25.
21. Clark JM, Freeman MAR, Witham D. The relationship of neck orientation to the shape of the proximal femur. *J Arthroplasty.* 1987;2:99–109.
22. Clemente CD. *Gray's Anatomy of the Human Body.* 13th ed. Philadelphia: Lea & Febiger; 1985:841.
23. Coventry MB, Beckenbaugh RD, Nolan DR, et al. 2,012 total hip arthroplasties: a study of postoperative course and early complications. *J Bone Joint Surg.* 1974;56A:273–284.
24. Crispin HA, Boghemans JPM. Thrombosis of the external iliac artery following total hip replacement. *J Bone Joint Surg.* 1980;62A:462–464.
25. Dai KR, An KN, Hein T. Geometric and biomechanical analysis of the femur. *Trans Orthop Res Soc.* 1985;10:99.
26. D'Ambrosia RD. *Musculoskeletal Disorders: Regional Examination and Differential Diagnosis.* 2nd ed. Philadelphia: JB Lippincott Co; 1986.
27. DeHart MM, Riley LH Jr. Nerve injuries in total hip arthroplasty. *J Am Acad Orthop Surg.* 1999;7(2):101–111.
28. Dorr L, Conaty JP, Kohl R, et al. False aneurysm of the femoral artery following total hip surgery. *J Bone Joint Surg.* 1974;56A:1059–1062.
29. Dorr LD. Structural and cellular assessment of bone quality of proximal femur. *Bone.* 1993;14:231–242.
30. Edwards BN, Tullos HS, Noble PC. Contributory factors and etiology of sciatic nerve palsy in total hip arthroplasty. *Clin Orthop.* 1987;218:136–141.
31. Edwards MS, Barbaro NM, Asher SW, et al. Delayed sciatic palsy after total hip replacement: case report. *Neurosurgery.* 1981;9:61–63.
32. Eftekhar NS, Kiernan HA, Stinchfield FE. Systemic and local complications following low-friction arthroplasty of the hip joint. *Arch Surg.* 1976;111:150–155.
33. Eriksson I, Erikson U, Johansson H, et al. Late hemorrhage produced by arterial erosion following orthopaedic surgery. *Injury.* 1971;3:104–106.
34. Eyscleshymer AC, Shoemaker DM. *A Cross-Section Anatomy.* 2nd ed. New York: Meredith; 1970:286–291.
35. Fabry G, MacEwen GD, Shands AR. Torsion of the femur: a follow-up study in normal and abnormal conditions. *J Bone Joint Surg.* 1973;55A:1726–1738.
36. Fiddian NJ, Sudlow RA, Browett. Ruptured femoral vein: a complication of the use of gentamicin beads in an infected excision arthroplasty of the hip. *J Bone Joint Surg.* 1984;66B:493–494.
37. Fleming RE, Michelsen CB, Stinchfield FE. Sciatic paralysis. *J Bone Joint Surg.* 1979;61A:37–39.
38. Gautier E, Ganz K, Krugel N, et al. Anatomy of the medial femoral circumflex artery and its surgical implications. *J Bone Joint Surg Br.* 2000;82:679–683.
39. Giacchetto J, Gallagher J. False aneurysm of the common femoral artery secondary to migration of a threaded acetabular component. *Clin Orthop.* 1988;231:91–96.
40. Gonzalez EJ, Hajdu M, Keim H, et al. Intraoperative somatosensory evoked potential monitoring. *Orthop Rev.* 1984;13:573.
41. Gonzalez EJ, Keim H, Hajdu M, et al. Quantification of intraoperative somatosensory evoked potentials. *Arch Phys Med Rehab.* 1984;65:721–725.
42. Goodfellow J, Fearn CB, Matthews JT. Iliacus hematoma: a common complication of hemophilia. *J Bone Joint Surg.* 1967;49B:748.
43. Gowitzke BA, Milner M. *Scientific Bases of Human Movement.* 3rd ed. Baltimore: Williams & Wilkins; 1988.
44. Gudmundsson GH, Pilgaard S. Prevention of sciatic nerve entrapment in trochanteric wiring following total hip arthroplasty. *Clin Orthop.* 1985;196:215–216.
45. Harty M. The calcar femorale and the femoral neck. *J Bone Joint Surg.* 1957;39A:625–630.
46. Hennessy OF, Timmis JB, Allison DJ. Vascular complications following hip replacement. *Br J Radiol.* 1983;56:275–277.

47. Heyes FLP, Aukland A. Occlusion of the common femoral artery complicating total hip arthroplasty. *J Bone Joint Surg.* 1985;67B:533–535.

48. Hirsch SA, Robertson H, Gorniowsky M. Arterial occlusion secondary to methylmethacrylate use. *Arch Surg.* 1976;111:204.

49. Hopkins NFG, Vangegan JAD, Jamieson CW. Iliac aneurysm after total hip arthroplasty. *J Bone Joint Surg.* 1983;65B:359–361.

50. Hoppenfeld S, deBoer P. *Surgical Exposures in Orthopaedics.* 3rd ed. Philadelphia: Lippincott Williams & Wilkins; 2003.

51. Inman VT, Ralston HJ, Todd F. *Human Walking.* Baltimore: Williams & Wilkins; 1981.

52. Jerosch J. Femoral nerve palsy in hip replacement due to pelvic cement extrusion. *Arch Orthop Trauma Surg.* 2000;120(9):499–501.

53. Johanson NA, Pellicci PM, Tsairis P, et al. Nerve injury in total hip arthroplasty. *Clin Orthop.* 1983;179:214–222.

54. Johnston RC, Fitzgerald RH, Harris WH, et al. Clinical and radiographic evaluation of total hip replacement. *J Bone Joint Surg.* 1990;72A:161–168.

55. Jones SJ, Edgar MA, Ransford AO, et al. A system for the electrophysiologic monitoring of the spinal cord during operations for scoliosis. *J Bone Joint Surg.* 1983;65B:134–139.

56. Kapandji IA. *The Physiology of the Joints.* Vol 2. Baltimore: Williams & Wilkins; 1970.

57. Kaplan EB. The iliotibial tract. *J Bone Joint Surg.* 1958;40A:825–832.

58. Keating EM, Merrill RA, Faris PM. Structures at risk from medially placed acetabular screws. *J Bone Joint Surg.* 1990;72A:509–511.

59. Kettlekamp DB, Powers SR. Femoral compression neuropathy in hemorrhagic disorders. *Arch Surg.* 1969;98:367–368.

60. Kingsley PC, Olmsted KL. A study to determine the angle of anteversion of the neck of the femur. *J Bone Joint Surg.* 1948;30A:745.

61. Kirkpatrick JS, Callaghan JJ, Vandemark RM, et al. The relationship of the intrapelvic vasculature to the acetabulum. *Clin Orthop.* 1990;258:183–190.

62. Koritke JG, Sick H. *Atlas of Sectional Human Anatomy.* Baltimore: Urban and Schwargenberg; 1989:93–100.

63. Korovesis P, Siablis D, Salonikidis P, et al. Abdominal-hip joint fistula. *Clin Orthop.* 1988;231:71–75.

64. Kroese A, Mollerud A. Traumatic aneurysm of the common femoral artery after hip endoprosthesis. *Acta Orthop Scand.* 1975;46:119–122.

65. Light TR, Keggi KJ. Anterior approach to hip arthroplasty. *Clin Orthop.* 1980;152:255–260.

66. Lozman H, Robbins H. Injury to the superior gluteal artery as a complication of total hip replacement arthroplasty. *J Bone Joint Surg.* 1983;65A:268–269.

67. Mallory TH. Rupture of the common iliac vein from reaming the acetabulum during total hip replacement. *J Bone Joint Surg.* 1972;54A:276–277.

68. Mallory TH. Sciatic nerve entrapment secondary to trochanteric wiring following total hip arthroplasty. *Clin Orthop.* 1983;180:198–200.

69. Matos MH, Amstutz HC, Machleder HI. Ischemia of the lower extremity after total hip replacement. *J Bone Joint Surg.* 1979;61A:24–27.

70. McLaughlin JR, Harris WH. Revision of the femoral component of a total hip arthroplasty with the Calcar-replacement femoral component. *J Bone Joint Surg.* 1996;78A:331–339.

71. Mears DC, Rubash HE. *Pelvic and Acetabular Fractures.* New York: Charles B Slack; 1986:107.

72. Middleton RG, Reilly DT, Jessop J. Occlusion of the external iliac vein by cement. *J Arthroplasty.* 1996;11(3):346–347.

73. Morrey BE, ed. *Joint Replacement Arthroplasty.* New York: Churchill Livingstone; 1991.

74. Mow VC, Flatow EL, Foster RJ. Biomechanics. In: Simon SR, ed. *Orthopaedic Basic Science.* Rosemont, IL: American Academy of Orthopaedic Surgeons; 1995.

75. Muller ME. Total hip prostheses. *Clin Orthop.* 1970;72:46–68.

76. Murray MP, Sepic SB. Maximum isotropic torque of hip abductor and adductor. *Phys Ther.* 1968;48:2.

77. Nachbur B, Meyer RP, Verkkala K. The mechanisms of severe arterial injury in surgery of the hip joint. *Clin Orthop.* 1979;141:122–133.

78. Neal J, Wachtel TL, Garza OT, et al. Late arterial embolization complicating total hip replacement. *J Bone Joint Surg.* 1979;61A:429–430.

79. Nemeth G, Ohlson H. In vivo moment arm lengths for hip extensor muscles at different angles of hip flexion. *J Biomech.* 1985;18:129–140.

80. Nercession OA, Gonzalez EG, Stinchfield FE. The use of somatosensory evoked potential during revision or reoperation for total hip arthroplasty. *Clin Orthop.* 1989;243:138–142.

81. Noble PC, Alexander JW, Lindahl LJ. The anatomic basis of femoral component design. *Clin Orthop.* 1988;235:148–165.

82. Norkin CC, White DJ. *Measurement of Joint Motion: A Guide to Goniometry.* Philadelphia: FA Davis Co; 1985.

83. Ovrum E, Dahl HK. Vessel and nerve injuries complicating total hip arthroplasty. *Arch Orthop Trauma Surg.* 1979;95:267–269.

84. Pai VS, Ortho D. Significance of the Trendelenburg test in total hip arthroplasty. *J Arthroplasty.* 1996;11(2):174–179.

85. Pansky B. *Review of Gross Anatomy.* 4th ed. New York: Macmillian; 1979.

86. Pare EB, Stern JT, Schwartz JM. Functional differentiation within the tensor fascia latae. *J Bone Joint Surg.* 1981;63A:1457–1471.

87. Pauwels F. *Biomechanics of the Normal and Diseased Hip.* Berlin: Springer-Verlag; 1976.

88. Pecina M, Lucijanic I, Rosie D. Surgical treatment of obturator nerve palsy resulting from extrapelvic extrusion of cement during total hip arthroplasty. *J Arthroplasty.* 2001;16(4):515–517.

89. Pereles TR, Stuchin SA, Kastenbaum DM, et al. Surgical maneuvers placing the sciatic nerve at risk during total hip arthroplasty as assessed by somatosensory evoked potential monitoring. *J Arthroplasty.* 1996;11(4):438–444.

90. Pess GM, Lusskin R, Waugh TR, et al. Femoral neuropathy secondary to pressurized cement in total hip replacement: treatment by decompression and neurolysis. *J Bone Joint Surg.* 1987;69A:623–625.

91. Petrera P, Trakru S, Mehta S, et al. Revision total hip arthroplasty with a retroperitoneal approach to the iliac vessels. *J Arthroplasty.* 1996;11(6):704–708.

92. Pick JW, Anson BJ, Ashley FL. The origin of the obturator artery. A study of 640 body halves. *Am J Anat.* 1942;70:317–344.

93. Pring ME, Trousdale RT, Cabanela ME, et al. Intraoperative electromyographic monitoring during periacetabular osteotomy. *Clin Orthop.* 2002;400:158–164.

94. Radin EL, Simon S, Rose R. *Practical Biomechanics for the Orthopedic Surgeon.* New York: John Wiley and Sons; 1979.

95. Ratliff AHC. Arterial injuries after total hip replacement. *J Bone Joint Surg.* 1985;67B:517–518.

96. Ratliff AHC. Vascular and neurological complications. In: Ling RSM, ed. *Complications of Total Hip Replacement.* New York: Churchill Livingstone; 1984:18–29.

97. Reikeras O, Bjerkreim I, Kolbenstvedt A. Anteversion of the acetabulum and femoral neck in normals and in patients with osteoarthritis of the hip. *Acta Orthop Scand.* 1983;54:18–23.

98. Reiley MA, Bond D, Branick RI, et al. Vascular complications following total hip arthroplasty. *Clin Orthop.* 1984;186:23–28.

99. Reitman RD, Emerson R, Higgins L, et al. Thirteen year results of total hip arthroplasty using a tapered titanium femoral component inserted without cement in patients with type C bone. *J Arthroplasty.* 2003;18:116–121.

100. Rothman RH, Hozak WJ. *Complications of Total Hip Arthroplasty.* Philadelphia: Saunders; 1988.

101. Rue JPH, Inoue N, Mont MA. Current overview of neurovascular structures in hip arthroplasty: anatomy, preoperative evaluation, approaches, and operative techniques to avoid complications. *Orthopedics.* 2004;27(1):73–81.

102. Ruff CB, Hayes WC. Subperiosteal expansion and cortical remodeling of the human femur and tibia with aging. *Science.* 1982;217:945–948.

103. Ryan JA, Johnson ML, Boettcher WG, et al. Mycotic aneurysm of the external iliac artery caused by migration of a total hip prosthesis. *Clin Orthop.* 1984;186:57–59.

104. Ryan W, Snyder W, Bell T, et al. Penetrating injuries of the iliac vessels. *Am J Surg.* 1982;144:642–645.

105. Salama R, Stavorovsky MM, Iellin A, et al. Femoral artery injury complicating total hip replacement. *Clin Orthop.* 1972;89:143–144.

106. Schmalzreid TP, Amstutz HD, Dorey FJ. Nerve palsy associated with total hip replacement. *J Bone Joint Surg.* 1991:73:1074–1080.

107. Schmalzried TP, Noordin S, Amstutz HC. Update on nerve palsy associated with total hip replacement. *Clin Orthop.* 1997;344:188–206.

108. Scullin JP, Nelson CL, Beven EG. False aneurysm of the left external iliac artery following total hip arthroplasty. *Clin Orthop.* 1975;113:145–149.

109. Shih C, Du Y, Lin Y, et al. Muscular recovery around the hip joint after total hip arthroplasty. *Clin Orthop.* 1994;302:115–120.

110. Shoenfeld NA, Stuchin SA, Pearl R, et al. The management of vascular injuries associated with total hip arthroplasty. *J Vasc Surg.* 1990;11(4):549–555.

111. Siliski JM, Scott RD. Obturator-nerve palsy resulting from intrapelvic extrusion of cement during total hip replacement. *J Bone Joint Surg.* 1985;67A:1225–1228.

112. Simmons C, Izant TH, Rothman RH, et al. Femoral neuropathy following total hip arthroplasty. *J Arthroplasty.* 1991;6:559–565.

113. Singh M, Nagrath AR, Maini PS. Changes in the trabecular pattern of the upper end of the femur as an index of osteoporosis. *J Bone Joint Surg.* 1970;52A:457–467.

114. Smith RW, Walker RR. Femoral expansion in aging women: implications for osteoporosis and fracture. *Henry Ford Hosp Med J.* 1980;28:168–170.

115. Smith-Petersen MN, Cave E, VanGorder G. Intracapsular fractures of the neck of the femur: treatment by internal fixation. *Arch Surg.* 1931;23:707–715.

116. Soderburg GL, Dostal WF. Electromyographic study of the three parts of the gluteus medius muscle during functional activities. *Phys Ther.* 1978;58:6.

117. Solheim LF, Hagen R. Femoral and sciatic neuropathies after total hip arthroplasty. *Acta Orthop Scand.* 1990;51:531–534.

118. Spotorno L, Schenk RK, Dietschi C. Personal experiences with uncemented prosthesis. *Orthopade.* 1987;16:225–238.

119. Stamatakis JD, Kakkar VV, Sagar S, et al. Femoral vein thrombosis and total hip replacement. *BMJ.* 1977;2:223–225.

120. Stone RG, Weeks LE, Hajdu M, et al. Evaluation of sciatic nerve compromise during total hip arthroplasty. *Clin Orthop.* 1985;201:26–31.

121. Stubbs DH, Dorner DB, Johnston RC. Thrombosis of the iliofemoral artery during revision of a total hip replacement. *J Bone Joint Surg.* 1986;68A:454–455.

122. Sunderland S. *Nerves and Nerve Injury.* Edinburgh: Churchill Livingstone; 1978.

123. Sutherland CJ, Miller DH, Owen JH. Use of spontaneous electromyography during revision and complex total hip arthroplasty. *J Arthroplasty.* 1996;11(2):206–209.

124. Tani Y, Miyawaki H. Femoral neuropathy caused by reinforcement ring malposition and extruded bone-cement after revision total hip arthroplasty. *J Arthroplasty.* 2002;17(4):516–518.

125. Tazawa A, Nakamura S, Otsuka K, et al. Transabdominal approach for intrapelvic migration of a total hip prosthesis component. *J Orthop Sci.* 2001;6(4):362–365.

126. Tkaczuk H. False aneurysm of the external iliac artery following hip endoprosthesis. *Acta Orthop Scand.* 1976;47:317–319.

127. Todd BD, Bintcliffe WL. Injury to the external iliac artery during hip arthroplasty for old central dislocation. *J Arthroplasty.* 1990;5:S53–55.

128. Vanhegan JAD, Sellu DP, Hopkins NFG. Iliac aneurysm in hip arthroplasty: surgical repair. *J R Soc Med.* 1981;74:841–843.

129. Waldman BJ. Advancements in minimally invasive total hip arthroplasty. *Orthopedics.* 2003;26:S833–836.

130. Walker PS, Robertson DD. Design and fabrication of cementless hip stems. *Clin Orthop.* 1988;235:25–34.

131. Wasielewski RC. Limitations in expanding the acetabulum during acetabular arthroplasty. Unpublished data. Ohio State University, Columbus, 1996.

132. Wasielewski RC, Cooperstein LA, Kruger MP, et al. Acetabular anatomy and the transacetabular fixation of screws in total hip arthroplasty. *J Bone Joint Surg.* 1990;72A:501–508.

133. Wasielewski RC, Cooperstein LA, Rubash HE. Radiographic analysis of intrapelvic transacetabular screws after acetabular arthroplasty. Presented at: American Academy of Orthopaedic Surgeons Annual Meeting poster exhibit; 1991.

134. Weber ER, Daube JR, Coventry MB. Peripheral neuropathies associated with total hip arthroplasty. *J Bone Joint Surg.* 1976;58A:66–69.

135. Wenz JF, Gurkan I, Jibodh SR. Mini-incision total hip arthroplasty: a comparative assessment of perioperative outcomes. *Orthopedics.* 2002;25:1031–1043.

136. Wheatly MD, Jahnke WD. Electromyographic study of the superficial thigh and hip muscles in normal individuals. *Arch Phys Med.* 1951;32:508.

137. Williams PL, Warwick R, eds. *Gray's Anatomy.* 37th ed. Philadelphia: WB Saunders; 1985.

138. Woodburn RT. *Essentials of Human Anatomy.* 6th ed. New York: Oxford University Press; 1978:544–546.

139. Wooten SL, McLaughlin RE. Iliacus hematoma and subsequent femoral nerve palsy after penetration of the medial acetabular wall during total hip arthroplasty. *Clin Orthop.* 1984;191:221–223.

140. Zechmann JP, Reckling FW. Association of preoperative hip motion and sciatic nerve palsy following total hip arthroplasty. *Clin Orthop.* 1989;241:197–199.

Arthroscopic Hip Anatomy

4

Bryan T. Kelly   Marc J. Philippon

Although arthroscopic surgery of the hip was first introduced by Burman in 1931, it did not begin to gain any popularity in North America until 1977 when Gross reported his experience with arthroscopy of congenitally dislocated hips (3,14). Anatomical constraints have made arthroscopy of the hip significantly more challenging than similar surgery around the shoulder and knee (Fig. 4-1). The femoral head is deeply recessed in the bony acetabulum and is convex in shape. The thick fibrocapsular and muscular envelopes around the hip joint decrease the amount of distention of the hip allowed during arthroscopy; the relative proximity of the sciatic nerve, lateral femoral cutaneous nerve, and remaining femoral neurovascular structures make portal placement more challenging (6,18). Nonetheless, over the past several years hip arthroscopy has begun to gain considerably more interest. The advent of better diagnostic tools, especially magnetic resonance imaging, has helped in the detection of intra-articular hip pathology in a more predictable fashion. New techniques and instrumentation have facilitated the visualization and treatment of these intra-articular lesions by hip arthroscopy. Most notably, the recent adaptation of arthroscopy equipment to create flexible scopes and instruments specifically designed for the hip has led to improved safety, visualization, and accessibility of this joint (Fig. 4-2) (32). With these improvements in technology a more detailed understanding of the arthroscopic anatomy of the hip has developed.

Hip arthroscopy offers a less invasive alternative for hip procedures that would otherwise require surgical dislocation of the hip. In addition, this procedure allows surgeons to address intra-articular derangements that were previously undiagnosed and untreated. Current indications for hip arthroscopy include management of labral tears, osteoplasty for decreased femoral head–neck junction offset, subtle rotational instability and capsular laxity, ligamentum teres injuries, lateral impact and chondral injuries, osteochondritis dissecans, internal and external snapping hip, removal of loose bodies, synovial biopsy, subtotal synovectomy, synovial chondromatosis, infection, and certain cases of mild to moderate osteoarthritis with associated mechanical symptoms. In addition, patients with long-standing, unresolved hip joint pain and positive physical findings may benefit from arthroscopic evaluation (7,11–13,15–17, 20,24,25,29,30,32). This chapter discusses the relevant arthroscopic anatomy of the hip and related pathologic and anatomic variations that are commonly encountered during this procedure.

GENERAL ANATOMIC CONSIDERATIONS

The articulation between the head of the femur and the acetabulum form the hip joint. This bony configuration is intrinsically stable except in situations where there is variation in the acetabular depth and femoral head geometry, which results in more reliance on the surrounding soft tissue. Version and inclination of the weight-bearing surface affect the joint capsule and ligaments of the hip, the labrum, and the ligamentum teres, as well as the suction effect of the hip (2,20). The femoral head normally forms two thirds of a sphere, and it is flattened in the area where the acetabulum applies its greatest load. In the neutral, anatomic position, the anterior part of the femoral head is not engaged in the acetabulum,

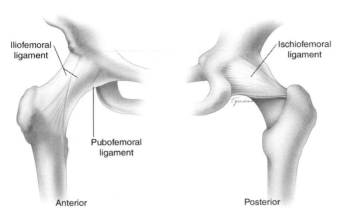

Figure **4-1** Anatomical constraints of the hip. The anterior ligamentous constraints of the hip seen in the anterior view include the iliofemoral and pubofemoral ligaments. The ischiofemoral ligament is the primary posterior restraint. (From *Am J Sports Med.* 2003;31, with permission.)

and the labrum augments the femoral head coverage by its extension from the bony acetabulum.

The hip joint is surrounded by a thick, fibrous capsule with three discreet thickenings that form the main capsular ligaments: the iliofemoral (Y-shaped ligament of Bigelow), the pubofemoral, and the ischiofemoral. These ligaments originate from the three named bones of the pelvis and insert on the intertrochanteric line, resulting in more than 95% of the femoral neck being intracapsular (Fig. 4-1). The iliofemoral ligament covers the anterosuperior portion of the joint. It is the thickest and strongest of the three ligaments and prevents anterior translation of the hip in the positions of

extension and external rotation. The zona orbicularis is the name of the terminal fibers of the iliofemoral ligament that form a deep circular orientation surrounding the femoral neck in a leashlike fashion (Fig. 4-3).

The labrum runs circumferentially around the acetabular perimeter to the base of the fovea and becomes attached to the transverse acetabular ligament posteriorly and anteriorly (Fig. 4-4) (32). Free nerve endings including proprioceptors and nociceptors have been identified within labral tissue, which may explain decreased proprioception and pain in an athlete with a torn acetabular labrum (21,23). Much like the meniscus, the labrum has its greatest healing potential at the peripheral capsulolabral junction. The vessels that penetrate the labrum are greatest at the outermost layer of the capsular surface, leaving the central articular margins less vascular (Fig. 4-5) (19). Arthroscopic visualization of injured labral tissue has demonstrated more extensive penetration of the vascular tissue throughout the entire substance of the labrum, suggesting an improved healing potential over what has been previously believed (Fig. 4-6).

The acetabular labrum is made of fibrocartilage and may enhance stability by maintaining negative intra-articular pressure in the hip joint (36). It also may act as a tension band to limit expansion during motion between the anterior and posterior columns during loading in the gait cycle (32). The intact labrum appears to have an important sealing function in the hip joint by limiting fluid expression from the joint space and protecting the cartilage layers of the hip (8,9). Ferguson et al. have found that the absence of the labrum significantly increased cartilage surface consolidation as well as contact pressure of the femoral head against the acetabulum (8–10). Ferguson et al. have further identified a stabilizing role of the labrum using a poroelastic finite

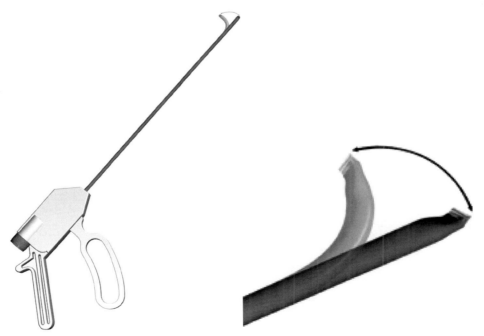

Figure **4-2** Flexible instruments allow for significantly improved access to most structures within the hip joint during routine arthroscopy. (From *Am J Sports Med.* 2003;31, with permission.)

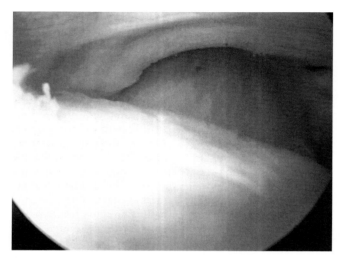

Figure 4-3 Arthroscopic view of the zona orbicularis. These circular fibers are an extension of the iliofemoral ligament and form a circular leash surrounding three quarters of the femoral neck. Its functional role is not well understood. See Color Plate.

element model to demonstrate that the labrum provided some structural resistance to lateral and vertical motion of the femoral head within the acetabulum (8,10). Since the labrum appears to enhance joint stability and preserve joint congruity, there is a significant concern about the potential for rotational instability or hypermobility of a hip associated with a deficiency of labral tissue. This instability may result in redundant capsular tissue and create a potential abnormal load distribution due to a transient incongruous joint resulting from subtle subluxation (32).

The ligamentum teres runs from the fovea capitis to the acetabular fossa and may have a secondary stabilizing effect on the hip joint, especially in the presence of a deficient labrum or a dysplastic hip (33). Arthroscopic examination of

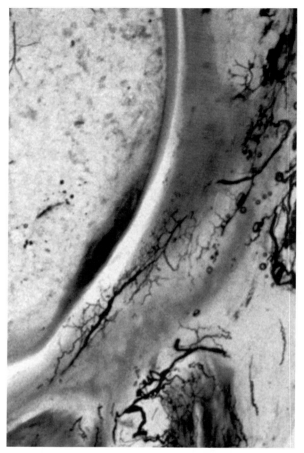

Figure 4-5 The hip labrum is relatively avascular; however, there is increased vascularity seen arising from the capsular attachments. This may have implication for arthroscopic repair of the labrum. See Color Plate.

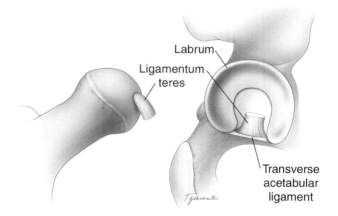

Figure 4-4 The labrum surrounds the rim of the acetabulum nearly circumferentially and is contiguous with the transverse acetabular ligament across the acetabular notch. The ligamentum teres arises from the margins of the acetabular notch and the transverse acetabular ligament. (From *Am J Sports Med.* 2003;31, with permission.)

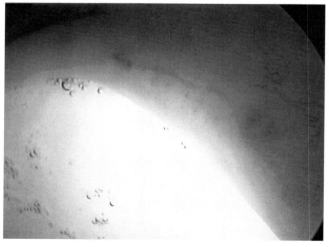

Figure 4-6 Arthroscopic view of the anterior superior labrum demonstrating vascular penetration through the substance of the labrum out to the central articular margin. See Color Plate.

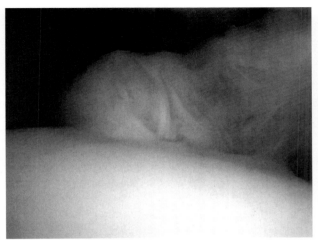
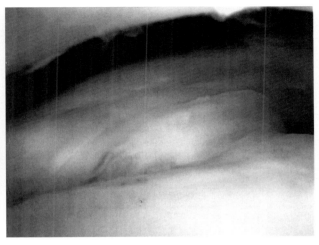

A   B

Figure 4-7 Dynamic hip arthroscopy demonstrates significant tightening of the ligamentum teres during external rotation **(B)** compared to internal rotation of the hip **(A)**. These findings support the biomechanical role of the ligamentum teres in the stabilization of the hip. (From *Am J Sports Med.* 2003;31, with permission.) See Color Plate.

the ligamentum teres demonstrates that it is composed of an anterior and posterior bundle. The anterior bundle tightens in external rotation of the hip (Fig. 4-7). The ligament originates from the fovea capitis, which is a small, depressed bare spot located at the medial aspect of the femoral head, and inserts adjacent to the transverse acetabular ligament in the acetabular fossa (Fig. 4-8). The pulvinar or fat pad fills the remainder of the acetabular fossa, which lies in the inferomedial portion of the acetabulum (Fig. 4-9). The psoas tendon crosses the front of the anteromedial aspect of the hip joint. The location of the tendon can be predictably located medial to an indentation in the anterior labrum known as the psoas U (Fig. 4-10). The psoas tendon helps to protect the anterior intermediate portion of the capsule and, by virtue of its anatomic location, can be subjected to increased load in athletic activities; such loads may be increased in athletes with

further intra-articular pathology. The psoas bursa communicates with the hip joint in the adult in approximately 20% of the population (31).

SURGICAL LANDMARKS

Accurate portal placement is essential for optimal visualization of all intra-articular structures and safe access to the hip joint. Typically, three basic portals are used: anterolateral, anterior, and posterolateral (Fig. 4-11). The vast majority of procedures performed within the joint can be accomplished with just two portals, the anterolateral and the anterior. Two accessory portals (proximal lateral and distal lateral) are useful for releases of the iliotibial band (ITB) and osteoplasty for decreased head–neck junction offset.

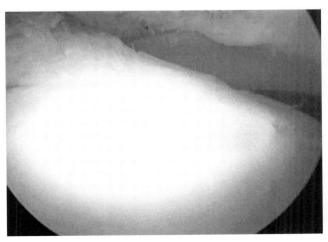
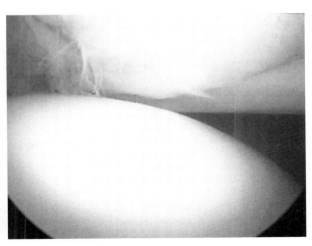

A   B

Figure 4-8 Arthroscopic picture of the fovea capitus where the ligamentum teres originates from the medial aspect of the femoral head **(A)** and the transverse acetabular ligament **(B)**. See Color Plate.

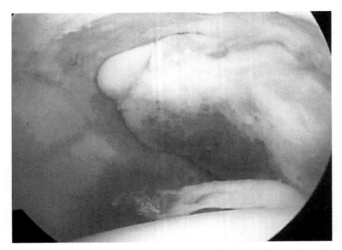

Figure 4-9 Arthroscopic view of the pulvinar or fat pad in the central aspect of the acetabular fossa. The fat pad likely plays a role in joint lubrication and should be treated cautiously during arthroscopic procedures. It is also highly vascular and has a propensity to bleed if it is débrided aggressively. See Color Plate.

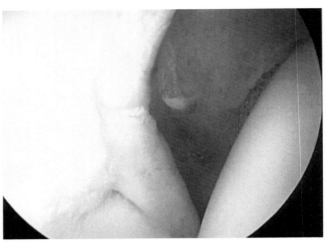

Figure 4-10 Arthroscopic view of the psoas U. This normal indentation in the labrum at the anteromedial aspect of the joint is a consistent landmark for identifying the location of the psoas tendon. In approximately 20% of patients the psoas tendon or bursae will lie intra-articularly at this level. See Color Plate.

Anterolateral Portal

The anterolateral portal has also been described as the anterior paratrochanteric portal, as it is referenced off of the greater trochanter. This portal is traditionally described as being approximately 1 to 2 cm superior and 1 to 2 cm anterior to the anterosuperior "corner" of the greater trochanter depending upon the patients weight and size. In our experience we have found the portal to be more useful if placed directly off of the anterosuperior portion of the greater trochanter. This portal allows for optimal visualization of the iliofemoral ligament, femoral head, anterior superior labrum, ligamentum teres, transverse ligament, and most of the

acetabulum. Typically a 70° scope is used through this portal for greatest visualization.

Anterior Portal

The anterior portal is typically the second portal to be established and allows for visualization of the posterior superior capsule, posterior superior labrum, posterior recess, femoral head, and ligamentum teres. This portal is also the optimal location for viewing the head–neck junction, anterior femoral neck, zona orbicularis, and distal insertion of the capsular ligaments on the intertrochanteric line. Again, use of the 70° arthroscope will allow for optimal visualization. The portal is established by

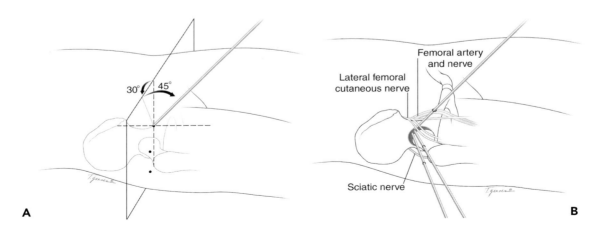

Figure 4-11 Three portals are traditionally used (anterolateral, posterolateral, and anterior). The anterior portal coincides with the intersection of a sagittal line drawn distally from the anterior superior iliac spine and a transverse line across the superior margin of the greater trochanter. **A:** The anterolateral and posterolateral portals lie anterior and posterior to the superior tip of the greater trochanter. **B:** Careful attention to proper portal placement is essential for avoidance of nearby neurovascular structures. (From *Am J Sports Med*. 2003; 31, with permission.)

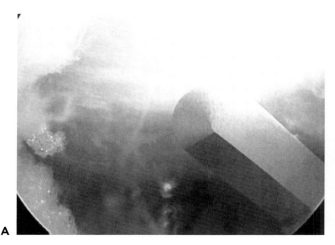
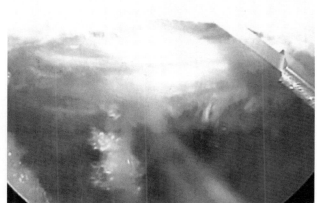

A   B

Figure 4-12 Arthroscopic view of the ITB. It is best visualized from the anterolateral portal with a 30° arthroscope **(A)**. Release of the band can be performed in patients with persistent external snapping hip through a proximal lateral accessory portal using a beaver blade knife **(B)**. See Color Plate.

identifying the intersection of the vertical line drawn from the anterior superior iliac spine distally and the horizontal line drawn from the superior surface of the femoral greater trochanter medially. This portal presents the greatest risk to the lateral femoral cutaneous nerve, which lies within several millimeters of the cannula. In addition, the lateral femoral circumflex artery and femoral neurovascular bundles must be protected (6). Care must be taken not to place this portal too anterior or deep, as this places the femoral neurovascular bundle at risk (5). The localization of the femoral pulse distal to the inguinal ligament helps prevent inadvertent injury to these structures.

Posterolateral Portal

The posterolateral portal is also described as the posterior paratrochanteric portal, as it is also referenced off of the greater trochanter. The entry site is 2 to 3 cm posterior to the tip of the greater trochanter at the same level as the anterolateral portal. Direct visualization of entry into the joint is possible with the scope in the anterolateral portal. The anterolateral and posterolateral portals should be established parallel to one another. The greatest risk with this portal is injury to the sciatic nerve, which lies approximately 3 cm away (5,35) Advancing the trocar with the femur in a neutral or slightly internally rotated position can protect the nerve, as this maneuver rotates the nerve away from posterior margin of the greater trochanter. This portal is used for visualization of the posterior aspect of the femoral head, posterior labrum, posterior capsule, and the inferior edge of the ischiofemoral ligament (6).

Proximal Lateral Accessory

The proximal lateral accessory portal is used for ITB releases. It is placed approximately 2 cm distal and in line with the anterolateral portal. The 30° arthroscope is placed in the anterolateral portal, and the accessory portal is established as a working portal for additional instruments required for

the release. The ITB can be clearly visualized through the anterolateral portal (Fig. 4-12A), and the release can be performed under direct visualization through the accessory portal (Fig. 4-12B).

Distal Lateral Accessory

The distal lateral accessory portal may be used for an osteoplasty performed in patients with decreased femoral head–neck junction offset (Fig. 4-13). It is placed at the midpoint between the anterior and anterolateral portals and approximately 4 cm distal. The portal typically enters the capsule at around the level of the zona orbicularis and allows for direct access to the anterior neck. This portal can be established under direct visualization with the 70° arthroscope placed in the anterior portal (Fig. 4-14).

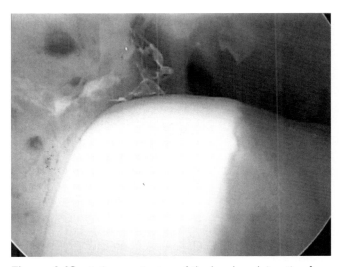

Figure 4-13 Arthroscopic view of the head–neck junction from the anterior portal. See Color Plate.

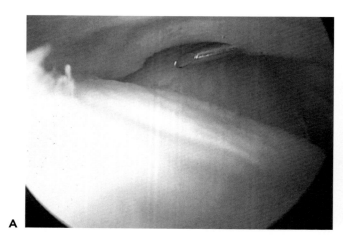
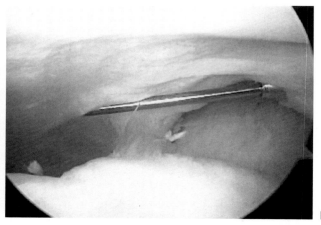

Figure 4-14 The distal lateral accessory portal is established under direct visualization. The entry point is at the level of the zona orbicularis and allows for direct access of the anterior femoral head–neck junction. See Color Plate.

SYSTEMATIC ARTHROSCOPIC EXAMINATION/NORMAL ANATOMY

We perform hip arthroscopy in the modified supine position in which the hip is placed in a position of 10° flexion, 15° internal rotation, 10° lateral tilt, and neutral abduction. However, the lateral position may also be used depending upon surgeon preference. In either case, distraction of the femoral head from the acetabulum must be performed to fully visualize the articular surfaces. A minimum of 8 to 10 mm of distraction is recommended to avoid any iatrogenic injury to the chondral surfaces or labrum. Adequate traction typically requires between 25 and 50 lb of force (4). Gentle countertraction is also applied to the contralateral limb. A thorough understanding of the anatomic relationships around the hip joint with special attention to neurovascular structures and tissue planes is of paramount importance. All of the intra-articular structures in the hip joint can be seen through the combined use of 70° and 30° arthroscopes, as well as the interchange of portals (20).

Once the traction is applied, the anterolateral portal is established under fluoroscopic guidance using the landmarks described above. Immediate visualization of the anterior triangle is established through this portal (Fig. 4-15). The anterior triangle represents the intra-articular portion of the lateral limb of the iliofemoral ligament. The anterior portal is established under direct visualization, as the spinal needle is directed between the lateral and medial limbs of the iliofemoral ligament (Fig. 4-16).

A systematic evaluation of the anterior structures of the joint can be performed with the arthroscope in the anterolateral portal. Starting anteromedially at the level of the psoas U (Fig. 4-10), the entire circumference of the labrum can be visualized (Fig. 4-17). The recess between the labrum and capsule can also be visualized in its entirety (Fig. 4-18). The anterior portion of the femoral head is completely inspected (Fig. 4-19), and this should include a complete evaluation of the fovea capitis (Fig. 4-8A). From this central position in the joint, the transverse acetabular ligament can be clearly seen (Fig. 4-8B),

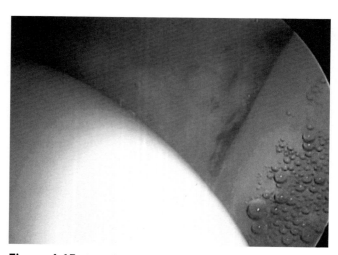

Figure 4-15 Visualization of the anterior triangle is achieved upon entry into the joint through the anterolateral portal. See Color Plate.

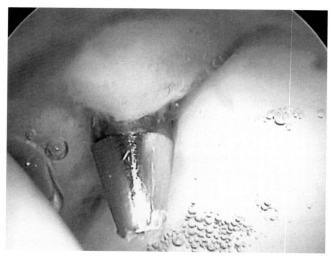

Figure 4-16 The anterior portal can be established under direct visualization from the anterolateral portal. The placement of the portal should be between the lateral and medial limbs of the iliofemoral ligament. See Color Plate.

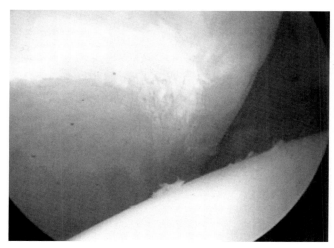

Figure 4-17 Nearly the entire circumference of the labrum can be visualized through the anterolateral portal. See Color Plate.

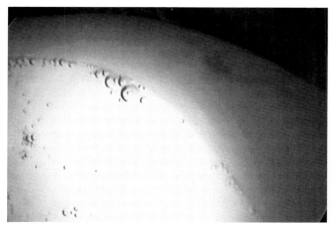

Figure 4-18 The recess between the labrum and the capsule can be clearly visualized through the anterolateral portal as well. See Color Plate.

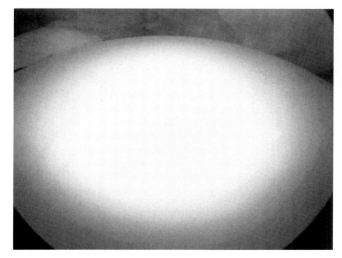

Figure 4-19 The anterior aspect of the femoral head should be inspected in its entirety to identify any chondral defects. See Color Plate.

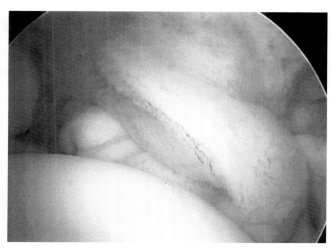

Figure 4-20 The ligamentum teres can be visualized by driving the arthroscope into the medial aspect of the joint. See Color Plate.

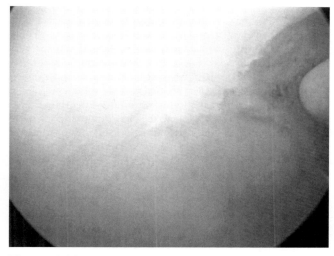

Figure 4-21 The medial aspect of the acetabulum can be viewed from the position in Figure 4.20 as well. See Color Plate.

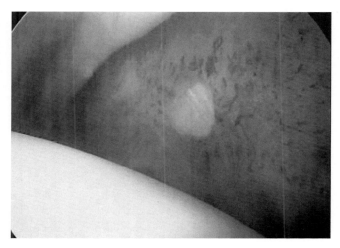

Figure 4-22 The location of the psoas tendon can be appreciated at the level of the psoas U and is found behind a thin veil of capsular tissue. See Color Plate.

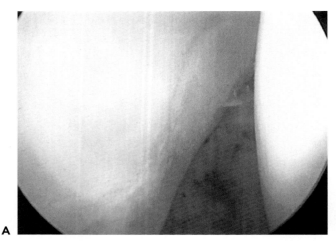
A

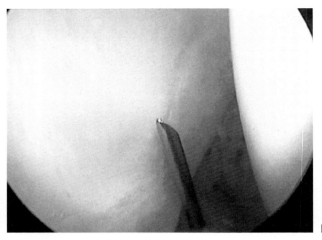
B

Figure 4-23   **A:** Complete view of the posterior labrum from the anterior portal. **B:** Direct visualization of needle entry into the posterior capsule. See Color Plate.

as well as the ligamentum teres (Fig. 4-20), the fat pad (Fig. 4-9), and the central aspect of the acetabulum (Fig. 4-21). The psoas tendon and/or bursae may be intra-articular in approximately 20% of people (Fig. 4-22); if it is extra-articular, the psoas tendon lies immediately medial to a thin veil of capsular tissue and can be easily palpated with a probe.

Once the inspection is complete from the anterolateral portal, the arthroscope is switched to the anterior portal for a more complete view of the posterior aspect of the joint. From this portal a more complete evaluation of the posterior labrum can be achieved (Fig. 4-23). The normal posterior sulcus of the labrum can be clearly seen from this vantage (Fig. 4-24). The posterior superior capsule can be inspected (Fig. 4-25). The posterior recess can be inspected for loose bodies; it is a common resting ground for any intra-articular debris. The posterior aspect of the femoral head can be more clearly evaluated with the arthroscope in this position (Fig. 4-26).

Once the intra-articular examination is complete, the scope is left in the anterior portal, and the traction is slowly released so that the head–neck junction can be evaluated. The anterior aspect of the hip may be adequately visualized with minimal traction. With hip flexion to 45° and external rotation to 30°, the anterior capsule becomes relatively patulous and can be distended with saline, making visualization of the head and neck relatively easy. As the traction is slowly released, an upward pressure must be maintained on the arthroscope to avoid articular cartilage injury. Once the traction is completely released, the arthroscope can be slid into the head–neck junction recess (Fig. 4-27). From this position, a clear view of the anterior femoral neck and the associated vincula (Fig. 4-28), and the normal labrum suction seal (Fig. 4-29) can be established. If any work needs to be performed in the head–neck junction recess, it is best accomplished through the distal lateral accessory portal described above (Fig. 4-14).

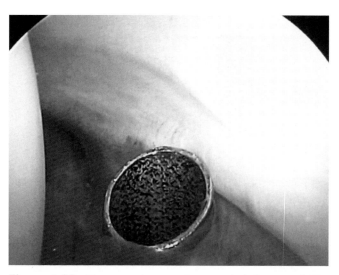

Figure 4-24   View of the normal posterior sulcus. This should not be misinterpreted as a labral tear. See Color Plate.

Figure 4-25   The posterior superior capsule is inspected. The location of the entry point for the anterolateral portal is evaluated from this view to confirm that the portal has not violated the labrum. See Color Plate.

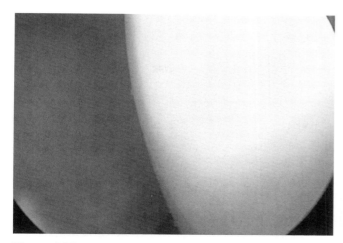

Figure 4-26 The posterior aspect of the femoral head should be completely evaluated to identify the presence of chondral lesions. See Color Plate.

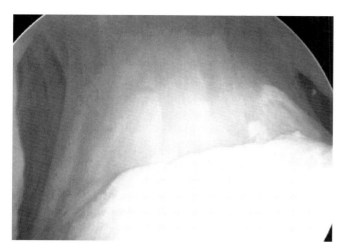

Figure 4-27 The head–neck junction recess is best visualized from the anterior portal with the traction released and the hip flexed to 45° and externally rotated. See Color Plate.

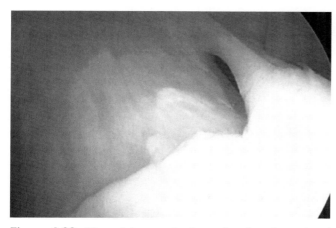

Figure 4-28 View of the anterior femoral neck and associated vincula. See Color Plate.

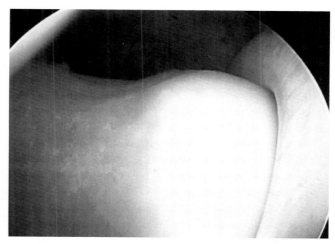

Figure 4-29 View of the normal suction seal of the labrum on the femoral head with the traction released. See Color Plate.

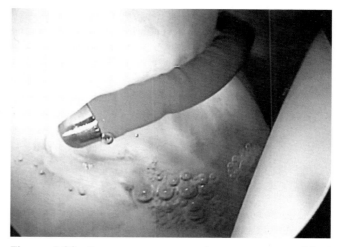

Figure 4-30 Common appearance of an anterosuperior labral tear. See Color Plate.

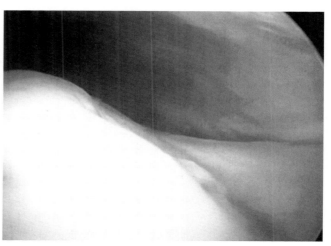

Figure 4-31 View of a large head–neck junction osteophyte resulting in femoroacetabular impingement. This has been previously described by Ganz as the CAM effect (1,22,34). See Color Plate.

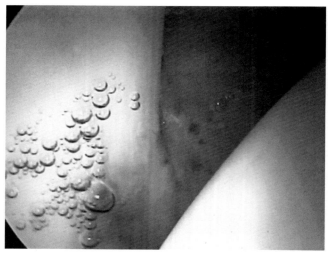

Figure 4-32 Labral bruising associated with excessive capsular laxity and pinching of the labrum between the anteriorly translated femoral head and acetabulum. See Color Plate.

If there is concern regarding pathology associated with the ITB, gluteus medius, or piriformis, a proximal lateral portal is established approximately 2 cm distal and in line with the anterolateral portal. A 30° arthroscope is placed in the antero-lateral portal, which allows for adequate visualization of the ITB (Fig. 4-12A). If the ITB is released, the arthroscope can be driven into the trochanteric bursae for evaluation and inspection of the gluteus medius and piriformis.

ARTHROSCOPIC PATHOLOGY/ ANATOMIC VARIANTS

A variety of common intra-articular soft tissue injuries are found during hip arthroscopy. One of the most common pathologic findings at the time of arthroscopy is the presence of an acetabular labrum tear (Fig. 4-30). Labral tears are

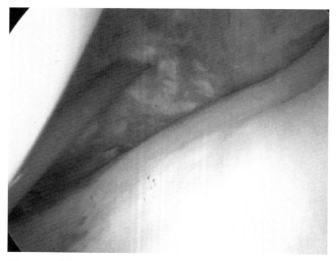

Figure 4-33 The hypoplastic labrum variant may be associated with loss of the normal suction seal and result in increased load across the capsular ligaments. See Color Plate.

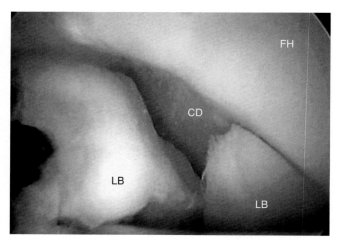

Figure 4-34 Chondral lesion to the femoral head. Image taken from the peripheral hip conpartment. FH, femoral head; LB, loose bodies; CD, Chondral defect. See Color Plate.

commonly associated with acetabular rim cartilage wear adjacent to the tear (26–28). The characteristics of these associated pathologies are clearly captured in the phrase "acetabular labrum articular disruption (ALAD)". Varying degrees of associated cartilage wear can be seen, ranging from softening of the adjacent cartilage (ALAD 1), to early peel back of the cartilage (ALAD 2), to a large flap of cartilage (ALAD 3), to complete loss of cartilage (ALAD 4). In our experience these types of lesions are oftentimes related to decreased offset at the femoral head–neck junction resulting in impingement of the femur against the anterior superior rim of the acetabulum, as has been previously described by Ganz (1,22,34) (Fig. 4-31).

Injury to the labrum may also result from joint hypermobility or associated capsular laxity. This condition results in abnormal loading of the anterior superior labrum. The most common arthroscopic finding in these patients is significant bruising of the labrum as it gets pinched by the anteriorly translated femoral head (Fig. 4-32). We have also noted in some symptomatic patients the presence of a hypoplastic labrum (Fig. 4-33). These patients do not have an adequate suction seal from the incompetent labrum, resulting in excessive loading on the capsular ligaments and the development of hip pain.

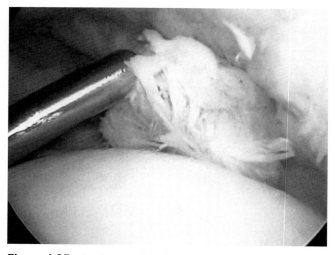

Figure 4-35 Partial tear of the ligamentum teres. See Color Plate.

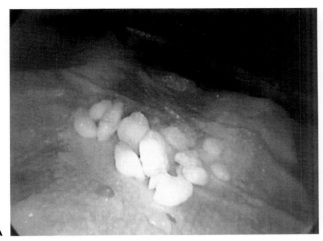
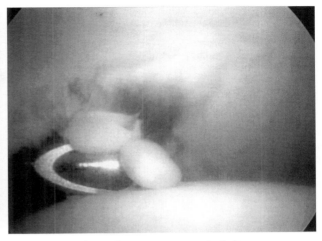

A   B

Figure 4-36   A: Complete exploration of the joint must be performed to assure removal of all fragments. **B:** Synovial chondromatosis results in numerous loose bodies. (From *Am J Sports Med.* 2003; 31, with permission.) See Color Plate.

Additional common intra-articular pathologic findings seen at the time of hip arthroscopy include chondral defects to the femoral head (Fig. 4-34); partial or complete tears of the ligamentum teres (Fig. 4-35); loose bodies or synovial chondromatosis (Fig. 4-36); and benign intra-articular tumors of the synovium, such as focal pigmented villonodular synovitis (PVNS).

CONCLUSION

The application of arthroscopic techniques to the hip joint for the minimally invasive management of intra-articular injuries is becoming increasingly more common within the orthopedic community. The recent advances in surgical techniques, advanced imaging modalities, and more versatile instrumentation have significantly improved the accessibility of the hip joint despite the numerous anatomic and technical constraints. Hip arthroscopy can now be performed safely and effectively as an outpatient procedure. A more thorough understanding of the normal, variant, and pathologic anatomy of this joint will further improve our ability to appropriately diagnose and treat these challenging intra-articular injuries.

REFERENCES

1. Beck M, Leunig M, Parvizi J, et al. Anterior femoroacetabular impingement: part II. Midterm results of surgical treatment. *Clin Orthop Relat Res.* 2004;418:67–73.
2. Bombelli R. *Structure and Function in Normal and Abnormal Hips.* New York: Springer-Verlag; 1993.
3. Burman M. Arthroscopy or the direct visualization of joints. *J Bone Joint Surg.* 1931;4:669–695.
4. Byrd JW. Hip arthroscopy. The supine position. *Clin Sports Med.* 2001;20:703–631.
5. Byrd JW, Pappas JN, Pedley MJ. Hip arthroscopy: an anatomic study of portal placement and relationship to the extra-articular structures. *Arthroscopy.* 1995;11:418–423
6. Dvorak M, Duncan CP, Day B. Arthroscopic anatomy of the hip. *Arthroscopy.* 1990;6:264–273
7. Edwards DJ, Lomas D, Villar RN. Diagnosis of the painful hip by magnetic resonance imaging and arthroscopy. *J Bone Joint Surg.* 1995;77B:374–376
8. Ferguson SJ, Bryant JT, Ganz R, et al. An in vitro investigation of the acetabular labral seal in hip joint mechanics. *J Biomech.* 2003;36:171–178.
9. Ferguson SJ, Bryant JT, Ganz R, et al. The acetabular labrum seal: a poroelastic finite element model. *Clin Biomech.* 2000;15:463–468
10. Ferguson SJ, Bryant JT, Ganz R, et al. The influence of the acetabular labrum on hip joint cartilage consolidation: a poroelastic finite element model. *J Biomech.* 2000;33:953–960.
11. Fitzgerald RH Jr. Acetabular labrum tears. Diagnosis and treatment. *Clin Orthop.* 1995;311:60–68.
12. Frich LH, Lauritzen J, Juhl M. Arthroscopy in diagnosis and treatment of hip disorders. *Orthopedics.* 1989;12:389–392.
13. Gondolph-Zink B. Current status of diagnostic and surgical hip arthroscopy. *Orthopade.* 1992;21:249–256.
14. Gross R. Arthroscopy in hip disorders in children. *Orthop Rev.* 1977;6:43–49.
15. Hawkins RB. Arthroscopy of the hip. *Clin Orthop.* 1989;249:44–47.
16. Ikeda T, Awaya G, Suzuki S, et al. Torn acetabular labrum in young patients. Arthroscopic diagnosis and management. *J Bone Joint Surg.* 1988;70B:13–16.
17. Janssens X, Van Meirhaeghe J, Verdonk R, et al. Diagnostic arthroscopy of the hip joint in pigmented villonodular synovitis. *Arthroscopy.* 1987;3:283–287.
18. Keene GS, Villar RN. Arthroscopic anatomy of the hip: an in vivo study. *Arthroscopy.* 1994;10:392–399.
19. Kelly BT, Shapiro GS, Digiovanni CW, et al. The vascularity of the hip labrum: a cadaveric investigation. *Arthroscopy.* 2005;21:3–11.
20. Kelly BT, Williams RJ 3rd, Philippon MJ. Hip arthroscopy: current indications, treatment options, and management issues. *Am J Sports Med.* 2003; 31:1020–1037.
21. Kim YT, Azusa H. The nerve endings of the acetabular labrum. *Clin Orthop.* 1995;310:60–68.
22. Lavigne M, Parvizi J, Beck M, et al. Anterior femoroacetabular impingement: part I. Techniques of joint preserving surgery. *Clin Orthop.* 2004;418:61–66.
23. Lephart S, Philippon MJ, Draovitch P. Golf injury prevention research models. Presented at: World Scientific Congress of Golf; 2002; St. Andrews, Scotland.
24. McCarthy JC, Busconi B. The role of hip arthroscopy in the diagnosis and treatment of hip disease. *Orthopedics.* 1995;18:753–756.
25. McCarthy JC, Lee JA. The role of hip arthroscopy: useful adjunct or devil's tool? *Orthopedics.* 2002;25:947–948.

26. McCarthy JC, Noble PC, Schuck MR, et al. The Otto E. Aufranc Award: the role of labral lesions to development of early degenerative hip disease. *Clin Orthop.* 2001;393:25–37.
27. McCarthy JC, Noble PC, Schuck MR, et al. The watershed labral lesion: its relationship to early arthritis of the hip. *J Arthroplasty.* 2001;16:81–87.
28. McCarthy JC, Wright J, Noble P, et al. The prevalence of lesions of the acetabular labrum and their association with articular cartilage pathology. (An arthroscopic analysis with cadaveric and vascular correlations). Presented at: American Academy of Orthopaedic Surgeons Annual Meeting; 2001; San Francisco.
29. Okada Y, Awaya G, Ikeda T, et al. Arthroscopic surgery for synovial chondromatosis of the hip. *J Bone Joint Surg.* 1989;71B:198–199.
30. O'Leary JA, Berend K, Vail TP. The relationship between diagnosis and outcome in arthroscopy of the hip. *Arthroscopy.* 2001;17:181–188.
31. Philippon MJ. Arthroscopy of the hip in the management of the athlete. In: *Operative Arthroscopy.* Philadelphia: Lippincott Williams & Wilkins; 2003:879–883.
32. Philippon MJ. The role of arthroscopic thermal capsulorrhaphy in the hip. *Clin Sports Med.* 2001;20:817–829.
33. Rao J, Zhou YX, Villar RN. Injury to the ligamentum teres. Mechanism, findings, and results of treatment. *Clin Sports Med.* 2001;20:791–799.
34. Siebenrock KA, Wahab KH, Werlen S, et al. Abnormal extension of the femoral head epiphysis as a cause of cam impingement. *Clin Orthop.* 2004;54–60.
35. Sweeney HJ. Arthroscopy of the hip. Anatomy and portals. *Clin Sports Med.* 2001;20:697–702.
36. Takechi H, Nagashima H, Ito S. Intra-articular pressure of the hip joint outside and inside the limbus. *J Jpn Orthop Assoc.* 1982;56:529–536.

Biomechanics of the Hip

5

James D. Johnston   *Philip C. Noble*   *Debra E. Hurwitz*   *Thomas P. Andriacchi*

An understanding of the biomechanics of the hip is vital to advancing the diagnosis and treatment of many pathologic conditions. Some areas that have benefited from advances in hip biomechanics include the evaluation of joint function, the development of therapeutic programs for treatment of joint problems, procedures for planning reconstructive surgeries, and the design and development of total hip prostheses. Biomechanical principles also provide a valuable perspective to our understanding of the mechanism of injury to the hip and the contributions of the capsule, labrum, and femoroacetabular impingement (FAI) to the etiology of degenerative hip disease.

The biomechanics of hip function may be described through reference to the kinematics or the kinetics of the hip joint or its prosthetic replacement. Joint kinematics is the description of the angular or translational motion of the joint in response to applied forces; kinetics refers to the forces and moments acting on the joint during motion, whether they arise from muscle activity, inertia, ligamentous restraints, or contact between the femur and pelvis and adjacent structures. Different approaches have been applied to study hip biomechanics. The kinematics of the joint may be quantified using motion analysis, especially in conjunction with analytical models of the musculoskeletal system. On the other hand, joint forces may be estimated from data derived from gait and force platform measurements, in combination with analytical models simulating the force of contraction and line of action of each of the hip muscles.

THE BIOMECHANICS OF INJURIES TO THE HIP JOINT

The Mechanical Role of the Soft Tissues of the Hip

Over the last decade, there has been increasing interest in the diagnosis and treatment of acute injuries of the hip joint, particularly those involving the labrum and the articular surfaces. This interest has arisen from the recognition that many events in the pathomechanics of degenerative joint disease occur early, and that soft tissue disruption is probably involved more frequently than had been recognized previously. In addition, advances in hip arthroscopy have allowed clinicians to examine the articular surfaces of the hip joint in patients with debilitating symptoms despite a normal radiographic appearance. In these patients, a frequent finding has been labral pathology, most commonly chondrolabral separation in the anterior aspect of the joint, with a disturbing prevalence of full-thickness articular lesions, often in communication with chondrolabral defects (53).

Given the significance of periarticular structures in the pathomechanics of hip disease, it is instructive to review the basic anatomy of the passive stabilizers of the hip joint, including the capsular ligaments and the acetabular labrum. The hip capsule (capsular ligament) is critical to the stability and proper function of the hip joint (78) and serves as a "check rein" preventing dislocation at the extremes of motion (38,46). This ligament is actually a complex structure consisting of three discrete ligaments: (a) the anteriorly located iliofemoral ligament, which restricts extension of the joint and limits internal rotation, (b) the femoral arcuate ligament, which limits abduction and external rotation and is also anteriorly located, and (c) the posteriorly located ischiofemoral ligament, which limits internal rotation and adduction when the hip is flexed (27,46). Mechanical testing of these ligaments has shown that the posterior ligament is much weaker than its anterior counterparts (37,78), which may explain why posterior dislocation occurs so much more frequently than anterior dislocation (62).

The acetabular labrum is a relatively stiff fibrocartilaginous tissue that forms an extension of the acetabular rim (25). The labrum increases the effective depth of the socket and the coverage of the femoral head and, so, has the potential to enhance the mechanical stability of the hip joint. Although the load-bearing function of the labrum was questioned by Konrath et al. (49), recent experimental studies have demonstrated that, due to its low permeability, the labrum acts as a seal, preventing fluid from flowing in and out of the intra-articular space (24,80). This increases the stability of the joint, as the seal must be broken to dislodge the femoral head from the acetabulum. Moreover the presence of the labrum elevates the intra-articular pressure during weight bearing, which is expected to enhance joint lubrication and minimize friction (23,24). Additionally, the removal of the labrum has been shown to increase strains within the cartilage matrix during weight bearing (23,24).

Clinical evidence has shown that labrum removal or pathology is closely linked to joint changes consistent with early osteoarthritis and joint disease (21,35,52–54), with the relative risk of significant cartilage erosion doubling in the presence of labral tears (53). It is hypothesized that a labral tear (occurring predominately anteriorly) disrupts the stability of the hip, especially at the extremes of joint motion. This leads to abnormal sliding of the articular surfaces under the dynamic torsional conditions often associated with sporting activities involving strenuous repetitive twisting and pivoting motions (such as ballet, football, soccer, basketball, and placekicking) (53). These motions accelerate degenerative changes and the progression of chondral involvement with time, leading to joint disease (44,53).

The Role of Mechanical Factors in the Etiology of Coxarthrosis

Osteoarthrosis is a disease involving the symptomatic loss of articular cartilage in a normal load-bearing area of a joint and is frequently associated with subchondral sclerosis and osteophyte formation (67). It is generally thought that the primary etiology is mechanical. Different authors have implicated excessive impulsive loading of the articular surface, leading to acute cartilage injury (64,68) and/or accumulated microtrauma of cartilage and subchondral bone in response to repetitive impulse loads (68). Articular cartilage is a viscoelastic material; its interstitial fluid component contributes to its bulk mechanical properties. When cartilage is loaded rapidly, the fluid does not have time to flow, resulting in increased tissue stiffness and high internal stresses (68). As the mechanical response of articular cartilage is mediated by both the permeability and the elastic modulus of the tissue, the pathologic response of joints to load bearing is highly dependent upon loading rate, in addition to load magnitude (68).

Previous experimental studies have demonstrated that osteoarthritic changes in weight-bearing joints occur in direct response to repetitive loading above threshold levels (69). An interesting study by Hadley et al. (33) showed that, provided

that mean pressures at the articular surface are kept below 2 MPa, articular cartilage is capable of tolerating repetitive loads almost indefinitely. Once pressures rose above 2 MPa, due to reduced or incomplete head coverage, degenerative changes were observed, depending upon the duration of exposure. Unsatisfactory outcomes were observed in 90% of the patients exposed to >10 MPa-yrs of articular loading, while in 81% of hips experiencing <10 MPa-yrs, satisfactory outcomes were observed.

Although joint loading or overloading can lead to cartilage degeneration, the precise mechanism remains controversial. Opinions differ concerning the relative contributions of direct mechanical trauma to articular cartilage versus elevation of articular stresses secondary to stiffening of the subchondral plate. Certainly, finite element studies have shown that localized increases in subchondral stiffness can lead to marked elevations of stresses in the overlying cartilage (12). However, there are no studies that allow us to directly separate the contributions of hydrostatic (i.e., direct compressive) and deviatoric (i.e., shearing) stresses generated by joint loading. Consequently, it is not known whether degenerative changes are primarily due to excessive loads applied during normal activities, or shearing of the cartilage during abnormal motions involving local instability. It is known that individuals performing heavy lifting or participating in elite sporting activities are at greater risk of osteoarthritis (39). It is hypothesized that acute injuries from trauma experienced during athletic activities, in addition to the strenuous twisting and pivoting motions, leads to recurrent microtrauma and eventual cartilage deterioration.

Femoro-Acetabular Impingement (FAI)

Clinical implications of Femoro-Acetabular Impingement (FAI) include acute hip pain (22,48), loss of motion (66), and chronic leveraging of the head in the acetabulum, possibly resulting in labral, cartilage, and chondral injury (51,66). Repeated contact between the femoral head–neck junction and the labrum can lead to progressive cartilage damage and labral tearing (22,45), thus influencing mechanical stability and the weight-bearing role of the joint (24,53). This in turn would accelerate degenerative changes and possibly lead to joint diseases such as osteoarthritis (44,54). The pathomechanics of FAI have been elucidated by Ganz and coworkers in many published studies. Impingement between the femoral neck and the acetabular rim results from reduced joint clearance (30,45,61) and possibly from forced articulation beyond the mechanical limits of joint motion (54). Joint clearance is compromised in the presence of abnormal morphologies of the acetabulum and/or proximal femur, including widening of the femoral neck, reduction in the head–neck offset, and overcoverage of the acetabulum, all of which reduce joint clearance, increasing the probability of impingement (30,45,58,61,66,84). Additional proximal femoral morphologies that potentiate impingement include abnormal head/neck configurations (e.g., a pistol-grip deformity) (57,66,75,81), reduction in femoral anteversion (45,81), reduced concavity at the femoral head–neck junction (61), subclinical displacement of the femoral epiphysis (head tilt or post slip) (31,45,57,66,75), malpositioned proximal fragments after neck fracture (22), and residual effects from childhood diseases such as Legg–Calvé–Perthes (30). On the acetabular side, the risk of impingement increases with acetabular retroversion, which results in a prominent anterolateral overcoverage, creating an obstacle for flexion and internal rotation (30). Other predisposing conditions are deepening of the acetabular socket (coxa profunda and protrusio acetabuli) and some posttraumatic deformities (30,48,73).

Two distinctive types of FAI have been recognized (Fig. 5-1). The first type is due to linear contact between the acetabular rim and the femoral head–neck junction, thus limiting range of motion (66). The first structure to fail is often the labrum, with continued impact resulting in deterioration of the labrum and ganglion formation, or ossification of the rim leading to additional acetabular deepening and over coverage. This type of impingement is seen more frequently in middle-aged women who participate in athletic activities involving hip motion (30,51). The second type or "cam" FAI is due to an abnormal femoral head with increasing radius in the anterolateral region (22,45,61). Motion of the abnormal head in the acetabulum results in high shear forces, producing abrasion of the acetabular cartilage and/or its avulsion from the labrum and the subchondral bone, often leading to tearing or detachment of the labrum. This type of impingement is most common in young and athletic males (30,51).

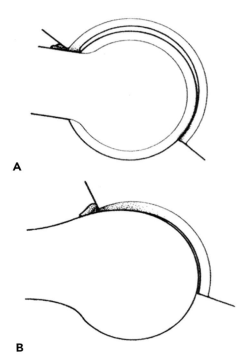

Figure 5-1 Mechanism of impingement caused by **(A)** direct linear contact between the labrum–acetabular rim and the head–neck junction, or **(B)** an increased head radius abutting against the acetabular rim (cam). (From Beck M, Leunig M, Parvizi J, et al. Anterior femoroacetabular impingement: part II. Midterm results of surgical treatment. *Clin Orthop.* 2004;418:67–73.)

FORCES TRANSMITTED BY THE HIP JOINT

In Vivo Measurements of Forces at the Hip Joint

The long-term integrity of both the normal and prosthetic hip is strongly influenced by the direction and magnitude of the force developed between the femoral head and the acetabulum during daily activities. As there is no method of directly measuring forces acting on the normal hip joint, the only in vivo measurements of forces or pressures at the joint surface have been provide by prostheses and endoprostheses instrumented with transducers (strain gauges) (Table 5-1). The earliest experiments utilizing a strain-gauged prosthesis were performed by Rydell, who measured peak forces of 3 body weights (BW) during gait (70). More extensive studies have been recently conducted by Bergmann et al. (3–6), who recorded peak forces that varied from 2.1 to 4.3 BW during gait (3,5,6), 2.3 to 5.5 BW during stair-climbing (3,6), to greater than 8 BW during accidental incidents of stumbling (4,5).

The magnitude of the peak resultant force generated during gait can vary from 1.6 to 4.3 BW (Table 5-1) and is affected by numerous factors, especially stride length and the speed of ambulation. During the stance phase of gait, the orientation of the load in the frontal plane is relatively constant and directed medially and inferiorly, while in the sagittal plane the orientation is more variable and is toward the posterior during the first part of the stance phase and anterior during the later part of the stance phase (Fig. 5-2). Analysis of data from several investigators indicates that the lateral, posterior, and inferior peak components during gait range from 0.4 to 1.7 BW, 0.2 to 1.0 BW, and 1.4 to 4.1 BW (3,5,6,16,70). In some cases, the determination of these force components was based on estimated anteversion angles and varus/valgus stem angles (4).

The magnitudes of the out-of-plane loads during daily activities can be substantial, with the anterior–posterior component of the hip reaction force reaching 20% to 25% of the force in the frontal plane during stair-climbing (6). In vivo force transducer data demonstrate that, during climbing up stairs, the torques generated about the implant longitudinal axis are 23% greater than in normal walking. Conversely, the axial torques recorded during walking and descending stairs were of similar magnitude (3,6). Moreover, the peak contact force and resulting torsional moment, and the posteriorly directed force component increase with walking speed. Out-of-plane loads, and the torques they generate about the femoral axis, are also affected by the anteversion angle (5). The largest torsional moments measured in vivo during activities of daily living reach the average experimental strength of implant fixation (33.1 N m), as determined from in vitro tests (65) (Fig. 5-3). Consequently, the moments generated during stair-climbing may be detrimental to the stability of implant fixation, especially in uncemented stems (8,28,34,65).

Contact pressures from a Moore-type endoprosthesis have been studied during numerous activities including walking, jogging, stair-climbing, and chair-rising (40,41,50,79). Peak pressures during gait occur between heel strike and early midstance and relate to increases in both ground reaction forces and

TABLE 5-1

HIP CONTACT FORCES MEASURED IN VIVO IN PATIENTS WITH INSTRUMENTED IMPLANTS

Activity	Typical Peak Force (BW)	Total Number of Patients	Time Since Surgery (Months)	References
Walking, slow	1.6–4.1	9	1–30	(3,5,6,70)
Walking, normal	2.1–3.3	6	1–31	(3)
Walking, fast	1.8–4.3	7	2–30	(3,5,6,70)
Jogging/running	4.3–5.0	2	6–30	(5,6)
Ascending stairs	1.5–5.5	8	6–33	(3,6,70)
Descending stairs	1.6–5.1	7	6–30	(3,6,70)
Standing up	1.8–2.2	4	11–31	(3)
Sitting down	1.5–2.0	4	11–31	(3)
Standing/2-1-2 legs	2.2–3.7	3	11–14	(3)
Knee bend	1.2–1.8	3	11–14	(3)
Stumbling	7.2–8.7	2	4–18	(4,5)

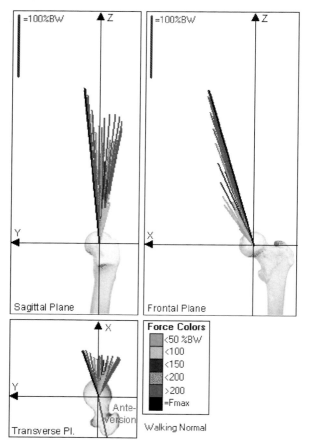

Figure 5-2 Force vectors and points of load transfer on the prosthetic head during level walking for a patient. Positive x is directed medially, positive y is in the direction of progression (anterior), and positive z is superior. (From Bergmann G, ed. *HIP98: Loading of the Hip Joint.* Berlin: Free University of Berlin; 2001, with permission. Compact disc, ISBN 3980784800.) See Color Plate.

abductor muscle activity. During gait, the maximum pressures (mean: 5.6 MPa) occur on the superior anterior femoral surface, which corresponds to the superior acetabular dome (79). Chair-rising triples pressures up to 9 to 15 MPa on the apex of the femoral head or superior posterior aspects of the acetabulum. The sites of high acetabular pressure on the superior posterior region of the acetabulum correspond to sites of frequent degenerative changes observed in cadaver specimens (40).

Although it is tempting to extrapolate data from instrumented prostheses to the physiology of the normal hip, some limitations of these experimental studies must be remembered. Firstly, because of their complexity, studies performed using instrumented prostheses have been limited to one or two subjects at most institutions. Early studies were frequently limited by equipment failure so that data were only collected during the early postoperative period, when the acute effect of surgical trauma may still have played a role. In some instances, assistive devices were routinely used for ambulation or subjects walked extremely slowly. Nonetheless, the consistency of peak loads measured by several different institutions seems to indicate that stems with similar features experience similar peak forces. In many instances, differences between the measured forces can be attributed to variations in the hip position during gait. For example, alterations in anteversion have a large effect on the out-of-plane loads in the transverse plane.

Analytical Estimates of Forces at the Hip Joint

Basic analytical approaches to the balance of forces and moments about the hip joint can be useful in estimating the effects of alterations in joint anatomy or different treatment modalities on the hip joint reaction force. The static loading of the hip joint has been frequently approximated with a simplified, two-dimensional analysis performed in the frontal (coronal) plane (Fig. 5-4). Several authors have used this

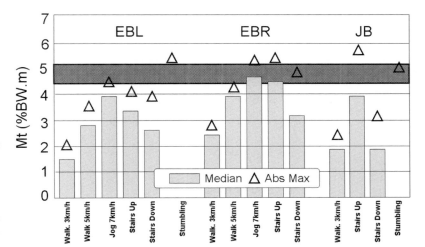

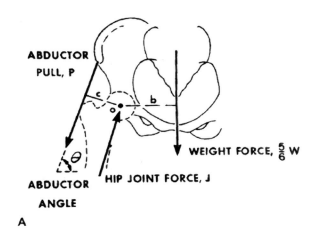

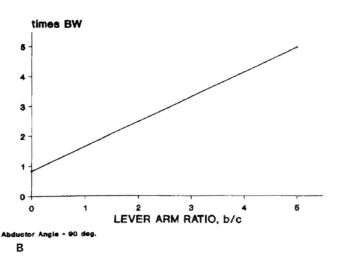

Figure 5-3 Torsional moments in the transverse plane: gray bar indicates fixation strength of cementless implants. (From Phillips TW, Nguyen LT, Munro SD. Loosening of cementless femoral stems: a biomechanical analysis of immediate fixation with loading vertical, femur horizontal. *J Biomech.* 1991;24:37–48, with permission. Bergmann G, Graichen F, Rohlmann A. Is staircase walking a risk for the fixation of hip implants? *J Biomech.* 1995;28:535–553, with permission.)

Figure 5-4 **(A)** Joint reaction force acting across the left hip during one-legged stance. **(B)** Variation of the Joint Reaction Force with changes in the ratio of the lever arms, band c. (From Greenwald AS. Biomechanics of the hip. In: Steinberg M, ed. *The Hip and Its Disorders.* Philadelphia: WB Saunders; 1991:49, with permission.)

approach to model the static forces during one-legged stance, both with and without a cane (13,26,59,60). In this analysis, it is assumed that the body is at rest, and that only the abductors are active. Thus, for equilibrium at the hip, the force of contraction of the abductors must generate a moment of equal magnitude, but opposite direction, to that produced by the weight of the body supported by the lower extremity, often called the effective body weight, acting on the head of the femur. During one-legged stance, the weight of the supporting extremity is distal to the hip joint and so does not contribute to the weight that must be supported. Thus the effective body weight is generally assumed to be five sixths that of the total weight of the body. The effective body weight acts vertically, in the direction of gravity, while the abductor muscle force has both a horizontal and a vertical component and is generally assumed to be oriented at 30° with respect to a vertical axis. Using this type of analysis, joint forces for one-legged stance of 2.75 BW (26) and 3.00 BW (60) have been calculated.

When estimates of hip mechanics are needed for dynamic activities, analytical approaches can be useful, as they are noninvasive and easily applied to a large number of patients. To calculate the forces and moments acting across the hip joint, several quantities must be measured or estimated, including the reaction forces developed between the ground and the foot (and any support devices) (Fig. 5-5), the inertial properties of moving limb segments, and the three-dimensional position of the joint centers during dynamic activities. Limb motions are measured with various types of optoelectronic methods, while the foot–ground reaction forces are measured using a force plate.

Once the net forces and moments acting across the hip have been calculated, it is possible to estimate the contributions of muscle contraction, passive soft tissue stretch, and articular reaction forces in a manner similar to that for the two-dimensional case, as described above. However, because so many muscles contribute to the joint reaction force, it is not possible to directly calculate the contribution of each of these components. Numerous authors have proposed methods of predicting the force of contraction of each muscle, based upon

TABLE 5-2
ANALYTICAL METHODS OF ESTIMATING PEAK HIP CONTACT FORCE

Activity	Magnitude (BW)	Method	Reference
Statically determinate methods			
Walking	4.2 after heel strike 4.8 before toe off	Reduction method	(63)
Stair-ascending Stair-descending	7.2 7.1	Reduction method	(63)
Statically indeterminate methods			
Walking slow with cane	2.2	Optimization:	(10)
Walking slow without cane	3.4	maximize	
Walking	5.0	endurance	(15)
Stair-climbing	7.4		
Chair-rising	3.3		
Walking	5.5	Quasi static: minimize muscle forces	(72)

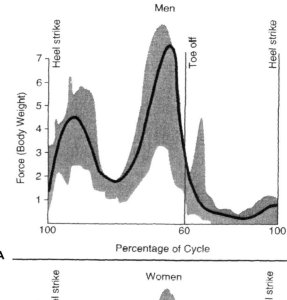

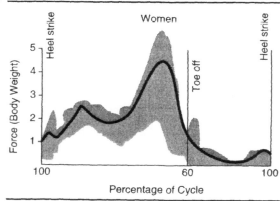

Figure 5-5   Hip joint reaction force during walking: shaded area represents subject variability. **A:** Normal men. **B:** Normal women. (Adapted from Paul JP. *Forces at the Human Hip Joint* [doctoral thesis]. Chicago: University of Chicago; 1967, with permission.)

electromyographic measurements and mechanical models of each muscle. Others have predicted the distribution of contraction force between muscles corresponding to the minimum value of force per cross-sectional area of each muscle, and other optimization criteria. These methods have been applied to estimate muscle forces and contact forces on the basis of externally measured forces during the activities of gait, stair-climbing, and chair-rising (Table 5-2) (10,15,63,72). A shortcoming of all of these methods is the fact that they are unable to account for the effect of cocontraction of muscles acting on opposite sides of the joint or the effect of capsular stiffness. These factors can be significant at the extremes of joint motion and in activities where the hip capsule contributed to joint stability. Studies involving both analytical estimates and in vivo load measurements have shown promising comparisons: Heller et al. (36) showed mean peak force differences of 12% during walking and 14% during stair-climbing, and Stansfield et al. (76) demonstrated load differences of approximately 16% during activities such as walking and sit-to-stand. A recent parametric model (Hurwitz et al., 2003) estimates the potential range in contact forces resulting from physiologically feasible muscle force distributions and thus allows for muscle co-contraction while not requiring an optimization criterion. For a representative subject, the peak contact force for a representative subject varied from 2.7 to 3.2 Body weights in the absence of antagonistic activity and increased approximately 0.2 Body weights for every 10% increase in antagonistic activity.

CLINICAL APPLICATIONS OF HIP BIOMECHANICS

The Impact of Walking Aids on the Hip Joint Force

Both analytical and in vivo studies have clearly shown that walking with a cane in the contralateral hand reduces the force acting across the hip joint (10,16). This is evident from the two-dimensional static analysis discussed earlier. The moment produced from both the cane and abductor muscles together produce a moment equal and opposite to that produced by the effective body weight. The two-dimensional static analysis indicates that the joint reaction force can be reduced by 50% (from 3.3 BW to 1.7 BW) when approximately 15% BW is applied to the cane (13). The substantial reduction in the joint reaction force, predicted when a cane is used for support, arises because the cane–ground reaction force acts at a much larger distance from the center of the hip than the abductor muscles. Thus, even when a relatively small load is applied to the cane, the contribution it makes to the moment opposing body weight is large enough to lead to significantly decrease the demand placed on the abductor muscles. Using the kinematics and kinetics of preoperative total hip replacement (THR) patients who routinely walked either with or without a cane, the three-dimensional analytical optimization models showed that those who walked with a cane had a contact force of only 2.2 BW—65% of those who walked without a cane (3.4 BW) (Table 5-2) (10).

The Effect of Hip Joint Geometry on the Forces at the Hip Joint

Alterations in joint anatomy, whether due to surgical intervention or a disease process, can dramatically affect the force acting across the joint and the stresses developed within the articular surfaces. These changes occur through alterations to the moment arms of the hip muscles and the area of contact between the femur and the acetabulum. A decreased head–neck angle (varus hip) increases the mechanical advantage of the abductors (Fig. 5-6). For a given neck length, joint contact forces decrease as the neck–shaft angle is reduced (i.e., as the neck becomes more horizontal) because of the corresponding increase in medial head offset (47). Lower neck–shaft angles also improve joint stability through increased coverage of the femoral head by the acetabulum. In addition, the mechanical advantage of the abductors may be increased by moving the greater trochanter laterally, and deepening the acetabulum. Clinically, increased abductor–adductor strength has been associated with increased neck length and a more distal position of the greater trochanter with respect to the joint center (32).

The length and inclination of the femoral neck also influence the bending moments generated within the proximal femur. A varus hip and an increase in neck length will both

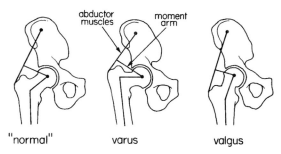

Figure 5-6 The abductor mechanism changes with head–neck angle or neck length. A valgus neck angle decreases the moment arm, while a varus neck angle or an increased neck length increases the moment arm. (Art by Judy Weik.)

increase the bending moment within the proximal femur by increasing the moment arm of the joint reaction force. After hip replacement, these bending moments will generate stresses within both the femoral stem and its interfaces, which, if excessive, can lead to loosening. Conversely, a shorter or more vertically inclined (valgus) femoral neck reduces the bending moment in the stem. However, the reduction in head offset means that larger abductor forces are needed to balance the weight of the body, leading to an increase in the joint reaction force. In practice, this leads to a significant increase in the wear rate of the artificial joint and a greater incidence of implant failure secondary to wear and osteolysis.

Previous investigators have developed mathematical models to calculate the effect of changes in the anatomic position of the hip center on the moment generating capacity of muscles crossing the joint (17,18,47). These analyses predict that the joint reaction force will be minimized when the joint center is moved medially, inferiorly, and anteriorly (Table 5-3). This position maximizes the moment generating capacity of the abductors and brings the joint center closer to the line of action of the foot–floor reaction force, thereby reducing the external moment that must be balanced by the muscle forces acting at the hip (18,47). This analysis also predicts that superior displacement of the hip center will reduce the moment generating capacity of the abductors, adductors, flexors, and extensors due to alterations in the resting lengths and moment arm of each muscle (18). Increasing the length of the neck of the prosthesis or advancing the greater trochanter partially compensates for these losses in muscle moment generating capacities (17). An increase in the hip joint forces with a

TABLE 5-3
THE EFFECT OF A 2-CM DISPLACEMENT IN THE HIP CENTER POSITION ON THE MOMENT GENERATING CAPACITY OF THE MUSCLES

	Superior	Inferior	Anterior	Posterior	Lateral	Medial
Abductors	−49%	26%	2%	1%	−3%	−8%
Adductors	−18%	11%	2%	0%	40%	−40%
Extensors	−7%	0%	36%	−36%	2%	−2%
Flexors	−22%	12%	−34%	22%	−3%	−3%

From Doehring TC, Rubash HE, Shelley FJ, et al. Effect of superior and superolateral relocations of the hip center on hip joint forces: an experimental and analytical analysis. *J Arthroplasty*, 1996;11:693–703, with permission.

superolateral joint center has also been identified using an experimental setup in which a loading fixture simulated the hip abductors, adductors, and extensors during one-legged stance and stair-climbing. In this experimental setup, purely superior displacement of the joint center did not substantially increase the hip joint force (20). The clinical application of these theoretical and experimental simulations assume that alterations in joint and femoral geometry do not alter the manner in which subjects perform the activities being simulated, and that antagonistic muscle contractions are not significant.

In general, the analytical and experimental results on the effect of joint geometry on hip joint forces are consistent with clinical studies performed on patients after THR. In these studies inferior functional outcomes have been associated with superior displacement of the joint center (9) and have associated decreases in abductor strength and loss of passive hip flexion motion with superior movements of the joint centers unless the superior movements are compensated for with increased neck length (32). In addition, higher rates of femoral loosening have been associated with neck lengthening (19) and superior and lateral displacement of the joint center with respect to the anatomical position (19,85), while increased wear of polyethylene cups has been correlated with a reduction in the medial offset of the femoral head and the abductor moment arm (71).

Gait and Functional Adaptations

Individuals with degenerative or artificial joints often alter how they accomplish activities of daily living. This change in function can be considered an adaptation to a stimulus such as pain, muscle weakness, or instability. For example, during the single-support phase of gait, the contraction of the abductors prevents the contralateral side of the pelvis from dropping as the weight of the swinging leg and upper body are supported by the weight-bearing extremity. If the abductors are compromised by reductions in either muscle strength or the length of the abductor moment arm, subjects may adopt a Trendelenburg gait pattern to lessen the demand on the hip abductor muscles.

Candidates for hip replacement typically display slower walking speeds with decreased cadence and shortened step length (56). Some of the reported abnormalities of the arthritic gait pattern may be a direct consequence of the reduction in walking speed (1,2). The customary increase in the duration of stance phase on the unaffected side corresponds to an increase in swing time on the affected side, which may be needed to bring the painful hip through its arc of motion (7). Decreased step lengths on the affected side occur from both a loss of hip extension during late stance phase, as well as a decrease in maximum knee flexion during swing phase and ankle extension at toe off (56).

Preoperatively, THR patients commonly demonstrate a loss of hip motion in flexion–extension and hesitation or reversal of motion as the hip goes into extension during stance phase (42,43,56,82). This hesitation or reversal of hip motion occurs in the presence of a flexion contracture and may be reflective of compensation for a lack of hip extension through increased lumbar lordosis. It may also serve as a pain avoidance mechanism by decreasing the hip joint force (56). In the coronal plane, subjects rotate the trunk laterally over the affected hip, increasing joint stability, while also reducing the demand on the abductors and the force on the hip joint. In the transverse plane, increased external rotation at heel strike may further increase lateral stability (82).

For the vast majority of patients, hip replacement eliminates pain and restores hip function; however, despite these achievements, normal function in performing activities of daily living is not always completely achieved (11,57,74). In general, following THR, gait velocity increases due to improved cadence, step length, and hip motion. Stance times become more symmetric with reductions in lateral lurching. Postoperatively, hip motion in the sagittal plane increases but is still less than normal (42,55,77,83). This decrease in hip motion may minimize the anterior and posterior components of the hip joint force, increasing implant stability by reducing the rotational moments about the implant stem (20).

Clinical experience suggests that a valgus stem position provides better function than a varus stem position, with fewer gait abnormalities (1,14,29,40). This may be indicative of biomechanical adaptation of gait in response to the increased bending moments or the increased implant micromotion associated with loading of varus stems.

REFERENCES

1. Andriacchi TP, Galante JO, Belytschko TB, et al. A stress analysis of the femoral stem in total hip prostheses. J Bone Joint Surg Am. 1976;58:618–624.
2. Andriacchi TP, Strickland AB. Lower limb kinetics applied to the study of normal and abnormal walking. In: Berme N, Engin AE, Correia Da Silva KM, eds. Biomechanics of Normal and Pathological Human Articulating Joints. Dordrecht: Martinus Nijhoff; 1985: 83–102.
3. Bergmann G, Deuretzbacher G, Heller M, et al. Hip contact forces and gait patterns from routine activities. J Biomech. 2001;34:859–871.
4. Bergmann G, Graichen F, Rohlmann A. Hip joint contact forces during stumbling. Langenbecks Arch Surg. 2004;389:53–59.
5. Bergmann G, Graichen F, Rohlmann A. Hip joint loading during walking and running, measured in two patients. J Biomech. 1993; 26:969–990.
6. Bergmann G, Graichen F, Rohlmann A. Is staircase walking a risk for the fixation of hip implants? J Biomech. 1995;28: 535–553.
7. Berman AT, Quinn RH, Zarro VJ. Quantitative gait analysis in unilateral and bilateral total hip replacements. Arch Phys Med Rehabil. 1991;72:190–194.
8. Berzins A, Sumner DR, Andriacchi TP, et al. Stem curvature and load angle influence the initial relative bone-implant motion of cementless femoral stems. J Orthop Res. 1993;11:758–769.
9. Box G, Noble PC. The position of the joint center and the functional outcome of total hip replacement. Transactions of the Orthopedic Research Society. 1993;18:525.
10. Brand RA, Crowninshield RD. The effect of cane use on hip contact force. Clin Orthop. 1980;147:181–184.
11. Brown M, Bahrke MS, Balke B. Walking efficiency before and after total hip replacement. Phys Ther. 1980;60:1259–1263.
12. Brown TD, DiGioia AM 3rd. A contact-coupled finite element analysis of the natural adult hip. J Biomech. 1984;17:437–448.
13. Cochran GVB. In: A Primer of Biomechanics. New York: Churchill Livingstone; 1982:240–250.
14. Collis DK. Femoral stem failure in total hip replacement. J Bone Joint Surg Am. 1977;59:1033–1041.
15. Crowninshield RD, Johnston RC, Andrews JG, et al. A biomechanical investigation of the human hip. J Biomech. 1978;11: 75–85.

16. Davy DT, Kotzar GM, Brown RH, et al. Telemetric force measurements across the hip after total arthroplasty. *J Bone Joint Surg Am.* 1988;70:45–50.
17. Delp SL, Komattu AV, Wixson RL. Superior displacement of the hip in total joint replacement: effects of prosthetic neck length, neck-stem angle, and anteversion angle on the moment-generating capacity of the muscles. *J Orthop Res.* 1994;12:860–870.
18. Delp SL, Maloney W. Effects of hip center location on the moment-generating capacity of the muscles. *J Biomech.* 1993;26:485–499.
19. Doehring TC, Rubash HE, Dore DE. Micromotion measurements with hip center and modular neck length alterations. *Clin Orthop.* 1999;362:230–239.
20. Doehring TC, Rubash HE, Shelley FJ, et al. Effect of superior and superolateral relocations of the hip center on hip joint forces: an experimental and analytical analysis. *J Arthroplasty.* 1996;11:693–703.
21. Dorrell JH, Catterall A. The torn acetabular labrum. *J Bone Joint Surg Br.* 1986;68:400–403.
22. Eijer H, Myers SR, Ganz R. Anterior femoroacetabular impingement after femoral neck fractures. *J Orthop Trauma.* 2001;15:475–481.
22a. English TA, Kilvington M. In vivo records of hip loads using a femoral implant with telemetric output (a preliminary report). *J Biomed Eng* 1979;1:111–115.
23. Ferguson SJ, Bryant JT, Ganz R, et al. An in vitro investigation of the acetabular labral seal in hip joint mechanics. *J Biomech.* 2003;36:171–178.
24. Ferguson SJ, Bryant JT, Ganz R, et al. The influence of the acetabular labrum on hip joint cartilage consolidation: a poroelastic finite element model. *J Biomech.* 2000;33:953–960.
25. Ferguson SJ, Bryant JT, Ito K. The material properties of the bovine acetabular labrum. *J Orthop Res.* 2001;19:887–896.
26. Frankel VH, Nordin M. *Basic Biomechanics of the Skeletal System.* Philadelphia: Lea & Febiger; 1980:xv, 303.
27. Fuss FK, Bacher A. New aspects of the morphology and function of the human hip joint ligaments. *Am J Anat.* 1991;192:1–13.
28. Galante JO. Causes of fractures of the femoral component in total hip replacement. *J Bone Joint Surg Am.* 1980;62:670–673.
29. Galante JO, Rostoker W, Doyle JM. Failed femoral stems in total hip prostheses. A report of six cases. *J Bone Joint Surg Am.* 1975;57:230–236.
30. Ganz R, Parvizi J, Beck M, et al. Femoroacetabular impingement: a cause for osteoarthritis of the hip. *Clin Orthop.* 2003;417:112–120.
31. Goodman DA, Feighan JE, Smith AD, et al. Subclinical slipped capital femoral epiphysis. Relationship to osteoarthrosis of the hip. *J Bone Joint Surg Am.* 1997;79:1489–1497.
32. Gore DR, Murray MP, Gardner GM, et al. Roentgenographic measurements after Muller total hip replacement. Correlations among roentgenographic measurements and hip strength and mobility. *J Bone Joint Surg Am.* 1977;59:948–953.
33. Hadley NA, Brown TD, Weinstein SL. The effects of contact pressure elevations and aseptic necrosis on the long-term outcome of congenital hip dislocation. *J Orthop Res.* 1990;8:504–513.
34. Hampton SJ, Andriacchi TP, Galante JO. Three dimensional stress analysis of the femoral stem of a total hip prosthesis. *J Biomech.* 1980;13:443–448.
35. Harris WH, Bourne RB, Oh I. Intra-articular acetabular labrum: a possible etiological factor in certain cases of osteoarthritis of the hip. *J Bone Joint Surg Am.* 1979;61:510–514.
36. Heller MO, Bergmann G, Deuretzbacher G, et al. Musculo-skeletal loading conditions at the hip during walking and stair climbing. *J Biomech.* 2001;34:883–893.
37. Hewitt JD, Glisson RR, Guilak F, et al. The mechanical properties of the human hip capsule ligaments. *J Arthroplasty.* 2002;17:82–89.
38. Hewitt J, Guilak F, Glisson R, et al. Regional material properties of the human hip joint capsule ligaments. *J Orthop Res.* 2001;19:359–364.
39. Hoaglund FT, Steinbach LS. Primary osteoarthritis of the hip: etiology and epidemiology. *J Am Acad Orthop Surg.* 2001;9:320–327.
40. Hodge WA, Andriacchi TP, Galante JO. A relationship between stem orientation and function following total hip arthroplasty. *J Arthroplasty.* 1991;6:229–235.
41. Hodge WA, Carlson KL, Fijan RS, et al., Contact pressures from an instrumented hip endoprosthesis. *J Bone Joint Surg Am.* 1989;71: 1378–1386.
42. Hurwitz DE, Chertack CC, Andriacchi TP. How gait changes in preoperative and postoperative patients with total hip replacements. *Proceedings of the second North American Congress on Biomechanics* 1992;313–314.
43. Hurwitz DE, Hulet CH, Andriacchi TP, et al. Gait compensations in patients with osteoarthritis of the hip and their relationship to pain and passive hip motion. *J Orthop Res.* 1997;15:629–635.
43a. Hurwitz DE, Foucher KC, Andriacchi TP. A new parametric approach for modeling hip forces during gait: a technical note. *J Biomechanics.* 2003;36(1):113–119.
44. Ikeda T, Awaya G, Suzuki S, et al. Torn acetabular labrum in young patients. Arthroscopic diagnosis and management. *J Bone Joint Surg Br.* 1988;70:13–16.
45. Ito K, Minka MA 2nd, Leunig M, et al. Femoroacetabular impingement and the cam-effect. A MRI-based quantitative anatomical study of the femoral head-neck offset. *J Bone Joint Surg Br.* 2001;83:171–176.
46. Jenkins DB, Hollinshead WH. *Hollinshead's Functional Anatomy of the Limbs and Back.* 6th ed. Philadelphia: Saunders; 1991:xxv,397.
47. Johnston RC, Brand RA, Crowninshield RD. Reconstruction of the hip. A mathematical approach to determine optimum geometric relationships. *J Bone Joint Surg Am.* 1979;61:639–652.
48. Klaue K, Durnin CW, Ganz R. The acetabular rim syndrome. A clinical presentation of dysplasia of the hip. *J Bone Joint Surg Br.* 1991;73:423–429.
49. Konrath GA, Hamel AJ, Olson SA, et al. The role of the acetabular labrum and the transverse acetabular ligament in load transmission in the hip. *J Bone Joint Surg Am.* 1998;80:1781–1788.
49a. Kotzar GM, Davy DT, Goldberg VM, et al. Telemeterized in vivo hip joint force data: a report on two patients after total hip surgery. *J Orthop Res* 1991;9:621–633.
50. Krebs DE, Elbaum L, Riley PO, et al. Exercise and gait effects on in vivo hip contact pressures. *Phys Ther.* 1991;71:301–309.
51. Lavigne M, Parvizi J, Beck M, et al. Anterior femoroacetabular impingement: part I. Techniques of joint preserving surgery. *Clin Orthop.* 2004;418:61–66.
52. McCarthy JC, Busconi B. The role of hip arthroscopy in the diagnosis and treatment of hip disease. *Orthopedics.* 1995;18:753–756.
53. McCarthy JC, Noble PC, Schuck MR, et al. The Otto E. Aufranc Award: The role of labral lesions to development of early degenerative hip disease. *Clin Orthop.* 2001;393:25–37.
54. McCarthy JC, Noble PC, Schuck MR, et al. The watershed labral lesion: its relationship to early arthritis of the hip. *J Arthroplasty.* 2001;16(8 suppl 1):81–87.
55. Murray MP, Brewer BJ, Zuege RC. Kinesiologic measurements of functional performance before and after McKee-Farrar total hip replacement. A study of thirty patients with rheumatoid arthritis, osteoarthritis, or avascular necrosis of the femoral head. *J Bone Joint Surg Am.* 1972;54:237–256.
56. Murray MP, Gore DR, Clarkson BH. Walking patterns of patients with unilateral hip pain due to osteo-arthritis and avascular necrosis. *J Bone Joint Surg Am.* 1971;53:259–274.
57. Murray RO. The aetiology of primary osteoarthritis of the hip. *Br J Radiol.* 1965;38(455):810–824.
58. Myers SR, Eijer H, Ganz R. Anterior femoroacetabular impingement after periacetabular osteotomy. *Clin Orthop.* 1999;363:93–99.
59. Neumann DA, Cook TM. Effect of load and carrying position on the electromyographic activity of the gluteus medius muscle during walking. *Phys Ther.* 1985;65:305–311.
60. Norkin C, Lavangie HW. *Joint structure and function. A comprehensive analysis.* Philadelphia: FA Davis Co; 2001.
61. Notzli HP, Wyss TF, Stoecklin CH, et al. The contour of the femoral head-neck junction as a predictor for the risk of anterior impingement. *J Bone Joint Surg Br.* 2002;84:556–560.

62. Offierski CM. Traumatic dislocation of the hip in children. *J Bone Joint Surg Br.* 1981;63-B(2):194–197.
63. Paul JP. Approaches to design: force actions transmitted by joints in the human body. *Proceeds Research Society London, Britain.* 1976;192:163–172.
64. Pauwels F. [Short survey of mechanical stress of bone and its importance for the functional adaptation (author's transl)]. *Z Orthop Ihre Grenzgeb.* 1973;111:681–705.
65. Phillips TW, Nguyen LT, Munro SD. Loosening of cementless femoral stems: a biomechanical analysis of immediate fixation with loading vertical, femur horizontal. *J Biomech.* 1991;24:37–48.
66. Rab GT. The geometry of slipped capital femoral epiphysis: implications for movement, impingement, and corrective osteotomy. *J Pediatr Orthop.* 1999;19:419–424.
67. Radin EL. Osteoarthrosis: the orthopedic surgeon's perspective. *Acta Orthop Scand Suppl.* 1995;266:6–9.
68. Radin EL, Burr DB, Caterson B, et al. Mechanical determinants of osteoarthrosis. *Semin Arthritis Rheum.* 1991;21(3 suppl 2):12–21.
69. Radin EL, Parker HG, Pugh JW, et al. Response of joints to impact loading. 3. Relationship between trabecular microfractures and cartilage degeneration. *J Biomech.* 1973;6:51–57.
70. Rydell NW. Forces acting on the femoral head-prosthesis. A study on strain gauge supplied prostheses in living persons. *Acta Orthop Scand.* 1966;37(suppl 88):1–132.
71. Sakalkale DP, Sharkey PF, Eng K, et al. Effect of femoral component offset on polyethylene wear in total hip arthroplasty. *Clin Orthop.* 2001;388:125–134.
72. Seireg A, Arvikar RJ. The prediction of muscular load sharing and joint forces in the lower extremities during walking. *J Biomech.* 1975;8:89–102.
73. Siebenrock KA, Wahab KH, Werlen S, et al. Abnormal extension of the femoral head epiphysis as a cause of cam impingement. *Clin Orthop.* 2004;418:54–60.
74. Skinner HB. Pathokinesiology and total joint arthroplasty. *Clin Orthop.* 1993;288:78–86.
75. Solomon L. Patterns of osteoarthritis of the hip. *J Bone Joint Surg Br.* 1976;58:176–183.
76. Stansfield BW, Nicol AC, Paul JP, et al. Direct comparison of calculated hip joint contact forces with those measured using instrumented implants. An evaluation of a three-dimensional mathematical model of the lower limb. *J Biomech.* 2003;36:929–936.
77. Stauffer RN, Smidt GL, Wadsworth JB. Clinical and biomechanical analysis of gait following Charnley total hip replacement. *Clin Orthop.* 1974;99:70–77.
78. Stewart KJ, Edmonds-Wilson RH, Brand RA, et al. Spatial distribution of hip capsule structural and material properties. *J Biomech.* 2002;35:1491–1498.
79. Tackson SJ, Krebs DE, Harris BA. Acetabular pressures during hip arthritis exercises. *Arthritis Care Res.* 1997;10:308–319.
80. Takechi H, Nagashima H, Ito S. Intra-articular pressure of the hip joint outside and inside the limbus. *Nippon Seikeigeka Gakkai Zasshi.* 1982;56:529–536.
81. Tonnis D, Heinecke A. Acetabular and femoral anteversion: relationship with osteoarthritis of the hip. *J Bone Joint Surg Am.* 1999;81:1747–1770.
82. Wadsworth JB, Smidt GL, Johnston RC. Gait characteristics of subjects with hip disease. *Phys Ther.* 1972;52:829–839.
83. White SC, Yack HJ, Lesswing AL. Pre and post surgical gait of a total hip replacement patient. Presented at: 7th Annual East Coast Gait Conference; 1992; Richmond, VA.
84. Yamaguchi M, Akisue T, Bauer TW, et al. The spatial location of impingement in total hip arthroplasty. *J Arthroplasty.* 2000;15:305–313.
85. Yoder SA, Brand RA, Pedersen DR, et al. Total hip acetabular component position affects component loosening rates. *Clin Orthop.* 1988;228:79–87.
86. Hurwitz DE, Foucher KC, Andriacchi TP: A new parametric approach for modeling hip forces during gait: A technical note. J Biomechanics 2003;36(1):113–119.
87. English TA, Kilvington M. In vivo records of hip loads using a femoral implant with telemetric output (a preliminary report) *J Biomed Eng.* 1979;1:111–115.
88. Ketzer GM, Devy DT, Goldberg VM, et al. Telemeterized in vivo hip joint force data: a report on two patients afetr total hip surgery. *J Orthop Res.* 1991;9:621–633.

Kinematics of the Hip

6

Richard D. Komistek *Douglas A. Dennis* *Mohamed R. Mahfouz*

Early failure mechanisms in total hip arthroplasty (THA) have included component loosening (17,33,46,47) or failure (3,18), infection (14), dislocation (7), osseous fracture (22,23), and neurovascular injury (3,7,17,18,21,33,45). More recently, premature polyethylene wear, particularly associated with modular acetabular components, has become prevalent (3,18). Only limited research has been conducted correlating polyethylene wear with the in vivo motions and forces occurring at the hip joint. Researchers have utilized both telemetry (1,2,9,15,46) and mathematical modeling (4,8,25,26,34,38,43,44) to predict in vivo forces across the hip joint. Data collected from these studies has been utilized in hip joint simulation devices to predict polyethylene wear patterns of acetabular components in THA (5,6,39,40,48). Unfortunately, actual polyethylene wear observed in THA simulator studies has not always produced wear patterns seen with retrieval analyses (5,6,12,31). Since discrepancies exist between wear patterns of simulated versus actual retrieval specimens, it can be assumed that variations exist between simulated and actual in vivo hip joint kinematics. These variations may be related, at least in part, to surgical alterations in the supporting soft tissue structures of the hip or to biomechanical alterations related to prosthetic geometry.

More recently, video fluoroscopy has been used to determine the in vivo kinematics of the hip joint (11,24,27). Initially, these studies assumed the motions of the normal and implanted hip joints would differ, since many of the soft tissue supporting structures of the hip joint are altered during THA. These previous fluoroscopic studies confirmed that after unconstrained metal-on-polyethylene (MOP) THA, the femoral head may separate (slide away) from the medial aspect of the acetabular component during both gait and during an active hip abduction–adduction activity (11,24,27). This separation phenomenon was not observed in either non-implanted normal hips or subjects implanted with a constrained THA device. It has also been reported that subjects having a metal-on-metal (MOM) THA experience less femoral head separation than subjects having a MOP THA (24). The objective of this review chapter is to comprise a comparative analysis of hip kinematics for subjects having a MOM, MOP, alumina-on-alumina (AOA), or alumina-on-polyethylene (AOP) THA. We compare the in vivo incidence of femoral head separation and the translational motion of five points fixed on the femoral head within the acetabular component.

METHODS

Forty subjects were analyzed under fluoroscopic surveillance while performing treadmill gait to determine the incidence and magnitude of hip separation in subjects implanted with various designs of THA. All 20 subjects having a metal femoral head and either a polyethylene or metal liner were implanted by a single surgeon. The other 20 subjects having an alumina head and either a polyethylene or alumina liner were implanted by a second surgeon. All patients completed an informed consent document, and approval for this study was granted through the Internal Research Review Board (IRRB) at HealthONE Rose Medical Center (IRRB #0445). Ten subjects were implanted with a MOM THA (Ultima; DePuy Orthopaedics, Warsaw IN), ten with a MOP THA (Ultima), ten with an AOP THA (Cerafit; Ceraver, Roissy, France), and ten with an AOA THA (Cerafit). None of the subjects reported any signs of hip instability, and none suffered a dislocation postoperatively. The average postoperative follow-up duration was 22 months (18 to 31 months) for patients with MOP THA,

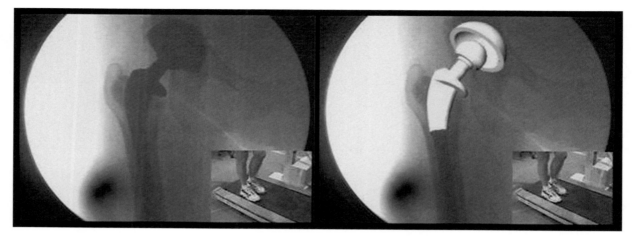

Figure 6-1   Example of the computer-automated 3D model-fitting process, where the femoral head, femoral stem, and acetabular component are overlaid onto the 2D fluoroscopic image.

and 19 months (3 to 30 months) for patients with MOM THA. Subjects in the MOM THA group were selected randomly from a group of patients participating in an investigational device evaluation (IDE) study (IRRB #0514). Inclusion criteria for all four groups included only those subjects with hip arthroplasties considered clinically to be highly successful (Harris hip scores [19] >90 points) without pain or functional deficits. Patients were matched as to follow-up periods within 1 year. No patient walked with a detectable limp, and all could actively abduct their operated hips against gravity without difficulty. Clinical and radiographic leg length measurements were performed for all subjects. None experienced shortening of their analyzed leg, while five subjects exhibited a slight lengthening of their operative extremity following operation.

Each subject performed normal walking while on a level treadmill, and the full gait cycle from first heel strike to second heel strike (stance phase and swing phase) was analyzed.

During stance phase, fluoroscopic video frames were analyzed at heel strike, toe off, and three other fluoroscopic images representing 25%, 50%, and 75% of stance phase. Then throughout the swing phase of gait, every third fluoroscopic video image was analyzed, including the image representing the second heel strike. The fluoroscopic images were then downloaded to a workstation computer for analysis. Three-dimensional (3D) kinematics for each THA were recovered from the two-dimensional (2D) fluoroscopic images using a previously described computer automated, 3D model fitting process (10,28,41) that determined the in vivo orientation of the femoral component relative to the acetabular component (Fig. 6-1). Using this process, the distance from the medialmost aspect of the acetabular component to the medial aspect of the femoral head was then measured to determine if separation of the femoral head from the acetabular component had occurred (Fig. 6-2).

No Separation   **Hip Separation**

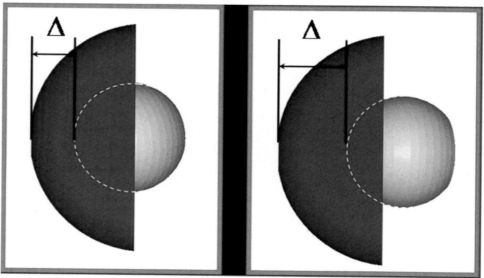

Figure 6-2   Under fully seated conditions, the distance between the femoral head and acetabular component liner is measured (Δ_1). During stance and swing phase, the distance between the femoral head and acetabular liner for each video frame is measured (Δ_2), and if Δ_2 is greater than Δ_1, then it is denoted that the femoral head has separated from the acetabular component liner.

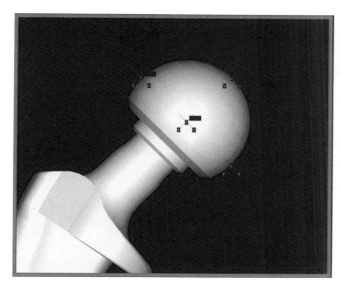

Figure 6-3 Location of the five femoral head loci contact positions utilized for development of acetabular component contact pathways. The first position (P1) is located at the superior pole of the femoral head and the other four positions (P2, P3, P4, P5) are equidistantly placed along the femoral head equator.

In an additional analysis, the translational motion patterns for five points fixed on the femoral head within the acetabular component for subjects having either a MOM or MOP THA were determined. Initially, reference frames were attached to both the femoral head and the acetabular component. Five

distinct points on the femoral head were designated and transformed into the acetabular component reference frame (Fig. 6-3). The femoral head contact patterns were then determined by analysis of sequential fluoroscopic video frames during both the swing and stance phases of gait. Of particular interest in the analysis of contact pathways was to determine the percentage of subjects exhibiting vector crossing pathways, as well as the length of excursion of individual loci contact pathways.

The same fluoroscopic images captured to determine the incidence of hip separation were reanalyzed to determine the in vivo vector pathways of the five predetermined femoral head loci. The acetabular component was separated into five areas: (a) center, (b) Q1, representing the inferior–posterior quadrant, (c) Q2, representing the inferior/anterior quadrant, (d) Q3, representing the superior/posterior quadrant, and (e) Q4, representing the superior/anterior quadrant (Fig. 6-4). Femoral head loci patterns were then critically analyzed within each of these five acetabular component regions.

An extensive error analysis was conducted using three different methods to verify the accuracy of the 3D model-fitting process. Initially, a mechanical apparatus that allows for two prosthetic components to be translated and rotated relative to each other was used. The known versus predicted implant positions were then compared (10). Using this process, the relative rotational error was $<0.75°$ and the translational error <0.5 mm. Next, the two components were similarly placed at known positions in space relative to each other. The fixated components were then rotated and translated while under dynamic fluoroscopic surveillance. The average error for this dynamic analysis was <0.5 mm in translation and $<0.5°$ in rotation (41). Finally, the two components were surgically

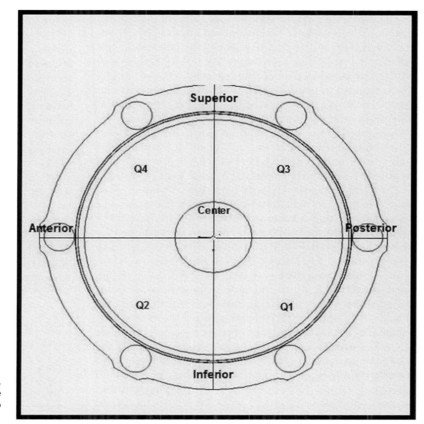

Figure 6-4 Location of the four quadrants (Q1, Q2, Q3, Q4) and the center region (C) of the acetabular component, which were analyzed to determine femoral head loci pathways.

TABLE 6-1

AVERAGE HIP JOINT SEPARATION VALUES FOR THE THA SUBGROUPS ANALYZED

	Metal on Poly (mm)	Metal on Metal (mm)	Alumina on Poly (mm)	Alumina on Alumina (mm)
Maximum	3.1	0.5	7.4	0.6
Minimum	0.8	0.3	0.3	0.1
Average	2.0	0.4	1.5	0.3

implanted into a fresh cadaver. Ninety relative orientations (translations and rotations) were captured using video fluoroscopy. An Opto-Track system (Northern Digital, Inc., Waterloo, Ontario, Canada), was used to determine the ground truth (known position of each component relative to a fixed reference frame). Then the model fitting process was used to predict relative orientation of the implanted components. The error of all 90 trials was <0.5 mm in translation and <0.5° in rotation. Therefore, femoral head separation was determined to occur if the femoral head–acetabular component distance was greater than our threshold error value of 0.5 mm (28).

An ANOVA statistical analysis was conducted to determine the differences in magnitudes of hip separation among hip replacements with differing articulating bearing surfaces as well as to detect differences in the incidences of vector crossing pathways.

RESULTS

During the swing phase of gait, no separation of the femoral head from the acetabular component was observed in subjects implanted with a MOM THA (maximum separation value was less than the error value of 0.5 mm) (Table 6-1). Only one of ten subjects (10%) implanted with an AOA THA experienced greater than 0.5 mm of femoral head separation, and this subject only experienced 0.6 mm. Separation of the femoral head from the acetabular component of at least 0.8 mm was observed during the swing phase of gait in all ten patients (100%) implanted with an unconstrained MOP articulation (Table 6-1). Six of ten subjects (60%) having an AOP THA experienced greater than 0.5 mm of femoral head separation.

The average amount of femoral head separation detected in subjects having a MOM THA or AOA THA was 0.4 mm (range 0.3 to 0.5 mm) and 0.3 mm (range 0.1 to 0.6 mm), which is less than our error value of 0.5 mm. The average separation for subjects having a MOP or AOP THA was 2.0 mm (range 0.8 to 3.1 mm) and 1.5 mm (range 0.3 to 7.0 mm), respectively.

All subjects having either an AOP or AOA THA were analyzed to determine if femoral head separation could occur during stance phase of gait. The results from this separate analysis revealed that no separation occurred for subjects having an AOA THA, but 50% (five of ten) of subjects having an AOP THA experienced femoral head separation from the acetabular component. The average amount of femoral head separation for these subjects was 1.5 mm. Also, the maximum amount of femoral head separation occurring at anytime during gait (stance or swing phase) was 7.4 mm, which occurred

for a subject having an AOP THA from midstance to toe off (Fig. 6-5). In all cases, separation was observed medially while a portion of the femoral head remained in contact with the acetabular component superolaterally, producing conditions where the femoral head typically pivoted on the superolateral lip of the acetabular liner. The differences in the separation profiles of MOM versus MOP THA, MOM versus AOP THA, AOA versus AOP THA, and AOA versus MOP THA patients were all statistically significant ($p <0.01$).

When analyzing femoral head loci contact pathways during the motion cycle (stance phase through swing phase of gait), the average number of vector crossing points (a point of the motion path crossing a previous point on the same path) was very similar for MOM versus MOP THA subjects ($p >0.05$) (Table 6-2). On average, subjects having a MOM THA experienced more vector crossing points in Q2 and Q3, while subjects having a MOP THA experienced more vector crossing points in the center zone and in Q3. Both groups, on average, experienced the same amount of crossing points in Q4. The largest number of crossing points was ten, occurring in Q4 for a subject having a MOP THA.

The percentage of subjects experiencing vector crossing pathways was also similar for subjects implanted with either MOM or MOP THA ($p >0.05$) (Table 6-3). At all five locations (center, Q1 through Q4), a high percentage of subjects in both THA groups experienced vector crossing pathways (>70%). All MOM THA subjects experienced at least one vector crossing pathway in Q3, while all MOP subjects experienced a vector crossing pathway in Q4. The lowest percentage of subjects experiencing a vector crossing pathway was 70%, occurring in Q1 for subjects having a MOP THA.

The main difference between MOP and MOM THA subjects, although not statistically significant ($p >0.05$), occurred

TABLE 6-2

NUMBER OF CROSSING POINTS OF FEMORAL LOCI VECTOR PATHWAYS

	Center	Q1	Q2	Q3	Q4
MOM average	2	3	3	2	3
MOM maximum	6	7	8	7	8
MOM minimum	0	0	0	1	0
MOP average	4	2	2	3	3
MOP maximum	8	8	5	6	10
MOP minimum	0	0	0	1	1

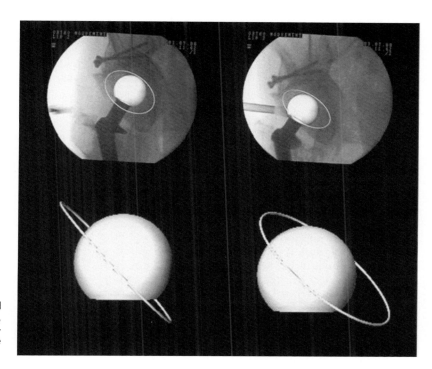

Figure 6-5 Fluoroscopic and computer-analyzed images of a subject implanted with an AOP THA, who experienced 7.4 mm of femoral head separation, occurring from the midstance to toe-off phase of the gait cycle.

in the length of excursion of the individual loci contact pathways (Table 6-4). The largest excursion length of a vector pathway, on average, was 72.2 mm, occurring in Q3 for subjects having a MOM THA. The smallest average excursion length was similar for both groups, occurring at the center (38.7 mm for MOM and 38.6 mm for MOP THA). In all four quadrants, the excursion length was greater for MOM THA subjects compared with MOP THA subjects. The vector pathway excursion lengths for MOM THA ranged from 13.1 to 22.2 mm longer than MOP THA. The lack of statistical significance may be related to the small sample size (ten in each group). Additionally, subjects having a MOM THA had a lower average length of follow-up, which may explain why two MOM subjects experienced much smaller vector pathway lengths than the other eight subjects having a MOM THA. Due to the limited follow-up of these two MOM THA subjects (<6 months), they may not have been able to perform a normal gait pattern with limited stride lengths.

High variability in contact pathways was observed for both groups (Figs. 6-6 through 6-9). The vector pathway patterns were quite different for each subject, with some subjects experiencing larger number of crossing points (Figs. 6-6, 6-7, and 6-10) and others exhibiting a minimal number of vector crossing points (Figs. 6-8 and 6-9). At times, depending on the hip

rotations, the vector pathway for the center zone crossed over into Q1 (Figs. 6-6 and 6-9). The other four vector pathways also crossed over from one quadrant to another, at times minimally (Fig. 6-6) and at other times substantially (Figs. 6-8 and 6-9). However, subjects having a MOM THA did experience more reproducible in vivo femoral loci patterns during gait than those subjects with MOP THA. In MOM THA subjects, the loci pathways would typically return to the origin position, while subjects having MOP THA designs experienced an open-loop loci pattern where the pathway often did not return to the origin position.

DISCUSSION

In an initial study analyzing subjects while performing a hip abduction–adduction maneuver, femoral head separation from the acetabulum was not observed in subjects with normal hip joints or those implanted with a constrained THA, but occurred in all subjects implanted with an unconstrained MOP THA (11). In a second early study, subjects having a MOP THA also experienced femoral head separation during gait, as had been noted during an abduction–adduction maneuver (27). These results lead to a hypothesis that patients implanted with

TABLE 6-3
PERCENTAGE OF MOM AND MOP THA SUBJECTS EXPERIENCING VECTOR CROSSING PATHWAYS

	Center	Q1	Q2	Q3	Q4
MOM	90% (9/10)	90% (9/10)	90% (9/10)	100% (10/10)	80% (8/10)
MOP	90% (9/10)	70% (7/10)	90% (9/10)	100% (10/10)	100% (10/10)

TABLE 6-4

AVERAGE EXCURSION LENGTH (MM) OF VECTOR PATHWAYS FOR MOM VERSUS MOP THA SUBJECTS

	Center	Q1	Q2	Q3	Q4
MOM	38.7	65.0	64.4	72.2	70.7
MOP	38.6	42.8	51.3	49.3	49.2

an unconstrained MOP THA are subjected to inertial forces that produce sliding of the femoral head from the acetabular component during several different dynamic activities.

In the normal hip joint, retention of the femoral head within the acetabulum is provided by numerous supporting soft tissue structures including the fibrous capsule, acetabular labrum, ligament of the head of the femur (LHF), and the iliofemoral, ischiofemoral, pubofemoral, and transverse acetabular ligaments. During THA, the LHF is surgically removed. Additionally, a portion of the remaining supporting soft tissue structures are transected or resected to facilitate surgical exposure. It is, therefore, logical to assume that the kinematics of the implanted hip may differ from the normal hip, since the stabilizing soft tissue envelope is altered at the time of operation. Hip joint separation is potentially detrimental and may play a role in complications observed with THA today, including premature polyethylene wear, prosthetic loosening and hip instability.

Although hip separation was initially only found (and thought to only occur) during the swing phase of gait, a high

incidence and magnitude of hip separation during stance phase of gait was also observed. It appears that during the stance phase of gait, the acetabular component slides away from the femoral head from 66% of stance phase to toe off. In the normal hip, as the momentum of the pelvis moves forward, the capsular and ligamentous structures of the hip joint help maintain the femoral head within the acetabular component, even while the lagging foot remains on the ground through toe off. We hypothesize that disturbance of capsuloligamentous structures during THA allows the femoral head to separate from the acetabulum as the pelvis thrusts forward and the opposite leg, moving through swing phase, moves forward and the lagging foot remains on the ground, completing stance phase through to toe off. The results from this analysis also revealed that femoral head separation did not occur during stance phase in the ten subjects having an AOA THA.

The presence of femoral head separation found in this analysis may contribute to premature polyethylene wear because of the increased amount of shear force placed on the polyethylene material during impulse loading cycles. The impulse generated by the collision of two objects has been shown to potentially compromise the structural integrity of mechanical components (44). A simplified kinetic analysis indicated a predicted average increase in hip forces of 289.5 N due to femoral head separation and secondarily due to the development of impulse loading conditions (31). These increased loads can potentially compromise implant fixation, resulting in premature component loosening. Additionally, during separation, the femoral head often remains in contact with and pivots on the polyethylene liner superolaterally, potentially creating excessive loads and accelerated polyethylene wear in this region (Fig. 6-11).

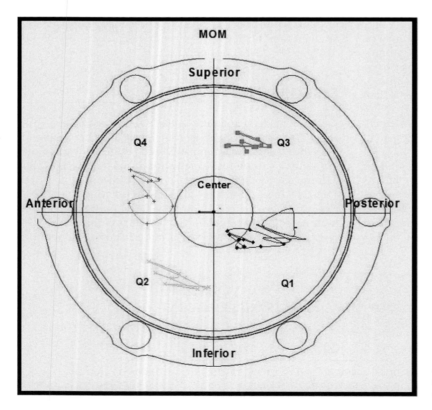

Figure 6-6 Example of the femoral head loci contact pathways of a MOM THA subject experiencing a significant number of points of vector crossing pathways.

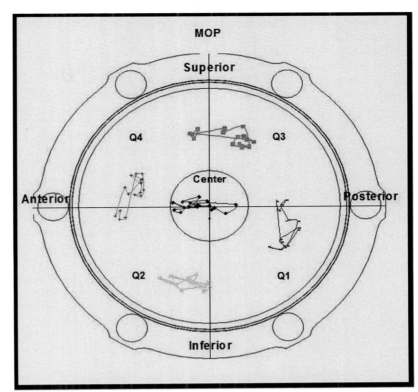

Figure 6-7 Example of the femoral head loci contact pathways of a MOP THA subject experiencing a significant number of points of vector crossing pathways.

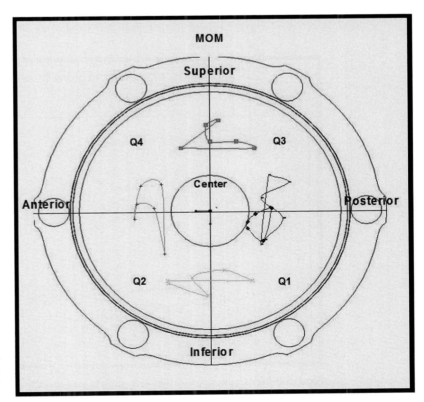

Figure 6-8 Example of the femoral head loci contact pathways of a MOM THA subject experiencing a minimal number of points of vector crossing pathways.

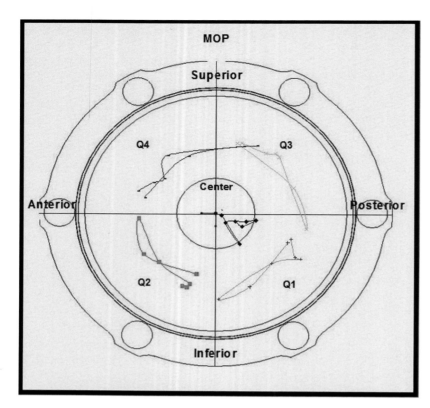

Figure 6-9 Example of the femoral head loci contact pathways of a MOP THA subject experiencing a minimal number of points of vector crossing pathways.

The hip separation noted may help describe the multidirectional wear vector patterns observed in retrieved acetabular components. Yamaguchi et al. (49) performed a 3D evaluation of wear vectors in 104 retrieved acetabular components and found that 31 (30%) demonstrated multidirectional wear vector patterns that were highly variable among different spec-

imens. Greater linear wear was observed in retrieved liners with multidirectional wear vectors than in those with unidirectional wear patterns. They hypothesized that the multidirectional wear pathways observed may result in accelerated polyethylene wear due to increased shear forces. Further study is required to define what role hip separation may play in

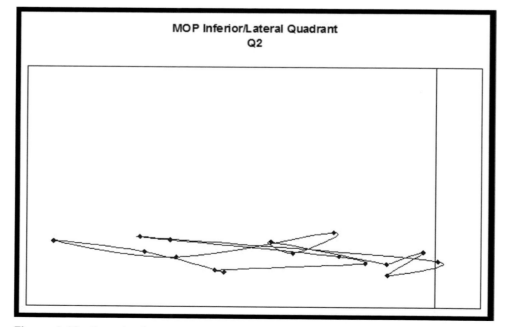

Figure 6-10 Example of a MOP THA subject demonstrating the most points of vector crossing pathways within a single quadrant.

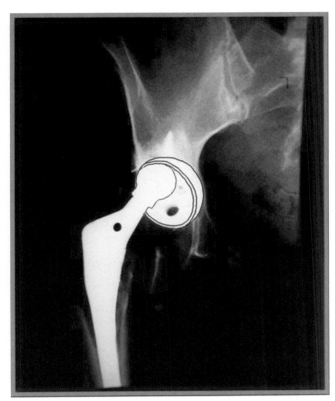

Figure 6-11 Anteroposterior radiograph of a subject implanted with a MOP THA demonstrating extensive polyethylene wear in the same region of the acetabular component liner where femoral head sliding (pivoting) is typically observed.

creation of multidirectional wear vectors and accelerated polyethylene wear.

While hip simulator experimentation has been valuable in providing information on polyethylene wear, in vivo wear has proven to be a complex and multifactorial process (12,13,20,30,31,40). Data from hip simulators has not always equated well with retrieval studies, with variations seen in wear rates and patterns as well as debris particulate size. These inconsistencies are likely related to multiple factors such as variations in the level of polyethylene oxidation, the rigidity of component fixation, the strength of periacetabular support (29), and hip kinematics of test versus retrieval specimens. Incorporation of hip separation into hip wear simulators may allow more accurate replication of in vivo conditions.

The significance of the hip separation findings in this study is supported by the recent report of Nevelos et al. (32), who conducted a hip simulator analysis to assess the significance of femoral head separation from the acetabular component in an AOA THA design. Their hip simulator was programmed to induce microseparation of the femoral head from the acetabular component during gait. Thereafter, they compared the simulated wear patterns to clinical retrievals for the same implant design. The wear damaged observed in the simulated analysis with microseparation was similar to the damage observed in clinical retrieval studies. Similar grain boundary fracture wear mechanisms were also found. Therefore, they concluded that microseparation during simulator testing reproduced, for the first time, clinically relevant wear rates, patterns, debris, and mechanics when compared with clinical THA retrievals.

Data collected from telemetric hip studies has demonstrated an increased force magnitude peak typically is present immediately after heel strike, compared to the force magnitude at toe off (1,2,20,36). It has been hypothesized that this increase in force is due to muscle contraction. Based on the present fluoroscopic evaluation, we theorize that the increased force seen immediately after heel strike results, at least in part, from the femoral head translating back into the acetabular component at heel strike, producing impulse loading conditions.

The narrow tolerance bands and high surface finishes of MOM and AOA THA components allow for a thin film of fluid to become entrapped between the femoral head and acetabular liner. Because of their precise surface finish, low diametral clearances, and the rheological properties of synovial fluid under physiological kinetics and kinematics, boundary and even thin-film microelectric hydrodynamic lubrication can be present. The tighter radial tolerances of MOM and AOA THA designs do not allow for discontinuities or voids between the femoral head and the acetabular liner, which, in turn, creates a fluid film cohesion with higher radial tension. We hypothesize that due to the increased wetability of the metal and ceramic surfaces, this film may effectively constrain the femoral head within the acetabular liner during gait. This cohesive force only needs to sufficiently overcome the inertial forces, causing the leg to separate from the body during the swing phase of gait. In MOP and AOP THA, larger diametral clearances between the femoral head and polyethylene liner exist. Additionally, wetability of polyethylene is less. We therefore suspect that the cohesiveness of the lubricating film of MOP and AOP THA components is reduced, allowing hip separation to occur. The absence of femoral head separation from the acetabular component in subjects having a MOM or AOA THA device leads to the hypothesis that patients implanted with these THA designs are subjected to more favorable mechanical environments and more uniform wear kinematics during gait.

The role of hip separation in instability following THA is unclear and deserves further evaluation. Coventry (7) reviewed a group of 32 patients who suffered late dislocations following Charnley THA. He postulated that stretching of the supporting soft tissue structures (i.e., pseudocapsule) over time and extremes of range of motion may lessen soft tissue constraints and allow for late dislocation. Continued study of our present patient group is indicated to see if the amount of hip separation increases over time, suggesting a role in late hip instability.

Previous studies of femoral head contact pathways, using computer simulations or hip simulator analyses, have reported that individual femoral head loci typically returned to their original starting point at the end of each gait cycle (36,37). Ramamurti et al. (36) tracked 20 selected femoral head loci pathways during a 3D computer simulation of gait motion. They observed most loci demonstrated quasi-elliptical contact pathways, which varied widely in both shape and length depending on their location on the femoral head. Contact pathways of neighboring loci often intersected each other, creating multidirectional shear forces on the acetabular component articulating surface. These authors hypothesized that the multidirectional wear pathways they observed in retrievals may result in accelerated polyethylene wear due to increased shear forces placed on the material. This hypothesis is supported by the work of Pooley and Tabor (35), who reported that when high-density polyethylene is subjected to unidirectional sliding, the polymer's molecules tend to align along the direction of sliding, resulting in lowering of the coefficient of friction, potentially reducing wear of the material. They observed when multidirectional wear patterns occur, polyethylene wear rates accelerate.

The results from the present in vivo analysis have determined that vector pathways experience a substantial number of vector crossing points for both MOM and MOP THA subjects. These results support the findings of Yamaguchi et al. (49) that multidirectional wear vector patterns are commonly present in THA. The number of crossing points varies considerably for each subject. The major difference in vector pathways between MOM and MOP THA subjects is the excursion length of the vector pathways. Subjects having a MOM THA experienced larger excursion lengths compared with implanted with a MOP THA. Therefore, it can be assumed that MOM THA subjects experience femoral head motion traversing a larger area of the acetabular component. The reduced wear rates observed in retrieval analysis of MOM versus MOP acetabular components (16) may be related to the presence of multidirectional motion patterns, which enhance wear of polyethylene. Interestingly, other data suggest wear of MOM articulations is reduced under conditions of multidirectional motion when compared to unidirectional wear patterns (42).

SUMMARY

The present study demonstrates that femoral head separation from the acetabular component can occur during weight-bearing gait in subjects having a MOP or AOP THA, but this did not occur in subjects having a MOM THA and for only one subject having an AOA THA. Potential detrimental effects resulting from hip joint separation include premature polyethylene wear secondary to creation of multidirectional motion pathways, component loosening secondary to the creation of impulse loading conditions, and late hip instability due to chronic pseudocapsular attenuation. Further research is necessary to determine if other subjects having different types of MOM or ceramic-on-ceramic THA implants experience hip joint separation.

REFERENCES

1. Bergmann G, Graichen F, Rohlmann A. Hip joint forces during load carrying. *Clin Orthop.* 1997;335:190–201.
2. Bergmann G, Graichen F, Rohlmann A. Hip joint loading during walking and running, measured in two patients. *J Biomech.* 1993;26:969–990.
3. Bono JV, Sanford L, Toussaint JT. Severe polyethylene wear in total hip arthroplasty. Observation from retrieved AML PLUS hip implants with an ACS polyethylene liner. *J Arthroplasty.* 1994;9:119–125.
4. Brand RA, Crowninshield RD, Wittock CE, et al. A model of lower extremity muscular anatomy. *J Biomech Eng.* 1982;104:304.
5. Clarke IC, Good V, Anissian L, et al. Charnley wear model validation of hip simulators-ball diameter versus polytetrafluoroethylene and polyethylene wear. *Proc Inst Mech Eng.* 1997;211:25–36.
6. Clarke IC, Kabo M. Wear in total hip replacement. In: Amstutz HC, ed. *Total Hip Arthroplasty.* New York: Churchhill Livingstone; 1991:535–570.
7. Coventry MB. Late dislocations in patients with Charnley total hip arthroplasty. *J Bone Joint Surg.* 1985;67A:832–841.
8. Crowninshield RD, Johnston RC, Andrews JG, et al. A biomechanical investigation of the human hip. *J Biomech.* 1978;11:75–85.
9. Davy DT, Kotzar GM, Brown RH, et al. Telemetric force measurements across the hip after total arthroplasty. *J Bone Joint Surg.* 1988;70A:45–50.
10. Dennis DA, Komistek RD, Hoff WA, et al. In vivo knee kinematics derived using an inverse perspective technique. *Clin Orthop.* 1996;331:107–117.
11. Dennis DA, Komistek RD, Northcut EJ, et al. In vivo determination of hip joint separation and the forces generated due to impact loading conditions. *J Biomech.* 2001;34:623–629.
12. Dowson D, Jobbins B. Design and development of a versatile hip joint simulator and preliminary assessment of wear and creep in Charnley total replacement hip joints. *Eng Med.* 1988;17:111–117.
13. Dumbleton JH, Miller DA, Miller EH. A simulator for load bearing joints. *Med Biol Eng.* 1972;8:37–43.
14. Eftekhar NS. Long term results of cemented total hip arthroplasty. *Clin Orthop.* 1987;225:207–217.
15. English TA. Measurement of hip load forces in vivo using a telemetric method design, method and results. *Brit Orthop Tes Soc* Bradford; 1978.
16. Firkins PJ, Tipper JL, Ingham E, et al. Influence of simulator kinematics on the wear of metal on metal hip prosthesis. *Proc Inst Mech Eng (H).* 2001;215:119–121.
17. Garcia-Cimbrelo E, Diez-Vazquez V, Madero R, et al. Progression of radiolucent lines adjacent to the acetabular component and factors influencing migration after Charnley low-friction total hip arthroplasty. *J Bone Joint Surg.* 1997;79A:1373–1380.
18. Gross AE, Dust WN. Acute polyethylene fracture in an uncemented acetabular cup. *Can J Surg.* 1997;40:310–312.
19. Harris WH, Sledge CB. Total hip and total knee replacement. *N Engl J Med.* 1990;323:725–731.
20. Hodge WA, Fijan RS, Carlson KL, et al. Contact pressures in the human hip joint measured in vivo. *Proc Natl Acad Sci USA.* 1986;83:2879–2883.
21. Ilchmann T. Radiographic assessment of cup migration and wear after hip replacement. *Acta Orthop Scand Suppl.* 1997;276:1–26.
22. Kavanagh BF. Femoral head fractures associated with total hip arthroplasty. *Orthop Clin North Am.* 1992;23:249–257.
23. Kavanagh BF, Ilstrup DM, Fitzgerald RH, et al. Revision total hip arthroplasty. *J Bone Joint Surg.* 1985;67A:517–526.
24. Komistek RD, Dennis DA, Haas BD, et al. An in vivo comparison of hip joint separation for after metal-on-metal or metal-on-polyethylene total hip arthroplasty. *J Bone Joint Surgery* 2002;84:1836–1841.
25. Komistek RD, Kane T, Mahfouz MR, et al. Knee mechanics: a review of past and present techniques to determine in vivo loads. *J Biomech.* 2005;38(2):215–228.
26. Komistek RD, Stiehl JB, Paxson RD, et al. Mathematical model of the lower extremity joint reaction forces using Kane's method of dynamics: a technical note. *J Biomech.* 1998;31:185–189.
27. Lombardi AV, Mallory TH, Dennis DA, et al. An in vivo determination of total hip arthroplasty pistoning during activity. *J Arthroplasty.* 2000;15:702–709.
28. Mahfouz MR, Hoff WA, Komistek RD, et al. A robust method for registration of three-dimensional knee implant models to two-dimensional fluoroscopy images. *IEEE Trans Med Imaging.* 2003;22:1561–1574.
29. Maxian TA, Brown, TD, Pederson DR, et al. 3-Dimensional sliding/contact computational simulation of total hip wear. *Clin Orthop.* 1996;333:41–50.
30. McKellop HA, Campbell P, Park SH, et al. The origin of submicron polyethylene wear debris in total hip arthroplasty. *Clin Orthop.* 1995;311:3–21.
31. McKellop HA, Clark IC. Evolution and evaluation of materials-screening machines and joint simulators in predicting in vivo wear phenomena. In: Duchyene P, Hastings GW, eds. *Functional*

Behavior of Orthopaedic Biomaterials. Applications. Vol 2. Boca Raton, FL: CRC Press; 1984:51–85.

32. Nevelos J, Ingham E, Doyle C, et al. Microseparation of the centers of alumina-alumina artificial hip joints during simulator testing produces clinically relevant wear rates and patterns. *J Arthroplasty.* 2000;15:793–795.

33. Numair J, Joshi AB, Murphy JC, et al. Total hip arthroplasty for congenital dysplasia or dislocation of the hip. Survivorship analysis and long term results. *J Bone Joint Surg.* 1997;79A: 1352–1360.

34. Paul JP. Approaches to design: force actions transmitted by joints in the human body. *Proc Res Soc Lond.* 1976;192:163–172.

35. Pooley C, Tabor D. Friction and molecular structure: the behavior of some thermoplastics. *Proc R Soc Lond.* 1972;329A:251.

36. Ramamurti BS, Bragdon CR, O'Connor DO, et al. Loci of movement of selected points on the femoral head during normal gait. Three-dimensional computer simulation. *J Arthroplasty.* 1996;11:845–852.

37. Ramamurti BS, Estok DM, Jasty M, et al. Analysis of the kinematics of different hip simulators used to study wear of candidate materials for the articulation of total hip arthroplasties. *J Orthop Res.* 1998;16:365–369.

38. Rydell NM. Forces acting on the femoral head-prosthesis. *Acta Orthop Scand Suppl.* 1996;88:113–124.

39. Saikko V, Paavolainen P, Kleimola M, et al. A five-station hip joint simulator for rate studies. *Proc Inst Mech Eng.* 1992;206:195–200.

40. Saikko VO, Paavolainen PO, Slatis P. Wear of the polyethylene acetabular cup. Metallic and ceramic heads compared in a hip simulator. *Acta Orthop Scand.* 1993;64:391–402.

41. Sarojak M, Hoff WA, Komistek RD, et al. An interactive system for kinematic analysis of artificial joint implants. *Biomed Sci Instr.* 1999;35:9–14.

42. Schmalzried TP, Peters PC, Maurer BT, et al. Long-duration metal-on-metal total hip arthroplasties with low wear of the articulating surfaces. *J Arthroplasty.* 1996;11:322–331.

43. Seireg A, Arvikar RJ. A mathematical model for evaluation of forces in lower extremities of the musculo-skeletal system. *J Biomech.* 1973;6:313–326.

44. Seireg A, Arvikar RJ. The prediction of muscular load sharing and joint forces in the lower extremities during walking. *J Biomech.* 1975;8:89–102.

45. Sochart DH, Porter ML. The long term results of Charnley low-friction arthroplasty in young patients who have congenital dislocation, degenerative osteoarthrosis, or rheumatoid arthritis. *J Bone Joint Surg.* 1997;79A:1599–1617.

46. Taylor SJ, Perry JS, Meswania JM, et al. Telemetry of forces from proximal femoral replacements and relevance to fixation. *J Biomech.* 1997;30:225–234.

47. Torchia ME, Klassen RA, Bianco AJ. Total hip arthroplasty with cement in patients less than twenty years old. *J Bone Joint Surg.* 1996;78A:995–1003.

48. Wright KWJ, Scales JT. The use of hip joint simulators for the evaluation of wear of total hip prosthesis. In: Winter GD, Leray JL, deGroot K, eds. *Evaluation of Biomaterials.* Chichester, UK: John Wiley and Sons; 1977:135–146.

49. Yamaguchi M, Bauer TW, Hashimoto Y. Three dimensional analysis of multiple wear vectors in retrieved acetabular cups. *J Bone Joint Surg.* 1997;79A:1539–1544.

Biomaterials Overview

7

Jonathan Black   Brett Levine   Joshua Jacobs

A biomaterial is "any substance, other than a drug, or combination of substances, synthetic or natural in origin, which can be used for any period of time, as a whole or as a part of a system which treats, augments, or replaces any tissue, organ or function of the body" (22). Therefore, when an engineer sets out to design a new implant to be used in total joint arthroplasty, and when a surgeon uses such a device to treat a patient, both are making use of a variety of biomaterials.

The selection of specific biomaterials for any device represents the result of a large number of interactions, but the most central recurring theme can be expressed in a reciprocal relationship: specific designs require specific materials; new materials enable new designs.

Some conclusions can be drawn directly from this reciprocal relationship. There can be no "best biomaterial" for the fabrication of a total hip replacement (THR) device, or even for the fabrication of any one component. The choices made for each part, including the composition, processing, and forming of the materials, represent a compromise between the ideals of the design and the realities of available biomaterials.

Because design is essentially an open-ended process, limited only by imagination, whereas fabrication requires the use of real materials, the process of designing and producing present and future THR components is properly described as "materials limited." Thus, it is easy to say, in contradiction of Charnley, who stated, "Objectives must be reasonable. Neither surgeon nor engineers can ever make an artificial hip-joint that will last thirty years and at some time in this period enable the patient to play football" (9), that we would indeed like a THR that would last for 30 years and permit the patient to play football. However, the problem becomes far more real when we then ask which biomaterials show satisfactory biologic performance (i.e., resistance to material degradation and acceptable host response to the material and its degradation products) so that they will perform as an articulating bearing pair in a THR for 30 years. As of today, we cannot answer this query definitively, despite the more than a third of a century of increasingly successful clinical application of THR since Charnley's 1961 paper (9) heralded the beginning of the new age of hip reconstruction arthroplasty.

Because design approaches and materials choices are reciprocally linked, design changes are more likely than not to require altered or different materials. Thus, if a THR device is optimized for a particular patient population, through engineering design, in vitro testing, and evolutionary clinical experience, significant changes in either the design or the design objectives probably require concomitant changes in materials selection and/or processing and forming, to provide optimum performance. The change of a fixation system, such as replacing polymethyl methacrylate (PMMA) ("bone cement") by a porous or structured surface coating to promote fixation by biologic ingrowth, has far more significance than the choice of an ice cream flavor, and it should be treated more seriously than is often the case. Although a specific design change may or may not result in improved clinical performance of one aspect of the device (in this case, the desired more reliable fixation of the component to the surrounding bone), it cannot be assumed that all other aspects of the device's performance remain unchanged. The recognition that porous or structured surfaces of femoral medullary stems are potential sources of third-body wear debris found associated with retrieved articular surfaces illustrates this point (18).

Because the properties of the materials strongly influence both initial design choices and eventual device performance, changes in these properties, both during fabrication and processing (including sterilization) and after implantation, may be expected to alter device performance. It is unfortunate that even today we know very little about such property changes during the now typically long life of a device within a patient's body. Serious consideration of the role that biomaterials play in the success or failure of surgical procedures involving permanent implants, such as THRs, should involve a greater sensitivity to the study of the properties both of clinically failed devices (removed and retrieved at revision) and of successful ones (recovered at autopsy) than has been shown to date.

Unfortunately, such studies are still rare, and they are sketchy at best, primarily because of a widespread inability to track and recover THR components with known "pedigrees" for materials analysis and study (17).

Nevertheless, biomaterials have contributed significantly to the stunning late 20th century medical success represented by THR arthroplasty. The latter portions of this chapter will discuss the generic (bio)materials requirements of THR devices and the choices of such materials in contemporary clinical practice and will reflect on some of the historical developments that have contributed to the present situation.

Much has been done and achieved, but real and challenging problems remain in the application of biomaterials to the alleviation of disease and disability of the adult hip. Later chapters deal specifically with various aspects of biomaterials selection and performance in THR arthroplasty.

THE TOTAL HIP REPLACEMENT PROSTHESIS AS A SYSTEM

Elements of the Total Hip Replacement Prosthesis

So-called replacement surgery of the hip is the result of a clinical decision, made jointly by the surgeon and patient, that dysfunction of the hip has progressed to a sufficient degree that such a radical procedure is the therapy of choice. The clinical hallmarks leading to this decision include pain, pain-limitation of active and passive motion (and, as a result, loss of function), physical reduction of passive range of motion, and x-ray or other imaging evidence of loss of joint space, deformation of the femoral head and/or acetabular socket, and significant change in bone quality or loss of bone stock. For the sake of this analysis, the etiology of such symptoms and diagnostic findings are of little importance. The engineer in association with the surgeon must deal with two significant physical deficits: loss of tribological quality and changes in physical configuration of the hip joint.

Therefore, the primary design goal for a THR device can be stated as follows: this permanent device will be used, as a part of a surgical implantation procedure, to alleviate pain and improve function of the hip joint through restoration of the geometry and bearing quality of the articulating interface. The general secondary design goals, in no particular order in the following list, are those sought in any engineering design solution:

■ Simplicity (in both design and use—in this case, surgical insertion)
■ Parsimony (expressed as a desire to sacrifice the minimum amount of healthy tissue)
■ Manufacturability
■ Cost (not traditionally considered in biomedical applications, but being rendered increasingly important by a general societal drive to restrain the rising costs of medical care)
■ Safety (especially with regard to potential malfunction and failure)
■ Durability
■ Serviceability (expressed through maximizing options and minimizing technical barriers to surgical replacement of failed THR components)

It is not possible to state specific secondary, but important, design goals for particular patient populations because of the many factors involved, including surgical philosophy; patient age, weight, and sex; causation of patient's disease; concurrent (pre-existing) disease conditions; patient expectations; job and family status; local standard of practice; and cultural and religious issues.

An example of the difficulty of generalizing secondary design goals arises from the use of the term "permanent" in the previous statement of the primary design goal. The act of removing the natural joint and replacing it with nonresorbing biomaterials implies that the THR device, like its natural predecessor, is implicitly expected to last for the remaining life of the patient. In fact, the use of the term "total joint replacement" conveys this assumption semantically. This may be a reasonable goal for a low-demand individual with a life expectancy of 10 years or less. However, it is currently an unrealistic goal for the high-demand patient (Charnley's sometime football player) with a life expectancy of 25 or more years. In the latter case, the primary goal of permanency has to yield grudgingly to secondary goals of safety (in modes of failure) and other features that will maximize surgical options during possible revision surgery. Similarly, even for age- and disease-matched patients, specific design goals probably should be different for devices intended for primary arthroplasty and those used in revision of failed primary (and secondary) arthroplasties.

However, the primary design goal of restoration of the geometry and bearing quality of the hip joint leads to the recognition that all THR devices involve two primary components (femoral and acetabular), each assembled from three elements (Fig. 7-1).

On the femoral side, the femoral component consists of the following:

■ An element to restore the articulating surface property and geometry of the femoral head (the articulation element)
■ An element to anchor (fix) the restored surface to the proximal femur (the fixation element)
■ An element to couple the articulation element and the fixation element, and to maintain an appropriate structural relationship between them (the structural element)

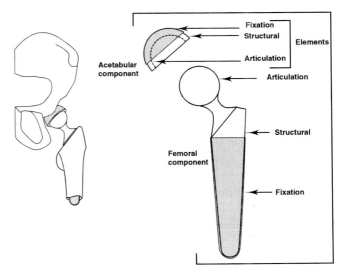

Figure 7-1 Generic total hip replacement device, showing components and elements.

Similarly, on the acetabular side, the acetabular component consists of the following:

- An element to restore the articulating surface property and geometry of the acetabular socket (the articulation element)
- An element to anchor (fix) the restored surface to the peri-acetabular pelvis (the fixation element)
- An element to couple the articulation element and the fixation element, and to maintain an appropriate structural relationship between them (the structural element)

While each of these two components may have more than one physical part, each of those parts may be assigned to one or more of the functional elements. Thus a PMMA-cemented all-metal one-piece (monoblock) femoral component contains the same three functional elements as a complex multipart modular device, with a metal stem, fixation pads, space-filling collars or wedges, a hydroxyapatite coating, and a ceramic femoral head. Therefore, the following discussion will focus on the requirements for femoral and acetabular components through a generic analysis of functional elements.

Materials Requirements

General

Materials used in THR device components are, by the previous definition, biomaterials. The primary requirement of a biomaterial, which sets it apart from materials used in all other engineering applications, is that it be biocompatible. Biocompatibility is defined as "the ability of a material to perform with an appropriate host response in a specific application" (2). On the negative side, this is to say that the material and its degradation products must evoke no more than a tolerable level of local, systemic, and remote side effects, consistent with the intended function of the device. On the positive side, the material (and its intrinsic structure) must evoke suitable (and intended) responses, such as adhesion and ingrowth. Space does not permit a full explication of this subject. The reader is referred to work by Black (2,5) for general principles, and to work by Friedman et al. (18) for more recent specific considerations.

In consideration of biocompatibility, it is extremely important to recognize both the initial interactions between the implanted biomaterials and the host (patient), and the later possible interactions involving released or altered materials. Materials that may arise from implanted THR components include monomer released by PMMA cement (27), corrosion products released by metals (4), and wear debris released by metals, polymers, and ceramics, by chemical degradation, direct articulation, and interfacial fretting (24).

Later chapters deal with biocompatibility in more detail. Suffice it to say here that considerations are usually given to the possibilities of causation or exacerbation of either local or remote site inflammatory, cytotoxic, infective, specific immune, and neoplastic transformation responses. The delicacy of homeostasis in human tissues is the major limiting factor in biomaterials selection. Thus, evaluation of present and new materials for specific designs tends to consider biocompatibility first, with engineering requirements addressed after these initial concerns are answered through theoretical analysis, cell culture screening studies in vitro, and nonfunc-

tional, as well as, in some cases, functional in vivo tests in animal models (2).

Femoral Component

The femoral component replaces the natural femoral head, portions or all of the femoral neck, and bony elements in the proximal femur between the greater and lesser trochanters. Furthermore, it supplants to some degree the load-carrying role of the proximal femur, because load sharing between remaining natural bone and the intramedullary portion of the femoral component occurs down to the distal limit of fixation. These anatomic considerations impose significant mechanical requirements on the structural element. Beyond being strong enough to not break under single peak loads, which may be as much as 5 times body weight (typically 3 to 3.5 kilonewtons [kN]), it must also not deform irreversibly (plastically) while resisting brittle (fatigue) fracture under dynamic loading of 1 to 2 million cycles per year. (5) This suggests that, so far as the structural aspect of the femoral stem is concerned, stronger is better. Unfortunately, this familiar catch phrase overlooks two important features of materials behavior.

First, the ability to resist fracture depends not just on strength but also on toughness, the ability to absorb energy elastically without failure. Thus, a weaker but tougher material will generally perform better under the bending loads imposed on the proximal stem and neck than a stronger but more brittle material. This has led to favoring metals as structural biomaterials in the femoral component.

Second, intrinsic stiffness, as described by the elastic modulus, increases with increasing strength. Thus a strong component is stiffer than a weaker one of the identical configuration. However, stiffer femoral components reduce peak stress in bone adjacent to the intramedullary stem, particularly in the proximal medial (or calcar) region of the femoral cortex. Interest in reducing this stress-shielding effect has tended in recent years to favor titanium alloys over stainless steels and cobalt-based alloys, because the former have elastic moduli about one half of the latter. This desire is also seen as one motivating factor in ongoing attempts to develop lower-modulus titanium-based alloys (the beta alloys) and still-lower-modulus fiber or particulate reinforced polymer matrix composites (see the section "Future Developments").

The bearing geometry favored in THR designs is a ball-and-socket arrangement of highly congruent, concentric articulating elements. This does not anatomically replace the relatively incongruent geometry of the natural hip, but it does permit restoration of a full range of motion. However, selection of such a geometry dictates the use of materials for the articulation surface that are hard, strong, and abrasion resistant, in contrast to normal articular cartilage, which is soft, weak, and abradable. It is also desirable to minimize the coefficient of friction of the bearing pair (at the femoral–acetabular interface), so as to reduce to a minimum the transmission of twisting forces (torques) to the fixation elements of both components. Despite historical concern for this problem (13), termed "stiction" friction, most modern materials pairs with satisfactory wear resistance and intrinsic strength apparently possess sufficiently low coefficients of friction in the reconstructed hip that it does not represent a selection criterion.

Far more critical is the desire to minimize wear. Except for early experience and occasional elevated wear during or subsequent to device failure, the problem is not of loss of bearing performance caused by wear but of adverse biologic response to the resulting debris. Thus, the selection criteria, with respect to the articulation element, are dominated by the desire to minimize the volume of resulting wear debris.

The aim of fixation is to mechanically join the structural element of the THR to the bone in a manner that preserves the integrity of both materials. Even with the best design and selection from among currently available biomaterials, the intramedullary portion of the femoral stem is structurally stiffer than the surrounding remaining corticocancellous shell of the proximal femur. There are three engineering approaches to solving the problem of stress transfer across such a stiffness discontinuity (5). The two materials may be joined by a direct, rigid bond, with a stiffer interposed member to limit deformation; they may be connected by an interposed material with a continuously varying or graded stiffness so as to reduce peak shear stresses; or they may be isolated by a very compliant later that can sustain high shear strain without failure. Of these three approaches, only two (graded and compliant) are currently invoked in THR arthroplasty. (The direct approach is rejected because it would necessarily lead to unacceptable levels of stress shielding.)

These engineering approaches have been resolved into four fixation designs:

Press-fitting. This is essentially fixation by absence of fixation, in which macrogeometrical features of the femoral component are secured by direct hard-tissue apposition. In this case, the design goal is to achieve and maintain local tissue stresses within a range that causes neither atrophy (by too low a stress) nor necrosis (by too high a stress). Press-fitting usually results, in the long term, in the production of an interposing soft tissue layer, and thus, despite absence of any real degree of component–tissue cohesion, it should be recognized as compliant bonding.

Cement. One of Charnley's contributions (8) to THR arthroplasty was the introduction of cure-in-situ PMMA which, although nonadhesive, is a space-filling agent that reduces peak stresses by distributing loads. Because the elastic moduli of the cements currently used (PMMA and its variants) are all less than those of cortical bone and of metallic biomaterials, this is also an example of compliant fixation. More recent experiments, with cements preadhered to the metal substrates ("precoat") and the addition of biologically active materials, such as hydroxyapatite, to the cement, introduce some elements of direct adhesion (see later) producing secondary graded bonds.

Ingrowth. In this case, fixation is brought about by configuring the surface of the structural element into an open porous layer so that bony tissue will grow into its interstices. This ingrown tissue then provides resistance to shear and, to a lesser degree, tensile displacement. Because such configured surfaces have a lower density (and thus are less stiff) than the metallic substrate, and because the bone frequently responds by remodeling to a more porous structure (cancellization), this form of fixation is regarded as a graded bond. An alternative, in which the substrate is merely roughened, without physically interlocking porosity, produces a similar result, but the biologic process is termed ongrowth rather than ingrowth and affords negligible tensile resistance. In both cases, the important selection criteria are that the surface be "friendly"

to in- or ongrowing osteoid and bone and that the features be large enough (75 to 100 μm minimum opening) (38) to permit the maturation of osteonal bone within the fixation element.

Adhesion. The final case is that of provision of a surface fixation element to which bone will actually adhere, presumably through some form of (as yet unclearly defined) chemical bonding process. Historically, only pure titanium and pure tantalum were known to evoke this response. However, recently calcium hydroxyapatite (CaHAP), as well as some chemically related crystalline and glassy materials, has been shown to produce direct adhesion. The principal design criterion appears to be good (strong) adhesion of the surface layer to the substrate. In the case of CaHAP and related materials, there is an interesting tradeoff of properties: the more crystalline materials are stronger but evoke more modest biologically responses, whereas the more amorphous materials are more biologically active but considerably weaker and more soluble (40). In any case, the cancellization of bone behind the bone–biomaterial interface produces an overall compliant bond structure, although the actual bonded biomaterial–tissue interface is probably quite stiff.

Acetabular Component

The requirements for the elements of the acetabular component are quite similar to those for the femoral component, with some slight but possibly significant differences. The articulation element requirements are identical, because the performance of the articulating (bearing) pair is defined by the combination of materials chosen for its two elements. The structural element requirements are somewhat less demanding, because the domed shape of the acetabular structural element provides some intrinsic stiffening, and the loads are more compressive and hooplike (tensile) in nature than in the femoral stem where bending (tension/compression) dominates. The fixation element requirements are very similar but less extreme than those on the femoral component, because loading across the fixation element–tissue interface is more compressive and demonstrates less shear than in the femoral medullary shaft.

Contemporary Materials Selection

General

The general requirements, taken with specific requirements for individual elements of components, have restricted the biomaterials used in contemporary designs of THR devices to little more than a dozen, including 15 metallic alloys, 3 polymers, and 4 ceramics (Table 7-1). Table 7-2 shows that, of the possible 132 applications (22 materials × 6 elements), less than half have been found to be successful.

Femoral Component

Figure 7-2 shows, with horizontal or inclined link lines, the materials choices and combinations thought to be in use today or that are currently considered technological feasible.

Fixation on the femoral side is now divided between PMMA-cemented components, and uncemented ones with or without surface features (e.g., porosity) and with or without CaHAP coatings. Choices for the metal for fabrication of the structural element are also varied; however, there appears to be a preference for titanium-based alloys for uncemented designs and cobalt-based (and stainless steel outside of the

TABLE 7-1

BIOMATERIALS USED IN CONTEMPORARY THR ARTHROPLASTY COMPONENTS

ASTM Designation[a]	Material[b]
F-67	Unalloyed (CP) titanium
F-75	Cast cobalt–chromium–molybdenum alloy (Co28.5Cr6Mo)[c]
F-90	Wrought cobalt–chromium–tungsten–nickel alloy (Co20Cr10Ni15W)
F-136	Wrought titanium alloy (Ti6Al4V–ELI)
F-451	Polymethyl methacrylate cement (PMMA)
F-560	Unalloyed tantalum
F-562	Wrought cobalt–nickel–chromium–molybdenum alloy (Co35Ni20Cr10Mo) [MP35N]
F-563	Wrought cobalt–nickel–chromium–molybdenum–tungsten–iron alloy (Co20Ni20Cr3.5Mo3.5W5Fe) [Syncoben]
F-603	Dense aluminum oxide [alumina]
F-648	Ultrahigh molecular weight polyethylene [UHMWPE]
F-1185	Calcium hydroxyapatite ($Ca_{10}(PO_4)_6(OH)_2$) [HA]
F-1295	Wrought titanium–aluminum–niobium alloy (Ti6Al7Nb)
F-1314	Wrought nitrogen containing stainless steel (Fe22Cr12.5Ni5Mn2.5Moo.4N) [Ortron 90]
F-1472	Wrought titanium alloy (Ti6Al4V)
F-1537	Wrought cobalt–chromium–molybdenum alloy (Co28Cr6Mo)
F-1579	Polyaryletherketone [PAEK]
F-1713	Titanium–niobium–zirconium alloy (Ti13Nb13Zr)
F-1813	Wrought titanium–molybdenum–zirconium–iron alloy (Ti12Mo6Zr2Fe)
F-1873	Dense yttria tetragonal zirconium oxide polycrystal [Y-TZP]
F-2066	Wrought titanium–molybdenum alloy (Ti15Mo)
F-2384	Zirconium–niobium (Zr2.5Nb) [Oxinium]
F-2393	Dense magnesia partially stabilized zirconium oxide [Mg-PSZ]

[a]ASTM specifications for biomaterials have the form "F NNNN-MM," where (19)MM is the year last revised; this suffix is omitted here for simplicity.
[b]Not title of standard: please see reference 1 for full title and latest revision date.
[c]Numbers preceding chemical symbol indicate nominal weight percent of element.
ASTM, American Society for Testing and Materials; CP, commercially pure; ELI, extra-low interstitial (high purity) grade; square brackets enclose commonly used (or trademark) abbreviations or names. Data from ref. (1).

United States) for cemented designs. The use of cast cobalt-chromium (CoCr) and stainless steel (SS) articulation elements is now mostly restricted to older monobloc designs. Newer designs, in which the head is separate from the stem and joined to it by a conical trunnion (structural element side) friction fitted into a mating bore (articulation element side), provide the option of using wrought cobalt-based alloys as well as alumina and zirconia. Ceramic articulation elements, while popular in European and worldwide markets, still constitute only quite a small percentage of U.S. usage.

Today in the United States, the most popular choices of materials for the femoral component are titanium-based or cobalt-based alloy structural elements, combined with wrought modular CoCr or CoCrMo articulation elements and a variety of fixation elements, with uncemented designs probably dominating.

Acetabular Component

Fixation on the acetabular side was, from the early 1960s through the 1980s, primarily by PMMA cementation. Within the last two decades, the use of uncemented designs, involving threaded, structured, or porous surfaces, in some cases including CaHAP coatings, has been growing rapidly, especially in light of the increasing evidence of the progressive loosening of PMMA-cemented all–ultrahigh molecular weight polyethylene (UHMWPE) designs, implanted with older, less sophisticated techniques than in use today, in the post-10-year time period. The choice for the structural element of acetabular components is still primarily UHMWPE, combined in most cases with a thin titanium, titanium-based, or cobalt-based alloy shell. This latter combination allows the use of a variety of uncemented fixation technologies, because UHMWPE performs poorly in direct contact with bone and has not as yet been successfully coated with CaHAP or other adhesion materials. UHMWPE is still the gold standard for the articulation element, but, as indicated above, there is increasing interest, within and outside the United States, in actual clinical use of alumina and wrought CoCrMo, each articulated on the femoral side and with itself, respectively.

Today in the United States, the most popular choices of materials for the acetabular component are titanium-based or cobalt-based alloy structural elements, combined with

TABLE 7-2

APPLICATION OF BIOMATERIALS TO CONTEMPORARY THR ARTHROPLASTY COMPONENTS

ASTM Designation	Common Name	Articular	Structural	Fixation	Articular	Structural	Fixation
Metals							
F-67	CP Ti	—	√	√[a]	—	—	√[a]
F-75	Cast CoCr	—	√	√	√	√	√
F-90	Wrt. CoCr	—	√	√	√	√	√
F-136	Ti6Al4VELI	—	√	√	—	√	√
F-560	Tantalum	—	√	√[a]	—	—	√[a]
F-562	MP35N	—	√	—	—	√	—
F-563	—	—	—	—	—	—	—
F-1295	Ti6Al7Nb	—	√	—	—	√	—
F-1314	High N SS	—	—	—	√[b]	√[b]	—
F-1472	Wrought Ti6Al4V	—	√	—	—	√	—
F-1537	Wrought CoCrMo	√	√	—	√	√	—
F-1713	Ti13Nb13Zr	—	√	√	—	√	√
F-1813	Wrought Ti12Mo6Zr2Fe	—	√	√	—	√	√
F-2066	Wrought Ti15Mo	—	√	√	—	√	√
F-2384	Zr2.5Nb	—	—	—	√[d]	√[c]	—
Polymers							
F-451	PMMA	—	—	√	—	—	√
F-648	UHMWPE	√	√	—	—	—	—
F-1579	PAEK	—	—	—	—	—	√[a]
Ceramics							
F-603	Aluminum oxide (alumina Al_2O_3)	√	√[b]	—	√	√[c]	—
F-1185	Hydroxylapatite (CaHAP)	—	—	√	—	—	√
F-1873	Zirconium oxide, yttria stabilized (zirconia-ZrO_2-Y-TZP)	√[b]	√[b]	—	√[b]	√[b]	—
F-2393	Zirconium oxide, magnesia stabilized (zirconia-ZrO_2-Mg-PSZ)	√[b]	√[b]	—	√[b]	√[b]	—

[a]Applied to a different metal alloy substrate (e.g., F-136, F-1472).
[b]Not in use in the United States, but in use elsewhere.
[c]Used as a modular component on metal alloy stem (e.g., F-90).
[d]Used in articulation only with UHMWPE.

UHMWPE articulation inserts and a variety of fixation elements, with uncemented technologies clearly dominating.

HISTORICAL DEVELOPMENT

Structural (Body) Materials

The history of THR replacement arthroplasty stretches back past the successes of Charnley to earlier eras of less successful total joint replacement, partial joint replacement, and, in the beginning, interposition arthroplasty. In these early experiments, there was no distinction between structural, articulation, and fixation elements, as a single material was used to fabricate each component, and few, if any, attempts were made to achieve fixation beyond physical retention of the component in the anatomic position in which it was placed. Early efforts to obtain useful synthetic interposition materials included chromization (tanning) or silver impregnation of tissues of human or animal origin, including epidermis, muscle, and fascia lata. More durable manufactured materials included zinc, silver, gold, magnesium, wax, lanolin, and rubber, in sheet or plate form (6).

Most of these efforts proved successful only in the short term until the clinical developments begun by Marius Smith-Petersen in 1923 (37). Being impressed by the pseudosynovial sheath surrounding a glass fragment that he had removed from a patient, Smith-Petersen had "mould" (cup) arthroplasties fabricated from a variety of glassy and polymeric materials. These were marginally successful until he began to use a cast cobalt-based alloy, Vitallium™. (*Note:* In the older literature, the term "vitallium" is used incorrectly to characterize all cobalt-based alloys. It is a registered trademark and can be used appropriately only to describe F-75 and F-90, when manufactured by a licensed vendor.) This alloy was developed in 1929 for dental applications and introduced into orthopedic surgery about 1938 (41). The cup arthroplasty was originally intended to be implanted temporarily to enable re-formation of cartilage on the head of the femur and within the acetabular cup. However, the excellent tolerance to the cobalt-based alloy cups, and the disappointing results after their surgical removal, led Smith-Petersen to leave them in place.

Cast CoCr (F-75 derived from Haynes 25) and low-carbon cast SS (F-55 derived from type 316) dominated the early days

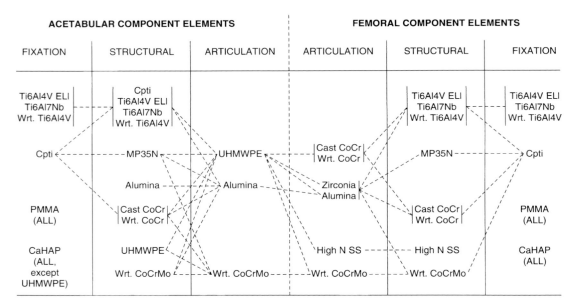

Figure 7-2 Combination of biomaterials in elements of THR components. Dashed horizontal and inclined link lines indicate known uses and/or presumed satisfactory combinations. Please refer to Table 7-2 for differences in U.S. usage. Wrt., wrought.

of THR arthroplasty. Improved versions of both alloys were produced over the years. Charnley in 1959 began to use a forged version of F-55 and later, sometime in the 1980s, adopted a still stronger high-nitrogen SS (F-1314) (36). In the cobalt-based alloys systems, later development included newer, high-strength CoNiCrMo (with nickel) (F-562), CoNiCrMoW (with tungsten) (F-563), and CoCrMo (F-1537) alloys.

Titanium-based alloys first came into use in the form of the well-known aviation alloy, Ti6A14V (F-136, originally not of high interstitial [ELI] purity) at the Royal National Orthopaedic Hospital (Stanmore, United Kingdom) in 1964 in the fabrication of femoral endoprostheses (12), and in femoral components articulating against UHMWPE by Sarmiento et al. in 1970 (34). Original components were of monobloc design, but concern about observations of poor wear behavior in vitro (21), and of significant tissue discoloration in vivo (metallosis) associated with loose THRs, led to the first significant adoption of modularity, with provision of, initially, cast CoCr (F-75) femoral heads. Later developments include improving alloy purity (development of ELI grades), devising forging variants (F-1471), and a vanadium-free alloy, Ti6A17Nb (F-1295).

Articular Surfaces

There is very little history to recount here. Thompson (39) and Moore (32) developed endofemoral versions of the cup arthroplasty with intramedullary stems, using both the cast CoCr and the less expensive SS. Early versions of two-component THRs, as we know them today, evolved through the combination of these and similar femoral endoprostheses with the Smith-Petersen cup and other designs. Thus, the original articulation in multicomponent THR devices was metal–metal.

McKee and Watson-Farrar (31), Ring (33), Hüggler et al. (42), and others developed specifically designed, mating acetabular and femoral components, but they retained, until very recently, the use of these two alloys, best described as ASTM F-75 and F-55.

The adoption of polyethylene (PE) (initially high density and then quite soon afterward ultrahigh molecular weight) by Charnley (after an abortive experience with a polytetrafluoroethylene material) marks the true beginning of the modern success of THR arthroplasty (10).

Many efforts have been made to provide articulation surfaces that are more satisfactory in the long run, primarily through reduction in annual production of wear debris and, as a presumed result, reduction in intermediate and late-term osteolysis. No polymers have been found that are superior to UHMWPE. In the late 1990s highly cross-linked UHMWPE was introduced as an alternative to "conventional" PE, with the promise of reduced wear and enhanced prosthesis survivorship. There are at least six new highly cross-linked PE variations currently available, all with slight variations in radiation dose, technique, and sequence; sterilization method; and extent of free radical extraction with thermal treatments. The overall effects of cross-linking include reductions in the wear rate and alteration of the mechanical properties of the PE so that with increased levels of radiation there is a decrease in the fracture toughness. While early results for modern highly cross-linked PE have been promising, long-term studies are still pending (28).

In 1970, Boutin (7) began to experiment with alumina–alumina articulations in patients, and in 1988, in a return to the past, Weber et al. (42) reintroduced the then almost completely abandoned metal–metal articulation with use of a wrought CoCrMo (F-1537) alloy. There are to date no long-term prospective, randomized clinical studies that compare the outcome of such promising articulations with that of conventional UHMWPE–metal articulations, uncomplicated by differences in structural and fixation element design, surgical technique, and patient selection.

Even more conservative changes, such as the pairing of alumina (since 1977) (35) and yttria-stabilized zirconia (late 1980s) (11) with UHMWPE, have been slow to be widely adopted. Despite evidence that alumina–UHMWPE probably shows a 25% to 50% or greater reduction in annual volumetric polymeric debris production in comparison to metal–UHMWPE (22), there also is no clinical proof of benefit as yet. Furthermore, high costs for modular ceramic femoral heads (in comparison to wrought cobalt-based alloy heads) and lingering concerns about brittle fracture retard their adoption in the United States. The recent withdrawal of zirconia heads from the U.S. market has also somewhat decreased the enthusiasm for use of ceramic bearings.

Fixation Systems

Initial efforts, from the era of interposition arthroplasty, through the use of Smith-Petersen cups and early metal–metal THRs, involved what we today call press-fit fixation. Charnley, utilizing a cure-in-situ PMMA that had been used as a space filler and internal fixation material, introduced the use of PMMA-cemented fixation in 1958 (9). Later developments included adding radiopacifiers, such as barium sulfate or zirconia, and modifying the polymeric chemistry.

Ingrowth fixation was originated clinically by Judet et al. (25) and by Lord and Bancel (29), who used casting technologies to form surface structures on SS and CoCr bases, respectively. Porous commercially pure (CP) titanium mesh was introduced by Galante and Rostocker in 1971 (20), while the more familiar modern multilayered sintered beaded surfaces (on cobalt-based alloys) were developed by Welsh et al. (43) and used clinically by Rayan and Booker (38) and by Engh and Bobyn (14) beginning in 1978.

Porous tantalum has also been recently introduced as a biocompatible and low modulus of elasticity metal that can be fashioned into various forms of orthopaedic implants. Tantalum is a transitional metal with a long history of biocompatibility, having been used in pacemaker electrodes, cranioplasty plates, and as radiopaque markers. (3) This metal represents an open-cell tantalum structure with repeating dodecahedrons that appears similar to trabecular bone upon direct visualization. Early reports of monoblock and modular components have shown promising results.

CaHAP was used as a bulk material to augment or replace bone in dental applications, beginning commercially in 1981 (30). It was first used clinically as an adhesion fixation material by Furlong and Osborne in 1985 (19), as a relatively thick (200 μm), low-crystallinity coating. The more modern, thinner (50 to 60 μm) coating was introduced clinically by Geesink in 1986 (15,23).

FUTURE DEVELOPMENTS

Hope springs eternal in the minds and hearts of orthopedic bioengineers and surgeons. With THR arthroplasty a highly successful procedure for the short and intermediate (10 to 15 years) term, the key to extension of this success to 20 to 25 years is widely regarded as improvement in the materials for construction of the mechanical components of the reconstruction. As a result, the late 1990s and early 2000s has been an era of remarkable innovation and development in orthopedic biomaterials. We will briefly summarize ongoing developments, with some comments on their strong and weak points. Citations are deliberately omitted here, because the field is evolving rapidly, and we do not wish to appear to favor one set of investigators over another in any area of development. A brief search of the current literature will provide suitable additional resources to expand upon these remarks.

Structural Materials

As previously mentioned, there is interest in two major areas. The titanium-based alloys, Ti6A14V and Ti6A17Nb, are called α–β alloys, because each contains a mixture of two physically and chemically different structures or phases. A group of new alloys that have a single uniform structure (called β alloys) is under development. These alloys have stiffnesses (elastic moduli) between two thirds and one half the stiffness of α–β alloys. As indicated, this is thought to be desirable because, in comparable designs, lower moduli could contribute to reduced stress shielding, especially in the proximal femoral shaft. However, these materials, lacking the internally stressed structure of α–β alloys, are apparently less strong, both in single-cycle and fatigue–failure modes.

Still less stiff (more flexible) materials have been produced by the use of polyaramide (Kevlar™) and carbon fibers and woven fabrics to reinforce polysulfone, polyether etherketone (PEEK), and polyaryletherketone (PAEK) thermoplastic polymer matrices. These composites are theoretically very attractive structural materials, as their elastic moduli are close to those of cortical bone. However, some have proven disappointing in early tests because of their lack of interphase bonding (between reinforcing and matrix phases) and their poor resistance to surface damage by bone and fixation materials. On the other hand, a composite of CoCr metal, PAEK, and CP Ti fiber metal has been approved for use in the United States and is currently in clinical use (26).

Fixation Materials

There are continuing efforts to modify PMMA cements by adding reinforcing phases, such as polymeric fibers, and in some cases, biologically active phases such as CaHAP granules. In either case, there is a trade off between enhanced strength and bonding ability and decreased handling and bone-penetration properties, respectively. There is some interest in nonpolymeric cements that would set in place (as do Portland cements in construction applications) and, perhaps, also be able to adhere directly to tissue. All of these developments are in very early stages and are too immature to evaluate critically.

Articulation Materials

Despite more than 30 years of effort, no polymeric materials superior to UHMWPE have yet been found. Current development efforts, focusing on evolutionary improvement of UHMWPE, through efforts to increase intermolecular bonding (cross-linking), have proven promising, in in vitro evaluation and in early clinical trials.

There is currently great interest in hard-on-hard bearing systems. The leading materials, alumina (F-603) for ceramic–ceramic systems and CoCrMo for metal–metal systems, are now well established in Europe, and efforts in this area are focusing more on bearing design and surface treatments than on further materials modifications. There continues to be interest in application of wear-resistant ceramic surface coatings, such as zirconia or pure-carbon diamondlike materials, to metallic substrates. Here again, early enthusiasm is tempered by recognition of accelerated wear, associated with film disruption, in in vitro studies. Recently, an oxygen diffusion–hardened zirconium–niobium alloy has been approved in the United States as a femoral articulating surface and is currently in clinical use. Long-term data on its clinical wear performance is not yet available (16).

CONCLUDING REMARKS

The following chapters expand on many of the points outlined here, providing substance and, in some cases, conflicting views. What all the authors would no doubt agree on is that, overall, THR arthroplasty is a remarkably successful procedure, both in comparison to other orthopedic procedures and to implantation procedures in other surgical specialties, such as cardiovascular and plastic surgery. All those who have contributed to this success should feel a great deal of satisfaction for a job (almost) well done.

The engineering, surgical, and legal environments have changed significantly since Charnley began to define the modern PMMA-cemented metal–polymer THR device in the late 1950s. The experience with many less successful and a very few perhaps more successful designs has encouraged both patients and medical professionals to enjoy heightened expectations of what is possible, both in terms of function and longevity, from THR arthroplasty. The reality is that for the current clinical population, highly satisfactory life-time results can be obtained for at least 75% of patients, with currently available components and reliable clinical histories (44). In the necessary pursuit of solutions for the remaining patients, largely younger and higher-demand individuals, in the desire to obtain improved and new biomaterials to optimize present designs and permit new designs of THR components, we must be careful not to seize failure from the jaws of success.

ACKNOWLEDGMENTS

This chapter is based on untold numbers of (and, in many cases, at least partly forgotten) discussions with students and colleagues over the past decades. We thank them for their insights and wish to recognize particularly the contributions of Howard Freese and Paul Serekian, who had an opportunity to review and comment on an early draft of portions of this chapter.

REFERENCES

1. ASTM. *2005 Annual Book of ASTM Standards. 13.01: Medical Devices; Emergency Medical Services.* West Conshohocken: American Society for Testing and Materials; 2005.
2. Black J. *Biological Performance of Materials: Fundamentals of Biocompatibility.* Boca Raton: Taylor and Francis; 2005.
3. Black J. Biological performance of tantalum. *Clin Mater.* 1994;16: 167–173.
4. Black J. Does corrosion matter? *J Bone Joint Surg Br.* 1988;70B: 517–520.
5. Black J. *Orthopaedic Biomaterials: Biomaterials in Orthopaedic Research and Practice.* New York: Churchill Livingstone; 1988.
6. Black J, Sholtes V. Biomaterial aspects of surface replacement arthroplasty of the hip. *Orthop Clin North Am.* 1982;13:709–728.
7. Boutin P. L'arthroplastie totale de la hanche par prothese en alumine. [Total hip arthroplasty with an alumina prosthesis.] *Acta Orthop Belg.* 1974;40:744–754.
8. Charnley J. *Acrylic Cement in Orthopaedic Surgery.* Baltimore: Williams & Wilkins; 1970.
9. Charnley J. Arthroplasty of the hip. A new operation. *Lancet.* 1961;1:1129–1132.
10. Charnley J. *Low Friction Arthroplasty of the Hip: Theory and Practice.* Berlin: Springer-Verlag; 1979:3.
11. Christel PS. Zirconia: the second generation of ceramics for total hip replacement. *Bull Hosp Joint Dis.* 1989;49:170–177.
12. Dobbs HS, Scales JT. Behavior of commercially pure titanium and Ti-318 (Ti-6Al-4V). In: Luckey HA, Kubli F Jr, eds. *Titanium Alloys in Surgical Implants.* ASTM STP 796. Philadelphia: American Society for Testing Materials; 1995:173–196.
13. Dumbleton JH. *Tribology of Natural and Artificial Joints.* Amsterdam: Elsevier; 1981:113.
14. Engh CA, Bobyn ID. *Biological Fixation in Total Hip Arthroplasty.* Thorofare, NJ: Slack; 1985.
15. Epinette J-A, Manley MT. *Fifteen Years of Clinical Experience with Hydroxyapatite Coatings in Joint Replacement.* Paris: Springer-Verlag; 2004.
16. Ezzet KA, Hermida JC, Colwell CW Jr, et al. Oxidized zirconium femoral components reduce polyethylene wear in a knee wear simulator. *Clin Orthop.* 2004;428:120–124.
17. Fielder JH, Black J. But it's my hip! The fate of failed medical devices. *Kennedy Inst Ethics J.* 1995;5:113–131.
18. Friedman RJ, Black J, Galante JO, et al. Current concepts in orthopaedic biomaterials and implant fixation. *Instr Course Lect.* 1994;43:233–255.
19. Furlong RJ, Osborn JF. Fixation of hip prostheses by hydroxyapatite ceramic coatings. *J Bone Joint Surg Br.* 1991;73:741–745.
20. Galante JO. New developments in hip arthroplasty. Overview of current attempts to eliminate methylmethacrylate. *Hip.* 1983;11: 181–189.
21. Galante JO, Rostoker WR. Wear in total hip prostheses. An experimental evaluation of candidate materials. *Acta Orthop Scand Suppl.* 1973;145:1–46.
22. Galletti PM, Boretos JW. Report on the consensus development conference on clinical applications of biomaterials, 1–3 November. *J Biomed Mater Res.* 1983;17:539–555.
23. Geesink RG. Hydroxyapatite-coated total hip prostheses. Two-year clinical and roentgenographic results of 100 cases. *Clin Orthop.* 1990;261:39–58.
24. Jacobs JJ, Shanbhag A, Glant TT, et al. Wear debris in total joint replacements. *J Am Acad Orthop Surg.* 1994;2:212–220.
25. Judet R, Siguier M, Brumpt B. A noncemented total hip prosthesis. *Clin Orthop.* 1978;137:76–84.
26. Karrholm J, Anderberg C, Snorrason F, et al. Evaluation of a femoral stem with reduced stiffness. A randomized study with use of radiostereometry and bone densitometry. *J Bone Joint Surg Am.* 2002;84A:1651–1658.

27. Keret D, Reis DR. Intraoperative cardiac arrest and mortality in hip surgery. Possible relationship to acrylic bone cement. *Orthop Rev.* 1980;9:51–56.

28. Kurtz SM. *The UHMWPE Handbook: Ultra-High Molecular Weight Polyethylene in Total Joint Replacement.* New York: Academic Press; 2004.

29. Lord G, Bancel P. The madreporic cementless total hip arthroplasty. New experimental data and a seven-year clinical follow-up study. *Clin Orthop.* 1983;176:67–76.

30. Manley MT. Calcium phosphate biomaterials: A review of the literature. In: Geesink GTR, Manley MT, eds. *Hydroxylapatite Coatings in Orthopaedic Surgery.* New York: Raven Press; 1993:1–24.

31. McKee GK, Watson-Farrar J. Replacement of arthritic hips by the McKee-Farrar prosthesis. *J Bone Joint Surg Br.* 1966;48:245–259.

32. Moore AT. The self-locking metal hip prosthesis. *J Bone Joint Surg Am* 1957;39A:811–827.

33. Ring PA. Total hip replacement. *Proc R Soc Med.* 1967;60:281–284.

34. Sarmiento A, Natarajan V, Gruen TA, et al. Radiographic performance of two different total hip arthroplasties. A survivorship analysis. *Orthop Clin North Am.* 1988;19:505–515.

35. Semlitsch M, Lehmann M, Weber H, et al. New prospects for a prolonged functional life-span of artificial hip joints by using the material combination polyethylene/aluminium oxide ceramic head. *J Biomed Mater Res.* 1977;11:537–552.

36. Semlitsch M, Willert H-G. Implant materials for hip endoprostheses; old proofs and new trends. *Arch Orthop Trauma Surg.* 1995; 114:61–67.

37. Smith-Petersen MN. Arthroplasty of the hip. A new method. *J Bone Joint Surg.* 1939;21:269–288.

38. Spector M. Historical review of porous-coated implants. *J Arthroplasty.* 1987;2:163–177.

39. Thompson FR. Two and a half years' experience with a vitallium intramedullary hip prosthesis. *J Bone Joint Surg Am.* 1954;36A: 489–502.

40. van Blitterswijk CA, Bovell YP, Flach JS, et al. Variations in hydroxylapatite crystallinity: effects on interface reactions. In: Geesnik GTR, Manley MT, eds. *Hydroxylapatite Coatings in Orthopaedic Surgery.* New York: Raven Press; 1993:33–47.

41. Venable CS, Stuck WG. *The Internal Fixation of Fractures.* Springfield, IL: CC Thomas; 1947.

42. Weber BG, Semlitsch M, Streicher R. Total hip joint replacement using a CoCrMo metal-metal sliding pairing. *J Jpn Orthop Assoc.* 1993;67:391–398.

43. Welsh RP, Pilliar RM, MacNab I. Surgical implants. The role of surface porosity in fixation to bone and acrylic. *J Bone Joint Surg Am.* 1971;53:963–977.

44. Williams DF, ed. *Definition in Biomaterials.* Amsterdam: Elsevier; 1987:67.

Ceramics

8

Jack E. Lemons

TERMINOLOGY AND DEFINITIONS

The classifications often used for synthetic-origin biomaterials utilized within the discipline of orthopaedic surgery include metallics, ceramics, polymerics, and mechanical mixtures and composites (different types of materials bonded together) (34). The ceramic biomaterials are often called "bioceramics," which are substances that are defined by properties and uses, rather than the more classical definition of a ceramic. For example, a ceramic is defined as a product made essentially from a nonmetallic mineral by firing in air at an elevated temperature. However, synthetic-origin bioceramics are often compounds not exposed to elevated temperature processing and may contain other materials such as carbon, carbon–silicon, calcium phosphates and sulfates, and diamondlike biomaterials. The broader use of the term "bioceramics" also extends to naturally occurring compounds that are utilized as fillers, carriers, and additions to bone grafts or substitutes and/or compounds for the controlled delivery of bioactive pharmaceuticals (growth factors, antibiotics, etc.) (46).

Overall, bioceramics have been subclassified (defined) in terms of their chemical–biochemical interactions within the host in vivo environment as those that are inert (biomaterials such as alumina and zirconia that are retained in vivo and now called biotolerant), bioactive (exchanged at the biological interface, and retained biomaterials such as

hydroxylapatite), and biodegradable (exchanged completely, such as tricalcium phosphate or calcium sulfate, to become active biological structures) (20,34). Within these definitions, specific applications influence this descriptive terminology. Therefore, when considering these terminologies and classifications, critical considerations are the physical, mechanical, chemical, electrical, and biological properties of the bioceramics, which exhibit unique properties as a class of materials. In general, bioceramics are strong on a relative basis under conditions of compressive-type loading but are brittle and weak related to mechanical fracture properties under conditions of tensile or shear loading. Bioceramics are nonconductors of heat and electricity (except carbon and carbon-silicon), normally have elastic moduli that are greater than bone (alumina and zirconia) or similar to bone (calcium phosphates), sometimes exhibit high indentation hardness and resistance to wear (alumina, zirconia, diamond, etc.), can be chemically and biochemically inert (biotolerants such as alumina and diamond), are relatively low density (compared to metallics), and are mostly off-white in color (like bone) except for the carbon-based materials (2).

As mentioned above, alumina and zirconia as bulk solids, in general, have elastic moduli that are considerably higher than compact bone. Therefore, surface features or porosities are often incorporated into the structures to decrease bulk elastic properties. However, the brittle nature of these types of materials and their "mechanical/notch sensitivity" under mechanical loading have sometimes been a limitation to longevity for porous- or rough-surfaced bioceramics.

HISTORY AND RATIONALE FOR CERAMICS

Interest in ceramic and ceramiclike materials (stones, minerals, and ivory) originated thousands of years ago, with practitioners of that period attempting to replace parts of the body (bones and teeth). For example, some gemstones found in ancient skulls showed occlusal wear facets indicating some stability at the bone interface and a period of in vivo function (36). Much of the interest in ceramiclike materials appears to have been based on availability, knowledge of relative chemical purity and inertness, aesthetics (tooth replacements), and the belief that the look, weight, and feel of the material was appropriate. Plus, nothing else was available, and materials for reconstructive surgery were needed (21,32).

The initial rationale for current-generation bioceramics (since the 1950s) evolved, in part, on the relative merit(s) of chemical–biochemical interactions. This was based on the idea that some ceramics could be chemotactic to biological cell and fluid products and could lead to osseous integration (direct biomaterial-to-bone contact and stability during functional loading) (24). Additionally, interest existed in enhanced attachment of prostheses to bone, and porous bioceramics were judged to be an advantage, specific to overall property characteristics (22). From the outset, it was recognized that bioceramics could be constituted and fabricated in a wide range of compositions and forms, leading to applications where biotolerants, bioactives, and biodegradables might be most appropriate. These initial beliefs have proven to be valid in many clinical circumstances, and hundreds of different types of bioceramics are now being used routinely in musculoskeletal surgical reconstructive procedures (45).

SCOPE AND INTENT OF CHAPTER

This chapter is intended to provide a brief summary of bioceramic-type biomaterials currently being utilized in orthopaedic surgery. The focus is on the relationships between some basic properties and the potential benefits gained from the utilization of these biomaterials and devices. In this regard, some experiences where the applications have not been completely favorable are briefly reviewed, specific to the importance of an evolving discipline and controlled studies for safety and efficacy of devices. References are cited for more detailed explanations within the various topic areas.

CERAMICS FOR ARTICULATING SURFACES

Aluminum Oxide (Alumina) Ceramics

Aluminum and other oxide ceramics can be processed as relatively inert (biotolerant), strong, hard, wear resistant, and nonconductive synthetic biomaterials for the ball and/or socket (liner) articulating regions of total hip arthroplasties (THAs). This area of interest started with some generally unfavorable clinical trials with low-strength glasses and related compounds (24,32). These experiences, in part, led to the realization that aluminum oxide (Al_2O_3) was routinely available within the industrial sector, and this material could be purified (96% to 99%), processed to reduce residual porosity (high-temperature sintering or hot isostatic pressing), and finished to dimensionally controlled and reproducible shapes with smooth surfaces (submicrometer) for total joint arthroplasty (TJA) (2,45).

Some initial interest existed in the overall devices being fabricated from alumina alone (all parts) for both enhanced articulation (reduced wear) and attachment (biointegration) with bone along the device-to-bone contact regions (21). Although ideal in theory, the overall mechanical properties of the alumina as a stem or threaded section proved to be a limitation (fracture) for the fully ceramic devices. These properties, in part, led to the increased interest in zirconia, which has enhanced mechanical toughness. However, the incorporation of alumina ceramic balls and liners within a modular THA system has proven to be an advantage specific to resistance to wear-related phenomena.

Initial alumina femoral ball and acetabular cup designs were, for the most part, processed from industrial grade materials. The early generation alumina bioceramics for femoral ball components (1970 and 1980) were processed by high-temperature sintering, thereby producing regions of larger material (microstructural) grain sizes (>5 μm dimensions), which resulted in less than ideal strength and wear resistance, on a relative basis. It was soon realized from laboratory and clinical studies that purity (residual oxide phases) and grain size (strength and wear resistance) needed to be further optimized (6,14,15,17). However, limited numbers of fractures and the transfer of grains (pull-out) into the articulating region during in vivo function had resulted in revisions due to breakage and abrasive (third-body) wear, causing localized tissue and host reactions. This early experience limited some applications of ceramics. Mechanical–biomechanical limitations were subsequently minimized by control of processing and finishing procedures. These processing–fabrication methodologies were improved significantly in the late 1980's and 1990's with increased strengths confirmed for all femoral balls by presterilization loading to assure properties (proof testing), plus applications of standardized quality assurance methodologies incorporating design and material considerations (2). Although very significant improvements have evolved related to alumina bioceramic properties, it is recognized that the technical–surgical aspects of clinical use require very controlled techniques (3,39).

Zirconium Oxide (Zirconia) Ceramics

Zirconium oxide (zirconia) bioceramics were recognized to offer potential advantages with respect to fracture toughness properties, based on the various in vitro studies and applications of chemically modified partially stabilized (toughened) materials (yttrium and magnesium oxide additions) (8,34,39,45). Early successes related to processing and finishing of toughened zirconia ceramics have resulted in extensive applications for femoral balls in THA (39). Processing and finishing of toughened zirconia, from the outset, presented unique considerations in that this type of bioceramics was produced in a metastable atomic arrangement (tetragonal structure) with possibilities for limited transformation over time, especially along wet external surfaces exposed to contact force and stress. This metastable atomic arrangement was known to be susceptible to some change with time and environmental exposure (tetragonal to monoclinic atomic arrangement). Localized atomic structure changes, therefore, could lead to a volume change within the bioceramic microstructure and, thereby, altered surface and/or bulk properties (e.g., increased roughness of the bioceramic surface and/or increased susceptibility to fracture) (11). Therefore, extensive in vitro testing was conducted, and it was proposed that these types of phase changes (atomic rearrangements) would not result in clinically significant surface/bulk alterations (9). These in vitro results are currently being questioned, based on limited results from longer-term retrieval and analysis investigations. Reports have recently presented theories and evaluations of explanted (revision surgery) femoral ball components where atomic phase changes have been associated with localized pitting and spalling (roughening) of the component surfaces. It has been proposed that these rougher surfaces could cause increased wear of the adjacent polyethylene liner surfaces and more particulate debris within the regional tissues (1,12,19). A recent report has shown limited changes in zirconia surfaces, but minimal influence on clinical outcomes after an eight-year assessment period (40).

The significantly increased fracture toughness and strength properties of stabilized zirconia strongly supported the merit of this biomaterial for TJA devices. Considerations of properties associated with industrial application have, in part, caused the ongoing interest in zirconia for orthopaedic and other medical–dental applications. Industrial processing of zirconia was established from experience, and it was recognized that mechanical characteristics could offer advantages of zirconia over alumina for femoral heads of total hips that utilized ultrahigh molecular weight polyethylene as the counterface within the acetabular component. Although this seems to be the result in general, some aspects of the industrial processing processes (e.g., phase change over time and a thermal exposure cycle used for densification and structural control, which was altered by one of the major manufacturers) has resulted in unanticipated in vivo roughening and fractures of some components from batches of THA femoral heads (31,37,43). This situation, leading to fractures, was corrected after the problem was identified, and the numbers of fractures were relatively small compared to the number of components being utilized.

These longer-term experiences, as with grain size control in alumina, demonstrate again the need for ongoing evaluation of any products where questions exist at the outset and where fabrication methods might be significantly altered, for any reason.

Ceramics within Modular and Composite Systems

In general, the femoral heads within modular THA systems have been attached to metallic femoral stems through a Morse taper connection. Control of the local geometry, dimensions, and roughness of the Morse taper regions were optimized to minimize loosening and femoral head ball fractures (2). In part because of the brittle properties, the ceramic head replacements have not been recommended for revision procedures where it is necessary to replace the ceramic THA femoral head along a damaged (roughened) metallic Morse taper zone (4,18,28,35).

Modularity and the necessary interconnections between ceramic and metallic parts often included assembly by mechanical connections. Concern continues about difficulties of precise alignments during surgery and avoiding chipping and/or incomplete seating during the in vivo assembly. Additional concerns have been specific to ball-to-cup edge contact during in vivo function (localized damage) and metallic transfers to the ceramic regions from unintended contacts with in vivo dislocation and relocation of the ball-liner articulating region. However, these considerations constitute relatively small numbers in terms of overall usage of the devices (3).

CERAMIC COATINGS

Experience in the industrial sector has previously demonstrated the value of ceramics for multiple applications as relatively thin coatings, primarily onto metallic substrates. The metallic substrate is intended to provide strength and toughness, while the ceramic surface offers opportunities for enhanced environmental tolerance, off-white color, and biointegration. A wide range of ceramic and diamondlike coatings have been tested in vitro and in vivo and applications continue to expand. One area where this has been popular is coatings of calcium-based compounds (hydroxylapatite, tricalcium phosphate, calcium sulfate, etc.). These coatings are intended to enhance bone healing (osteointegration) and longer-term attachment between the device and the supporting bone. Although concerns have been raised about added cost, limited mechanical strength (debonding), and longer-term biodegradation, numerous favorable reports exist in the orthopaedic and related literature (26,33). Devices remain available commercially where calcium-based compounds are applied to roughened, macrofeatured, and porous metallic devices.

Carbon, Carbon-Silicon, and Diamondlike Systems

Vitreous (glassy) carbon (C), and carbon-silicon (C-Si) materials were investigated and subsequently utilized for musculoskeletal devices starting in the late 1960s (5,13,30). Of special note was the capacity of these materials to form direct contact interfaces with bone (like alumina and zirconia). However, in contrast to alumina and zirconia, the elastic moduli properties of C and C-Si were very similar to compact bone. Some have suggested advantages for longer-term biointegration of devices due to the more similar elastic properties of C and C-Si biomaterials. Also, similar composition biomaterials, when polished, were proposed for articulating surface applications (41). The carbon-based biomaterials were lower strength, on a relative basis compared to alumina and zirconia, and were conductors of heat and electricity. In some situations for modular combinations with stainless steel, the devices were subject to increased corrosion of the metallic areas (galvaniclike effects) (29).

The carbon- and graphite-based biomaterials have found extensive applications as parts for heart valves and surface coatings for contact with blood and tissue fluids (34). Longer-term biocompatibility profiles have been associated with the in vivo stability (inertness) of this class of biomaterials, as well as enhanced surface wetting, physical–mechanical properties and abilities to be polished to a very smooth condition. Some suggest that detailed knowledge of mechanical properties (strength modulus toughness, brittleness, hardness, etc.) must be understood in depth to properly design and utilize these biomaterials and devices for orthopaedic applications (5,13,30,41).

The black color of C and C-Si has sometimes been considered an issue (concern) for near-skin location of device surfaces. However, interest continues in this class of biomaterials, and the importance of appropriate design and manufacturing continues to be emphasized (41).

Diamondlike materials have been proposed as biomaterials for TJA, with specific interests in coatings and in some cases bulk form products (10,25,42). These compounds are often combined with metallics (composites) and offer potential advantages related to strength, hardness, and wear resistance for articulating surface (hard–hard) combinations. Clinical trials are anticipated as the control of properties and fabrication methods continues to evolve. At this time, some are proposing that strength and wear resistance offer special properties (enhancement) for total joint articulating surfaces (42).

BIOCERAMICS FOR BONE APPLICATIONS

Bioceramic Forms and Shapes for Bone Replacement

Most of the biotolerant and bioactive ceramics have been investigated for space filling or augmentation applications specific to treatments of injury, pathology, and aging-related bone alterations (27). In many situations, the compatibility properties of the ceramic surfaces and opportunities for local biointegration along ceramic-to-bone interfaces and/or ingrowths of bone into macrofeatures or porosities have been intended outcomes. These types of products remain available for selected applications, although concerns have been raised about the longer-term strength and fracture properties of bulk (larger) sizes under in vivo conditions where tensile and/or shear loading might exist (2). Therefore, some have proposed ceramic particulates versus bulk forms for bone implants, in order to minimize possibilities of longer-term biomechanical breakdown. Examples exist from retrieval studies where biointegration of ceramics and bone have been maintained for years (23).

Many of the early studies on biodegradable ceramics were based on macro- and microporous tricalcium phosphates (TCP) used alone or in combination with autogenously grafting substances (16,27). The TCP was subsequently combined with bovine collagen and then with growth factors (e.g., bone morphogenic proteins [BMPs], platelet-derived growth factors [PDGFs], etc.). A similar pathway was followed for hydroxylapatite (ceramic), hydroxyapatites (HA-other), other calcium phosphate compounds, and calcium sulfates (44). One extensive investigative series utilized a biphasic HA/TCP as a porous block for stem cell delivery and standardized assessments of cellular/product osteo activity (7).

Bone Substitutes and Tissue-Engineered Medical Products

Bioceramics are popular as solid, porous, particulate, or mixture forms for bone graft substitute products (16). In general, the bioceramics are added to natural or organic-based grafting materials for enhancing strength and handling characteristics. In many situations the ceramic also serves as a scaffold and/or as a carrier for controlled delivery of active biological or chemical compounds to enhance healing and/or to treat infections (antibiotics). These tissue-engineered medical products most often utilize the biodegradable forms of bioceramics (calcium phosphates and sulfates), although calcium aluminates and other compounds have been evaluated (38).

SUMMARY

Bioceramics for applications in orthopaedic surgery have evolved over time and experience, with large numbers in clinical use for components of prostheses, coatings, bone graft substitutes, and tissue-engineered medical products. Ongoing research and development strongly support significant advantages for this class of biomaterials for future applications within musculoskeletal surgical reconstructive procedures.

REFERENCES

1. Allain J, LeMouel S, Goutallier D, et al. Eight year survival of cemented zirconia-polyethylene total hip replacement. *J Bone Joint Surg Br.* 1999;81:835–842.
2. American Society for Testing and Materials. Vol 13.01. Philadelphia: ASTM; 2003.
3. Bierbaum B, Nairus J, Kuesis D, et al. Ceramic-on-ceramic bearings in total hip arthroplasty. *Clin Orth Rel Res.* 2002;405:158–163.
4. Bobyn JD, Dujovne AR, Krygier JJ, et al. Surface analysis of the taper junctions of retrieved and in vitro tested modular hip prostheses. In: Morrey BF, ed. *Biological, Material, and Mechanical Considerations of Joint Replacement.* Bristol-Myers Squibb/Zimmer Orthopaedic Symposium Series. New York: Raven Press; 1993:287–301.
5. Bokros J, Gott V, Lagrange C, et al. Correlation between tissue biocompatibility and heparin absorptivity for an impermable isotropic pyrolytic carbon. *J Biomed Mater Res.* 1969;3:497.
6. Boutin P, Christel P, Dorlot J-M, et al. The use of dense alumina-alumina ceramic combination in total hip replacement. *J Biomed Mater Res.* 1988;22:1203–1232.
7. Bruder S, Kraus K, Goldberg V, et al. The effect of implants loaded with autologous mesenchymal stem cells in the healing of segmental bone defects. *J Bone Joint Surg.* 1998;80A:985–996.
8. Cales B. Zirconia as a sliding material: histologic, laboratory and clinical data. *Clin Orthop.* 2000;379:94–112.
9. Cales B, Stefani Y, Lilley E. Long-term in vivo and in vitro aging of a zirconia ceramic used in orthopaedics. *J. Biomed Mater Res* 1994;28:619–624.
10. Catledge S, Fries M, Vohra Y, et al. Nanostructured ceramics for biomedical implants. *J Nanosci Nanotechnol.* 2002;2:3.
11. Christel P, Dorlot J-M, Meunier A. On the specifications for the use of bioinert ceramics in total hip replacement. In: Oonishi H, Aoki H, Sawai K, eds. *Bioceramics.* St. Louis: Euroamerica, Inc; 1989:262–266.
12. Clark I, Manaka M, Green D, et al. Current status of zirconia used in total hip implants. *J Bone Joint Surg Am.* 2003;85(suppl 4):73–84.
13. Cook S, Beckenbaugh R, Redondo J, et al. Long-term follow-up on pyrolytic carbon metacarpophalengeal implants. *J Bone Joint Surg.* 1999;81A:635–647.
14. Dorlot JM. Long-term effects of alumina components in total hip prostheses. *Clin Orthop.* 1992;282:47–52.
15. Dorlot JM, Christel P, Neunier A. Wear analysis of retrieved alumina heads and sockets of hip prosthesis. *J Biomed Mater Res.* 1989;23(A3 suppl):229–310.
16. Ducheyne P, Lemons J, eds. bioceramics: material characteristics versus in vivo behavior. New York: New York Academy of Science; 1988.
17. Fruh HJ, Willmann G, Pfaff HG. Wear characteristics of ceramic-on-ceramic for hip endoprostheses. *Biomaterials.* 1997;18:873–876.
18. Goldberg JR, Gilbert JL, Jacobs JJ, et al. A multicenter retrieval study of the taper interfaces of modular hip prostheses. *Clin Orthop.* 2002;401:149–161.

19. Haraguchi K, Sugano N, Nishii T, et al. Phase transformation of a zirconia ceramic head after a total hip arthroplasty. *J Bone Joint Surg Br.* 2001;83:996–1000.

20. Hench L, Best S. Ceramics, glasses and glass-ceramics. In: Ratner B, Hoffman A, Schoen F, et al, eds. *Biomaterials Science.* New York: Elsevier; 2004;153–170.

21. Hench L, Wilson J, eds. *An Introduction to Ceramics,* Hackensack, NJ: World Scientific; 1989.

22. Hench L, Wilson J. *Science.* 1984;226:630–636.

23. Horting-Hansen E, Worsaae N, Lemons J. Histologic response after implantation of porous hydroxyapatite ceramics in humans. *Int J Oral Maxillo Implants.* 1990;5:255–263.

24. Hulbert S, Cooke F, Klawitter J, et al. Attachment of prosthesis to the musculoskeletal system by tissue ingrowth and mechanical locking. *J Biomed Mater Res.* 1974;4:1–23.

25. Huo M. What's new in hip arthroplasty. *J Bone Joint Surg.* 2002;84A:157–167.

26. Jones D. Coating of ceramics on metals. In: Ducheyne P, Lemons J, eds. *Bioceramics: Material Characteristics versus In Vivo Behavior.* New York: New York Academy of Science; 1988:19–38.

27. Laurencin C, ed. *Bone Graft Substitutes.* W. Conshohocken, PA: ASTM Press; 2003.

28. Lieberman JR, Rimnac CM, Garvin KL, et al. An analysis of the head-neck taper interface in retrieved prostheses. *Clin Orthop.* 1994;300:162–167.

29. Lemons J. Dental implant retrieval analyses. *J Dent Ed.* 1988;52: 748–756.

30. More R, Haubold A, Bokros J. Pyrolytic carbon for long-term medical implants. In: Ratner B, Hoffman A, Schoen F, et al, eds. *Biomaterials Science.* San Diego: Elsevier; 2004:170–181.

31. Norton MR, Yarlagadda R, Anderson GH. Catastrophic failure of the elite plus total hip replacement, with hylamer acetabulum and zirconia ceramic femoral head. *J Bone Joint Surg Br.* 2002;84: 631–635.

32. Oonishi H, Aoki H, Sawai K, eds. *Bioceramics.* St. Louis: Euroamerica, Inc; 1989.

33. Parr J, Horowitz M, eds. *Characterization and Performance of Calcium Phosphate Coatings for Implant.* STP 1196. Philadelphia: American Society for Testing and Materials; 1994.

34. Ratner B, Hoffman A, Schoen F, et al, eds. *Biomaterials Science.* 2nd ed. New York: Elsevier; 2004.

35. Richter HG, Burger W, Osthues F. Zirconia for medical implants: the role of strength properties. In: Anderson GH, Yli-Urpo A, eds. *Bioceramics.* Vol. 7. London: Butterworth; 1994:401–406.

36. Ring M. *Dentistry and Illustrated History.* New York: Abradale Press, Mosby Year Book; 1985:14–17.

37. Saint-Gobain Desmarquest. Report of unprecedented fracture rate of Th-zirconia balls in patients in France and the United States; 2002; www.prozyr.com.

38. Schuttle E, Kaplan D, Picciolo G. *Tissue Engineered Medical Products.* STP 1452. W. Conshohocken, PA: ASTM Press; 2004.

39. Skinner H. Ceramic bearing surfaces. *Clin Orthop.* 1999;369: 135–141.

40. Stewart T, Flemming N, Siney P, et al. The stability and durability of zirconia femoral heads [abstract]. Presented at: 51st AAOS/ORS Meeting; February 2005; Washington, DC.

41. Strzepa P, Klawitter J. Ascension pyrocarbon hemisphere wear testing against bone [abstract]. Presented at: 51st AAOS/ORS Meeting; February 2005; Washington, DC.

42. Taylor J, Pope B, Gardinier C, et al. The development of polycrystalline diamond compact (PDC) for arthroplasty bearing applications. Presented at: Seventh World Biomaterials Congress; 17–21 May 2004; Sydney, Australia.

43. Values for ball fracture ratios in seven lots of Th-zirconia manufactured by Saint-Gobain Desmarquest; 2003; www.prozyr.com.

44. Walsh W, Morberg P, Yu Y, et al. Response of a calcium sulfate graft substitute in a confined cancellous defect. *Clin Ortho Rel Res.* 2003;406:228–236.

45. Wright T, Maher S. The articulation. In: *Joint Replacement Arthroplasty.* Morrey B, ed. Philadelphia: Churchill Livingstone; 2003:34–35.

46. Yamamura T, Hench L, Wilson J. *Handbook of Bioactive Ceramics.* Vols 1 and 2. Boca Raton, FL: CRC Press; 1990.

Polyethylene in Total Hip Replacement

9

Roy D. Crowninshield   Orhun K. Muratoglu   Michael Hawkins

Clinical success and implant durability in total hip replacement is a multifactorial-dependent accomplishment that includes patient-, surgical-, and implant-related factors. From an engineering and material science perspective, success in total hip replacement is enhanced by the achievement of implant component fixation, maintenance of implant component structural integrity, and limitation of articular surface wear. Early in the history of total hip replacement, it was appreciated that there existed a strong interdependence of these components of durable joint reconstruction (10,58). Motion at the articular surface of total hip replacement produces particulate wear products (30). These particulate byproducts of wear can initiate an inflammatory response of the tissues that surround and support prosthetic joint components (51). The loss of periprosthetic bone can in turn compromise both implant fixation and prosthetic component structural support. This cascade of events that can follow from articular surface wear can contribute alone or with other factors to limitation in reconstructive implant durability. Advancement in the success of total hip replacement continues to result from improved understanding of the role and limitations of patient factors, surgical achievement, prosthetic component design, and implant material properties.

THE BEARING MATERIAL OF CHOICE

Nearly from its onset and throughout its history, total hip replacement has utilized a variety of articular surface materials mated in many combinations. Metal-on-metal bearing couples were utilized in the first total hip replacement in the late 1930s in the form of stainless steel components (1). These earliest metal-on-metal devices were followed by cobalt–chromium alloy metal-on-metal articular surface devices in the 1940s and 1950s (29). After evolving through many design changes, metal-on-metal articular surface devices remain in use today (53). Ceramic-on-ceramic prosthetic hip articulation components emerged in the 1970s and also remain in use today (40). Despite their long history and their demonstrated clinical utility, these so-called hard-on-hard bearings have not dominated total hip reconstruction. The predominant wear couples in total hip replacement over that last 40 years utilize a polymer acetabular surface articulating against either a metal or ceramic femoral head.

In the late 1950s John Charnley first began clinical utilization of a polymer acetabular component made of polytetrafluoroethylene (PTFE) articulating against a stainless steel femoral component head (8–10,58,59). PTFE was chosen for this application because of it softness and low coefficient of friction. However, PTFE proved to be a poor choice, as clinical failure due to wear-induced implant loosening and associated pain became apparent within a just few years in the approximately 300 patients who received implants of this material. An additional 20 of John Charnley's patients received an acetabular component made from another polymer (Fluorosint-Polypenco), which also proved to be unsuccessful (58).

117

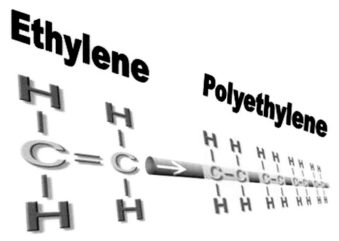

Figure 9-1 The ethylene monomer combines to form the polymer polyethylene.

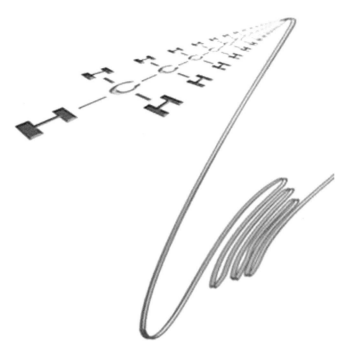

Figure 9-2 UHMWPE is a simple linear molecule of enormous length.

In 1962 John Charnley was introduced to a new polymer material in the form of high molecular weight polyethylene (HMWP) (9,10,58). This material performed much better in laboratory wear tests than did the previous polymers. Encouraged by these laboratory results, he began clinical use of polyethylene in total hip replacement in late 1962. By 1965 John Charnley had implanted several hundred total hip replacements utilizing polyethylene as an articular surface. Many of these earliest polyethylene acetabular devices were implanted utilizing bone cement, John Charnley's other significant polymer introduction to total joint surgery (58).

In addition to materials innovation, other aspects of John Charnley's approach to implant science and medical education helped polyethylene become established as the material of choice for total hip replacement. Charnley recognized early on that the outcome of total hip surgery was highly dependent on the achievement of surgical skill. Up until the early 1970s Charnley restricted the manufacturer of his total hip prostheses from selling devices to surgeons other than those that he personally trained (58). Charnley also emphasized the value of documenting and reporting the outcome of clinical treatment. Some of the best document long-term clinical outcomes of total hip replacement have come from Charnley's original experience (59). As a result, both the general utility and specific limitations of polyethylene based total joint replacement became appreciated in the 1970s. Since that time, the surgical procedure, prosthetic component designs, and implant materials used in polymer articular surface total hip replacement have continued to evolve and to improve.

Polyethylene has established itself as the bearing material of choice in total joint replacement. To date approximately 20 million polyethylene total joint replacements have been implanted, 15 million are likely still in service, and 1.2 million new ones will be implanted this year.

POLYETHYLENE IN ORTHOPAEDICS

The ethylene molecule (Fig. 9-1) has a molecular weight of 28 g/mole. It is one of the simplest organic compounds, having only two carbon and four hydrogen atoms. Ultrahigh molecular weight polyethylene (UHMWPE) is a linear semicrystalline polymer of extreme length (Fig. 9-2). Older discussions of UHMWPE, to include Charnley's reference to the material, have sometimes characterized the material as high-density polyethylene (HDPE) (58,59). While the two materials that we know today as UHMWPE and HDPE are both polyethylenes, the properties of the materials are very different. UHMWPE is slightly less dense, much more chemically resistant, and has better mechanical properties than HDPE. The defining difference in properties between HDPE and UHMWPE can be attributed to the molecular weight of the polymer. The molecular weight influences the arrangement of the polymer chain, which in turn affects the material's properties. UHMWPE is arranged in two phases, a crystalline phase and an amorphous phase (Fig. 9-3). The crystalline phase comprises molecular chains folded back and forth in a layered or lamellar structure typically 10 to 50 nm in thickness and 10 to 50 μm in length. Evidence of the crystalline phase of UHMWPE can be seen in transmission electron microscopy imaging of UHMWPE (Fig. 9-3). The presence of the crystalline phase confers important properties to the material. The amorphous phase of UHMWPE comprises polymer chains, chain ends extending from crystals, and smaller molecules that do not exhibit long-range order.

UHMWPE has undergone evolutionary changes since Charnley's first use of the material. Much of the early polyethylene use in total hip replacement was RCH 1000, a compression-molded resin manufactured at the time by Hoechst. This material had a molecular weight of approximately 1 million g/mole (47). Although over time the basic material remained the same, the molecular weight, cleanliness, and material consistency of UHMWPE used in orthopaedics have improved. As typically used in orthopedics today, UHMWPE has molecular weight of approximately 5 to 6 million g/mole. The orthopaedic UHMWPE depicted in Figure 9-1 would thus today have

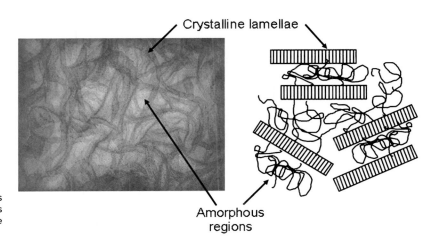

Figure 9-3 The long-chain polyethylene molecules assume a random orientation in the amorphous regions. In the crystalline lamellae, the molecules are oriented in a long-range order.

approximately 200,000 repeating monomer units. The wear of UHMWPE is reported to be influenced by molecular weight, with less wear associated with higher molecular weight material (47). Other mechanical properties of polyethylene, including its strength, can also be molecular weight dependant (49).

Unlike metals, polymer crystals do not have distinct grain boundaries. The crystals can be described as "fuzzy," with polymer chains hanging off and entangled with other chains from other crystals. The formation of and disorganization of the crystalline phase of UHMWPE is thermally influenced, with the crystalline phase melting (becoming amorphous) at temperatures above about 137°C. The extent of crystallinity in UHMWPE is thus dependent on thermal history during synthesis and further processing. Crystallinity in finished orthopaedic devices has typically ranged between about 35% and 55%. The crystallinity of UHMWPE and the presence of amorphous regions within the polymer affect mechanical and chemical properties of the material (57).

The biphasic physical arrangement of the UHMWPE is one of the keys to its success as an implant material. In an orthopaedic application, polyethylene is placed in an active chemical environment. The close packing of molecular chains in the crystalline phase of UHMWPE inhibits movement of materials into the crystalline region of the polymer. As such, the crystallinity of UHMWPE imparts significant chemical resistance to the material. The crystalline regions are resistant to attack by liquids in the body, as well as dissolved gases such as oxygen. The pathway for chemical sensitivity in UHMEPE is largely though the materials' amorphous phase. The polymer in the amorphous regions is less tightly packed and is more susceptible to chemical attack. These amorphous regions tend to allow more movement of liquids and gases into the polymer. The high level of bulk UHMWPE biocompatibility is in part the result of the material's resistance to solvents and the resulting difficulty in extraction or release of polymer elements from these large and densely packed polymer chains.

The biphasic structure of UHMWPE is also responsible for much of the material's physical properties. Subject to loading, the crystalline regions are mechanically more rigid, while the amorphous regions are more easily distorted. Crystallinity and the cross-linking of polyethylene, discussed later, tend to provide a more rigid and less ductile polymer structure. Highly amorphous UHMWPE tends to be highly ductile and weaker than more crystalline material. Through a balance of crystalline and amorphous phases UHMWPE can have the strength, ductility, and toughness suitable for orthopaedic implant use.

UHMWPE resin is polymerized as a fine powder (Fig. 9-4) or flake with a particle size typically ranging from approximately 50 to 300 μm in diameter. The UHMWPE resins historically available and currently used in the manufacture of orthopaedic devices are listed in Table 9-1.

These resins can be characterized by manufacturer, their molecular weight, and the presence or absence of added calcium

TABLE 9-1
UHMWPE RESINS USED IN ORTHOPAEDIC IMPLANTS

Material	Manufacturer	Approximate Dates of Use	Molecular Weight	Calcium Stearate
RCH 1000	Hoechst	1960–1985	1×10^6	
H 1900	Himont (Montel)	1972–present	$2–4 \times 10^6$	None added
GUR 412	Hoechst (Ticona)	1985–1995	$3–4 \times 10^6$	500 ppm
GUR 415	Hoechst (Ticona)	1985–1995	$4–6 \times 10^6$	500 ppm
GUR 4150	Hoechst (Ticona)	1985–present	$4–6 \times 10^6$	500 ppm
GUR 1020	Hoechst (Ticona)	1996–present	$3–4 \times 10^6$	None added
GUR 1050	Hoechst (Ticona)	1996–present	$4–6 \times 10^6$	None added

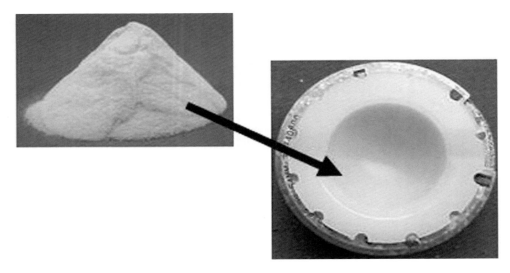

Figure 9-4 Polyethylene flake prior to consolidation into an acetabular component.

stearate $(C_{36}H_{70}CaO_4)$. The resin type and its method of consolidation, discussed later, can affect the performance of UHMWPE components (29,33). Calcium stearate was historically added to many polyethylene resins to help prevent processing equipment corrosion and to aid in resin flow during the ram extrusion process of powder consolidation into a polyethylene form useful in orthopaedic implants. The identification of specific polyethylene resins historically used in orthopaedic devices can be confusing. Some producers of UHMWPE have changed ownership, experienced name changes, or changed resin designations over the history of orthopaedic use. As an example, the company Ticona, which currently produces GUR 4150 and GUR 4120 resins, was formerly Hoechst, the company that produced the similar 415 and 412 UMMWPE resins. This family of UHWMPE resins is the material from which most orthopaedic implants have been produced over the last several decades. Another polymer used in orthopaedics is H 1900 resin, from Montel Basell, which was HiFax 1900, formerly from the Himont and Hercules companies. The H 1900 resin is produced with little or no added calcium stearate. The most commonly used UHMWPE resins in orthopaedic implant production currently include GUR 1050 and GUR 1020 from Ticona. These materials came into use in the mid 1990s and they do not have added calcium stearate.

UHMWPE CONSOLIDATION

UHMWPE flake (Fig. 9-4) must be consolidated into solid shapes in order to be useful in an orthopaedic implant. The consolidation of polyethylene flake into a solid polyethylene form requires controlled application of pressure and elevated polymer temperature. The two commonly utilized methods of polymer consolidation used on orthopaedic polyethylene are ram extrusion and compression molding. Ram extrusion (Fig. 9-5) is a discontinuous flow process where the UHMWPE resin powder is heated in a chamber while subject to pressure from a reciprocating ram. In this process the time, temperature, and pressure history of the material is controlled as the polymer powder is heated and compressed. The UHMWPE flows through an open extrusion die and emerges as a continuous bar of consolidated material. Calcium stearate was added to some UHMWPE resins to facilitate the ram extrusion process. Compression molding (Fig. 9-6) is a static process wherein the time, temperature, and pressure history of the UHMWPE resin is controlled as the material is contained within a mold cavity. Compression molding can be used to produce large sheets of bulk consolidated UHMWPE. Direct compression molding can produce consolidated polyethylene of the shape defined by the mold design geometry. Most compression molded UHMWPE is from resins free of added calcium stearate.

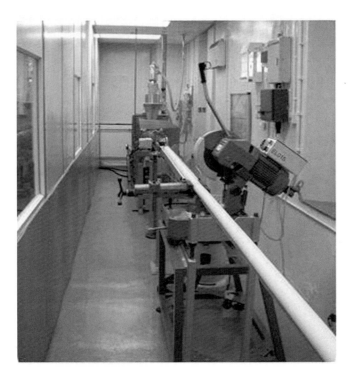

Figure 9-5 Equipment used in ram extrusion to produce UHMWPE bar. (Courtesy of Perplas Medical, Bacup, Lancashire, England.)

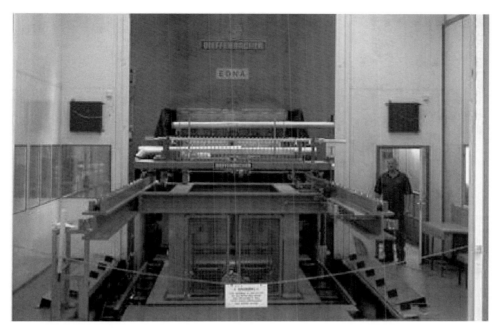

Figure 9-6 Equipment used in compression molding to produce UHMWPE sheet. (Courtesy of Perplas Medical, Bacup, Lancashire, England.)

IMPLANT SHAPING

The geometry of an UHMWPE orthopaedic implant is commonly produced by machining of consolidated UHMWPE bar stock or sheet material that may have been produced by either ram extrusion or compression molding. Ram extrusion produces bar stock directly, while large-scale compression molding can be used to produce thick sheets of UHMWPE that can then be reduce by cutting or machining to rectangular or round bars, depending on the product to be produced. Since UHMWPE is a tough but relatively soft material, the manufacture of precision orthopaedic requires special machining processes. Machining of orthopaedic implants from UHMWPE stock offers the advantage of speed and efficiency in the production process. With current machining processes, a high level of dimensional control, production of complex implant shapes, and achievement of smooth articulating surface finishes can be achieved.

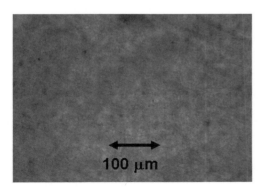

Figure 9-7 The microstructure of a compression-molded GUR 1050 acetabular component.

Final implant shapes can also be produced by direct compression molding. In the direct compression molding process the flake is simultaneously consolidated and shaped into the implant geometry. In this process the geometry of the mold used in polymer consolidation is matched to the desired final implant geometry. Implants shaped in this manner can be entirely polymer or can include integrated metal components inserted within the mold. Direct compression molding can also be used to produce a preform of UHMWPE incorporating some aspects of the final implant geometry. That preform can be subsequently machined to provide other aspects of the finished implant geometry. The partial machining of otherwise direct-compression-molded components may be performed due to requirement of dimensional or geometric features that are difficult to achieve in the molding process.

The forms of orthopaedic UHMWPE implants in common used include direct-compression-molded components, components partially or fully machined from compression molded stock, and components machined from ram-extruded stock. In considering both the historical and currently available UHMWPE implants it may be important to correctly identify the methods of implant shaping as molded, molded/machined, and ram-extruded/machined. Each of these processes can produce well-consolidated UHMWPE components of complex geometry and high dimensional tolerance. The microstructural appearance of compression-molded GUR 1050 components is shown in Figure 9-7.

PACKAGING AND STERILIZATION

Thermal sterilization is not suitable for polyethylene components, since autoclaving temperatures are typically in the same range as the melting temperature of polyethylene. Exposing

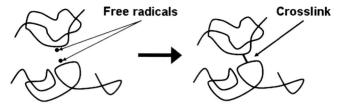

Figure 9-8 During irradiation, carbon–hydrogen bonds are broken, forming free radicals along the backbone of the polyethylene molecule. The reaction of two free radicals in two separate molecules results in the formation of a cross-link.

polyethylene to autoclave temperatures results in thermal distortion of components. Almost from the onset of its use and to the present time, most UHMWPE components used in orthopaedics have been sterilized by exposure to ionizing radiation. Sterilization of polyethylene components by exposure to 25 to 40 kGy of gamma radiation is the most common form of sterilization used for UHMWPE orthopaedic implants. Gamma rays penetrate entirely through the component and packaging and can result in both component surface and subsurface sterilization. Gamma radiation can also be used to sterilize UHMWPE components that incorporate or are packaged with metal implant components.

In addition to sterilization, radiation exposure also can alter the structure of the UHMWPE molecule. During irradiation, the bond between carbon atoms in the polymer can be broken, producing shorter polymer chains, and the bond between the carbon and hydrogen atoms can also be broken. These alterations of the polymer produce free radicals (unpaired electrons) within the material. These free radicals are reactive chemical species that can form branched chains, combine with other nearby elements, or simply recombine to re-establish the polymer chain. The formation of branch chains is generally referred to as cross-linking and results from the formation of interchain covalent bonds (Fig. 9-8). Cross-linking of UHMWPE has been shown to affect some mechanical properties of UHMWPE, including improving its wear performance (34), and is discussed in detail later. Free radicals that do not recombine or result in cross-links can provide sites on the polymer chain where available oxygen can attach to the polymer. Since oxygen is a relatively small molecule it can diffuse into UHMWPE over time (44,45). The oxidization of polyethylene, which can occur in any oxidized environment including the in vivo environment, can be associated with changes the material's mechanical properties (55). To reduce the effects of oxidation in the implant storage environment, most gamma-radiation-sterilized UHMWPE components are now provided in packaging with low oxygen content (4,5,13, 16,27,34,52,55). Low oxygen exposure can be achieved by implant packaging in an inert gas, vacuum, or oxygen-scavenged condition. Sterilization and shelf storage of polyethylene components in low-oxygen packaging has been demonstrate to reduce the oxidation of the material during storage (13). However, when removed from an oxygen protected environment and placed in an oxygen containing environment such as body fluids, oxidation of the polyethylene will occur (5). Although low-oxygen packaging of radiation-sterilized polyethylene has demonstrated lower initial material oxidation, poststerilization oxidation of polyethylene is

dependent on many factors including resin type (16), method of consolidation (16), crystallinity (46), molecular weight (46), and radiation exposure (34). Polyethylene implants packaged and stored in low-oxygen environments may result in improved clinical performance due to a possibly higher level of cross-linking and low level of oxidation present at the time of implantation. However, concerns related to the lack of clinical performance data, changes in mechanical properties, and changes in the oxidative degradation for these oxygen-protected components have been expressed (13,44).

Sterilization by other methods has been used on UHMWPE components, including exposure to ethylene oxide or gas plasma. These methods provide surface sterilization of components and do not result in the generation of free radicals. Since these methods are limited to surface sterilization only, they may not be applicable to implant components packaged or assembled with gas-tight interfaces. These methods of sterilization avoid of the generation of free radicals and thus the increased potential for oxidization. However, these methods of sterilization also do not provide an opportunity for potentially beneficial cross-linking (34).

MATERIAL STANDARDS

There are a number of standards that have been developed that are applicable to the implant use of UHMWPE. These standards are the product of standard-setting organizations such as the American Society for Testing and Materials (ASTM) and the International Standards Organization (ISO). The basic standards for UHMWPE are ASTM F-648 and ISO 11542/2 (2,3,21). These standards cover subjects such as basic chemical and physical properties of the flake and consolidated forms, as well as methods of material testing and analysis. These standards are developed to help guide industry in the use of UHMWPE and continue to evolve through the participation of material producers, implant manufacturers, orthopaedic surgeons, academic researchers, and government regulators.

EXTENSIVE CROSS-LINKING

In the late 1990s the deliberate cross-linking of UHMWPE by radiation exposure combined with thermal treatment emerged as a technology to improve the wear and oxidation resistance of UHMWPE acetabular components (32,35,37). The development of this technology led to a series of new alternate polyethylene bearing materials with varying cross-link densities.

The deliberate cross-linking of UHMWPE utilizes the effect of radiation on polyethylene that was previously discussed relative to sterilization. Following radiation exposure, free radical recombination takes place mainly in the amorphous phase of the polymer, where the molecules are in close enough proximity to allow the formation of the interchain carbon–carbon bonds that constitute cross-links (7,18). In the crystalline phase, and because of the increased distance between the molecules, cross-linking is not favored. As a result, the free radicals generated in the crystalline regions are postulated not to take part in the cross-linking reaction and become trapped, mainly

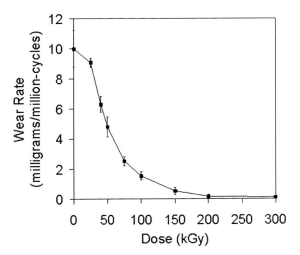

Figure 9-9 Average wear rate of cylindrical pins as a function of radiation dose level. The pins were machined from GUR 1050 UHMWPE blocks that were first irradiated to the indicated radiation dose level and subsequently melted. The wear rate decreases with increasing radiation dose level. (Reprinted from Muratoglu OK, Bragdon CR, O'Connor DO, et al. Unified wear model for highly cross-linked ultra-high molecular weight polyethylenes [UHMWPE]. *Biomaterials.* 1999;20:1463–1470, with permission.)

in the crystalline–amorphous interfaces (22,24,43). These residual free radicals are precursors of oxidation following radiation exposure (12,37). To deliberately cross-link the material, thermally treatment of UHMWPE after radiation exposure can encourage cross-linking and can reduce the concentration of free radicals (32,35,37).

Many orthopedic implant manufacturers offer acetabular liners fabricated from highly cross-linked UHMWPEs. Table 9-2 lists the current manufacturing techniques used for the fabrication of highly cross-linked acetabular liners. These radiation cross-linking techniques include variations in the radiation source, radiation dose, radiation temperature, postirradiation thermal treatment, and sterilization method.

Commercially available cross-linked acetabular components can differ in their source of radiation exposure. Gamma irradiation sources are commonly based on the artificial isotope of cobalt (^{60}Co) that generates gamma photons. These photons have no practical limitations in the penetration of UHMWPE, such that thick sections of material can be uniformly exposed. However, gamma sources typically have a low activity level, which limits the radiation dose rate and extends the time for radiation dose achievement. Electron beam irradiation utilizes accelerated charged particles. The penetration of the effects of e-beam radiation is limited by the kinetic energy of the electron beam, typically measured in million electron volts (MeV). With a 10 MeV electron beam incident on a polyethylene surface, radiation penetrates about 4 to 4.5 cm. Through double-sided exposure, uniform radiation exposure of a 9-cm-thick UHMWPE stock is possible. Compared to gamma radiation exposure, a commercial e-beam accelerator provides about two orders of magnitude greater radiation dose, which results in relatively short times for radiation dose achievement.

Commercially available cross-linked acetabular components can also differ in their level of radiation exposure. Components are available with radiation dose of between

50 and 100 kGy. The level of wear improvement increases with radiation level up to about 100 kGy, where cross-linking saturation tends to occur (Fig. 9-9). Some researchers have proposed that lower levels of radiation exposure and cross-linking are sufficient to produce components that will produce wear below the lysis threshold (32). Others have, however, demonstrated that exposure at about 100 kGy results in cross-linked UHMWPE that generates minimal wear debris (14,35,37) and preferable wear particle morphology (50).

Perhaps, the most important processing step difference in the manufacture of cross-linked acetabular components is the thermal treatment used following irradiation. These thermal treatments are used to eliminate or reduce the residual free radical population within the UHMWPE. The most effective method of reducing free radicals is to raise the temperature of polyethylene above its peak melting transition (about 137°C) to eliminate the crystalline domains and liberate the residual free radicals trapped within the crystals. Above the melt temperature the rapid removal of the residual free radicals will occur through recombination reactions. Upon cooling, polyethylene crystallizes, reforming most of the crystalline domains, now in the presence of cross-links. Postirradiation melting is used in conjunction with a gas sterilization method, resulting in a sterile, free radical–free and oxidation resistant implant. In contrast, when radiation-exposed UHMWPE is heated (annealed) to a temperature below the point where the crystalline domains become amorphous, some of the free radicals may engage in cross-linking, while other free radicals will remain. This postirradiation annealing below the melt temperature, thus, partially cross-links and only reduces the concentration of residual free radicals in radiation-exposed UHMWPE. Gamma sterilization in nitrogen after cross-linking and annealing below the melt temperature may increase the concentration of the residual free radicals to above that of conventional UHMWPE (39).

The concentration of residual free radicals is typically measured by electron spin resonance (ESR). With state-of-the-art ESR equipment, the lowest detection limit is 10^{14} residual free radicals per gram of material. Postirradiation melting of UHMWPE has been reported to result in no detectable residual free radicals with this technique (11,39). In contrast, postirradiation annealing below the melt temperature followed by gamma sterilization can produce a material with a residual free radical concentration greater than that of some conventional gamma-sterilized UHMWPE (11,39). The residual free radicals can lead to changes in the mechanical and chemical properties of polyethylene. The chemical changes resulting from oxidation can result in reduced strength, reduced ductility, and increased modulus of elasticity (32,35,37).

WEAR AND MECHANICAL PROPERTIES

The wear of UHMWPE in total hips is mainly adhesive and abrasive in nature, and it results in the generation submicron-size particulate debris (30). The wear mechanisms of acetabular liners have been described based on the analysis of the articular surface morphology of explanted components (23). Elongated fibrils, oriented in the flexion–extension direction of the hip, form on the articulating surfaces of the acetabular

TABLE 9-2
CURRENT APPLICATIONS OF HIGHLY CROSS-LINKED POLYETHYLENES IN TOTAL HIP REPLACEMENT

	Manufacturer	Radiation Temperature	Radiation Dose (kGy[a])	Radiation Type	Postirradiation Thermal Treatment	Sterilization Method	Total Radiation Dose Level (kGy)	Residual Free Radicals Present?
Longevity™	Zimmer	~40°C	100		Melted at 150°C for 6 hours	Gas plasma	100	No
Durasul™	Sulzer	~125°C	95	E-beam	Melted at 150°C for 2 hours	EtO	95	No
Marathon™	Depuy/JJ	RT	50		Melted at 155°C for 24 hours	Gas plasma	50	No
XLPE™	Smith & Nephew	RT	100		Melted at 150°C for a proprietary duration	EtO	100	No
Crossfire™	Stryker/Osteonics/ Howmedica	RT	75	Gamma	Annealed at 120°C for a proprietary duration	Gamma (30 kGy) in nitrogen	105	Yes
Aeonian™	Kyocera	RT	35		Annealed at 110°C for 10 hours	Gamma (25–40 kGy) in nitrogen	60–75	Yes

RT, room temperature.
[a]10 kilogray (kGy) = 1 megarad (Mrad).

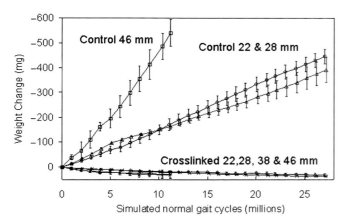

Figure 9-10 Average weight change of acetabular liners as a function of simulated gait cycles. Control liners were machined from GUR 1050 resin and gamma sterilized in nitrogen. Cross-linked liners were machined from GUR 1050 resin with the electron beam at a dose level of 95 kGy and subsequent melting. (Reprinted from Muratoglu OK, Bragdon CR, O'Connor DO, et al. Larger diameter femoral heads used in conjunction with a highly cross-linked ultra-high molecular weight polyethylene: a new concept. *J. Arthroplasty.* 2001;16(8 suppl):24–30, with permission.)

liner. These oriented fibrils strain harden the material in the sliding direction and weaken it in the transverse direction. As a result, crossing motions induced by the rotation and abduction–adduction of the hip cause the fibrils to break up into submicron-size particulate debris.

The reduction in the wear rate of UHMWPE associated with cross-linking is likely the result of the *above-described* mechanism of orientation and weakening of the articular surface. The cross-links act as constraints on UHMWPE molecules and reduce its ductility. Consequently, cross-linking reduces the extent of articular surface orientation in the principal direction of motion and the secondary weakening in the transverse direction. At high cross-link densities, this effect is more prominent, and the wear resistance of the polymer is significantly improved (26,37).

Extensive data are available from hip simulator studies (Fig. 9-10) showing significant improvement in the wear resistance of UHMWPE with cross-linking (14,32,34–37). Other reports of in vitro hip simulator studies lubricated with bovine serum and added third-body particles (e.g., bone cement particles) provide evidence that the wear rate of highly cross-linked UHMWPE can be significantly lower than that of conventional UHMWPE even in the presence of clinically relevant third-body particles (6,14,31,48).

The mechanical properties of UHMWPE can be affected by the radiation technologies used to improve its wear resistance (37). In general, increased cross-link density results in a decrease in the ductility of the polymer. The postirradiation melting can reduce the polymer's crystallinity and hence the elastic modulus and yield strength. The postirradiation annealing below the melting temperature results in a slight increase in the crystallinity, yield strength, and elastic modulus, and a decrease in the strength of the polymer (56). However, embrittlement secondary to long-term oxidation of the residual free radicals in UHMWPE irradiated and annealed below the melt temperature may further reduce the strength of the polymer (39).

The improved wear properties associated with highly cross-linked polyethylene has in some cases lead to the use of larger femoral heads to help reduce the incidence of dislocation or to provide additional stability in a hip with a history of dislocation. The combination of thinner polyethylene associated with larger femoral heads, acetabular component malposition, and the intrinsic mechanical properties of cross-linked polyethylene can produce an environment of elevated stress and associated fracture of a polyethylene component rim (15,20). Such occurrences demonstrate the need to fully consider the mechanical properties as well as the wear properties when choosing utilize highly cross-linked polyethylene in total hip replacement.

CLINICAL STUDIES

There are a number of historical, retrospective evaluations of experimental UHMWPEs with increased cross-link density. These studies each involved a small number of patients without matched control groups (19,42,60). The methods of UHMWPE cross-linking included high-dose (1000 kGy) gamma radiation in air by Oonishi et al. (42), gamma radiation (100 kGy) in the presence of acetylene by Grobbelaar et al. (19), and silane chemistry by Wroblewski (60). The radiographic wear measurements of Oonishi et al. showed a decreased average rate of femoral head penetration (0.072 to 0.076 mm/year) for the 1000-kGy-irradiated UHMWPE, in comparison with the control UHMWPE (0.098 to 0.25 mm/year) that had been gamma sterilized in air (42). Grobbelaar and coworkers used acetylene gas to increase the efficiency of cross-linking, and they reported on two different clinical follow-up series where all patients received a highly cross-linked acetabular liner (19). With follow-up as long as 22 years, the vast majority of patients demonstrated no measurable wear, and the average wear was 0.011 mm/year. In another study, Wroblewski reported on the wear behavior of 22-mm-diameter, silane cross-linked polyethylene acetabular components with a mean clinical follow-up of 10 years and 6 months of 14 patients (60). After an initial "bedding-in" penetration, the subsequent average penetration rate (or wear rate) was measured as 0.02 mm/year. In all of these historical follow-up studies (19,42,60) of three different types of early highly cross-linked polyethylene acetabular liners, the in vivo femoral head penetration rate was reported to be markedly lower than that with the conventional polyethylene.

Several total hip acetabular components made using contemporary cross-linking technologies have been in clinical use in since 1998. Early radiographic follow-up studies including high-precision measurement utilizing radiostereometric analysis (17,28,41) show a significant decrease in the femoral head penetration into the highly cross-linked polyethylene acetabular liners compared with the contemporary conventional UHMWPE liners. These in vivo findings confirm the in vitro tests that showed increased wear resistance with cross-linked UHMWPE (14,35). In addition, analysis of both conventional and highly cross-linked polyethylene acetabular liners surgically retrieved after short in vivo durations also showed a significant reduction in adhesive/abrasive wear with cross-linking (38).

POLYETHYLENE PAST, PRESENT, AND FUTURE

The use of polyethylene has enabled the successful restoration of hip function for millions of patients worldwide. From the onset of it use to the present day, UHMWPE has remained the bearing material of choice in total hip replacement. John Charnley first popularized polyethylene total hip replacement with the early use of a compression-molded and machined material with a relatively low molecular weight. This material has demonstrated durable implant function in clinical follow-up of as long as 30 years (54). The more extensive use of UHMWPE in ram-extruded and molded forms sterilized in air by exposure to gamma irradiation has also demonstrated durable implant function for at least 25 years (25). Over the history of it use, changes in resin selection and improved resin consolidation have been implemented in implant manufacture. The improved understanding of the effects of cross-linking and oxidation on UHMWPE has lead to the common use of oxygen-protected packaging during radiation sterilization and shelf storage. Most recently, methods to deliberately and more extensively cross-link UHWMPE while reducing the material's potential to oxidize have been develop in the form of extensively cross-linked UHMWPE.

Although laboratory data may suggest that new preparations of UHMWPE possess improvements, the utility of specific preparations of UHMWPE in total hip replacement can only be determined in well-controlled and carefully conducted long-term clinical trials. Several such trials are ongoing, and their results will in time improve our understanding of the utility of evolutionary changes in the manufacture of UHMWPE total hip components.

REFERENCES

1. Amstutz HC, Grigoris P. Metal on metal bearings in hip arthroplasty. *Clin Orthop Relat Res.* 1996;329S:S11–S34.
2. ASTM. *Standard F 648-00. Standard Specification for Ultra-High-Molecular-Weight Polyethylene Powder and Fabricated Form for Surgical Implants.* West Conshohocken, PA: American Society for Testing and Materials; 2000.
3. ASTM. *Standard F2003-00. Standard Guide for Accelerated Aging of Ultra-High Molecular Weight Polyethylene.* West Conshohocken, PA: American Society for Testing and Materials; 2000.
4. Bargmann LS, Bargmann BC, Collier JP, et al. Current sterilization and packaging methods for polyethylene. *Clin Orthop Relat Res.* 1999;369:49–58.
5. Bostrom MP, Bennett AP, Rimnac CM, et al. The natural history of ultra high molecular weight polyethylene. *Clin Orthop Relat Res.* 1994;309:20–28.
6. Bragdon CR, Jasty M, Muratoglu OK, et al. Third-body wear of highly cross-linked polyethylene in a hip simulator. *J Arthroplasty.* 2003;18:553–561.
7. Brandrup J, Immergut EH. Cross-linking with radiation. In: Brandrup J, Immergut EH, Grulke E, et al., eds. *Polymer Handbook.* New York: John Wiley & Sons; 1989:218–219.
8. Charnley J. Arthroplasty of the hip: a new operation. *Lancet.* 1961;(May 27):1129–1132.
9. Charnley J. Evolution of total hip replacement. *Ann. Chirurg. Gynaecol.* 1982;71:103–107.
10. Charnley J. *Low Friction Arthroplasty of the Hip.* Berlin: Springer-Verlag; 1979.
11. Collier J, Currier BH, Kennedy FE, et al. Comparison of cross-linked polyethylene materials for orthopaedic applications. *Clin Orthop Relat Res.* 2003;414:289–304.
12. Collier JP, Sperling DK, Currier JH, et al. Impact of gamma sterilization on clinical performance of polyethylene in the knee. *J Arthroplasty.* 1996;11:377–389.
13. Collier JP, Sutula LC, Currier BH, et al. Overview of polyethylene as a bearing material: comparison of sterilization methods. *Clin Orthop Relat Res.* 1996;333:76–86.
14. Crowninshield R, Laurent M, Yao JQ, et al. Cross-linking to improve THR wear performance. *Hip Int.* 2002;12(2):103–107.
15. Crowninshield RD, Maloney WJ, Wentz DH. Biomechanics of large femoral heads: what they do and don't do. *Clin Orthop Relat Res.* 2004;429:102–107.
16. Currier BH, Currier JH, Collier JP, et al. Effect of fabrication method and resin type on performance of tibial bearings. *J Biomed Mater Res.* 2000;53:143–151.
17. Digas G, Karrholm J, Malchau H, et al. RSA evaluation of wear of conventional versus cross-linked polyethylene acetabular components in vivo. Presented at: 49th Annual Meeting of the Orthopaedic Research Society; 2003; New Orleans, LA.
18. Dole M. Cross-linking and crystallinity in irradiated polyethylene. *Polym Plastics Technol Eng.* 1979;13:41–64.
19. Grobbelaar CJ. Clinical experience with gamma irradiation-cross-linked polyethylene: a 14 to 20 year follow-up report. *S Afr Bone Joint Surg.* 1999;11:140–147.
20. Halley D, Glassman A, Crowninshield RD. Recurrent dislocation of a total hip following treatment with a large prosthetic femoral head. *J Bone Joint Surg.* 2004;86A:827–830.
21. ISO. *5834. Implants for Surgery: Ultra-High Molecular Weight Polyethylene.* Geneva: International Standards Organization; 2005.
22. Jahan MS, Wang C, Schwarts G, et al. Combined chemical and mechanical effects on free radicals in UHMWPE joints during implantation. *J Biomed Mater Res.* 1991;25:1005–1017.
23. Jasty MJ, Goetz DD, Bragdon CR, et al. Wear of polyethylene acetabular components in total hip arthroplasty. An analysis of 128 components retrieved at autopsy or revision operation. *J Bone Joint Surg.* 1997;79:349–358.
24. Kashiwabara H, Shimada S, Hori Y. Free radicals and cross-linking in irradiated polyethylene. *Radiat Phys Chem.* 1991;37:43–46.
25. Keener JD, Callaghan JJ, Goetz DD, et al. Long-term function after charnley total hip arthroplasty. *Clin Orthop Relat Res.* 2003;417:148–156.
26. Kurtz SM, Pruitt LA, Jewett CW, et al. Radiation and chemical cross-linking promote strain hardening behavior and molecular alignment in ultra high molecular weight polyethylene during multi-axial loading conditions. *Biomaterials.* 1999;20:1449–1462.
27. Kurtz SM, Rimnac CM, Bartel DL. Degradation rate of ultra-high molecular weight polyethylene. *J Orthop Res.* 1997;15:57–61.
28. Martell JM, Incavo SJ. Clinical performance of a highly cross-linked polyethylene at two years in total hip arthroplasty: a randomized prospective trial. Presented at: 49th Annual Meeting of the Orthopaedic Research Society; 2003; New Orleans, LA.
29. McKee GK. Total hip replacement: past, present and future. *Biomaterials.* 1982;3:130–136.
30. McKellop HA, Campbell PA, Park SH, et al. The origin of submicron polyethylene wear debris in total hip arthroplasty. *Clin Orthop Relat Res.* 1995;311:3–20.
31. McKellop H, Shen F, DiMaio W, et al. Wear of gamma-cross-linked polyethylene acetabular cups against roughened femoral balls. *Clin Orthop Relat Res.* 1999;369:73–82.
32. McKellop H, Shen F, Lu B, et al. Development of an extremely wear resistant ultra-high molecular weight polyethylene for total hip replacements. *J Orthop Relat Res.* 1999;17:157–167.
33. McKellop H, Shen FW, Lu B, et al. Effect of molecular weight, calcium stearate, and sterilization method on the wear of ultra-high molecular weight polyethylene acetabular cups in a hip joint simulator. *J Orthop Res.* 1999;17:329–339.
34. McKellop H, Shen FW, Lu B, et al. Effect of sterilization method and other modifications on the wear resistance of acetabular cups made of ultra-high molecular weight polyethylene. *J Bone Joint Surg.* 2000;82A:1708–1725.
35. Muratoglu OK, Bragdon CR, O'Connor DO, et al. A novel method of cross-linking UHMWPE to improve wear, reduce oxidation and retain mechanical properties. *J Arthroplasty.* 2001;16:149–160.

36. Muratoglu OK, Bragdon CR, O'Connor DO, et al. Larger diameter femoral heads used in conjunction with a highly cross-linked ultra-high molecular weight polyethylene: a new concept. *J Arthroplasty.* 2001;16(8 suppl):24–30.

37. Muratoglu OK, Bragdon CR, O'Connor DO, et al. Unified wear model for highly cross-linked ultra-high molecular weight polyethylenes (UHMWPE). *Biomaterials.* 1999;20:1463–1470.

38. Muratoglu OK, Greenbaum E, Larson S, et al. Surface analysis of early retrieved acetabular polyethylene liners: a comparison of standard and highly cross-linked polyethylenes. Presented at: 48th Annual Meeting of the Orthopaedic Research Society; 2002; Dallas, TX.

39. Muratoglu OK, Merrill EW, Bragdon CR, et al. Effect of radiation, heat, and aging on in vitro wear resistance of polyethylene. *Clin Orthop Relat Res.* 2003;417:253–262.

40. Nich C, Ali EHS, Hannouche D, et al. Long-term results of alumina-on-alumina hip arthroplasty for osteonecrosis. *Clin Orthop Relat Res.* 2003;417:102–111.

41. Nivbrant B, Roerhl S, Hewitt BJ, et al. In vivo wear and migration of high cross-linked poly cups: a RSA study. Presented at: 49th Annual Meeting of the Orthopaedic Research Society; 2003; New Orleans, LA.

42. Oonishi H, Takayama Y, E. Tsuji. The low wear of cross-linked polyethylene socket in total hip prostheses. In: Wise DL, Trantolo DJ, Altobelli DE, et al, eds. *Encyclopedic Handbook of Biomaterials and Bioengineering. Part A: Materials.* New York: Marcel Dekker Inc; 1995:1853–1868.

43. Randall JC, Zoepfl FJ, Silverman J. A 13C NMR study of radiation-induced long-chain branching in polyethylene. *Makromol Chem Rapid Commun.* 1983;4:149–157.

44. Rimnac CM, Klein RW, Betts F, et al. Post-irradiation aging of ultra-high molecular weight polyethylene. *J Bone Joint Surg.* 1994; 76A:1052–1056.

45. Rimnac CM, Wright TM, Klein RW, et al. Characterization of material properties of ultra high molecular weight polyethylene before and after implantation. Presented at: Society of Biomaterials Symposium; St. Charles, Illinois Sept 17–20, 1992.

46. Roe RJ, Grood ES, Shastri R, et al. Effect of radiation sterilization and aging on ultrahigh molecular weight polyethylene. *J Biomed Mater Res.* 1981;15:209–230.

47. Rose RM, Goldfarb HV. On the pressure dependence of the wear of ultrahigh molecular weight polyethylene. *Wear.* 1983;92: 99–111.

48. Saikko V, Calonius O, Keranen J. Wear of conventional and cross-linked ultra-high-molecular-weight polyethylene acetabular cups against polished and roughened CoCr femoral heads in a biaxial hip simulator. *J Biomed Mater Relat Res (Appl Biomater)* 2002;63: 848–853.

49. Sauer JA, Foden E, Morrow DR. Influence of molecular weight on fatigue behavior of polyethylene and polystyrene. *Polym Eng Sci.* 1977;17(4):246–250.

50. Scott M, Morrison M, Mishra SR, et al. A method to quantify wear particle volume using atomic force microscopy. Presented at: 48th Annual Meeting of the Orthopaedic Research Society; 2002; Dallas, TX.

51. Schmalzried TP, Kwong LM, Jasty M, et al. The mechanism of loosening of cemented acetabular components in total hip arthroplasty. *Clin Orthop Relat Res.* 1992;274:60–78.

52. Shen FW, McKellop HA. Interaction of oxygen and cross-linking in gamma-irradiated ultrahigh molecular weight polyethylene. *J Biomed Mater Res.* 2002:430–439.

53. Sieber HP, Rieker CB, Kottig P. Analysis of 118 second-generation metal-on-metal retrieved hip implants. *J Bone Joint Surg.* 1999; 81-B:46–50.

54. Sochart BH, Porter ML. Long-term results of cemented Charnley low-friction arthroplasty in patients aged less than 30 years. *J Arthroplasty.* 1998;13:123–131.

55. Sutula LC, Collier JP, Saum KA, et al. Impact of gamma sterilization on clinical performance of polyethylene in the hip. *Clin Orthop Relat Res.* 1995;319:28–40.

56. Taylor SK, Serekian P, Bruchalski P, et al. The performance of irradiation-cross-linked UHMWPE cups under abrasive conditions throughout hip joint simulation wear testing. *Trans Orthop Res Soc* 1999;45:252.

57. Trainor A, Haward RN, Hay JN. The effect of density on the properties of high molecular weight polyethylenes. *J Polym Sci Polym Phys Ed.* 1977;15:1077–1088.

58. Waugh W. *John Charnley: The Man and the Hip. The Plan Fullfilled 1959–1969.* London: Springer-Verlag; 1990.

59. Wroblewski BM, Siney PD. Charnley low-friction arthroplasty of the hip: long-term results. *Clin Orthop Relat Res.* 1993;292: 191–201.

60. Wroblewski B, Siney P, Fleming P. Low-friction arthroplasty of the hip using alumina ceramic and cross-linked polyethylene: A ten-year follow-up report. *J Bone Joint Surg.* 1999;81-B:54–55.

Metals

10

Jeremy L. Gilbert

ORTHOPEDIC ALLOYS

The history of arthroplasty and the use of orthopedic alloys has been reviewed by Dowson (39) and by Friedman et al. (44). In the early 1920s and 1930s, interpositional arthroplasty was investigated; with this technique, a material was interposed between the two sides of the joint to inhibit arthrodesis. A variety of materials were considered for this application. The metals investigated consisted of gold foil and cobalt-chromium-molybdenum (Co-Cr-Mo) alloy (Vitallium, Howmedica, Inc.), which was then in use as a dental material. Use of steels in fracture fixation was reported as early as 1804 (44). Stainless steel (18% chromium, 8% nickel) was not introduced until 1926. However, its corrosion resistance was not adequate for long-term implantation until it was later found that 2% to 3% molybdenum would reduce pitting and crevice corrosion attack.

The modern age of joint replacement appears to be based, in part, on the work of Wiles, who introduced a stainless steel total joint replacement in 1938 (73). In the 1950s, McKee and Ferrar (60) introduced the first metal-on-metal total joint, initially using stainless steel but later switching to the Co-Cr-Mo alloy (Vitallium). These prostheses were used well into the 1970s. The concept of metal-on-metal articulating surfaces is seeing increased use and will be discussed in later sections on wear and corrosion.

It is generally accepted that Co-Cr-Mo–based alloys were initially used in dentistry and were adopted later by the orthopedics community. These alloys were developed by E. Haynes in the early 1900s (Haynes Stellite-21). By the 1930s, Vitallium (see Table 10-3 later in the chapter for the composition of ASTM F-75) was in use as an alloy for partial dentures (38). These alloys were not developed by the aircraft industry, despite what many have stated; rather they were adapted to high-temperature aircraft engine use in 1941. Consequently, cobalt-based alloys are thought of as superalloys.

Titanium alloys were developed primarily for the aircraft industry and were adopted by the biomaterials community in the late 1950s and early 1960s. In recent years, they have come to be among the most heavily used alloys in orthopedics for several reasons, including their high strength, low modulus, and excellent corrosion resistance.

The alloys used today in orthopedic applications primarily include iron-based (stainless steel), cobalt-based, and titanium-based alloys. Recently, other alloys including zirconium (Zr) and tantalum alloys have gained in use. In total joint replacements, the primary alloy systems used are the Co-Cr-Mo alloys and the titanium alloys, in particular, titanium, 6 aluminum, 4 vanadium (Ti-6Al-4V ELI). In some regions of the world, stainless steel prostheses are utilized (e.g., in the United Kingdom), with newer formulations of these alloys coming into use. Each of these alloys has a particular set of physical and mechanical properties that make it highly successful in orthopedic applications.

This chapter reviews the basic science of orthopedic alloys and identifies the bulk and surface structures and the properties that result in the highly successful materials in use today. It also touches upon the basic mechanisms of degradation in orthopedic alloys, including corrosion, wear, and fatigue. Alternative surface treatments to enhance the surface properties of alloys (wear and corrosion resistance) are reviewed, and clinical findings related to alloy degradation are discussed. Also, some future possibilities for alloys and surface treatments are presented.

BASIC SCIENCE OF METALS

As is true for any class of materials, the properties and performance of metals and alloys are dependent on the composition and structure of the material. In a classic materials science sense, processing–structure–property relationships will dictate metal behavior. That is, how a material is fabricated will affect the resulting structure (e.g., grain size, alloy composition, carbide distribution), and subsequently these structural features will dictate, to a large extent, the resultant mechanical and physical properties (e.g., fatigue strength and corrosion resistance). If one can gain an appreciation of these structure–property relationships, one will be in a better position to assess alternative materials or treatments.

ATOMIC STRUCTURE AND DEFECTS

Metals are made up of crystals. That is, metal atoms are positioned in a three-dimensional periodic array within a single crystal. A typical implant is composed of many metal crystals (i.e., it is polycrystalline) joined together at grain boundaries (Fig. 10-1). Many of the physical and mechanical properties of metals are governed by these crystals. There are several different possible relationships between atoms within a crystal (i.e., its crystal structure). These include body-centered cubic (BCC), face-centered cubic (FCC), and hexagonal close-packed (HCP) (Fig. 10-2). There are 14 different ways atoms can be arrayed in a crystal (so-called Bravais lattices [26]). However, most of the implant alloys used in orthopedics are either BCC (e.g., β-Ti), FCC (e.g., 316L stainless steel), or HCP (e.g., α-Ti, Co-Cr).

It is important to note that metal crystals are not defect free. In fact, there are several types of defects in metals that, it turns out, are the primary factors affecting properties. These defects can be classified according to their spatial dimension (i.e., point defect, line defect, area defect, and volume defect).

Point defects are known as vacancies. These defects occur when a lattice site in the crystal is not occupied by a metal atom (see Fig. 10-1). These defects are present in all metals and alloys and provide a mechanism for diffusion in solids.

a. Face Centered Cubic   b. Body Centered Cubic

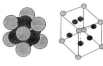

c. Hexagonal Close Packed

Figure 10-2 Three common crystal structures found in implant alloys: face-centered cubic (FCC) **(a)**, body-centered cubic (BCC) **(b)**, and hexagonal close-packed (HCP) **(c)** crystal structures.

Line defects, also known as dislocations, are the major defect affecting the mechanical properties of metals. A dislocation is the result of an extra half-plane of atoms in a crystal (see Fig. 10-1). That is, when a plane of atoms terminates within the middle of the crystal, it locally distorts the crystal structure. This distortion or internal strain energy is experienced only in the immediate vicinity of the end of the extra half-plane of atoms; hence, a dislocation is a line defect where the line represents the end of the half-plane. When a stress of sufficient magnitude is applied, these dislocations can move through the lattice, resulting in a permanent change in the shape of the crystal, and the metal is said to plastically deform. When a metal is deformed plastically (i.e., there is a permanent deformation that remains after the loading is removed), the cause was the creation and movement of dislocations.

Grain boundaries can be thought of as area defects. That is, the region where two metal crystals come together is the grain boundary (see Fig. 10-1), and it is a region of higher disorder in the metal than the internal grain regions.

Finally, volume defects, known as voids or cracks, are well-known and more easily understood forms of defects that can affect the mechanical performance of a metal or alloy. Even small scratches on the surface of a metal may significantly affect the behavior of the alloy (e.g., lower the fatigue strength).

Each of these forms of defects can have a profound effect on the behavior of the alloy. In particular, the mechanical behaviors of the alloy (e.g., its strength, ductility, fracture toughness, and fatigue resistance) are all dependent on how the structure of the alloy affects its deformation mechanisms (primarily dislocation generation and motion). In fact, the key to understanding how and why metals and alloys are strengthened is based on an understanding of dislocations. Those processes or structures within the polycrystalline metal that tend to impede the motion of dislocations will act to strengthen the metal. There are other deformation mechanisms possible in metal alloy systems, including twinning and grain boundary sliding. These alternative deformation mechanisms are not as prevalent (typically) as dislocation motion and will not be discussed here.

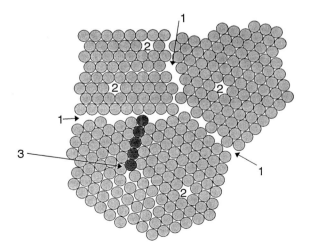

Figure 10-1 Schematic representation of three grains of a metallic crystal structure. Note the presence of grain boundaries **(1)**, vacancies (hole in crystals) **(2)**, and dislocations **(3)**; dark atoms represent the extra half-plane. Note the distortion of the lattice below the extra half-plane.

STRENGTHENING MECHANISMS IN ORTHOPEDIC ALLOYS

Orthopedic alloys rely on several different mechanisms for improvements in strength. These strengthening mechanisms are based on the concept of impeding dislocation motion. That is, if there are methods (such as alloying—adding other atoms to the crystal, heat treating—heating and cooling the metal to induce specific changes in the alloy, cold working—deforming the metal to create and entangle dislocation; see below for more details) that make it more difficult for dislocations to move, then alloys that have undergone these processes will be stronger. The following is a brief description of the most common strengthening mechanisms.

Solid Solution Strengthening

Solid solution strengthening, both interstitial and substitutional, results when one or more elements (which make up the so-called solute) are added to the primary metal (the so-called solvent metal) to form an alloy (a mixture of two or more elements). The solute atoms can reside in one of two possible sites within the lattice, either substituting for a solvent atom on a lattice site or sitting in an interstitial site between solvent atoms (see Fig. 10-1). Substitutional atoms are typically of a size similar to that of the solvent, whereas interstitial atoms are typically much smaller (e.g., C, O, N, or B). Both interstitial and substitutional atoms contribute to the strength of a metal. However, interstitial atoms are typically more effective. For example, the addition of less than 0.1% carbon to iron results in a steel with about a 10-fold increase in strength. Similarly, in titanium, the addition of small amounts of oxygen (an interstitial solute atom) will significantly increase strength. Solid solution strengthening can result in several modifications of microstructure that will affect strength. The main effect is to pin dislocations by developing locally solute rich regions in the vicinity of the dislocation line. These so-called dislocation atmospheres increase the strain energy needed to break the dislocation free and move it (i.e., induce plastic deformation), thus raising the strength of the alloy.

Cold and Hot Working

Cold working is a process whereby deformation of a metal results in an increase in strength. On a microstructural level, deformation of the metal or alloy results in a significant increase in the dislocation density (the amount of dislocation line per unit volume) and entangles these dislocations into tight bundles. This results in a structure in which it is much more difficult to continue to move dislocations within the lattice. Thus, the strength can increase substantially as a result of cold working. Cold working typically increases both yield strength and ultimate strength, but it decreases ductility. Cold working is often performed on 316L stainless steel as a strengthening mechanism. The metal may be cold worked by rolling, by compression between two platens, by drawing through a die (for wire and rod), or by another deformation mechanism.

To remove some or most of the dislocations created during cold working, a heat treatment process called "annealing" is performed. In this process, the alloy is heated to a sufficiently high temperature (but below any transformation tempera-

ture), and, over a period of time, new grains of dislocation-free material will nucleate and grow into the previously cold-worked grains. This process is called "recrystallization," and it causes the alloy to return to its pre-cold-worked structure and properties. Other processes also take place during the heating of cold-worked alloys. These include a process called "recovery" and another called "grain growth." Both have some effect on mechanical properties but not to the extent that recrystallization does. Annealing is performed for several possible reasons, including restoring the ductility of the material, relieving internal (or residual) stresses, and reducing the grain size of the material (see later).

Very often, alloys are hot worked (deformed at a high temperature). These high-temperature deformation processes fall into the category of thermomechanical processes. *Wrought* (deformed into shape) and *forged* (high-temperature deformation to form a shape) are both terms describing thermomechanical processes. Often, high-temperature deformation processes are performed to form a shape (i.e., a hip prosthesis), but these processes can also alter the microstructure of the alloy. For example, in the ASTM standard for Ti-6Al-4V (ASTM F-136, ASTM F-1481), a "bimodal" $\alpha + \beta$ microstructure is called for. This microstructure results from the deformation of Ti-6Al-4V at a temperature high in the $\alpha + \beta$ phase region but still below the β transus temperature (about 930°C).

Grain size reduction can also be attained during hot working. In this process, the deformation of the grains increases the internal strain energy by the generation and entanglement of dislocations. This strain energy can be eliminated by a process known as "recrystallization" (described above) during which new grains that are relatively dislocation free nucleate and grow into the old, heavily deformed grains. Depending on the temperature, time, and extent of prior deformation, the grain size of the structure can be refined by this process. See one of several good references on this subject (64).

Grain Size Effects

Grain size affects the strength of an alloy. This again is the result of the interaction of the grain boundaries with the dislocations in the grains. Grain boundaries prevent dislocations from easily passing from one grain to another. Thus they impede dislocation motion. If there are more grain boundaries per unit volume (which results when grains are smaller), then it will be more difficult to move dislocations (i.e., to plastically deform). Therefore, increases in strength can be obtained if one makes smaller grains (assuming no other process intervenes).

Precipitation Hardening

Precipitation hardening is a mechanism that relies on the presence of a second phase dispersed in the parent microstructure to inhibit dislocation motion. This mechanism can operate only in those materials in which second-phase particles or grains can exist. Examples of where precipitation hardening can occur are in Co-Cr-Mo alloys and in Ti-6Al-4V. Typically, metal carbides can form in Co-Cr-Mo alloys, and if these carbides are uniformly dispersed through the structure, they can pin dislocations and make it more difficult to deform. Variations in the size and distribution of precipitates within the structure will alter the mechanical properties. Precipitates will grow over time when the alloy is subjected to high temperatures, as in an annealing or homogenization treatment. When precipitation-strengthened alloys are heated, this process is called "aging." There is typically an optimal aging treatment for an alloy, which represents an optimal distribution of precipitates through the structure.

It should be pointed out that orthopedic implants are manufactured in several ways, including casting (for cobalt-based prostheses), machining from forged or wrought bar stock, and forging into near net shape. Cast Co-Cr-Mo alloy prostheses may have large variations in grain size as well as very large grains, up to 2 to 5 mm in diameter. Large grain sizes and variability can reduce strength, and hence cast Co-Cr-Mo microstructures are typically lower in strength than fine-grained wrought Co-Cr-Mo microstructures (see Table 10-4 later in this chapter for examples).

Other manufacturing processes include hot isostatic pressing (HIP'ing) of powders. Here, the alloy is first made into fine powders (on the micron scale) by spraying droplets of molten alloy into a chamber and letting the drops solidify. Once collected, these fine powders are placed in a shaped mold and heater and pressed to allow sintering or diffusion bonding and consolidation to occur. This is done by heating and pressing adjacent powder beads so that atoms on the surface can interdiffuse and bond together. HIP'ing is also used to attach a porous surface coating to prostheses. Other surface coating methods include plasma spraying of either metal or hydroxyapatite and precipitation of calcium phosphates from solution.

MECHANICAL PROPERTIES

When discussing strengthening mechanisms in metals, it is important to understand what is meant (or not meant) by strength. Figure 10-3 is a typical stress–strain curve for a metal. In it are defined the terms used to describe the mechanical behavior of a metal (or other material). In the low-stress/low-strain region, there is typically a linear relationship between stress and strain. This proportionality is known as the modulus, Young's modulus, or elastic modulus. This property reflects the stiffness of the material, which is dependent on the ease or difficulty of stretching atoms from their equilibrium position in the crystal lattice. Modulus is relatively insensitive to the presence of defects such as dislocations.

The stiffness of a prosthesis is the result of a combination of geometry and modulus. For hip stems, the main deformation mode is bending, and the stiffness concept for beam bending is known as "flexural rigidity" (EI), where I is known as the second moment of area and is a measure of the spread of the cross-sectional area about its center axis. This concept is exploited in some hip stems by, for example, reducing the flexural rigidity by putting a slot in the distal stem shaft. This effectively lowers the distal stem rigidity and allows for less stress shielding to occur.

Returning to the tensile test curve of Fig. 10-3, as the stress increases beyond the elastic range, there is a point at which dislocations begin to be created and to move through the grains and impart some plastic deformation. When this occurs, there is no longer a linear relationship between stress and strain. The material is said to reach the proportional limit. When the permanent deformation reaches 0.2%, the stress at this arbitrary permanent strain defines the yield stress of the material. The ultimate stress of the material is the highest stress reached during testing; the percent elongation is the amount of plastic strain imparted prior to failure and is a measure of the ductility of the material. Other measures of ductility include the reduction of area, which is the percent change in the cross-sectional area in a tensile sample before testing and after failure.

There are other material properties that are important to consider for implant applications. A primary mechanical property of interest to total joint replacements is the fatigue strength. Fatigue is a process whereby a cyclic stress or strain is applied to a material and, over the course of many cycles (up to 10^7 cycles or more), a crack is initiated and propagated to failure. Most people load their hips on average 2 to 5 million times per year, clearly a high-cycle fatigue condition. The *fatigue strength* of a material is the cyclic stress required to cause failure at some number of cycles. *Fatigue life* is another term often used to describe fatigue behavior. The fatigue life of a material is the number of cycles that will cause failure at a fixed cyclic stress. Fatigue strength and fatigue life are related to each other in a classic cyclic-stress versus number-of-cycles-to-failure curve (also known as a *Wohler curve* or an *S-N curve*). This is a plot of the cyclic stress versus the log of the number of cycles to failure (Fig. 10-4). As a general rule, the fatigue strength of an implant alloy will scale with the tensile strength of the alloy. For example, for high-cycle/low-stress fatigue

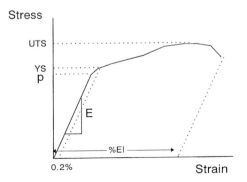

Figure 10-3 Schematic stress–strain curve for a typical metal. Note the elastic region with Young's modulus (E), proportional limit (P), yield strength (YS), ultimate tensile strength (UTS), and percent elongation (%El).

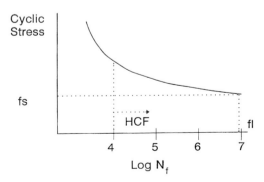

Figure 10-4 Schematic of a fatigue curve. Wohler diagram: cyclic stress versus log number of cycles-to-failure curve (S-N curve) for fatigue evaluation; fs, fatigue strength at 107 cycles; fl, fatigue life at fs; HCP, high-cycle fatigue regime.

situations, the fatigue strength (at 10^7 cycles) is about 0.3 to 0.5 of the ultimate tensile strength (UTS) (63). High-cycle fatigue is when the number of cycles required to cause failure is about 10^4 or greater. In metals during high-cycle fatigue, most of the fatigue life is spent initiating a fatigue crack, and only a small percentage is spent propagating that crack to failure. Thus, those material properties that will inhibit crack initiation will be more successful in enhancing the fatigue life of the material. These include creating smooth surfaces, since fatigue cracks tend to initiate at the surface; imparting compressive residual stresses at the surface (e.g., ion implantation); and raising the cold work level, or hardness, of the surface (e.g., shot peening or ion implantation).

SPECIFIC IMPLANT ALLOYS

Stainless Steels

Stainless steels are iron-carbon–based alloys and are covered by ASTM specifications F-138, F-139, F-621, F-745, F-899, F-1314, F-1586, and F-2229 (7,8,12,14,16,21). In general, these alloys contain approximately 18% to 22% by weight Cr, 12% to 14% by weight Ni, 2.5% by weight Mo, 2% to 5% by weight Mn, and 0.03% to 0.08% by weight C (Table 10-1). The steels described in ASTM F-899 are for use as surgical instruments rather than surgical implants and include both 300 series (austenitic) and 400 series (martensitic) steels. The latter steels are heat-treatable steels (i.e., they will vary their mechanical properties with different heat treatment procedures), whereas 300 series steels (e.g., 316) are not heat treatable but can be cold worked.

The most common steels used for implants (e.g., bone plates, screws) are the 316 stainless steels, which are austenitic (i.e., they have an FCC crystal structure). There are two grades, grade 1 (316) and grade 2 (316L), with the L designating a lower carbon content. Other alloys include a nitrogen-strengthened, manganese-containing alloy (ASTM F-1314). An example of the microstructure of stainless steel is shown in the scanning electron micrograph (SEM) in Figure 10-5. Newer steel alloys include F-2229, which has a lower Ni content and tends to be more pitting corrosion resistant than standard 316L stainless steel.

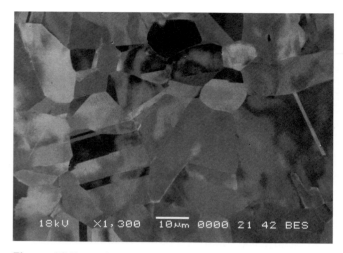

Figure 10-5 Backscattered electron image (BEI) of a 316L stainless steel alloy that has been electropolished. Backscattered electrons provide contrast in the image as a result of crystallographic orientation differences between grains. (Backscattered electron imaging is also known as electron channeling contrast imaging.) Note that the grains also show evidence of twins, which are structures in the grains that result from deformation.

The austenitic (316 series) alloys are typically used in fracture-fixation devices, such as bone plates, intramedullary rods, and bone screws. They have been used for total joint replacements in the past and are seeing increased use in Europe (particularly the United Kingdom). In the past they were found to be less reliable than the current alloys used in these applications (cobalt-based and titanium-based alloys), although newer steel alloys appear to be much more capable of withstanding the loading and environment of the body. They are solid solution strengthened and can be cold (or hot) worked to increase strength. Hot working can also be performed to reduce the grain size of the material. They are not typically precipitation strengthened, with the exception of F-1314, which may contain small dispersions of carbonitrides within the grains. The low carbon content in grade 2 was meant to minimize the potential for forming metal carbides, the presence of which may adversely affect the corrosion resistance of the alloy by a process known as sensitization (37). The mechanical

TABLE 10-1

CHEMICAL COMPOSITION OF MOST USED IRON-BASED ALLOYS

ASTM Designation	Fe	Cr	Ni	Mo	Mn	C	Si	N	Cu	P	S	Others
					Composition (wt%)							
F-138 (316L)	Bal	17.00–19.00	13.00–15.00	2.25–3.00	2.00	0.030	0.75	0.10	0.50	0.025	0.010	—
F-1314	Bal	20.50–23.50	11.50–13.50	2.00–3.00	4.00–6.00	0.030	0.75	0.20–0.40	0.50	0.025	0.010	0.10–0.30 Nb 0.10–0.30 V
F-1586	Bal	19.50–22.00	9.00–11.00	2.00–3.00	2.00–4.25	0.08	0.75	0.25–0.50	0.25	0.025	0.010	0.25–0.80 Nb
F-2229	Bal	19.00–23.00	0.10	0.50–1.50	21.00–24.00	0.08	0.75	0.90 min	0.25	0.03	0.010	—

TABLE 10-2
MECHANICAL PROPERTIES OF STAINLESS STEELS

	UTS (MPa)	YS (MPa)	%El
ASTM F-138 (316/316L)[a]	480–860	170–690	40–12
ASTM F-745	480	205	30
ASTM F-1314	690–1035	380–862	35–12

MPa, megapascal; UTS, ultimate tensile strength; YS, yield strength; %El, percent elongation.
[a]Annealed to heavily cold worked.
Values are minimum acceptable levels for ASTM standards.

properties of the steel alloys used in orthopedics are listed in Table 10-2.

Cobalt-based Alloys

The cobalt-based alloys typically contain chromium, molybdenum, carbon, and other elements such as nickel, silicon, and iron. Table 10-3 summarizes the ASTM-designated cobalt-based alloys used in medical devices. Cobalt-based alloys in use today include ASTM F-75, F-90, F-562, F-563, F-688, F-799, F-1058, F-1091, F-1377, and F-1537 (3,5,9,10,13,15,17,18,22,25). Some of these specifications have compositions similar to others, or they do not address alloy composition. The only difference between F-1537 and F-75 is the presence of a higher nitrogen concentration in the former. Cobalt alloys can be either an FCC (α) structure (typically at temperatures higher than 400°C) or an HCP (ε) structure (T lower than 400°C) (34).

Cobalt-based alloys are used primarily in total joint replacement applications where high strength and corrosion resistance are necessary. These alloys are strengthened by solid-solution strengthening and, to some extent, precipitation hardening resulting from the precipitation of carbides. A

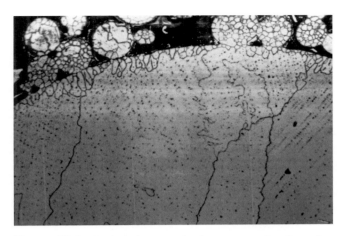

Figure 10-6 Optical photograph of a cross section through a porous-coated Co-Cr-Mo prosthesis, etched electrolytically in phosphate-buffered saline at about 800 mV (SCE) for 20 hours. Note the large grains indicative of a cast structure and the carbides dispersed throughout each grain. The grains in the surface region and in the porous-coating beads are much smaller than in the bulk alloy.

typical microstructure of a cast Co-Cr-Mo hip prosthesis is shown in cross section in the optical micrograph in Figure 10-6. Note the very large grains present as a result of the casting as well as the smaller grains near the porous coating on the surface. Also shown in this micrograph are the dispersed carbides present within the grains (and at the grain boundaries), which provide some precipitation strengthening. The as-cast structure of Co-Cr-Mo is one of a dendritic (treelike) structure with a highly varying chemistry across the dendrite (called "coring") (33,57). There are interdendritic carbides present as well. The chemistry and phase structure of Co-Cr-Mo alloys are not well understood. A backscattered electron micrograph of a cast structure is shown in Figure 10-7. The carbide region (bright and dark region) is complex in structure and chemistry.

TABLE 10-3
ASTM DESIGNATION AND CHEMICAL COMPOSITIONS FOR COBALT-BASED ALLOYS

ASTM Designation	Composition (wt%)											
	Co	Cr	Ni	Mo	Fe	C	Si	Mn	W	P	S	Others
F-75, cast	Bal	27.0–30.0	1.00	5.0–7.0	0.75	0.35	1.00	1.00	0.20	0.020	0.010	0.25N; 0.30Al; 0.01 B
F-90, wrought	Bal	19.0–21.0	9.0–11.0	—	3.00	0.05–0.15	0.40	1.00–2.00	14.00–16.00	0.040	0.030	—
F-562[a], wrought	Bal	19.0–21.0	33.0–37.0	9.0–10.5	1.00	0.025	0.15	0.15	—	0.015	0.010	1.0 Ti
F-563	Bal	18.0–22.0	15.00–25.00	3.00–4.00	4.00–6.00	0.05	0.50	1.00	3.00–4.00	—	0.010	0.50–3.50 Ti
F-799	Bal	26.0–30.0	1.0	5.0–7.0	0.75	0.35	1.0	1.0	—	—	—	0.25 N
F-1058	42	21.5	18	7.5	Bal	0.15	1.2	2.0	—	0.015	0.015	0.001 Be
F-1537	Bal	30.0	1.0	7.0	0.75	0.35	1.0	1.0	—	—	—	0.25 N

[a]Also known as MP35N: Multiphase, 35% Ni; Bal: Balance.

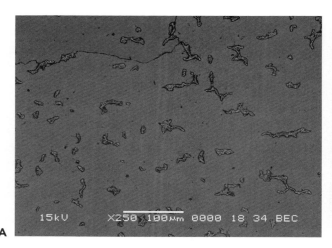 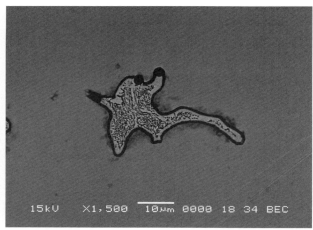

Figure 10-7 Backscattered electron micrographs of cast Co-Cr-Mo alloy (ASTM F-75) showing the complex carbide structure present in these alloys. Bright and dark spots represent the carbide regions, and the varying contrast is in part due to compositional differences between regions; low magnification **(A)** and higher magnification **(B)** image of a carbide.

Wrought Co-Cr-Mo has a microstructural appearance very different from that of cast Co-Cr-Mo. This material typically has much smaller grains that are more equiaxed (i.e., of approximately equal diameter in all directions), as can be seen in Figure 10-8. This is an SEM of a retrieved wrought Co-Cr-Mo femoral head (ASTM F-799) inside the modular taper after retrieval from a patient. The surface has been etched by body solutions, causing fretting crevice corrosion attack in the body (46). Figures 10-9A and 10-9B show examples of currently used high-carbon–forged Co-Cr-Mo alloy microstructure. Note the numerous dispersed carbides present and the small grains (about 10 μm or less) that make these alloys very strong and wear resistant.

Cobalt-based alloys have several properties that make them excellent alloys for total joint prostheses. They are high-strength materials and have a high hardness (resistance to surface deformation). A summary of the mechanical properties of the above alloys is shown in Table 10-4. Furthermore, as a result of several factors, they work-harden very rapidly. That is, a small amount of plastic deformation results in a large increase in the strength. This property of cobalt-based alloys gives them a high wear resistance and makes them ideally suited for articulating surface applications. The presence of carbides on the surface (as well as throughout the alloy) also enhances the wear resistance of these materials by providing a dispersion of very hard carbides embedded in a matrix of metal alloy upon which surface contact is made. A downside of the high work hardening of this material is the difficulty in machining and deformation processing of the alloy. These cobalt-based alloys also have very good corrosion resistance in chloride-containing solutions (58).

Titanium-Based Alloys

There are several titanium-based alloy systems in use or under consideration. Commercially pure titanium (cP-Ti) (see

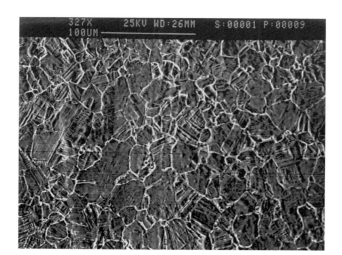

Figure 10-8 Scanning electron micrograph (SEM) of a wrought Co-Cr-Mo head after etching by body solutions in the modular taper region. The exposure of this microstructure was most likely the result of fretting crevice corrosion within the taper recess of the modular connection, and it is an indicator of the severity of the attack that may take place inside these tapers.

TABLE 10-4

MECHANICAL PROPERTIES OF COBALT-BASED ALLOYS (MINIMUM ACCEPTABLE LEVELS)

Alloy	UTS (MPa)	YS (MPa)	%El
ASTM F-75	655	450	8
ASTM F-90	860	310	30
ASTM F-562[a]	793–1793	241–1586	50–8
ASTM F-563[a]	600–1586	276–1310	50–12
ASTM F-799	1172	827	12
ASTM F-1058[b]	895–1795	—	—
ASTM F-1537[c]	897–1172	517–827	20–12

[a]Annealed, or cold worked and aged, respectively.
[b]Cold worked strip.
[c]Either annealed or hot worked, respectively.
MPa, megapascal; UTS, ultimate tensile strength; YS, yield strength; %El, percent elongation.

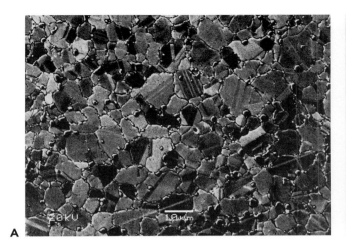
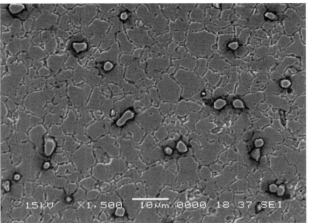

A   B

Figure 10-9 Scanning electron micrographs (SEMs) of high-carbon–forged Co-Cr-Mo alloy microstructure. Note the carbides and small grains present. **A:** Backscattered electron image. Note the twinning in the structure. **B:** Secondary electron image of a wrought high-carbon Co-Cr-Mo alloy. Note the extremely small grains present (2 to 5 μm).

Fig. 10-10) and an alloy typically containing aluminum and vanadium (Ti-6Al-4V; see Fig. 10-11) are the common alloy compositions for titanium in use in the United States. Alternate alloys are being considered in the United States or are in use in other parts of the world (e.g., Ti-6Al-7Nb in Europe). Titanium-based materials are among the most intensely studied implant alloy systems for orthopedic applications. There are many alternative titanium alloys under investigation, including β-Ti alloys. Titanium alloys are known to be highly biocompatible and have several other properties that make them suitable for implant applications, such as high strength and fatigue resistance. There are several ASTM specifications for titanium alloys, including ASTM F-67, F-136, F-620, F-1108, F-1295, F-1472, F-1580, F-1713, F-2066, and F-2063 (2,6,11,19,20,23,24). The compositions of some of these alloys are listed in Table 10-5.

Commercially pure titanium has a single-phase HCP crystal structure; it comes in four grades that, as can be seen in Table 10-5, vary primarily in their oxygen concentration. Titanium has a very large affinity for oxygen and will absorb it in high concentrations at high temperatures. Oxygen can serve as an interstitial solid-solution–strengthening element, and at very small concentrations, it can have a significant effect on mechanical properties. Too high an oxygen concentration can result in a so-called α-case, in which the high oxygen levels result in an α-stabilized continuous grain structure at the surface, which lowers the fatigue strength and surface ductility (65). The yield strength for cP-Ti varies from about 150 MPa (grade 1) to 480 MPa (grade 4). Table 10-6 summarizes the mechanical properties of some currently used orthopedic titanium alloys. Commercially pure titanium does not have the strength required to carry the large stresses associated with total joint replacements, and it is usually used in orthopedics only as a material for porous coatings or in low-stress applications.

Ti-6Al-4V is the primary implant alloy in use today. It has high strength and fatigue resistance. The microstructure of Ti-6Al-4V (Fig. 10-11) consists of small, approximately 10- to

20-μm α grains (HCP structure [gray areas in Fig. 10-11]), surrounded by regions of transformed β phase (a mixture of retained β [BCC phase] and acicular α [whiter regions in Fig. 10-11]). This so-called bimodal microstructure results from the deformation of the alloy high in the two-phase temperature region of the alloy (where both α and β phases are stable). This thermomechanical process causes the acicular α to be disrupted and to form the equiaxed bimodal microstructure shown in Figure 10-11. If this alloy is heated above the region where both phases are stable (into the β phase field), then the microstructure will revert to the acicular structure and will lose some of its fatigue resistance. This bimodal microstructure results in a high-strength, high-fatigue-crack-initiation-resistant alloy. These changes in the shape of the α grains in Ti-6Al-4V significantly affect the material's mechanical properties.

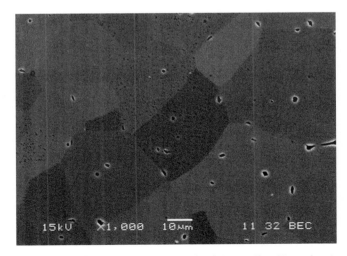

Figure 10-10 Electron micrograph of CP-Ti alloy. Note that it does not have precipitates (dark spots are etching artifacts). Also, it is a single-phase structure that differs from the structure of Ti-6Al-4V (see Fig. 10-11).

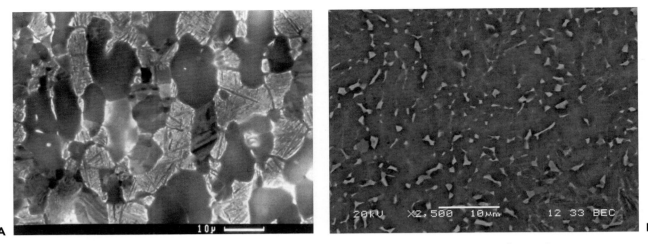

Figure 10-11 SEM of Ti-6Al-4V microstructure. **A:** Backscattered electron image. White regions are the β grains, and the gray/darker regions are the α HCP phases. **B:** Secondary electron image showing another microstructure for Ti-6Al-4V. Here the β phase is more blocky (raised regions) and the α phase surrounds them.

Rounded, globular (equiaxed) α grains present in a bimodal microstructure have strength properties that are very different from the acicular (needlelike) α grains in the transformed β structure. This is an excellent example of how microstructure affects mechanical properties. One property of interest in titanium alloys is its low elastic modulus compared to other implant alloys. It is about one half the value found for Co-Cr-Mo or 316L stainless steel. This reduced modulus will lower the flexural rigidity and is thought to aid in stress transfer from implant to bone and to minimize the potential for stress shielding and bone resorption.

More recent work has focused on a class of titanium alloys known as beta-titanium (β-Ti). There several alloy compositions that are being investigated for use as orthopedic alloys. The primary reason for this development work is the potential to further reduce the elastic modulus of β-Ti compared to Ti-6Al-4V (modulus, E, is 110 GPa for Ti-6Al-4V versus 70–90 for β-Ti). Some of the β-Ti alloys and their properties are listed in Table 10-7. The term *beta-titanium* refers to the fact that these alloys are primarily in the β crystal structure (i.e., BCC) or near-beta (α + β), as opposed to the α crystal structure (HCP) or near-alpha (α + β). These alloys are further divided into

TABLE 10-5
ASTM DESIGNATION AND CHEMICAL COMPOSITION FOR TITANIUM-BASED ALLOYS (MAXIMUM COMPOSITIONS IN WT %)

ASTM Designation	Composition (wt%)											
	Ti	Al	V	C	Ni	N	H	O	Nb	Fe	Zr	Others
F-67, CP-Ti grade 1	Bal	—	—	0.10	—	0.03	0.015	0.18	—	0.20	—	—
CP-Ti grade 2	Bal	—	—	0.1	—	0.03	0.012	0.25	—	0.3	—	—
CP-Ti grade 3	Bal	—	—	0.1	—	0.05	0.012	0.35	—	0.3	—	—
CP-Ti grade 4	Bal	—	—	0.1	—	0.05	0.012	0.4	—	0.5	—	—
F-136, wrought, ELI	Bal	5.5–6.5	3.5–4.5	0.08	—	0.05	0.012	0.13	—	0.25	—	—
F-1295	Bal	5.5–6.5	—	0.08	—	0.05	0.009	0.2	6.5–7.5	0.25	—	0.5 Ta
F-2146	Bal	2.50–3.50	2.0–3.0	0.05	—	0.020	0.015	0.12	—	0.30	—	—
F-1713	Bal	—	—	0.08	—	0.05	0.012	0.15	12.5–14.0	0.25	12.5–14.0	
F-2066	Bal	—	—	0.10	—	0.05	0.015	0.20	—	0.10	—	14.00–16.00 Mo
F-2063, wrought, SMA	Bal	—	—	0.070	54.5–57.0	—	0.005	0.050	0.025	0.050	—	0.050 Co, 0.010 Cu, 0.01 Cr,

SMA, shape memory alloy.
ELI, extra-low interstitial; Bal: Balance.

TABLE 10-6

MECHANICAL PROPERTIES OF SELECT TITANIUM ALLOYS

Composition	UTS (MPa)	YS (MPa)	%El
F-67, cP-Ti grade 1	240	170	24
F-67, cP-Ti grade 2	345	275	20
F-67, cP-Ti grade 3	450	380	18
F-67, cP-Ti grade 4	550	483	15
F-136, Ti-6Al-4V ELI	860	795	10
F-1108, cast Ti-6Al-4V	860	758	8
F-1295, Ti-6Al-6Nb	900	800	10
F-1472, Wr Ti-6Al-4V	930	860	10

MPa, megapascal; UTS, ultimate tensile strength; YS, yield strength; %El, percent elongation.
Note: These are minimum required strengths and ductilities for meeting ASTM specifications.

stable β (isomorphous β) and metastable β (eutectoid β) alloys. Metastable beta-titanium alloys can be age hardened (i.e., precipitation hardened: they increase in strength with heating).

Although these materials have not been accepted for use in the United States to date, there is an extensive effort by the implant community to gain acceptance of these alloys.

Zirconium and Tantalum Alloys

Other alloy systems gaining in use include Zr alloys (Zr-2.5 Nb) and tantalum (which has been used in craniofacial plates and pacemaker leads). Zr is somewhat similar to Ti in terms of its properties and behavior. A particular use of these alloys in knee implants exploits an interesting characteristic they possess. When heated under controlled conditions, the surface of the Zr alloy oxidizes into ZrO_2, which is highly wear and corrosion resistant.

Tantalum is also finding increased use in orthopedics as a "trabecular metal." Trabecular metal is a metal mesh that appears geometrically similar to bone. It is being used as a bone ingrowth substrate for porous coated surfaces and appears to have excellent biocompatibility and ingrowth characteristics (29,30).

TABLE 10-7

MECHANICAL PROPERTIES OF SELECTED BETA-TITANIUM ALLOYS

Alloy	UTS (MPa)	E (GPa)	%El	Fatigue Strength (MPa)
Ti-13Nb-13Zr (aged) (55)	1000	81	13	500
Ti-11Mo-7Zr-2Fe (65)	1100	88	13	550
Ti-15Mo	874	78	21	—
Ti-6Al-4V	930	115	10	480–590

TABLE 10-8

FATIGUE STRENGTH (AT 10^7 CYCLES) FOR SOME MEDICAL ALLOYS

Alloy	Fatigue Strength (MPa)
Ti-6Al-4V (68)	480–590
316L stainless steel (63)	180–300[a]
ASTM F-75	310
Grade 3 cP-Ti	330

[a]Annealed and cold worked, respectively.

FATIGUE BEHAVIOR OF MEDICAL ALLOYS

Table 10-8 is a summary of the fatigue strength of cobalt-based, titanium-based, and iron-based medical alloys. It can be seen that Ti-6Al-4V has the highest fatigue strength of all alloys reported. This is true for the bimodal α + β microstructure. Beta microstructures of titanium, in which the α grains are acicular, result in lower fatigue strengths (68). These fatigue strengths were measured on smooth, polished surfaces with few surface defects. Some alloys, in particular titanium, are sensitive to surface flaws during fatigue. That is, they are notch sensitive. Thus, if a notch or scratch is present on a surface during fatigue, it may accelerate the fatigue failure process (i.e., result in failure for a set stress in fewer cycles). Similarly, sharp changes in geometry, such as at porous coating junctions, may locally raise the stress because of the stress-concentrating effect of the changing geometry. This, in turn, can reduce the fatigue life for the material if the porous coating is present in the high-stress region.

ALLOY SURFACE STRUCTURE

The surface structure of orthopedic alloys includes the presence of an oxide film, also known as a passive film. Passive films are the result of the oxidation of the outermost metal atoms on the surface. These films are extremely thin, on the order of 2 to 10 nm, and they are thermodynamically stable in air and in saline under normal conditions. These films provide the corrosion resistance associated with orthopedic alloys. Passive films serve as kinetic barriers to the release of metal ions (54). The driving force for corrosion (the free energy driving oxidation) is very high for orthopedic alloys. That is, these alloys would corrode rapidly in the absence of the passive oxide film that forms (either spontaneously in air, thermally during high-temperature processing, or in solution) on their surface. The nature and structure of the oxides may change over time in solution, and they are susceptible to hydration (53), the presence of ions in solution, and the potential across the alloy–solution interface. Most studies of oxide films have required high-vacuum methods of analysis such as x-ray photoelectron spectroscopy or Auger spectroscopy. However, the nature of the oxide may be dramatically different in solution. Similarly, the structure of oxides, analyzed with transmission electron microscopy (TEM), requires significant processing, which may alter the oxide film structure.

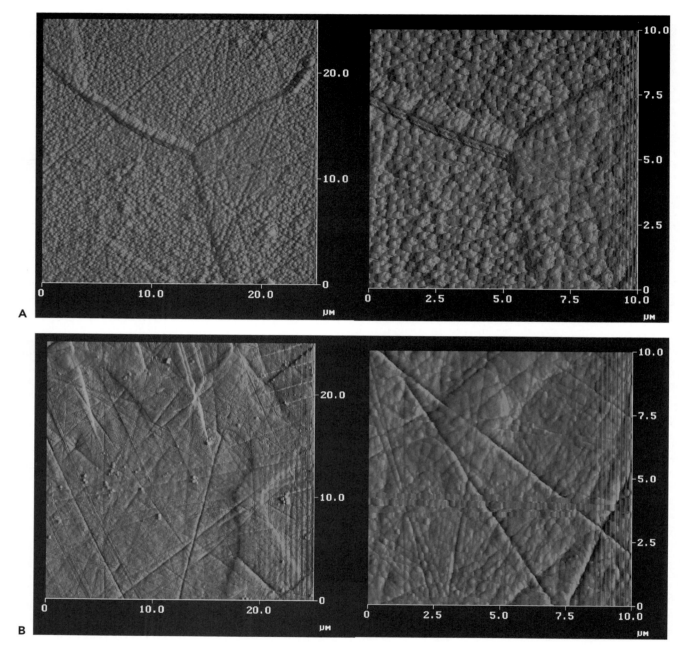

Figure 10-12 Atomic force microscopy deflection image pairs at two different magnifications of different alloys in air after polishing and etching. Deflection images highlight surface oxide topography and reveal the morphology of the oxide films on these metals. Shown are the surface oxides of 316L stainless steel (**A**), Co-Cr-Mo (F-75) (**B**), Ni-Ti SMA alloy (**C**), and CP-Ti (**D**).

Figure 10-12 includes a set of atomic force microscopy images of the surface oxides on several typical orthopedic alloys. Shown are the domelike films associated with the surface of Co-Cr-Mo (F-75), Cp-Ti (grade 2), Ni-Ti SMA alloy, and 316L stainless steel. These images demonstrate that the so-called passive oxide films are actually more complex in geometry and chemistry (not shown) than previously understood. These domes are much more dynamic than had previously been thought and are likely to interact to a much greater extent with the surrounding environment.

Several researchers have studied the structure and chemistry of oxide films formed on orthopedic alloys. Stainless steels, for example, have oxide films that contain primarily Cr_2O_3, with some FeO and Fe_2O_3. The majority of the corrosion resistance, however, comes from the presence of a chromium oxide.

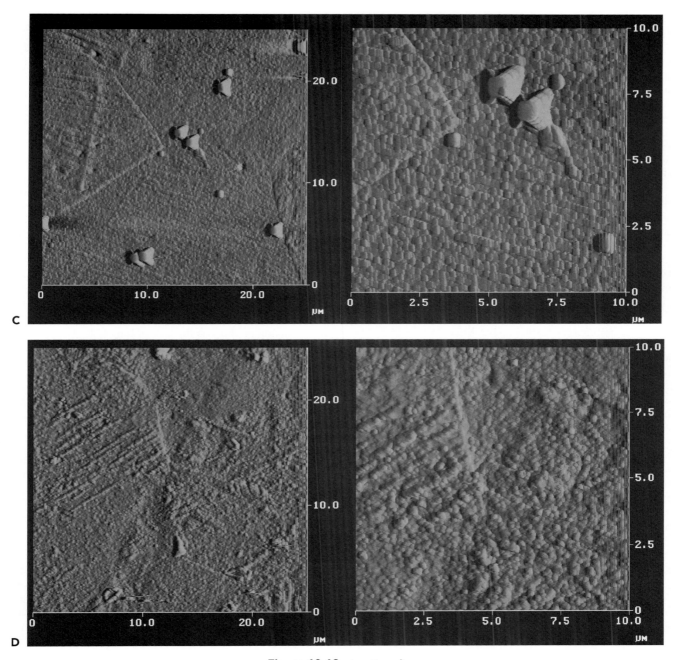

Figure 10-12 *(continued)*.

For Co-Cr-Mo alloys, the surface oxide is primarily Cr_2O_3, with some cobalt- and molybdenum-based oxides present as well. Not much information exists about the structure or chemistry of surface oxides of Co-Cr-Mo. Ohnsorge and Holm (62) investigated the surface chemistry of Co-Cr alloys and found that the chemistry of the oxide film is dependent on the history of the surface. Immersion-induced hydration of the oxide and thermal treatments above 400°C could induce Cr to diffuse to the surface and enrich the oxide layer. Also, they showed that the surface oxide may be mixed in chemistry, containing Cr, Mo, and Co oxides.

Titanium and titanium alloys form TiO_2 films, which are thought to be amorphous (without structure) but may undergo crystallization over time (41). Oxides of titanium also appear to undergo hydration, with significant hydroxides attaching to the outer oxide surface (53). Fraker and Ruff (43), using TEM, have shown that needlelike oxides of titanium oxide (TiO_2) are formed. Effah et al. (41), also using TEM methods, demonstrated that the oxide film changes its structure over the time of immersion. There appears to be an increase in the size of the TiO_2 oxide domes, and the electron diffraction patterns appear to become more distinct. These results are interesting because they point to the fact that oxide films of titanium are not static structures. They are responsive to the environment and may be susceptible to solution chemistry and sample potential effects. Brown et al. (31) and Bearinger et al. (27,28), using atomic force microscopy methods, also showed that oxide films of titanium will change as a function of the potential of the alloy in solution. They studied titanium in oxalic acid and found that when the potential of the alloy was increased, the oxide dome size increased and the density of the domes decreased.

Thus, the results of these studies of oxide films indicate that their surface layers are dynamic and susceptible to changes in history. Also, they will tend to change with immersion and sample potential.

There is a high thermodynamic driving force for the formation of oxide films. However, in solution, factors such as solution chemistry and sample potential can reduce the driving force for oxide formation and may, under certain circumstances, result in instability of the oxide. For example, 316L stainless steel can be induced to undergo crevice, pitting, or fretting corrosion in vivo (40). Similarly, Co-Cr alloys have been demonstrated to be susceptible to crevice attack in the presence of mechanical stress and fretting (35,36,46,59).

Oxide film surfaces are important in the wear processes associated with articulating alloy surfaces. Besides being thermodynamically stable, oxide films must also be resistant to abrasion. High oxide film adhesion to the substrate and good oxide mechanical strength are prerequisites to good wear resistance. It has recently been shown that the abrasive contact loads required to induce oxide fracture are extremely low for titanium alloy compared to Co-Cr alloys (48,49). This is further supported by work with all-titanium alloys, in which severe wear processes were found with titanium articulating against polyethylene (1). Similarly, sample potential was found to significantly affect the formation of oxide films. Specifically, oxides of Ti would not form in physiological saline solutions at potentials below –500 to –700 mV SCE (saturated calomel electrode). Above these potentials, oxide films will form but the thickness of the reformed oxide (after about 10 msec) varies linearly with potential. Similar results were seen with Co-Cr alloy oxides. However, oxide films did not start to form until –400 to –500 mV, and these oxides undergo a breakdown reaction starting at about 300 to 500 mV (SCE) where the oxide films are thinner and/or do not form the tightly adherent passive films needed for corrosion resistance (51).

The surfaces of orthopedic alloys are typically treated with a passivation treatment (ASTM F-86) (4) that involves immersion of the alloy in an aqueous nitric acid bath for a period of time. This method has been shown to be useful for treating chromium-containing alloys that form Cr_2O_3, in particular, 316L stainless steel. There is little evidence that this passivation treatment performs any significant function on alloys of titanium or Co-Cr. For 316L stainless steel, the effect of passivation is to ensure that the oxide film is fully formed on the surface and that any surface regions where impurities exist will be dissolved away to leave an oxide film-covered surface.

SURFACE MODIFICATIONS

The goal of surface modification methods for metals is to create a surface that is resistant to wear and corrosion processes. Recently, surface modification technologies have been investigated for enhancing the surface properties of orthopedic alloys. These surface treatments are widely varied in processing and include ion implantation (42), chemical and physical vapor deposition (32), nitriding, and oxygen diffusion hardening (67). These processes have some similarities in that they result in a local region of the surface that is high in strength and hardness. How they create this hardened region varies. In ion implantation, high velocity ions (e.g., N^+) are accelerated toward the surface. These ions penetrate the surface, colliding with the near-surface atoms and creating a surface region high in dislocations and other defects. Typical thicknesses of ion-implanted surfaces are on the order of 0.5 µm or less.

Chemical vapor deposition (CVD) and physical vapor deposition (PVD) processes usually result in a new coating that attaches to the surface. These coatings include CrN or TiN, very high hardness coatings. One potential problem with these coating methods is the lack of long-lasting adhesion to the substrate alloy. Coatings of this type are about 1 µm thick. Another CVD process under consideration is the use of diamondlike films (DLCs). Here, a carbon layer is deposited on the surface of a material in which the carbon atoms have, at least partially, an sp^3 hybrid-type character indicative of a diamond structure. These coatings are also very hard and represent an overlayer placed on top of the metal or alloy.

Other processes under investigation include diffusion hardening (67,74) and thermal nitriding processes (66), which result in a diffusion of atoms in from the surface and which harden by means of interstitial solid-solution strengthening.

PERFORMANCE OF ORTHOPEDIC ALLOYS

Most of the issues surrounding the use of alloys in orthopedics relate to mechanical strength, wear processes, and corrosion behavior. These are somewhat distinct, but they are also interrelated. That is, very often corrosion events can be dramatically accelerated by mechanical factors such as wear or fretting. Similarly, mechanical failure modes can be accelerated dramatically if the appropriate chemical or electrochemical factors (e.g., corrosion fatigue) are present.

Corrosion processes are always present in orthopedic alloys. Their rate is limited by the presence of the passive films previously discussed. If this rate is low enough for the body to eliminate the generated corrosion debris, then this ionic and particulate release may not have any clinical significance. However, there are circumstances in which corrosion can become a significant risk. Recent evidence of mechanically assisted crevice corrosion (i.e., fretting crevice corrosion) has been reported on modular connections of femoral hip prostheses (35,36,46,59). This corrosion process is a conjoint effect of mechanical abrasion of the oxide film covering the surface of the alloy in the taper plus the restricted crevice environment. These two factors combine to dramatically accelerate the corrosion process. For a more detailed discussion of the corrosion process, see Gilbert et al. (45,46). Urban et al. (71) demonstrated that corrosion products from the taper crevices are associated with osteolytic lesions as well as other inflammatory processes. Jacobs et al. (55) demonstrated that systemic levels of Cr and Co are elevated in patients who were later found to have severe corrosion in tapers, unlike the levels in those with little or no evidence of corrosion. In some cases, modular taper corrosion appeared to contribute to the fatigue failure of Co-Cr stems inside the taper (47). In any region of the prosthesis where mechanical abrasion can occur, either as fretting or as wear, significant conjoint corrosion effects are possible.

Mechanically assisted corrosion has been demonstrated to occur in stainless steel IM rods and Co-Cr and Ti-6Al-4V alloys regardless of the material combination (45,56,70). This corrosion attack has been demonstrated to result in osteolysis (56) and can even result in etching and pitting attack of titanium in the human body. This latter observation implies that the pH within the restricted solution environment must undergo changes that dramatically acidify the solution. For titanium to be attacked in this fashion, pH values below 1 must be reached in the human body. Evidence of etching of Ti-6Al-4V alloy tapers in S-ROM devices was recently reported (70).

Fatigue failures of orthopedic implants are less common than they once were, primarily because of improved materials and processing. However, fatigue failures do still occasionally occur. Fatigue in orthopedic applications is typically dominated by high-cycle fatigue processes, and fatigue crack initiation plays an important role in such processes. Most fatigue cracks begin at the surface of the implant; thus, the surface conditions (e.g., roughness, residual stress, and degree of cold work) play an important role. Fatigue failures of tibial trays (50), acetabular components (69), and femoral stems (47) (in the distal stem region as well as the neck region) have all been reported within the past 10 years. Many factors contribute to the failure of prostheses beyond the material and its processing history. Patient factors such as activity and weight, the presence of bony defects requiring bone grafts, and progressive bone loss with age, as well as other unknown or uncontrollable factors, can contribute to fatigue failures.

Wear processes at the articulating surfaces of knee and hip prostheses do affect the metal components of total joint replacements. Metal debris is still generated during articulation and walking, although perhaps not at the volume that is seen with polymeric debris. Recent work on metal-on-metal prostheses has further raised the concern of conjoint effects of corrosion and wear on the metal–metal contact region, and further study is needed to assess the risks and benefits of this approach to articulating couples.

This chapter has tried to present a basic summary of metal structure–property relationships for currently used and potential orthopedic alloys. Some of the issues related to these alloys and their use in the human body have been presented, including mechanical properties, surface properties, corrosion, fatigue, and wear. Although this has by no means been an exhaustive treatment of the subject, it is hoped that some basic concepts have been relayed to the reader that will provide a basis for understanding the complex and multifaceted milieu in which these alloys operate.

ACKNOWLEDGMENTS

I would like to thank Rob Gettens, Zhijun Bai, and Spiro Megremis for their assistance in this revision of the manuscript and Dr. Debra Wright-Charlesworth and Mr. Robert Urban for their original assistance with photography.

REFERENCES

1. Agins HJ, Alcock NW, Bansal M, et al. Metallic wear in failed titanium-alloy total hip replacements: a histological and quantitative analysis. *J Bone Joint Surg.* 1988;70A(3):347–356.
2. ASTM F-67-95: standard specification for unalloyed titanium for surgical implant applications. In: *ASTM Annual Book of Standards.* Philadelphia: American Society for Testing and Materials; 1995; 13.01:1–3.
3. ASTM F-75-92: standard specification for cast cobalt-chromium-molybdenum alloy for surgical implant applications. In: *ASTM Annual Book of Standards.* Philadelphia: American Society for Testing and Materials; 1995;13.01:4–5.
4. ASTM F-86-91: standard practice for surface preparation and marking of metallic surgical implants. In: *ASTM Annual Book of Standards.* Philadelphia: American Society for Testing and Materials. 1995;13.01:6–8.
5. ASTM F-90-92: standard specification for wrought cobalt-chromium-tungsten-nickel alloy for surgical implant applications. In: *ASTM Annual Book of Standards.* Philadelphia: American Society for Testing and Materials; 1995;13.01:9–11.
6. ASTM F-136-92: standard specification for wrought titanium 6Al-4V ELI alloy for surgical implant applications. In: *ASTM Annual Book of Standards.* Philadelphia: American Society for Testing and Materials; 1995;13.01:19–21.
7. ASTM F-138-92: standard specification for stainless steel bar and wire for surgical implants. In: *ASTM Annual Book of Standards.* Philadelphia: American Society for Testing and Materials; 1995; 13.01:22–24.
8. ASTM F-139-92: standard specification for stainless steel sheet and strip for surgical implants. In: *ASTM Annual Book of Standards.* Philadelphia: American Society for Testing and Materials; 1995; 13.01:25–27.
9. ASTM F-562-95: standard specification for wrought cobalt-35 nickel-20 chromium-10 molybdenum alloy for surgical implant applications. In: *ASTM Annual Book of Standards.* Philadelphia: American Society for Testing and Materials; 1995;13.01:89–91.
10. ASTM F-563-95: standard specification for wrought cobalt-nickel-chromium-molybdenum-tungsten-iron alloy for surgical implant applications. In: *ASTM Annual Book of Standards.* Philadelphia: American Society for Testing and Materials; 1995; 13.01:92–94.
11. ASTM F-620-92: standard specification for titanium 6Al-4V ELI alloy forgings for surgical implants. In: *ASTM Annual Book of Standards.* Philadelphia: American Society for Testing and Materials; 1995;13.01:116–117.
12. ASTM F-621-92: standard specification for stainless steel forgings for surgical implants. In: *ASTM Annual Book of Standards.* Philadelphia: American Society for Testing and Materials; 1995; 13.01:118–119.
13. ASTM F-688-95: standard specification for wrought cobalt-35 nickel-20 chromium-10 molybdenum alloy plate, sheet and foil for surgical implants. In: *ASTM Annual Book of Standards.* Philadelphia: American Society for Testing and Materials; 1995; 13.01:166–168.
14. ASTM F-745-95: standard specification for 18 chromium-12.5 nickel-2.5 molybdenum stainless steel for cast and solution annealed surgical implant applications. In: *ASTM Annual Book of Standards.* Philadelphia: American Society for Testing and Materials; 1995;13.01:189–191.
15. ASTM F-799-95: standard specification for cobalt-28 chromium-6 molybdenum alloy forgings for surgical implants. In: *ASTM Annual Book of Standards.* Philadelphia: American Society for Testing and Materials; 1995;13.01:230–232.
16. ASTM F-899-94: standard specification for stainless steel billet, bar, and wire for surgical instruments. In: *ASTM Annual Book of*

Standards. Philadelphia: American Society for Testing and Materials; 1995;13.01:261–263.

17. ASTM F-1058-91: standard specification for wrought cobalt-chromium-nickel-molybdenum-iron alloy for surgical implant applications. In: *ASTM Annual Book of Standards.* Philadelphia: American Society for Testing and Materials; 1995;13.01:355–357.

18. ASTM F-1091-91: standard specification for wrought cobalt-chromium alloy surgical fixation wire. In: *ASTM Annual Book of Standards.* Philadelphia: American Society for Testing and Materials; 1995;13.01:372–373.

19. ASTM F-1108-92: standard specification for Ti6Al4V alloy castings for surgical implants. In: *ASTM Annual Book of Standards.* Philadelphia: American Society for Testing and Materials; 1995; 13.01:398–400.

20. ASTM F-1295-92: standard specification for wrought titanium-6 aluminum-7 niobium alloy for surgical implant applicationss. In: *ASTM Annual Book of Standards.* Philadelphia: American Society for Testing and Materials; 1995;13.01:687–689.

21. ASTM F-1314-94: standard specification for wrought nitrogen strengthened-22 chromium-12.5 nickel-5 manganese-2.5 molybdenum stainless steel bar and wire for surgical implants. In: *ASTM Annual Book of Standards.* Philadelphia: American Society for Testing and Materials; 1995;13.01:690–691.

22. ASTM F-1377-92: standard specification for cobalt-chromium-molybdenum powder for coating of orthopedic implants. In: *ASTM Annual Book of Standards.* Philadelphia: American Society for Testing and Materials; 1995;13.01:722–723.

23. ASTM F-1472-93: standard specification for wrought Ti-6Al-4V alloy for surgical implant applications. In: *ASTM Annual Book of Standards.* Philadelphia: American Society for Testing and Materials; 1995;13.01:828–831.

24. ASTM F-1580-95: standard specification for titanium and titanium − 6% Aluminum − 4% Vanadium alloy powders for coatings of surgical implants. *ASTM Annual Book of Standards.* Philadelphia: American Society for Testing and Materials; 1995; 13.01:913–915.

25. ASTM F-1537-94: standard specification for wrought cobalt-28 chromium-6 molybdenum alloy for surgical implants. In: *ASTM Annual Book of Standards.* Philadelphia: American Society for Testing and Materials; 1995;13.01:865–867.

26. Avaroff LV. *Elements of X-Ray Crystallography.* New York: McGraw-Hill; 1968;50.

27. Bearinger JP, Orme CA, Gilbert JL. Direct observation of hydration of TiO_2 on Ti using AFM: freely corroding versus potentiostatically held. *Surface Sci.* 2001;491:370–387.

28. Bearinger JP, Orme CA, Gilbert JL. In-situ imaging and impedance measurements of titanium surfaces using AFM and SPIS. *Biomaterials.* 2003;24:1837–1852.

29. Bobyn JD, Stackpool GJ, Hacking SA, et al. Characteristics of bone ingrowth and interface mechanics of a new porous tantalum biomaterial. *J Bone Joint Surg [Br].* 1999;81:907–914.

30. Bobyn JD, Toh KK, Hacking SA, et al. Tissue response to porous tantalum acetabular cups: a canine model. *J Arthroplasty.* 1999;14: 347–354.

31. Brown GM, Thundat T, Allison DA, et al. Electrochemical and in situ atomic force microscopy investigations of titanium in oxalic acid solutions, *J Vac Sci Tech.* 1992;10(5):3001–3006.

32. Bunshah RF. PVD and CVD coatings. In: *ASM Handbook: Friction, Lubrication and Wear Technology.* Warrendale, OH: ASM International; 1992;18:840.

33. Clemow AJT, Daniell BL. Solution treatment behavior of Co-Cr-Mo alloy. *J Biomed Mater Res.* 1979;13:265–279.

34. *Cobalt Monograph.* Brussels: Centre d'Information du Cobalt; 1960:170–177.

35. Collier JP, Surprenant VA, Jensen RE, et al. Corrosion at the interface of cobalt-alloy heads on titanium-alloy stems. *Clin Orthop.* 1991;271:305–312.

36. Collier JP, Surprenant VA, Jensen RE, et al. Corrosion between the components of modular femoral hip prostheses. *J Bone Joint Surg.* 1992;74B:511–517.

37. *Corrosion.* Metals Park, OH: ASM International; 1987:11. Metals Handbook No. 13.

38. Craig RG. *Restorative Dental Materials.* 8th ed. New York: Mosby; 1989:362.

39. Dowson D. Friction and wear of medical implants and prosthetic devices. In: *ASM Handbook: Friction, Lubrication and Wear Technology.* Warrendale, OH: ASM International; 1992:18:656.

40. Ducheyne P. *J Biomed Mater Res.* 1980;14:31.

41. Effah EAB, Bianco PD, Ducheyne P. Crystal structure of the surface oxide layer on titanium and its changes arising from immersion. *J Biomed Mater Res.* 1995;29:73–80.

42. Fenske GR. Ion implantation. In: *ASM Handbook: Friction, Lubrication and Wear Technology.* Metals Park, OH: ASM International; 1992;18:850.

43. Fraker AC, Ruff AW. Studies of oxide film formation on titanium alloys in saline water. *Corrosion Sci.* 1971;11:763–765.

44. Friedman DW, Orland PJ, Greco RS. Biomaterials: an historical perspective. In: Greco RS, ed. *Implantation Biology: The Host Response and Biomedical Devices.* Boca Raton, FL: CRC Press; 1994;1–12.

45. Gilbert JL. Mechanically assisted corrosion of biomedical alloys. In *Corrosion.* Materials Park, OH: ASM International. In press. American Society for Materials Handbook 13C.

46. Gilbert JL, Buckley CA, Jacobs JJ. In vivo corrosion of modular hip prosthesis components in mixed and similar metal combinations: the effect of crevice, stress, motion and alloy coupling. *J Biomed Mater Res.* 1993;27:1533–1544.

47. Gilbert JL, Buckley CA, Jacobs JJ, et al. Intergranular corrosion-fatigue failure of cobalt-alloy femoral stems. *J Bone Joint Surg.* 1994;76A(1):110–115.

48. Gilbert JL, Buckley CA, Lautenschlager EP. Titanium oxide film fracture and repassivation: the effect of potential, pH and aeration. In: Lemons JE, SA Brown, eds. *Medical Applications of Titanium, and Its Alloys: The Materials and Biological Issues.* Philadelphia: American Society for Testing and Materials; 1996:199–215. ASTM Special Technical Publication 1272.

49. Gilbert JL, Jacobs JJ. The mechanical and electrochemical processes associated with taper fretting crevice corrosion: a review. In: Parr JE, Mayor MB, Marlowe DE, eds. *Modularity of Orthopedic Implants.* Philadelphia: American Society for Testing and Materials; 1996. ASTM Special Technical Publication 1301.

50. Gilbert JL, Stulberg SD. Fatigue fracture of titanium alloy (Ti-6Al-4V) knee prostheses in vivo. In: *ASM Handbook of Case Histories in Failure Analysis.* Vol 2. Metals Park, OH: ASM International; 1994:2.

51. Goldberg JR, Lautenschlager EP, Gilbert JL. Electrochemical behavior of Co-Cr-Mo alloy after mechanical fracture of the surface oxide film. *Trans Soc Biomater.* 1995;18:206.

52. Gruen TA. *J Biomed Mater Res.* 1975;9:465.

53. Healy KE, Ducheyne P. Hydration and preferential molecular adsorption of titanium in vitro. *Biomaterials.* 1992;13:553–561.

54. Jacobs JJ, Gilbert JL, Urban RM. Corrosion of metallic implants. In: Stauffer N, et al., eds. *Advances in Operative Orthopaedics.* St. Louis, MO: Mosby; 1994:2:279–312.

55. Jacobs JJ, Urban RM, Gilbert JL, et al. Local and distant products from modularity. *Clin Orthop.* 1995;319:94–105.

56. Jones D, Marsh JL, Nepola JV, et al. Focal osteolysis at the junctions of a modular stainless steel femoral intramedulary nail. *J Bone Joint Surg.* 2001;83A:537–548.

57. Kilner T, Pilliar RM, Weatherly GC. Phase identification and incipient melting in a cast Co-Cr surgical implant alloy. *J Biomed Mater Res.* 1982;16:63–79.

58. Kuhn AT. Corrosion of Co-Cr alloys in aqueous environments *Biomaterials* 1981;2:68–77.

59. Mathiesen EB, Lindgren JU, Blomgren GA, et al. Corrosion of modular hip prostheses. *J Bone Joint Surg.* 1991;73B:569–575.

60. McKee, Ferrar. *J Bone Joint Surg.* 1966;48B(2):245.

61. Mishra AK, Davidson JA, Kovacs P, et al. Ti-13Nb-13Zr: a new low modulus, high strength corrosion resistant near-beta alloy for orthopedic implants. In: Eylon D, Boyer RR, Koss DA, eds. *Beta Titanium Alloys in the 1990s.* Warrendale, PA: Minerals, Metals, and Materials Society; 1993;61–72.

62. Ohnsorge J, Holm R. Surface investigations of oxide layers on cobalt-chromium alloyed orthopedic implants using ESCA technique. *Med Prog Technol.* 1978;5:171–177.

63. Pohler OEM. *Study of the Initiation and Propagation Stages of Fatigue and Corrosion Fatigue of Orthopedic Implant Materials* [dissertation]. Columbus: Ohio State University; 1983.

64. Reed-Hill R. *Physical Metallurry Principles.* 2nd ed. New York: Van Nostrand; 1973;267–321.

65. Reinsch WA. Terminology for titanium microstructure. In: *Titanium and Titanium Alloys: Source Book, ASM.* Metals Park, OH: American Society for Metals; 1982;47.

66. Shetty R, Ottersberg WH. Method of surface hardening cobalt-chromium based alloys for orthopedic implant devices. U.S. Patent No. 5,308,412, May 1994.

67. Streicher RM, Weber H, Schon R, et al. New surface modification for Ti-6Al-7Nb alloy: oxygen diffusion hardening (ODH). *Biomaterials.* 1991;12:125–129.

68. Stubbington CA. Metallurgical aspects of fatigue and fracture in titanium alloys. *Titanium and Its Alloys: Source Book, ASM.* Metals Park, OH: American Society for Metals; 1982;140–158.

69. Trousdale RT, Berry DJ, Jacobs JJ, et al. Fracture of a non-cemented acetabular component: a case report. *J Bone Joint Surg.* 1997; 79A(6):901–905.

70. Urban RM, Gilbert JL, Jacobs JJ. Corrosion of modular titanium alloy stems in cementless hip replacement. In: *Titanium, Niobium, Zirconium, and Tantalum for Medical and Surgical Applications.* Vol. 2, No. 10. West Conshohocken, PA, ASTM International, 2005;1–10. ASTM Special Technical Publication.

71. Urban RM, Jacobs JJ, Gilbert JL, et al. Migration of corrosion products from modular hip prostheses. *J Bone Joint Surg.* 1994;76A(9): 1345–1359.

72. Wang K, Gustovson L, Dumbleton J. The characterization of Ti-12Mo-6Zr-2Fe: a new biocompatible titanium alloy developed for surgical implants. In: Eylon D, Boyer RR, Koss DA, eds. *Beta Titanium Alloys in the 1990s.* Warrendale, PA: Minerals, Metals, and Materials Society; 1993;49–60.

73. Wiles P. The surgery of the osteo-arthritic hip. *Br J Surg.* 1957; 45:488.

74. Yun YH, Slack SM, Turitto VT, et al. Initial biocompatibility of novel titanium and zirconium alloys for cardiovascular applications: compatibility of biomedical implants. *Proc Electrochemical Soc.* 1995;94(15):105–112.

Orthopedic Bone Cement

Anuj Bellare

HISTORY

For over 40 years, poly(methylmethacrylate) (PMMA)–based bone cement, commonly referred to as acrylic bone cement, has been used for fixation of total joint replacement prostheses to periprosthetic bone tissue. Today, most PMMA cements on the market consist of a liquid and powder component, which are mixed in the operating room until they become doughlike and are then applied to the tissue prior to insertion of the metallic component of the joint replacement prosthesis. The primary purpose of cements is to fix the joint replacement prosthesis to the periprosthetic bone tissue.

The basic component of acrylic bone cements is methylmethacrylate (MMA), which is an ester of methacrylic acid. Large-scale chemical synthesis of MMA was achieved in the 1920s in the laboratories of Rohm and Haas, and one of the first biomedical applications of PMMA was the fabrication of dentures (31). In the 1930s it was discovered that the mixing of prepolymerized PMMA powder with MMA monomer and benzoyl peroxide initiator resulted in the formation of a doughlike material that slowly hardens into a glassy polymer. This two-component cement was used to close cranial defects. In 1951, Kaier and Jansen in Copenhagen were the first to use PMMA bone cement for the fixation of acrylic cups to the subchondral bone of the femoral head. In 1953, Haboush used bone cement as a seating material for femoral head replacements without inserting it into the medullary canal. In 1958, Sir John Charnley used PMMA bone cement to anchor femoral head prostheses in the femur, as is done in modern-day joint arthroplasty. Charnley used a self-curing PMMA cement called Nu-Life, which was a pink-colored denture repair material obtained from the Turner Dental School at Manchester University. These early total hip replacements had a high incidence of failure, not because of the cemented stems but because of the use of polytetrafluoroethylene (PTFE) acetabular cups. In 1962, ultra high molecular weight polyethylene acetabular cups were used for the first time, and both the cup and the stem were cemented using Nu-Life, manufactured by CMW Laboratories. In 1966, CMW began supplying the first sterilized bone cement specifically formulated for fixation of total joint replacement prostheses. Recently, uncemented total hip replacement prostheses designs have been introduced in the orthopedic market, but acrylic cements continue to be the primary method of fixation of joint replacement prostheses, especially for total knee replacement prostheses. In addition, new injectable formulations of acrylic bone cements are being developed and investigated for applications in vertebroplasty, increasing the applicability and importance of bone cements as an orthopedic biomaterial.

Several material properties and process factors affect the clinical performance of bone cements, such as their chemical composition, viscosity, porosity, radiopacifiers and antibiotic additives, mixing methods, sterilization, temperature during handling, mechanical properties, and biocompatibility. Acrylic bone cements have been extensively studied, and several review articles present various issues related to their use in total joint replacement prostheses (28,31,62,98).

COMPOSITION AND CHEMISTRY

The MMA monomer comprises two carbon atoms that are covalently linked, with one of the carbon atoms covalently bonded to two hydrogen atoms and the other covalently bonded to a methyl and acrylic group, as shown in Figure 11-1. Polymerization of MMA monomer converts it into PMMA, which is a polymer or a macromolecule, terms used for long-chain molecules made up of monomeric units. Hardened acrylic bone cement consists of linear, uncross-linked PMMA macromolecules of various lengths ranging from a few tens of thousands to a few million grams per mole, but their length can vary widely depending on the manufacturer (12,40,93,106).

Acrylic bone cements comprise two components: (a) a powder component, usually in a 40 g package, and (b) a liquid component, in a 20 mL ampoule, as shown in Figure 11-2. There are several reasons for using a two-component bone cement instead of simply polymerizing pure MMA monomer. First, the polymerization of MMA monomer is too slow compared with the duration of the surgery and can take several hours or days, depending on the type and amount of reaction initiator used. Second, pure MMA monomer has a very low viscosity and can easily diffuse into the blood stream, which can lead to cardiorespiratory and vascular complications. Even with bone cement, some of the MMA monomer can escape into the periprosthetic tissue, causing some of these effects (11,16,29,51,74,87,90,108). Third, it is much easier to shape the doughy cement to fill the space between the prosthesis and periprosthetic bone over a reasonable time period. Fourth, the heat of polymerization can easily increase the temperature of the cement to over 100°C (boiling point for MMA = 100.3°C), which could lead to boiling of the volatile MMA monomer. The use of less monomer and the presence of prepolymerized PMMA beads in the powder decreases the amount of released heat and assists in heat dissipation, decreasing the overall temperature. Lastly, pure MMA, upon polymerization into PMMA, has a volumetric shrinkage of 21% due to differences in the density of the MMA monomer and the PMMA polymer. This amount of shrinkage is unacceptable and would lead to a large gap at the cement–bone interface, compromising the fixation of the prosthesis.

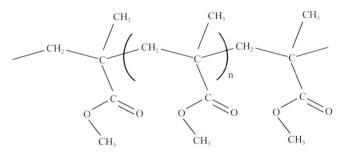

Figure 11-1 Schematic of the molecular structure of polymethylmethacrylate.

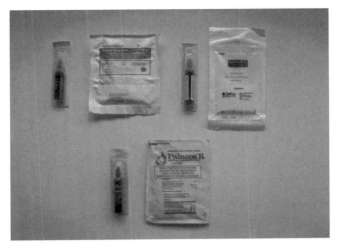

Figure 11-2 Typical commercial cements, with a powder component accompanied by a liquid component contained in a glass ampoule.

The powder component primarily consists of prepolymerized PMMA beads of 10 to 150 μm diameter. The prepolymerized beads of some bone cements include copolymers of MMA with styrene, methyl acrylate, or butyl methacrylate comonomers. The MMA monomer can self-polymerize with long exposure to heat and light. However, this reaction is very slow. Therefore, dibenzoyl peroxide (BPO) reaction initiator in powder form is also included in the powder component. BPO can also be present in the prepolymerized PMMA beads. Finally, radiopacifier particles of either barium sulfate or zirconium oxide are also present in the powder component to make the cement mantle visible in x-ray radiographs. Several cements also include an antibiotic, such as gentamicin sulphate, in powder form to provide prophylaxis against infections, which can occur during surgery. The initiator, radiopacifier, and antibiotic powders are all approximately 1 μm in diameter.

The liquid component is primarily MMA monomer. A small amount of a reaction accelerator, usually N,N-dimethyl-para-toluidine (DMPT), is also present to speed up the polymerization and setting of the cement. In addition, a stabilizer, usually hydroquinone, is included in the liquid component, since MMA can spontaneously polymerize during storage. The overall composition of a few common commercial bone cements is present in Table 11-1.

MMA polymerizes using the mechanism of free radical polymerization, which comprises three steps: initiation, propagation, and termination (35). In the case of polymerization of MMA monomer in bone cements, the initiation step involves decomposition of BPO monomer into radicals at room temperature. Upon mixing of the two components, the DMPT in the liquid component decomposes BPO into a benzoyl radical and a benzoate anion as follows:

$$(C_6H_5COO)_2 + CH_3C_6H_4N(CH_3)_2 \rightarrow C_6H_5COO\bullet + \\ C_6H_5COO^- + CH_3C_6H_4N(CH_3)_2\bullet^+ \rightarrow \\ CH_3C_6H_4NCH_3CH_2\bullet + H^+$$

where BPO = $(C_6H_5COO)_2$, DMPT = $CH_3C_6H_4N(CH_3)_2$, benzoyl radical = $C_6H_5COO\bullet$, and benzoate anion = $C_6H_5COO^-$. The radical cation of DMPT is then converted into a neutral

TABLE 11-1

BONE CEMENT COMPOSITIONS IN PERCENTAGE (W/W) UNLESS STATED OTHERWISE

Constituent	CMW1	CMW3	Palacos R	Simplex P	Zimmer Regular	Zimmer LVC
Powder component						
BPO	2.60	2.20	0.5–1.6	1.19	0.75	0.75
$BaSO_4$	9.10	10.00	—	10.00	10.00	10.00
ZrO_2	—	—	14.85	—	—	—
Chlorophyll	—	—	200 ppm	—	—	—
PMMA	88.30	87.80	—	16.55	89.25	89.25
P(MMA/MA)	—	—	83.55–84.65	—	—	—
P(MMA/S)	—	—	—	82.26	—	—
Liquid component						
N,N-DMPT	0.40	0.99	2.13	2.48	2.73	2.75
Hydroquinone	15–20 ppm	15–20 ppm	64 ppm	75 ppm	75 ppm	75 ppm
MMA	98.66	98.07	97.87	97.51	97.27	97.25
Ethanol	0.92	0.92	—	—	—	—
Ascorbic acid	0.02	0.02	—	—	—	—
Chlorophyll II	—	—	267 ppm	—	—	—

BPO, benzoyl peroxide; PMMA, poly(methylmethacrylate); P(MMA/MA), poly(methylmethacrylate-co-methyl acrylate); P(MMA/S), poly(methylmethacrylate-co-styrene); N,N-DMPT, N,N-dimethyl-para-toluidine; MMA, methylmethacrylate.
Reproduced from Lewis G. Properties of acrylic bone cement: state of the art review. *J Biomed Mater Res.* 1997;38:155–182.

radical by removal of a proton. The second step of the free radical polymerization is chain propagation in which the benzoyl radical reacts with the MMA monomer as follows:

$$C_6H_5COO\bullet + CH_2{=}CCH_3COOCH_3 \rightarrow C_6H_5COO\text{-}CH_2\text{-}CCH_3COOCH_3\bullet + CH_2{=}CCH_3COOCH_3 \rightarrow C_6H_5COO\text{-}CH_2CCH_3COOCH_3\text{-}CH_2CCH_3COOCH_3\bullet \rightarrow etc.$$

Basically, the free radical attacks one of the double bonds of the MMA monomer. One electron of the double bond pairs up with the electron of the free radical to form a bond between the oxygen of the benzoyl free radical and one of the carbon atoms of the MMA monomer while the second electron of the double bond shifts to the other carbon atom, which then turns into a free radical. This free radical then attacks another MMA monomer and the chain propagates until a PMMA of relatively high molecular weight, on the order of 100,000 to 1,000,000 g/mol, is achieved.

Finally, chain termination can be achieved by chain coupling as follows:

$$\text{-}CH_2CXCH_3\bullet + \bullet CXCH_3CH_2\text{-} \rightarrow \text{-}CH_2CXCH_3\text{-}CXCH_3CH_2\text{-}$$

or, to a lesser extent, by disproportionation via transfer of a hydrogen atom as follows:

$$\text{-}CH_2CXCH_3\bullet + \bullet CXCH_3CH_2\text{-} \rightarrow \text{-}CH_2CXCH_2 + CXH{=}CH\text{-}$$

where X refers to the substituent $COOCH_3$.

The glass transition temperature of PMMA is about 105°C, but the glass transition temperature of hardened PMMA-based bone cement can be lower due to plasticization effects of residual monomer and water (81). As the polymerization proceeds, the growing polymer chains slowly turn into a hard, glassy material, and it becomes difficult for the monomer to diffuse through the hardened PMMA matrix to continue chain propagation. Thus the final cement contains some residual monomer embedded in the PMMA matrix. The hardened acrylic bone cement consists primarily of linear, uncross-linked PMMA macromolecules of various lengths, but their length (or molecular weight) can vary widely depending on the manufacturer (12,40,93,106), as shown in Table 11-2. The molecular weight of the hardened cement depends on several factors, such as (a) the molecular weight of the monomer used (usually MMA), (b) the molecular weight of the prepolymerized beads (which are sometimes copolymers of MMA and styrene), (c) the ratio of the initiator and the accelerator (if the concentration of the initiator is low, fewer chains will grow simultaneously to a high molecular weight until almost all of the monomer is used up), (d) the presence of stabilizers,

TABLE 11-2

WEIGHT AVERAGE AND NUMBER AVERAGE MOLECULAR WEIGHT OF SELECTED BONE CEMENTS

Bone Cement	Weight Average MW	Number Average MW
Zimmer	256,000	58,700
Simplex	240,000	89,700
Palacos	872,000	170,000

Reproduced from Rimnac CM, Wright TM, McGill DL. The effect of centrifugation on the fracture properties of acrylic bone cements. *J Bone Joint Surg [Am].* 1986;68:281–287.

(e) the ambient temperature during polymerization (which alters the reaction kinetics), and (f) the sterilization method (gamma radiation can degrade the PMMA, especially in the long term [37,42,64]).

PROCESSING AND HANDLING OF BONE CEMENT

The handling characteristics and setting times of acrylic cements receive a great deal of attention by orthopedic surgeons since they are very important in planning the surgery and directly impact the duration of surgery. There are four basic stages in the setting of acrylic cements when the liquid component comes into contact with the powder component: (a) the mixing period, (b) The waiting period, (c) the working period, and (d) the hardening or setting period.

When the liquid and powder components of a cement are mixed together, the MMA liquid wets the surface of the prepolymerized PMMA powder. PMMA is a polymer that dissolves in its monomer, which is not necessarily the case for all polymers. Thus the prepolymerized beads swell, and some of them dissolve completely during mixing. The dissolution of PMMA into MMA results in a substantial increase in the viscosity of the mixture compared with the viscosity of the MMA monomer. However, at this stage the viscosity is still relatively low compared with the later stages of polymerization. A general rule of thumb is that after approximately 3 minutes of mixing the intrinsic viscosity is approximately 100 Pa·s (82). New cements containing additives, new polymers, or other chemicals that influence the polymerization rate must have similar mixing characteristics to ensure easy implementation in cemented joint arthroplasties.

At the end of the mixing period, the cement is a homogeneous mass that is transferred to a cement gun. At this stage, the cement is sticky and has a toothpastelike consistency. This period is followed by a waiting period to permit further swelling of the beads and allow the polymerization to proceed, leading to an increase in viscosity. At this stage, the cement turns into a sticky dough.

The start of the working period occurs when the cement is no longer sticky but of sufficiently low viscosity to enable the surgeon to easily apply the cement to the femur. During this period, the chain propagation continues, along with an increase in viscosity. In addition, the reaction exotherm associated with the free radical polymerization leads to the generation of heat in the cement. This heat, in turn, results in thermal expansion of the cement, while there is a competing volumetric shrinkage of the cement as the MMA monomer converts into the denser PMMA polymer. The viscosity of the cement must be carefully monitored during the working period because with a very low viscosity the cement would not be able to withstand the bleeding pressure in the femur. This would result in blood lamination in the cement, which can weaken the cement (9,34,39).

The final stage is the hardening period, when the polymerization terminates and leads to a hardened cement. The temperature of the cement continues to be elevated and then slowly decreases to body temperatures. During the course of this period, the cement continues to undergo volumetric shrinkage along with thermal shrinkage as the cement cools

down to body temperature. While the manufacturer can define the hardening period using in vitro measurements at a controlled temperature and humidity in a laboratory environment, it is difficult to predict the hardening period with accuracy due to variations in the ambient environment in the operating room, the body temperature, and thickness of the cement mantle, all of which can alter the setting times of the cement.

Several factors, such as the type of mixing method used, the viscosity of the cement, the precooling of the monomer and/or powder, the preheating of the powder component, and the preheating of the femoral stem, can also significantly alter the times associated with some of the handling phases. Thus it is important for the surgeon to be familiar with each of the factors that can alter the duration of each phase.

CEMENT RHEOLOGY

The enormous importance of the handling characteristics of bone cement places much attention on the variation in viscosity of bone cement, which increases at different rates after mixing of the powder and liquid components. The mixed cement begins as a viscous liquid, then turns into a viscoelastic material, and finally hardens into a predominantly elastic solid. Thus, it is important to monitor both the dynamic viscosity as well as the viscoelastic parameters, such as storage modulus (G'), loss modulus (G''), and tanδ (their ratio). A high storage modulus indicates that the material is more solidlike whereas a high loss modulus shows that the material is more viscous. Figure 11-3 shows that the viscosity of commercial bone cements are different at the start of setting, and the differences in viscosity can change over the course of setting due to differences in setting rates. For example, Farrar and Rose (32) showed that Palacos R had the highest viscosity among the cements studied and that Zimmer LVC, which has the smallest prepolymerized beads and low molecular weight (33), had the lowest viscosity. The low molecular weight of Zimmer LVC continues to maintain a low viscosity even after the other

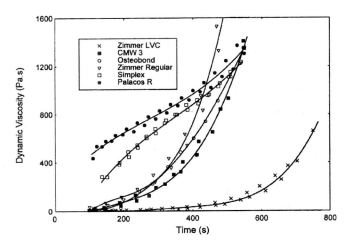

Figure 11-3   Plot of dynamic viscosity as a function of time for commercial bone cements at room temperature. (Reproduced with permission from Farrar DF, Rose J. Rheological properties of PMMA bone cements during curing. *Biomaterials.* 2001;22: 3005–3013.)

TABLE 11-3
VISCOELASTIC PARAMETERS OF BONE CEMENT AT DOUGH TIME

Cement	Dough Time(s)	G′ (kPa)	G″ (kPa)	|G*| (kPa)	tanδ
Palacos R	240	34.8	21.4	40.9	0.61
Simplex P	360	26.0	26.0	36.8	1.0
Zimmer Regular	540	71.0	69.0	99.0	1.0
Osteobond	390	16.5	17.8	24.3	1.1
CMW3	330	7.8	11.3	13.7	1.4

G′, storage modulus; G″, loss modulus; \|G*\|, $(G'^2 + G''^2)^{1/2}$; tanδ, G″/G′.
Reproduced from Farrar DF, Rose J. Rheological properties of PMMA bone cements during curing. *Biomaterials*. 2001;22:3005–3013.

cements have transformed into a viscoelastic solid. In contrast, Palacos R, which is known to have a high molecular weight (see Table 11-2), had a much higher viscosity, since higher molecular weight polymer melts have a higher viscosity.

All bone cements generally define a setting time and a dough time. The setting time of bone cement is the time at which the reaction exotherm heats the cement to a temperature that is exactly halfway between the ambient and maximum temperature. Dough time is defined as the time when the cement no longer sticks to a latex glove. Commercial bone cements have their own unique dough time, as shown in Table 11-3. The characterization of the rheological state of bone cement using viscosity is inadequate when it achieves the doughy state, since the cement is no longer a viscous liquid. Farrar and Rose characterized the rheology of a few commercial bone cements as a function of time using a parallel-plate rheometer, and they measured the storage modulus, loss modulus, and their ratio, as shown in Table 11-3 (32). As expected, the storage modulus increases with setting, as the cement converts from a viscous liquid into a viscoelastic solid. In general, the ratio of the storage and loss modulus approached 1 when the dough time was attained, which is not surprising, since it is an intermediate state between an elastic solid and a viscous fluid.

The viscosity of bone cement has an enormous influence on the working period, which is of great importance to the orthopedic surgeon. Some bone cements have a long working period but their viscosity can be very high during this period so that application of cement and fixation can be more difficult. In some low-viscosity cements, the working time is long but the increase in viscosity during this period is large, making the time of application of the cement relatively short. Low-viscosity cements have the advantage that they mix to form a homogeneous mixture more easily than high-viscosity cements. Second, modern cementing techniques emphasize the importance of the flow of cements into the interstices of the bone by pressurization, which can be more easily achieved using low-viscosity cements (53). However, some low-viscosity cements may have a lengthy waiting period before dough time is attained. If there is rapid increase of viscosity during the working period, the surgeon has very little time to apply the cement. Furthermore, if the dough is inserted too quickly, then the viscosity is too low to resist the bleeding pressure, leading to blood being mixed into the cement. Blood lamination can weaken the cement–bone interface (39). It is also important to note that vacuum mixing of low-viscosity cement must be conducted at low vacuum levels compared to

medium- and high-viscosity cements, since the low vapor pressure may promote boiling of the MMA monomer. This makes it more difficult to eliminate microporosity in low-viscosity cements. Prechilling of the monomer could conceivably decrease this problem, but it may lead to unreasonably long setting times, since some low-viscosity cements already have a longer setting time than high-viscosity cements. It is also important to note that temperature significantly affects viscosity and thus handling characteristics. Thus, prechilling or preheating the cement or monomer (43,71), the temperature of the operating room (80), and the use of a preheated or precooled femoral stem (44,95), among other things, can significantly affect the handling period.

CEMENT MORPHOLOGY: PORES AND RADIOPACIFIERS

The morphology of hardened cement comprises prepolymerized beads of PMMA or their copolymers fused with the polymerized MMA monomer, which also contains radiopacifiers and additives, such as powders of antibiotics, as well as pores or voids and residual initiator. Figure 11-4 shows that rapid

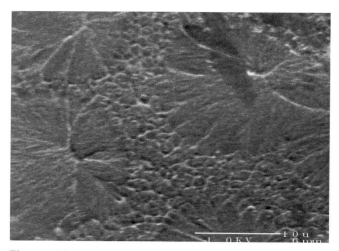

Figure 11-4 Low-voltage scanning electron micrograph of freeze-fractured cross section of radiopaque bone cement showing prepolymerized beads embedded in hardened MMA matrix containing radiopacifiers.

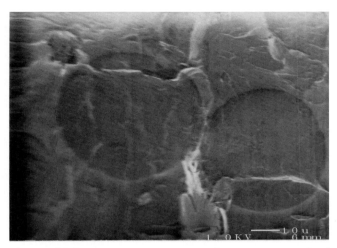

Figure 11-5 Low-voltage scanning electron micrograph of freeze-fractured cross section of radiolucent bone cement showing impressions of unfused prepolymerized powder particles that were expelled upon fracturing the cement.

fracture of the cement moves smoothly across the prepolymerized beads containing no additives. However, a large number of fracture features are observed surrounding the prepolymerized beads, which are due to cracks deviating from their path when they encounter flaws in their path associated with pores and radiopacifier particles, a process referred to as crack blunting (105). Thus, the fracture surface appears to be rougher in the interbead matrix region of bone cement.

One of the most common sources of flaws in bone cement is the presence of pores. These flaws occur due to the following possible causes: (a) air dissolved within the powder particles; (b) air entrapment during mixing of powder and liquid monomer; (c) incomplete fusion of prepolymerized PMMA beads with the setting MMA, as shown in Figure 11-5, which shows impressions of unfused beads on the fracture surface; (d) evaporation of the volatile monomer due to the heat of reaction during setting; (e) air entrapment during transfer of the dough to the gun; and (f) air entrapment during introduction of cement into the medullary canal (10). The major problem associated with the presence of flaws due to pores and additives is that when a critical flaw size is achieved, the flaws act as sites of stress concentration, leading to weakening of the cement (7,40,46,73). The Griffith crack criterion stipulates that there exists a critical flaw size unique to each material above which its fracture strength is compromised (38). For PMMA, the critical flaw size is 70 μm. Thus, porosity alone would not compromise the fracture strength of bone cement, especially if all the pores were smaller than the critical flaw size for PMMA. But the size of the pores and their distribution are expected to strongly affect the fracture strength if some of the pores exceed the critical flaw size for PMMA. It is generally well known that hardened bone cement contain macropores (pore diameter greater than 1 mm) and micropores (pore diameter 0.1–1.0 mm) (113,114). Based on the Griffith theory, elimination of the macropores would be more important than elimination of the micropores, especially the pores much smaller than 70 μm in diameter. The most common method of eliminating pores is to use centrifugation and vacuum mixing methods

(discussed in the next section). In addition to pores in the bulk cement, pores at the interface between the cement and femoral stem can also act as sites of stress concentration, with the potential for crack initiation; the number of these pores can be decreased by preheating the femoral stem (43,44).

Several techniques have been used to measure bulk porosity in bone cements. The apparent density method or the flotation technique is the simplest method of measuring the total volume fraction of pores (101). However, this method does not monitor the size of the pores, which have a direct bearing on the fracture strength. The size of large pores or macropores is commonly measured using x-ray radiographs along with image analysis techniques (15,46).

Another source of flaws that can be potential sites of high stress concentration are radiopacifier powder particles. A radiopacifier powder, usually barium sulfate or zirconium oxide, consists of particles with a broad range of sizes, from approximately 0.2 to 2 μm in diameter (Fig. 11-6). These particles are necessary for the orthopedic surgeon to monitor cracks in bone cement and associated loosening using x-ray radiographs. All cements contain approximately 8% to 15% by weight of opacifiers. Zirconium oxide is a more radiopaque material than barium sulfate, but it is a harder material. Thus, if there is loosening, there could be concerns related to third-body abrasive wear in the bearing surface of the joint replacement. Barium sulfate is generally insoluble, but there are concerns about toxic barium ion release, which, again, would only be significant upon loosening of the implant (4,109).

Poor dispersion of radiopacifier particles in the region between the prepolymerized cement beads can affect both crack initiation as well as crack propagation, especially if they are larger than the critical flaw size for PMMA (8,83,105). The radiopacifier particles do not bond with PMMA and instead reside loosely within pores. The pores surrounding radiopacifier particles or their aggregates occur because the polymerizing MMA monomer shrinks away from the radiopacifier particles. The lack of a strong interaction or bond between the hard radiopacifier particles and the matrix PMMA means that they do not provide any mechanical reinforcement. Despite the

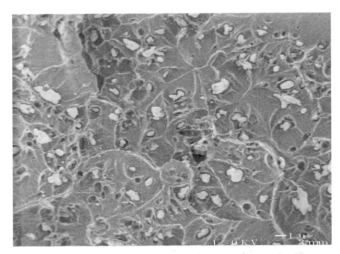

Figure 11-6 Low-voltage scanning electron micrograph of freeze-fractured cross section of radiopaque bone cement showing barium sulfate radiopacifier particles dispersed in the cement matrix.

lack of a strong interaction between radiopacifiers and the matrix polymer, it has been shown that radiopacifiers strongly affect the mechanism of crack propagation. In their absence, fatigue cracks propagate through both the prepolymerized PMMA beads as well as the interbead matrix regions. However, the cracks proceed primarily through the interbead matrix regions when radiopacifier particles are present in the cement. In addition, the presence of the radiopacifier particles decreases the rate of propagation of fatigue cracks, possibly by deflection of cracks (83). That barium sulfate radiopacifiers lead to mechanical reinforcement is corroborated by a recent study showing that an increased amount of barium sulfate required for higher opacity enhanced the mechanical properties of bone cement (56). Another plausible explanation for the mechanical reinforcement effect of hard radiopacifier particles is that the presence of such inhomogeneities, especially the particles that are submicrometer in size, could promote crazing. Crazes, which are ellipsoidal-shaped, pre-microcrack structures that can form ahead of a crack tip, are known to occur in glassy polymers, such as PMMA, under tensile stresses. The two elliptical surfaces of a craze encompassing the void space are held together by thin microfibrils, which are energy absorbing in that they must be fully stretched to he point of fracturing before the crack can propagate any further. Thus, inhomogeneities that promote the formation of crazes would decrease the rate of propagation of cracks in bone cement. Regardless, new, nonparticulate radiopacifiers utilizing organo-bismuth compound (26) and iodine-based monomers (5,36,67,77) are being studied as potential replacements for barium sulfate and zirconium oxide.

MIXING TECHNIQUES AND POROSITY REDUCTION

Mixing techniques are of prime importance in determining the content and size of flaws that can compromise fracture toughness. Historically, three methods of mixing of cement have been employed: (a) hand mixing in air (73); (b) hand mixing followed by centrifugation (14,17,21,45,46); and (c) hand mixing in an evacuated mixing device (3,55,59,60, 65,66,70,71,113,114,116), commonly known as "vacuum mixing."

Hand mixing involves mixing of the liquid and powder components in an open bowl using a spatula at a speed of 1 to 2 Hz for a period of duration of approximately 2 minutes (62,63). The most important concern during mixing of cements is that a large number of voids can be introduced into the cement and compromise clinically relevant mechanical properties. The hand-mixing method can introduce a porosity of 7% or higher (101). Charnley demonstrated that excessive mixing can lead to increased porosity, later confirmed by another study (40,46). Careful mixing by decreasing the number of beats and waiting for a short duration after wetting the powder component with the monomer can decrease the porosity to approximately 5%.

Centrifugation was later introduced as a method to eliminate pores (14,17,22,24,45,46,76,93,101,103,115). In this method, the liquid and powder components are initially hand mixed and then placed in a tube and subjected to centrifugation at a speed of 2300 to 4000 rpm for a duration of 0.5 to

3 minutes. This method results in a dramatic decrease in total porosity since the air-filled pores have a much lower density than the components of bone cement and consequently rise to the surface of the cement. The total porosity decreases to 1% or less, which is significantly lower than the porosity observed in hand mixing. More importantly, centrifugation increases several clinically significant mechanical properties associated with the presence of macropores in cement, such as fatigue strength, as compared with hand mixing. It has been shown that for centrifugation to be effective, the viscosity of the cement must be relatively low, allowing the air bubbles to flow to the surface of the cement under the centrifugal force. One way to assist centrifugation is to chill the MMA monomer prior to mixing to maintain a low viscosity by decreasing the rate of polymerization (14). One potential drawback of the centrifugation mixing technique is that it can lead to an inhomogeneous distribution of radiopacifier particles in the centrifuged cement, due to the sedimentation of these particles, which are denser than PMMA and MMA monomer (102). Despite this potential drawback, centrifugation mixing vastly decreases the amount of porosity and significantly improves the bulk quality of bone cement.

The third type of mixing technique is vacuum mixing, in which the two components of bone cements are placed in a mixing bowl and are mixed after subjecting the bowl to vacuum conditions. Several vacuum-mixing devices have been developed (a few examples are shown in Fig. 11-7), and these have proven to substantially decrease porosity in cements to less than 1% and consequently to increase their fatigue properties (3,20,59,71,72,76,79,101,115,116). It has been shown, however, that very high vacuum levels can lead to excessive shrinkage of cement and also have been associated with the presence of cracks in the cement (30). Thus using moderate levels of vacuum applied to the cement while mixing is generally recommended for decreased porosity and the associated higher fatigue strength. Another compelling reason for using vacuum mixing is that MMA monomer is contained within the mixing bowl, which limits exposure to its vapors (11,100). Toxicology information obtained from materials safety data sheets (MSDSs) show that MMA monomer is harmful if

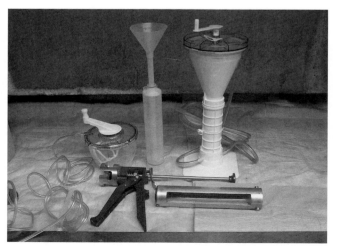

Figure 11-7 Three typical commercial vacuum mixers and a cement gun.

inhaled, swallowed, or absorbed through the skin. Thus, vacuum mixing has an advantage over centrifugation mixing in that it combines the advantages of low porosity and low exposure to vapors without the possibility of a variation in the distribution of radiopacifier additives. It must be noted that not all vacuum mixers can be used indiscriminately with all types of cements. For example, low-viscosity cements require lower vacuum levels than medium- and high-viscosity cements. Otherwise, the low vapor pressure can promote boiling of the monomer, resulting in pore formation. While prechilling of the monomer could alleviate such problems in low-viscosity cements, it would also increase the setting times substantially. Thus, cements and mixers must be appropriately chosen so that the mixers are effective for the particular type of cement.

THERMAL EXPANSION AND VOLUMETRIC SHRINKAGE

Volumetric shrinkage of bone cement is to be expected since the difference in the density of the MMA monomer (0.943 g/cc) and the PMMA polymer (1.20 g/cc) translates into a 21% volumetric shrinkage upon complete polymerization of MMA into PMMA. In a typical bone cement, approximately one third of the total volume of the cement is the MMA monomer. Therefore, no more than 7% volumetric shrinkage is expected. The amount of shrinkage is expected to be slightly lower than this number due to loss of the volatile MMA monomer and incomplete polymerization (40). In addition, thermal expansion of the cement is expected due to the heat of polymerization, which is an exothermic reaction (6,68,86,107). The temperature of bone cement has been found to rise to between 66°C and 82.5°C, depending on the cement composition (41). This temperature rise is followed by cooling and thermal shrinkage, which has the potential to induce residual stresses and cracks in the cement (86). The volumetric shrinkage is also closely related to the total porosity present in bone cement. A larger number of pores would result in a lower amount of shrinkage since only the bulk material shrinks. It has been proposed that porosity may be beneficial for fixation since cement shrinkage would lead to a gap at the interface between the cement and the bone and consequently incomplete fixation (25). Also, the presence of a gap at this interface could lead to micromotion-related fretting of the cement against bone and contribute to loosening and shedding of particulate debris. However, if the cement tightly adhered to the bone and metal interface, it is expected that there would be more efficient transfer of stresses across the cement. It is not clear whether bone cement in its current state could endure elevated stresses to a larger extent. Vacuum mixing and centrifugation mixing decrease porosity and consequently lead to further shrinkage in bone cement. However, the geometry of the cement mantle dictates that diametral shrinkage is more important for fixation than overall volumetric shrinkage, and diametral shrinkage is much lower than volumetric shrinkage (18). In addition, it should be noted that some polymerization has already occurred prior to insertion of the cement, which further decreases the amount of shrinkage in the cement within the medullary canal. New bone cement formulations for vertebroplasty applications require a higher ratio of monomer to polymer to lower their viscosity and to make them injectable. These cements are expected to shrink to more than bone cement used in total joint replacement prostheses.

ANTIBIOTICS

Buchholz and Engelbrecht were the first to add gentamicin antibiotic to a bone cement, Palacos R, in order to treat infected joints and provide prophylaxis against infective organisms in the case of primary joint replacement (13). Later, it was shown that oxacillin, cefazolin, and gentamicin are all stable in PMMA bone cement and were released in active form. The largest release of antibiotics occurred in the first 24 hours, but high bactericidal concentrations of the antibiotics were measured in the periprosthetic bone for up to 21 days after implantation (78). A small amount of antibiotic elution is observed even after 5 years (112). Bone cement without any antibiotics had no bacteriostatic effect on *Staphylococcus aureus*, *Escherichia coli*, and *Pseudomonas aeruginosa* organisms. Antibiotics are added in the form of powder, which is unable to diffuse through a hard, glassy polymer. So the mechanism of elution of the antibiotics is believed to be closely related to water-absorbing properties of the cement with respect to time and distance from the surface of the cement. The diffusion rate of the antibiotics depends on several factors, such as the chemical composition of the cement, the surface area at the cement–bone interface, and cement handling. For example, Palacos cement containing prepolymerized beads of P(MMA-co-MA) were shown to elute gentamicin at more rapidly than Simplex containing prepolymerized beads of P(MMA-co-S) (78). In addition, vacuum mixing, which decreases the porosity in bone cement, can also alter the kinetics of the elution of antibiotics and was shown to decrease their rate of elution by 50% (54).

In Europe, several bone cements containing antibiotics such as gentamicin, tobramycin, erythromycin, and colistin have been commercially available. In fact, in Norway and Sweden, over 97% of cemented hip replacements are fixed with antibiotic bone cement (1,2). Until recently, the US Food and Drug Administration (FDA) had not cleared antibiotic-containing cement in the United States for clinical practice. Therefore, it has been common practice in the United States for the surgeon to add antibiotics to bone cement in the operating room. In 2003, the first antibiotic-containing cement (incorporating tobramycin) became available in the market in the United States. This occurred in part because of the reclassification of bone cement by the FDA as a class II device, making it possible for antibiotic-containing cements to be approved. Antibiotics premixed into the cement by the manufacturer can be advantageous since the addition of antibiotic powder manually can lead to agglomeration and a decrease in the mechanical strength of the cement (27).

Antibiotics are added to cement in the powdered form since it was demonstrated that the addition of liquid antibiotics resulted in a decrease in mechanical strength due to interference with the early stages of polymerization of the MMA monomer (57). The amount of antibiotic powder required for a therapeutic level of elution is approximately 0.5 to 2 g in a standard 40-g package of prepolymerized PMMA powder. Note that antibiotic powder, like radiopacifiers and pores, also results in defects or flaws in bone cement.

The flexural strength of antibiotic-containing cement was shown to be lower than that of cement without antibiotics, and the toughness of antibiotic-containing cement decreased further with excessive amounts of antibiotics (13,58). A likely reason for this is that excess amounts of undissolved antibiotics agglomerate into aggregates exceeding the critical flaw size for PMMA. However, doses of 2 g of well-dispersed antibiotic powder may not have any adverse effect on the mechanical properties of bone cement if the size of the inclusions remain below the critical flaw size for PMMA (19,23).

MECHANICAL PROPERTIES

The tensile, compressive, shear, fracture toughness, creep deformation, and fatigue properties of PMMA bone cement have been studied in great detail and are presented in several reviews (52,61,89,98). All of these mechanical properties have relevance to the loading history experienced by bone cement. For example, the cement mantle experiences tensile stress, although small, due to bending stresses, especially on the lateral side. A more obvious example is compressive stress experienced due to the patient's body weight. The compressive stress would also depend on the stem design. For example, a tapered stem with a smooth finish is expected to exert more compressive stress distally than a stem that has less taper and a roughened surface (85). The fixation of the cement to the stem, along with the compressive stress associated with the patient's body weight, would also result in shear stress experienced by the cement mantle. This would also depend on the surface roughness of the stem and the quality of fixation. Although this appears to be an important mechanical test, there are few reports on the measurement of ultimate shear strength of cement. Tensile, compressive, shear, and flexural (which combines the first three types of loading) properties of bone cement obtained from previous studies are summarized in Table 11-4. The variation in these properties is related to differences in composition, mixing methods, aging, temperature and viscosity during cement application and other factors. PMMA is a material of high modulus and low ductility compared with other polymers used for implants, such as ultra high molecular weight polyethylene. Figure 11-8 shows that polyethylene undergoes large plastic strain prior to failure, while bone cement fails upon reaching the yield stress. The slope of the initial linear region, representing the modulus or

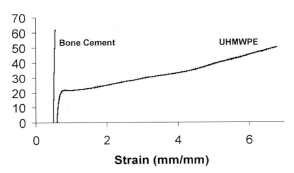

Figure 11-8 Tensile stress-strain curve for PMMA bone cement and ultra high molecular weight polyethylene.

stiffness, is higher for PMMA bone cement. Both high modulus and high toughness are difficult to achieve in polymers. The high stiffness of PMMA bone cement is more important for this application since high modulus is usually associated with low creep deformation.

Permanent deformation is undesirable in bone cement since it can lead to implant subsidence. PMMA is a viscoelastic polymer and can therefore undergo creep deformation over time under both static and dynamic loads (111). When the applied stress exceeds the yield stress, deformation in polymers occurs via plastic deformation. However, when the applied stress is below the yield stress, permanent deformation occurs via creep deformation. In the case of the cement mantle, the applied stress is generally below the yield stress of PMMA, and consequently permanent deformation occurs via creep deformation. Creep deformation can be influenced by several factors, such as cement composition, porosity, additives, and molecular weight (84,88,106). Studies have reported that creep may not play a large role in implant subsidence and that other factors such as bone remodeling may influence implant subsidence (76,110). Other studies, though, have reported that creep dominates fatigue damage at the cement–bone interface, contributing to loosening of the implant (47,48). The contribution of cement creep may also vary depending on the roughness of the metallic stem, for greater roughness would distribute stresses more evenly along the length of the stem (85). In general, creep can be decreased by choosing an implant design and a mantle thickness that reduce the applied stress on the cement.

TABLE 11-4
SELECTED MECHANICAL PROPERTIES OF BONE CEMENT

Test Method	Yield Strength (MPa)	Modulus (MPa)	Strain to Break (%)
Tensile	25.0–49.2	1583–4120	0.86–2.49
Compressive	72.6–114.3	1950–3000	—
Shear	37.0–69.0	—	—
3-point flexural	49.9–125.0	1290–2916	—
4-point flexural	12.1–74.0	1950–3160	—

Reproduced from Lewis G. Properties of acrylic bone cement: state of the art review. *J Biomed Mater Res.* 1997;38:155–182.

Fatigue failure testing is the most important mechanical test since it relates more closely than other tests to the cyclic loading experienced by bone cement during the physiological gait of the patient. Morphological studies show that fatigue failure and fatigue crack propagation are the primary mechanisms of failure of bone cement associated with prosthetic loosening (105). These studies show that fracture occurs in the regions of the cured MMA monomer containing pores and agglomerated radiopacifier fillers. A major difficulty in comparing the results of the extensive literature on fatigue testing reviewed by Krause and Mathis (52) and later by Lewis (62) is that investigators have used a variety of test conditions, sample preparation techniques, and methods of data analysis. Lewis recommends the use of the linearized form of the three-parameter Weibull equation or the Ogilvie-type equation for the analysis of fatigue data (62,63). Also recommended is the use of at least five specimens per stress amplitude to enable reasonable statistics for comparing different types of cement or different methods of cement mixing. While appropriate test conditions for fatigue tests are being developed and standardized, the current test methods continue to assist in evaluating the quality of bone cement. For example, fatigue tests combined with mixing techniques have been instrumental in demonstrating the role of pores, radiopacifiers, and antibiotic powders in the fatigue life of cements and showing that appropriate mixing techniques can substantially improve this clinically relevant material property of bone cements (21–23,56). One of the limitations, however, is that, though highly successful in evaluating the role of flaws in the bulk cement, these tests do not evaluate the role of surface flaws present at the cement–bone interface and especially the cement–metal interface, which has been implicated in early loosening.

COMPOSITE BONE CEMENTS

PMMA-based bone cement has a high modulus but low toughness compared with ductile polymers. In order to address the lack of fracture toughness and fatigue strength, many investigators who have developed new composite PMMA cements use the concept of fiber reinforcement and incorporate a low-volume fraction of chopped fibers of approximately 1% to 2%. Several types of fibers, such as fibers made of carbon (91,94,97,99), polyethylene terephthalate, oriented PMMA (117,118), ultra high molecular weight polyethylene (92), titanium (104), aramid (96), Kevlar (103), graphite (49), and steel (50) have been used to reinforce PMMA-based bone cement. While these composites have displayed improved fatigue failure properties, biocompatibility concerns and complications of processing have prevented their implementation in the manufacture of PMMA bone cement.

SUMMARY

PMMA-based bone cements have been used effectively for the fixation of total joint replacement for over 4 decades now. Although new cement formulations based on other monomers and bioactive cements are being developed, PMMA-based bone cements remain the most effective

cements for fixation of total joint replacement prostheses. It is important for the surgeon to have knowledge of the material properties of various bone cements and understand how factors such as mixing technique, the temperature of the components of bone cement or implant, the ratio of powder to monomer, and the addition of antibiotics affect these properties, since they have a direct bearing on the handling characteristics of the cement and the choice of cementing technique and implant design. Today, the demand for improved fixation of joint replacements will likely be even greater than previous years because of the development of extremely low wear alternative bearing surfaces and the expectation of longer clinical lifetimes for the implant and the cement mantle. Until new formulations of cement become available in the market, PMMA-based bone cements will continue to play an important role in the fixation of total joint replacement in the years to come.

REFERENCES

1. Annual Report. In: *Swedish Hip Arthroplasty Register*. Göteborg, Sweden; 2002.
2. Annual Report. In: *Norwegian Arthroplasty Registry*. Bergen, Norway; 2002.
3. Alkire MJ, Dabezies EJ, Hastings PR. High vacuum as a method of reducing porosity of polymethylmethacrylate. *Orthopedics*. 1987;10:1533–1539.
4. Artola A, Goni I, Gil J, et al. A radiopaque polymeric matrix for acrylic bone cements. *J Biomed Mater Res B Appl Biomater*. 2003; 64:44–55.
5. Artola A, Gurruchaga M, Vazquez B, et al. Elimination of barium sulphate from acrylic bone cements: use of two iodine-containing monomers. *Biomaterials*. 2003;24:4071–4080.
6. Baliga BR, Rose PL, Ahmed AM. Thermal modeling of polymerizing polymethylmethacrylate, considering temperature-dependent heat generation. *J Biomech Eng*. 1992;114:251–259.
7. Bayne SC, Lautenschlager EP, Compere CL, et al. Degree of polymerization of acrylic bone cement. *J Biomed Mater Res*. 1975;9: 27–34.
8. Beaumont PW. Fracture processes in acrylic bone cement containing barium sulphate dispersions. *J Biomed Eng*. 1979;1:147–152.
9. Benjamin JB, Gie GA, Lee AJ, et al. Cementing technique and the effects of bleeding. *J Bone Joint Surg [Br]*. 1987;69:620–624.
10. Berger RA, Steel MJ, Schleiden M, et al. Preventing distal voids during cementation of the femoral component in total hip arthroplasty. *J Arthroplasty*. 1993;8:323–329.
11. Bettencourt A, Calado A, Amaral J, et al. The influence of vacuum mixing on methylmethacrylate liberation from acrylic cement powder. *Int J Pharm*. 2001;219:89–93.
12. Brauer GM, Termini DJ, Dickson G. Analysis of the ingredients and determination of the residual components of acrylic bone cements. *J Biomed Mater Res*. 1977;11:577–607.
13. Buchholz HW, Engelbrecht H. Uber die Depotwirkung einiger Antibiotica bei Vermischung dem Kunstharz Palacos. *Chirurg*. 1970;41:511–515.
14. Burke DW, Gates EI, Harris WH. Centrifugation as a method of improving tensile and fatigue properties of acrylic bone cement. *J Bone Joint Surg [Am]*. 1984;66:1265–1273.
15. Chao EY, Chin HC, Stauffer RN. Roentgenographic and mechanical performance of centrifuged cement in a simulated total hip arthroplasty model. *Clin Orthop Relat Res*. 1992;285:91–101.
16. Dahl OE. Cardiorespiratory and vascular dysfunction related to major reconstructive orthopedic surgery. *Acta Orthop Scand*. 1997;68:607–614.
17. Davies JP, Burke DW, O'Connor DO, et al. Comparison of the fatigue characteristics of centrifuged and uncentrifuged Simplex P bone cement. *J Orthop Res*. 1987;5:366–371.
18. Davies JP, Harris WH. Comparison of diametral shrinkage of centrifuged and uncentrifuged Simplex P bone cement. *J Appl Biomater*. 1995;6:209–211.

19. Davies JP, Harris WH. Effect of hand mixing tobramycin on the fatigue strength of Simplex P. *J Biomed Mater Res.* 1991;25:1409–1414.

20. Davies JP, Harris WH. Optimization and comparison of three vacuum mixing systems for porosity reduction of Simplex P cement. *Clin Orthop Relat Res.* 1990;No. 254:261–269.

21. Davies JP, Jasty M, O'Connor DO, et al. The effect of centrifuging bone cement. *J Bone Joint Surg [Br].* 1989;71:39–42.

22. Davies JP, O'Connor DO, Burke DW, et al. Comparison and optimization of three centrifugation systems for reducing porosity of Simplex P bone cement. *J Arthroplasty.* 1989;4:15–20.

23. Davies JP, O'Connor DO, Burke DW, et al. Influence of antibiotic impregnation on the fatigue life of Simplex P and Palacos R acrylic bone cements, with and without centrifugation. *J Biomed Mater Res.* 1989;23:379–397.

24. Davies JP, O'Connor DO, Greer JA, et al. Comparison of the mechanical properties of Simplex P, Zimmer Regular, and LVC bone cements. *J Biomed Mater Res.* 1987;21:719–730.

25. De Wijn JR, Driessens FC, Slooff TJ. Dimensional behavior of curing bone cement masses. *J Biomed Mater Res.* 1975;9:99–103.

26. Deb S, Abdulghani S, Behiri JC. Radiopacity in bone cements using an organo-bismuth compound. *Biomaterials.* 2002;23:3387–3393.

27. DeLuise M, Scott CP. Addition of hand-blended generic tobramycin in bone cement: effect on mechanical strength. *Orthopedics.* 2004;27:1289–1291.

28. Demian HW, McDermott K. Regulatory perspective on characterization and testing of orthopedic bone cements. *Biomaterials.* 1998;19:1607–1618.

29. Eggert A, Huland H, Ruhnke J, et al. Der Einfluβ der Anruhrzeit des Knochenzements auf hypotone Kreislaufreaktionen bei Huftgelenksersatzoperationen. *Chirurg.* 1975;46:236–239.

30. Eveleigh R. The preparation of bone cement. *Br J Perioper Nurs.* 2001;11:58–62.

31. Eveleigh R. Temperature and its effect on bone cement. *Br J Perioper Nurs.* 2001;11:164–168.

32. Farrar DF, Rose J. Rheological properties of PMMA bone cements during curing. *Biomaterials.* 2001;22:3005–3013.

33. Ferracane JL, Greener EH. Rheology of acrylic bone cements. *Biomater Med Devices Artif Organs.* 1981;9:213–224.

34. Flivik G, Yuan X, Ryd L, et al. Effects of lamination on the strength of bone cement. *Acta Orthop Scand.* 1997;68:55–58.

35. Flory PJ. *Principles of Polymer Chemistry.* Ithaca: Cornell University Press; 1953.

36. Ginebra MP, Albuixech L, Fernandez-Barragan E, et al. Mechanical performance of acrylic bone cements containing different radiopacifying agents. *Biomaterials.* 2002;23:1873–1882.

37. Graham J, Pruitt L, Ries M, et al. Fracture and fatigue properties of acrylic bone cement: the effects of mixing method, sterilization treatment, and molecular weight. *J Arthroplasty.* 2000;15:1028–1035.

38. Griffith AA. The phenomena of rupture and flow in solids. *Mech Eng.* 1920;A221:163–198.

39. Gruen TA, Markolf KL, Amstutz HC. Effects of laminations and blood entrapment on the strength of acrylic bone cement. *Clin Orthop Relat Res.* 1976;No. 119:250–255.

40. Haas SS, Brauer GM, Dickson G. A characterization of polymethylmethacrylate bone cement. *J Bone Joint Surg [Am].* 1975;57:380–391.

41. Hansen D, Jensen JS. Prechilling and vacuum mixing not suitable for all bone cements: handling characteristics and exotherms of bone cements. *J Arthroplasty.* 1990;5:287–90.

42. Hughes KF, Ries MD, Pruitt LA. Structural degradation of acrylic bone cements due to in vivo and simulated aging. *J Biomed Mater Res A.* 2003;65:126–135.

43. Iesaka K, Jaffe WL, Kummer FJ. Effects of the initial temperature of acrylic bone cement liquid monomer on the properties of the stem-cement interface and cement polymerization. *J Biomed Mater Res B Appl Biomater.* 2004;68:186–190.

44. Jafri AA, Green SM, Partington PF, et al. Pre-heating of components in cemented total hip arthroplasty. *J Bone Joint Surg [Br].* 2004;86:1214–1219.

45. James SP, Jasty M, Davies J, et al. A fractographic investigation of PMMA bone cement focusing on the relationship between porosity reduction and increased fatigue life. *J Biomed Mater Res.* 1992;26:651–662.

46. Jasty M, Davies JP, O'Connor DO, et al. Porosity of various preparations of acrylic bone cements. *Clin Orthop Relat Res.* 1990;No. 259:122–129.

47. Kim DG, Miller MA, Mann KA. Creep dominates tensile fatigue damage of the cement-bone interface. *J Orthop Res.* 2004;22:633–640.

48. Kim DG, Miller MA, Mann KA. A fatigue damage model for the cement-bone interface. *J Biomech.* 2004;37:1505–1512.

49. Knoell A, Maxwell H, Bechtol C. Graphite fiber reinforced bone cement: an experimental feasibility investigation. *Ann Biomed Eng.* 1975;3:225–229.

50. Kotha SP, Li C, Schmid SR, et al. Fracture toughness of steel-fiber–reinforced bone cement. *J Biomed Mater Res A.* 2004;70:514–521.

51. Kraft J. Polymethylmethacrylate: a review. *J Foot Surg.* 1977;16:66–68.

52. Krause W, Mathis RS. Fatigue properties of acrylic bone cements: review of the literature. *J Biomed Mater Res.* 1988;22:37–53.

53. Krause WR, Miller J, Ng P. The viscosity of acrylic bone cements. *J Biomed Mater Res.* 1982;16:219–243.

54. Kuechle DK, Landon GC, Musher DM, et al. Elution of vancomycin, daptomycin, and amikacin from acrylic bone cement. *Clin Orthop Relat Res.* 1991;No. 264:302–308.

55. Kurdy NM, Hodgkinson JP, Haynes R. Acrylic bone-cement: influence of mixer design and unmixed powder. *J Arthroplasty.* 1996;11:813–819.

56. Kurtz SM, Villarraga ML, Zhao K, et al. Static and fatigue mechanical behavior of bone cement with elevated barium sulfate content for treatment of vertebral compression fractures [erratum appears in *Biomaterials.* 2005;26:5926]. *Biomaterials.* 2005;26:3699–3712.

57. Lautenschlager EP, Jacobs JJ, Marshall GW, et al. Mechanical properties of bone cements containing large doses of antibiotic powders. *J Biomed Mater Res.* 1976;10:929–938.

58. Lautenschlager EP, Marshall GW, Marks KE, et al. Mechanical strength of acrylic bone cements impregnated with antibiotics. *J Biomed Mater Res.* 1976;10:837–845.

59. Lewis G. Effect of mixing method and storage temperature of cement constituents on the fatigue and porosity of acrylic bone cement. *J Biomed Mater Res.* 1999;48:143–149.

60. Lewis G. Effect of two variables on the fatigue performance of acrylic bone cement: mixing method and viscosity. *Biomed Mater Eng.* 1999;9:197–207.

61. Lewis G. Fatigue testing and performance of acrylic bone-cement materials: state-of-the-art review. *J Biomed Mater Res B Appl Biomater.* 2003;66:457–486.

62. Lewis G. Properties of acrylic bone cement: state of the art review. *J Biomed Mater Res.* 1997;38:155–182.

63. Lewis G, Austin GE. Mechanical properties of vacuum-mixed acrylic bone cement. *J Appl Biomater.* 1994;5:307–314.

64. Lewis G, Mladsi S. Effect of sterilization method on properties of Palacos R acrylic bone cement. *Biomaterials.* 1998;19:117–124.

65. Lewis G, Nyman J, Trieu HH. The apparent fracture toughness of acrylic bone cement: effect of three variables. *Biomaterials.* 1998;19:961–967.

66. Lewis G, Nyman JS, Trieu HH. Effect of mixing method on selected properties of acrylic bone cement. *J Biomed Mater Res.* 1997;38:221–228.

67. Lewis G, van Hooy-Corstjens CS, Bhattaram A, et al. Influence of the radiopacifier in an acrylic bone cement on its mechanical, thermal, and physical properties: barium sulfate-containing cement versus iodine-containing cement. *J Biomed Mater Res B Appl Biomater.* 2005;73:77–87.

68. Li C, Mason J, Yakimicki D. Thermal characterization of PMMA-based bone cement curing. *J Mat Sci Mater Med.* 2004;15:85–89.

69. Li C, Schmid S, Mason J. Effects of pre-cooling and pre-heating procedures on cement polymerization and thermal osteonecrosis in cemented hip replacements. *Med Eng Phys.* 2003;25:559–564.

70. Lidgren L, Bodelind B, Moller J. Bone cement improved by vacuum mixing and chilling. *Acta Orthop Scand.* 1987;58:27–32.

71. Lidgren L, Drar H, Moller J. Strength of polymethylmethacrylate increased by vacuum mixing. *Acta Orthop Scand.* 1984;55: 536–541.

72. Linden U. Fatigue properties of bone cement: comparison of mixing techniques. *Acta Orthop Scand.* 1989;60:431–433.

73. Linden U. Porosity in manually mixed bone cement. *Clin Orthop Relat Res.* 1988;No. 231:110–112.

74. Linder L. Tissue reaction to methyl methacrylate monomer: a comparative study in the rabbit's ear on the toxicity of methyl methacrylate monomer of varying composition. *Acta Orthop Scand* 1976;47:3–10.

75. Lu Z, McKellop H. Effects of cement creep on stem subsidence and stresses in the cement mantle of a total hip replacement. *J Biomed Mater Res.* 1997;34:221–226.

76. Macaulay W, DiGiovanni CW, Restrepo A, et al. Differences in bone-cement porosity by vacuum mixing, centrifugation, and hand mixing. *J Arthroplasty.* 2002;17:569–575.

77. Manero JM, Ginebra MP, Gil FJ, et al. Propagation of fatigue cracks in acrylic bone cements containing different radiopaque agents. *Proc Inst Mech Eng [H].* 2004;218:167–172.

78. Marks KE, Nelson CL, Lautenschlager EP. Antibiotic-impregnated acrylic bone cement. *J Bone Joint Surg [Am].* 1976;58: 358–364.

79. Mau H, Schelling K, Heisel C, et al. Comparison of various vacuum mixing systems and bone cements as regards reliability, porosity and bending strength. *Acta Orthop Scand* 2004;75: 160–172.

80. Meyer PR Jr, Lautenschlager EP, Moore BK. On the setting properties of acrylic bone cement. *J Bone Joint Surg [Am].* 1973;55:149–156.

81. Migliaresi C, Fambri L, Kolarik J. Polymerization kinetics, glass transition temperature and creep of acrylic bone cements. *Biomaterials.* 1994;15:875–881.

82. Miller J, Krause WR, Krug WH, et al. Low viscosity cement. 1981. *Clin Orthop Relat Res.* 1992;No. 276:4–6.

83. Molino LN, Topoleski LD. Effect of BaSO4 on the fatigue crack propagation rate of PMMA bone cement. *J Biomed Mater Res.* 1996;31:131–137.

84. Norman TL, Kish V, Blaha JD, et al. Creep characteristics of hand- and vacuum-mixed acrylic bone cement at elevated stress levels. *J Biomed Mater Res.* 1995;29:495–501.

85. Norman TL, Thyagarajan G, Saligrama VC, et al. Stem surface roughness alters creep induced subsidence and "taper-lock" in a cemented femoral hip prosthesis. *J Biomechanics.* 2001;34: 1325–1333.

86. Orr JF, Dunne NJ, Quinn JC. Shrinkage stresses in bone cement. *Biomaterials.* 2003;24:2933–2940.

87. Orsini EC, Byrick RJ, Mullen JB, et al. Cardiopulmonary function and pulmonary microemboli during arthroplasty using cemented or non-cemented components: the role of intramedullary pressure. *J Bone Joint Surg [Am].* 1987;69:822–832.

88. Pal S, Saha S. Stress relaxation and creep behaviour of normal and carbon fibre reinforced acrylic bone cement. *Biomaterials.* 1982;3:93–96.

89. Park JB. Acrylic bone cement: in vitro and in vivo property-structure relationship: a selective review. *Ann Biomed Eng.* 1983; 11:297–312.

90. Petty W. Methyl methacrylate concentrations in tissues adjacent to bone cement. *J Biomed Mater Res.* 1980;14:427–434.

91. Pilliar RM, Blackwell R, Macnab I, et al. Carbon fiber-reinforced bone cement in orthopedic surgery. *J Biomed Mater Res.* 1976;10:893–906.

92. Pourdeyhimi B, Wagner HD. Elastic and ultimate properties of acrylic bone cement reinforced with ultra-high-molecular-weight polyethylene fibers. *J Biomed Mater Res.* 1989;23:63–80.

93. Rimnac CM, Wright TM, McGill DL. The effect of centrifugation on the fracture properties of acrylic bone cements. *J Bone Joint Surg [Am].* 1986;68:281–287.

94. Robinson RP, Wright TM, Burstein AH. Mechanical properties of poly(methyl methacrylate) bone cements. *J Biomed Mater Res.* 1981;15:203–208.

95. Rodop O, Kiral A, Arpacioglu O, et al. Effects of stem design and pre-cooling prostheses on the heat generated by bone cement in an in vitro model. *J Int Med Res.* 2002;30:265–270.

96. Saha S, Pal S. Improvement of mechanical properties of acrylic bone cement by fiber reinforcement. *J Biomechanics.* 1984;17: 467–478.

97. Saha S, Pal S. Mechanical characterization of commercially made carbon-fiber–reinforced polymethylmethacrylate. *J Biomed Mater Res.* 1986;20:817–826.

98. Saha S, Pal S. Mechanical properties of bone cement: a review. *J Biomed Mater Res.* 1984;18:435–462.

99. Saha S, Pal S. Strain-rate dependence of the compressive properties of normal and carbon-fiber–reinforced bone cement. *J Biomed Mater Res.* 1983;17:1041–1047.

100. Schlegel UJ, Sturm M, Ewerbeck V, et al. Efficacy of vacuum bone cement mixing systems in reducing methylmethacrylate fume exposure: comparison of 7 different mixing devices and hand-mixing. *Acta Orthop Scand.* 2004;75:559–566.

101. Schreurs BW, Spierings PT, Huiskes R, et al. Effects of preparation techniques on the porosity of acrylic cements. *Acta Orthop Scand.* 1988;59:403–409.

102. Skinner HB, Murray WR. Variations in the density of bone cement after centrifugation. *Clin Orthop Relat Res.* 1986;No. 207:263–269.

103. Topoleski LD, Ducheyne P, Cuckler JM. The effects of centrifugation and titanium fiber reinforcement on fatigue failure mechanisms in poly(methyl methacrylate) bone cement. *J Biomed Mater Res.* 1995;29:299–307.

104. Topoleski LD, Ducheyne P, Cuckler JM. The fracture toughness of titanium-fiber–reinforced bone cement. *J Biomed Mater Res.* 1992;26:1599–1617.

105. Topoleski LD, Ducheyne P, Cuckler JM. Microstructural pathway of fracture in poly(methyl methacrylate) bone cement. *Biomaterials.* 1993;14:1165–1172.

106. Treharne RW, Brown N. Factors influencing the creep behavior of poly(methyl methacrylate) cements. *J Biomed Mater Res.* 1975;9:81–88.

107. Turner RC, Atkins PE, Ackley MA, et al. Molecular and macroscopic properties of PMMA bone cement: free-radical generation and temperature change versus mixing ratio. *J Biomed Mater Res.* 1981;15:425–432.

108. Urist MR. Acrylic cement stabilized joint replacements. *Curr Probl Surg.* 1975;1–54.

109. van Hooy-Corstjens CS, Govaert LE, Spoelstra AB, et al. Mechanical behaviour of a new acrylic radiopaque iodine-containing bone cement. *Biomaterials.* 2004;25:2657–2667.

110. Verdonschot N, Huiskes R. Acrylic cement creeps but does not allow much subsidence of femoral stems. *J Bone Joint Surg [Br].* 1997;79:665–669.

111. Verdonschot N, Huiskes R. Creep behavior of hand-mixed Simplex P bone cement under cyclic tensile loading. *J Appl Biomater.* 1994;5:235–243.

112. Wahlig H, Dingeldein E. Antibiotics and bone cements: experimental and clinical long-term observations. *Acta Orthop Scand.* 1980;51:49–56.

113. Wang JS, Franzen H, Jonsson E, et al. Porosity of bone cement reduced by mixing and collecting under vacuum. *Acta Orthop Scand.* 1993;64:143–146.

114. Wang JS, Toksvig-Larsen S, Muller-Wille P, et al. Is there any difference between vacuum mixing systems in reducing bone cement porosity? *J Biomed Mater Res.* 1996;33:115–119.

115. Wixson RL. Do we need to vacuum mix or centrifuge cement? *Clin Orthop Relat Res.* 1992;No. 285:84–90.

116. Wixson RL, Lautenschlager EP, Novak MA. Vacuum mixing of acrylic bone cement. *J Arthroplasty.* 1987;2:141–149.

117. Wright DD, Lautenschlager EP, Gilbert JL. Bending and fracture toughness of woven self-reinforced composite poly(methyl methacrylate). *J Biomed Mater Res.* 1997;36:441–453.

118. Wright DD, Lautenschlager EP, Gilbert JL. Interfacial properties of self-reinforced composite poly(methyl methacrylate). *J Biomed Mater Res.* 1998;43:153–161.

Engineering Techniques for Implant Design and Evaluation

12

Thomas D. Brown

Mechanical measurements and mechanical analyses form much of the information base for contemporary hip reconstruction. Orthopedists often are called on to make decisions that draw heavily on data that have been collected using advanced mechanical engineering techniques. Unfortunately, orthopedic training normally includes little or no exposure to the operational principles of contemporary mechanical engineering instrumentation, so it sometimes is difficult for surgeons to appreciate the limitations of data collected from complex laboratory models that use these technologies. The purpose of this chapter is to outline the technical basis for the major classes of mechanical measurements and analyses currently utilized to plan and/or evaluate hip reconstructions.

In laboratory physical testing, many experimental preparations involve application of functionally representative loadings at the whole-construct level, together with the use of sensors to measure deformations, strains, loads, and stresses at specific sites. As a practical matter, the development of construct-level load application systems represents a compromise between clinical realism and cost/complexity, usually resolved in favor of the latter. Logistical compromises also often govern the choice of mechanical sensors, compounded by size constraints, measured complexity, and signal transduction artifact. Finally, differing levels of abstraction are employed to represent the host bone or joint, including the use of human cadaver material, artificial bone surrogates of several types, and other species in the case of in vivo models.

Mathematical analyses also have found broad application in the study of hip implants, because the underlying physical principles of Newtonian mechanics lend themselves well to description in mathematical terms. The main advantage of the mathematical approach is that, once the model has been developed and (hopefully) validated, individual variables can be very easily isolated and perturbed, allowing systematic and economical study of how constructs respond to changes of individual physical or material factors. Digital computational approaches—especially finite element models—have proven especially useful in that regard. However, mathematical models can be no more realistic than the input data (geometry, material properties, loading conditions) with which they are supplied. And, although physical spot checks and clinical validation are very reassuring when available, it is important to appreciate the major simplifications and limitations of the underlying theoretical framework.

Sometimes it is possible to make the pertinent mechanical measurements directly from patient materials, such as clinical imaging studies or autopsy retrievals. Here, clinical realism is seldom an issue, but a trade-off is that the nature of the available information often compromises mechanical measurement rigor. And, there normally is a much greater degree of variability than occurs under controlled laboratory conditions.

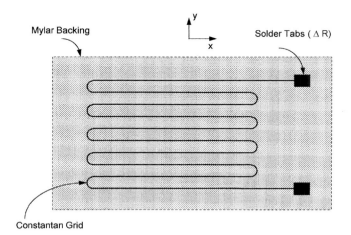

Mylar Backing

Solder Tabs (Δ R)

Constantan Grid

Figure 12-1 Schematic diagram of a bonded resistance strain gauge. A multiply looped metal grid (usually constantan, a copper–nickel alloy) is deposited on a plastic backing. When the gauge is attached to a substrate whose strain is to be measured, the metal grid undergoes the same deformation as the substrate. If the gauge is stretched in its longitudinal direction (here, denoted by x), its electrical resistance increases. This resistance increase Δ R (measured between the solder tabs) can be sensitively detected by means of a Wheatstone bridge circuit.

MECHANICAL SENSORS

Probably the most widely used sensor, either for direct application by the end user or as the functional element in manufactured transducers, is the bonded resistance strain gauge. Originally devised in the 1930s (22), these are expendable units that consist of patterned films, usually of copper or constantan (a copper–nickel alloy), deposited by a photoetching process on a thin plastic backing. Typical footprint sizes of the functional portion of the gauge (gauge width and gauge length) (Fig. 12-1) range from 2 to 6 mm. The underside of the gauge is glued (usually by cyanoacrylate) directly to the substrate whose strain is to be measured. Therefore, as the substrate surface deforms during load application, the foil pattern of the gauge deforms with it. The functional portion of the grid of the gauge consists of a multiple elongated S pattern, typically with several dozen repetitions transversely. As the gauge is stretched longitudinally (x direction in Fig. 12-1) by substrate deformation, each of the strands becomes slightly longer and thinner, thereby very slightly increasing the total electrical resistance.

When connected to a simple resistance imbalance detection (Wheatstone bridge) circuit, gauge strain can be converted to an analog voltage, and it can be subsequently amplified for recording or display. Gauges as manufactured are in effect precalibrated, in that their ratio of relative resistance change to relative length change (known as the gauge factor) is supplied by the vendor on a batch-specific basis (42). Given known settings of the Wheatstone bridge electrical parameters, knowledge of the gauge factor allows the user to read absolute strain values of the substrate surface without the need for in situ calibration. Of course, since single-element strain gauges are intended to measure strain in the direction of their S legs (x direction in Fig. 12-1), the user must take considerable care in appropriately aligning the gauge if absolute

strain levels are to be read without additional physical calibration. Situations requiring multidirectional strain measurement are addressed using "rosette" gauges, which consist of multiple individual gauge elements oriented in specific directions (usually either 120° increments or a 0°–45°–90° arrangement).

Strain measurement accuracy depends on factors such as the meticulousness of the gauge mounting on the substrate, appropriate compensation for thermal sensitivity artifact, the quality of the bridge and amplifier electronics, and the adequacy of connector cable noise shielding. In routine biomechanics laboratory usage, absolute errors in strain readings from metal-film gauges are typically of the order of 1 to 10 μm (i.e., 1 to 10 parts in 1,000,000). When used as the sensing element in high-quality instruments such as extensometers or pressure transducers, even more precise strain measurements are the norm. In applications requiring especially high sensitivity, semiconductor films are substituted for metal films.

Besides direct strain measurements by the end user, bonded resistance strain gauges are the basic sensing element in most commercial load cells and extensometers and in many fluid pressure transducers (23). The functional elements within the load cells used in familiar laboratory devices such as materials testing systems (MTS) or Instron machines are precision-machined metal members (e.g., beams), on whose surfaces strain gauges are bonded. By making appropriate internal electrical connections between individual gauges, it is possible to isolate axial versus flexural versus torsional strains in these precision internal members. And, knowing the size and elastic modulus of these mounting substrates, strains can be converted to point forces on the internal members. By this means, the load cell can transduce one or more specific force or moment components, with very little cross talk from extraneous load or moment components. Depending on design, load cells can be configured to sense anywhere from a single channel (i.e., one force or one moment component) up to a full six channels (three force components and three moment components). Accuracy of 0.1% of the full scale force or moment reading is typical.

Most extensometers are based on a related concept, in that they monitor flexural strains of a springlike, internally housed precision substrate. Normally, extensometers measure point-to-point displacements by means of two external arms that are connected to the strain-gauged substrate in an outrigger-like arrangement. Usually, the extensometer arms are lightly attached (commonly by rubber band clamp-on) to the member whose pointwise displacements are being monitored. In the case of fluid pressure transducers, strain gauges are bonded to one side of a thin diaphragm that undergoes drum-like flexural deformation as a result of a transwall pressure differential.

Another frequently encountered mechanical sensor is the linear variable differential transformer (LVDT). These devices take advantage of inductance effects of a metal core sliding inside a transformer coil, which in turn is electrically excited by alternating current. LVDTs can be extremely precise, with measurement error on the order of tenths of a micrometer (22). They can transduce motions over a wide range of frequencies, from static up into the tens of kHz. However, LVDTs require specialized excitation/conditioning circuitry, and they are more expensive than strain-gauge-based extensometers. LVDTs and their rotary cousins, RVDTs, are usually the built-in sensing elements that report displacements (linear and rotational) in materials testing machines.

Electromagnetic field effects are also used to measure displacements in various noncontact devices. One type frequently encountered in biomechanical applications is the eddy current transducer (also sometimes known as a proximeter). Here, the operational principle is that radiofrequency excitation of a source coil induces eddy currents at the surface of a nearby conductive target, typically a piece of thin metal foil. These passive target eddy currents, in turn, feed back to slightly change the impedance of the source coil, an effect that can be calibrated against coil-to-target distance by means of appropriate demodulation circuitry. Depending on their design parameters, eddy current transducers can sense uniaxial motions at typical accuracy ratings in the range of a few micrometers, over sensing lengths of a few millimeters up to approximately 1 to 2 cm (31).

Conceptually related electromagnetic tracking systems are widely used to monitor displacements and rotations occurring on a larger motion scale, such as in locomotion or in gross motions of joints or limb segments (4). In these systems, small orthogonally oriented excitation coils mounted within a movable module cause perturbations in the electromagnetic behavior of a fixed coil in a base module. These instruments can transduce multiaxial motions (three components of displacement and three of rotation) of multiple moving modules. Disadvantages are that their accuracy (typically rated in the tenths of millimeters) is far less than that of eddy current transducers, that the size (several cubic centimeters) and weight (several grams) of the movable coil modules may be significant in some applications, and that the movable coil modules must receive electrical excitation by means of direct wire connection to the instrument's circuitry. Also, the accuracy of noncontact sensors that use electromagnetic field effects may be influenced by nearby metallic objects and by ambient electrical or magnetic fields.

Other physical modalities are also applied to specialty displacement measurements. Various ultrasound devices correlate displacement with change of the time of flight between an emitted and back-reflected impulse. Ultrasound sensors are especially useful for detecting motions where the point or interface of interest does not lie on an externally accessible surface. However, their precision is somewhat limited by the fact that the back-reflected signals cannot usually be localized to a single site. Also, in some designs, the available frequency range is limited by the time necessary for the impulse to propagate and reflect back. Laser displacement sensors employing triangulation require an externally accessible target surface, and they operate on the principle that the beam reflected from a target will fall at a different position on an eccentric sensor surface, depending on the distance from the target to the sensor. Provided that the orientation of the target surface relative to the sensor does not change, extremely high spatial and temporal resolution can be obtained (2). Optical marker triangulation is widely employed for segmental motion tracking in gait analyses, using either passively reflective or actively energized (e.g., light-emitting or infrared-emitting diode) arrays mounted externally on limb or torso segments.

Unlike displacement measurements, the measurement of interfacial contact stress (e.g., the pressure across an interface such as an articular surface or a press-fit junction) poses special difficulties for which no precision instrumentation is as yet commercially available. Any physical sensor inserted between the contacting surfaces necessarily disturbs the local contact configuration (56), often to the point of involving largely artifactual recordings. Special purpose techniques have been devised to circumvent this difficulty in select circumstances, such as retrorecessed transducers machined in the inner wall of a hollowed head of a femoral hemiprosthesis (29), or cartilage-isocompliant miniature load cells recessed in the articular surface of natural cadaver femoral heads (13). Most frequently, however, investigators have used thin pressure-sensitive sheets that span the entire contact surface. This approach, although in principle still disturbing the pre-existing contact pattern, at least avoids the major local stress redistributions occurring around discrete indwelling sensors.

The two primary sheet-measurement approaches currently in use are pressure-sensitive film and multiplexed conductor arrays. Of the various pressure-sensitive films, the acetate product marketed by Fuji (under the trade name PresSensor) has become virtually synonymous with contact stress measurements in orthopedics. When subjected to pressure, the initially white acetate substrate stains red, the staining intensity correlating (nonlinearly) with pressure magnitude. Pressure transduction is achieved mechanochemically via rupture of reactant-containing microcapsules deposited on the film surface (Fig. 12-2). Quantitation is typically performed by means of digital image analysis (50). The film is limited to making static measurements, of modest accuracy (15% errors are typical), and it is subject to crinkling artifact over bicurvilinear surfaces (15). Nevertheless, the film is widely employed because it is inexpensive, easy to use, relatively thin (~0.2 mm), and provides whole-surface mappings at a spatial resolution that is adequate for most purposes (25). Mutliplexed conductor arrays (Fig. 12-3) function by sampling either the electrical resistance or the electrical capacitance between alternative combinations of parallel conductor arrays situated in a row/column arrangement on opposite sides of a filler sheet (45). By means of electronic switching, the local pressure at individual conductor row/column intersections can be sampled rapidly enough (many thousands of times per second) to allow computational display of full-field transient pressure distributions in near real time (12). Although initially introduced for low-resolution applications such as foot–floor pressure, miniaturization of the conductor arrays has recently achieved sampling pixel sizes on the order of 0.7 mm^2, thus inviting application to more demanding measurements such as contact stresses in articular joints. The principal disadvantages are that the technology is moderately expensive, that the conductor arrays are vulnerable to damage under harsh loading conditions, and that difficulties can arise in calibration because of nonlinearity and time dependency of the mechanoelectrical behavior of the filler sheets.

MATERIALS TESTING MACHINES

Materials testing machines, sometimes known as load frames, lie at the heart of most biomechanical setups used to make mechanical measurements on total hip arthroplasty (THA) constructs or materials. Two basic classes of machines are in common use: screw-driven and servohydraulic. Screw-driven

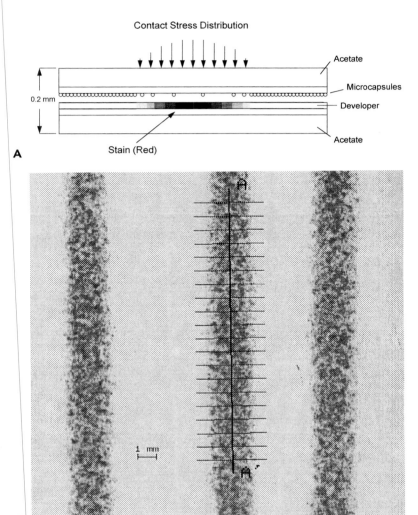

Figure 12-2 **A:** Functional schematic of PresSensor contact film, consisting of paired acetate layers, each approximately 0.1 mm thick. One layer is coated with reactant-filled microcapsules, and the other is coated with developer. When subjected to contact stress, some of the microcapsules rupture, liberating liquid reactant that turns red when it contacts the developer. The greater the contact stress, the greater the fraction of the microcapsules that rupture, and hence the denser the stain. **B:** Typical PresSensor patterns, magnified to show the discrete nature of the microstains resulting from individual microcapsule ruptures. Quantitation is usually by means of densitometry, and it is facilitated by digital image analysis. Here, an overlain coordinate axis *(line A–A8)* is used to define a series of sampling profiles *(transverse parallel lines)*. The three stains are from three repetitions of edge contact of a cylinder against a flat surface. Note that the staining pattern is reproducible on the global level, even though the distribution of microstains differs stochastically within each of the global stains.

machines use a precision gear drive to control rotational motions of two large and very stiff power screws, which in turn drive unidirectional motions of a massive transverse crosshead with which they mesh. Control circuitry allows the machine operator to program from a menu of input waveform choices (e.g., ramps, square waves), usually with the input being the imposed motion of the crosshead. Load developed in the specimen in response to the imposed displacement input is sensed by a load cell, normally user-mountable either on the traveling crosshead or on the fixed machine base. Advantages of screw-driven machines are their (relative) inexpense, and the fact that very large crosshead displacements are feasible, in principle spanning the full length of the power screws. Disadvantages are that maximum crosshead displacement speeds tend to be slow (on the order of a few centimeters per second), that it is difficult to precisely maintain/input specific load histories, and that torsional loading is feasible only with specialized additional fixturing.

Servohydraulic machines are far more elaborate in terms of internal complexity and testing capability. These devices involve one or more hydraulically powered actuators, whose pistoning motions are modulated by electronically controlled servovalves (Fig. 12-4). In most currently manufactured

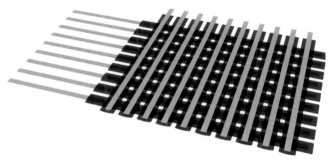

Figure 12-3 Schematic diagram of multiplexed conductor arrays used to measure transient contact stress. Piezoresistive filler material separates two orthogonal arrays of parallel conductors. To measure pressure at a specific junction, termed a "sensel," the measurement circuitry samples the electrical resistance between the corresponding row and column of the respective conductor arrays. Because electronic switching permits very rapid scanning over many hundreds of such individual row–column combinations, two-dimensional contact stress distributions can be assembled computationally and displayed transiently.

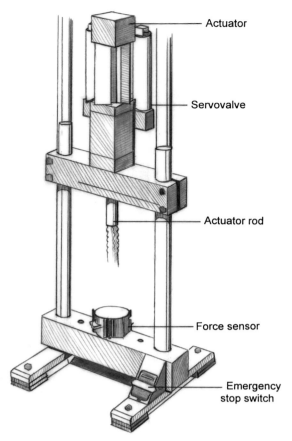

Figure 12-4 Schematic diagram of the load frame of a typical materials testing system. The actuator rod of this particular instrument is capable of applying both a vertical force and a torque about the vertical axis. The impetus for these inputs is high-pressure hydraulic fluid, controlled by means of a servovalve, which in turn is under computer control, programmed by the machine user. The specimen of interest is inserted between the actuator rod and the force sensor. (Diagram from handout notes of the TestStar II Operations Course given by MTS, 14000 Technology Drive, Eden Prairie, MN 55344-2290.)

machines, the servovalves are controlled by digital signals, although older instruments used analog control circuitry. Operators can program inputs either under stroke (i.e., displacement) or under load control, for which closed-loop feedback control circuitry ensures that the stroke or load developed by the actuator stays close to the programmed command signal. These instruments are capable of high displacement speeds, and they are especially advantageous for fatigue studies requiring many rapid load reversals. Both linear and rotational actuators can be employed, so as to give biaxial testing capability. Additional (non-built-in) hydraulic actuators can usually also be accommodated for specialty applications, using the same control circuitry. Modern servohydraulic systems typically operate under computer control in multiwindow graphic user interface environments, and they offer great flexibility for input control. Turnkey collection and recording of load and stroke data are the norm, and many instruments offer a user-friendly computer interface for multichannel signal acquisition from ancillary sensors such as strain gauges,

extensometers, or LVDTs. One major disadvantage is cost (often in excess of $100,000), although these instruments are regarded as a necessary capital expense in most contemporary orthopedic biomechanics laboratories. Smaller capacity loading frames, actuated either pneumatically or electromagnetically, have recently emerged to provide an intermediate cost/performance compromise.

Testing of THA implants or constructs typically involves mounting a specimen within fixtures that interface with a test frame, and then applying an appropriate loading while transducing mechanical signals of interest (e.g., surface strains, interfacial motions) at one or more sites on the specimen (Fig. 12-5). Many hundreds of such experiments have been reported in the biomechanics literature, and a detailed review is beyond the scope of this chapter. When interpreting the data from such experiments, the reader should consider the degree of simplification of the loading protocol adopted, the geometric and material realism of the test specimen, and the adequacy of the mechanical sensors employed. Parameters of importance in loading protocols include the magnitude, direction, waveform and rate of application, use of single versus cyclic loading events, and use of pointwise versus distributed surface loadings. Also, because the fixturing for specimen attachment to the load frame disturbs stress/strain distributions in adjacent regions of the specimen (St. Venant's principle), local signals acquired in the near vicinity of grips may not be meaningful.

As regards material realism, the choice of bone model is the primary concern. Human cadaver bone has been the material of choice in most laboratory studies. The literature is equivocal as to whether or not embalming appreciably alters

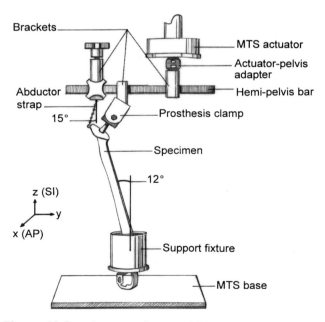

Figure 12-5 Schematic of a typical laboratory biomechanical specimen test. In this particular instance, a THA femoral component is mounted in a cadaver femur; it is loaded through a surrogate hemipelvis that permits application of both articular contact force and abductor tension. The surrogate hemipelvis is connected to the MTS actuator, and the distal femur is potted in PMMA within a support fixture that is in turn attached to a base plate situated atop a force sensor. (Courtesy of Frank Barich, Ph.D.)

the strength and stiffness of cortical bone (35), although most investigators agree that embalmed material is undesirable in applications where trabecular bone load carriage is important. Fresh or fresh-frozen cadaver bones are subject to degradation under room conditions in lengthy experiments. Also, many of the cadaver specimens available for laboratory testing purposes tend to be from individuals who were very aged, and/or whose underlying systemic diseases, medical regimens, or inactivity patterns involved appreciable osteopenia. Artificial bone surrogates of many types have been employed, frequently involving simplified shapes (e.g., circular tubes) for ease of fabrication and data analysis. Anatomically realistic fiberglass bone replicas are in increasing use, having been demonstrated to reasonably mimic the mechanical behavior of cadaver material while minimizing interspecimen variability (28). Certain dense polymeric foams have been shown to approximate the mechanical properties of trabecular bone (53), and formal testing standards employing such materials have been introduced.

A number of special-purpose testing systems have been developed to study processes of polyethylene wear in acetabular liners. These systems supplement simplified tribologic material screening protocols such as pin-on-disk wear testing (10), and they offer varying degrees of realism with regard to hip joint motion and force application histories. Motion inputs have included reciprocal uniaxial rotations (mimicking pure flexion–extension) (48), biaxial rocking (41) (Fig. 12-6), and most recently, programmable multiaxial rotations (44). The input force histories used typically mimic human level walking, as estimated from gait analyses (46). Hip simulator testing is very demanding technically, and there exist several areas of controversy (e.g., appropriate fluid lubrication) as to how best to mimic the in vivo situation. Large interspecimen variability is the norm, even under seemingly identical testing conditions. Measured wear rates in most hip simulator series tend to underestimate those occurring clinically, most likely because of the absence of third-body particles (40).

COMPUTER MODELING

Most phenomena in the field of mechanics involve physical principles that are well understood on a formal quantitative basis. For that reason, mathematical analysis has long been an important part of the practice of mechanical engineering. In the area of biomechanics, however, usefully accurate mathematical analyses have historically been hindered by factors such as the complex material behavior of musculoskeletal tissues, the highly irregular geometries involved, and uncertainties regarding loadings. For most biomechanical problems, obtaining realistic solutions of the governing equations of Newtonian mechanics is tractable only by using approximation techniques that rely on high speed digital computers. Foremost among these is finite element analysis (FEA), an approach originally introduced in the structural mechanics community in the 1950s and first applied to musculoskeletal mechanics in 1972 (30).

Rigorous description of the mathematical basis of FEA is typically the subject of semester-long courses at the advanced engineering undergraduate level and therefore lies beyond the scope of the present discussion. A brief summary of the major

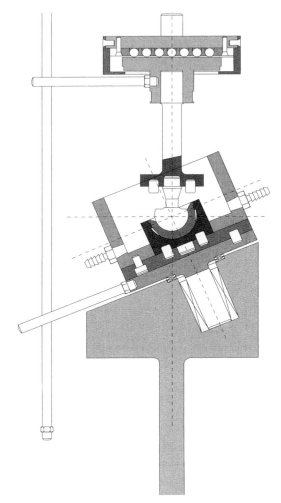

Figure 12-6 Schematic diagram of physical test configuration used for laboratory wear simulation of an acetabular component. The cup is mounted on bearings that are recessed perpendicular to the surface of a (23°) beveled platform. A gearing system induces this beveled platform to rotate about a vertical axis at approximately 1 revolution per second. An outrigger arm affixed to the cup housing partially constrains cup rotation, leading to a bobblinglike motion frequently described as biaxial rocking. Simultaneously, a time-variant vertical load is applied, simulating the force pattern of level walking (maximum = 2 kN). (Diagram from an in-house technical report from MTS, 14000 Technology Drive, Eden Prairie, MN 55344-2290: Mejia LC, Brierly TJ. A hip wear simulator for the evaluation of biomaterials in hip arthroplasty components. Presented at: ISABE 93 International Symposium on Advanced Bio-Materials and Engineering; September 1–4, 1993; Utsunomiya, Japan.)

aspects, as pertinent to clinical biomechanical applications, is available elsewhere (11). The basic idea behind FEA is that over small discretized domains (elements) of a continuous region, the actual distribution of physical variables such as displacement, strain, stress, and temperature can be approximated by simplified mathematical expressions, usually taking the form of polynomials (6). Provided that appropriate continuity of these approximation expressions is enforced between adjacent elements, the overall system's behavior can be modeled accurately, especially if the overall system is discretized into a very large number of very small domains. Obtaining stress distributions

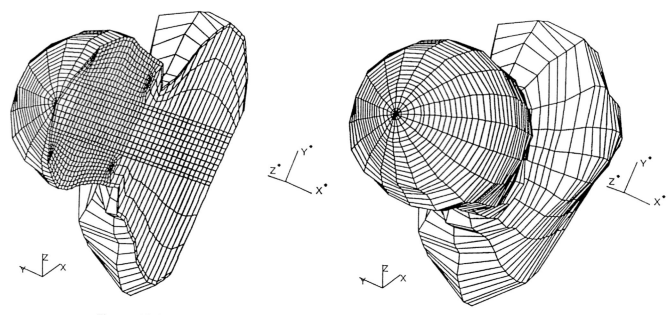

Figure 12-7 Finite element mesh of the natural proximal femur. This particular mesh is used to study stress redistributions in femoral head osteonecrosis, caused by insertion of a fibular strut graft. A coronal midsection of the mesh is shown at left to illustrate internal detail; the exterior surface is shown at right. (Courtesy of Jim Rudert, Ph.D.)

involves the solution of large numbers of simultaneous algebraic equations, typically one equation per direction of possible motion (degree of freedom) for each nodal point in the discretized mesh. In the early days of digital computation, finite element models were necessarily crude and therefore not very realistic, because computer processor speeds and memory limits restricted tractable problem sizes to a few hundred degrees of freedom. Usually, these problem sizes were small enough that they lent themselves to manual zoning of the discretization mesh, which of course almost always was two dimensional. Over the years, steady improvements in computation speed and storage have led to a steady increase in the number of elements that can be considered. Easy-to-use analysis programs are now widely available commercially, mesh generation is highly automated, and fully three-dimensional stress analysis problems involving tens or hundreds of thousands of elements are commonplace (Figs. 12-7 and 12-8). In a few specialized research problems involving custom-written computer programs, orthopedic problem sizes in the million-degrees-of-freedom range have recently been successfully solved (55). As with physical testing, finite element studies in the orthopedic literature now number well in the hundreds, and a thorough review is beyond the scope of this chapter.

When interpreting the results of a finite element analysis in THA, several factors merit attention. First, is the geometry realistic? Typical source data for modern three-dimensional models are CT scans and physical sections, with other imaging modalities—especially magnetic resonance imaging (MRI)—being increasingly used in specialized applications (5). In the past, two-dimensional meshes were often zoned from plane film radiographs. However, the utility of simple planar models has progressively diminished to the point where they now appear only infrequently in major peer-reviewed journals. If specific THA hardware is being modeled, it is desirable that its geometry be directly grounded in manufacturer data. If, instead, generic hardware is being modeled, the rationale for the geometry employed should be evident. Increasingly commonly, voxel image sources are directly converted to finite element meshes [i.e., 1:1 correspondence between image voxels and hexahedral

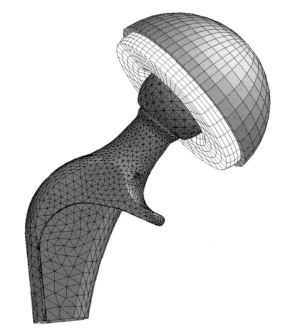

Figure 12-8 Finite element mesh of THA femoral and acetabular components. This model was used to study acetabular polyethylene stresses accompanying subluxation and dislocation of the femoral component. Elements encompassing the metal backing shell of the acetabular component are shaded light gray.

finite elements (34)], sometimes with supplemental surface smoothing operations to reduce local stress computation artifacts arising from "stair-step" image edges (24).

Second, are the material properties realistic? This is seldom a problem with metal implants: their behavior for most purposes is linearly elastic, and the pertinent coefficients (Young's modulus and the Poisson ratio) are well documented. Material treatment is less straightforward for other orthopedic biomaterials, especially soft polymers—ultrahigh molecular weight polyethylene (UHMWPE) being an important case in point)—because some applications involve stress levels that exceed the linearly elastic range (37). Commercial FEA algorithms typically include elements that are mathematically capable of addressing complexities such as large deformations, strain-dependent elastic material behavior, plastic flow, poroelastic behavior, and creep and stress relaxation. However, appropriate input coefficients for many orthopedic biomaterials are lacking and require state-of-the-art research.

For biologic tissues, there is a wide range of treatment sophistication. Bone is usually represented as being linearly elastic, sometimes with homogeneous material coefficients and sometimes with material coefficients linked to the anatomic density distribution [e.g., with modulus regressed upon CT Hounsfield number (51)]. Direction-dependence of elastic modulus is nowadays often included, especially for diaphyseal cortical bone (1) and for highly oriented trabecular regions (14). Studies in which articular cartilage must be represented are more problematic, because the material behavior has a strong time dependence resulting from fluid–solid interplay at the intrinsic tissue level (43). Linear elastic treatment of cartilage nevertheless is widely encountered, it often being argued that rate dependence is inappreciable under very slow (i.e., all fluid flow has ceased) and very fast (i.e., no flow has begun) loading regimes. More complex finite element treatments have recently been introduced, with fluid–solid interactions being addressed either by customized finite element formulations implementing specialized mixture theory models (52), or alternatively, by assuming that cartilage behavior is well approximated by conventional poroelastic theory (54).

Third, are the loading conditions realistic? There is a fair degree of consensus on hip joint contact forces during level walking gait, based on data from instrumented prostheses (7,19) and from multisegmental Newtonian gait analyses (9). Rather less information is available for other activities of daily living, although recent awareness of torsion as a failure mode in THA has sparked interest in hip loadings from stair-climbing and chair-rise activities (36). In laboratory models specifically involving muscle loadings, there remains little alternative to relying on indirect estimates (18), because direct recordings from humans have been blocked by technical and ethical hurdles. Usually, the complex muscle and joint loading patterns occurring during the duty cycle are neglected in favor of simply addressing the worst-case instant of peak joint loading magnitude. The realism of a worst-case loading approach obviously depends on context: it may be very reasonable if one is studying frank failure processes such as polymethyl methacrylate (PMMA) fracture, whereas a more complex set of inputs is appropriate if one is studying history-dependent processes such as adaptive bony remodeling (57).

Fourth, are material interface conditions treated realistically? The simplest class of finite element problems is that in which all interfaces remain fully and rigidly bonded, regardless of construct load distribution. Such interfaces can freely transmit all components of stress (compression, tension, and shear) regardless of the stress magnitudes involved. This is a very reasonable approximation in many circumstances, such as for well-fixed cemented THA. In constructs involving biologic ingrowth fixation, however, more sophisticated interface treatment can be a matter of considerable importance (33), because ingrowth tends to occur on only a small fraction of the available surface area (17). Areas of the interface that are not ingrown can transmit compression but not tension, and they have only limited ability to transmit shear.

Computationally, the simplest treatment for such interfaces involves so-called gap elements (available in most commercial FEA packages), which assume that the local gap between sets of specific nodal point pairs on opposite sides of an interface is either closed or open. If the gap is closed, compression and (limited) shear stress can be transmitted, whereas tension cannot; if the gap is open, then no stress components whatsoever can be transmitted. The mathematical solution process in gap element models is computationally more burdensome than in bonded-interface problems, because the simultaneous equation system must be iteratively re-solved many times, until a stress distribution is arrived at that identifies the particular combination of gap element openings and closures that sustains the externally applied load with minimum overall energy storage. Yet further complexity exists across interfaces that can locally slide (e.g., articular surfaces, press-fit interfaces). In such instances, the node-to-node "sticky" behavior implicitly assumed for gap elements is inapplicable. The treatment instead requires use of yet-more-complex elements known as contact elements (21). These again are available in many commercial finite element programs, although the degree of rigor of the contact treatment varies substantially, depending on the mathematics involved. For example, some very robust contact elements allow several sets of nodes to slide past one another during load uptake, whereas other more simple versions require that a given node's contact remain within a small target area. As with gap elements, contact elements require computationally intensive iterative solutions. Also, finite element contact problems are notoriously ill behaved computationally and therefore place great demands on the technical skill of the analyst. Fully three-dimensional contact treatments are still a relative rarity (39), although they are now appearing with increasing frequency.

ANIMAL MODELING

In situations where active biologic response is an important factor, animal models play a pivotal role. Whereas background issues such as material biocompatibility have typically been addressed in rodent screening models, the use of larger animals—most frequently canine or sheep models—is usually necessary for hip implant studies on the whole-construct level. By far, the bulk of THA animal work has involved canine models, which hold considerable attraction in terms of availability, activity level, ease of training, longevity, reasonably large bone size, well-developed veterinary and maintenance infrastructure, and the large information base concerning, for example, functional anatomy and habitual loading (3). The anatomic size of sheep hips more closely approximates that of the human, but sheep are relatively difficult to work with experimentally, availability of animals and maintenance facilities are restricted in many research centers, and knowledge of habitual activity and joint loading patterns is fairly primitive (47). Besides their morphologic differences from the human, a major limitation of canine and sheep models—and quadruped models in general—is that a painful operated limb can be fully or partially spared from loading during ambulation. This makes it very difficult to ensure that quadruped hip reconstructions experience postoperative loading protocols that mimic clinical circumstances. Despite these limitations, however, bipedal (i.e., primate) models are almost never used to study hip reconstructions because the expense is prohibitive. Recently, emus have shown strong promise as a more economical bipedal alternative, in studies of femoral head necrosis (16).

CLINICALLY DERIVED MATERIALS

Conventional patient imaging studies, especially plain film radiographs, computed tomography (CT), and dual energy x-ray absorptiometry (DEXA), constitute a widely used information source for quantitative engineering analyses. Frequently, however, measurements of biomechanical interest require specialized techniques that go beyond the simple manual measures that usually suffice for routine clinical purposes. Many mechanical models involving patient radiographs require collecting precise coordinates of large numbers of points (typically dozens or even hundreds) to quantitate, for example, orientations, bony landmarks, and surface contours. This process is facilitated by digitizing equipment, of which two main classes are in widespread use. The first type is stylus digitizers, which require that an operator manually position a stylus, a hand-held cursor, or some other such instrument over the film point whose coordinates are to be encoded. The operator then provides an electronic cue to the instrument circuitry

or host computer, to record the location. Most frequently, the location is quantitated either by a conductive pad or by triangulating time-of-flight measurements of an acoustic or ultrasound impulse to multiple microphones. Intrinsic instrument accuracy ratings are in the tenths of millimeters, although as a practical matter the figure typically approaches a millimeter when one allows for operator-dependent matters such as positioning judgment and hand unsteadiness. The second approach to digitizing involves encoding the whole film in digital form, followed by image analysis. For plain radiographs or other hardcopy films, this requires an intermediate imaging step, using a flatbed scanner or similar device. Typical spatial resolutions obtained are in the tens of thousands of pixels per square centimeter, with each pixel being assigned an integer gray-scale value. Most commonly, gray-scale resolution is 8-bit (range from 0 to 255), but several high-end instruments now offer 12-bit (0 to 4095) resolution. Of course, if absolute density is of interest, graded calibration phantoms need be included in the view field, because digitized optical density is a strong function of many film exposure parameters. The intermediate scanning step is unnecessary if the image data are already available in digital format (e.g., CT, digital radiograph, or MRI), although spatial resolution is then inherently limited by the source image, typically only several hundred to a few thousand pixels per square centimeter. Once the image is formatted digitally, it can be rendered on a computer screen and the operator can make the measurements of interest. This can be done by manually positioning an electronic cursor, by invoking a computer program that automatically detects image features, or by some combination of the two (Fig. 12-9). Illustrative contemporary applications involve tracking component orientations and migrations (26,32), measuring polyethylene wear (20,38,49), detecting and quantitating radiolucencies (8), and measuring adaptive bony density changes (27).

Another important clinical information source is autopsy retrievals. Here the focus is usually on the fate of implant

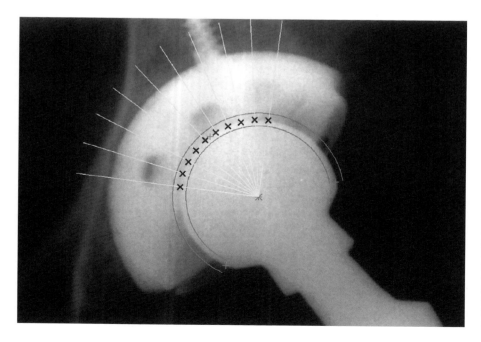

Figure 12-9 Illustration of digital imaging analysis of a clinical radiograph. Here, a conventional AP radiograph of the hip has been encoded in digital form and is displayed as background against which computer-constructed measurement lines are drawn. This particular application involves an acetabular wear measurement, based on automated gray-scale detection of the head and cup backing margins.

components, although tissue characteristics are often also of interest. Typical follow-up laboratory measurements include metrology (e.g., surface contours in acetabular liners, indicative of wear patterns), interface characteristics (e.g., ingrowth patterns in porous-anchorage implants), identification of failure processes (e.g., PMMA fracture surfaces) or adverse tissue response (e.g., granuloma, osteolysis), detection of degradation products (corrosion, wear debris), and quantitation of adaptive bony changes. Because there are two very distinct sources of retrieval materials (failed implants versus successfully functional postmortem specimens), one must always bear in mind the final clinical status of the reconstruction when interpreting the severity of the measured parameter changes.

ACKNOWLEDGMENTS

Financial assistance was provided by NIH grants AR46601, AR47653, and AR49919, and by a grant from DePuy, Incorporated.

REFERENCES

1. Adams DJ, Pedersen DR, Brand RA, et al. Three-dimensional geometric and structural symmetry of the turkey ulna. *J Orthop Res.* 1995;13:690–699.
2. Adsens Technology Inc. *Laser Analog Displacement Sensors.* Technical publication 93/7/30000. La Puente, CA: Adsens Technology; 1993.
3. Alexander RM. The mechanics of jumping by a dog *(Canis familiaris)*. *J Zool.* 1974;173:549–573.
4. An K-N, Jacobsen MC, Berglund LJ, et al. Application of a magnetic tracking device to kinesiologic studies. *J Biomech.* 1988;21: 613–620.
5. Baker KJ, Brown TD, Brand RA. MRI-based finite element stress distributions in femoral head osteonecrosis: a parametric study of factors influencing reproducibility. *Pittsburgh Orthop J.* 1991;2: 101–106.
6. Bathe K-J. *Finite Element Procedures.* Englewood Cliffs, NJ: Prentice Hall; 1996.
7. Bergmann G, Graichen F, Rolhmann A. Hip joint loading during walking and running, measured in two patients. *J Biomech.* 1993;26:969–990.
8. Boys GB, Callaghan JJ, Park JB, et al. Use of edge detection to characterize femoral loosening in cemented total hip replacement. In: *Transactions of the 42nd Annual Meeting of the Orthopaedic Research Society.* Rosemont, IL: Orthopaedic Research Society; 1996:240.
9. Brand RA, Pedersen DR, Davy DT, et al. Comparison of hip force calculations and measurements in the same patient. *J Arthroplasty.* 1994;9:45–51.
10. Briscoe BJ, Stolarski TA. The influence of contact zone kinematics on wear processes of polymers. In: *Wear of Materials.* Fairfield, NJ: ASME Press; 1991:187–192.
11. Brown TD. Finite lement modeling in musculoskeletal biomechanics. *J Appl Biomech.* 2004;20:336–366.
12. Brown TD, Rudert MJ, Grosland NM. New methods for assessing cartilage contact stress after articular fracture. *Clin Orthop.* 2004;423:59–63.
13. Brown TD, Shaw DT. A Technique for measuring instantaneous in vitro contact stress distributions in articular joints. *J Biomech.* 1982;15:329–333.
14. Brown TD, Way ME, Ferguson AB. Stress transmission anomalies in femoral heads altered by aseptic necrosis. *J Biomech.* 1980;13: 687–699.
15. Caldwell NJ, Hale JE, Rudert MJ, et al. An algorithm for approximate crinkle artifact compensation in pressure-sensitive film recordings. *J Biomech.* 1993;26:1001–1010.
16. Conzemius MG, Brown TD, Zhang Y, et al. A new animal model of femoral head osteonecrosis: one that progresses to human-like mechanical failure. *J Orthop Res.* 2002;20:303–309.
17. Cook SD, Thomas KA, Haddad RJ. Histologic analysis of retrieved human porous-coated total joint components. *Clin Orthop.* 1988;234:90–101.
18. Crowninshield RD, Johnston RC, Andrews JG, et al. A biomechanical investigation of the human hip. *J Biomech.* 1978;11: 75–85.
19. Davy DT, Kotzar GM, Brown RH, et al. Telemetric force measurements across the hip after total arthroplasty. *J Bone Joint Surg.* 1988;70A:45–50.
20. Devane PA, Bourne RB, Rorabeck CH, et al. Measurement of polyethylene wear in metal-backed acetabular cups. II: Clinical application. *Clin Orthop.* 1995;319:317–326.
21. Eterovic AL, Bathe KJ. On the treatment of inequality constraints arising from contact conditions in finite element analysis. *Comput Struct.* 1991;40:203–209.
22. Figliola RS, Beasley DE. *Theory and design for mechanical measurements.* New York: John Wiley & Sons; 1995.
23. Grindy SS. Force and torque measurement: a technology overview. *Exp Tech.* 1985;9:28.
24. Grosland NM, Brown TD. A voxel-based formulation for contact finite element analysis. *Comput Methods Biomech Biomed Eng.* 2002;5:21–32.
25. Hale JE, Brown TD. Contact stress gradient detection limits of PresSensor Film. *ASME J Biomech Eng.* 1992;114:352–357.
26. Hardinge K, Swanson SAV, Joines PR, et al. Measurement of hip prostheses using image analysis. The maxima hip technique. *J Bone Joint Surg.* 1991;73B:724–728.
27. Harrigan TP, Biegler FB, Reuben JD. Bone adaptation to total hip femoral components: effects of multiple loads and comparison to clinical follow-Up. In: *Transactions of the 42nd Annual Meeting of the Orthopaedic Research Society.* Rosemont, IL: Orthopaedic Research Society; 1996:261.
28. Heiner AD, Brown TD. Structural properties of a new design of composite replicate femurs and tibias. *J Biomech.* 2001;34: 773–783.
29. Hodge WA, Carlson KL, Fijan RS, et al. Contact pressures from an instrumented hip endoprosthesis. *J Bone Joint Surg.* 1989;71A: 1378–1386.
30. Huiskes R, Chao EYS. A survey of finite element analysis in orthopaedic biomechanics: the first decade. *J Biomech.* 1983;16: 385–409.
31. Kaman Instruments Corporation. *Multi-VIT Multi-purpose Position Sensing.* Tech publ 860103-000, Rev. A. Colorado Springs, CO: Kaman Instruments Corporation; 1994.
32. Karrholm J, Thanner J, Malchau H, et al. Migration of porous acetabular cups with hydroxyapatite and tricalcium-phosphate coating. In: *Transactions of the 42nd annual meeting of the Orthopaedic Research Society.* Rosemont, IL: Orthopaedic Research Society; 1996:239.
33. Keaveny TM, Bartel DL. Mechanical consequences of bone ingrowth in a hip prosthesis inserted without cement. *J Bone Joint Surg.* 1995;77A:911–923.
34. Keyak JH, Skinner HB. Three-dimensional finite element modeling of bone: effects of element size. *J Biomed Eng.* 1992;14:483–489.
35. Kim YS, Callaghan JJ, Ahn PB, et al. Fracture of the acetabulum during insertion of an oversized hemispherical component. *J Bone Joint Surg.* 1995;77A:111–117.
36. Kotzar GM, Davy DT, Berilla J, et al. Torsional loads in the early postoperative period following total hip replacement. *J Orthop Res.* 1995;13:945–955.
37. Kurtz SM, Bartel DL, Rimnac CM. The effects of post-irradiation aging on the stresses and strains in UHMWPE tibial components for TKR. In: *Transactions of the 2nd Combined Meeting of the Orthopaedic Research Societies of USA, Japan, Canada and Europe.* Rosemont, IL: Orthopaedic Research Society; 1995:70.
38. Livermore J, Ilstrup D, Morrey BF. Effect of femoral head size on wear of the polyethylene acetabular component. *J Bone Joint Surg.* 1990;72A:518–528.
39. Maxian TA, Brown TD, Pedersen DR, et al. A sliding-distance-coupled finite element formulation for wear in total hip arthroplasty. *J Biomech.* 1996;29:687–692.

40. McKellop HA, Campbell P, Park S, et al. The origin of sub-micron polyethylene wear debris in total hip arthroplasty. *Clin Orthop.* 1995;311:3–20.
41. McKellop HA, Clarke IC. Evolution and evaluation of materials: screening machines and wear simulators in predicting in vivo wear phenomena. In: Ducheyne P, Hastings GW, eds. *Functional Behavior of Orthopaedic Biomaterials. Vol II: Applications.* Boca Raton, FL: CRC Press; 1984.
42. Micro-Measurements Division, Measurements Group Inc. *Strain Gage Selection: Criteria, Procedures, Recommendations.* Technical note 505-1. Raleigh, NC: Measurements Group Inc; 1989.
43. Mow VC, Holmes MH, Lai WM. Fluid transport and mechanical properties of articular cartilage: a review. *J Biomech.* 1984;17:377–394.
44. O'Connor DO, Bragdon CR, Burke DW, et al. *A 12-Station, Upright Hip Simulator Wear Machine Employing Oscillating Motion Replicating the Human Gait Cycle.* Unpublished technical report. Massachusetts General Hospital; 1995.
45. Otto JK, Brown TD, Callaghan JJ. Static and dynamic response of a multiplexed-array piezoresistive contact sensor. *Exp Mech.* 1999;39:317–323.
46. Paul J. Loading on normal hip and knee joints and on joint replacements. In: Schaldach M, Hohman D, eds. *Engineering in Medicine. Vol 2: Advances in artificial hip and knee joint technology.* New York: Springer-Verlag; 1976.
47. Radin EL, Orr RB, Kelman JL, et al. Effect of prolonged walking on concrete on the knees of sheep. *J Biomech.* 1982;15:487–492.
48. Saikko V, Paavolainen P, Kleimola M, et al. A five-station hip joint simulator for wear rate studies. *Proc Inst Mech Eng.* 1992;206:195–200.
49. Shaver SM, Brown TD, Hillis SL, et al. Digital edge detection measurement of polyethylene wear in total hip arthroplasty. *J Bone Joint Surg.* 1997;79A:690–700.
50. Singerman RJ, Pedersen DR, Brown TD. Quantitation of pressure-sensitive film using digital image scanning. *Exp Mech.* 1987;27:99–105.
51. Skinner HB, Kim AS, Keyak JH, et al. Femoral prosthesis implantation induces changes in bone stress that depend on the extent of porous coating. *J Orthop Res.* 1994;12:553–563.
52. Spilker RL, Almeida ES, Clutz CJ, et al. Three dimensional automated biphasic finite element analysis of soft tissues from stereophotogrammetric data. In: Tarbell JM, ed. *1993 Advances in Bioengineering (BED).* Vol. 26. New York: ASME Press; 1993:15–18.
53. Szivek JA, Thompson JD, Benjamin JB. Characterization of three formulations of a synthetic foam as models for a range of human cancellous bone types. *J Appl Biomater.* 1995;6:125–128.
54. Van Der Voet AF. *Finite Element Modelling of Load Transfer through Articular Cartilage* [Ph.D. thesis]. Alberta: Department of Civil Engineering, University of Calgary; 1992.
55. Van Rietbergen B, Weinens H, Huiskes R, et al. Determination of tissue loading in a trabecular bone specimen, using a full scale FE-model. In: *Transactions of the 40th Annual Meeting of the Orthopaedic Research Society.* Rosemont, IL: Orthopaedic Research Society; 1994:58.
56. Walker PS, Erkman M. The role of the menisci in force transmission across the knee. *Clin Orthop.* 1975;109:184–192.
57. Weinens H, Huiskes R, Grootenboer HJ. Effects of fit and bonding characteristics of femoral stems on adaptive bone remodelling. *ASME J Biomech Eng.* 1994;116:393–400.

Failure Scenarios and the Innovation Cycle

Rik Huiskes   Nico Verdonschot

Total hip prostheses were traditionally developed using trial-and-error processes. Ideas materialized and were tried in patients; if an innovation was not successful, the clinical results would tell, and the prosthesis would be adapted to avoid the problems met. This approach was necessary at a time when no satisfactory, reproducible cure for the conditions concerned was available. The degree of success was determined against the pain of the untreated patient. Presently, however, a reproducible cure is available, in the form of the cemented fixation of a metal femoral stem and a polyethylene cup. The results of innovative prosthetic designs can now be measured relative to those provided by this gold standard; exposing patients to a trial-and-error process is no longer necessary. Many failed innovations of the past have illustrated the validity of this thesis (1,13,18,29,57,82), as illustrated by the example of the Capital hip prosthesis.

We have studied aseptic loosening of the femoral component in 76 patients with primary total hip replacement using the Capital prosthesis. The mean follow-up was 26 months (10 to 37). Twelve femoral components (16%) were definitely and eight (10%) were possibly loose. They were characterized by a thin cement mantle ($p < 0.001$) and excessive residual cancellous bone in the proximo-medial region ($p < 0.01$). We recommend that the cement mantle around the prosthesis should be 2 to 3 mm and that further long-term studies are needed to evaluate the wear properties of titanium-nitride-coated titanium femoral heads (64).

In the United Kingdom this resulted in guidelines for hip implants, set by the National Institute for Clinical Excellence (NICE). This institute published guidance for the selection of prostheses for primary total hip arthroplasty (THA) in April 2000. This was followed in June 2002 by guidance on the use of metal-on-metal hip resurfacing arthroplasty. The NICE guidelines set an acceptable revision rate at 10% or less for a given prosthesis at 10 years, or performance compatible with that benchmark at 3 years. Prostheses unable to satisfy these requirements should be the subject of rigorous research or observational study if the implant is already clinically used.

However, further development of prostheses is still necessary. Both cement and polyethylene have problems, and the younger patients can still expect one or more revisions in their lifetimes. The challenge is to promote progress while limiting the exposure of patients to risks of failed innovations. Although orthopaedic innovators and industry are the principal participants in promoting this progress, and some form of government regulation is indispensable, it is the individual surgeon who is best positioned to protect the individual patient by the selection of implants and operational procedures. This chapter presents the pitfalls in prosthesis design innovation and the preclinical and clinical design evaluation methods presently available, and addresses what information the surgeon should use to select the appropriate device to ensure that the patient achieves optimal benefit from innovative efforts with the least risk of failure.

THE INNOVATION CYCLE AND QUALITY ASSURANCE

The prosthetic innovation cycle is described in Figure 13-1 (13). Ideas for new designs tend to be based on clinical research in which particular problems are identified, or on experimental research with new concepts or materials for total hip arthroplasty (THA). Before manufacturing begins on a

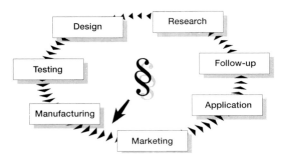

Figure 13-1 The prosthetic innovation "life cycle"; the *paragraph symbol* represents market introduction. (Adapted from Faro LM, Huiskes R. Quality assurance of joint replacement. Legal regulation and medical judgement. *Acta Orthop Scand Suppl.* 1992;250:1–33, with permission.)

large scale, tests are carried out to establish the safety and efficacy of the new design. These assessments may involve several kinds of experimental tests and clinical trials.

Tests and trials may be subject to government regulations concerning market approval. Regulatory systems in several countries were analyzed by Faro and Huiskes (13). Federal Food and Drug Administration (FDA) regulation in the United States depends on whether a new prosthesis is essentially equivalent to other devices currently available, or whether it has aspects that are new. In the first case, market approval may be given immediately, but in the latter, safety and efficacy must be established in documented trials with a follow-up of at least 2 years. The FDA may also require particular experimental design confirmation tests. Despite the time and money necessary to pass FDA inspection and to introduce a new device, there is no direct proof that quality assurance regulation is better in the United States than in other countries with seemingly less strict rules. The approval of the Mittelmeier prosthesis by the FDA just prior to the appearance of reports from Europe about excessive failures suggests that 2 years of clinical trials cannot guarantee endurance in the longer term. Conversely, acrylic cement, which triggered the success of THA at large, did not enter the U.S. market until long after being introduced in Europe (13).

Several different kinds of regulatory systems for orthopedic implants were used in European countries, including some of total freedom (13). As a result of the Directive on Medical Devices of the European Union in 1995, however, since June 1998, prostheses were allowed on the EU market if they obtained a CE mark. A CE mark means that the implants meet the EU requirements for safety, efficacy, toxicity, biocompatibility, chemical and physical stability, sterility, and product information. European (CEN) standards were developed to specify these requirements for particular products. A manufacturer can either test its products according to these standards or use alternative methods. In any case, the appropriateness of the CE mark is inspected by Notified Bodies, testing institutes certified by the European Union, of which there are a number in each member country. Once the CE mark is obtained in one country, the product can be freely marketed in all member states. The EU regulatory system is different from the American FDA-controlled one in that it leaves initiatives, responsibilities, and the associated costs to the private sector. The only government involvement is in the approval of the CEN standards and the certification of the Notified Bodies.

Whatever the regulatory situation, it does not discharge the orthopaedic community—or the individual surgeon—from responsibility for the selection of sensible prostheses. The importance of this responsibility was emphasized in an article by Murray et al. (70), who analyzed the THA market in the United Kingdom and found that of the 24 brands of noncemented hip prostheses available, only three had been subject to survival analysis in peer-reviewed journals, and of those only one for longer than 5 years. Typical also for the optimism that tends to motivate surgeon-innovators is the frequency of recurring ideas for prosthetic-design concepts that failed earlier, but resurrected with design adaptations and marketed widely after limited clinical trials. The example below concerns hip surface replacement, which results in the 1980s were disastrous, but not just due to wear debris, as the authors suggest.

> The historical failure of surface replacement has been due to the production of wear debris with subsequent bone resorption, loosening, and failure. To avoid these problems, a surface replacement using a metal on metal bearing allowing thin components and femoral design and instrumentation to avoid varus alignment has been designed. Two hundred thirty-five joints have been resurfaced with this prosthesis in almost 5 years. There have been no femoral neck fractures and no dislocations. There have been 4 designs differing in the method of fixation. In the press fit group, 6 of 70 hips had to be revised for aseptic loosening. In the cemented group, debonding of the cup occurred in 3 of 43 cases. Six patients had hydroxyapatite coated components and have had excellent clinical outcomes. The current design uses a peripherally expanded hydroxyapatite coated cup and a cemented metal head; 116 of this design have been implanted during a 19-month period with excellent outcome. Despite short follow-up the authors are hopeful that the combination of a polar metal on metal bearing with appropriate fixation will yield a method of preserving bone stock in the younger patient requiring arthroplasty (66).

To determine what kind of information should be used to select a prosthesis we shall consider four sources: (a) postmarketing surveillance to remove unsafe or ineffective devices from the market, (b) prospective clinical trials to prevent unsafe or ineffective devices from becoming freely available on the market, (c) preclinical tests to prevent unsafe or ineffective devices from being tried in patients, and (d) design confirmation studies to validate principles and expectations on which designs are based.

METHODS TO ASSESS SAFETY AND EFFICACY

Postmarketing Surveillance

In the United States, the FDA monitors the safety of implants and requires failures with medical devices to be reported as a matter of law. In some other countries, postmarketing surveillance (PMS) is organized by the orthopedic community itself to monitor (safety and efficacy) on a voluntary basis. The most advanced system is that of the Swedish National Hip Arthroplasty Register (23,59), which is discussed elsewhere in this book. In this register, all primary THA reconstructions and

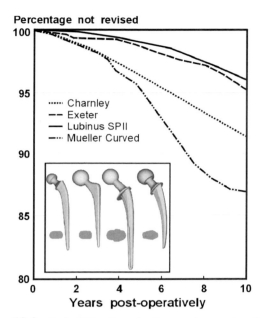

Figure 13-2 Probability of survival (percentage not revised) of four cemented total hip replacements. The stems of these replacements are shown on the inset; from left to right: Charnley, Exeter, Lubinus SPII, Mueller Curved. The data are taken from the Swedish National Hip Arthroplasty Register containing a total of 92,675 patients who received a THR between 1978 and 1990. (Adapted from Herberts P, Malchau H. Long-term registration has improved the quality of hip replacement: a review of the Swedish THR Register comparing 160,000 cases. *Acta Orthop Scand.* 2000;71:111–121.)

revisions are stored by patient, surgeon, and device specifications, complete with information about indications and surgical parameters. Because of the large number of patients and cases stored, the well-delineated population, identifiable by a unique national patient number, and the collaboration of virtually all surgeons, statistically significant information can be obtained about individual design-, surgeon-, and patient-related factors influencing the success of THA, with time-to-revision as the outcome parameter. Figure 13-2 gives an example of how the average endurance of a prosthesis can be evaluated relative to a control after long term service. Hip registers have now developed into powerful tools for the long-term assessment of prosthetic safety and efficacy. Other countries, or regions, that have now developed registers as well, following the success of Sweden, include Norway (22), New Zealand (78), Denmark (55), Finland (77), and, regionally, the United Kingdom (61).

Restricted Clinical Trials

Although restricted trials produce useful information about the feasibility of a new design, they cannot guarantee its long-term safety and efficacy in an absolute sense because of two limitations. First, the trials are usually conducted by a limited group of surgeons, and often they are the innovators themselves and well aware of the design philosophy, or at least they are individuals highly experienced in THA. Their results are likely to be superior to those from a general population of surgeons. Second, these trials are not normally extended long enough to assess the long-term results with time-to-revision as the outcome parameter before the device is introduced to the market.

When revision is not taken as the indicator of failure, postoperative studies in patient series are less conclusive. Rating systems to score function and pain mostly rely on patient interviews and are not objective (113). Longitudinal postoperative radiographs are another source of information for the quality of hip reconstructions. However, radiographic exposure procedures are not standardized, hence, morphological and bone-density parameters tend to be variable. In addition, conventional radiographs are two-dimensional reductions of a three-dimensional reality. As a result, measurements based on their use tend to be imprecise and inconclusive (38,60,112).

Since the introduction of modern hip prostheses, methods have been developed that allow for more precise determinations of prosthetic behavior and, consequently, for earlier detection of problems. It was shown that aseptic loosening of prosthetic components is virtually always preceded by migration (17,43,107). Using roentgen stereophotogrammetric analysis (RSA), these migrations can be detected with an accuracy of 50 to 100 μm (42,68,88). The use of this method allows significant predictions of pending loosening of THA even 6 months after surgery (43). In view of its mounting prominence as a tool for timely detection of deficient prostheses, RSA is described briefly below.

Dual-energy x-ray absorptiometry (DEXA) is a radiographic method to measure bone mass in vivo, with an accuracy of about 5%. This method can be used to detect loss of bone around a prosthesis and predict pending problems, or to assess the effectiveness of particular prostheses in their bone-preserving potential (2,8,12). Gait analysis, finally, is another method for objectively measuring the quality of THA and detecting problems at an early stage (25,52,54,72,74,91).

Dual energy x-ray absorptiometry was used to measure periprosthetic, distal femoral, and proximal tibial bone mass in the affected and contralateral limbs of eight patients 10 years after unilateral total hip arthroplasty with a cementless, porous-coated titanium alloy femoral stem. Gait analyses to assess the presence of asymmetries in loading of the lower extremities were also performed 10 years postoperatively. The patients had excellent clinical results and no other significant lower extremity pathology. On the basis of comparison of the affected and unaffected proximal femora, bone loss adjacent to the proximal medial aspect of the femoral stem was determined to be 34% (p <0.001). However, the patients also had 16% less bone in the ipsilateral proximal tibia (p = 0.003) and 15% less bone in the ipsilateral femur 3 cm distal to the prosthesis (p = 0.007) compared with the contralateral limb. When normalized to the asymmetry in tibial bone mineral content, the estimated proximal medial periprosthetic bone loss was still statistically significant, but the magnitude was reduced from 34 to 17% (p = 0.009). The gait analyses indicated that several measures that influence the loads at the hip and knee joints were reduced in the involved limb compared with the contralateral limb. Furthermore, the bilateral difference in the vertical component of the external force acting on the proximal tibia was correlated with the bilateral difference in tibial bone mineral content (r = 0.80, p = 0.02). These data suggest that two mechanical factors, the local stress-shielding effect of the prosthesis and the global effect of decreased loading of the limb, can both make significant contributions to periprosthetic bone loss. It is apparent that the magnitude of the periprosthetic bone loss related to stress-shielding has been overestimated by as much as 50% in retrospective studies (5).

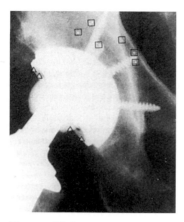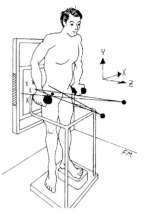

Figure 13-3 RSA uses tantalum pellets (*left*) and stereoradi-ograms (*right*) to determine micromotions and migrations of THA components in vivo. (From (*left*) Kärrholm J, Snorrason F. Migration of porous coated acetabular prostheses fixed with screws. *J Orthop Res.* 1992;10:826–835, with permission, and (*right*) Ryd L. Roentgen stereophotogrammetric analysis of prosthetic fixation in the hip and knee joint. *Clin Orthop.* 1992;276:56–65, with permission.)

Roentgen Stereophotogrammetric Analysis

The late Dr. Göran Selvik developed roentgen stereopho-togrammetric analysis (RSA) (86). The method is based on the principle that a change in relative position of an implant can be monitored by the migration of at least three of its identifi-able points, and that the spatial coordinates of points in the body can be reconstructed from two radiographic images. To create identifiable points in bone and implants, highly radio-dense tantalum pellets are inserted (Fig. 13-3A) (42).

Before the position of a point in space can be determined, the space has to be defined with a laboratory coordinate sys-tem. When the positions of the two x-ray foci and the radi-ographic plates are known, the position of an object point can be reconstructed by calculating the intersection of the x-ray beams. The laboratory coordinate system is defined by a calibration cage containing high-density markers (tantalum) of which the relative positions are known. From a stereocali-bration exposure of the cage, and the known cage-marker coordinates, the positions of the foci relative to the laboratory coordinate system are reconstructed. After this procedure, the position of any point in space can be reconstructed by calcula-tion of the intersection of the two lines between the foci and the projections of the object point on the films (Fig. 13-3B). Because of measuring errors, the two lines representing the beams do not usually intersect exactly, which leads to inaccu-racies in the results. The accuracy can be optimized by using a redundant system of markers. Using this technique, the three-dimensional coordinates of an object point can be recon-structed with an accuracy of about 25 μm (86).

When detecting migration of implants, one is interested in the position of one rigid body (the prosthesis) relative to another one (bone), and how it changes over time. The posi-tion of each of these rigid bodies can be determined from at least three marked points in the bodies. When two or more pairs of radiographs in a particular time sequence are avail-able, the migration of one rigid body relative to the other over time can be determined, in terms of three rotations and three translations. To minimize errors, more than three markers

should be used, particularly when it is expected that the bodies will not remain ideally rigid. A computer program is used to determine the relative kinematics of the two rigid bodies, from which gradual migrations of implant relative to bone along three perpendicular axes, and rotations about those axes, are determined.

Although originally developed as a method to accurately determine three-dimensional motion patterns between bone segments, such as in human joints, RSA was eventually applied to study permanent displacements (migration) and induced relative motions between prosthetic components and bone in vivo (42–45,69,79). These studies have shown that early excessive migration of components is correlated with early revision, and that the RSA technique has appropriate sensitiv-ity to detect these early micromotions. Kärrholm et al. (43) could identify a migration threshold already after only 6 months, beyond which time there was an increased risk of early loosening and revision (Fig. 13-4).

The advantage of RSA is that it can provide significant infor-mation about the quality of THA designs even early after surgery (at 6 to 24 months). The RSA technique is very precise and reliable, and it provides the real three-dimensional relative motions between implant and bone, which is impossible to obtain with other techniques. On the negative side, the evalua-tion tends to be rather tedious and time-consuming. Once the radiograms are digitized, further processing of the data is fully computerized. Because of the program's high precision, sig-nificant information about the migration of a new prosthesis can be obtained already with a group of 10 to 20 patients, rel-ative to a control group, if both groups are relatively homoge-neous and comparable in bone anatomy and other patient and surgical factors. One should carefully reflect the migration

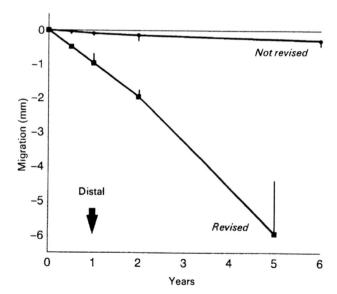

Figure 13-4 In vivo proximal–distal migration (millimeters) of the center of the femoral head (mean and standard error) determined with RSA techniques in a series of 80 cemented THA reconstruc-tions. The reconstructions that were revised within 6 years due to failure and those that were not could be significantly discriminated within 1 year postoperatively by using RSA. (Reproduced from Kärrholm J, Borssén B, Löwenhielm G, et al. Does early micro-motion of femoral stem prostheses matter? *J Bone Joint Surg.* 1994;76B:912–917, with permission.)

patterns to the design philosophy of the implant. If an implant is designed to remain bonded to the cement mantle (like a rough-surfaced stem), a small migration might indicate early failure. However, if an implant is designed such that it can accommodate stem-cement debonding (like a highly polished stem), higher migration values may be acceptable.

In recent years the use of RSA was simplified by the development of intelligent measuring tools. For example, the positions of the bone and prosthetic markers can now be measured automatically from digitized radiographs (73), and the markers themselves can be based on prosthetic characteristics.

> Roentgen stereophotogrammetric analysis (RSA) was developed to measure micromotion of an orthopaedic implant with respect to its surrounding bone. A disadvantage of conventional RSA is that it requires the implant to be marked with tantalum beads. This disadvantage can potentially be resolved with model-based RSA, whereby a 3D model of the implant is used for matching with the actual images and the assessment of position and rotation of the implant. In this study, a model-based RSA algorithm is presented and validated in phantom experiments. To investigate the influence of the accuracy of the implant models that were used for model-based RSA, we studied both computer aided design (CAD) models as well as models obtained by means of reversed engineering (RE) of the actual implant. The results demonstrate that the RE models provide more accurate results than the CAD models. If these RE models are derived from the very same implant, it is possible to achieve a maximum standard deviation of the error in the migration calculation of 0.06 mm for translations in x- and y-direction and 0.14 mm for the out of plane z-direction, respectively. For rotations about the y-axis, the standard deviation was about 0.1 degrees and for rotations about the x- and z-axis 0.05 degrees. Studies with clinical RSA-radiographs must prove that these results can also be reached in a clinical setting, making model-based RSA a possible alternative for marker-based RSA (41).

Design Confirmation Studies and Preclinical Tests

It must be assumed that some form of preclinical testing was conducted by manufacturers in the past for new prostheses, if only to check whether they would fit the bones. However, there is no generally accepted or obligatory set of tests other than the International Standard Organization (ISO) standard test (ISO7206-4) for fatigue strength of femoral stems, and the biocompatibility tests for new materials. Nevertheless, the following preclinical evaluation methods have been developed and tested in recent years in orthopedic research (33).

Geometric Analysis

The long-term success of THA may depend largely on how well the components fit the bones. For noncemented components, interface fit is crucial for timely and extensive osseus integration or bony ingrowth. Cemented components rely on complete cement mantles with adequate thickness, to avoid early mechanical damage and cement degradation. Placement of the components also determines the position of the femoral head, which in turn affects the hip joint forces as they result from the dynamics of hip motion. Malplacement may cause excessive forces to be generated (3,50), with lack of osseus integration or mechanical failure as a result.

Component dimensions are based on anatomical data, in combination with the particular design philosophy concerning placement and fit. Innovators or design engineers use populations of postmortem bones to establish anatomical dimensions, either directly or from databases. Eventually, the question will be whether the design, in combination with the surgical instruments, is adequate in this respect for a typical patient population, when placed by any surgeon. Although such tests are probably performed by companies in some form, they are rarely reported.

Preclinical testing of new prostheses for adequacy of placement and fit can be done using postmortem bones in laboratory experiments (71,83). After placement, the reconstructions can be sectioned and measured for position and interface fit. In an early stage of the design process, computer simulation can be applied, using three-dimensional graphic models of bone populations obtained from computed tomography (CT) scans (Fig. 13-5). In both cases, it is crucial that the series of bones tested adequately represents the patient population at large (49).

Laboratory Bench Tests

Laboratory experiments to investigate the mechanical behavior of THA reconstructions can grossly be divided into micromotion and migration tests, stress and strain analyses, dynamic endurance tests, and wear tests (33).

Micromotion and Migration Tests

These tests are aimed at determining the relative motions and migrations of the components under dynamic loading (6,10,56,85,96,108). The amount of micromotion between implant and bone is a critical factor in the fixation mechanism of cementless prostheses. These implants require minimal motions at the implant–bone interface, to allow bony ingrowth into porous surfaces or osseus integration with hydroxylapatite coatings (76). Hence, it is important for noncemented stems to have adequate initial stability, which can be established in laboratory bench tests. High relative motions may also cause bone to resorb at the interface and create a fibrous-tissue membrane (89). Micromotion and migration analyses applied to cemented THA reconstructions are meant to test whether motion between the stem and the cement mantle is produced when the structure is dynamically loaded. The detection of relative motion would indicate that the stems had debonded from the cement.

> The long-term clinical success of cemented hip stems is influenced both by the implant design, and by the surgical procedure. A methodology is proposed for discriminating between implant designs with different clinical outcomes. The protocol was designed with industrial pre-clinical validation in mind. Two cemented stem types were tested, one (Lubinus SPII) having good and the other (Muller Curved) having poor clinical outcomes. Three implants for each type were subjected to a mechanical in vitro test of one million loading cycles. Each cycle reproduced the load components of stair climbing. Interface shear micromotion was measured during the test in the direction of rotation and along the stem axis. The stem roughness before and after the test was compared. After the test, the cement mantles were retrieved and inspected through dye penetrants to detect evidences of micro-damage. For each specimen, the events of the loosening process were examined, based on the in vitro data available, so as to analyze the whole failure mechanism. The protocol developed was sensitive to the implant design, with significantly different results being found for the two stem types, both in terms of stem-cement micromotions, surface roughness alteration, and cement mantle damage. The information yielded by

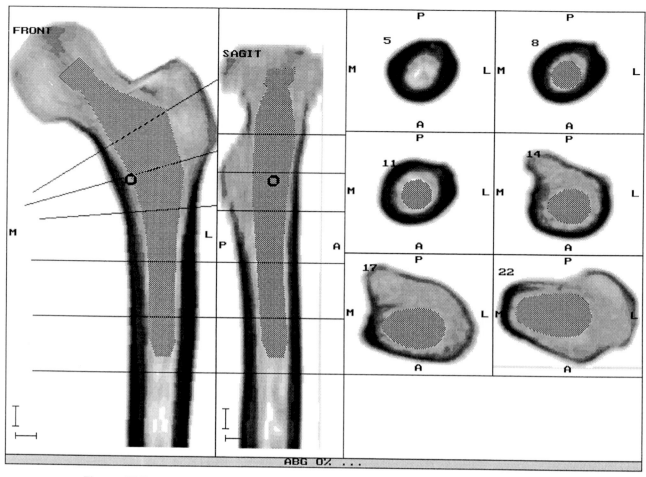

Figure 13-5 Example of a three-dimensional graphics computer program in which a CT-scanned bone image can be imported, as well as the implant geometry. The implant can be moved relative to the bone in order to find the desired position and investigate the prosthetic fit. In this way, fit and placement of a new design can be preclinically tested in a computer simulation.

the three different investigation techniques was consistent for each of the two groups of specimens tested, allowing a better understanding of the failure process. In vitro inducible micromotion and permanent migration measurements, together with cement-stem interface fretting damage and cement fatigue damage, can help predicting the clinical performance of cemented stems (10).

To perform these analyses, the structure is (dynamically) loaded and the motions of the components are recorded using sensors that measure the displacements at one or more points of the prosthesis, relative to the bone. Sometimes, only particular motion components are measured, such as subsidence in axial or rotation in torsional loading of femoral stems (56).

The loads in laboratory bench tests are usually simplified. Muscle forces are often absent or restricted to the representation of the abductor muscles only. A problem may arise when different prosthetic designs are tested relative to each other. Ideally, the points of application of the loads relative to the bone should be equal in all cases. However, because of the different prosthetic shapes and implantation procedures, the position of load application may vary considerably (e.g., because of a different offset). This can affect the local loading conditions considerably (a smaller offset results in a reduction

of the bending moment), and it obscures the interpretation of the results obtained with the various designs.

Laboratory studies with series of postmortem femurs are hampered by the variety in geometrical and mechanical properties of human femurs. Bone quality is often very poor, as the bones come from relatively old donors. This makes them less suitable for testing noncemented implants, which are clinically used in patients with good bone quality. To overcome this problem, synthetic composite femurs can be used. It was shown that the mechanical properties of these femurs, such as the bending stiffness, are similar to those of bones (67). This indicates that the cortical bone is adequately represented. However, the inside of the synthetic bone consists of porous polyurethane that is somewhat dissimilar to trabecular bone in mechanical properties.

Stress and Strain Analyses

The second type of laboratory bench tests are the ones that focus on stress analysis in the bone-implant composite (14,15,26,33,40,106). Information about stresses in the THA reconstruction are important to assess the probability of mechanical failure or bone resorption. If the stresses in polyethylene or metal components, or at the interfaces, are excessive as compared to the strength of the materials, or their bonds, mechanical failure might occur. Periprosthetic stresses in bone should be moderate compared with its strength, so as not to generate cracks, but not too low in comparison with natural values, so as to prevent stress shielding and associated bone resorption (33).

Laboratory stress analyses are usually applied on laboratory models, using bone specimens or bone substitutes. In all cases, deformations (strains) are actually measured and then either visually interpreted or used to calculate the stresses, utilizing elasticity theory. The common methods used to measure deformations in biomechanics are strain-gauge analysis, holography, photoelastic analysis (with photoelastic models, coatings, or films) and thermography.

The most popular method is strain-gauge analysis, whereby an electrical gauge is glued to a free surface of an object (33). The gauge contains one or more electrical filaments that deform with the surface to which they are attached. A strain gauge works on the principle that a deformation of the filament is proportional to a change in its electrical resistance, thus the strain of the material at the point where the gauge is applied can be measured by simply monitoring the electrical resistance. When the elastic properties of the object are known, the stresses can be calculated using the theory of elasticity.

Strain gauges were applied mostly to assess deformation patterns at periosteal bone surfaces, for instance, to assess strain patterns in the bone before and after prosthetic fixation. Strain gauges applied for this purpose have some limitations, however. First, the deformation patterns, and therefore stress patterns, at the outside bone surface are not very sensitive to the details of stress transfer far away within the structure at implant–bone interfaces. Further, from the surface measurements, no information exists about the stress state within the structure. Hence, this method lacks the required sensitivity to assess the probability of prosthetic, cement or interface failure. Second, strains are obtained in a particular region of finite dimensions. The number of spots to be sampled is limited by space, instrumentation, and cost restrictions. Hence, to obtain a good representation of the stress patterns, one must either know a priori where the values of interest might occur or have a method of interpolating the data.

Continuous strain patterns on the outside surface of bone specimens can be visualized by using photoelastic coatings (115). The deformations in the coating, which is thin and flexible, follow precisely those of the bone surface and can be visualized as optical fringe patterns when viewed under polarized light. Photoelastic coatings have limitations similar to those of strain gauges with regard to information obtained at the outside surface of the bone only. They have the additional disadvantage of being difficult to quantify accurately. However, they do give continuous strain patterns that provide easy qualitative interpretation. Methods with similar results, advantages, and limitations are holography and thermography. These methods also display continuous deformation patterns at the outside surface of structures. Holography was used to provide very accurate measurements of deformation, whereas thermography usually provides rough qualitative pictures only.

Dynamic Endurance Tests

Because experimental stress analysis does not reliably predict the probability of failure inside the THA reconstruction, alternative methods must be used to preclinically test new components. One method is to use laboratory models in which the components are fixed, and load them to failure. However, there are two problems with such a scheme. First, mechanical failure of cement or implant–bone interfaces is not a matter of "static" strength in the sense that the materials will break as a result of a single, excessive force. The hip joint forces occurring in normal functioning are simply not high enough to accomplish that. Failure is caused by gradual accumulation of microcracks in repetitive, dynamic loading. Such a process is called material fatigue. So the question is, rather, how many cycles a THA reconstruction can endure at a particular load level, before it fails. Such endurance tests can take a long time, as 1 year of loading (some 1 million cycles) at the natural frequency of 1 Hz takes more than 11 days of continuous testing in a dynamic loading machine. Hence, to simulate a reasonable long-term endurance of 10 years takes almost 4 months! The potential validity of tests at higher frequencies has not really been explored yet. These tests could be performed with fewer cycles if, for instance, migration is used as an indicator for endurance, in the same way as this is done in clinical RSA studies. However, the second problem is the difficulty of keeping postmortem bones fresh for a prolonged period of time. So the tests should be limited to a relatively short time period or must be performed with bone substitutes, which provide less reliable results because the polyurethane material they are made from has properties somewhat different from trabecular bone. Particularly in recent years, methods for dynamic endurance tests were developed that lack the deficiencies discussed above, because they monitor prosthetic migration, rather than failure propagation (4,10). Another alternative is to use computer simulation methods for these tests, as discussed later.

This study examined the effect of including muscle forces in fatigue tests of cemented total hip arthroplasty reconstructions. An experimental device capable of applying the joint reaction force, the abductor force, the vastus lateralis force, and the tensor fasciae latae force to the implanted femur is described. Current in vitro fatigue tests of cemented total hip arthroplasty reconstructions do not apply physiological muscle loads. Experimental and numerical studies report significant differences in stresses obtained in the cement mantle depending on the loads applied. The differing stresses may alter the outcome of an in vitro test. Ten femoral components were reproducibly implanted into proximal composite femurs. Five of these femoral components were tested using a load profile which included muscle loading, five were tested without muscle loading. The migration of each femoral component was monitored continuously during dynamic fatigue tests. Clinically comparable migration amounts were found for both sets of femoral components, with the femoral components tested with muscle loading experiencing lower mean migration, lower mean inducible displacement, and less experimental scatter. The inclusion of muscle forces seems to stabilize the femoral component during the test. In vitro fatigue tests of cemented total hip arthroplasty reconstructions should include muscle loading to provide increased confidence in the results obtained. This study examined how the migration of cemented femoral hip prostheses is influenced by muscle forces. Hip prostheses are one of the few medical devices for which pre-clinical testing protocols have emerged, and this study ascertains whether or not the inclusion of muscle forces is necessary for pre-clinical tests. The conclusion is that muscle loading should be included, and that it is important for the development of a new generation of standardized tests to provide enhanced patient protection against functionally poor prostheses (10).

Wear Tests

The wear resistance of articular surfaces and modular connections of THA components, and the production of wear particles, can, in principle, be preclinically tested in hip simulators (16,65,80). The importance of this ability was reemphasized in the late 1980s, when a new heat treatment method for polyethylene was approved by the FDA and subsequently led to failures on a large scale (97,114). It must be noted that hip simulators may be used to quantify wear-particle production, but they do not give information about the ease of particle transport provoked by a particular prosthesis. An important prosthetic feature such as that should be preclinically tested as well. Wear and hip simulators are described extensively elsewhere in this book.

Finite-Element Computer Simulation Analysis

Computer simulation based on finite-element analysis (FEA) can be useful for the purpose of research in THA, preclinical testing, and design. Particularly in the last 20 years, their applicability has been improved tremendously through research and developments in computer hardware and software (31,33). The possibilities and limitations of FEA, however, must be correctly understood, and this is more difficult for computer than for laboratory methods, because the former are more abstract. As tools of research for THA failure processes, computer simulation experiments are conceptually similar to laboratory, animal, and clinical experiments in that models (or populations) are applied representing reality in a particular way. In any investigation, one must consider how close to reality the model is, compared to the experimental control (Fig. 13-6). When a patient is used as a clinical model for investigative purposes, one is dealing with reality but has very little control over experimental parameters. Conversely, a computer simulation provides virtually absolute experimental control but is remote from reality. Other models can be positioned between these two extremes (Fig. 13-6).

When using computer simulation models, one can investigate pure cause–effect relationships for well-defined sets of parameters. A single design parameter can be varied to estimate its role in a particular failure scenario. Another advantage is that computer simulation is relatively cheap. For example, new THA designs can be tested from the drawing board without prototypes. These advantages can be exploited and weighted against the limitations of remoteness from reality.

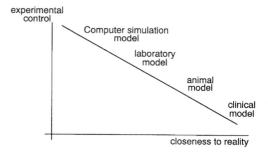

Figure 13-6 Models used for an investigation are subject to requirements of closeness to reality and control over the experimental parameters. Which to choose depends on the scientific question posed.

FEA is suitable for determining stresses and strains at any given point inside a structure of arbitrary geometrical and material complexity, given the loads applied to it and the mechanical properties of the materials (33). The shape of the structure to be analyzed is divided into small elements. Groups of elements are defined as they represent the components in the structure (e.g., metal, bone, acrylic cement, polyethylene), and the appropriate mechanical properties are allocated. Each element has nodal points, usually at its corners. Forces and displacements are prescribed at these nodal points, and FEA produces information about the deformations, stresses, and relative micromotions at those points. It is virtually impossible to obtain this information with any other method of stress analysis. FEA can be effectively utilized for parametric analysis (11,19,24,33,46,47,50,63,75,90,92,101, 105), which means that structural parameters can be altered and their effects established rapidly. The stress values determined are compared to known values of material strength, which indicates whether failure is likely.

An FEA model relies on accurate data for material properties, geometry, loading characteristics, and boundary and interface conditions. With regard to the analysis of THA reconstructions, the models are usually simplified for practicality. The materials are generally assumed to be linear elastic, isotropic, and constant in time, without imperfections, and usually only a few loading cases are considered out of the many possible ones. As a consequence of these assumptions, the results of FEA are indicative rather than precise, and conclusions should be limited to general trends and qualitative effects of the design parameters that are varied in the model. In the case of preclinical tests, analyses of new designs should always be done on a relative basis, using a control.

CT data is now commonly used to create anatomic three-dimensional models, and multiple loading cases are taken into account. In addition, FEA has been expanded by taking time-dependent processes into account. This has led to FE simulations of material damage processes, debonding and micromotion simulations, and simulations of periprosthetic bone-remodeling processes. Below, examples of these FEA simulations are briefly discussed.

Accumulated Damage Analysis

Because of the long-term, dynamic loads applied to THA reconstructions, they may fail mechanically as a result of fatigue of the materials or their interfaces. Fatigue involves the gradual accumulation of microcracks (damage), which coalesce into large cracks. The amount of damage accumulated in a material can be measured by a reduction in stiffness, strength, or residual life time. The effects of accumulated damage in a THA reconstruction can be analyzed by application of the theory of continuum damage mechanics in combination with FEA (33,93–95,102,103). In this case, FEA is used iteratively in a stepwise manner, simulating the cyclic loading process. In each simulation step, FEA determines the stresses in the materials and compares those to known data on material fatigue strength. Where stresses surpass strengths, damage is allocated in the finite-element model, and the computer turns to the next step. This process continues until the material is predicted to be fully damaged, or until an adequate number of cycles is simulated (Fig. 13-7).

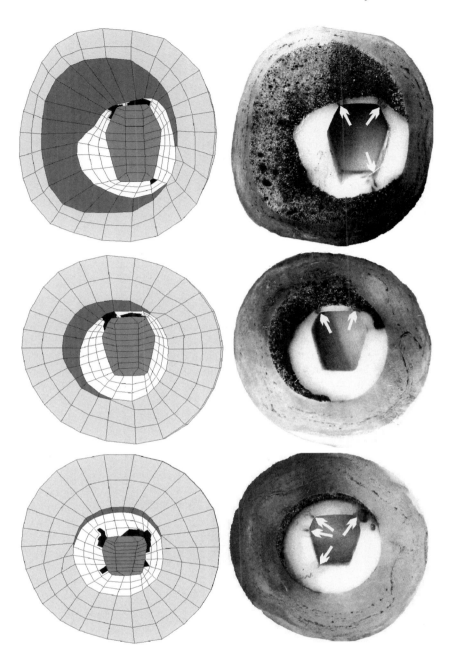

Figure 13-7 Crack patterns around the Mueller curved stem as found (*left*) in three transverse sections of experimental reconstructions tested in a dynamic loading rig and (*right*) in a three-dimensional finite-element simulation of damage accumulation. (Stolk et al., Ref. 92)

Rigorous preclinical testing of cemented hip prostheses against the damage accumulation failure scenario will reduce the incidence of aseptic loosening. For that purpose, a finite element simulation is proposed, that predicts damage accumulation in the cement mantle, and prosthetic migration. If the simulation is to become a convincing preclinical test, it should be able to distinguish between implants in a clinically relevant way, based on accurate predictions of long-term failure mechanisms of cemented hip prostheses. The algorithm was used to simulate long-term fatigue experiments on femoral reconstructions with Mueller Curved and Lubinus SPII stems. Clinically, the Mueller Curved system performs inferior to the Lubinus SPII system. The finite element simulation predicted much more cement damage around the Mueller Curved stem and showed that the entire cement mantle was involved in the failure process, which was not the case around the Lubinus SPII

stem. In addition, the Mueller Curved stem was predicted to migrate more than the Lubinus SPII. The predictions showed excellent agreement with the experimental findings: similar damage locations in the cement, more damage for the Mueller Curved, similar prosthetic migration directions, and more migration for the Mueller Curved stem. This is the first time that a finite element simulation is able to differentiate between a clinically superior and an inferior implant, based on accurate simulation of the long-term failure mechanisms in a cemented reconstruction. Its use for preclinical testing purposes is corroborated (92).

Debonding and Micromotion Analysis

Loosening of THA components is often accompanied by disruption or non-ingrowth of interfaces. FEA has been used to study the effects of interface debonding and micromotion processes (33). It became evident from these studies that nothing alters the load-transfer mechanism in a THA so drastically as a change from bonded to debonded interfaces. Hence, of all the relevant design parameters, the bonding characteristics are the most prominent ones affecting stresses.

Computer simulation of a debonding process with FEA is analogous to simulation of damage processes, in that the computer treats it in an iterative, stepwise manor. After every step, debonding is locally implemented where stresses surpass fatigue strengths of the bond, and the simulation is continued until the interface is completely debonded, or an adequate number of loading cycles has been considered. If a connection (between cement and implant, or implant and bone) is (locally) debonded, the parts move apart when tensile stress is applied. Also, the parts will slide when sheared, provided that friction is overcome. The FEA program will calculate these relative interface motions in every iteration and monitor the migration of the implant for the duration of the test.

In cemented THA, the stem is likely to debond from the cement, which creates subsidence and increases cement stresses (20,30,39,103). In noncemented THA, the implant–bone interface is unbonded until ingrowth or osseus integration occurs. The interface micromotions that result from the repetitive hip joint forces may hamper the process of integration itself, if they are too extensive. These motions depend not only on the loading magnitudes, but also on the shape of the implant, the coefficient of interface friction, and even on the elastic modulus of the prosthetic material, as illustrated in Figure 13-8 (51).

dynamic interface motions (µm)

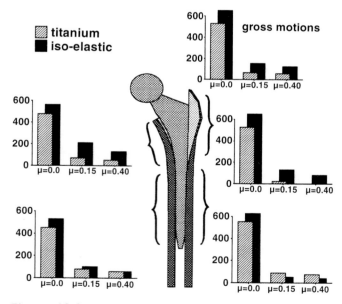

Figure 13-8 Amplitudes of cyclic movements along the implant–bone interface for a noncemented stem, determined by FEA computer simulations. The average rigid-body motion (gross motion) is shown, as well as the motions in four locations. The motions depend mostly on interface friction characteristics, but also on the stiffness of the stem material. (Adapted from Kuiper JH, Huiskes R. Friction and stem stiffness affect dynamic interface motion in total hip replacement. *J Orthop Res.* 1996;14:36–43, with permission.)

Also in this case the FEA model represents an idealized reality; it ignores surgical inaccuracies, such as lack of fit and interface gaps. As a result, the motions predicted by the analyses tend to be less than those found in laboratory tests. However, the results using laboratory tests tend to correlate with those of FEA simulation for different prostheses, indicating that relative to a control, they produce the same conclusions (92,104).

Strain-Adaptive Bone Remodeling Analysis

When a metal stem is fixed within the femur, the stresses within the bone change, even if the external loads remain the same. In accordance with Wolff's Law, a process of strain-adaptive bone remodeling then emerges, changing the shape and internal structural organization to adapt to the new mechanical requirements. The load, which was earlier carried by the bone alone, is now shared with the stem. This phenomenon causes stress shielding of the bone; that is, the bone is shielded by the stem from the stress it is normally subjected to. As a result, the bone stresses are subnormal and the bone resorbs to adapt to this new situation.

It was only in the mid 1970s that a first quantitative form of Wolff's law emerged (9). Later, mathematical remodeling rules were combined with finite-element models to enable practical applications of strain-adaptive bone remodeling analysis to orthopaedic problems, using computer simulation of the remodeling processes to predict results (7,21,32,36).

These computer simulation models can be applied to study bone remodeling around joint replacements, for instance to evaluate the relationships between prosthetic design characteristics and the extent of resorption. Figure 13-9 is a schematic outline of how such a simulation is conducted. The distribution of local load in the periprosthetic bone, in the form of the strain energy to which the bone tissue is subjected by the external hip and muscle loads, is compared to their values in the intact bone, in the same location and for the same external loads. The amount of bone to be added or subtracted in the model after every iterative remodeling step is calculated in the mathematical remodeling rule, which is shown graphically in Figure 13-9. Bone becomes denser locally (up to a certain level) where the strain energy surpasses the natural value, and less dense where it is below that value. The simulation process continues until a new equilibrium is reached, in which bone mass is again adapted to the loads applied to it (Fig. 13-10).

We asked the question whether the excellent clinical results recently reported for the Hydroxyapatite-coated ABG hip are consistent with results of pre-clinical computer simulation methods for the prediction of strain-adaptive bone remodeling patterns around implants. We also investigated whether a further improvement of the results can be expected if complete proximal load transfer is enforced by reducing the ABG stem length. Resorption patterns predicted by the computer simulation study were in very good agreement with radiographic clinical findings. Mechanical failure of the bone-implant interface was judged based on a Hoffman interface stress criterion, which was very low, indicating that no bone-implant interface failure is expected. Reducing the stem length did not reduce proximal bone resorption. We conclude that the proximal load transfer for the Hydroxyapatite-ABG Hip Stem is favorable for the present design and is not improved by further stem-length reduction (98).

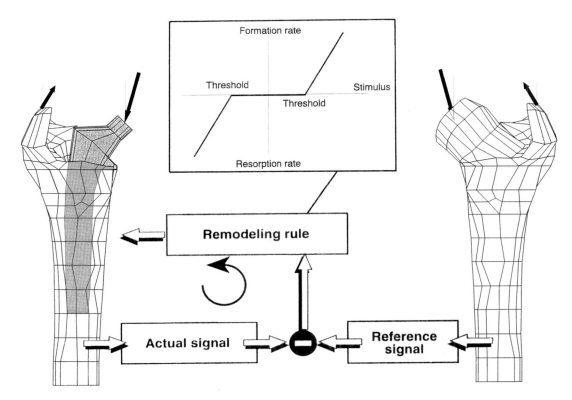

Operated Femur　　　　　　　　　　　　　　**Intact Femur**

Figure 13-9 Schematic representation of an iterative computer simulation model of periprosthetic bone remodeling. The strain energy around the prosthesis resulting from the external load (actual signal) is compared to the strain energy in the intact bone for the same load. The difference between the values is the mechanical stimulus for the bone remodeling process. The relationship between mechanical stimulus and remodeling—the remodeling rule—is described by a nonlinear function, featuring a threshold dead zone (*inset*). Beyond this threshold, bone will be formed with a high positive mechanical stimulus, and it will resorb with a negative stimulus. The iterative simulation process continues until a new equilibrium signal distribution is obtained. (Reproduced from Huiskes R. Bone remodeling around implants can be explained as an effect of mechanical adaptation. In: Galante JO, Rosenberg AG, Callaghan JJ, eds. *Total Hip Revision Surgery.* New York: Raven Press; 1995:159–171, with permission.)

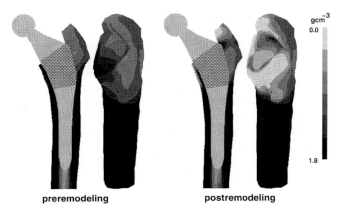

preremodeling　　　　postremodeling

Figure 13-10 Immediate postoperative density distribution around a cementless prosthesis, as based on CT data (*left*) and density distribution after long-term remodeling simulation (*right*), as determined in a bone remodeling simulation study using a three-dimensional FEA model. (Adapted from van Rietbergen B, Huiskes R. Load transfer and stress shielding of the hydroxyapatite-ABG hip: a study of stem length and proximal fixation. *J Arthroplasty.* 2001;16(8 suppl 1):55–63, with permission.)

The simulation equations were validated relative to bone mass density distributions in the normal femur (35,110), series of canine experiments with different types of hip prostheses (99,111), and retrievals of human THA (28,48). The simulation model has been used to study the effects of various design, surgical and patient factors on periprosthetic bone loss (34,35,37,109,110). One important finding was that the amount of eventual bone loss in the femur caused by stress shielding grossly depends on its preoperative density. The less bone mass to start with, the more will disappear. The influence of this factor is more prominent than any of the other prosthetic-design parameters (27). Strain-adaptive bone remodeling analyses are now often used to estimate the qualities of joint prostheses relative to their potential to create bone resorption (53,75).

FAILURE SCENARIOS

Of all the sources of information about prosthetic safety and efficacy listed earlier, only postmarketing surveillance is based on revision—hence endurance—as the outcome parameter. In all other cases of restricted clinical trials or laboratory studies, parameters must be defined to determine the safety and efficacy of an implant. These parameters must be derived from the failure mechanisms known. These failure mechanisms are not easily delineated, however, and commonly a subject of controversy. Pain and functional disabilities, the clinical signs of failure, are usually associated with fibrous tissue interfaces containing wear particles, and migration of implants relative to bone. Although these signs are clear, they do not inform us about the causes of the loosening, which is the result of a process, hardly ever an event. Different causes, such as inadequate biocompatibility, mechanical damage, or reactions to wear particles, produce similar histomorphologic, radiographic, and clinical effects, in the end. How are these processes initiated, how do they propagate, and how can they be related to implant factors? These are crucial questions for the application and interpretation of short-time clinical and preclinical tests. As yet, there is no definite answer; most suggestions in the literature are hypothetical, not least because failure processes are likely to have multifactorial causes.

A way around this problem is to direct clinical and preclinical tests at separate failure scenarios, rather than at complex failure mechanisms (29). A failure scenario is a paradigm for a failure mechanism, a particular course of events that is hypothetical but latent. The question addressed in a test or a trial is then how likely it is that a prosthetic device may provoke failure according to a particular failure scenario.

An example of a failure scenario for cemented THA stems is illustrated in Figure 13-11 (100). It is proposed that, as a result of the weakness of the metal–cement bond, debonding is likely to occur early after surgery. This promotes, on the one hand, stem subsidence in cement, cement stress increase, and crack formation (compare Fig. 13-7). On the other hand, the debonded stem will rub against the cement and produce wear particles. Both mechanisms in this scenario are likely to cause cement–bone interface resorption and clinical failure of the reconstruction. In this scenario, there are several questions to assess a new prosthesis: Will the stem easily debond? If

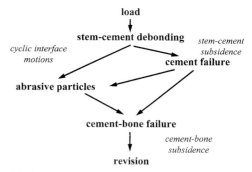

Figure 13-11   A detailed failure scenario for cemented THA stems. According to this scenario, the failure process is initiated by stem–cement debonding. This allows relative motions between the stem and the cement, thereby producing abrasive wear particles. Stem–cement debonding leads also to prosthetic subsidence and to increased cement stresses, resulting in cement failure. The wear products and the failed cement mantle promote failure of the cement–bone interface and induce cement–bone subsidence, leading to gross loosening of the implant. (Adapted from Verdonschot N. *Biomechanical Failure Scenarios for Cement Total Hip Replacement* [PhD thesis]. Nijmegen, The Netherlands: University of Nijmegen; 1995, with permission.)

debonded, to what extent does that increase cement stresses and the probability of mechanical failure? If debonded, what metal–cement relative motions does that produce, and will it promote excessive production of wear particles? Such a detailed failure scenario is a mixture of two generic scenarios, concerning mechanical damage on the one hand, and reactions to wear particles on the other.

A number of such generic failure scenarios for THA are known and can be summarized as follows (29).

Accumulated Damage

The accumulated damage scenario is based on gradual accumulation of mechanical damage in materials and interfaces as a result of repetitive dynamic loading. The damaging process proliferates to eventual disruption of the implant from the bone, interface micromotion, bone resorption, fibrous interposition, and, finally, gross loosening. As a generic scenario, it is certainly relevant not only for cemented stems, as in the previous example, but also for cemented acetabular cups and for noncemented components at both sides (e.g., it may lead to disruption of prosthetic coatings). The fact that cemented stems are more sensitive than other types of components for this scenario is not the issue here. The whole point of failure scenarios is how easily they could be provoked by a particular new design. Prostheses can be tested for their susceptibility to this failure scenario by laboratory endurance tests or by computer simulation, using damage-accumulation analysis, as discussed.

Particulate Reaction

Wear particles from articulating surfaces, debonded interfaces, or modular-component connections can migrate into the cement–bone (cemented) or implant–bone (noncemented) interfaces. These small particles activate microphages at the interface into inflammatory responses of local bone resorption (lysis), thereby gradually debonding cement and bone (84). Eventually this process produces relative interface motions and proliferates to gross loosening, in much the same way as the final stage of the accumulated-damage scenario described above. This means that one can usually not discriminate these two scenarios by studying radiograms or retrieved specimens, since their eventual results are similar. In addition to wear-particle production, the elements of the particulate-reaction scenario include particle transport and biologic bone reactions. Although the latter is a factor of the patient rather than implant design, the characteristics of wear particles in terms of material, size, and shape are certainly relevant for this scenario (62,87). This can be tested preclinically using hip simulators (e.g., 56).

Failed Bonding

The failed-bonding scenario is valid for noncemented components only. It implies that ingrowth or osseous integration does not occur because of gaps and relative motions at the implant–bone interface (27,81,89). The biological bonding, or ingrowth, processes require a certain quiescence at the interface to succeed. If relative motions occur beyond about 150 μm (76), ingrowth will be prevented and motions will be enhanced, provoking bone resorption, fibrous-tissue formation, and, eventually, loosening. The elements of this scenario are initial fit, osseus induction (the capacity of a coating material to induce bony adhesion and fill gaps), initial relative interface motions, and interface-motion-induced bone resorption. Relevant tests for this scenario are geometric analyses of fit, laboratory micromotion studies or computer simulations, and animal experiments to test the osseoinductive capacity of the implant surface.

Stress Shielding

Stress shielding involves particularly the bone around the femoral stem. Because the bone is stress shielded by the stem, the bone stresses are subnormal. In accordance with Wolff's Law, resorption develops. Although this does not automatically lead to prosthetic loosening, it may enhance bone or stem fracture, and it may complicate a possible revision operation. The potential of a particular stem design to provoke excessive bone resorption can now be preclinically tested with computer simulation methods with good accuracy, as discussed above. Laboratory stress analyses to measure bone stresses can also be used.

Stress Bypass

Stress bypass is similar to the stress-shielding scenario but develops through another route, when proximal load transfer in the noncemented femoral THA is bypassed in favor of distal load transfer. As a result, the proximal bone is again understressed. Its cause can be inadequate proximal fit, either initially as an effect of inadequate fit or bone preparation, or gradually after surgery as an effect of stem subsidence (99). Preclinical tests for this scenario should include geometric analyses of trial implantations, and laboratory stress analyses or computer simulation.

Destructive Wear

The destructive-wear scenario implies that articulating surfaces or modular component connections (e.g., cone connections between metal head and stem of the femoral component, or connections between polyethylene liner and metal backing in the acetabulum) simply wear out, to the extent that mechanical integrity can no longer be maintained. The sensitivity of a design for this scenario can be preclinically tested in hip simulators (65,80).

INTRODUCTION AND SELECTION OF PROSTHESES

In an ideal world, no implant would be used in patients if its long-term quality could not be guaranteed. However, the reality is that no THA reconstruction lasts forever, that the ideal would be prohibitive for industry with respect to innovation times and costs, and that patients would be denied the benefit of improvements for a very long time. Hence, compromises are inevitable, coupling acceptable risks to reasonable costs and development times. We believe that the guidelines for a system in which this is realized should be laid down by the orthopaedic community. The system we propose is based on stepwise introduction of new designs (13,29,57). This implies

that a number of questions will have to be answered consecutively before an innovative design would be fit for admission to on the market. A suggestion for such a system is the following.

Stepwise Introduction of THA Designs into the Market

Step 1: Design Rationale

The question to be answered explicitly in this step is why a new design was initiated; in other words, this is a statement of intent. This implies the description of a problem known to occur with other prostheses already on the market, which this new design is supposed to solve. The statement will include an explicit description of the new design features and the reasons why they are assumed to solve the problem.

Step 2: Design Confirmation

This step is the conceptual validation of the preceding assumption. Although certainty can be obtained only after many years of clinical service, there are ways to substantiate certain claims. If, for example, the rationale for a new design is the reduction of wear, and the feature to realize that is a new material, substantiation could be achieved by laboratory tests using hip simulators.

This type of validation may seem trivial, but many examples from the past show that it is not. Hip surface replacement, for instance, was introduced based on expectations of better revisability and more natural bone stresses than intramedullary stems. A simple FEA to test the latter hypothesis, however, would have shown it to be invalid: the bone in the femoral head is dramatically stress shielded (36). Even today, some prostheses admitted to the market are based on claims that are in no way substantiated. To overcome this omission, the orthopedic community must insist that all claims be substantiated.

Which techniques are to be used for design confirmation studies depends, as in all scientific investigations, on the problem the new design is supposed to solve. All the previously mentioned methods could be considered. Computer simulation is attractive particularly in this stage, because it requires only a conceptual design and not an actual product or prototype; but the criterion for a suitable test must be met if a reasonable answer is to be expected from the methodology applied.

Step 3: Preclinical Testing

Whereas design confirmation studies are performed to investigate the particular hypothesis on which new design features are based, preclinical testing is meant to test the design as a whole. Discriminating between design confirmation studies and preclinical testing will not always be necessary, but the possibility still exists that a design feature that solves one problem, introduces another. Design objectives for THA are often incompatible (30). For example, reduced stiffness of a stem decreases stress shielding in the periprosthetic bone, but it increases the probability for interface motions and mechanical loosening, or failed bonding. The question addressed in preclinical testing is how likely the new design would be to fail, according to any of the failure scenarios known, in comparison to other types of prostheses, of which the long-term results are known.

A definite answer to this question can be given only after long-term clinical application, but the tests may reveal weaknesses or predict problems that can be avoided in this stage. Several examples come to mind. All THA components should be tested for placement and fit in a postmortem bone population of adequate generality. Stems should be tested for fatigue strength in the laboratory, according to the ISO standard, particularly when they are relatively slender. Modular components, including metal-backed acetabulae, should be tested for fatigue and wear endurance. All noncemented components could undergo micromotion and migration tests to check for the failed-bonding scenario. Cemented femoral reconstructions can be tested for interface holding power, subsidence, and mechanical endurance of the cement. Noncemented stems should be checked for their potential to provoke periprosthetic bone loss due to stress shielding, using bone remodeling analyses or other suitable methods, as discussed.

Several prostheses with inferior clinical endurance were marketed in the past; their shortcomings would have been revealed in preclinical tests (13,30,57). However, preclinical tests can reveal weaknesses in designs only relative to failure scenarios that are known, and even then a test may not be effective, producing a false negative result. Hence, preclinical tests can only be a first sieve for unsafe or ineffective devices; they cannot replace clinical trials. The results cannot proof that a particular design will be successful; but they may indicate potential problems associated with a new prosthesis, from which patients involved in trials could be protected.

Step 4: Restricted Clinical Trials

The issue to be addressed here is whether the new prosthesis creates unexpected problems in the short term in clinical use, and to estimate its safety and efficacy for the long term. These trials should be performed by surgeons not involved with the development of the prosthesis. They should be prospective, well documented, and preferably randomized. Short-term clinical trials are of little use where detection of long-term endurance is concerned, if subjective clinical or imprecise radiographic parameters are used to evaluate results. Highly recommended, or even indispensable, is the application of DEXA for bone remodeling evaluations and RSA for migration and inducible micromotion. RSA, particularly, has shown to be a dependable and powerful tool to predict prosthetic loosening in the longer term as soon as 6 months to 1 year after placement, for cemented and noncemented, femoral and acetabular components alike.

A new prosthesis should not be on the market until steps 1 through 4 are finalized and the results readily available in well-documented reports or, preferably, peer-reviewed articles. Even then, however, there is no certainty that the new design will do better, clinically, than those already on the market; it may even cause a disaster as a result of failure scenarios hitherto unknown. To monitor its performance continuously, the prosthesis should preferably be entered in a national or regional register, such as the one in Sweden.

The system we propose here may seem tedious, expensive, and time-consuming, and it is. Such a system, however, is meant to protect the patients, not to stimulate industrial activity. At a time when a particular, cemented design produces 96.9% endurance after a 10-year follow-up in the Swedish register, which include virtually all patients and surgeons in Sweden using that prosthetic type (58), it may be asked whether new designs are required at all. It seems logical to demand any new claim for improvement in THA to be substantiated in the most complete sense possible (1,18,82).

The Responsibility of the Individual Surgeon

Only the orthopaedic field itself could consent to organize an introduction system as described here. Companies will perform extensive preclinical tests, provide well-documented information, and put restraints on market introduction only if forced to do so, either by the law or by their customers. There is no reason, however, why individual customers should not apply a scheme themselves, when considering whether to use another design.

The safest method for selecting a prosthesis is to take one that has been documented in a register by reasonable numbers for an adequate amount of time, and that shows good results relative to other prostheses. If there are reasons to select one not covered in a register, one can ask manufacturers to provide information about tests and trials for which the description given here provides guidelines. There are no formal standards for the trials and the tests yet. This means it is difficult for a surgeon to judge whether they were conducted correctly. Nevertheless, the first objective is to check whether they were done at all and to what extent.

It must be pointed out, once again, that THA safety and efficacy is not purely a matter of product quality characteristics (13), but rather of service quality characteristics. This is determined by patient and surgical factors as well. The prosthesis may not even be the most important factor; it may even be better to have a bad prosthesis from a superb surgeon than vice versa. But still, the best solution is to optimize all three factors. The issue is the patient; the surgeon is the only guard between failure and success. Knowing what prosthesis to use is part of the job.

REFERENCES

1. Bauer GCH. Editorial: what price progress? *Acta Orthop Scand.* 1992;63:245–246.
2. Bobyn JD, Mortimer ES, Glassmann AH, et al. Producing and avoiding stress shielding. Laboratory and clinical observations of noncemented total hip arthroplasty. *Clin Orthop.* 1992;274:79–96.
3. Brand RA, Pedersen DR. Computer modeling of surgery and a consideration of the mechanical effects of proximal femoral osteotomies. In: Welch RB, ed. *The Hip.* St. Louis: Mosby; 1984:193–210.
4. Britton JR, Walsh LA, Prendergast PJ. Mechanical simulation of muscle loading on the proximal femur: analysis of cemented femoral component migration with and without muscle loading. *Clin Biomech Bristol Avon.* 2003;18:637–646.
5. Bryan JM, Sumner DR, Hurwitz DE, et al. Altered load history affects periprosthetic bone loss following cementless total hip arthroplasty. *J Orthop Res.* 1996;14:762–768.
6. Burke DW, O'Connor DO, Zalenski EB, et al. Micromotion of cement and uncemented femoral components. *J Bone Joint Surg.* 1991;73B:22–37.
7. Carter DR, Fyhrie DP, Whalen RT. Trabecular bone density and loading history: regulation of connective tissue biology by mechanical energy. *J Biomech.* 1987;20:785–794.
8. Cohen M., Rushton N. Accuracy of DEXA measurement of bone mineral density after total hip arthroplasty. *J Bone Joint Surg.* 1995;77B:479–483.
9. Cowin SC, Hegedus DH. Bone remodeling. I: Theory of adaptive elasticity. *J Elasticity.* 1976;6:313–326.

10. Cristofolini L, Teutonico AS, Monti L, et al. Comparative in vitro study on the long term performance of cemented hip stems: validation of a protocol to discriminate between "good" and "bad" designs. *J Biomech.* 2003;3611:1603–1615.

11. Dalstra M, Huiskes R, Van Erning L. Development and validation of a three-dimensional finite element model of the pelvic bone. *J Biomech Eng.* 1995;117:272–278.

12. Engh CA, Hooten JP Jr, Zettl-Schaffer KF, et al. Porous-coated total hip replacement. *Clin Orthop.* 1994;298:89–96.

13. Faro LM, Huiskes R. Quality assurance of joint replacement. Legal regulation and medical judgement. *Acta Orthop Scand Suppl.* 1992;250:1–33.

14. Finlay JB, Bourne RB, Landsberg RPD, et al. Pelvic stresses in vitro. I: Malsizing of endoprostheses. *J Biomech.* 1986;19:703–714.

15. Finlay JB, Rorabeck CH, Bourne RB, et al. In vitro analysis of proximal femoral strains using PCA femoral implants and a hip-abductor muscle simulator. *J Arthroplasty.* 1989;4:335–345.

16. Fisher J, Hu XQ, Stewart TD, et al. Wear of surface engineered metal-on-metal hip prostheses. *J Mater Sci Mater Med.* 2004;15:225–235.

17. Freeman MAR, Plante-Bordeneuve P. Early migration and late aseptic failure of proximal femoral prostheses. *J Bone Joint Surg.* 1994;76B:432–438.

18. Goodfellow J. Editorial: knee prostheses—one step forward, two steps back. *J Bone Joint Surg.* 1992;74B:1–2.

19. Harrigan T, Harris WH. A three-dimensional non-linear finite element study of the effect of cement-prosthesis debonding in cemented femoral total hip components. *J Biomech.* 1991;24:1047–1058.

20. Harris WH. Is it advantageous to strengthen the cement-metal interface and use a collar for cemented femoral components of total hip replacement? *Clin Orthop.* 1992;285:67–72.

21. Hart RT, Davy DT, Heiple KG. A computational method of stress analysis of adaptive elastic materials with a view toward application in strain induced remodeling. *J Biomech Eng.* 1984;106:342–350.

22. Havelin L, Espehaug B, Vollset SE, et al. The Norwegian arthroplasty register. *Acta Orthop Scand.* 1993;64:245–251.

23. Herberts P, Malchau H. Long-term registration has improved the quality of hip replacement: a review of the Swedish THR Register comparing 160,000 cases. *Acta Orthop Scand.* 2000;71:111–121.

24. Hertzler J, Miller MA, Mann KA. Fatigue crack growth rate does not depend on mantle thickness: an idealized cemented stem construct under torsional loading. *J Orthop Res.* 2002;20:676–682.

25. Hodge WA, Andriacchi TP, Galante JO. A relationship between stem orientation and function following total hip arthroplasty. *J Arthroplasty.* 1991;6:229–235.

26. Hua J, Walker PS. Closeness of fit of uncemented stems improves the strain distribution in the femur. *J Orthop Res.* 1995;13:339–346.

27. Huiskes R. Biomechanics of noncemented total hip arthroplasty. *Curr Orthop.* 1996;7:32–37.

28. Huiskes R. Bone remodeling around implants can be explained as an effect of mechanical adaptation. In: Galante JO, Rosenberg AG, Callaghan JJ, eds. *Total Hip Revision Surgery.* New York: Raven Press; 1995:159–171.

29. Huiskes R. Failed innovation in total hip replacement. *Acta Orthop Scand.* 1993;64:699–716.

30. Huiskes R. Mechanical failure in total hip arthroplasty with cement. *Curr Orthop.* 1993;7:239–247.

31. Huiskes R, Hollister SJ. From structure to process, from organ to cell: recent developments of FE-analysis in orthopaedic biomechanics. *J Biomech Eng.* 1993;115:520–527.

32. Huiskes R, Ruimerman R, van Lenthe GH, et al. Effects of mechanical forces on maintenance and adaptation of form in trabecular bone. *Nature.* 2000;405:704–706.

33. Huiskes R, Stolk J. Biomechanics and preclinical testing of artificial joints. In: Mow VC, Huiskes R, eds. *Basic Orthopaedic Biomechanics and Mechano-Biology.* 3rd ed. New York: Lippincott Williams & Wilkins; 2005.

34. Huiskes R, Van Rietbergen B. Preclinical testing of total hip stems. *Clin Orthop.* 1995;319:64–76.

35. Huiskes R, Weinans H, Dalstra M. Adaptive bone remodeling and biomechanical design considerations for noncemented total hip arthroplasty. *Orthopedics.* 1989;12:1255–1267.

36. Huiskes R, Weinans H, Grootenboer HJ, et al. Adaptive bone-remodeling theory applied to prosthetic-design analysis. *J Biomech.* 1987;20:1135–1150.

37. Huiskes R, Weinans H, Van Rietbergen B. The relationship betweeen stress shielding and bone resoption around total hip stems and the effects of flexible materials. *Clin Orthop.* 1992;272:124–134.

38. Ilchmann T, Franzén H, Mjöberg G, et al. Measurement accuracy in acetabular cup migration. A comparison of four radiologic methods versus roentgen stereo-grammetric analysis. *J Arthroplasty.* 1992;7:121–127.

39. Jasty M, Maloney WJ, Bragdon CR, et al. The initiation of failure in cemented femoral components of hip arthroplasties. *J Bone Joint Surg.* 1991;73B:551–558.

40. Jasty M, O'Connor DO, Henshaw RM, et al. Fit of the uncemented femoral components and the use of cement influence the strain transfer to the femoral cortex. *J Orthop Res.* 1994;12:648–656.

41. Kaptein BL, Valstar ER, Stoel BC, et al. A new model-based RSA method validated using CAD models and models from reversed engineering. *J Biomech.* 2003;36:873–882.

42. Kärrholm J. Roentgen stereophotgrammetry. Review of orthopaedic applications. *Acta Orthop Scand.* 1989;60:491–503.

43. Kärrholm J, Borssén B, Löwenhielm G, et al. Does early micromotion of femoral stem prostheses matter? *J Bone Joint Surg.* 1994;76B:912–917.

44. Kärrholm J, Nivbrant B, Thanner J, et al. Radiosstereometric evaluation of hip implant design and surface finish. Presented at: Scientific Exhibition, AAOS Meeting; 2000; Orlando, FL.

45. Kärrholm J, Snorrason F. Migration of porous coated acetabular prostheses fixed with screws. *J Orthop Res.* 1992;10:826–835.

46. Keaveny TM, Bartel DL. Effects of porous coating and collar support on early load transfer for a cementless hip prosthesis. *J Biomech.* 1993;26:1205–1216.

47. Keaveny TM, Bartel DL. Mechanical consequences of bone ingrowth in a hip prosthesis inserted without cement. *J Bone Joint Surg.* 1995;77A:911–923.

48. Kerner J, Huiskes R, van Lenthe GH, et al. Correlation between pre-operative periprosthetic bone density and post-operative bone loss in THA can be explained by strain-adaptive remodelling. *J Biomech.* 1999;32:695–703.

49. Khang G, Choi K, Kim CS, et al. A study of Korean femoral geometry. *Clin Orthop Relat Res.* 2003;406:116–122.

50. Kleemann RU, Heller MO, Stoeckle U, et al. THA loading arising from increased femoral anteversion and offset may lead to critical cement stresses. *J Orthop Res.* 2003;21:767–774.

51. Kuiper JH, Huiskes R. Friction and stem stiffness affect dynamic interface motion in total hip replacement. *J Orthop Res.* 1996;14:36–43.

52. Kyriazis V, Rigas C. Temporal gait analysis of hip osteoarthritic patients operated with cementless hip replacement. *Clin Biomech Bristol Avon.* 2002;17:318–321.

53. Lengsfeld M, Gunther D, Pressel T, et al. Validation data for periprosthetic bone remodelling theories. *J Biomech.* 2002;3512:1553–1564.

54. Loizeau J, Allard P, Duhaime M, et al. Bilateral gait patterns in subjects fitted with a total hip prosthesis. *Arch Phys Med Rehabil.* 1995;76:552–557.

55. Lucht U. The Danish Hip Arthroplasty Register. *Acta Orthop Scand.* 2000;71:433–439.

56. Maher SA, Prendergast PJ. Discriminating the loosening behaviour of cemented hip prostheses using measurements of migration and inducible displacement. *J Biomech.* 2002;35:257–265.

57. Malchau H. *On the Importance of Stepwise Introduction of New Hip Implant Technology* [PhD thesis]. Göteborg, Sweden: Göteborg University; 1995.

58. Malchau H, Herberts P. Prognosis of total hip replacement. Presented at: Scientific Exhibit, 57th AAOS Meeting; 22–26 February 1996; Atlanta, GA.

59. Malchau H, Herberts P, Ahnfelt L. Prognosis of total hip replacement in Sweden. Follow-up of 92,675 operations performed 1978–1990. *Acta Orthop Scand.* 1993;64:497–506.

60. Malchau H, Kärrholm J, Wang YX, et al. Accuracy of migration analysis in hip arthroplasty. *Acta Orthop Scand.* 1995;66: 418–424.

61. Malik MH, Gambhir AK, Bale L, et al. Primary total hip replacement: a comparison of a nationally agreed guide to best practice and current surgical technique as determined by the North West Regional Arthroplasty Register. *Ann R Coll Surg Engl.* 2004;86: 113–118.

62. Maloney WJ, Smith RL, Schmalzried TP, et al. Isolation and characterization of wear particles generated in patients who have had failure of a hip arthroplasty without cement. *J Bone Joint Surg.* 1995;77A:1201–1210.

63. Mann KA, Bartel DL, Wright TM, et al. Coulomb frictional interfaces in modeling cemented total hip replacements: a more realistic model. *J Biomech.* 1995;28:1067–1078.

64. Massoud SN, Hunter JB, Holdsworth BJ, et al. Early femoral loosening in one design of cemented hip replacement. *J Bone Joint Surg Br.* 1997;79:603–608.

65. McKellop H, Campbell P, Park SH, et al. The origin of submicron polyethylene wear debris in total hip arthroplasty. *Clin Orthop.* 1995;311:3–20.

66. McMinn D, Treacy R, Lin K, et al. Metal on metal surface replacement of the hip. Experience of the McMinn prothesis. *Clin Orthop.* 1996;329(suppl):S89–98.

67. McNamara BP, Cristofolini L, Toni A, et al. Evaluation of experimental and finite element models of synthetic and cadaveric femora for pre-clinical design-analysis. *Clin Mater.* 1995;17: 131–140.

68. Mjöberg B. Fixation and loosening of hip prostheses. A review. *Acta Orthop Scand.* 1991;62:500–508.

69. Mjöberg B, Hanson LI, Selvik G. Instability, migration and laxity of total hip prostheses. A röntgen stereophotogrammetric study. *Acta Orthop Scand.* 1984;55:504–506.

70. Murray DW, Carr AJ, Bulstrode CJ. Which primary total hip replacement? *J Bone Joint Surg.* 1995;77B:520–527.

71. Noble PC, Alexander JW, Granberry ML, et al. The myth of "press-fit" in the proximal femur. Presented at: Scientific Exhibit, 55th AAOS Meeting; 4–9 February 1988; Atlanta, GA.

72. Olsson E. Gait analysis in hip and knee surgery. *Scand J Rehabil Med Suppl.* 1986;15:1–55.

73. Ostgaard SE, Gottlieb L, Toksvig-Larsen S, et al. Roentgen stereophotogrammetric analysis using computer-based image-analysis. *J Biomech.* 1997;30:993–995.

74. Perrin T, Dorr LD, Perry J, et al. Functional evaluation of total hip arthroplasty with five- to ten-year follow-up evaluation. *Clin Orthop.* 1985;195:252–260.

75. Peter B, Ramaniraka N, Rakotomanana LR, et al. Peri-implant bone remodeling after total hip replacement combined with systemic alendronate treatment: a finite element analysis. *Comput Methods Biomech Biomed Eng.* 2004;7:73–78.

76. Pilliar RM, Lee JM, Maniatopoulos C. Observation on the effect of movement on bone ingrowth into porous-surfaced implants. *Clin Orthop.* 1986;208:108–113.

77. Puolakka TJ, Pajamaki KJ, Halonen PJ, et al. The Finnish Arthroplasty Register: report of the hip register. *Acta Orthop Scand.* 2001;72:433–441.

78. Rothwell AG. Development of the New Zealand Joint Register. *Bull Hosp Joint Dis.* 1999;58:148–160.

79. Ryd L. Roentgen stereophotogrammetric analysis of prosthetic fixation in the hip and knee joint. *Clin Orthop.* 1992;276:56–65.

80. Saikko VO, Pavolainen PO, Slätis P. Wear of the polyethylene acetabular cup. Metallic and ceramic heads compared in a hip simulator. *Acta Orthop Scand.* 1993;64:391–402.

81. Sandborn PM, Cook SD, Spires WP, et al. Tissue response to porous-coated implants lacking initial bone apposition. *J Arthroplasty.* 1988;3:337–346.

82. Sarmiento A. Staying the course. *J Bone Joint Surg.* 1991;73A: 479–483.

83. Schimmel JW, Huiskes R. Primary fit of the Lord cementless total hip. A geometric study in cadavers. *Acta Orthop Scand.* 1988;59: 638–642.

84. Schmalzried TP, Kwong LM, Jasty M, et al. The mechanism of loosening of cemented acetabular components in total hip arthroplasty. Analysis of specimens retrieved at autopsy. *Clin Orthop.* 1992;274:60–78.

85. Schneider E, Eulenberger J, Steiner W, et al. Experimental method for the in vitro testing of the initial stability of cementless hip prostheses. *J Biomech.* 1989;22:735–744.

86. Selvik G. Roentgen stereophotogrammetry. A method for the study of the kinematics of the skeletal system. *Acta Orthop Scand Suppl.* 1989;232:1–51.

87. Shanbhag AS, Jacobs JJ, Glant TT, et al. Composition and morphology of wear debris in failed uncemented total hip replacement. *J Bone Joint Surg.* 1994;76B:60–67.

88. Snorrason F, Kärrholm J. Primary stability of revision total hip arthroplasty: a roentgen stereophotogrammetric analysis. *J Arthroplasty.* 1990;5:217–229.

89. Søballe K, Hansen ESB, Rasmussen H, et al. Tissue ingrowth into titanium and hydroxyapatite-coated implants during stable and unstable mechanical conditions. *J Orthop Res.* 1992;10:285–299.

90. Spears IR, Pfleiderer M, Schneider E, et al. The effect of interfacial parameters on cup-bone relative micromotions. A finite element investigation. *J Biomech.* 2001;34:113–120.

91. Steens W, Rosenbaum D, Goetze C, et al. Clinical and functional outcome of the Thrust Plate prosthesis: short- and medium-term results. *Clin Biomech Bristol Avon.* 2003;18:647–654.

92. Stolk J, Maher SA, Verdonschot N, et al. Can finite element models detect clinically inferior cemented hip implants? *Clin Orthop.* 2003;409:138–150.

93. Stolk J, Verdonschot N, Huiskes R. Hip-joint and abductor-muscle forces adequately represent in vivo loading of a cemented total hip reconstruction. *J Biomechanics.* 2001;34:917–926.

94. Stolk J, Verdonschot N, Christofolini L, et al. Finite element and experimental models of cemented hip joint reconstructions can produce similar bone and cement strains in pre-clinical tests. *J Biomechanics.* 2002;35:499–510.

95. Stolk J, Verdonschot N, Murphy BP, et al. Finite element simulation of anisotropic damage accumulation and creep in acrylic bone cement. *Eng Fracture Mech.* 2004;71:513–528.

96. Sugiyama H, Whiteside LA, Kaiser AD. Examination of rotational fixation of the femoral component in total hip arthroplasty. *Clin Orthop.* 1989;249:122–128.

97. Tulp NJA. Polyethylene delamination in the PCA total knee. Material analysis in two failed cases. *Acta Orthop Scand.* 1992;63: 262–266.

98. van Rietbergen B, Huiskes R. Load transfer and stress shielding of the hydroxyapatite-ABG hip: a study of stem length and proximal fixation. *J Arthroplasty.* 2001;16(8 suppl 1):55–63.

99. van Rietbergen B, Huiskes R, Weinans H, et al. ESB Research Award 1992. The mechanism of bone remodeling and resorption around press-fitted THA stems. *J Biomech.* 1993;26:369–382.

100. Verdonschot N. *Biomechanical Failure Scenarios for Cement Total Hip Replacement* [PhD thesis]. Nijmegen, The Netherlands: University of Nijmegen; 1995.

101. Verdonschot N, Huiskes R. The cement debonding process of THA stems and its effects on cement stresses. *Clin Orthop.* 1997;336:297–307.

102. Verdonschot N, Huiskes R. The effects of cement-stem debonding in THA on the long-term failure probability of cement. *J Biomech.* 1997;30:795–802.

103. Verdonschot N, Huiskes R. The mechanical effects of stem-cement interface characteristics in total hip replacement. *Clin Orthop.* 1996;329:326–336.

104. Verdonschot N, Huiskes R, Freeman MAR. Pre-clinical testing of hip prosthetic designs: a comparison of finite element calculations and laboratory tests. *J Eng Med.* 1993;207: 149–154.

105. Viceconti M, Pancanti A, Dotti M, et al. Effect of the initial implant fitting on the predicted secondary stability of a cementless stem. *Med Biol Eng Comput.* 2004;42:222–229.

106. Waide V, Cristofolini L, Stolk J, et al. Modelling the fibrous tissue layer in cemented hip replacements: experimental and finite element methods. *J Biomech.* 2004;37:13–26.

107. Walker P, Mai SF, Cobb AG, et al. Prediction of clinical outcome of THR from migration measurements on standard radiographs. *J Bone Joint Surg.* 1995;77B:705–714.

108. Walker PS, Schneeweis D, Murphy S, et al. Strains and micromotions of press-fit femoral stem prostheses. *J Biomech.* 1987;20:693–702.

109. Weinans H, Huiskes R, Grootenboer HJ. Effects of fit and bonding characteristics of femoral stems on adaptive bone remodeling. *J Biomech Eng.* 1994;116:393–400.

110. Weinans H, Huiskes R, Grootenboer HJ. Effects of material properties of femoral hip components on bone remodeling. *J Orthop Res.* 1992;10:845–853.

111. Weinans H, Huiskes R, Van Rietbergen B, et al. Adaptive bone remodeling around bonded noncemented total hip arthroplasty: a comparison between animal experiments and computer simulation. *J Orthop Res.* 1993;11:500–513.

112. West JD, Mayor MB, Collier JP. Potential errors inherent in quantitative densitometric analysis of orthopaedic radiographs. *J Bone Joint Surg.* 1987;69A:58–64.

113. Wiklund I, Romanus B, Hunt SM. Self-assessed disability in patients with arthrosis of the hip joint. Reliability of the Swedish version of the Nottingham Health Profile. *Int Disabil Stud* 1988;10:159–163.

114. Wright TM, Rimnac CM, Stulberg SD, et al. Wear of polyethylene in total joint replacement: observations from retrieved PCA implants. *Clin Orthop.* 1992;276:126–134.

115. Zhou XM, Walker PS, Robertson DD. Effect of press-fit femoral stems on strains in the femur. *J Arthroplasty.* 1990;5:71–82.

Fixation by Methyl Methacrylate

14

Andrew D. MacDowell   *Donald W. Howie*

Polymethyl methacrylate, otherwise known as "bone cement," has been used in the fixation of hip implants since the early 1960s. Sir John Charnley, the pioneer of modern day hip replacement, incorporated the use of cement in the development of low frictional torque hip arthroplasty.

Since then, the use of acrylic bone cement has become recognized as a highly reliable method of fixation. Cement does not act as an adhesive, as sometimes thought, but relies on an interlocking fit to provide mechanical stability at the cement–bone interface, while at the prosthesis–cement interface it achieves stability either by optimizing the fit of the implant in the cement mantle, such as in a tapered femoral stem, or by interlocking with the surface of a component such as in a cemented acetabular component.

Fixation using cement has evolved with development of improved cementing methods, changes in cement preparation, and a better understanding of how prosthesis design and surface finish can significantly improve outcome. Improved knowledge of the interrelationship between wear, periprosthetic osteolysis and aseptic loosening, and the observation that loosening also occurs in uncemented hip arthroplasty, has allayed concerns about "cement disease," and in fact, has led some to conclude that an optimally designed cemented femoral stem will decrease the problems of periprosthetic femoral osteolysis. In this chapter, the con-

cepts of femoral stem design and fixation, clinical results, and advances in understanding of the optimal use of cement are reviewed.

CEMENTED FEMORAL STEM DESIGN

The design of femoral stem clearly influences the clinical result either by effects at the prosthesis–cement interface, or how the stem transfers load to cement and thereby to bone. Increasingly it is recognized that it is a combination of shape and surface finish of the stem that significantly influences long-term results. Based largely on the surface finish of the stem, and also on the way the stem interacts with the cement mantle, two main philosophies of fixation have evolved, one based around a polished stem surface, the other based on a rough stem surface, with or without adjuvant fixation features.

Polished Stems Designed to Subside

The first approach uses the highly polished surface in concert with the shape of the metal stem to optimize fit of the stem within the cement mantle and ensure that wear due to micromotion at the prosthesis–cement interface is minimized. This approach recognizes the problem of relying on a rough surface to achieve and maintain adherence between a rigid metal stem and a self-polymerizing acrylic polymer.

Of the polished stems, there are essentially three types, some of which have been successful over a number of decades. There are, first, those modeled on the original polished Charnley stem (DePuy International Ltd., Leeds, U.K.), which have a rounded stem proximally with relatively rounded edges in cross section, especially medially, and a small collar; second, the collarless double-tapered stems, characterized by tapers from proximal to distal in the sagittal and frontal planes and a predominantly rectangular cross section proximally; and

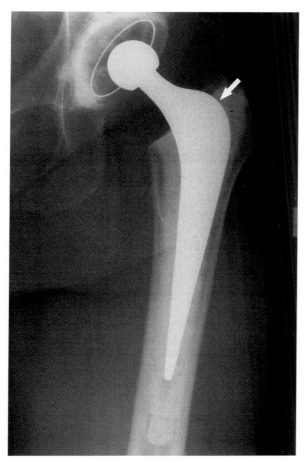

Figure 14-1 AP hip radiograph of a primary CCDT hip arthroplasty 1 year postoperatively, showing controlled subsidence (*arrow*).

third, and more recently, collarless triple-tapered stems, which have an additional taper from lateral to medial. The developers of the concept of the cemented collarless double-tapered (CCDT) stems, Ling and Lee, popularized the advantages of polished stems. Initially they had proposed optimizing loading of the cement by use of a double-tapered wedge-shaped stem. Later they appreciated the importance of controlled microsubsidence of the polished stem in the cement mantle to achieve and maintain intimate contact between stem and cement and to optimize loading of the cement and, thereby, the bone (Fig. 14-1). Further, it became apparent that the collarless design and polished surface combined with the viscoelastic properties of cement could allow for stress relaxation within cement, so preserving these optimal loading conditions.

It is likely the other types of polished stems share a number of the attributes of the polished CCDT stems, and this explains the good results. However, there are some subtle differences. The small collar of the more proximally rounded stems might interfere with subsidence, so preventing intimate contact of the stem within cement, especially in suboptimal cementing conditions. Also, these designs of stem and the recent triple-tapered stems have a less-pronounced rectangular cross section proximally and so may be less resistant to posterior rotation, a now-recognized important mechanism of stem loosening.

The proposed reason for the excellent clinical results of the polished CCDT stems is that they subside within the cement mantle, usually by a few millimeters, and this mainly occurs over the first few years following insertion. Simply put, and remembering that stems are subject to considerable anteroposterior forces, this ensures the stem wedges itself tightly into the cement mantle, thereby ensuring optimal contact between the stem and cement. Under load, axial forces are converted by the taper in the cement to radially compressive forces at the cement–bone interface. During periods of reduced load, tensile hoop strains remain within the cement, but stress relaxation can occur, with the taper maintaining the strain. Hughes et al. suggest that when load is reapplied, further controlled subsidence occurs again until a new equilibrium is reached (30). On the other hand, should a design aim for bonding between a rough-surfaced stem and cement, stress relaxation within the construct will not occur unless the interface is disrupted.

A proposed advantage of polished stems is that there is minimal wear of the cement and metal, should micromotion occur at the stem–cement interface. Thus wear-particle production is minimized, and any gap due to wear between the stem and cement is minimized. This, and maintenance of maximal contact by controlled subsidence, minimizes the access of wear-particle-containing joint fluid and attendant transmission of joint pressure to the femur via any defects in the cement mantle.

Anthony et al. (3) described four cases of localized endosteal bone lysis related to defects in the cement mantle in patients with otherwise radiologically well-fixed cemented matte Exeter (Stryker Howmedica Osteonics, Berkshire, U.K.) stems. They concluded that such defects in the cement mantle allow a route through which joint fluid could reach the cement–bone interface, subsequently leading to localized osteolysis and, ultimately, frank loosening. Fowler et al. showed that localized endosteal bone osteolysis is very rare when a polished tapered stem that can subside in its cement mantle is used (22).

Polished CCDT stems have been very successful. Williams et al. reported survivorship of 100% at 8 to 12 years for the Exeter modular stem (61), with the end point of revision for aseptic loosening. Yates et al. reported no aseptic loosening of the CPT stem at 5 years follow-up (64). The 2002 Swedish National Hip Arthroplasty Register report (58) shows a survivorship of 96% for Exeter stems at 10 years, and the 2002 Danish Hip Arthroplasty Register report describes a survivorship for CPT (Zimmer Inc., Warsaw IN, USA) stems of more than 98% at 6 years (17).

Rougher Stems Designed to Bond with Cement

The other philosophy of stem design aims to achieve rigid interlock between the stem and cement and thereby nullify movement at this interface. This includes matte, grit-blasted and beaded or porous surfaces and those with indentations. A further development of this philosophy includes those stems manufactured with a precoat of cement applied to the stem with the aim of improving bonding between the stem and cement.

It is proposed that the implant–cement–bone construct acts as a "composite beam," and the intention is to prevent movement at each of the interfaces. For this composite beam to be effective, there needs to be perfect bonding at both interfaces, with good support from the cement (53). If the construct is unable to withstand the stresses passing through it during loading, then either the cement mantle will fracture or undesirable movement will occur between implant and cement, leading to debonding at the interface. With this type of system, separation of the stem from cement, termed debonding, is thought to be an important event in the development of aseptic loosening. Harrigan and Harris, in a finite-element study of a stem designed to achieve bonding of the stem with cement, predicted a tripling of critical cement stress levels in the debonded construct compared to when bonding was present (24). Analysis of cemented stems of the rough type retrieved post-mortem has demonstrated separation of these stem types from cement and fractures within the cement (32,33). Thus, debonding of this design of stem is considered a predictor of failure, but this must be distinguished from the designed subsidence of polished tapered stems, which in fact is proposed to optimize fixation.

The post-mortem and other findings with rough or bonded stems has lead to an emphasis on obtaining a complete cement mantle, which lessens the chance of cement cracks and failure due to mechanical reasons and also access of joint fluid to the bone of the femur, resulting in osteolysis.

Rough or Smooth Stem? How Changes in Design and Surface Finish Affect Fixation

Interestingly, during the evolution of the cemented collarless double-tapered system, there were design changes that altered the way in which the implant behaved. When the double-tapered Exeter stem was inadvertently changed from its early polished design to a matte surface finish, the clinical results were far inferior to the early polished stems and those used for almost the last two decades.

Howie et al. compared the incidence of aseptic loosening of 20 polished nonmodular tapered Exeter stems with 20 stems that were identical apart from having a matte surface finish. At 9 years, 4 of the matte stems had been revised for aseptic loosening, while all of the polished stems were well fixed (28). Middleton and Howie showed that matte and polished Exeter stems behave differently in the cement mantle. Polished stems subsided in the cement mantle an average of 1 mm at 2 years following insertion but did not go on to loosen up to 12 years following surgery, while early debonding at the matte stem to cement interface was associated with early loosening (40).

The Charnley stem is another prosthesis that has undergone changes in its design over the past 40 years. In a number of studies, this prosthesis has been shown to have excellent long-term results. Wroblewski et al. demonstrated that even in high-demand young patients under the age of 51, the survivorship of the Charnley stem was 93% at 10 years, 74% at 20 years and 55% at 27 years following surgery (63). The initial design from the early 1960s was the polished, flat-backed stem, and long-term results using this implant have been impressive, with reports of survivorship of 85% at 20 years (52). In 1976, the second-generation stem was introduced with a satin surface finish and round-backed geometrical profile. All further design changes have maintained the satin finish. Interestingly, Dall et al. reported a 4- to 17-year clinical and radiological follow-up and found an 11% incidence of stem loosening in second- and subsequent-generation Charnley prostheses but only a 3% incidence when the original design had been inserted (16). Schulte noted that in his series of first-generation smooth flat-backed Charnley stems, a radiographic lucent line was commonly noted superolaterally between stem and cement, indicating debonding (52). Despite this, other features of aseptic loosening did not develop, the lucent lines did not progress, and the overall survivorship of the series was 85% at 20 years despite first-generation cementing techniques. Similarly, Berry et al. found that in a series of 279 consecutive smooth Charnley stems followed up for 20 years, early radiographic debonding did not have an effect on the long-term survival of the implant (5). However, when excessive migration with radiolucent lines of greater than 2 mm at the superolateral border of the stem was noted, there was significantly increased risk of aseptic loosening requiring revision.

These findings may support Shen's suggestion that the original smooth flat-backed design subsided in a controlled manner (53), while design changes including the satin finish and change in profile prevent this.

Crowninshield suggests that the fate of the debonded stem may depend in part on the surface roughness of the implant (15). While a rougher surface finish increases the interlock between stem and cement, if debonding does occur, motion at the interface can produce increased amounts of abrasion with cement debris production. This would be unfavorable as it might accelerate the adverse biological process of osteolysis and contribute to loosening.

Collis et al. demonstrated that in a single surgeon's extensive experience over a 27-year period, femoral stems with a rough surface were associated with higher rates of osteolysis and loosening than smooth stems (14). More recently, the same author compared clinical outcomes using rough and polished Iowa (Zimmer Inc., Warsaw IN, USA) stems with essentially the same geometrical profile and found that over a relatively short-term follow-up of just over 5 years, there was a significantly higher rate of revision and impending revision of the stem when a roughened grit-blasted implant was used compared to a polished implant (13). Similarly, Sporer et al. found a higher rate of aseptic loosening with the rougher grit-blasted Iowa stem compared to the smoother bead-blasted version (54).

The issue of whether to use a cemented polished or roughened stem is hotly debated among hip surgeons. Harris argues that it is impossible to look at surface finish as an independent variable when looking at failure of cemented implants (25). He states that aseptic loosening is multifactorial in etiology and refers to several series reported in the literature of roughened stems with good results (4,42,62).

Precoating of stems with polymethyl methacrylate has been used to try to improve the bond between implant and cement, as failure at this interface is thought to be the catalyst for the development of aseptic loosening. There have been reports of high loosening rates using this technique (19,45), but other groups have demonstrated good clinical outcomes. Clohisy et al. prospectively followed up a consecutive series of 121 hip arthroplasties using a precoated stem for an average of

10 years and reported that only 1 stem needed revising for aseptic loosening (12). Dowd et al. found that failure was more likely if there was a thin or deficient cement mantle or if the stem was not properly centralized within the canal (19). It may be that using precoated stems is technique dependent and works well when the stem is centralized within a good cement mantle of adequate thickness but is in danger of failure if these criteria are not met.

Stem Metallurgy

Stem metallurgy is probably as important as stem design and surface finish in determining how a cemented stem fares following insertion. Most stems inserted with cement in current practice are made of alloys of cobalt chrome or stainless steel. Historically, titanium alloys have been used with cement, with the proponents stating that the lower stiffness promotes less stress shielding of the proximal femur. This is probably beneficial in the uncemented stem scenario but has provided unique problems when combined with cement. Willert et al. revised 28 cemented Muller (Protek AG, Berne, Switzerland) straight titanium alloy stems for pain at an average of 25 months following insertion. At surgery they reported finding large amounts of titanium alloy, cement, and polyethylene debris together with evidence of crevice corrosion (60). Scalloping osteolysis was found secondary to debris particle-induced foreign body granulomas, and pain was explained by the crevice corrosion occurring in a highly acidic environment, confirmed by pH measurements. Willert et al. concluded that titanium alloys could no longer be recommended for cementing. Other authors have had similar experiences with titanium stems. Massoud et al. looked at 76 cemented titanium Capital (3M Health Care Ltd., Leicestershire, U.K.) stems with a mean follow-up of 26 months and found a 16% incidence of "definitely" loose stems and 10% that were "probably" loose (38). This, and other reports, led to the Medical Devices Agency in the United Kingdom issuing a hazard warning regarding the use of this product (39). Recently, Bowditch and Villar have suggested that the results of cemented titanium stems may not be as bad as previously reported, quoting their series of 122 arthroplasties using the cemented Howse II/Ultima (DePuy, Leeds, U.K.) stem with a survivorship of 97% at 7.5 years (9). However, the authors accept that these are only midterm results and that longer-term analysis is required.

RSA Studies of Cemented Stems

Improved technology has allowed more accurate assessment of how prostheses behave following insertion. Roengten stereophotogrammetric analysis (RSA) is a sensitive tool in measuring migration of prostheses. Karrholm et al. used RSA to study the migration of the femoral head in cemented Lubinus SP I (Waldemar Link, Hamburg, Germany) hip arthroplasties (34). At 4 to 7 years following implantation, 55 hips had not been revised, while 7 had been revised for symptomatic aseptic loosening. Interestingly, 49 of the 55 hips not revised showed some migration of the femoral head in a medial, posterior, or distal direction, or a combination thereof. This indicates that even in the clinically asymptomatic stable hip prosthesis designed to bond with cement, there is a small amount of migration of the stem. However, in the group requiring revision, RSA analysis demonstrated significantly more migration in all 7 hips, the femoral head translating in a medial, posterior, and distal direction, with the total translation ranging from 4.6 to 24.4 mm. The best predictor of medium-term survivorship of the stem was found to be the amount of migration measured on the 2-year assessment, with the probability of revision being greater than 50% if the total subsidence was 1.2 mm or more.

Alfaro-Adrian et al. have compared migration of the Exeter smooth-polished double-tapered stem with the satin finish modular Charnley Elite prosthesis, the latest-generation Charnley stem, using RSA (1). They concluded that migration of the tip of the Exeter stem was an average of 1 mm after 1 year, with movement entirely at the cement–prosthesis interface. This would be expected with a smooth-polished double-tapered stem designed to subside in a controlled manner and is comparable with the findings of Yates et al. with the CPT stem (64). With the Charnley Elite stem, the average distal migration was 0.3 mm at 1 year, with migration occurring at both the prosthesis–cement and cement–bone interfaces. For both designs, the stems stabilized after 1 year. In a subsequent study, the same group elaborated on the different patterns of subsidence occurring with the two systems (2); the Exeter migration subsidence was predominantly distal with slight tilt into valgus, while the Charnley Elite stem had slow distal migration but a tendency to rapid posterior head migration. While the authors point out that the results should only be applied to the two stems they studied, it is apparent that migration patterns differ quite markedly between different stems. One potential advantage of a collarless double-tapered stem, such as the Exeter or CPT, is that the predominantly rectangular cross-sectional profile provides additional torsional stability and prevents rotational migration into retroversion. One concern with certain bonded stems is that the biomechanical forces passing through the hip will take the whole construct into retroversion with movement at the cement–bone interface, and this will predispose to failure.

When analyzing the fixation achieved with cemented femoral stems, it is clear from these and other studies that differentiation should be made between the likely behavior of a collarless double-tapered stem and a bonded stem. However, it seems clear that for all types of design, early excessive migration is a predictor of failure by aseptic loosening. With the introduction of new implants on to the market, it is imperative to monitor migration closely using accurate measurement tools such as RSA.

Importance of a Good Cement Mantle

Over the past 30 years there has been increasing emphasis placed on improving the cement mantle around the prosthesis and so optimizing the fixation with cement. Refinements in cementing technique have been incorporated in an attempt to produce uniform, even cement mantles, without deficiencies or voids. Defects in the cement mantle can contribute to aseptic loosening, as they act as stress risers predisposing to mechanical failure ,and they can also allow joint fluid to reach the cement–bone interface and trigger the biological cascade responsible for osteolysis.

Barrack has described a radiographic grading system of the adequacy of the cement mantle around the femoral component (4). In this grading system from A through to D, a grade A is defined as a uniform, even "white-out" around the whole of the implant, while a grade D indicates a radiolucency of 100% at the cement–bone interface. Chambers et al. demonstrated that an inadequate cement mantle was predictive of poor clinical outcome, with radiographs showing Barrack grades C and D being more likely to progress to aseptic loosening than those with better cement mantles (10).

It is, however, interesting to note that CCDT stems have been used by many surgeons of varying experience and technical ability, but the results remain excellent. This suggests that, while the cement mantle is important, the CCDT stem is very forgiving of poor cement mantles, and this does not seem to be the critical issue as it is with rough stems.

Surgeons using CCDT stems, such as the Exeter and CPT, aim to leave a few millimeters of cancellous bone during preparation of the canal to obtain a good interlock at the cement–bone interface, allowing a 2- to 3-mm mantle of cement proximally, while the taper provides a thicker mantle distally with less risk of deficiency (Fig. 14-2). This technique is generally well accepted by CCDT users. Traditionally, users of rougher stems have adopted a similar aim of obtaining a mantle of at least 2 mm around the implant, as thin and deficient mantles have been associated with adverse results (10). Recently, this viewpoint has been challenged by Langlais et al., who have fashioned the phrase "the French paradox" to describe their finding that certain French-designed straight stems, which maximally fill the medullary canal with the intention of leaving thin or even incomplete mantles in places, have good medium- and long-term results (35). The authors of this paper challenge the traditionally accepted understanding of why cemented stems succeed or fail. Of note, some of these stem designs were polished, which likely contributed to the good results. It is also important to note that in two of the papers referenced to in this article, patients lost to follow-up exceeded 10%, and a worst-case analysis would not have yielded as convincing an argument. Be that as it may, these observations are interesting. However, it seems that current mainstream opinion, certainly in non-Francophone countries, continues to be one of attempting to obtain a complete mantle, approximately 2 mm thick, around the whole of the implant.

OPTIMIZING FIXATION WITH CEMENT

Cementing Technique

Initial cementing techniques relied on finger-packing cement into the medullary cavity. Modern-generation cementing techniques were developed with the introduction of cement plugs to prevent cement distalizing in the femur, retrograde cement insertion using guns and pulsed lavage to clean the cancellous bony interface, and the use of proximal seals with pressurization to allow better intrusion of cement into the trabecular bone. Further suggested refinements, so called third generation, involve mixing the cement in a centrifuge or vacuum during preparation.

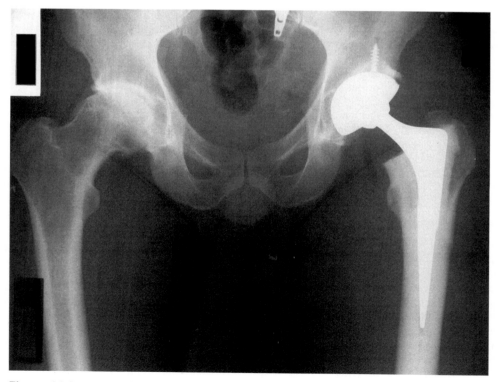

Figure 14-2   AP pelvis radiograph of a primary CCDT stem taken immediately postoperatively. Modularity of this system allows anatomical correction of the offset and leg length.

Modern cementing techniques have been reflected in the improved survivorship of implants. The Swedish Hip Arthroplasty Register annual report for 2002 reflects this improvement (58); in the period 1979 to 1991 when a variety of cementing techniques were incorporated, the survivorship of all cemented primary hip arthroplasty for osteoarthritis was 92% at 10 years when revision for aseptic loosening was used as an end point. This is still a satisfactory performance, but in the more recent cohort of patients from 1992 to 2002, in whom modern cement insertion techniques have been used, the survivorship is 95% at 10 years following surgery. This change may seem fairly moderate but perhaps reflects that even with early implant designs and cementing techniques, fixation with cement has been reliable. It will be interesting to see whether the reduction in revision rates for aseptic loosening becomes more pronounced in the 10- to 20-year reviews. To put these figures into perspective, the survivorship of all uncemented primary arthroplasty in the period 1992 to 2002 is 83% at 10 years with revision for aseptic loosening as the end point.

Modern generation techniques appear to have been near universally accepted as being the gold standard when inserting a cemented implant. The Swedish National Hip Arthroplasty Register reports that in 2002, of more than 12,000 primary cemented arthroplasties performed, in all cases a distal femoral plug and pulsed lavage were used, while in 85% a proximal femoral seal was used to pressurize the cement (58). The authors of the report state that regression analysis reveals clear advantages of pressurizing cement on the femoral side, and it is associated with a significantly reduced risk of revision for aseptic loosening.

Cement Preparation

While pressurization is well accepted, the issue of whether to vacuum-mix or hand-mix the cement during its preparation is more controversial. Theoretically, vacuum mixing may produce less-porous cement and hence produce a cement mantle with fewer voids due to trapped air bubbles. However, the 2000 report from the Swedish National Hip Arthroplasty Register showed that up to 5 years following surgery, there is an increased risk of early revision of vacuum-mixed cemented total hip replacements compared to manual hand-mixing (57). Muller et al. suggest that this may be explained by dynamic volume changes occurring during polymerization of the cement (41). They showed that hand-mixed porous cement undergoes a transient volume expansion before solidification, occurring at the critical time of microinterlock at the cement–prosthesis and cement–bone interfaces, and hence possibly improving fixation. Conversely, vacuum-mixed cement undergoes a progressive volume reduction throughout the polymerization process and may interfere with fixation. However, after 5 years the relative risk of revision using vacuum-mixed cement becomes less than manual mixing and continues to reduce with continued follow-up, and overall its use seems to be justified.

Timing of Insertion of Stem and Cement

The timing of cement introduction and implant insertion may affect the quality of fixation. Stone et al. investigated how the viscosity of cement at its insertion affects the bone–cement interface fixation (55). They found that cement introduced at an early, less-viscous stage produced higher failure strengths in push-out tests than cement inserted later. While cement should be injected as soon as it is manageable, the prosthesis should be inserted when the cement is in a more viscous state. Dayton et al. compared stem insertion in cadaveric femora early in the cement cure process to when the implant was introduced later (18). Radiographs showed significantly less radiolucency at the cement–bone interface in Gruen zones 2 and 6, with similar trends in the other zones, when the stems were inserted later in the cement curing process. This finding correlates with earlier work from the same group in which stem insertion into late cure stage, high-viscosity cement resulted in significantly higher intramedullary pressures and cement intrusion and suggests that delaying introduction of the implant can minimize voids at the cement–bone interface (11).

Preheating Stem

Preheating of the stem prior to its insertion is another technique used by some surgeons. During polymerization, cement reduces in volume. Curing of the cement starts at the warmer cement–bone interface, and so during volume reduction of the cement, shrinkage away from the implant may occur, causing voids at the cement–prosthesis interface. Theoretically, preheating the stem may cause some reversal of the direction of polymerization and prevent shrinkage of cement away from the stem. Bishop et al. looked at the effect of preheating stems prior to insertion into cadaveric femora and found that the area of porosity at the cement–stem interface was dramatically reduced compared to when stems at room temperature were inserted (6). They showed that the stem had to be preheated to at least 44°C to have an effect on the polymerization process.

Cement Brand

There are several different commercial brands of acrylic cement available for use in hip arthroplasty. Although each may be a polymer of methyl methacrylate, the precise chemical and physical properties may vary subtly, causing differences in the biomechanical properties of the cement.

This has been reflected in clinical outcome studies. There have been several reports of unacceptably high early failures due to aseptic loosening with the use of Boneloc (Biomet Inc., Warsaw IN, USA) cement (44,59), ultimately leading to the withdrawal of this product from sale. Using data from the Norwegian hip registry, Espehaug et al. assessed the survivorship of 17,323 primary Charnley arthroplasties and reported significantly increased rates of failure for prostheses inserted with CMW (DePuy International Ltd., Leeds, U.K.) cement compared to Palacos G (Schering–Plough, Welwyn, U.K.) (20). Havelin et al. had previously reported better survivorship with high-viscosity cement brands such as Palacos and Simplex (Howmedica Inc., London, U.K.), than low-viscosity preparations such as CMW3 (26).

Antibiotics in Cement

One potential advantage of using cement as the mode of fixation in hip arthroplasty is that antibiotics may be added for use as prophylaxis against deep infection. More recently, some centers have started impregnating the cement with much higher doses of antibiotic in revisions for septic loosening. However, there are issues regarding how this might affect the biomechanical properties of the cement, and these discussions are outside the scope of this chapter.

ACETABULAR COMPONENT

Clinical Results of Cemented Acetabular Components

Fixation of the acetabular prosthesis remains a challenge to hip surgeons. While long-term survivorship of well-designed stems up to 20 years and beyond is well documented, obtaining a reliable long-lasting acetabular fixation has proved more problematic. Fixation of the socket with cement is a well-established technique, and there are several studies reporting excellent medium to long-term survivorship. In an 8- to 12-year follow-up after insertion of a cemented cup, of which 94% were metal backed, Williams et al. report a survivorship of 97% of the socket with regard to revision for aseptic loosening (61).

However, although survivorship at 10 years appears satisfactory, particularly in the older age group, it seems that the fixation thereafter is less secure. Mulroy et al. reported an average 15-year follow-up of cemented primary hip arthroplasties (42); despite using second-generation cementing techniques for both the socket and stem, 10% of the all polyethylene cups had been revised for aseptic loosening, while 42% of the cups were radiographically loose according to Harris's criteria. In the same group of patients, the stems fared much better.

Bos et al. have analyzed the cement–bone interface in 25 autopsy specimens of acetabulae with apparently well-fixed cemented sockets (8); they found that with the exception of some focal direct cement–bone contacts, the bone and cement were separated by a soft tissue membrane. This membrane increased in thickness the longer the implant had been in situ and contained abundant infiltrates of histiocytes containing wear particles of cement and polyethylene.

Ritter et al. found that when the initial radiograph after surgery showed a radiolucency in DeLee and Charnley zone 1 following insertion of an all polyethylene Charnley cup, this was highly predictive of aseptic loosening (50). Hence, every effort must be made to try to obtain a good cement mantle around the cup with no radiolucent lines evident on the postoperative radiographs. As with the stem, care should be taken with cementing and insertion of the socket. The cancellous bony bed should be clean and dry prior to cement insertion, key holes need to be created, and cement should be pressurized in an attempt to improve intrusion of the cement and optimize interlocking fixation.

It should be noted that, while there is increasing use of cementless acetabular components, the reoperation incidence for these designs is high, and higher than good results with cemented components. Reoperation for liner exchange or osteolysis is much the same in terms of clinical insult to the patient as a simple cemented cup revision, with the same incidence of general complications, and is approximately the same complexity for an experienced revision surgeon. Therefore, it could be argued that the place for cementless acetabular components is not yet established and will not be until there is convincing evidence that the increased wear and massive osteolysis around cementless components have been overcome with new articulations and designs.

FIXATION WITH CEMENT IN REVISION HIP ARTHROPLASTY

Fixation with cement alone or with impaction grafting has been used for both the femoral and acetabular components in revision hip arthroplasty and should be considered an important part of the armamentarium of the hip surgeon. Also, cement offers the opportunity to undertake simple cement within cement femoral revision, cementing a component into a retained cup, into a reconstruction shell or cage, or into trabecular metal cups, as well as being used to fix augments to acetabular components. Importantly, cement can be used as a carrier for antibiotics during either one- or two-stage revision.

Cement in Acetabular Revision

Cemented Revision
On the acetabular side, revision using cement as the mode of fixation probably has limited indications. Certainly, if there are large bone deficiencies present, simply filling the area with cement is likely to give a tenuous fixation and the likelihood of early failure.

Cementing into Retained Components, Reconstruction Cages, and Revision Shells
Cementing a polyethylene acetabular component or liner into a retained component is a useful option available during socket revision. For example, during revision for recurrent dislocation, the surgeon may encounter a well-fixed but malaligned acetabular shell. Rather than remove the shell and risk creating further bony deficiencies during extraction, a polyethylene cup or liner can be cemented into the shell in the correct alignment.

When extensive acetabular deficiencies are present, structural augmentation is often indicated. Traditionally this has been managed with varying types of reconstruction cages supported by allograft, although more modern designs include trabecular metal shells with augmentation, which have promising early results. In both scenarios, cemented polyethylene cups are inserted following reconstruction of the socket.

Acetabular Impaction Grafting
A cemented acetabular component is also used in more complex acetabular revisions, where segmental defects are present that need reconstruction using techniques such as impaction grafting or reconstruction cages with bone grafting. In these scenarios, cement is currently the best mode of fixation available. Schreurs et al. reported an extensive experience of acetabular reconstruction with impaction grafting and a cemented cup and demonstrated a survivorship of over 90% at greater than 10 years follow-up in both primary and revision arthroplasty when revision for aseptic loosening was the end point (51).

Cement in Femoral Revision

Long-Stem Cemented Revision
Historically, early series of femoral revisions using cement had mixed results, but first-generation cementing techniques

together with the use of standard-length prostheses may have contributed to these outcomes (48,56).

More recently, there have been series using better-designed implants, including long stems, with modern cementing techniques, which have been very encouraging. The advantages of using cemented long-stem revision include immediate primary fixation, which allows full weight bearing and early rehabilitation, and it is particularly valuable in middle-aged and elderly patients who do not cope well with partial weight bearing. Other potential advantages of cemented long-stem revision are that the stem and cement combination acts as a custom device that fits the damaged femur exactly and can be used to fit femoral deficiency and deformity, without the need for aggressive bone removal or extended trochanteric or other corrective osteotomy; in this way the revision arthroplasty is simplified. Cemented fixation is along the whole of the stem, so that most types of proximal bone loss can be ignored, thus minimizing the risk of early subsidence that can be a problem with some cementless designs. If a polished collarless long stem with a continuous taper or consecutive dual taper is used, stem removal from the cement is relatively straightforward in cases of re-revision for instability or infection. Furthermore, these cemented long stems are relatively inexpensive compared to uncemented implants.

Hultmark et al. reported on a series of cemented revision stems with a survivorship of 92% at 10 years following surgery when re-revision for aseptic loosening was used as an end point (31). They noted that when long stems were used, the survivorship was 98% at 10 years. Using radiological criteria for aseptic loosening, this difference was exaggerated with a 65% survivorship for standard-length stems and 93% when long stems were used.

Recently, Howie et al. have reported a series of 190 revision hip replacements having either a standard- or long-stem cemented collarless double-tapered implant (29). They reported a survivorship to femoral re-revision for aseptic loosening at 8 years of 96% for long stems and 96% for standard stems, with no patients lost to follow-up. Of note is the excellent results with long-stem revision at up to 16 years follow-up This compares favorably with other series in terms of clinical outcome, and the authors report a low incidence of complications. Importantly, with regard to fixation, none of the surviving long stems had subsided more than 5 mm, indicating that the implants were stable. Also, it is interesting that the standard-length stems, while no longer recommended for revision without additional impaction grafting, had better survivorship than most reports of revision using other designs of standard stems even with third-generation cementing (21), suggesting that the collarless double-tapered polished stem is an optimal design for use with cement.

In comparing the clinical and radiological outcomes of revision total hip replacement using cemented, cementless, and hybrid fixation, Howie et al. concluded that the technique of cemented long-stem revision is successful at long term and is applicable for the majority of routine revisions (27) (Fig. 14-3). Long-stem revisions are increasingly used rather than standard-length stems as bone strains can be reduced to near normal levels if the revision stem passes beyond cortical diaphyseal defects by 1.5 femoral canal diameters (46), and finite-element analysis (37) shows a significant improvement in the relative motion and cement–bone interface stresses.

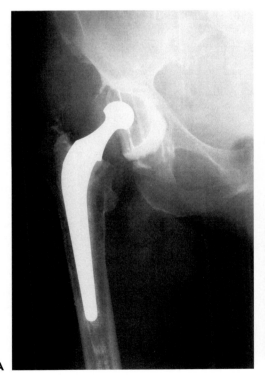
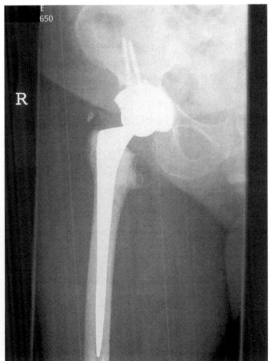

Figure 14-3   A: Preoperative radiograph of a patient with femoral osteolysis and loose acetabular component. **B:** Immediate postoperative radiograph of a long stem CCDT revision with a cementless acetabular component.

Given these findings it has been our practice to bypass cortical defects by 2 canal diameters and to extend the femoral stem 5 cm past the areas of major endocortical damage.

Cement in Cement Femoral Revision

"Cement into cement" stem revision is a relatively simple procedure that can be used when the femoral prosthesis has to be changed but the cement mantle is otherwise intact following removal of the component. It is particularly useful when a smooth-polished double-tapered prosthesis is in situ, since removal of the component is simply performed. This scenario may occur, for example, during revision for recurrent dislocation with a malaligned femoral prosthesis. Following extraction of the prosthesis, cement is inserted, and a correctly orientated but smaller-sized implant introduced. This technique relies on careful radiological assessment of the cement mantle preoperatively, but its advantage is that of simplifying the surgery yet maintaining good fixation.

Femoral Impaction Grafting

In younger patients where restoration of bone stock is a priority, or in cases of major bone loss, a cemented stem can be combined successfully with impaction grafting. Impaction grafting of the femur is a complex, technically demanding procedure, and, in some early reports, complications such as major early subsidence and periprosthetic fracture were a problem (47). However, it is recognized that there are unique advantages of the technique, with preservation of bone and remodeling of impacted graft to living bone (43). In many cases a standard-length stem can be used, thereby not transgressing the isthmus of the femur, and so minimizing problems of stress shielding, thigh pain, and the problems of re-revising a long stem in the future.

Impaction grafting can be used routinely for revision, and the clinical results when the technique is used for first revision are excellent (7,36,49), or it can be used selectively when other techniques are contraindicated, such as the large canal with osteoporotic bone that will not support a large cementless stem, in cases of angular deformity, where there is a distal TKR stem, or in patients having their third or fourth revision.

The polished CCDT stem in combination with impaction grafting incorporates a philosophy based on fundamental engineering principles represented by key design features of the prosthesis and the properties of polymethyl methacrylate bone cement. Recently, there have been very encouraging series with excellent clinical outcomes at long-term. Halliday et al. report a series of 226 hips revised with femoral impaction grafting techniques with survivorship of 99% at 10 years with femoral reoperation for symptomatic aseptic loosening as the end point (23). Development of improved and simplified techniques for impaction grafting, including modular tamping systems, aim to make the technique simpler for surgeons and avoid some of the earlier technical problems.

SUMMARY

Fixation with cement provides a very reliable form of fixation in both primary and revision hip arthroplasty. Long-term survivorship studies of primary hip arthroplasty indicate that when a well-designed femoral prosthesis is inserted with cement, the clinical results are excellent. Surgeons should be aware that a smooth, polished stem is designed to subside in a controlled manner within the cement, whereas rougher stems are designed to bond to the cement. Both these designs have good results, but increasing clinical, and now RSA evidence suggests the use of polished stems designed with a proximal shape that resists posterior rotational forces may be the optimum design. On the acetabular side, cement provides good clinical results at 10 years following insertion, especially in the elderly; however, in the second decade following surgery the rate of clinical and radiological loosening increases.

In revision hip arthroplasty, cement can usefully be used to fix new polyethylene liners into existing well-fixed acetabular shells and into reconstruction cages and newly designed reconstruction shells. Cemented collarless polished tapered long stems are successful at long-term follow-up and can be used in the majority of routine revisions. In the younger patient in whom restoration of bone stock is a consideration, impaction grafting with cement fixation has excellent results.

ACKNOWLEDGMENTS

The authors would like to acknowledge Kerry Costi for her assistance with the preparation of this chapter, and the support of the Royal Adelaide Hospital.

REFERENCES

1. Alfaro-Adrian J, Gill HS, Murray DW. Cement migration after THR. A comparison of Charnley Elite and Exeter femoral stems using RSA. *J Bone Joint Surg.* 1999;81B:130–134.
2. Alfaro-Adrian J, Gill HS, Murray DW. Should total hip arthroplasty femoral components be designed to subside? A radiostereometric analysis study of the Charnley Elite and Exeter stems. *J Arthroplasty.* 2001;16:598–606.
3. Anthony PP, Gie GA, Howie CR, et al. Localised endosteal bone lysis in relation to the femoral components of cemented total hip arthroplasties. *J Bone Joint Surg.* 1990;72B:971–979.
4. Barrack RL, Mulroy RD, Harris WH. Improved cementing techniques and femoral component loosening in young patients with hip arthroplasties: a 12-year radiographic review. *J Bone Joint Surg.* 1992;74B:385–389.
5. Berry DJ, Harmsen WS, Ilstrup DM. The natural history of debonding of the femoral component from the cement and its effect on long-term survival of Charnley total hip replacements. *J Bone Joint Surg.* 1998;80A:715–721.
6. Bishop NE, Ferguson S, Tepic S. Porosity reduction in bone cement at the cement-stem interface. *J Bone Joint Surg.* 1996;78B: 349–356.
7. Boldt JG, Dilawari P, Agarwal S, et al. Revision total hip arthroplasty using impaction bone grafting with cemented nonpolished stems and Charnley cups. *J Arthroplasty.* 2001;16(8):943–952.
8. Bos I, Fredebold D, Diebold J, et al. Tissue reactions to cemented hip sockets. Histological and morphometric autopsy study of 25 acetabula. *Acta Orthop Scand.* 1995;66:1–8.
9. Bowditch M, Villar RN. Is titanium so bad? Medium-term outcome of cemented titanium stems. *J Bone Joint Surg.* 2001;83B: 680–685.
10. Chambers IR, Fender D, McCaskie AW, et al. Radiological features predictive of aseptic loosening in cemented Charnley femoral stems. *J Bone Joint Surg.* 2001;83B:838–842.
11. Churchill DL, Incavo SJ, Uroskie JA, et al. Femoral stem insertion generates high bone cement pressurization. *Clin Orthop Relat Res.* 2001;393:335–344.
12. Clohisy JC, Harris WH. Primary hybrid total hip replacement, performed with insertion of the acetabular component without

cement and a precoat femoral component with cement: an average ten-year follow-up. *J Bone Joint Surg.* 1999;81A:247–255.

13. Collis DK, Mohler CG. Comparison of clinical outcomes in total hip arthroplasty using rough and polished cemented stems with essentially the same geometry. *J Bone Joint Surg.* 2002;84A:586–592.

14. Collis DK, Mohler CG. Loosening rates and bone lysis with rough finished and polished stems. *Clin Orthop Relat Res.* 1998;355:113–122.

15. Crowninshield RD, Jennings JD, Laurent ML, et al. Cemented femoral component surface finish mechanics. *Clin Orthop Relat Res.* 1998;355:90–102.

16. Dall DM, Learmonth ID, Solomon MI, et al. Fractures and loosening of Charnley femoral stems: comparison between first-generation and subsequent designs. *J Bone Joint Surg.* 1993;75B:259–265.

17. Danish Hip Arthroplasty Register. *2002 Annual Report.* Aarhus, Denmark: Danish Hip Arthroplasty Register; 2002.

18. Dayton MR, Incavo SJ, Churchill DL, et al. Effects of early and late stage cement intrusion into cancellous bone. *Clin Orthop Relat Res.* 2002;405:39–45.

19. Dowd JE, Cha CW, Trakru S, et al. Failure of total hip arthroplasty with a precoated prosthesis: 4 to 11 year results. *Clin Orthop.* 1998;355:123–136.

20. Espehaug B, Fumes O, Havelin LI, et al. The type of cement and failure of total hip replacements. *J Bone Joint Surg.* 2002;84B:832–838.

21. Eisler T, Svensson O, Iyer V, et al. Revision total hip arthroplasty using third-generation cementing technique. *J Arthroplasty.* 2000;15:974–981.

22. Fowler JL, Gie GA, Lee AJC, et al. Experience with the Exeter total hip replacement since 1970. *Orthop Clin N Am.* 1988;19:477–489.

23. Halliday BR, Rnglish HW, Timperley AJ, et al. Femoral impaction grafting with cement in revision total hip replacement. Evolution of the technique and results. *J Bone Joint Surg.* 2003;85B:809–817.

24. Harrigan TP, Harris WH. A three-dimensional non-linear finite element study of the effect of cement-prosthesis debonding in cemented femoral total hip components. *J Biomechanics.* 1991;24:1047–1058.

25. Harris WH. Long term results of cemented femoral stems with roughened precoated surfaces. *Clin Orthop Relat Res.* 1998;355:137–143.

26. Havelin LI, Espehaug B, Lie SA, et al. Prospective studies of hip prostheses and cements: a presentation of the Norwegian Arthroplasty Register 1987–1999. Presented at: 67th AAOS Meeting; 15–19 March 2000: Orlando, FL.

27. Howie DW, McGee M, Costi K, et al. Comparison of clinical and radiological outcomes of revision total hip replacement using cemented, cementless and hybrid fixation. Presented at: SICOT/SIROT 2002 World Congress, 212f; August 2002; San Diego.

28. Howie DW, Middleton RG, Costi K. Loosening of matt and polished cemented femoral stems. *J Bone Joint Surg.* 1998;80B:573–576.

29. Howie DW, Wimhurst JA, McGee M, et al. Mid to long term results of revision total hip replacement using cemented collarless double tapered stems. Presented at: 71st AAOS Meeting; 10–14 March 2004: San Francisco.

30. Hughes N, Gie GA, Lee AJC, et al. The time-dependent properties of bone cement and femoral component. *J Bone Joint Surg.* 1997;79B(suppl 3):367.

31. Hultmark P, Karrholm J, Stromberg C, et al. Cemented first-time revisions of the femoral component. Prospective 7 to 13 years' follow-up using second-generation and third-generation cementing technique. *J Arthroplasty.* 2000;15:551–561.

32. Jasty M, Maloney WJ, Bragdon CR, et al. Histomorphological studies of the long term skeletal responses to well fixed cemented femoral components. *J Bone Joint Surg.* 1990;72A:1220–1229.

33. Jasty M, Maloney WJ, Bragdon CR, et al. The initiation of failure in cemented femoral components of hip arthroplasties. *J Bone Joint Surg.* 1991;73B:551–558.

34. Karrholm J, Borssen B, Lowenhielm G, et al. Does early micromotion of femoral stem prostheses matter? *J Bone Joint Surg.* 1994;76B:912–917.

35. Langlais F, Kerboull M, Sedel L, et al. Annotation: The "French Paradox." *J Bone Joint Surg.* 2003;85B:17–20.

36. Ling RSM. Revision total hip arthroplasty. Cemented revision for femoral failure *Orthopedics.* 1996;19:763.

37. Mann KA, Ayers DC, Damron TA. Effects of stem length on mechanics of the femoral hip component after cemented revision. *J Orthop Res.* 1997;15:62–68.

38. Massoud SN, Hunter JB, Holdsworth BJ, et al. Early femoral loosening in one design of cemented hip replacement. *J Bone Joint Surg.* 1997;79B:603–608.

39. Medical Devices Agency. *Hazard Notice HN9801.* London: MDA; 1998.

40. Middleton RG, Howie DW, Costi K, et al. Effects of design changes on cemented tapered femoral stem fixation. *Clin Orthop Relat Res.* 1998;355:47–56.

41. Muller SD, Green SM, McCaskie AW. The dynamic volume changes of polymerizing polymethylmethacrylate cement. *Acta Orthop Scand.* 2002;73:684–687.

42. Mulroy WF, Estok DM, Harris WH. Total hip arthroplasty with use of so-called second generation cementing techniques. A fifteen-year average follow-up study. *J Bone Joint Surg.* 1995;77A:1845–1852.

43. Nelissen RGHH, Bauer T, Weidenhielm LRA, et al. Revision hip arthroplasty with the use of cement and impaction grafting. *J Bone Joint Surg.* 1995;77A:412–422.

44. Nilsen AR, Wiig M. Total hip arthroplasty with Boneloc: loosening in 102/157 cases after 0.5–3 years. *Acta Orthop Scand.* 1996;67:57–59.

45. Ong A, Wong KL, Lai M, et al. Early failure of precoated femoral components in primary total hip arthroplasty. *J Bone Joint Surg.* 2002;84A:786–792.

46. Panjabi MM, Trumble T, Hult JE, et al. Effect of femoral stem length on stress raisers associated with revision hip arthroplasty. *J Orthop Res.* 1985;3:447–455.

47. Pekkarinen J, Alho A, Lepisto J, et al. Impaction bone grafting in revision hip surgery. A high incidence of complications. *J Bone Joint Surg.* 2000;82B:103–107.

48. Pellicci PM, Wilson PD, Sledge CB, et al. Long-term results of revision total hip replacement. A follow-up report. *J Bone Joint Surg.* 1985;67:513–516.

49. Piccaluga F, Gonzalez Della Valle A, Encinas Fernandez JC, et al. Revision of the femoral prosthesis with impaction allografting and a Charnley stem. A 2- to 12-year follow-up. *J Bone Joint Surg.* 2002;84B:544–549.

50. Ritter MA, Zhou H, Keating EM, et al. Radiological factors influencing femoral and acetabular failure in cemented Charnley total hip arthroplasties. *J Bone Joint Surg.* 1999;81B:982–986.

51. Schreurs BW, Slooff TJ, Gerdeniers JW, et al. Acetabular reconstruction with bone impaction grafting and a cemented cup: 20 years' experience. *Clin Orthop Relat Res.* 2001;393:202–215.

52. Schulte KR, Callaghan JJ, Kelley SS, et al. The outcome of Charnley total hip replacement with cement after a minimum twenty year follow-up. The results of one surgeon. *J Bone Joint Surg.* 1993;75A:961–975.

53. Shen G. Femoral stem fixation. An engineering interpretation of the long-term outcome of Charnley and Exeter stems. *J Bone Joint Surg* 1998;80B:754–756.

54. Sporer SM, Callaghan JJ, Olejniczak JP, et al. The effects of surface roughness and polymethylmethacrylate precoating on the radiographic and clinical results of the Iowa hip prosthesis. A study of patients less than 50 years old. *J Bone Joint Surg.* 1999;81A:481–492.

55. Stone JJ, Rand JA, Chiu EK, et al. Cement viscosity affects the bone-cement interface in total hip arthroplasty. *J Orthop Res.* 1996;14:834–837.

56. Stromberg CN, Herberts P. A multicentre 10-year study of cemented revision total hip arthroplasty in patients younger than 55 years old. A follow-up report. *J Arthroplasty.* 1994;9:595–601.

57. Swedish Arthroplasty Register. *2000 Annual Report.* Göteborg, Sweden: Swedish Arthroplasty Register; 2000.

58. Swedish Arthroplasty Register. *2002 Annual Report.* Göteborg, Sweden: Swedish Arthroplasty Register; 2002.

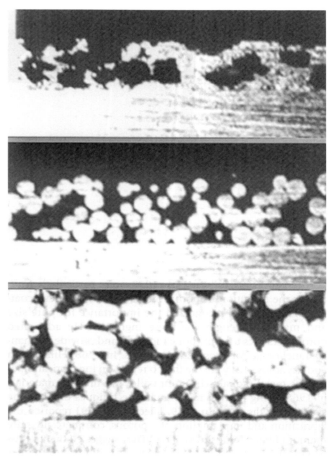

Figure 15-1 Cross section through some of common porous coatings. **Top:** Plasma-sprayed coating. **Middle:** Sintered sphere coating. **Bottom:** Fiber mesh coating.

porous ceramic materials (16) did not become as popular as the clinical application of porous metal materials.

Current metallurgical techniques allow the fabrication of a wide variety of porous-surfaced implants with a variety of materials, pore sizes, pore geometries, and attachments of porous coatings to solid metal substrates of the implants (Fig. 15-1). The majority of total joint prosthesis used today employ the biologic fixation methods using porous-surfaced metal implants. The subsequent sections in this chapter discuss requirements and the results in the clinical use of these implants as load-bearing members in total joint replacements.

BASIC REQUIREMENTS FOR INGROWTH

The principal requirements for osseointegration (6,40) and bone ingrowth (111,113) are now well understood. The term *osseointegration* refers primarily to the attachment of implants to bone where the implants become part of the bone by bone ingrowth into the porous surfaces or by bone ongrowth onto the surface of an implant that is not porous but rough or textured on a microscopic scale (5,6). The term *bone ingrowth* refers to actual bone formation within the porous surface structure of an implant and the interconnection of ingrown

bone spicules within the porous coating. This chapter primarily discusses the latter phenomenon, although there is evidence from animal experimental studies that a textured surface (i.e., a surface roughening by grit blasting) also is excellent for bone implant attachment (31,35). Thus *bone ingrowth* in this context refers to interconnecting bone within the porous coating that is a three-dimensionally interconnecting porous layer.

The physiologic response to a porous-coated implant inserted into bone after rasping or reaming the bone resembles the healing cascade of cancellous defects, with the newly formed tissues occupying the void spaces of the porous material. Repair of a hole drilled within the medullary canal of a long bone or a cavity created by reaming the subchondral bone of the acetabulum is associated with the formation of a hematoma and development of mesenchymal tissue, which is replaced by woven bone. Intramembranous bone formation is seen in and around the porous coating in as little as a week after surgery, and extensive woven bone is seen in the porous coating by 3 weeks. Lamellar bone remodeling soon follows, as does re-establishment of the bone marrow usually by around 6 weeks. As in primary fracture healing with stable osteosynthesis (73), no intermediate fibrocartilaginous stage occurs. However, rare areas of callus and endochondral bone formation can be seen with porous-coated implants, probably reflecting the small amount of micromovements that occur at the bone–porous coating interface. Consequently, the clinical success of biologic fixation by bone ingrowth depends on a stable implant–bone interface. Implants that obtain only fibrous tissue ingrowth rather than bone ingrowth can function well on occasion but not as reliably and consistently as those that obtain bone ingrowth.

BIOCOMPATIBILITY OF IMPLANT MATERIALS

Various metallic, ceramic, and polymeric implant materials have been introduced in joint replacements over the years. These implant materials are known to demonstrate different patterns of biocompatibility.

Based on animal experimental studies, the reactive new bone formation adjacent to the material surfaces can be categorized, according to Osborn (79), as distance osteogenesis, contact osteogenesis, and bond osteogenesis, with subsequent classification of the extent of biocompatibility (Table 15-1). However, transmission electron microscopy studies have demonstrated that the implant–bone ultrastructures for chemically pure (CP) titanium (Ti), Ti6Al4V, cobalt–chromium (Co-Cr) alloy, and stainless steel were comparable.

Accordingly, various porous surface technologies were developed, including porous metals (titanium [33,69], cobalt-chromium-molybdenum alloy [15,42,125], and stainless steel [29,98]), porous polymers (Teflon, polyethylene, polysulfone, and polypropylene [8,17,64,104–106]), porous carbon (17,76), and porous ceramics (8,43,64). Only the porous coatings of titanium, cobalt-chromium-molybdenum, Teflon, polysulfone, and polyethylene have been used clinically. Presently, the porous materials that are most commonly used are porous metal coatings because of their excellent biocompatibility and strength. These coatings are applied by sintering techniques (Co-Cr microspheres, Co-Cr

TABLE 15-1
BIOCOMPATIBLE MATERIALS AND THEIR REACTIVE BONE FORMATION

Materials	Extent of Biocompatibility	Reactive Bone Formation
PMMA	Biotolerant	Distance osteogenesis
Stainless steel	Biotolerant	Distance osteogenesis
Al_2O_3 ceramic	Bioinert	Contact osteogenesis
Carbon	Bioinert	Contact osteogenesis
Ti-based alloys	Bioinert	Contact osteogenesis
Co-Cr–based alloys	Bioinert	Contact osteogenesis
Ca-P ceramics	Bioactive	Bond osteogenesis
Surface-active glass	Bioactive	Bond osteogenesis

PMMA, polymethlmethacrylate.

fiber–metal composites, CP Ti fiber–metal composites, and CP Ti microspheres). One of the sintering techniques is diffusion bonding, where metal titanium fibers are pressed to a solid titanium substrate under pressure and temperature so as to weld the fibrous porous coatings onto the metal substrate. More recently, trabecular metal surfaces made of tantalum materials, which have greater porosity than sphere or fiber coatings, have also become popular.

EXPERIMENTAL MODELS FOR THE ASSESSMENT OF BONE INGROWTH

Numerous animal models have been used to assess bone ingrowth. Models using rodents appear to have the disadvantage of a comparatively high bone formation rate. The bone formation rates of primates, canines, sheep, and pigs are closer to human bone formation rates. Therefore, the majority of experimental studies were done using the later models and employed quantitative means to assess bone ingrowth and strength of fixation (11,26,48,110,115). A recent study comparing primate and canine models for bone ingrowth experimentation found no significant difference in bone growth into the experimental plugs between the two animal models, indicating the acceptability of cross-species interpretation of existing data from dogs (95). Most models were used for both weight-bearing and non-weight-bearing study designs. In both types of models, either the implants are placed in a press fit fashion to ensure intimate contact with the host bone or interfacial gaps are created by overdrilling or over-reaming.

A more complicated though clinically more relevant approach is to use a weight-bearing revision model. In this model, an initial implant is fixed by bone cement in a manner predisposing to loosening of the implant. The loosening process is accompanied by and presumably caused by a histiocytic response and bone resorption. Once the cemented implant is loose, it is surgically removed, and the failed prosthesis is replaced with a cementless porous-coated revision implant. Because of the loosening process, the medullary cavity in the region of the implant is devoid of normal marrow, and gaps are present between the revision implant and the host bone.

In the press-fit model, the control is usually an untreated press-fit implant. In the gap studies, a negative control is provided by an untreated gap, and a positive control is provided by a press-fit implant. In the revision studies, a negative control is provided by untreated implants. The negative control is needed to determine if the graft material has an enhancing effect (i.e., to determine if it improves the amount of bone ingrowth or the strength of fixation of the implant). A positive control is useful in that it indicates the maximal amount of bone ingrowth or fixation strength that can reasonably be expected.

PORE SIZE AND SHAPE AND POROSITY

In order for bone ingrowth into the porous coating to occur, appropriate pore size must be provided. Bone trabeculae and osteons are on the order of tens of micrometers thick, and pore size should be at least on this order; otherwise bone ingrowth would not occur. A pore size of greater than 100 μm would allow structural organization to the ingrown bone (trabecular and osteonal spaces) and would be desirable. However, a pore size greater than 500 μm up to a millimeter would resemble a macrotextured surface rather than a three-dimensionally interconnecting porous surface and theoretically would lead to loss of interface shear strength. The effect of pore size on the strength of fixation has been investigated in canine models using pore sizes ranging from less than 50 μm to 800 μm. In studies examining pore sizes less than 100 μm, increased pore size was associated with increased strength of fixation (88,125). Most studies analyzing pore sizes in the range 150 to 400 μm have shown no relationship between pore size and strength of fixation (2,25,66), although one study suggested a decrease of bone ingrowth and strength of fixation (19) when the pore size was increased (in the range 175 to 325 μm). In a weight-bearing canine total hip replacement model, however, it has been reported that more bone ingrowth was observed in acetabular components with 450-μm and 200-μm pores than in those with 140-μm pores (48). From these studies, it can be concluded that the optimal range for pore sizes is 100 to 400 μm. Most of the porous-coated prostheses currently in use have pore sizes in this range (56).

The porosity of the porous-coating layer is also an important parameter governing the fixation of porous-coated implants. Sintering techniques in current clinical use provide porosities of around 30% to 50%. The wire mesh and cancellous structured porous coatings generally provide greater degrees of porosity without compromising the structural integrity of the porous coatings than do the plasma-sprayed or sintered sphere porous coatings. Some of the early implants with plasma-sprayed and sintered sphere coatings had problems with the coating separations, but most coatings used today have adequate strength and porosity to be successful in clinical use.

Another important parameter determining the mechanics at the bone–porous coating interface is the interconnecting pore size. This is the size of the pore where one pore interconnects to another pore within the porous coating. Larger numbers of interconnecting pores with adequate interconnecting pore sizes lead to better strength at the bone–porous coating interface, particularly in tension, owing to the three-dimensional

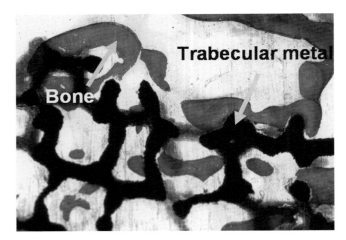

Figure 15-2 Bone ingrowth into tantalum trabecular metal porous coating. See Color Plate.

interconnectivity of the ingrown bone. The interconnecting pore sizes are partly dependent on the techniques used to fabricate the porous surface. In general, the connecting pores are larger in fiber metal and trabecular metal porous coatings and wire mesh porous coatings than the connecting pores in sintered porous coatings, which in turn are larger than the connecting pores in plasma-sprayed or corundum roughened surfaces. This is because the porous surface geometry can be better controlled with the meshes than it can be with spheres or sprayed coatings. For example, the pore geometry and size are determined by the diameter of the spheres and their spacing in sintered sphere coatings. Excessively increasing the size of the spheres or packing them too loosely in order to increase the interconnecting pore sizes would lead to loss of the interconnections (or welds) between the spheres and thus to loss of porous coating strength. Current sintering techniques, however, are able to provide adequate strength of porous coatings and of the bone–porous coating interface to maintain firm and long-lasting fixation of implants to the skeleton with any of the porous coatings in clinical use. Some of the newer porous coatings, such as the trabecular metal porous coating, are thought to have the advantage of providing increased porosity and interconnecting pore sizes while retaining high strength of the porous coating (Fig. 15-2).

IMPLANT STABILITY OR MICROMOTION

Uncemented porous-coated implants require bone ingrowth for long-term stability. Rigid initial fixation by mechanical means is necessary for these implants to allow bone ingrowth that provides long-term stability. The initial fixation is provided by a variety of surgical techniques, such as ancillary fixation with screws, ancillary fixation with projections from the implants (e.g., spikes and pegs), or press-fit fixation where the implant is driven into a cavity that is slightly undersized compared with the dimensions of the implant. The particular method of initial fixation employed depends on the types of implants and the location of their use as well as the philosophy of the designers. Most acetabular components are fixed by press-fitting a hemispherical component into a slightly undersized hemispherical cavity and

by supplemental fixation employing screws inserted through the component into the adjacent bone. Most femoral components are fixed by press-fitting a cylindrical or conical implant into the femoral canal, which is prepared to be slightly smaller than the implant either in the diaphysis or the metaphysis.

The implants that are designed to have bone grow into the porous surface rely on a tight initial fit in the bone. Over time, bone is expected to grow into the interconnected pores and firmly incorporate and fix the implant to the bone. If the bone grows into and remains in the pores, these implants should theoretically provide a stable and permanent fixation. Unfortunately, even the very slightest motion between the implant and bone may inhibit, prevent, or delay the growth of bone into the pores. There is evidence that too much relative motion between the implant and host bone leads to ingrowth of fibrous connective tissue rather than bone. The extent of implant stability contributes to a reduction in relative motion between the implant and host bone (7,97,108,122). It has been demonstrated in experimental studies in which fixed micromotions were applied to porous-coated implants in vivo that micromotions of 150 μm induce fibrous tissue ingrowth (11,44). Micromotions of 150 μm did allow the formation of woven bone within a porous titanium wire surface (Fig. 15-3). However, there appeared to be no osseous continuity between the woven bone within the coating and the trabecular bone adjacent to the implant. The interface formed under displacements of 40 μm was composed of a mixture of bone and fibrous tissue. The interface formed under displacements of 0 μm and 20 μm consisted predominantly of bone ingrowth without intervening fibrous tissue or fibrocartilage. In another animal study, bone ingrowth was observed in situations where the relative displacements were less than 28 μm, but when the displacements were greater than 150 μm, only mature connective tissue provided the fixation (83).

Although the studies just described employed fixed displacements to implant plugs in bone, other studies measured the initial stability of femoral components in canine femurs and compared that to the femoral component stability in vivo after bone ingrowth had taken place (51). These studies showed that an average initial micromotion of around 60 μm was found immediately after femoral component insertion, but excellent bone ingrowth occurred with this degree of motion. The bone ingrowth markedly increased the stability of the femoral component, which measured less than 10 μm after bone ingrowth had taken place.

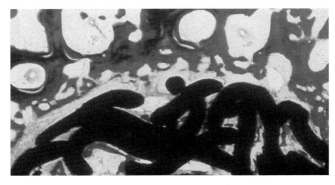

Figure 15-3 Fibrous tissue formation at the interface of a porous-coated plug that had induced motion of 150 μm in vivo. See Color Plate.

Recent roentgen stereophotogrammetric analysis (RSA) in vivo studies in porous-coated THA and total knee arthroplasty (TKA) components have demonstrated that in many cases the analyzed micromotions were well above the limits of bone ingrowth compatibility (54,55,58,77,91). Bone ingrowth can occur even with such movements.

It is difficult to define accurately the initial stability require for bone ingrowth in terms of micromotion, however. This is because the implants are subjected to fixed loads and not fixed displacements in vivo. During the days and weeks following implantation, an implants is gradually further stabilized by enchondral or intramembranous bone formation, maturation of the ingrown bone, and remodeling, each of which reduce the micromotion under a given load. Although all of this is going on, the amount of initial press-fit decreases, due to relaxation of surrounding bone and its remodeling. Thus it is difficult to determine accurately the initial micromotion below which bone ingrowth occurs and above which fibrous tissue ingrowth occurs. In a canine total hip arthroplasty (THA) model, bone ingrowth has been observed in femoral components that had an initial micromotion of 56 μm (51). It is generally assumed, however, that initial stability of the prosthetic component with micromotions less than about 100 μm should be maintained for bone ingrowth to occur.

Additional hydroxyapatite (HA) coating demonstrated an effect on the architecture of fibrous tissue formation in a weight-bearing canine gap model, allowing controlled micromovements of 150 μm. In this study (103), both the HA-coated and the titanium porous-coated implants had only fibrous tissue ingrowth. However, there was a stronger fibrous anchorage of the HA-coated implants, together with the presence of fibrocartilage, higher collagen concentration, and radiating orientation of the collagen fibers.

It can be concluded that bone ingrowth depends on an optimal primary stability. From a clinical perspective, this primary stability can vary depending on implant design variables (cross-sectional geometry, means of additional fixation, mismatch in implant–bone stiffness), implantation technology variables (accuracy of tools for rasping, reaming, drilling, sawing), surgical technique variables (accuracy of utilization of the implantation technology), and patient variables (bone quality, bone defects). Most of the contemporary implants and current surgical techniques are adequate to achieve bone ingrowth fixation of porous-surfaced implants consistently and reliably.

INTERFACE DISTANCES

The lack of a direct and continuous interface contact between the porous surface and the host bone has a negative effect on bone ingrowth and strength of fixation in both weight-bearing and non-weight-bearing models. Numerous gap models with a controlled gap and a stable implant have demonstrated the inhibiting effect of gap size on bone ingrowth and strength of fixation.

Laboratory animal studies employing canine total hip models have shown that in weight-bearing porous-coated acetabular components, gaps between the bone and porous coatings as little as 0.5 mm at the time of implantation adversely effect the bone ingrowth and lead to fibrous tissue formation (48). Current surgical techniques, instruments, and

implants allow this degree of precision in primary surgery, though some gaps are unavoidable in revision surgery.

A 2-mm non-weight-bearing gap model with a Ti porous-coated implant was used to analyze the effect of an additional HA coating. After an in situ duration of 3 weeks, the amount of bone ingrowth was 6 times higher for the press-fit inserted implants than for the contralateral 2-mm gap control (56,61). Other studies have also demonstrated that gaps at the interface of 2 mm and less impair bone ingrowth (3,15,48,72,93).

In two studies, bone ingrowth was impaired by a 3-mm gap (60,116). Compared to a similar press-fit model with intimate bone implant contact, the amount of bone ingrowth was reduced sixfold (115). In one canine non-weight-bearing study, gap sizes of 2, 1, and 0.5 mm were compared with a press-fit situation. The increase of the gap size led to a decrease in both bone ingrowth and strength of fixation (26).

Clinically, these studies imply the importance of accomplishing direct implant bone contact by employing precise surgical techniques, instruments, and implants.

STRESS SHIELDING

Major bone loss of the proximal femoral cortex due to stress shielding has been a problem in using uncemented, porous-coated femoral components, particularly when very large, stiff prosthetic components are used. This is due to the fact that a normal bone, such as the femur, deforms under load but that metallic prosthetic components larger than about 14 mm in diameter are much stiffer than the cortical bone and prevent the bone from deforming (bending) under load if firmly attached to the bone by bone ingrowth. The proximal femur is thus exposed to much lower levels of stress, which leads to disuse osteopenia. The more extensively the prosthesis is porous coated, the greater this stress protective effect. The stress protective effect is also greater with larger prostheses.

Canine studies have demonstrated this stress protective effect. Extensively porous femoral components (porous coating in the diaphysis as well metaphysis) fixed to the metaphysis and diaphysis produced extensive cortical thinning and porosis as early as 6 months after surgery. Hollow femoral components produced less proximal cortical atrophy than solid stems owing to the reduced stiffness of the hollow components. Prostheses with the porous coatings confined to the proximal portions also showed less proximal cortical atrophy than fully porous coated components.

Reducing the stiffness of the femoral component by employing composite plastic femoral components with small diameter metal cores (for strength) has been investigated in animal studies. A composite plastic stem containing a central carbon fiber core surrounded by molded poly-etheretherketone (PEEK) with a titanium fiber metal porous coating has been investigated in a canine study. The stiffness of the composite femoral stems was approximately 25% that of the metal stems. In spite of the lower modulus, excellent bone ingrowth into the porous layer of this stem occurred; further, there was no significant difference in the amount of bone ingrowth or the quality of ingrown bone compared with the fully metal stems, while proximal femoral cortical atrophy was lessened. The composite plastic femoral stems are in clinical use and are advocated by some for patients with large femoral canals.

Femoral components with porous coatings confined to the proximal aspects are preferred by many surgeons over fully porous coated femoral components. It is believed that they cause less proximal bone atrophy as well as less thigh pain. The decrease in thigh pain is attributed to a decrease in stress concentration at the tip of the femoral component. Even though the proximally porous coated femoral components contain less porous coating than the fully porous coated femoral components, the amount of bone ingrowth in these devices appears sufficient to provide the necessary stability for clinical use in almost all patients.

ENHANCEMENT OF BONE INGROWTH

Although excellent biologic fixation by bone ingrowth can now be achieved consistently with proper implants and surgical techniques, there was a need to enhance bone ingrowth in the early postoperative periods through biologic means, especially in the more vigorous patients, those with poor bone stock, and those undergoing revision surgery. A variety of means were tried to achieve bone ingrowth earlier and in greater amounts. Autogenous or allogenic bone grafts, demineralized bone, electromagnetic irradiation, systemic anti-bone-resorbing agents, osteoconductive calcium phosphates, and osteoinductive bone-stimulating proteins with different

TABLE 15-2
EFFECT OF LOCAL FACTORS ON BONE INGROWTH/STRENGTH OF FIXATION

| Author (Ref.) | Non-Weight-Bearing Model | | Weight-Bearing Model | | | | | | |
	pf	Gap	pf	Gap	Revision	Species	Time Interval (Weeks)	Control	Comment
Autogenous bone graft									
Rivero (85)	o					Dog	2, 4, 6	ut	
Lewis (67)		+				Dog	4, 8, 16	ut, pf	pf after 4 weeks
Kienapfel (59)		+				Dog	4, 8	ut	
Shen (96)		(+)				Rabbit	4, 8, 12	ut	pf after 8 weeks
Kang (53)				+		Dog	6, 12	ut	
McDonald (72)					+	Dog	12	ut	
Turner (120)					+	Dog	24	ut	
Hofmann (43)	+					Human	6–49	ut	
Fresh-frozen allogenic bone graft									
Lewis (67)		+				Dog	4, 8, 16	ut, pf	pf after 4 weeks
Soballe (103)		+				Dog	6	ut	
McDonald (72)					+	Dog	12	ut	
Freeze-dried allogenic bone graft									
Kienapfel (59)		(−)				Dog	4, 8	ut	
Demineralized bone matrix									
McLauglin (74)	+					Dog	6	ut	
Rivero (85)	−					Dog	2, 4, 6	ut	
Shen (96)		(+)				Rabbit	4, 8, 12	ut	pf after 8 weeks
Demineralized bone matrix mixed with fibrin adhesive system									
Shen (96)		(−)				Rabbit	4, 8, 12	ut	
Bone morphogenetic protein									
Kozinn (65)	(−)					Rabbit	1–8	ut	
Hermens (41)				(−)		Dog	3–8	ABG	
Transforming growth factor-beta (together with HA/TCP coating)									
Sumner (116)		+				Dog	4	ut	
Prostaglandin F$_{2\alpha}$									
Trancik (118)	+					Rabbit	2, 4, 8	ut	
Fibrin adhesive system									
Pflüger (81)		+				Dog	1	ut	very small gap
Kienapfel (60)		(−)				Dog	4, 8	ut	
Roy (89)					(−)	Dog	12	ABG	no homog. gap

+, enhancement of bone ingrowth and/or strength of fixation; −, inhibition of bone ingrowth and/or strength of fixation; (o), no enhancement or inhibition; (+), possible enhancement but no negative control (untreated gap); (−), possible inhibition but no negative control; ABG autogenous bone graft; HA, hydroxyapatite; pf, press fit; rev, revision model; TCP, tricalcium phosphate; ut, untreated control.
This table excludes Ca-P ceramics.

carriers have been investigated as means to stimulate bone ingrowth into porous-surfaced implants in experimental studies. These studies as well as studies on local factors that interfere with bone ingrowth are summarized in Tables 15-2 to 15-5.

Until recently, autogenous bone graft appeared to be the gold standard of bone graft materials for enhancement of bone ingrowth. Although the mechanisms are not well defined, it appears that autogenous bone combines osteoconductive properties, osteoinductive properties, and the stimulation of an inflammatory response accompanied by the release of cytokines.

Osteoconduction is a phenomenon that includes the ingrowth of sprouting capillaries, perivascular tissues, and osteoprogenitor cells from the recipient host bed into the three-dimensional structure of an implant or graft (122). Calcium phosphate ceramic coatings are used both on porous and nonporous implant surfaces for this osteoconductive effect. With respect to the latter, critical questions about the long-term durability have to be addressed, whereas the ideal characteristics of a calcium phosphate coating for enhancement of bone ingrowth into a metal porous or metal-textured surface have yet to be analyzed. As the use of calcium phosphates has been demonstrated to enhance bone ingrowth, a combined calcium phosphate–metal porous coating, with the mechanical interlocking of the

ingrown bone with the porous surface, might well have long-term clinical advantages. However, this has yet to be demonstrated.

Osteoinduction is a process that supports the mitogenesis of undifferentiated perivascular mesenchymal cells, leading to the formation of osteoprogenitor cells with the capacity to form new bone (121). The results of a recent study (116) have demonstrated that enhancement of bone ingrowth in implants that have been treated with a combination of a local osteoconductive factor (hydroxyapatite-tricalcium phosphate coating) and a local osteoinductive factor (transforming growth factor β-1) exceeds the effect of autogenous bone graft alone.

Osteoconductive calcium phosphate coatings (plasma-sprayed partially resorbable hydroxyapatite/tricalcium phosphate) applied to the porous coatings were shown to enhance the bone ingrowth into the porous coatings of the acetabular components in canine total hip models by about 20% at 3 weeks. However, the coatings did not enhance the bone ingrowth when good apposition between the bone and the porous surface was not present. In addition, the enhancement was not present at 6 weeks after surgery.

Osteoinductive materials made possible by genetic engineering techniques showed great promise in enhancing fracture healing in the recent past and thus are believed to be of great benefit in improving prosthetic fixation by bone ingrowth as well. These

TABLE 15-3
EFFECT OF LOCAL FACTORS ON BONE INGROWTH/STRENGTH OF FIXATION: CA-P CERAMICS

Author (Ref.)	Non-Weight-Bearing Model		Weight-Bearing Model		Revision	Species	Time Interval	Control	Comment
	pf	Gap	pf	Gap					
Calcium phosphate granules									
Lewis (85)	+					Dog	4, 8, 16	ut, pf	TCP, pf
Kang (53)				−		Dog	12	ut	HA/TCP/ABG
Greis (37)				−		Dog	12, 24	ut	HA/TCP/BM/Co
Rusotti (90)			(−)			Dog	12	ut	HA/TCP
Turner (120)					+	Dog	24	ut	HA/TCP
Spivak (107)		+				Dog	6, 12	ut	HA/blood
Calcium phosphate coatings									
Ducheyne (28)	+					Dog	2, 4, 12	ut	HA slurry
Rivero (86)	(+)					Dog	1, 2, 4, 6	ut	HA plsp
Mayor (71)	(−)					Rabbit	3	ut	TCP plsp
Soballe (102)		+				Dog	6	ut	HA plsp
Soballe (100)		+				Dog	4–16	ut	HA plsp
Jasty (52)			+			Dog	3	ut	HA/TCP plsp
Greis (37)				(+)		Dog	12	ut	HA/TCP plsp
Spivac (107)	+					Dog	6, 12	ut	HA sputtercoat
Tisdel (117)	+					Rabbit	1, 2, 3, 4, 6, 12, 24	ut	HA/TCP plsp
Cook (24)	+					Dog	2, 4, 6, 8, 12	ut	HA plsp
Orth (78)	+					Mini-pig	4, 8, 12, 24	ut	HA plsp
Kienapfel (62)		+				Sheep	3	ut	HA plsp
Moroni (75)	+					Dog	12	ut	HA plsp

+, enhancement of bone ingrowth and/or strength of fixation; −, inhibition of bone ingrowth and/or strength of fixation; (o), no enhancement or inhibition; (+), possible enhancement but no negative control (untreated gap); (−), possible inhibition but no negative control; BM, bone marrow; HA, hydroxyapatite; pf, press fit; plsp, plasma sprayed; rev, revision model; TCP, tricalcium phosphate; ut, untreated control.

TABLE 15-4

EFFECT OF LOCAL FACTORS ON BONE INGROWTH/STRENGTH OF FIXATION: ELECTROMAGNETIC AND RADIATION FACTORS

Author (Ref.)	Non-Weight-Bearing Model		Weight-Bearing Model		Revision	Species	Time Interval (Weeks)	Control	Comment
	pf	Gap	pf	Gap					
Electric stimulation									
Rivero (87)	(−)					Dog	4	ut	icpemf
Schutzer (94)			(−)			Dog	6	ut	ccpemf
Park (80)	+					Dog	2–6	ut	des
Weinstein (124)	+					Dog	1–8	ut	des
Colella (20)	+					Dog	1, 2, 3	des	
Berry (1)	+					Dog	1–10	des	
Irradiation									
Sumner (115)	(−)					Dog	2, 4, 6	ut	500 rad
Sumner (115)	−					Dog	2, 4, 6	ut	1000 rad
Chin (18)	−					Dog	12	ut	5500 rad

+, enhancement of bone ingrowth and/or strength of fixation; −, inhibition of bone ingrowth and/or strength of fixation; (o), no enhancement or inhibition; (+), possible enhancement but no negative control (untreated gap); (−), possible inhibition but no negative control; ccpemf, capacitively coupled electric field; des, direct electric stimulation; icpemf, inductively coupled pulsed electromagnetic field; pf, press fit; ut, untreated control. Deutsche Forschungsgemeinschaft grant KI 354/1-1.

agents applied locally over implants or in the prepared bone cavities may provide appropriate local environments to stimulate bone formation in primary as well as revision surgery. However, the various parameters in the optimal use of these materials, such as the dose, physical composition, and appropriate carrier systems, have not been defined adequately.

In one canine total hip replacement study employing 2-cm diameter head and 2-mm defects behind the acetabular component, recombinant BMP-2 with a calcium phosphate carrier (BSM) stimulated the bridging of a bony gap adjacent to a porous coating (5). In addition, consistent uniform bone ingrowth into the porous coating adjacent to the gap was also noted, even though no increase in bone ingrowth into the porous implant in areas of intimate bone–implant contact occurred. Quantitative measurements confirmed these observations.

Thus it appears that bone ingrowth can be enhanced by synthetic osteoinductive materials and recombinant bone morphogenic proteins. The latter seem to be particularly useful and can promote bone ingrowth even when there are defects between bone and porous coatings. Although very expensive and investigational at this time, these techniques may be extremely useful in revision surgeries in the future.

CLINICAL AND RETRIEVAL STUDIES

Studies of implants retrieved at revision surgery and at autopsy have validated the concepts of bone ingrowth fixation in humans. Early retrieval studies have shown variable and inconsistent bone ingrowth into implants that were mostly retrieved during revision surgery (21,23). As the parameters required for bone ingrowth have been delineated, surgical techniques and implant designs have improved. Later studies have shown marked improvements in the rate and amount of bone ingrowth (Fig. 15-4) (112). Bone ingrowth in up to 35% of available porous surface in acetabular components and up to 65% in femoral components was shown in retrieval studies. Even though there had been wide variations in the amount of bone ingrowth in these studies due to variations in implant designs, patient selection, surgical techniques, and the reason for revision surgery, the ingrowth of bone was found to be consistent. Radiographic appearance suggesting bone ingrowth is found in 90% of implants of contemporary design inserted with current surgical techniques. Such has not been the case with total knee replacement, however. Two studies of porous-coated tibial components of total knee replacements in animals and human retrievals showed that bone ingrowth was consistently found within and near the fixation pegs but was variable elsewhere (58,114).

Intermediate and long-term clinical studies of patients undergoing total hip replacements with uncemented porous-coated prosthetic components are now available, showing success rates well above 90% at greater than 10 years follow-up (1,39,62,70). Implant survival rates are greater than 95% at 10 years for acetabular components and proximally porous coated and fully porous coated femoral components. Obtaining bone ingrowth into the porous coating had not been a problem with total hip replacements.

LATE FAILURE OF BONE INGROWTH

Although firm and long-lasting fixation can be provided by bone ingrowth into porous-coated implants, late failure of bone ingrowth can occur and can lead to implant loosening (47). This can be a result of fatigue fractures of the bridging trabeculae, which can lead to failure of fixation in femoral

TABLE 15-5
EFFECT OF SYSTEMIC FACTORS ON BONE INGROWTH/STRENGTH OF FIXATION

Author (Ref.)	Non-Weight-Bearing Model pf	Gap	Weight-Bearing Model pf	Gap	Revision	Species	Time Interval (Weeks)	Control	Comment
						Indomethacin			
Cook (22)	(−)					Dog	3, 6, 8, 12, 24	ut	
						Disodium (1-hydroxythylidene) diphosphonate			
Kitsugi (63)	(−)					Rabbit	8	ut	0.1–1 mg/d
Kitsugi (63)	+					Rabbit	8	ut	2.5–5 mg/d
						Factor XIII			
Kienapfel (61)	+					Sheep	3	ut	FXIII conc
Kienapfel (61)	(−)					Sheep	3	ut	rec FXIII
						Estrogen			
Shaw (95)	(−)					Monkey	22	ut	oox
Shaw (95)	(−)					Dog	22	ut	oox
						Warfarin			
Callahan (12)	−					Goat	3, 6, 12	ut	
						Hydrocortisone acetate			
Guyton (38)	(−)					Goat	3, 6, 12, 26, 52	ut	5 mg/kg SQ
						Methotrexate			
Lisecki (68)	−					Goat	3, 6, 12, 26, 52	ut	
						Coumadin			
Lisecki (68)	(−)					Goat	3, 6, 12, 26, 52	ut	
						Cisplatin			
Young (126)	−					Dog	12	ut	postop med
Young (126)	(−)					Dog	12	ut	preop med

+, enhancement of bone ingrowth and/or strength of fixation; −, inhibition of bone ingrowth and/or strength of fixation; (o), no enhancement or inhibition; (+), possible enhancement but no negative control (untreated gap); (−), possible inhibition but no negative control; FXIII conc, human factor XIII concentrate (Fibrogammin, Behringwerke Marburg, FRG); HA, hydroxyapatite; oox, oophorectomy; pf, press fit; rec FXIII, recombinant factor XIII (Behringwerke Marburg); SQ, subcutaneous; ut, untreated control.

stems even in the presence of bone ingrowth. Most often this occurs when there is a substantial amount of bone loss surrounding implants from periprosthetic osteolysis. This periprosthetic osteolysis is due to the biologic foreign body reaction to particulate implant debris that most often results from wear of the polyethylene at the articulation (45). The wear at the articulation produces billions of wear particles that are very small in size (micron and submicron in diameter), many of which find their way into the bone–porous coating interface under hydrostatic pressure present in the joint. The foreign body response mounted in response to these wear particles (primarily consisting of macrophages and giant cells) leads to a cascade of cellular and biochemical events, some of which cause the resorption of adjacent bone. Late failure of fixation can occur when there is not sufficient bone remaining to support the prosthetic component. Many of the failures of the early generations of cementless total hips were due to this periprosthetic osteolysis and late failure of fixation.

Studies of mechanisms by which the polyethylene undergoes wear and how the micron and submicron wear particles are liberated have led to many advances in improving the wear performance of polyethylene in the past decade (50). Radiation cross-linking the polyethylene and eliminating the free radicals produced during radiation by heating has resulted in a polyethylene that is highly wear resistant in laboratory studies. Early clinical studies are confirming the very low wear rates of these materials and a substantial reduction in the rate of periprosthetic osteolysis (52).

CONCLUSION

Biologic fixation of prosthetic components with porous surfaced implants has been considerably improved over the past two decades. The characteristics of the porous coatings and the design features of the prosthetic components necessary to obtain reliable and consistent fixation to the skeleton by bone ingrowth have been elucidated. Total joint replacements using uncemented prosthetic components fixed biologically with bone ingrowth into porous coatings have now become commonplace operations, with excellent intermediate-term

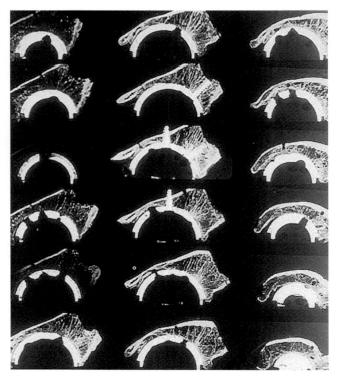

Figure 15-4 Serial sections through an acetabular component retrieved at autopsy from a patient who had undergone uncemented total hip replacement. The sections show extensive ingrowth.

success rates. Wear of the polyethylene at the articulation and the wear debris associated with periprosthetic osteolysis had been the major factors limiting the longevity of these procedures until recently. It is hoped that the development of new wear-resistant, cross-linked polyethylenes and alternate bearing materials will further increase the success rates of these procedures.

REFERENCES

1. Archibeck MJ, Berger RA, Jacobs JJ, et al. Second-generation cementless total hip arthroplasty: eight to eleven-year results. *J Bone Joint Surg [Am].* 2001;83:1666–1673.
2. Bobyn JD, Pilliar RM, Cameron HU, et al. The effect of porous surface configuration on the tensile strength of fixation of implants by bone ingrowth. *Clin Orthop.* 1980;149:291.
3. Bobyn JD, Pilliar RM, Cameron HU, et al. The optimum pore size for the fixation of porous-surfaced metal implants by the ingrowth of bone. *Clin Orthop.* 1980;150:263.
4. Bobyn JD, Pilliar RM, Cameron HU, et al. Osteogenic phenomena across endosteal bone–implant spaces with porous surfaced intramedullary implants. *Acta Orthop Board.* 1981;52:145.
5. Bragdon CR, Doherty AM, Rubash HE, et al. The efficacy of BMP-2 to induce bone ingrowth in a total hip replacement. *Clin Orthop Relat Res.* 2003;No. 417:50–61.
6. Branemark PI, Zarb GA, Albrektason T. *Tissue Integrated Prostheses: Osseointegration in Clinical Dentistry.* Chicago: Quintessence; 1985.
7. Branson PJ, Steege JW, Wixson RL, et al. Rigidity of initial fixation with uncemented tibial knee implants. *J Arthroplasty.* 1989;4:21.
8. Brown SD, Drummond JL, Feber MK, et al. In vitro and in vivo evaluation of meltsprayed alumina coatings on 316L and T16A14V alloy substrated. In: Williams DF, Hastings G, eds. *Mechanical Properties of Biomaterials.* New York: Wiley, 1980.
9. Bryan RS, Janes HM, Grindlay JH. The effect of polyvinyl-formal (Ivalon) sponge on cortical bone healing. *Proc Staff Mtg Mayo Clin.* 1958;35:453.
10. Burke DW, Bragdon CR, Lowenstein L. Mechanical aspects of the bone porous surface interface under known amounts of implant motion [abstract]. *Trans Orthop Res Soc.* 1993;18:470.
11. Burke DW, Bragdon CR, O'Connor DO, et al. Dynamic measurement of interface mechanics in vivo and the effect of micromotion on bone ingrowth into a porous surface device under controlled loads in vivo [abstract]. *Trans Orthop Res Soc.* 1991;16:103.
12. Callahan BC, Lisecki EJ, Banks RE, et al. The effect of warfarin on the attachment of bone to hydroxyapatite-coated and uncoated porous implants. *J Bone Joint Surg Am.* 1995;77:225.
13. Cameron HU, Macnab I, Pilliar RM. A porous metal system for joint replacement surgery. *Int J Artif Organs.* 1978;1:104.
14. Cameron HU, Pilliar RM, Macnab I. The effect of movement on the bonding of porous metal to bone. *J Biomed Mater Res.* 1973;7:301.
15. Cameron HU, Pilliar RM, Macnab I. The rate of bone ingrowth into porous metal. *J Biomed Mater Res.* 1976;10:295.
16. Camerot H, Rlev J, Bouaquet G, et al. Alumina plasma spray coatings on stainless steel and titanium alloys for prostesis anchorage. In: Helmke G, ed. *Bioceramics.* Oxford: Butterworth-Heinemann; 1989:211.
17. Cestero HJ Jr, Salyer KE, Toranto IR. Bone growth into porous carbon, polyethylene, and polypropylene prostheses. *J Biomed Mater Res.* 1975;9:1.
18. Chin HC, Frassica FJ, Markel MD, et al. The effects of therapeutic doses of irradiation on experimental bone graft incorporation over a porous-coated segmental defect endoprosthesis. *Clin Orthop.* 1993;289:254.
19. Clemow AJ, Weinstein AM, Klawitter JJ, et al. Interface mechanics of porous titanium implants. *J Biomed Mater Res.* 1981;15:73.
20. Colelia SM, Miller AG, Stang RG, et al. Fixation of porous titanium implants in cortical bone enhanced by electrical stimulation. *J Biomed Mater Res.* 1981;15:37.
21. Collier JP, Bauer TW, Bioebaum RD, et al. Results of implant retrieval from postmortem specimens in patients with well-functioning, long-term total hip replacement. *Clin Orthop.* 1992;274:97.
22. Cook SD, Barraok RL, Dalton JE, et al. Effects of indomethacin on biologic fixation of porous-coated titanium implants. *J Arthroplasty.* 1995;10:351.
23. Cook SD, Thomas KA, Barraok RL, et al. Tissue growth into porous-coated acetabular components in 42 patients: effects of adjunct fixation. *Clin Orthop.* 1992;289:163.
24. Cook SD, Thomas KA, Dalton JE, et al. Hydroxylapatite coating of porous implants improves bone ingrowth and interface attachment strength. *J Biomed Mater Res.* 1992;26:989.
25. Cook SD, Walsh KA, Hadded RJ Jr. Interface mechanics and bone growth into porous Co-Cr-Mo alloy implants. *Clin Orthop.* 1985;193:271.
26. Dalton JE, Cook SD, Thomas KA, et al. The effect of operative fit and hydroxyapetite coating on the mechanical and biological response to porous implants. *J Bone Joint Surg Am.* 1995;77:97.
27. Ducheyne P, De Meester P, Asmoudt E. Influence of a functional dynamic loading on bone ingrowth into surface pores of orthopedic implants. *J Biomed Mater Res.* 1977;11:511.
28. Ducheyne P, Hench LL, Kagan A II, et al. Effect of hydroxyapatite impregnation on skeletal bonding of porous coated implants. *J Biomed Mater Res.* 1980;14:231.
29. Ducheyne P, Mariena M, Aemoudt E, et al. Skeletal fixation by metal fiber coating of the implant. *Acta Orthop Belg.* 1974;40:799.
30. Engh CA, Bobyn JD, eds. *Biologic Fixation in Total Hip Arthroplasty.* Thorofare, NJ: Slack; 1965.
31. Feighan JE, Goldberg VM, Davy D, et al. The influence of surface-blasting on the incorporation of titanium-alloy implants in a rabbit intramedullary model. *J Bone Joint Surg.* 1995;77A:1380.
32. Friedenberg AB, Simon WH. Bone ingrowth in Teflon sponge. *Surg Gynecol Obstet.* 1983;116:588.
33. Galante JO, Rostoker W, Lucok R, et al. Sintered fiber metal composites as a basis for attachment of implants to bone. *J Bone Joint Surg.* 1971;53A:101.

34. Glimer WS, Tooms RS, Salvatore JE. An experimental study of the influence of implanted polyurethane sponges upon subsequent bone formation. *Surg Gynecol Obstet.* 1981;113:143.

35. Goldberg VM, Stevenson S, Feighan J, et al. Biology of grit-blasted titanium alloy implants. *Clin Orthop.* 1995:122.

36. Greenfield EJ. Mounting of artificial teeth [abstract]. 1909.

37. Greis PE, Kang JD, Silvaggio V, et al. A long-term study on defect filling and bone ingrowth using a canine fiber metal total hip model. *Clin Orthop.* 1992;274:47.

38. Guyton JL, Sumner DR, Rudert J, et al. The effect of corticosteroids on bone ingrowth in a canine model [abstract]. *Trans Orthop Res Soc.* 1991;16:32.

39. Harris WH. Results of uncemented cups: a critical appraisal at 15 years. *Clin Orthop Relat Res.* 2003;417:121–125.

40. Heimke G, ed. *Osseointegrated Implants.* Boca Raton: CRC Press; 1990.

41. Herrmens KA, Kim WC, O'Caroll PF, et al. Bone morphogenetic protein and cancellous graft use in porous surfaced interface voids [abstract]. *Trans Orthop Res Soc.* 1988;11:343.

42. Hirachhom JS, Reynolds JT. Powder metallurgy fabrication of cobalt alloy surgical implant materials. In: Korstoff E, ed. *Research in Dental and Medical Materials.* New York: Plenum Press; 1989.

43. Hulbert SF, Cooke FW, Klawitter JJ, et al. Attachment of prostheses to the musculoskeletal system by tissue ingrowth and mechanical interlocking. *J Biomed Mater Res.* 1973;7:1.

44. Jasty M, Bragdon C, Burke D, et al. In vivo skeletal responses to porous-surfaced implants subjected to small induced motions. *J Bone Joint Surg [Am].* 1997;79:707–714.

45. Jasty M, Bragdon C, Jiranek W, et al. Etiology of osteolysis around porous-coated cementless total hip arthroplasties. *Clin Orthop Relat Res.* 1994;No. 308:111–126.

46. Jasty M, Bragdon CR, Maloney WJ, et al. Bone ingrowth into a low-modulus composite plastic porous-coated canine femoral component. *J Arthroplasty.* 1992;7:253–259.

47. Jasty M, Bragdon CR, Maloney WJ, et al. Ingrowth of bone in failed fixation of porous-coated femoral components [see comments]. *J Bone Joint Surg.* 1991;73A:1331.

48. Jasty M, Bragdon CR, Schulzer S, et al. Bone ingrowth into porous coated canine total hip replacements: quantification by backscattered scanning electron microscopy and image analysis. *Scanning Microsc.* 1989;3:1061.

49. Jasty M, Bragdon CR, Zalenski E, et al. Enhanced stability of uncemented canine femoral components by bone ingrowth into the porous coatings. *J Arthroplasty.* 1997;12:106–113.

50. Jasty M, Goetz DD, Bragdon CR, et al. Wear of polyethylene acetabular components in total hip arthroplasty: an analysis of one hundred and twenty-eight components retrieved at autopsy or revision operations. *J Bone Joint Surg [Am].* 1997;79:349–358.

51. Jasty M, Krushell R, Zalenski EB, et al. The contribution of the nonporous distal stem to the stability of proximally porous-coated canine femoral components. *J Arthroplasty.* 1993;8:33.

52. Jasty M, Rubash HE, Muratoglu O. Highly cross-linked polyethylene: the debate is over—in the affirmative. *J Arthroplasty.* 2005;20(4 Suppl 2):55–58.

53. Jasty M, Rubash HE, Paiement GD, et al. Porous-coated uncemented components in experimental total hip arthroplasty in dogs. Effect of plasma-sprayed calcium phosphate coatings on bone ingrowth [see comments]. *Clin Orthop.* 1992;280:300.

54. Karrhoim J, Malchau H, Snorrason F, et al. Micromotion of femoral stems in total hip arthroplasty: a randomized study of cemented, hydroxyapatite-coated, and porous-coated stems with roentgen stereophotogrammetric analysis. *J Bone Joint Surg.* 1994; 76A:1692.

55. Karrholm J, Snorrason F. Migration of porous coated acetabular prostheses fixed with screws: roentgen stereophotogrammetric analysis. *J Orthop Res.* 1992;10:826.

56. Kienapfel H, Klenapfel H, eds. *Grundiagen der zementfrelen Endoprothetik: Der Einfluss von lokalen und systemischen Faktoren auf das Knocheneinwachsverthalten und die Verankerungsfestigkeilt von metallporoösen Oberflachenimplantaten.* Grateffing, Munich: Damater Verlag; 1994.

57. Kienapfel H, Martell J, Rosenberg A, et al. Cementless Gustillo-Kyle and BIAS total hip arthroplasty: 2- to 5-year results. *Arch Orthop Trauma Surg.* 1991;110:179.

58. Kienapfel H, Sprey S, Meuct P, et al. The effect of hydroxyapatite coating on the implant micromotion in non-cemented porous coated total knee arthroplasty. In: Niwa S, Yoshino S, Kurosaka M, et al. eds. *Reconstruction of the Knee Joint.* Tokyo: Springer-Verlag, 1996.

59. Kienapfel H, Sumner DR, Turner TM, et al. Efficacy of autograft and freeze-dried allograft to enhance fixation of porous coated implants in the presence of interface gaps. *J Orthop Res.* 1992;10:423.

60. Kienapfel H, Sumner DR, Turner TM, et al. Efficacy of autograft, freeze-dried allograft, and fibrin glue to enhance fixation of porous coated implants in the presence of interface gaps [abstract]. *Trans Orthop Res Soc.* 1990;15:432.

61. Kienapfel H, Swain R, Hettel A, et al. Recombinant and non-recombinant factor XIII and its effect on bone ingrowth and strength of fixation. *Arch Orthop Trauma Surg.* 1997;116:239–243.

62. Kim YH, Kim JS, Cho SH. Primary total hip arthroplasty with the AML total hip prosthesis. *Clin Orthop Relat Res.* 1999;No. 360: 147–158.

63. Kitsugi T, Yamamuro T, Nakamura T, et al. Influence of disodium (1-hydroxythylidene) diphosphonate on bone ingrowth into porous, titanium fiber-mesh implants. *J Arthroplasty.* 1995;10:245.

64. Klawitter JJ. Applications of porous ceramics for the attachment of load-bearing internal orthopedic applications. *J Biomed Mater Res.* 1971;2:161.

65. Kozinn SC, Hedley AK, Urist MR. Augmentation of bone ingrowth: ingrowth into bone morphogenetic protein (BMP) impregnated porous implants [abstract]. *Trans Orthop Res Soc.* 1981;6:181.

66. Lambert E, Galante JO, Rostoker W. Fixation of skeletal replacement by fiber metal composites. *Clin Orthop.* 1972;No. 87:303.

67. Lewis CG, Jones LC, Connor KM, et al. An evaluation of grafting materials in cementless arthroplasty [abstract]. *Trans Orthop Res Soc.* 1987;12:319.

68. Lieecki EJ, Cook SD, Dalton JE, et al. Attachment of HA coated and uncoated porous implants is influenced by methotraxate and coumadine [abstract]. *Trans Orthop Res Soc.* 1992;17:368.

69. Lueck RA, Galante JO, Rostoker W, et al. Development of an open pore metallic implant to permit attachment to bone. *Surg Forum.* 1969;20:456.

70. Mallory TH, Lombardi AV, Leith JR, et al. Why a taper? *J Bone Joint Surg [Am].* 2002;84:S81–89.

71. Mayor MB, Collier JP, De Cheryl D, et al. Enhanced early fixation of porous coated implants using TCP [abstract]. *Trans Orthop Res Soc.* 1987;12:483.

72. McDonald DJ, Fitzgerald RH Jr, Chao EY. The enhancement of fixation of a porous-coated femoral component by autograft and allograft in the dog. *J Bone Joint Surg.* 1988;70A:728.

73. McKibbin B. The biology of fracture healing in long bones. *J Bone Joint Surg.* 1978;60B:150.

74. McLaughlin RE, Reger SI, Bolander M, et al. Enhancement of bone ingrowth by the use of bone matrix as a biologic cement. *Clin Orthop.* 1984;No. 183:258.

75. Moroni A, Caja VL, Egger EL, et al. Histomorphometry of hyroxyapatite coated and uncoated porous titanium bone implants. *Biomaterials.* 1994;15:926.

76. Nilies JL, Lapitsky M. Biomechanical investigations of bone–porous carbon and porous metal interfaces. *J Biomed Mater Res.* 1973;7:63.

77. Nilsson KQ, Karrholm J, Ekelund L, et al. Evaluation of micromotion in cemented vs uncemented knee arthroplasty in osteoarthrosis and rheumatoid arthritis: randomized study using roentgen stereophotogrammetric analysis. *J Arthroplasty.* 1991;8:285.

78. Orth J, Kautzmann J, Griss P. Bone tissue response to porous HA and wire mesh of stainless steel with and without coatings of HA and titanium nitrate. *Adv Biomater.* 1990;9:283.

79. Osborn JF. Biowerkstoffe und ihre Anwendung bel implantation [Biomaterials and their application to implantation]. *SSO Schwalz Monstsechr Zahnheikd.* 1979;89:1138.

80. Park JB, Salman NN, Kenner GH, et al. Preliminary studies on the effects of direct current on the bone/porous implant interfaces. *Ann Biomed Eng.* 1980;8:93.

81. Pfluger G, Bosch P, Grundsohober F, et al. Untersuchungan uber des Elnwachsen von Kochangewebe in poroes Metallimplantate [Investigation of bone growth into porous metal implants]. *Wien Klin Wochenachr.* 1979;91:482.

82. Pilliar RM, Cameron HU, Macnab I. Porous surface layered prosthetic devices. *Biomed Eng.* 1975;10:126.

83. Pilliar RM, Lee JM, Manistopouios C. Observations on the effect of movement on bone ingrowth into porous surfaced implants. *Clin Orthop.* 1988;108.

84. Popoviol AF. Polyvinyl plastic sponge in experimental orthopaedic surgery: a preliminary report. *Bull Georgetown Univ Med Cent.* 1954;7:177.

85. Rivero DP, Fox J, Skipor AK, et al. Calcium phosphate-coated porous titanium implants for enhanced skeletal fixation. *J Biomed Mater Res.* 1988;22:191.

86. Rivero DP, Fox J, Skipor AK, et al. Effect of calcium phosphates and bone grafting materials on bone ingrowth in titanium fiber metal [abstract]. *Trans Orthop Res Boc.* 1985;10:191.

87. Rivero DP, Landon GC, Skipor AK, et al. Effect of pulsing electromagnetic fields on bone ingrowth in a porous material [abstract]. *Trans Orthop Res Soc.* 1988;11:492.

88. Robertson DM, Pierre L, Chehal F. Preliminary observations of bone ingrowth into porous materials. *J Biomed Mater Res.* 1976; 10:335.

89. Roy RG, Markel MD, Lipowitz AJ, et al. Effect of homologous fibrin adhesive on callus formation and extracortical bone bridging around a porous-coated segmental endoprosthesis in dogs. *Am J Vet Res.* 1993;54:1185.

90. Rusotti GM, Okada Y, Fitzgerald RHJ, et al. Efficacy of using bone graft substitute to enhance biological fixation of a porous metal femoral component. In: *The Hip.* St Louis: Mosby; 1987:120.

91. Ryd L, Lindstrand A, Stenstrom A, et al. The influence of metal backing in unicompartmental tibial component fixation: an in vivo roentgen stereophotogrammetric analysis of micromotion. *Arch Orthop Trauma Surg.* 1992;111:143.

92. Sadr B, Arden GP. A comparison of the stability of Proplast-coated and cemented Thompson prostheses in the treatment of subcapital femoral fractures. *Injury.* 1977;8:234.

93. Sandborn PM, Cook SD, Spires WP, et al. Tissue response to porous-coated implants lacking initial bone apposition. *J Arthroplasty.* 1988;3:337.

94. Schutzer BF, Jasty M, Bragdon CR, et al. A double-blind study on the effects of a capacitively coupled electrical field on bone ingrowth into porous-surfaced canine total hip prostheses. *Clin Orthop.* 1990;260:297.

95. Shaw JA, Wilson SC, Bruno A, et al. Comparison of primate and canine models for bone ingrowth experimentation, with reference to the effect of ovarian function on bone ingrowth potential. *J Orthop Res.* 1994;12(2):268.

96. Shen WJ, Chung KC, Wang GJ, et al. Demineralized bone matrix in the stabilization of porous-coated implants in bone defects in rabbits. *Clin Orthop.* 1993:348.

97. Shimagaki H, Bechtold JE, Sherman RE, et al. Stability of initial fixation of the tibial component in cementless total knee arthroplasty. *J Orthop Res.* 1990;8:64.

98. Skinner HB, Davis CM, Shackelford JF, et al. Evaluation of a commercial, porous stainless steel as a prosthetic implant material. *Biomater Med Devices Artif Organs.* 1979;7:141.

99. Smith L. Ceramic–plastic material as bone substitute. *Arch Surg.* 1983;87:137.

100. Soballe K. Hydroxyapatite ceramic coating for bone implant fixation: mechanical and histological studies in dogs. *Acta Orthop Scand Suppl.* 1993;255:1.

101. Soballe K, Hansen ES, Brockstedt Rasmussen H, et al. Bone graft incorporation around titanium-alloy- and hydroxyapatite-coated implants in dogs. *Clin Orthop.* 1992;272:282.

102. Soballe K, Hansen ES, Brockstedt Rasmussen H, et al. Gap healing enhanced by hydroxyapatite coating in dogs. *Clin Orthop.* 1991;272:300.

103. Soballe K, Hansen ES, Brockstedt Rasmussen H, et al. Tissue ingrowth into titanium and hydroxyspatite-coated implants during stable and unstable mechanical conditions. *J Orthop Res.* 1992;10:285.

104. Spector M, Flemming WR, Kreutner A. Bone growth into porous high-density polyethylene. *J Biomed Master Res.* 1978;10:595.

105. Spector M, Harmon SL, Kreutner A. Characteristics of tissue growth into Proplast and porous polyethylene implants in bone. *J Biomed Mater Res.* 1979;13:877.

106. Spector M, Michno MJ, Smarook WH, et al. A high-modulus polymer for porous orthopedic implants: biomechanical compatability of porous implants. *J Biomed Mater Res.* 1978;12:665.

107. Spivak JM, Ricci JL, Blumenthal NC, et al. A new canine model to evaluate the biological response of intramedullary bone to implant materials and surfaces. *J Biomed Mater Res.* 1990; 24:112.

108. Strickland AB, Chan KH, Andriacchi TP, et al. The initial fixation of porous coated tibial components evaluated by the study of rigid body motion under static load [abstract]. *Trans Orthop Res Soc.* 1988;13:476.

109. Struthers AM. An experimental study of polyvinyl sponge as a substitute for bone. *Plast Reconstr Surg.* 1955;15:27.

110. Sumner DR, Bryan JM, Urban RM, et al. Measuring the volume fraction of bone ingrowth: a comparison of three techniques. *J Orthop Res.* 1990;5:448.

111. Sumner DR, Galante JO. Bone ingrowth. In: Evarts CM, ed. *Surgery of the Musculoskeletal System.* New York: Churchill Livingstone; 1990:151.

112. Sumner DR, Jasty M, Jacobs JJ, et al. Histology of porous-coated acetabular components: 25 cementless cups retrieved after arthroplasty. *Acta Orthop Scand.* 1993;84:619.

113. Sumner DR, Klenapfel H, Galante JO. Metallic implants. In: Habal MB, Reddi AH, eds. *Bone Grafts: From Basic Science to Clinical Application.* Philadelphia: WB Saunders; 1992:252.

114. Sumner DR, Klenapfel H, Jacobs JJ, et al. Bone ingrowth and wear debris in well fixed cementless porous-coated tibial components removed from patients. *J Arthroplasty.* 1996;10:157.

115. Sumner DR, Turner TM, Pierson RH, et al. Effects of radiation on fixation of non-cemented porous-coated implants in a canine model. *J Bone Joint Surg Am.* 1990;72A:1527.

116. Sumner DR, Turner TM, Purchio AF, et al. Enhancement of bone ingrowth by transforming growth factor-beta. *J Bone Joint Surg.* 1995;77A:1135.

117. Tisdel CL, Goldberg VM, Parr JA, et al. The influence of a hydroxyapatite and tricalcium-phosphate coating on bone growth into titanium fiber–metal implants. *J Bone Joint Surg.* 1994;76A:159.

118. Trancik T, Vinson N. The effect of prostaglandin F2-alpha on bone ingrowth into a porous coated implant [abstract]. *Trans Orthop Res Soc.* 1990;15:167.

119. Tullos HS, McCaskill BL, Dickey R, et al. Total hip arthroplasty with a low modulus porous coated femoral component. *J Bone Joint Surg.* 1984;66A:866.

120. Turner TM, Urban RM, Sumner DR, et al. Revision, without cement, of aseptically loose, cemented total hip prostheses: quantitative comparison of the effects of four types of medullary treatment on bone ingrowth in a canine model [see comments]. *J Bone Joint Surg.* 1993;75A:845.

121. Urist MR. Bone: formation by autoinduction. *Science.* 1965; 150:893.

122. Urist MR. Bone transplants and implants. In: Urist MR, ed. *Fundamental and clinical bone physiology.* Philadelphia: Lippincott; 1980:331.

123. Volz RG, Nisbet JK, Lee RW, et al. The mechanical stability of various noncemented tibial components. *Clin Orthop.* 1988;226:38.

124. Weinstein AM, Klawitter JJ, Cleveland TW. Electrical stimulation of bone growth into porous A1203. *J Biomed Mater Res.* 1976;10:23.

125. Weish RP, Pilliar RM, Macnab I. Surgical implants. The role of surface porosity in fixation to bone and acrylic. *J Bone Joint Surg.* 1971;53A:963.

126. Young DR, Shih DY, Rock MG, et al. Effects of perioperative cisplatin chemotherapy on biologic fixation of a model limb salvage prosthesis [abstract]. *Trans Orthop Res Soc.* 1994;19:250.

Bone Remodeling Around Hip Implants

16

Charles A. Engh · Christi J. Sychterz · James Keeney · William Maloney

It is well accepted that bone adapts to the forces acting upon it, changing its structure to best resist those forces. Areas of bone experiencing high stress will respond by increasing bone mass (9,14). Areas under lower stress will respond by decreasing bone mass, either by becoming more porous (internal remodeling), or by getting thinner (external remodeling) (9,14). This well-known observation, termed Wolff's Law, forms the basic orthopaedic understanding of bone remodeling.

In the case of hip arthroplasty, the load (and hence stress) in the proximal femur—normally transferred from the femoral head through the cortical and cancellous bone of the femoral neck to the femoral diaphysis—is drastically altered. The femoral head is removed and an endoprosthesis is inserted in the femoral canal, which then shares the load originally carried by the bone alone. As a result of decreased stress, the bone remodels in accordance with Wolff's Law, and the femur undergoes architectural changes.

Although the exact mechanism of bone remodeling remains uncertain, clinical and autopsy studies have taught us much about the physical characteristics, quality, and magnitude of the skeletal response to an implanted femoral endoprosthesis. This chapter attempts to summarize information gained about bone remodeling from studies of cementless and cemented femoral prostheses.

DIFFERENTIATING BETWEEN THE CAUSES OF BONE RESORPTION

Prior to detailed discussion of changes in bone architecture following hip arthroplasty due to changing stress distributions, one must recognize the presence of bone adaptation due to alternate causes. Bone resorption can be induced by the body's inflammatory response to particulate debris (15,16,23,29). These changes in bone architecture are often classified as pathologic rather than adaptive. Particulate debris, usually metal or polyethylene, is created by the articulation of implant surfaces and/or by in vivo metallic corrosion. Bone resorption caused by this granulomatous response to particulate debris usually occurs at the location where debris collects. Because the bulk of debris originates from the articular surface and has easy access to the proximal medial femoral cortex and trochanteric region of the hip, localized osteolysis is common in these areas. Osteolysis remote from the articulation can also occur, however, when debris gains access to distal sites (23). For uncemented femoral components, this can occur with noncircumferentially coated devices or when the femoral implant is not osseointegrated and is able to move within the bone, allowing particulate debris to be pumped toward the tip of the stem (1,2,16). For cemented components, focal lysis remote from the joint can occur at the site of a cement mantle defect which allows direct communication between the joint and lesion through the stem–cement interface (1,20).

207

It is important to differentiate between bone loss caused by granuloma and bone loss caused by the response to an altered stress state, because the consequences of each etiology are very different. Although in general bone atrophy is felt to be undesirable, the bone atrophy that occurs when an uncemented femoral prosthesis becomes osseointegrated rarely results in adverse consequences. In the case of a porous-coated femoral endoprosthesis, bone atrophy can be a desirable sign indicating implant fixation. Conversely, bone loss caused by a granulomatous response is usually a progressive process and is more likely to result in bone fracture or prosthetic loosening (1,15,16).

HOW BONE REMODELING DEFINES CEMENTLESS PROSTHETIC FIXATION

Direct bonding of bone to a cementless prosthesis is termed osseointegration. Until recently, confirmation of osseointegration required removing the implant, sectioning it, and microscopically evaluating the implant–host interface. It could then be determined whether bone was directly bonded to the implant or whether fibrous tissue was interposed between the bone and the implant. By studying postmortem-retrieved femoral prostheses and comparing histology with radiographs we have learned that it is possible, with uncemented implants such as the Anatomic Medullary Locking prosthesis (AML, DePuy, Warsaw, IN), to determine the histological type of fixation by its radiographic appearance. We found that when serial radiographs showed that the position of an implant had

shifted within the femur, examination of autopsy specimens revealed the implant to be separated from the bone by fibrous tissue. This fibrous encapsulation of the implant allowed it to be easily removed from the femur. Conversely, if serial radiographs showed that the implant's position within the femur had remained stable over time, examination of autopsy specimens revealed that the implant was fixed to the bone with tissue. Consequently, the stem could not be easily extracted from the femur.

We also learned that the radiographic pattern of bone remodeling was different when the implant was fixed to the bone by osseointegration rather than fibrous tissue ingrowth. The differentiating radiographic features between the two types of fixation included (a) changes in the appearance of the cortical bone, (b) changes within the intramedullary canal, and (c) changes directly at the implant surface.

When an implant is osseointegrated, the cortical bone adjacent to the upper portion of the prosthesis typically becomes porous (Fig. 16-1). In areas where the implant contacts the cortices, particularly near the termination of the porous coating, cortical densification also occurs (Fig. 16-1). Such localized areas of bone bridging between the surface of the implant and the femoral cortex have been termed spot welds. These changes typically occur in the first postoperative year. Additionally, when the stem is osseointegrated, serial radiographs show that both the size of the intramedullary canal and the appearance of the bone–implant interface usually remain unchanged.

When the endoprosthesis is not osseointegrated, however, the pattern of bone remodeling differs. Proximal cortical bone

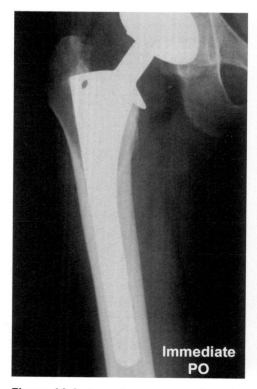
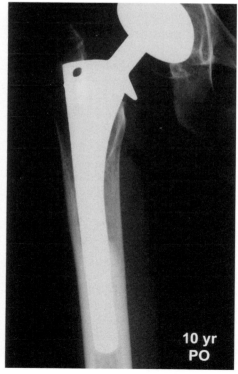

Figure 16-1 Immediate postoperative radiograph of a femur implanted with a porous-coated AML stem (*left*). 10 year postoperative radiograph of the same femur showing bone remodeling (*right*). There has been atrophy of the cortical bone adjacent to the medial proximal side of the stem. Near the termination of the porous coating, the cortex appears denser and thicker.

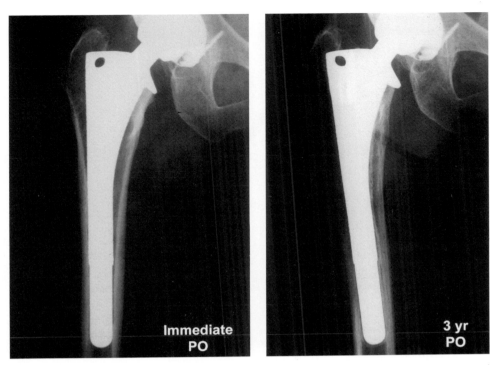

Figure 16-2   Immediate postoperative radiographs of a femur implanted with a porous-coated AML stem (*left*). 3 year postoperative radiograph of the same femur showing that the cortical bone adjacent to the proximal part of the prosthesis has not atrophied (*right*). White line surrounding the prosthesis indicates failed osseointegration.

atrophy is not observed (Fig. 16-2), and the intramedullary canal often widens. In addition, a bridge of new bone, termed a pedestal, often forms within the intramedullary canal just beneath the tip of the prosthesis. This hypertrophy of the proximal cortex and obliteration of the intramedullary canal beneath the stem are interpreted as signs that weight-bearing loads are being transferred from the implant to the femur at these two areas, and not to the cortical bone adjacent to the sides of the porous-coated prosthesis. The appearance of the bone–implant interface also differs when osseointegration does not occur. White radiographic demarcation lines develop in areas where the implant is encapsulated by fibrous tissue (Fig. 16-2). These white radiographic lines are the walls of a covering layer of new bone surrounding the implant like a cocoon. The translucent space between this white bone cover and the implant is fibrous tissue.

Understanding these radiographic signs allows physicians who care for patients with femoral endoprostheses to confirm osseointegration based on radiographic information rather than on microscopic evaluation of the implant surface. This ability to differentiate between osseointegrated and fibrous-encapsulated prostheses is important because often fibrous-encapsulated endoprostheses become loose and painful, whereas osseointegrated implants rarely loosen or require revision.

BONE REMODELING AROUND CEMENTED PROSTHESES

A radiographic and morphologic study of femora retrieved at autopsy described the qualitative changes that occur in femora

implanted with stable cemented femoral prostheses (17). In an analysis of 13 femora in situ from 3.3 to 17.5 years, Jasty et al. found that the bone remodeling response to a cemented stem included the creation a dense shell of substantial new bone around the cement mantle (Fig. 16-3). This shell resembled a new cortex and was attached to the outer cortex by new trabecular struts (17). In the adjacent femoral cortex, there was substantial osteoporosis and cortical thinning. Jasty et al. reported that the cement mantle was well supported by the extensive medullary bone remodeling and formation of a dense shell of new bone. The internal bone remodeling helped to maintain the cemented femoral components over time and did not cause loosening of the prosthesis.

QUANTIFYING THE REMODELING RESPONSE: DUAL-ENERGY X-RAY ABSORPTIOMETRY

Although plain radiographs can clearly demonstrate bone remodeling changes, radiographic bone density can change dramatically with small variations in x-ray technique; thus, radiographs alone cannot be used to quantify the magnitude of the bone remodeling response. With the development of dual-energy x-ray absorptiometry (DEXA), a noninvasive method of measuring bone mineral content, quantifying bone remodeling changes has become possible.

Several clinical studies have used DEXA analysis to examine the remodeling response to cementless femoral prostheses. In 1993, Kilgus et al. used this technology to assess the

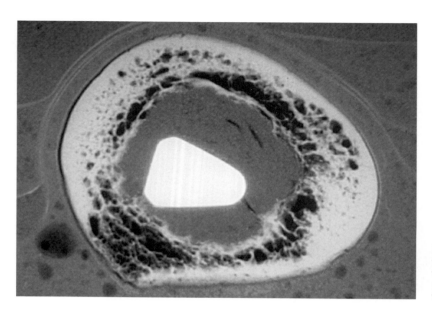

Figure 16-3 Contact radiograph of a femoral section containing a cemented prosthesis demonstrating the formation of a second medullary canal around the cement mantle as well as hypertrophy of the circumferential trabeculae.

changes in bone mineral density in patients with unilateral hip disease treated by implanting a porous-coated AML prostheses (18). The study documented that the greatest decrease in bone density (34.8%) occurred in the most proximal 1 cm of the medial cortex of the implanted femur. The next most severe decrease (20% to 25%) occurred in the next most proximal 6 cm of the medial femoral cortex. In other studies, Kiratli et al. and Venesmaa et al. used DEXA analysis to prospectively assess changes in bone density after cementless total hip arthroplasty (19,28). Evidence of rapid initial bone loss in the first six postoperative months followed by a plateau of little further change was reported. Venesmaa et al. further reported that the magnitude of postoperative bone loss was inversely related to preoperative bone mineral density (28).

DEXA analysis has also been used to examine well-functioning cementless prostheses in femora retrieved at autopsy. Like the aforementioned clinical studies, these studies demonstrated three consistent principles of bone remodeling in response to stable cementless femoral components (12,22,26). First, there is an overall mean decrease in bone mineral content of femora implanted with cementless stems. The mean reported bone loss in the autopsy studies was 23%, ranging from 5.4% to 47.4% (12,26). On average, females experienced a greater decrease in bone mineral content (31%) than males (12%). Second, bone loss occurs on a gradient (Fig. 16-4), with the greatest loss occurring adjacent to the proximal third of the implant (mean, 42.1%) and the least bone loss occurring distally (mean, 5.5%) (26). Third, and most importantly, the amount of bone loss is related to preoperative bone density levels. In the autopsy studies, the percentage decrease in bone mineral content was highly correlated with the bone mineral content of the contralateral, normal hip ($r^2 = 0.94$) (22,28). No other clinical factor, including stem size ($r^2 = 0.18$), duration of implantation ($r^2 = 0.11$), patient weight ($r^2 = 0.38$), or patient age ($r^2 = 0.08$) was a strong predictor of postarthroplasty bone loss (26). Femora with low control bone mineral content (<30 g) were associated with pronounced bone loss (>30% loss), even when the smallest diameter stem was used. Conversely, femors with high control bone mineral content (>45 g) did

not experience appreciable bone resorption (<10% loss), even with the largest-sized stem.

DEXA analysis has also been used to examine bone remodeling around cemented stems, but to a much more limited extent. In a prospective analysis of 20 hips implanted with

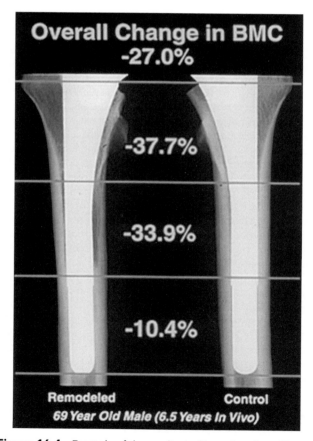

Figure 16-4 Example of the gradient of bone loss for a 69 year-old man following unilateral hip arthroplasty. At 5.5 years post arthroplasty, there was a 37.7% loss of bone mineral content (BMC) proximally, a 33.9% loss of bone in the mid section, and a 10.4% loss of bone adjacent to the distal portion of the implant.

cemented Charnley components, Cohen et al. documented a mean 6.7% reduction in bone density in the calcar and a mean 5.3% increase in bone density in the femoral shaft distal to the tip of the implant (7). Similar to that noted with cementless stems, this change in periprosthetic bone mineral content is consistent with a pattern of reduced stress in the proximal femur and increased stress around the tip of the prosthesis.

THREE-DIMENSIONAL ANALYSIS OF BONE REMODELING

Although DEXA analysis is an important tool for quantifying changes in bone mineral content, it is limited to a two-dimensional assessment of bone remodeling. DEXA analysis can provide information regarding variations in bone mineral content over time but cannot differentiate between the causes of these variations, including changes in cortical bone area or changes in cortical porosity or both. Moreover, DEXA analysis of changes in bone mineral content around cemented stems is difficult. As previously mentioned, Jasty et al. described the formation of an internal cortex around the cement mantle of stable cemented stems that is indistinguishable from cement on clinical x-rays (17). This results in a problem of identifying the boundary between the cement

and the bone, limiting the application of DEXA in femora with cemented components.

To analyze the three-dimensional nature of the bone remodeling response to both cemented and cementless prostheses, a large analysis of 24 pairs of autopsy-retrieved femora was undertaken (21). With this analysis, cross-sectional femoral slabs from the autopsy-retrieved femora were radiographed, digitized, and subsequently analyzed using custom-designed software. Cortical thickness, cortical bone area, and bone mineral content were assessed in four quadrants at five discrete femoral levels. A note of caution should be made, however, that direct comparison of the magnitudes of bone loss between cemented and cementless groups in this study is not appropriate because the specimens were obtained from unselected groups of patients and were not matched on variables known to affect the remodeling process (such as age, gender, weight, diagnosis, disease state, etc.).

The detailed analysis of cross-sectional femoral slabs confirmed the results of DEXA studies and added additional three-dimensional remodeling information. The analysis showed that the histomorphologic pattern of bone remodeling was characterized by cortical thinning and a decrease in cortical bone area and bone mineral density. For cementless components, a marked decrease (averaging 53%) in the thickness of the femoral cortex in the medial quadrant of the most

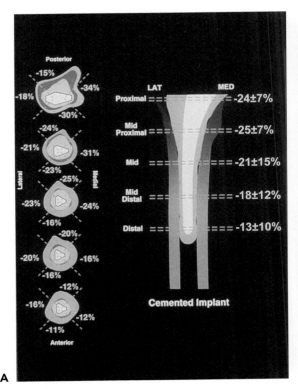
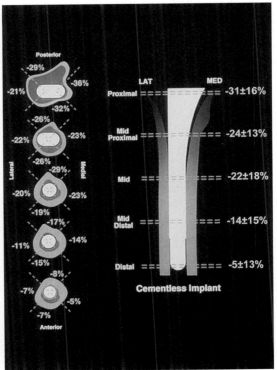

Figure 16-5   A: Mean percentage change in bone mineral density comparing remodeled with control femur by quadrant and level for 13 autopsy-retrieved cemented specimens. **B:** Mean percentage change in bone mineral density comparing remodeled with control femur by quadrant and level for 11 autopsy-retrieved cementless specimens. The metaphyseal levels showed greatest loss of cortical bone mineral density for both types of fixation. The magnitude of loss decreased from proximal to distal levels. (Reprinted from Maloney WJ, Sychterz C, Bragdon C, et al. The Otto Aufranc Award. Skeletal response to well fixed femoral components inserted with and without cement. *Clin Orthop.* 1996;333:15–26, with permission.)

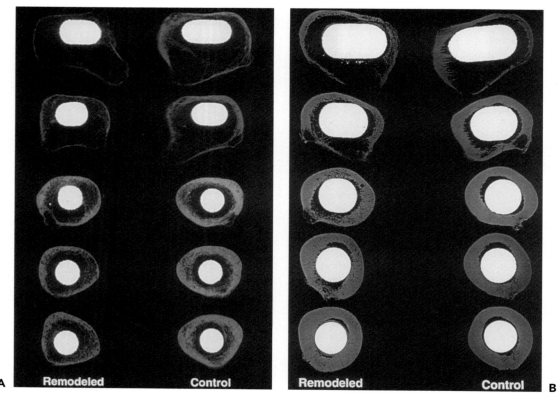

Figure 16-6 **A:** Cross-sectional radiographs from a patient who had a cementless total hip arthroplasty 2.8 years before death (remodeled, *left;* control, *right*). Note the isolated spot welds and absence of an inner cortex in the remodeled specimens. **B:** Cross-sectional radiographs from a patient who had cementless total hip arthroplasty 4.2 years before death (remodeled, *left;* control, *right*). Despite a relatively small stem (10.5-mm AML prosthesis) the remodeled femur shows marked bone loss compared with the control femur. (Reprinted from Maloney WJ, Sychterz C, Bragdon C, et al. The Otto Aufranc Award. Skeletal response to well fixed femoral components inserted with and without cement. *Clin Orthop.* 1996;333:15–26, with permission.)

proximal femoral section was found. Cortical thickness loss of 53% also was observed at the anterior quadrant of the mid-proximal section. Interestingly, there also were marked decreases of cortical thickness in the posterior quadrants of the diaphyseal region of the femur (middle, middistal, and distal femoral sections). Similar to DEXA analysis, a gradient in bone loss was observed. The largest decrease in bone density occurred in the medial quadrant of the proximal level (39%); decreases in density became less pronounced moving toward the distal tip of the prosthetic (Fig. 16-5).

For cemented components, the formation of an internal cortex similar to that described by Jasty et al. was found (17). Cemented specimens also demonstrated marked decreases in the thickness of the femoral cortex at the proximal medial quadrant (averaging 40%) and at the posterior quadrants of the diaphyseal region of the femur (range, 25% to 39%). A gradient of bone density decreases proximally to distally was observed (Fig. 16-5). The greatest levels of bone density loss occurred at the proximal (mean 24%) and midproximal (mean 25%) levels, and the least loss occurred adjacent to the tip of the stem (mean 13%). The largest loss of density in any one quadrant occurred in the proximal medial cortex (mean 34%). For changes in bone area, the middle level displayed the maximum amount of bone loss (mean 27%) for the cemented specimens.

Although the study showed that for both groups the remodeled femur had thinner cortices, less cortical bone area, and lower bone mineral density as compared to the control femora, there was a tremendous variability in the amount of bone loss from individual to individual, regardless of implant fixation (Figs. 16-6 and 16-7). Moreover, a strong correlation between the bone mineral density of the control femur and the percentage decrease in bone density of the remodeled femur was reported. In this study, stem stiffness did not correlate well with decreases in bone mineral density of the remodeled femur.

CORRELATION OF MECHANICAL FACTORS AND BONE LOSS

Finite-element and animal studies have indicated that bone remodeling is related to the ratio of stem stiffness to femoral stiffness: the stiffer the stem in relation to the femur, the less stress carried by the femur, and the greater the subsequent bone loss (3,8,25). Some clinical studies have confirmed the importance of stem stiffness in predicting bone loss (10,11), whereas other studies have found little relationship between the two variables (21,26). The studies that have examined the

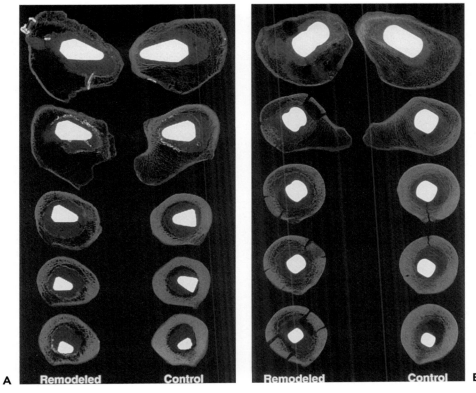

Figure 16-7   **A:** Cross-sectional radiographs from a patient who had a cemented total hip arthroplasty 15 years before death (remodeled, *left*; control, *right*). Note the inner cortex around the cement mantle in the remodeled sections. Note the thinning of the cortex in the remodeled femur even in the diaphyseal sections compared to the control femur. Also note the marked thinning of the posterior cortex. **B:** Cross-sectional radiographs from a patient who had a cemented total hip arthroplasty 4 years before death (remodeled, *left*; control, *right*). When compared to Figure 16-7A, the remodeling response is less dramatic with less cortical thinning and change in cortical bone area. (Reprinted from Maloney WJ, Sychterz C, Bragdon C, et al. The Otto Aufranc Award. Skeletal response to well fixed femoral components inserted with and without cement. *Clin Orthop.* 1996;333:15–26, with permission.)

relationship between femoral stiffness and bone remodeling around cementless components, however, have assumed a constant modulus for human cortical bone and have calculated femoral stiffness solely from changes in femoral geometry (3,8,10). Because the elastic modulus of cortical bone is related directly to its density (4–6), variations in modulus of different femora would be expected for the range of bone densities seen in patients having hip replacements. In bone remodeling studies, therefore, it is important for femoral stiffness calculations to account for changes in modulus resulting from variations in patient bone mineral density as well as to account for variations in femoral geometry. Two final studies discussed here have investigated the relationships between bone loss and the material and cross-sectional properties of the implant and bone, accounting for patient differences in cortical modulus and geometry.

In an investigation of 20 pairs of cadaveric femora from patients with unilateral cementless hip replacements, Sychterz et al. used femoral and stem stiffness values to model periprosthetic bone loss (27). Femoral stiffness calculations accounted for variations in modulus attributable to patient differences in bone mineral density and geometric properties attributable to differences in the shape of individual femora. The study found that axial bone stiffness was the strongest

individual predictor of bone loss; increased axial stiffness of the femur was associated with decreased bone loss. Individual implant stiffness terms were not significantly correlated with bone loss. Furthermore, multiple linear regression analysis, using stem-to-bone stiffness ratios as independent variables, accounted for 46% of the variance in bone loss data. In the regression analysis, axial stem-to-bone stiffness ratio was the strongest correlate with bone loss.

In a similar study of 13 pairs of cadaveric femora, Silva et al. examined the correlation between mechanical parameters and bone remodeling around cemented femoral implants (24). Similar to the study on cementless implants, Silva et al. found a strong correlation between stiffness parameters of the femur and bone loss and found no correlation between implant parameters and bone loss. In contrast to the cementless study, however, Silva et al. did not find that femoral axial parameters were more strongly correlated with bone loss than femoral bending or torsional parameters; all the parameters were associated equally with bone loss. The difference in results may be because cemented femoral implants are on average smaller and less stiff than uncemented femoral components. Therefore, the difference between the axial stiffness of the implant and that of the femur would be much smaller for a cemented femoral component than for an uncemented component.

Results from these studies suggest that the characteristics of the femur into which the stem is implanted may be more important than stem stiffness in determining the extent of bone loss following hip replacement surgery. As reiterated by Maloney et al., this is not to imply that stem stiffness is not an important factor influencing bone loss; however, with the great variations in bone parameters occurring in the hip replacement population, stem stiffness seems not as important as femoral parameters (bone mineral content, femoral stiffness) in governing the amount bone loss (21). It is likely that as sample sizes increase, permitting the evaluation of patients with similar cortical bone mass, the relationship between stem stiffness and adaptive bone remodeling will become evident.

SUMMARY

Clinical and autopsy studies have demonstrated that following implantation of a femoral endoprosthesis, a femur experiences a mean overall decrease in bone mineral density compared to the contralateral side. In accordance with Wolff's Law, the decrease in density mirrors the gradient of strain reduction also quantified from autopsy studies (13). DEXA analyses have quantified these decreases as between 5% and 39% loss of bone mineral density in different regions of the femur (18,21,22,26,28). Moreover, studies have demonstrated that bone loss occurs on a gradient, with the most loss proximally and the least loss distally (18,21,26). Studies also demonstrate that bone loss is more related to the characteristics of the femur into which a stem is implanted than any other variable (21,24,26,27).

The patterns of bone loss noted from well-fixed cementless and cemented femoral hip replacements have similarities and differences. In both groups, the remodeled femur had thinner cortices, less cortical bone area, and lower bone mineral density as compared to the control femora (21). With cemented stems, the bone remodeling response includes the creation a dense shell of substantial new bone around the cement mantle (17,21). This shell resembles a new cortex and is attached to the outer cortex by new trabecular struts. With cementless implants, the bone remodeling response is characterized by proximal bone atrophy, distal bone hypertrophy the presence of spot welds, and localized areas of bone bridging between the surface of the implant and the femoral cortex. Because this femoral pattern of bone remodeling is readily recognized radiographically, it can be used as a clinical tool for identifying bone-ingrown components on plain radiographs.

REFERENCES

1. Anthony PP, Gie GA, Howie CR, et al. Localised endosteal bone lysis in relation to the femoral components of cemented total hip arthroplasties. *J Bone Joint Surg Br.* 1990;72:971–979.
2. Bobyn JD, Jacobs JJ, Tanzer M, et al. The susceptibility of smooth implant surfaces to periimplant fibrosis and migration of polyethylene wear debris. *Clin Orthop.* 1995;311:21–39.
3. Bobyn JD, Mortimer ES, Glassman AH, et al. Producing and avoiding stress shielding: laboratory and clinical observations of noncemented total hip arthroplasty. *Clin Orthop.* 1992;274:79–96.
4. Burstein AH, Wright TM: Mechanical behavior of bone. In: *Fundamentals of Orthopaedic Biomechanics.* Baltimore: Williams & Wilkins; 1994:173–179.
5. Carter DR, Hayes WC. The compressive behavior of bone as a two-phase porous structure. *J Bone Joint Surg.* 1977;59A:954–962.
6. Carter DR, Spengler DM. Mechanical properties and composition of cortical bone. *Clin Orthop.* 1978;135:192–217.
7. Cohen B, Rushton N. Bone remodelling in the proximal femur after Charnley total hip arthroplasty. *J Bone Joint Surg Br.* 1995;77:815–819.
8. Dujovne AR, Bobyn JD, Krygier JJ, et al. Mechanical compatibility of noncemented hip prosthetics with the human femur. *J Arthroplasty.* 1993;8:7–22.
9. Dunn MG, Maxian SH. Biomaterials used in orthopaedic surgery. In: Greco RS, ed. *Implantation Biology, the Host Response and Biomedical Devices.* Boca Raton, FL: CRC Press; 1994.
10. Engh CA, Bobyn JD. The influence of stem size and extent of porous coating on femoral bone resorption after primary cementless hip arthroplasty. *Clin Orthop.* 1988;231:7–28.
11. Engh CA, Bobyn JD, Glassman AH. Porous-coated hip replacement. The factors governing bone ingrowth, stress shielding, and clinical results. *J Bone Joint Surg Br.* 1987;69B:45–55.
12. Engh CA, McGovern TF, Bobyn JD, et al. A quantitative evaluation of periprosthetic bone-remodeling after cementless total hip arthroplasty. *J Bone Joint Surg Am.* 1992;74A:1009–1020.
13. Engh CA, O'Connor D, Jasty M, et al. Quantification of implant micromotion, strain shielding, and bone resorption with porous-coated anatomic medullary locking femoral prostheses. *Clin Orthop.* 1992;285:13–29.
14. Fung YC. *Biomechanics: Mechanical Properties of Living Tissues.* New York: Springer-Verlag; 1981.
15. Harris WH. The problem is osteolysis. *Clin Orthop.* 1995;311:46–53.
16. Jacobs JJ, Shanbag A, Glant TT, et al. Wear debris in total joint replacements. *J Am Acad Orthop Surg.* 1994;2:212–220.
17. Jasty M, Maloney WJ, Bragdon CR, et al. Histomorphological studies of the long-term skeletal responses to well fixed cemented femoral components. *J Bone Joint Surg Am.* 1990;72:1220–1229.
18. Kilgus DJ, Shimaoka EE, Tipton JS, et al. Dual-energy X-ray absorptiometry measurement of bone mineral density around porous-coated cementless femoral implants. Methods and preliminary results. *J Bone Joint Surg Br.* 1993;75:279–287.
19. Kiratli BJ, Checovich MM, McBeath AA, et al. Measurement of bone mineral density by dual-energy x-ray absorptiometry in patients with the Wisconsin hip, an uncemented femoral stem. *J Arthroplasty.* 1996;11:184–193.
20. Maloney WJ, Jasty M, Rosenberg A, et al. Bone lysis in well-fixed cemented femoral components. *J Bone Joint Surg Br.* 1990;72:966–970.
21. Maloney WJ, Sychterz C, Bragdon C, et al. The Otto Aufranc Award. Skeletal response to well fixed femoral components inserted with and without cement. *Clin Orthop.* 1996;333:15–26.
22. McAuley JP, Sychterz CJ, Engh CA Sr. Influence of porous coating level on proximal femoral remodeling. A postmortem analysis. *Clin Orthop.* 2000;371:146–53.
23. Schmalzried TP, Jasty M, Harris WH. Periprosthetic bone loss in total hip arthroplasty: polyethylene wear debris and the concept of the effective joint space. *J Bone Joint Surg.* 1992;74A:849–863.
24. Silva MJ, Reed KL, Robertson DD, et al. Reduced bone stress as predicted by composite bone theory correlates with cortical bone loss following cemented total hip arthroplasty. *J Orthop Res.* 1999;17:525–531.
25. Skinner HB, Kilgus DJ, Keyak J, et al. Correlation of computed finite element stresses to bone density after remodeling around cementless femoral implants. *Clin Orthop.* 1994;305:178–189.
26. Sychterz CJ, Engh CA Sr. The influence of clinical factors on periprosthetic bone remodeling. *Clin Orthop.* 1996;322:285–292.
27. Sychterz CJ, Topoleski LD, Sacco M, et al. Effect of femoral stiffness on bone remodeling after uncemented arthroplasty. *Clin Orthop.* 2001;389:218–227.
28. Venesmaa PK, Kroger HP, Jurvelin JS, et al. Periprosthetic bone loss after cemented total hip arthroplasty: a prospective 5-year dual energy radiographic absorptiometry study of 15 patients. *Acta Orthop Scand.* 2003;74:31–36.
29. Willert HG. Reactions of the articular capsule to wear products of artificial joint prostheses. *J Biomed Mater Res.* 1977;11:157–64.

Tribology

17

Markus A. Wimmer   Alfons Fischer

HISTORY OF TRIBOLOGY

Tribology, whose name derives from the Greek terms for rubbing (τριβειν) and science (λογοσ), has been defined as "the science and technology of interacting surfaces in relative motion." Tribology comprises scientific and technical aspects of friction, wear, and lubrication and has made its appearance in many scientific branches, including orthopedics.

For several millennia, humankind has been aware of friction and wear. Cavemen used friction to light a fire by rubbing sticks on a piece of wood. The Egyptians and Sumerians (3500–35 BC) used leather belts to reduce friction between the axle and wheel of their carriages (29). Water, oil, fat, and bitumen served as early lubricants, the use of which permitted the transport of the stone blocks needed to build the pyramids. The first scientific approaches to analyze friction and wear were made by Italian Leonardo da Vinci (1452–1519). Da Vinci measured the frictional forces of bodies sliding on horizontal and inclined planes. He found that the friction force depended on the normal load but was independent of the apparent contact area. He also studied the wear on technical bearings in particular and recommended an alloy of three parts copper and seven parts tin as the material of choice.

Two centuries later, in France, Guillaume Amontons (1663–1705) independently confirmed the work of Leonardo da Vinci that the friction force depends on the normal load but not on the apparent area of contact. His observations on dry friction of solid bodies, in addition to those of his French compatriot Charles Augustin Coulomb (1736–1806), are commonly referred to as Coulomb's laws. Also the Englishman Sir Isaac Newton (1646–1727) was active in this branch of science. He became aware of the favorable influence of lubricants in reducing friction and wear and described their viscosity by means of fluid mechanics.

Two centuries later, the German Richard Striebeck (1861–1950) determined that adhesion, deformation, and lubrication were the principal portions of friction. With these newly developed laws, it became possible to describe the sliding frictional behavior of both lubricated and nonlubricated metal-on-metal joints. Because of the complex nature of friction and wear and the required interdisciplinary approach, a commission was founded by the British Department of Education and Science in 1966 and assigned the task of defining the scientific evaluation of friction, wear, and lubrication and of introducing the necessary interdisciplinary tools needed to solve the related problems (47). This commission defined the term "tribology" in 1966.

In contrast to natural synovial joints, which have excellent characteristics of low friction, high load carrying capacity, high shock absorption, and long endurance, many total joint prostheses have shown serious problems such as component failure and joint loosening due to wear. It was Sir John Charnley who introduced tribological thinking to the medical community as a result of his early clinically unsuccessful experience with Teflon (22). This well-known low friction material had extremely poor wear characteristics when articulating against a metallic counterbody in vivo. Large amounts of generated debris caused severe inflammatory reactions, which rapidly led to loosening of the artificial devices. This emphasized the need to carefully consider all the characteristics of a material under tribological stresses prior to implantation in humans.

SYSTEMIC ASPECTS OF TRIBOLOGY

Definitions, Terms, and Structure of a Tribological System

Friction arises from the interaction between moving solids in contact and hinders (sliding friction) or prevents (static friction) motion. Friction is the introduction, transformation, and dissipation of energy and may lead to loss of material. This (progressive) loss of particulate debris from the surface of a solid body due to mechanical action has been defined as *wear*. While mechanical fracture of the component may also occur in extreme contact cases, wear typically results in dimensional and

215

topographical changes as well as in surface damage. This can cause secondary problems such as misalignment or insufficient motion of the joint. The generation of wear debris, however, is in many cases even more detrimental than the actual dimensional change of components. Entrapped particles act as an interfacial medium and may change the acting wear mechanism. The effect of entrapped particles is, therefore, as important as their generation. While the mechanical properties of engineering materials can be described in terms of strength and toughness, friction and wear are not intrinsic material properties. Wear and friction are characteristic of a specific tribosystem and incorporate the physical (e.g., Young's modulus or thermal conduction) as well as the chemical properties (e.g., reactivity) of surfaces (25). A tribosystem consists of four principal elements: body, counterbody, interfacial medium, and environment (25,26). The operating variables load, relative speed, ambient temperature, and loading time bring about motion and work as an input to the system, resulting in motion and work as output. The loss of the system can be defined in terms of energy (heat or sound) and material (wear debris). Figure 17-1 shows a schematic of a tribosystem.

Since wear and friction arise from conditions at the interface, the properties of the surfaces in contact need to be looked at. Technical surfaces are far from being smooth and exhibit varying degrees of roughness, ranging from the nanometer to millimeter scale. Figure 17-2 highlights the differences between apparent and real area of contact on the micrometer scale. The irregularities of the surface usually consist of broad-based hills with angles of inclination of less than $15°$ from the base (104). The ratio of real to apparent area of contact changes constantly during motion and can range from $<10^{-4}$ to 1. This is dependent on the statistical distribution of topographical irregularities; the acting shear and normal contact forces; and the mechanical, physical, and chemical properties of the materials in contact, which might be distinctly different from the bulk properties.

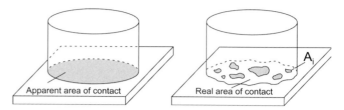

Figure 17-2 Apparent and real area of contact.

Because of the complex nature of friction and wear, the problems of tribology are difficult to assess by any simple model. The system approach as depicted in Figure 17-1 is an easy-to-use approach that can be applied to any tribological problem from an engineering point of view. In order to define the limits of this approach as well as its possibilities, it is mandatory to analyze worn surfaces under real operating conditions (e.g., hip joints from patients with complete medical history and clinical follow-up). Of course, this is a time-consuming and expensive process. A suitable wear-testing apparatus should reflect the structure of the tribosystem and the type of dynamic interaction between its elements. It should be considered that the proper modeling of the input parameters (e.g., loading and motion of the joint) will determine the acting wear mechanisms, while in turn a suitable wear-resistant material must be chosen with respect to them (32). In other words, the key to any solution of a tribological problem is inextricably linked to knowledge of the wear mechanisms as well as the sequence and interdependence of their acting. The authors stress the importance of knowing the acting wear mechanisms, since it is known that even for the same *wear mode* different design or material modifications are appropriate. For example, the parameters of the wear mode "three-body abrasion" of a metal-on-metal bearing with incorporated mineral particles can change in such a way that either the mechanism "adhesion" (cold welding of surface spots by plastic deformation of surface asperities), "abrasion" (grooving of surfaces by plastic flow), or "surface fatigue" (predominantly cyclic elastic and/or plastic deformation) apply. Thus, a successful plan to improve the characteristics of the materials in contact demands an exact understanding of the structure of the tribosystem and the interaction of its elements.

Initially, information on prosthesis design, joint kinematics, and kinetics in the physiological situation is requested. In the following subsections we introduce the relevant terminology regarding friction and wear on the basis of the historical development of today's available systematic, empirical approaches. Knowledge of the acting wear mechanism is essential to identify precise and purposeful measures for wear reduction and, thus, to go beyond simple trial-and-error methods. Theoretical models based on mechanical finite-element or chemical molecular-dynamics computer simulations will not be considered here, because, to date, they only investigate a very small area of interest and do not incorporate the entire tribosystem. Nevertheless, these models are very helpful in guiding the way from the systematic engineering approaches to the atomistic, theoretical level and facilitate a better understanding of specific single effects on friction and wear (40,53).

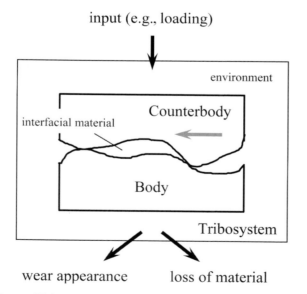

Figure 17-1 General description of the tribosystem, which consists of four principal elements: the two bodies in contact, the interfacial material, and the environment. All these elements can affect each other and change the mechanism of interaction.

Friction

Friction is generally understood as the introduction, transformation, and dissipation of energy. The introduction of friction is accomplished by cyclic elastic or plastic deformation of contact spots of the real contact area. Then it is transformed into elastic or plastic deformation energy within interlocking surface asperities (33,36) and/or leads to crack initiation and propagation (7,24). This describes the contribution of deformation to friction, which might also be responsible for the generation of particles. Another contribution comes from the adhesion of the surface atoms and molecules of body and counterbody. The probability of adhesion depends on mechanical properties (10) and the tendency of atoms and molecules to react chemically (73,76). Both the deformation and adhesion contributions to friction can be distinctly lowered by means of surface modifications or coatings as well as by lubrication. At least 90% of the introduced energy is dissipated by transformation into heat (8,44,50–52), leading to an increase of the temperature within the contact zone. Depending on local normal forces and the relative velocity, the average as well as the so-called flash temperatures may rise. Although the average temperature is primarily governed by the normal force, the flash temperature depends mostly on the relative velocity and lasts for only a few nanoseconds or milliseconds. The remaining 10% is dissipated by storing mechanical energy within lattice defects generated by cyclic elastic and plastic deformation (75), phase transformation (97), or chemical reaction of body, counterbody, interfacial medium, and environment (37).

Lubrication

Friction can be reduced by lubrication. The principal idea behind lubrication is to interpose a material between two contacting solids to minimize interaction between them. For example, wetting of the surfaces reduces adhesion. The extent of fluid film formation plays an important role in the wear process of artificial joints in vivo. It has been pointed out that under wet conditions the wear rate of UHMWPE decreases steadily with decreasing counterface roughness, whereas under nonlubricated (dry) conditions an optimum roughness exists (due to the competing mechanisms adhesion and abrasion) (30). Hence, adequate surface finishing of the counterface (at least $R_a < 0.05$ µm) without imperfections is recommended when prosthetic head materials are paired with UHMWPE (61).

The effectiveness of a lubricant film can be defined by the specific film thickness h which is dependent on the viscosity of the lubricant, the relative velocity between body and counterbody, the pressure across the interface, and, last but not least, the roughness of the mating surfaces. h can be used to estimate the occurrence of different lubrication regimes, as shown in Figure 17-3. In the case of boundary lubrication, the lubricant adheres chemically to one of the surfaces, and there is full contact between the solids, in contrast to hydrodynamic lubrication, where a total separation of the two bodies takes place. Elastohydrodynamic (EHD) lubrication occurs when the pressure in the fluid film is sufficiently high to deform the asperities of the solid surfaces. Thus, even if the thickness of the fluid film is less than the heights of the asperities of body and counterbody, a total separation may be still achieved.

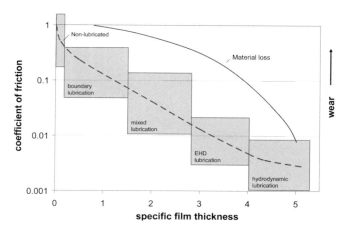

Figure 17-3 Coefficient of friction and wear resistance in rolling–sliding contact as a function of the specific lubricant film thickness. (Adapted from Zum Gahr K-H. *Microstructure and Wear of Materials*. Amsterdam: Elsevier; 1987. Tribology Series vol. 10.)

Under realistic loads and in the presence of synovial fluid, metal-on-polyethylene hip joints articulate in the mixed film (67) or boundary (31) lubrication regime. Hard-on-hard bearings primarily work in the elastohydrodynamic and mixed film lubrication regime (45); however, with increasing femoral head size (>28 mm), a shift toward full fluid film (hydrodynamic) lubrication can be observed as well (86).

Wear

Wear has been defined as removal of material from the body in contact as a consequence of mechanical action; thus, creep and plastic deformation are not forms of wear per se because they do not produce wear debris but dimensional changes of the contacting surfaces. Also, corrosion is not directly related to wear because it can take place without any mechanical activation at all. In order to be able to describe wear phenomena unequivocally, it is strongly suggested to distinguish between *wear modes*, *wear appearances*, and *wear mechanisms* (104).

Wear Mode

The wear mode defines the general mechanical conditions under which the bearing is functioning when wear occurs. Wear modes are defined by two sets of criteria: first by the macroscopic structure of the tribosystem and the kinematic interaction of its elements and second by the combination of acting wear mechanisms. Table 17-1 displays a selection of relevant wear modes that have been put together based on *Tribology: Definitions, Terminology, Testing* (93). It should be noted that the wear mode is not a steady-state condition and can change from one form to another. For example, particulate debris generated by two-body abrasion may function as an interfacial medium and turn the problem into a particle-related (third-body) phenomenon. Depending on the circumstances, this may reduce or increase the wear rate.

Wear Mechanisms

The wear mechanisms describe the mechanical, physical, and chemical interaction of the elements of a tribosystem. Today,

TABLE 17-1
A SYNOPSIS OF WEAR MODES

Systemic Structure	Tribological Operating Condition		Wear Mode	Acting Mechanism (Single or Combined)			
				Adhesion	Abrasion	Surface Fatigue	Tribo-Chemical Reactions
Solid body – lubricant – (total separation) Solid body	Sliding, rolling, impact		—			●	○
Solid body — Solid body	Sliding		Sliding wear	●	○	○	●
	Rolling		Rolling wear	○	○	●	○
	Oscillating		Fretting wear	●	●	●	●
			Impact wear	○	○	●	○
Solid body — Particles			Impact erosion		●	●	○
Solid body — Solid body + Particles	Sliding		Three-body abrasion	○	●	●	○
	Rolling		Rolling abrasion	○	●	●	○

Note: The prevalent wear mechanisms are shown for each mode. Please note that this table is based on "general" observation. Also, other combinations of wear mechanisms may apply for the specific wear mode.
Adapted from *Tribology: Definitions, Terminology, Testing.* Moers, Germany: German Society of Tribology; 2002. GfT Arbeitsblatt 7.

four major wear mechanisms are distinguished: abrasion, surface fatigue, adhesion, and tribochemical reactions. Whereas abrasion and surface fatigue are mechanically dominated, adhesion and tribochemical reactions are mechanically and chemically driven.

Nearly all implants that have been removed from patients exhibit grooves and/or scratches; thus, *abrasion* is one of the most obvious wear mechanisms. Abrasion may be induced by foreign particles (contaminants from outside the wear system, such as bone cement) or by system inherent particles (e.g., fractured carbides, wear debris). Depending on the local contact situation (e.g., attacking angle, sharpness) and the properties of the bodies in contact (e.g., hardness, fracture toughness, strength, ductility), abrasion may reveal four different submechanisms—microploughing, microcutting, microcracking, and microfatigue—that reflect the cyclic elastic and/or plastic nature of the contact (104). Although the main wear loss is attributed to abrasion in many references, it is often questionable whether this wear mechanism initiated the failure sequence.

Surface fatigue acts during repeated sliding or rolling over the same wear track. The repeated loading and unloading can induce the initiation and propagation of microcracks parallel and orthogonal to the surfaces for mechanical (88) or material-related (14,79) reasons. As a result, shallow pits and filaments (delaminations) are generated.

During *adhesion*, material from both surfaces adheres to each other within the contact spots. This process is similar to friction welding. During mechanical action, these microjunctions are torn off, and fragments may become particles or be transferred from body to counterbody and vice versa, bringing about surface damage in the form of flakes and pitting. If the generated flakes and particles are bigger than the clearance of the bearing, they may act as abrasive particles or even block the joint. In particular, metals with high ductility in a self-mating contact situation experience adhesion (13,85).

Tribochemical reactions occur when surfaces in mechanical contact react with the interfacial medium and the environment, resulting in the alternating formation and removal of

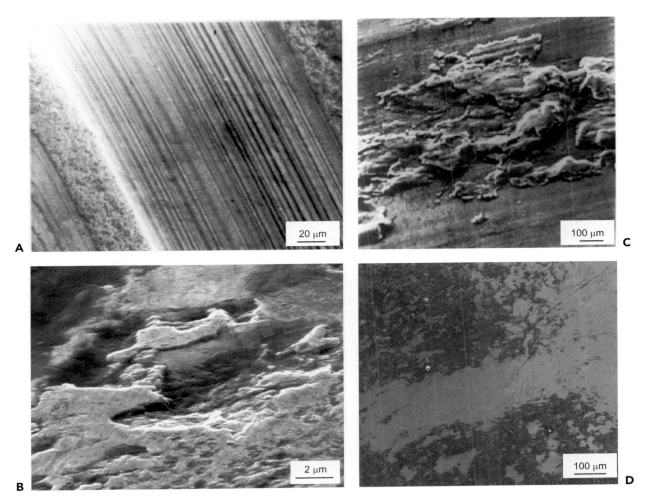

Figure 17-4 Typical appearance of the four major wear mechanisms. **A:** Abrasion: grooves on a metal surface. **B:** Surface fatigue: delamination on the surface of a metallic component. **C:** Adhesion: transferred metal flakes. **D:** Tribochemical reactions: chromium-rich, denatured protein layers on the head of a metal-on-metal articulation. Note the differences in scale.

chemical reaction products at the surfaces. Mechanical and thermal activation of the surfaces due to friction leads to contact spots with an increased chemical reactivity (9) such that, for example, oxidized islands are generated (72). These oxide layers spall off the surfaces after reaching a critical thickness. It is also possible that the interfacial medium (e.g., synovial fluid) is directly involved in the generation of tribochemical reaction layers, with sustained effects to friction and wear of the bearing (103). This process is similar to the action of so-called extreme-pressure (EP) additives in high-performance lubricants for the motors of passenger cars or trucks.

Wear Appearance

The wear appearances describe the visible changes of a surface structure as a consequence of wear. "Wear pattern" or "wear damage" are synonyms that can be found in the literature. Wear appearances are characteristic signs of the wear mechanisms (Fig. 17-4) that have been acting on the contacting bodies and that are responsible for the resultant changes in surface texture and shape.

At this point it is worth mentioning that retrieved components show primarily those appearances of wear related to

mechanisms acting immediately before removal. Since most removals are conducted because of a preceding prosthesis failure, the steady-state wear mode might be obscured by a secondary wear mode taking place *after* failure initiation. Further, it is likely that wear marks are being introduced during the explantation procedure itself. In the past, we have been repeatedly confronted with grooves with distinct piles at their edges that cannot stem from a steady-state action of abrasion. In those cases, the piles at the rims would have brought about adhesion and led to an extremely severe wear loss.

Clearly, within the system there are many sharp and blunt particles of different origin[1] that are capable of inducing abrasion or a certain form of surface fatigue during steady-state wear (e.g., bone cement [PMMA], x-ray contrast particles [ZrO_2], remains of sandblast cleaning [Al_2O_3], and wear particle agglomerates [fused nanometer-size metal particles]). Surface fatigue appears as small indentations and can be easily identified, but abrasion produces grooves of different depths and widths that become very difficult to attribute to a

---

[1] It should be noted that very small particles in the nanometer range are not necessarily harmful but could act as solid lubricant.

particular wear mode unambiguously. It is therefore important to understand the sequence of acting mechanisms as well as their contribution to the behavior of the entire tribosystem. Also, the mechanisms should always be investigated relative to the specific physiological conditions and materials involved. Specific supplementary biomechanical and biochemical dispositions of the patient should be recognized and included in the analysis. Then it will be possible to state clear recommendations regarding the wear improvement of the device.

TRIBOLOGY OF THE ARTIFICIAL HIP JOINT

System Analysis

The human hip joint is a tribological system and should be looked at using the system analysis methodology discussed later in this chapter. With respect to Figure 17-1, the ball is the body and the cup is designated as the counterbody. The interfacial medium is the synovial fluid, which maintains a temperature of 37°C during function. The environment (oxygen pressure, temperature, etc.) is regulated by the human body. The loads and motions during daily activity determine the input to the system, and the moment of friction and the generation of particulate debris and/or metal ions characterize the output.

System Input

Daily Activities

A recent study of the frequency and duration of daily activities in patients after total hip arthroplasty demonstrated that the most frequent patient activity was sitting (44.3% of the time), followed by standing (24.5%), walking (10.2%), lying (5.8%), and stair climbing (0.4%) (60). The average patient performed 6048 steps per day, which adds up to approximately 1.1 million gait cycles per year. In addition, 164 stairs were climbed on average.

As we all experienced personally, wear is a function of use, and Schmalzried et al. (82) reported a significant correlation between the progression of wear of the implant and patient-specific activity (measured in steps per day). Without three recognized outliers, wear was highly significant but moderately correlated to use ($r^2 = 0.3$), suggesting additional system factors that influence the output.

The activity of human beings is highly variable, and it recently became obvious that resting periods make up a substantial part of daily activity (64). Resting phases as long as 30 seconds' duration with the patient in the upright position were found to represent a frequent component of daily activities. For example, 10- to 30-second standstills occurred up to 26 times per hour. Shorter resting periods of 2 to 5 seconds have been found to occur even more frequently (100 times per hour). Resting periods may be detrimental because they can cause a disruption of lubrication. Interestingly, metal-on-metal bearings showed the highest increase in friction after motion initiation (64).

Load and Motion

Because of its frequency and load demand, gait is the most important activity for the purpose of wear testing and analysis.

There were a few patients whose load and motion profile was directly measured using instrumented hip prostheses (4,6,27,39,77); however, much of our current knowledge about the kinematics and kinetics of hip joints has been derived from gait analysis.

Relative motion of the hip joint during gait involves all three angular degrees of freedom. At heel strike, the hip is in a flexed position and extends throughout the stance phase. During the time period from initial swing through midswing, the hip moves from extension into flexion and stays flexed until heel strike. For a typical, normal male the flexion–extension range of motion during stance spans from +30° (flexion) to −10° (extension), accompanied by a coronal arc movement of approximately 10° and a transverse plane motion of approximately 15° (70,94). It should be noted that total hip patients often show an abnormal gait pattern with decreased range of motion (62,69).

Ground reaction forces, arising during human locomotion, impose *external forces* and *external moments* at the hip joint, which must be balanced by a set of internal forces (1). These internal forces are generated by muscles, the hip joint contact force, and soft-tissue constraints. The muscles are in the best position to resist the external moments because they have lever-arms of sufficient length, defined from their lines of action to the point of contact at the joint.

At heel strike, the external moment tends to flex the hip joint, reaching a maximum value just before midstance. In order to balance this moment internally, the extensor muscles are active. The pattern reverses direction just before midstance to a moment tending to extend the joint. This sinusoidal flexion-extension pattern is accompanied by an adduction moment, which acts almost throughout the entire period of stance. The internal–external rotation moment is much lower in value and thus has less contribution in the generated contact force at the hip joint. Typical moment values for a total hip population are listed in Table 17-2.

TABLE 17-2

MINIMUM, MAXIMUM, MEAN AND STANDARD DEVIATION FOR EXTERNAL PEAK HIP JOINT MOMENTS DURING STANCE, FLEXION–EXTENSION HIP RANGE OF MOTION DURING STANCE, AND WEAR RATE FOR 13 TOTAL HIP PATIENTS

	Minimum	Maximum	Mean	Standard Deviation
Flexion (Nm)	44.7	200.2	110.0	44.1
Extension (Nm)	28.8	123.8	62.3	30.21
Adduction (Nm)	14.2	101.3	60.5	24.0
Abduction (Nm)	1.6	29.3	10.7	9.0
Internal rotation (Nm)	2.0	12.0	4.3	2.8
External rotation (Nm)	1.1	60.5	13.4	15.2
Range of motion (degrees)	16.8	33.2	24.4	5.0
Wear rate (mm/a)	0.009	0.395	0.163	0.095

It is important to note that the measured moments during gait can only be interpreted in terms of "net muscle" demand, because of antagonistic and synergistic muscle activity during gait. Still, using the correct physiological rules that put limits on the force a muscle can generate, plus finding the right criteria for the in vivo optimization process, it is possible to predict hip joint contact forces using musculoskeletal models (38,41).

Contact Forces

Bergmann et al. published the most recent measured contact force data during various activities using a telemetric transmission system (4,5). From the four patients analyzed during routine activities, the average peak load at the hip was approximately 2.4 times the body weight (BW) when walking at a "normal" speed of 1.1 m/s. This was slightly more than standing in single-leg stance. When going upstairs, the joint contact force was 2.5 BW, and going downstairs, 2.6 BW. The peak contact forces during all other common daily activities were comparably small, except for stumbling. Peak forces during unanticipated stumbling were as high as 8 BW (5), which is considerably larger than the impact during jogging of 5.5 BW (6).

These forces have been measured directly and can therefore be regarded as accurate. Nevertheless, it should be noted that there is an enormous intra- and intervariability of forces during daily activities among total hip patients that is not reflected by the numbers given above. The applied force has an effect on the tribological behavior of the system. Thus, a recent study showed that the peak external joint moments (as a measure for the joint contact force) and the hip range of motion during the stance phase (assuming equal head sizes) predicted the wear rates in total hip patients (102). Six male and seven female patients were included in this study. By the time of surgery, these patients were 54 years old. All patients were tested at least once in the biomotion laboratory. A self-selected "normal" speed for each of the subjects was chosen to represent that subject's daily walking pattern. A computer-assisted vector wear technique for digital radiographs was used for the determination of linear polyethylene wear of the cup. On average, seven radiographs, acquired every 1 to 2 years during follow-up visits, were used. It was found that the sagittal plane motion, as well as the external moments at the hip, was very variable among patients during the stance phase (Table 17-2). Similarly, the linear wear rates for the 13 patients varied between 0.009 and 0.395 mm per year, which is an inconsistent finding, given the fact that all patients wore the same prostheses with the same ball diameter implanted in a single institution. Interestingly, the combination of joint moments and sagittal plane motion was significantly correlated with the wear rates of these patients (according to Archard's equation [2], where the generated wear volume is proportional to the applied force times the sliding distance). Regression analysis indicated that 43% of the variance in the wear rate was explained by the product of added joint moments and hip range of motion (Fig. 17-5). Eliminating recognized outliers further increased the strength of the relationship to $r^2 = 0.65$.

Overall the above findings suggest that the patient-specific contact force (and motion) during gait is highly variable and indicative of the progression of wear. Many studies have reported that total hip patients *do not* achieve a "normal" walking pattern as compared with age-matched control subjects (12,57,63,68). Yet, most wear tests are based on motion

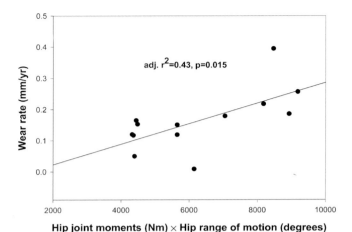

Figure 17-5 Relationship between wear rate and the complex of loads acting on the component. Hip moments (as a surrogate marker for joint load) and the range of motion during flexion–extension (as a marker for sliding distance) explain nearly half of the variability in wear.

and force input data derived from normal gait (e.g., ISO Hip and Knee Wear Testing standards [42,43] and ASTM Hip and Knee Wear Testing standard and proposals respectively [3,96]). This should be born in mind when performing tribological analyses.

Wear Path

Ramamurti et al. (74) performed an analysis of the wear path during human locomotion on the acetabular bearing surface. It was revealed that the wear tracks form quasi-elliptical to rectangular paths. The paths varied widely in shape as well as in length over the contact area, but all crossed each other during the cyclic motion pattern of gait. It was therefore suggested that the surface experiences multidirectional shear forces disturbing the structural alignment of UHMWPE. Additional experimental studies verified the concept of "multidirectional wear" in that the crossing of the wear tracks accelerated the formation of particulate debris (11).

Saikko and Calonius (78) repeated the analysis of Ramamurti et al. (74) but used a new computation method based on Euler angles (Fig. 17-6). Their findings were different from those of Ramamurti et al., and they showed that there are distinct differences between the shapes of the wear tracks generated by contemporary hip simulator designs (18,78). In a subsequent paper, the authors focused on the track drawn by the resultant contact force (17). Taking published motion data from a normal subject (46), they plotted the length of the so-called force track and its related velocities. For a 28-mm head, the length of the force track was 23.2 mm. The relative speed between head and cup ranged from 0.6 to 49.6 mm/s, with an average of 20.5 mm/s. Following Archard's equation, the product of the instantaneous load and increment of sliding distance was numerically integrated and determined to be 22.3 Nm for one completed gait cycle. Plotting the same product for 11 contemporary hip simulators demonstrated that already the motion and load input may account for the large interlaboratory range

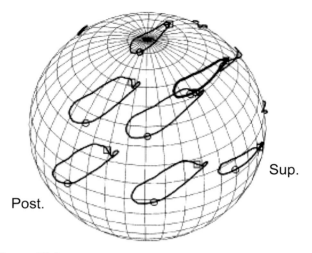

Post.

Sup.

Figure 17-6 Slide tracks of selected points on the femoral head computed from the three angular motions of the hip during gait. The "force track" is drawn with a *thicker line*. The *square* indicates heel-strike and the *circle* toe-off. (Reproduced with permission from Saikko V, Calonius O. Slide track analysis of the relative motion between femoral head and acetabular cup in walking and in hip simulators. *J Biomech* 2002;35:455–464.)

of measured wear rates: the track length–force integral ranged from 17.4 to 43.5 Nm.

Wear Mode

In conclusion, by and large, the wear mode in a human hip joint can be designated as multidirectional sliding wear because the wear paths of the forward and backward stroke do not lie on identical geometrical lines. However, there are time intervals during the gait cycle where the strokes match. In these circumstances, the wear mode is attributed solely to reciprocating sliding wear. Thus, the wear mode is a mixture of reciprocating and multidirectional sliding wear. Nevertheless, in both wear modes all known major wear mechanisms—adhesion, abrasion, surface fatigue, and tribochemical reactions—may act at the same time (93). Hence, it becomes imperative to identify those dominating the tribological behavior.

Wear Mechanisms with Respect to System Output

Characteristic wear appearances for all four major wear mechanisms have been observed on the articulating surfaces of total hip prostheses and are documented in an extensive body of literature. Often, particle nature, size, and shape can help in identifying the particular mechanism as well.

Adhesion

Appearances of adhesion have been found on the surface of polyethylene cups matched with a metallic ball (58). Microscopic welding between cup and ball generated fibrils on the surface of the polymeric material. These fibrils may become torn off and pulled away as loose particles. Note their characteristic elongated shape in Figure 17-7. Without sufficient

lubrication, bigger fragments may be transferred from counterbody to body and vice versa.

As reviewed in one of the previous chapters, metal-on-metal bearings are successfully used in a self-mating contact despite the fact that this violates a principle of tribology engineering, which is never to allow surfaces of high ductility to slide on each other. Taking the face-centered cubic microstructure of these cobalt–chromium alloys into account, flakelike particles with a diameter of several microns should be expected (85). However, metal-on-metal wear debris has been reported smaller than 250 nm, with a prevalence 50-nm particles (19,28). Investigating this paradox more closely, the authors indeed found no appearances of adhesion in a collection of 42 McKee-Farrar prostheses from 13 male and 29 female patients with an average time in situ of 11.7 years (103).

Abrasion

Abrasion is an often-reported mechanism in metal-on-metal and other hip joint bearings, because scratches and grooves are always obvious (20,21,59,83,84,95,99). As commented earlier, abrasion may be induced by many sources from outside and inside the system. System-inherent abrasive bodies include fractured carbides, compacted wear debris, and large flakes generated as a consequence of adhesion. Figure 17-8 shows grooves and scratches on a polyethylene cup due to third-body influence.

Surface Fatigue

Surface fatigue is typically associated with repetitive loading, and its wear appearances, such as pitting and delamination, are often reported for the polyethylene liner of the artificial knee joint but less frequently for the polyethylene cup (23,54). In postmortem liners (and thus in implants still in a well-functioning condition by the time of retrieval), pitting occurred with a low severity (90) and was mostly found in the transition zone from contact area to noncontact area. This may be an indication for the influence of extrinsic third

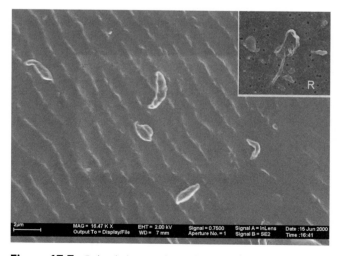

Figure 17-7 Polyethylene surface of a worn hip cup. The surface ripples are most likely an effect of the crystalline structure of polyethylene. "Shreds" and "fibrillar" particles are generated because of adhesion of the articulating bodies. The small window shows captured polyethylene particles on a 0.1 μm filter.

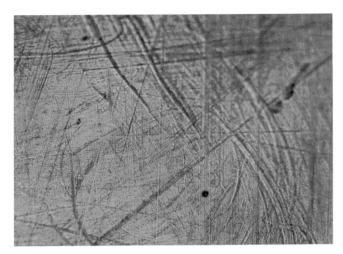

Figure 17-8 Light microscope image showing typical scratches and grooves on the dome of a polyethylene cup (original magnification 100×).

bodies (bone cement, bone chips) during the early part of service life (34). Delamination appeared occasionally in polyethylene cups but was mostly limited to heavily oxidized liners (89).

Surface fatigue is introduced by direct solid contact of surface asperities or by foreign and system-inherent third bodies that repeatedly slide or roll within the wear track. The authors showed that the so-called indentations or micropits in metal-on-metal joints (Fig. 17-9) are generated by fractured carbides and agglomerated wear particles forced to roll over the articulating surfaces (101). These small particles separate the metal surfaces from each other, preventing adhesion (and thus a potential catastrophic breakdown of the tribosystem). However, at the same time, these third bodies cause wear loss by surface fatigue, whereby this loss is several orders of magnitude smaller than that caused by adhesion or abrasion (80). The situation changes with bigger and/or sharper particles. Those typically get

stuck on either one of the two bearing surfaces and generate grooves on the countersurface. As a consequence, abrasion takes place. In particular, in the case of ductile face-centered cubic metals, appearances of the submechanisms microcutting and microploughing are prevalent (101,104).

Tribochemical Reactions

In most systems, tribochemical reactions distinctly alter the chemical properties of surfaces, hindering or preventing adhesion. For that reason, they are beneficial for the tribological behavior of technical applications. For polyethylene components, tribochemical reactions are not yet described, while for metal-on-metal implants, there have been indications of the beneficial influence of tribochemical reactions on the wear behavior (101,103). Organic tribochemical reaction layers that consist predominantly of decomposed proteins stuck rigidly to the oxide layers on the metal surfaces of the previously described McKee-Farrar prostheses (Fig. 17-10). It is believed that they are generated in the contact spots due to flash temperatures reaching more than 60°C. By reducing the probability of solid metal-on-metal contact, the reaction layers act as a solid lubricant (87). In addition, surface fatigue was also reduced effectively. Scanning electron microscopy (SEM) with energy-dispersive spectroscopy (EDS) and X-ray photoelectron spectroscopy (XPS) indicated that the layers were made up of carbon, oxygen, sodium, magnesium, calcium, nitrogen, sulfur, phosphorus, and chlorine. These elements are available from proteins within the physiological environment. The layers were proven to be of protein origin by the Bradford dye-binding method (103).

"Foreign layers" have been observed in vivo and in vitro by several authors (20,56,59,71,83,91,95) and have been described as "(calcium phosphate) precipitates" and/or "deposits." However, they were not believed to participate in the wear process directly. Due to the fact that they disturbed the weight and profile measurements (59), ethylene-diamine-tetra-acetic acid (EDTA) has been used as a serum additive to minimize calcium phosphate deposits in vitro. Interestingly, the effects on wear of using EDTA as a serum additive are negligible (21). This

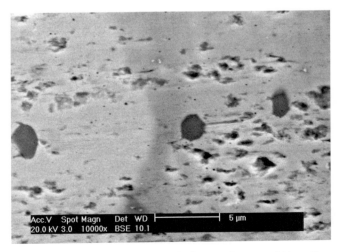

Figure 17-9 Pitting on the head of a metal-on-metal hip articulation. Note the arrangement of the pits, which point toward surface fatigue as major wear mechanism. The BSE detector allows the differentiation between matrix and carbides. Due to the lower atomic number, the carbides appear dark in the micrograph.

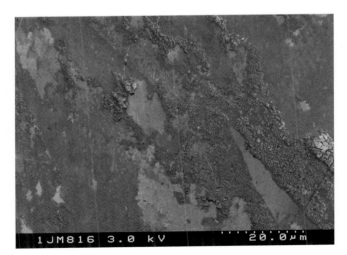

Figure 17-10 Tribochemical reaction layers as seen on explanted McKee-Farrar prostheses. The carbon rich layers are of varying thickness and are firmly attached to the cobalt–chromium matrix.

finding supports the opinion of the authors that the deposits are generated by tribochemical reactions and are not due to chemical attack. Such a possibility had been at first ruled out by Semlitsch et al. (83), but the consequences with respect to wear sequence and interaction of wear mechanisms were not further investigated.

OUTLOOK FOR OTHER HIP TRIBOSYSTEMS AND CONCLUSIONS

In wrapping up this chapter, it should be mentioned that artificial hip prostheses involve more than one tribosystem with specific characteristics. The above described ball-and-cup system is characterized by a stroke length exceeding the dimensions of the Hertzian contact area. This wear mode is called sliding wear. The surface of at least one body is always in direct contact with the interfacial medium and/or with the environment. In the case of a metal-on-metal component, this gives rise to tribochemical reactions (low wear) that hinder surface fatigue (more wear) and prevent adhesion (high wear). Other nonarticulating surfaces like those between bone cement and shaft or between components of modular junctions can show very small strokes caused by stiffness differences between the bodies in contact. If these strokes are smaller than the dimensions of the Hertzian contact area, the wear mode is designated as fretting. Typically, the contacting surfaces of body and counterbody are barely exposed to the interfacial medium and to the environment. Thus, tribochemical reactions and their protecting effect diminish, giving rise to surface fatigue and adhesion and ultimately to severe wear. In addition, it is possible for the environmentally truncated contact area to undergo oxygen depletion, triggering crevice corrosion and other corrosive effects (98). Thus, surface cracks can further propagate into the bulk and may bring about fatigue failure of the stem.

Returning to the ball-and-cup system, one of the most important tasks of the tribologist is to prevent adhesion, which is typically present when the same materials are paired. Assuming that the tribological data for a bearings system are unknown, catastrophic adhesion can be securely prevented with non-self-mating couples (e.g., metal–polymer and ceramic–polymer). Also non-chemically-active self-mating couples (e.g., ceramic–ceramic) are a safe choice. Despite of the reported low in vivo wear rates of ceramic–ceramic couples (66,81,100), there is little information about the in vivo acting mechanisms from clinical applications. Until recently, it was not possible to replicate clinically relevant wear rates, patterns, and particles for ceramic–ceramic couples in hip simulators. More realistic wear has been achieved by inducing microseparation between ball and cup during the swing phase of the gait cycle (35,65,92). This purposeful malpositioning of ball and cup increases the contact stress (55) and, thus, increases the possibility of surface fatigue—probably the dominant wear mechanism of ceramic–ceramic couples in vivo. In addition to mechanical stress cycles, ceramics undergo distinct thermal cycles within contact spots because of their low thermal conductivity. The acting temperatures could lead to thermoshock or phase transformation, especially with zirconia (48,49). Other ceramics like alumina have more favorable physical and chemical properties and are claimed to withstand thermal stress cycles better (48).

To summarize the above cited investigations of hip joints, it appears that moderate adhesion dominates in polymer–metal couples, is reduced in polymer–ceramic couples, and disappears completely in metal-on-metal bearings. As a first macroscopic approximation on the basis of the geometrical and biomechanical study of the tribosystem, this might look inconclusive, but by adding a second microscopic one based on an understanding of the acting wear mechanisms, a sound analysis is acquired. Thus, large wear particles of a polymer stuck to the surface of a metal ball (adhesion) result in rougher surfaces and increase local contact pressures. Mechanically activated surfaces do react with the interfacial medium and the environment, resulting in protective ceramic (oxidic passive layers) or organic (decomposed proteins) tribochemical reaction layers. In addition, the nanometer-size wear particles act as some kind of solid lubricant. These small particles stem from a nanocrystalline layer generated during the run-in period by recrystallization in combination with mechanical mixing of the surface material with the interfacial medium. Now it is important that the bulk is able to support this layer sufficiently. Co-base alloys bring about such a beneficial gradient of microstructures under physiological stresses (15,16), whereas, for example, UHMWPE polymers or 316L-type steels do not (14) and therefore generate much larger wear particles.

Obviously the floating equilibrium between the wear mechanisms acting on the surface and the microstructural changes of the materials underneath stabilize the tribosystem. Thus, any focused optimization can only be carried out on the basis of a complete and sound analysis of the macroscopic mechanical and chemical loading, an analysis of the microscopic mechanisms acting on and underneath the surface, and an understanding of their interaction.

REFERENCES

1. Andriacchi TP, Natarajan RN, Hurwitz DE. Musculoskeletal dynamics, locomotion and clinical applications. In: Mow VC, Hayes WC, eds. *Basic Orthopaedic Biomechanics.* 2nd ed. Philadelphia: Lippincott-Raven; 1997:37–68.
2. Archard JF. Contact and rubbing of flat surfaces. *J Appl Phys* 1953;24.981–988.
3. *ASTM F 2025: Standard Practice for Gravimetric Measurement of Polymeric Components for Wear Assessment.* West Conshohocken, PA: ASTM; 2000.
4. Bergmann G, Deuretzbacher G, Heller M, et al. Hip contact forces and gait patterns from routine activities. *J Biomech* 2001; 34:859–71.
5. Bergmann G, Graichen F, Rohlmann A. Hip joint contact forces during stumbling. *Langenbecks Arch Surg* 2004;389:53–59.
6. Bergmann G, Graichen F, Rohlmann A. Hip joint loading during walking and running, measured in two patients. *J Biomech* 1993;26:969–990.
7. Bethune B. The surface cracking of glassy polymers under a sliding spherical indenter. *J Mater Sci* 1976;11:199–205.
8. Blok H. General discussion on lubrication. *Proc Inst Mech Eng* (London) 1937;2:121.
9. Bowden FP, Hughes TP. Physical properties of surfaces, IV: polishing, surface flow and the formation of Beilby layer. *Proc R Soc Lond A* 1937;160:575–587.
10. Bowden FP, Tabor D. *The Friction and Lubrication of Solids.* Vols. 1, 2. Oxford: Clarendon Press, 1964.
11. Bragdon CR, O'Connor DO, Lowenstein JD, et al. The importance of multidirectional motion on the wear of polyethylene. *Proc Inst Mech Eng [H]* 1996;210:157–165.
12. Bryan JM, Sumner DR, Hurwitz DE, et al. Altered load history affects periprosthetic bone loss following cementless total hip arthroplasty. *J Orthop Res* 1996;14:762–768.

13. Buckley D. *Surface Effects in Adhesion, Wear and Lubrication.* Amsterdam: Elsevier; 1984. Tribology Series vol. 5.
14. Büscher R, Fischer A. Metallurgical aspects of sliding wear of fcc materials for medical applications. *MATWER* 2003;34: 966–975.
15. Büscher R, Täger G, Gleising B, et al. Subsurface microstructure of metal-on-metal hip joints and its relationship to wear particle generation. *J Biomed Mat Res* 2005;72B:206–214.
16. Büscher R, Wimmer MA, Täger G, et al. The origin of nanometer sized debris in metal-on-metal hip joints. *Transactions of the 50th Annual Meeting of the Orthopaedic Research Society* 2004; 29:1511.
17. Calonius O, Saikko V. Force track analysis of contemporary hip simulators. *J Biomech* 2003;36:1719–1726.
18. Calonius O, Saikko V. Slide track analysis of eight contemporary hip simulator designs. *J Biomech* 2002;35:1439–1450.
19. Catelas I, Bobyn JD, Medley JB, et al. Effects of digestion protocols on the isolation and characterization of metal-metal wear particles, I: analysis of particle size and shape. *J Biomed Mater Res* 2001;55:320–329.
20. Chan FW, Bobyn JD, Medley JB, et al. Engineering issues and wear performance of metal on metal hip implants. *Clin Orthop* 1996;333:96–107.
21. Chan FW, Bobyn JD, Medley JB, et al. Wear and lubrication of metal-on-metal hip implants. *Clin Orthop* 1999;(369):10–24.
22. Charnley J. *Low Friction Arthroplasty of the Hip.* New York: Springer Verlag; 1979.
23. Collier JP, Bargmann LS, Currier BH, et al. An analysis of Hylamer and polyethylene bearings from retrieved acetabular components. *Orthopedics* 1998;21:865–871.
24. Conway JC, Kirchner HP. The mechanics of crack initiation and propagation beneath a moving sharp indenter. *J Mater Sci* 1980;15:2879–2883.
25. Czichos H. *Tribology: A Systems Approach to the Science and Technology of Friction, Lubrication and Wear.* Amsterdam: Elsevier;1978.
26. Czichos H, Habig KH. *Tribologie Handbuch.* 2nd ed. Munich: Carl Hanser Verlag; 2003.
27. Davy DT, Kotzar GM, Brown RH, et al. Telemetric force measurements across the hip after total hip arthroplasty. *J Bone Joint Surg* 1988;70A:45–50.
28. Doorn PF, Campbell PA, Worrall J, et al. Metal wear particle characterization from metal on metal total hip replacements: TEM study of periprosthetic tissues and isolated particles. *J Biomed Mater Res* 1998;42:103–111.
29. Dowson D. *History of Tribology,* London: Longman, 1975.
30. Dowson D, El-Hady Diab MM, Gillis BJ, et al. Influence of counterface topography on the wear of ultra high molecular weight polyethylene under wet or dry conditions. In: Lee L-H, ed. *Polymer Wear and Its Control.* Washington, DC: American Chemical Society; 1985:171–187.
31. Dumbleton JH. *Tribology of Natural and Artificial Joints.* Amsterdam: Elsevier; 1981. Tribology Series vol. 3.
32. Fischer A. Well-founded selection of materials for improved wear resistance. *Wear* 1995; 194:238–245.
33. Greenwood JA, Williamson, JBP. The contact of nominally flat surfaces. *Proc R Soc A* 1966;295:300–319.
34. Hall RM, Unsworth A, Siney P, et al. Wear in retrieved Charnley acetabular sockets. *Proc Inst Mech Eng [H]* 1996;210:197–207.
35. Hatton A, Nevelos JE, Nevelos AA, et al. Alumina-alumina artificial hip joints, I: a histological analysis and characterisation of wear debris by laser capture microdissection of tissues retrieved at revision. *Biomaterials* 2002;23:3429–3440.
36. Heilmann P, Rigney DA. Running-in process affecting friction and wear. In: Dowson D, et al., eds. *The Running-In Process in Tribology.* Guildford: Butterworth-Heinemann; 1982:25–32.
37. Heinicke G. *Tribochemistry.* Munich: Carl Hanser Verlag; 1984.
38. Heller MO, Bergmann G, Deuretzbacher G, et al. Musculo-skeletal loading conditions at the hip during walking and stair climbing. *J Biomech* 2001;34:883–893.
39. Hodge WA, Carlson KL, Fijan SM, et al. Contact pressures from an instrumented hip endoprosthesis. *J Bone Joint Surg* 1989;71A: 1378–1386.
40. Homola AM, Israelachvili JN, McGuigan PM, et al. Fundamental experimental studies in tribology: the transition from "interfacial" friction of undamaged molecularly smooth surfaces to "normal" friction with wear. *Wear* 1990;136:65–83.
41. Hurwitz DE, Foucher KC, Andriacchi TP. A new parametric approach for modeling hip forces during gait. *J Biomech* 2003;36:113–119.
42. *Implants for Surgery: Wear of Total Hip-Joint Prostheses.* Pt. 1. *Loading and Displacement Parameters for Wear-testing Machines and Corresponding Environmental Conditions for Test.* Geneva: International Organization for Standardization; 2002. ISO 14242.
43. *Implants for Surgery: Wear of Total Knee-Joint Prostheses.* Pt. 1. *Loading and Displacement Parameters for Wear-testing Machines with Load Control and Corresponding Environmental Conditions for Test.* Geneva: International Organization for Standardization; 2002. ISO 14243.
44. Jaeger JC. Moving sources of heat and the temperature of sliding surfaces. *Proc R Soc NSW* 1942;66:203–224.
45. Jin ZM, Dowson D, Fisher J. Analysis of fluid film lubrication in artificial hip joint replacements with surfaces of high elastic modulus. *Proc Inst Mech Eng [H]* 1997;211:247–256.
46. Johnston RC, Smidt GL. Measurement of hip-joint motion during walking: evaluation of an electrogoniometric method. *J Bone Joint Surg* 1969;51A:1083–1094.
47. Jost PH. Tribology: origin and future. *Wear* 1990;136:1–17.
48. Kloss H, Willmann G, Woydt M. Calculation on the temperature at the articulating surfaces in artificial hip joints. *MATWER* 2001;32:200–210.
49. Kloss H, Woydt M, Willmann G. Calculation of flash temperatures of microcontacts in artificial hip joints by using the contact model of Greenwood-Williamson *MATWER* 2002;33:534–543.
50. Kong HS, Ashby MF. Friction heating maps and their application. *MRS Bull* 1991;16(10):41–48.
51. Kuhlmann-Wilsdorf D. Demystifying flash temperatures, I: analytical expressions based on a simple model. *Mater Sci Eng* 1987;93:107–117.
52. Kuhlmann-Wilsdorf D. Demystifying flash temperatures, II: first order approximation for plastic contact spots. *Mater Sci Eng* 1987;93:119–133.
53. Landmann U, Luedtke WD, Ribarsky MW. Micromechanics and microdynamics via atomistic simulations. In: Pope L, Fehrenbacher LL, Winer WO, eds. *New Material Approaches to Tribology: Theory and Application.* Pittsburgh, PA: MRS; 1989:101–117. MRS Symposium Proceedings vol. 140.
54. Magnissalis EA, Eliades G, Eliades T. Multitechnique characterization of articular surfaces of retrieved ultrahigh molecular weight polyethylene acetabular sockets. *J Biomed Mater Res* 1999;48:365–373.
55. Mak MM, Besong AA, Jin ZM, et al. Effect of microseparation on contact mechanics in ceramic-on-ceramic hip joint replacements. *Proc Inst Mech Eng [H]* 2002;216:403–408.
56. McCalden RW, Howie DW, Ward L, et al. Observations on the long-term wear behaviour of retrieved McKee-Farrar total hip implants. *Transactions of the 41st Annual Meeting of the Orthopaedic Research Society* 1995;20:242.
57. McCrory JL, White SC, Lifeso RM. Vertical ground reaction forces: objective measures of gait following hip arthroplasty. *Gait Posture* 2001;14:104–109.
58. McKellop HA, Campbell P, Park SH, et al. The origin of submicron polyethylene wear debris in total hip arthroplasty. *Clin Orthop* 1995;(311):3–20.
59. McKellop H, Park S-H, Chiesa R, et al. In vivo wear of 3 types of metal on metal hip prostheses during 2 decades of use. *Clin Orthop* 1996;No. 329(suppl):128–140.
60. Morlock M, Schneider E, Bluhm A, et al. Duration and frequency of every day activities in total hip patients. *J Biomech* 2001;34:873–881.
61. Murakami T. The lubrication in natural synovial joints and joint prostheses. *JSME Int J* 1990;33:465.
62. Murray MP, Brewer BJ, Gore DR, et al. Kinesiology after McKee-Farrar total hip replacement. *J Bone Joint Surg* 1975;57A:337–342.
63. Murray MP, Brewer BJ, Zuege RC. Kinesiologic measurements of functional performance before and after McKee-Farrar total hip replacement. *J Bone Joint Surg* 1972;54A:237–256.
64. Nassutt R, Wimmer MA, Schneider E, et al. The influence of resting periods on friction in the artificial hip. *Clin Orthop* 2003;No. 407:127–138.

65. Nevelos J, Ingham E, Doyle C, et al. Microseparation of the centers of alumina-alumina artificial hip joints during simulator testing produces clinically relevant wear rates and patterns. *J Arthroplasty* 2000;15:793–795.

66. Nich C, Ali el-HS, Hannouche D, et al. Long-term results of alumina-on-alumina hip arthroplasty for osteonecrosis. *Clin Orthop* 2003;No. 417:102–111.

67. O'Kelly J, Unsworth A, Dowson D, et al. An experimental study of friction and lubrication in hip prostheses. *Eng Med* 1979;8:153.

68. Perrin T, Dorr LD, Perry J, et al. Functional evaluation of total hip arthroplasty with five- to ten-year follow-up evaluation. *Clin Orthop* 1985;No. 195:252–260.

69. Perron M, Malouin F, Moffet H, et al. Three-dimensional gait analysis in women with a total hip arthroplasty. *Clin Biomech* 2000;15:504–515.

70. Perry J. *Gait Analysis: Normal and Pathological Function.* Thorofare, NJ: Slack Inc; 1992.

71. Plitz W, Huber J, Refior HJ. Experimentelle Untersuchungen an Metall-Metall-Gleitpaarungen und ihre Wertigkeit hinsichtlich eines zu erwartenden in-vivo-Verhaltens. *Orthopäde* 1997;26: 135–141.

72. Quinn TFJ. NASA interdisciplinary collaboration in tribology: a review of oxidational wear. 1983. NASA Contractor Report 3686.

73. Rabinowicz E. Practical uses of the surface energy criterion. *Wear* 1964;7:9–22.

74. Ramamurti BS, Bragdon CR, O'Connor DO, et al. Loci of movement of selected points on the femoral head during normal gait: three-dimensional computer simulation. *J Arthroplasty* 1996;11: 845–852.

75. Rigney DA, Hirth JP. Plastic Deformation and sliding friction of metals. *Wear* 1979;53:345–370.

76. Roy-Chowdhury SK, Pollock HM. Adhesion between metal surfaces: the effects of surface roughness. *Wear* 1981;66:307–321.

77. Rydell NW. Forces acting on the femoral head-prosthesis: a study on strain gauge supplied prostheses in living persons. *Acta Orthop Scand* 1966;37(suppl 88):1–132.

78. Saikko V, Calonius O. Slide track analysis of the relative motion between femoral head and acetabular cup in walking and in hip simulators. *J Biomech* 2002;35:455–464.

79. Saleski WJ, Fisher RM, Ritchie RO, et al. The nature and origin of sliding wear debris from steels. In: Ludema KC, ed. *Wear of Materials '83* (conference proceedings). Reston, VA: ASME; 1983:434–445.

80. Sasada T, Emori N, Oike M. The effect of abrasive grain size on the transition between abrasive and adhesive wear. In: Ludema KC, ed. *Wear of Materials '83* (conference proceedings). Reston, VA: ASME; 1983:26–31.

81. Sauer WL, Anthony ME. Predicting the clinical performance of orthopedic bearing surfaces. In: Jacobs JJ, Craig TL, eds. *Alternative Bearing Surfaces in Total Joint Replacement.* West Conshohocken, PA: ASTM; 1998:1–29. ST1346.

82. Schmalzried TP, Shepherd EF, Dorey FJ, et al. Wear is a function of use, not time. *Clin Orthop* 2000;No. 381:36–46.

83. Semlitsch M, Streicher RM, Weber H. Verschleißverhalten von Pfannen und Kugeln aus CoCrMo-Gußlegierung bei langzeitig implantierten Ganzmetall Hüftprothesen. *Orthopäde* 1989;18: 377–381.

84. Sieber HP, Rieker CB, Kottig P. Analysis of 118 2nd generation metal-on-metal retrieved hip implants. *J Bone Joint Surg [Br]* 1999;81:46–50.

85. Sikorski ME. The adhesion of metals and factors that influence it. *Wear* 1964;7:144–162.

86. Smith SL, Dowson D, Goldsmith AA. The effect of femoral head diameter upon lubrication and wear of metal-on-metal total hip replacements. *Proc Inst Mech Eng [H]* 2001;215:161–170.

87. Sprecher C, Hauert R, Grad S, et al. Solid lubrication: a relevant wear mechanism for reducing wear in metal-on-metal THA components? *Transactions of the 49th Annual Meeting of the Orthopaedic Research Society* 2003;28:1391.

88. Suh NP. The delamination theory of wear. *Wear* 1973;25:111–124.

89. Sutula LC, Collier JP, Saum KA, et al. Impact of gamma sterilization on clinical performance of polyethylene in the hip. *Clin Orthop* 1995;No. 319:28–40.

90. Sychterz CJ, Moon KH, Hashimoto Y, et al. Wear of polyethylene cups in total hip arthroplasty: a study of specimens retrieved post mortem. *J Bone Joint Surg [Am]* 1996;78:1193–1200.

91. Täger KH. Untersuchungen an Oberflächen und Neogelenkkapseln getragener McKee-Farrar-Endoprothesen. *Arch OrthopUnfall-Chir* 1976;86:101–113.

92. Tipper JL, Hatton A, Nevelos JE, et al. Alumina-alumina artificial hip joints, II: characterisation of the wear debris from in vitro hip joint simulations. *Biomaterials* 2002;23:3441–3448.

93. *Tribology: Definitions, Terminology, Testing.* Moers, Germany: German Society of Tribology; 2002. GfT Arbeitsblatt 7.

94. Vaughan CL, Davis BL, O'Connor JC. *Dynamics of Human Gait.* 2nd ed. Cape Town: Kibhho Publishers; 1999.

95. Walker PS, Salvati E, Hotzler RK. The wear on removed McKee-Farrar total hip prostheses. *J Bone Joint Surg [Am]* 1974;56:92–100.

96. Wear assessment of prosthetic hip designs in simulator devices [document under consideration by the ASTM F-04 technical committee (status February 2003)]. West Conshohocken, PA: ASTM.

97. Whitehead JR. Surface deformation and friction of metals at light loads. *Proc R Soc A* 1949;201:109–124.

98. Willert HG, Broback LG, Buchhorn GH, et al. Crevice corrosion of cemented titanium alloy stems in total hip replacements. *Clin Orthop* 1996;No. 333:51–75.

99. Willert HG, Buchhorn GH, Göbel D, et al. Wear behavior and histopathology of classic cemented metal on metal hip protheses. *Clin Orthop* 1996;No.329S:160–186.

100. Willmann G, Kalberer H, Pfaff HG. Ceramic acetabulum cup inserts for hip endoprotheses. *Biomed Tech* (Berl) 1996;41: 98–105.

101. Wimmer MA, Loos J, Heitkemper M, et al. The acting wear mechanisms on metal-on-metal hip joint bearings: in-vitro results. *Wear* 2001;250:129–139.

102. Wimmer MA, Moisio KC, Genge R, et al. Hip joint moments predict polyethylene wear in total hip arthroplasty. Paper presented at the 50th Annual Conference of the Orthopaedic Research Society; San Francisco; March 7–10, 2004.

103. Wimmer MA, Sprecher C, Hauert R, et al. Tribochemical reaction on metal-on-metal hip joint bearings: a comparison between in-vitro and in-vivo results. *Wear* 2003;255:1007–1014.

104. Zum Gahr K-H. *Microstructure and Wear of Materials.* Amsterdam: Elsevier; 1987. Tribology Series vol. 10.

Wear Assessment: Mechanical

18

Orhun K. Muratoglu

The total hip arthroplasty provides pain relief and improvement in function to millions of patients with end-stage arthritis of the hip (10,12). Charnley pioneered the development of total hip surgery and first used a femoral head with a diameter of 41.5 mm (11). Initially Charnley observed a high acetabular loosening rate, which he attributed to rapid wear of the plastic material available at the time and also to the frictional torque induced by the large head size despite the use of a low friction material, poly(tetrafluoro-ethylene) (Teflon™). Subsequently, Charnley began using a femoral head with a 22.2-mm diameter in an effort to reduce frictional torque and prevent early aseptic loosening. He also began using increased liner thickness and ultrahigh-molecular-weight polyethylene (UHMWPE) as the articulating surface material. This has been the long-standing gold standard of total hip replacement surgery and has achieved outstanding clinical outcomes.

In late 1970s and early 1980s, the pioneering work of Willert et al. (54–56) and Harris et al. (19,20,24,49) showed that aseptic loosening of the acetabular components is not induced primarily through frictional torque but rather through periprosthetic osteolysis, which is secondary to the particulate debris generated in the joint space. Adhesive and abrasive wear of the polyethylene articular surface generates the majority of the particulate debris. Therefore, research in total joint replacement has focused on the discovery of materials with improved wear resistance to replace the conventional polymers.

For the past 2 decades, research in this field centered on studying the fundamental wear mechanisms that are involved in the failure of total joint replacement surgery, creating new means to critically evaluate candidate materials with greater wear resistance, and discovering new polyethylene materials with improved wear resistance. Radiation and heat treatment of polyethylene proved to be an important advance and resulted in the discovery of a number of highly cross-linked polyethylenes with improved wear resistance (29,32–34,36,38). Some of these improved polyethylenes have been in clinical use since 1998, and early clinical studies showed markedly reduced wear rates with the new polyethylenes in comparison with conventional polyethylenes (16,28,39). These novel polyethylene materials are showing promise of reversing the limitations of conventional polyethylene and possibly reducing osteolysis, which remains the number one long-term complication in total hip replacements. These novel materials are also leading to major innovations in implant design.

In this chapter, I review the basics of polyethylene cross-linking, discuss the laboratory wear studies that were used during the development of highly cross-linked polyethylene formulations for total hips, and describe the early in vivo wear behavior of these new polymers.

BASICS OF CROSS-LINKED UHMWPE TECHNOLOGY

In the late 1990s radiation cross-linking combined with thermal treatment emerged as a technology capable of improving

227

Crystalline lamellae

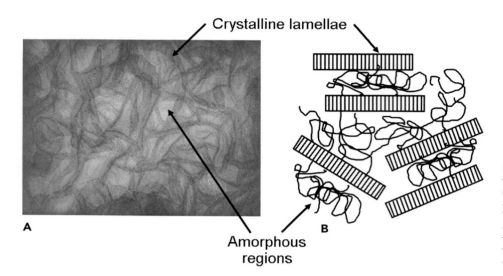

A

B

Amorphous
regions

Figure 18-1 A transmission electron micrograph **(A)** and a schematic **(B)** of UHMWPE shows the lamellae embedded in an amorphous matrix. The long-chain polyethylene molecules assume a random orientation in the amorphous regions. In the crystalline lamellae, the molecules are oriented in a long-range order.

the wear and oxidation resistance of UHMWPE acetabular components (29,32–34,36,38). The development of this technology led to a series of new alternate polyethylene bearing materials with various cross-link densities. These materials with improved wear resistance have been in clinical use in total hips since 1998. To date, the clinical follow-up studies (16,28,39) and analyses of surgically retrieved acetabular liners show a significant reduction in adhesive and abrasive wear of highly cross-linked acetabular liners in vivo (38), thus confirming the in vitro tests that showed increased wear resistance with cross-linked polyethylenes (14,29,32–34,36,38).

Polyethylene is a semicrystalline material with crystalline domains of lamellae embedded in an amorphous matrix (Fig. 18-1). Cross-linking of polyethylene can be achieved either through the use of ionizing radiation (9) or by chemical methods using peroxides (15) or silanes (1–3). The cross-links are formed by the reaction of the free radicals generated by these methods, leading to the creation of predominantly interchain covalent bonds. Peroxide chemistry leads to unstable cross-linked networks (29,35), and therefore it is not a desirable method for the manufacture of medical

devices. On the other hand, the cross-linked networks formed by ionizing radiation are stable provided that the residual free radicals are stabilized (29,36). With ionizing radiation, free radicals are formed through the radiolytic cleavage of C-H and C-C bonds in polyethylene (Fig. 18-2a,b). These free radicals recombine with each other and form cross-links in the amorphous portion of the polymer (Fig. 18-3). The free radicals generated in the crystalline phase become trapped primarily at the crystalline–amorphous interface and adversely affect the long-term oxidative stability of the material. The effects of residual free radicals on the long-term induced embrittlement have been well documented in the case of in-air gamma sterilization of polyethylene components (13,51).

Oxidative embrittlement of polyethylene is initiated when the residual free radicals react with oxygen. A complex cascade of events leads to the formation of peroxy free radicals, hydroperoxides, and ultimately carbonyl species, mainly ketones, esters, and acids. The formation of the carbonyl species can be accompanied by chain scission, reducing the molecular weight of the polymer. This eventually leads to recrystallization, increase in stiffness, and embrittlement of the UHMWPE.

A thermal treatment step typically follows the radiation cross-linking of UHMWPE to decrease the concentration of the residual free radicals and to minimize or eliminate the adverse effects of the residual free radicals on the properties of UHMWPE (29,36,38). The most effective method is to melt

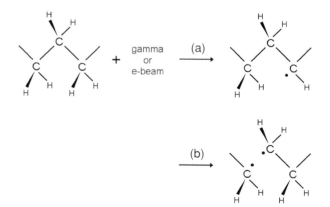

Figure 18-2 When polyethylene is exposed to ionizing radiation such as gamma or e-beam, free radicals are formed through radiolytic cleavage of C-H **(a)** and C-C **(b)** bonds.

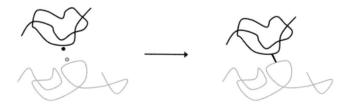

Figure 18-3 During irradiation, carbon-hydrogen bonds are broken, forming free radicals along the backbone of the polyethylene molecule. The reaction of two free radicals in two separate molecules results in the formation of a cross-link.

TABLE 18-1

CONTEMPORARY HIGHLY CROSS-LINKED POLYETHYLENES IN CLINICAL USE IN TOTAL HIP REPLACEMENTS

	Manufacturer	Radiation Temperature	Radiation Dose (kGy)[a]	Radiation Type	Postirradiation Thermal Treatment	Sterilization Method	Total Radiation Dose Level (kGy)	Residual Free Radicals Present?
Longevity	Zimmer	~40°C	100	E-beam	Melted at 150°C for 6 hours	Gas plasma	100	No
Durasul	Zimmer	~125°C	95		Melted at 150°C for 2 hours	EtO	95	No
Marathon	Depuy/JJ	RT	50	Gamma	Melted at 155°C for 24 hours	Gas plasma	50	No
XLPE	Smith & Nephew	RT	100		Melted at 150°C for a proprietary duration	EtO	100	No
Crossfire	Stryker/ Osteonics/ Howmedica	RT	75		Annealed at 120°C for a proprietary duration	Gamma (30 kGy) in nitrogen	105	Yes
Aeonian	Kyocera	RT	35		Annealed at 110°C for 10 hours	Gamma (25–40 kGy) in nitrogen	60–75	Yes

RT, room temperature.
[a]10 kilogray (kGy) = 1 megarad (Mrad).

the irradiated UHMWPE, which reduces the concentration of the residual free radicals to undetectable levels. Polyethylene components machined from irradiated and melted UHMWPE are sterilized with gas sterilization techniques utilizing gas plasma or ethylene oxide gas, neither of which has known adverse effects on the oxidative stability of UHMWPE.

Another method used to lower the free radical concentration is annealing, which involves heating the irradiated UHMWPE to a temperature below its peak melting transition. UHMWPE is partially molten at the annealing temperature, and therefore this technique results in a partial reduction of the residual free radicals. UHMWPE acetabular liners annealed below the melt are typically gamma sterilized, which increases the concentration of the residual free radicals in the material and can compromise long-term properties through oxidation (32).

The manufacturing practices used in the fabrication of highly cross-linked polyethylene acetabular liners (Table 18-1) are discussed in more detail in Chapter 10.

WEAR MECHANISMS IN THR

The primary mechanism of polyethylene wear in total hip is adhesive and abrasive in nature. Polyethylene's long-chain molecules play a major role during wear of the articular surfaces. During articulation, the long-chain molecules elongate in the primary direction of motion, which is the arc of motion created by flexion–extension, resulting in the formation of elongated fibrils on the articulating surface of the acetabular liner (25). An example of a surgically retrieved acetabular component with this fibril formation on the articular surface is shown in Figure 18-4. The long-chain molecules of the polyethylene are highly oriented along the axis of the fibrils, which hardens the material in

the direction of the flexion–extension motion. However, this orientation also causes weakening of the polyethylene surface in the transverse direction. In turn, abduction and adduction shears the surface of the polyethylene in the weakened transverse direction and liberates micron and submicron wear particles from the surface (25,53). Investigations into the effect of crossing motions on wear of polyethylene (6,7,41,44,53) and the evolution of polyethylene microstructure near the articulation (17,38) are providing further evidence of the dominating role of this wear mechanism in the total hip.

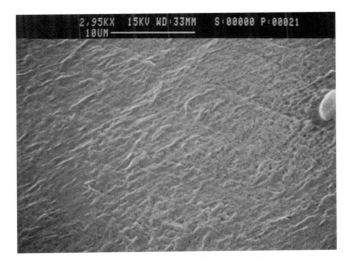

Figure 18-4 The articular surface of a surgically retrieved conventional polyethylene showing surface deformation and fiber formation that results in the wear of the material. The explant shown was retrieved after 124 months.

Because of the described mechanism of adhesive–abrasive wear, cross-linking is likely to improve the wear resistance of polyethylene. Cross-linking the long-chain molecules of polyethylene would hinder the surface orientation of the material during articulation. This would in turn reduce the weakening of the surface in the transverse direction and decrease the amount of wear debris liberated from the polyethylene surface during in vivo use. The effect of cross-linking on the wear resistance of polyethylene has been investigated using both pin-on-disk wear testers and hip simulators (14,29,32–34,36,38,47).

PIN-ON-DISK WEAR TESTING OF UHMWPE AND THE EFFECT OF CROSS-LINKING ON WEAR

Pin-on-disk (POD) wear testing is a common screening tool to quantify the wear rate of polyethylene load-bearing materials used in orthopedics. The polyethylene test sample is machined typically in the form of a cylindrical pin and is articulated against a smooth counterface, such as an implant-finish flat surface of a metallic disk. Prior to early 1990s, water or saline solution was commonly used as lubricants in POD tests; also, the pin motion with respect to the disk was unidirectional in nature. Later studies showed that more physiologically relevant lubricants (4,26,42–44,52) and rubbing motions (6,7,41,44,53) were needed to better stimulate polyethylene wear in POD experiments.

Proteins play an important role in the wear of polyethylene (4,26,42–44,52). The nonspecific binding of proteins on the surface of the polyethylene alters the lubrication process. When water is used as a lubricant, a transfer film of the polyethylene forms on the counterface, resulting on polyethylene-on-polyethylene articulation, which is not present in vivo. In contrast, when the lubricant contains proteins, transfer film does not form. Today, bovine serum instead of water or saline solution is used to lubricate the POD wear testers.

The in vivo motion of the hip is not unidirectional in nature at the articulating interface (40). In the hip, the flexion–extension motion creates unidirectional rubbing of the femoral head on the acetabular liner, and the abduction–adduction as well as internal–external rotation create multidirectional motions at the articulating interface. The wear rate of the polyethylene increases substantially when the articular motion is changed from a unidirectional to a multidirectional path (7). Therefore, to properly simulate the in vivo wear mechanisms, all state-of-the-art POD wear testers follow a multidirectional motion path. One such POD wear tester was developed in our laboratory with a bidirectional rectangular motion, where the polyethylene pin articulates on a rectangular path against a metallic disk (7). The articulation is lubricated by undiluted bovine serum. Testing is carried out at a frequency of 2 Hz. The wear rate is determined by the linear regression of the weight loss as a function of number of cycles. Typically the first 200,000 cycles are discounted in the linear regression, as this portion of the testing eliminates the surface asperities on the polyethylene. Beyond 200,000 cycles the wear reaches a steady state unless there are imperfections in the polyethylene pin, such as the presence of subsurface oxidation.

Using the bidirectional POD wear tester, we investigated the effect of cross-linking on the wear rate of UHMWPE (38).

The UHMWPE stock material was cross-linked by electron beam irradiation at different dose levels ranging from 25 to 200 kGy. The irradiated UHMWPE samples were melted to eliminate the residual free radicals and improve the oxidative stability of the material. Test pins were machined from the irradiated and melted UHMWPE stocks. The wear test was carried out for 2 million cycles at different radiation dose levels. The wear rate decreased progressively as a function of increasing radiation dose (Fig. 18-5). Beyond the 100-kGy radiation dose, the rate of decrease in the wear rate of cross-linked polyethylene decreased with increasing radiation dose level. Therefore, we determined the optimum radiation dose to be 100 kGy (10 Mrad) achieved with electron beam irradiation and followed by the melting process. At this dose level, the mechanical properties of the irradiated and melted polyethylene were within the ranges specified by the ASTM standard and FDA guidance documents for surgical grade polyethylene.

We also examined the wear surfaces of the irradiated and melted polyethylene pins after 2 million cycles of testing on the bidirectional POD tester as a function of radiation dose (38). The surfaces exhibited formation of ripples, commonly observed in explanted polyethylene acetabular components, perpendicular to the direction of the two motions. As seen in Figure 18-6, two groups of parallel ripples that were orthogonal to each other were present on the articular surfaces, similar to the bidirectional motion used during testing. The distance between the ripples decreased with increasing radiation dose level (Fig. 18-6). This change on the articular surfaces presented strong evidence for the reduction of surface deformation of polyethylene during articulation with increasing cross-linking density.

Other POD wear studies (45) with highly cross-linked UHMWPE corroborated the findings from our laboratory. Saikko et al. (46) studied the effects of counterface roughness on the wear of conventional and highly cross-linked UHMWPE with a multidirectional POD device. The highly cross-linked polyethylene in their study was 100-kGy irradiated and melted UHMWPE. The wear resistance of the highly cross-linked UHMWPE was significantly greater than that of conventional

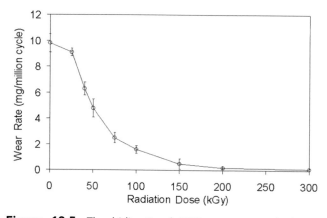

Figure 18-5 The bidirectional POD wear rate of electron beam–irradiated and melted UHMWPE as a function of increasing dose level is shown here. At higher dose levels, the wear rate decreased and asymptotically approached an undetectable wear level. (Reproduced with permission from Muratoglu OK, et al. Unified wear model for highly crosslinked ultra-high molecular weight polyethylenes (UHMWPE). *Biomaterials.* 1999;20:1463–1470.)

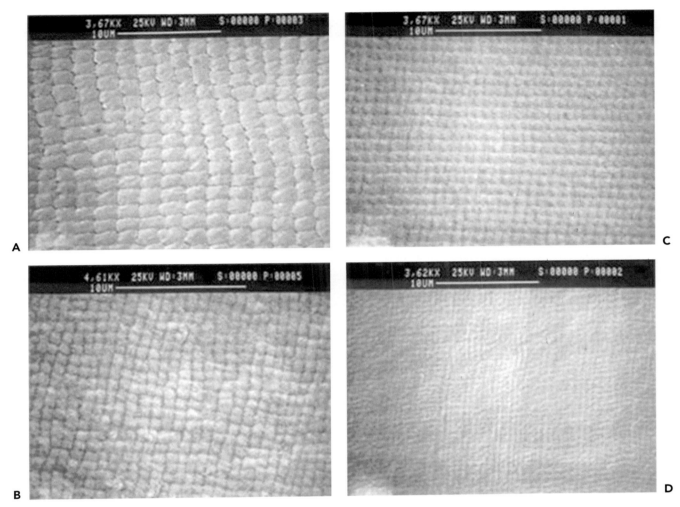

Figure 18-6 The photomicrographs show typical morphologies on the wear surfaces of the pins tested in POD study shown in Figure 18-5. The micrographs **(A)**, **(B)**, **(C)**, and **(D)** correspond to dose levels of 25, 50, 100, and 200 kGy, respectively, following 2 million cycles of bidirectional rubbing action against an implant-finish Co-Cr disk. Note that the increase in the radiation dose results in an increase in the cross-link density, which leads to a decrease in the amount of surface orientation accumulated during the wear test.

polyethylene when tested against smooth counterfaces. The same observation was made with roughened counterfaces; the wear of the highly cross-linked polyethylene against roughened counterfaces was even lower than the wear of conventional polyethylene against polished counterfaces. The wear tester used by Saikko et al. achieved multidirectional motion by circularly translating the pin on the disk counterfaces (46). The researchers also used bovine serum as a lubricant and conducted the tests for 3 million cycles. Their studies used diluted bovine calf serum to match the protein concentration found in synovial fluid.

The reduction in UHMWPE wear by cross-linking can be explained by the decreased surface deformation that occurs on the wear surfaces of cross-linked polyethylenes (17,38). This decrease in surface deformation was apparent on the wear surfaces of the pins that we have tested on bidirectional POD testers (38). A later study by Edidin et al. (17) examined the crystalline structure of the polyethylene near the wear surfaces of acetabular liners following wear testing on a hip simulator. They found a layer of polyethylene, the so-called plasticity-

induced damage layer, at the wear surface where the crystalline lamellae were primarily oriented parallel to the articular surfaces. The formation of this damage layer is postulated to cause strain hardening of the polyethylene surface. The thickness of the damage layer decreased with increasing cross-link density. This observation highlights the importance of the constraint established by the chemical cross-links on the polyethylene and how that decreases the ability of the material to deform during the rubbing action of the counterface and as a result improves the wear resistance of polyethylene (17,38).

HIP SIMULATOR WEAR STUDIES WITH HIGHLY CROSS-LINKED POLYETHYLENES

Extensive data are available from hip simulator studies showing the improvement in the wear resistance of polyethylene with cross-linking (14,29–31,34,36), even in the presence of clinically relevant third-body particles (8,31,47). The state-of-the-art hip simulators used in the development of highly cross-linked polyethylenes have been designed to closely simulate the in vivo polyethylene wear mechanisms in terms of rate of wear, debris size and shape, and wear surface morphology. Although most of the reported hip simulator studies were able to replicate the wear mechanisms of conventional polyethylene, there still are differences in a number of parameters used by different research groups. The multidirectional motion of the articulating pairs is common to most of these studies, but some achieve this by simulating normal gait kinematics (14,36) and others by artificial motions, such as biaxial rocking (29). As a result, the distance that a point on the femoral head travels on the acetabular liner differs with different types of simulators. For instance, the distance traveled on the Boston Hip Simulator, which is modeled after normal gait, is about one third the distance traveled on the Biaxial Rocking Machine during one cycle of testing (40). The wear rate is expected to be greater with longer distance traveled per cycle. The extent to which the bovine serum is diluted also varies among laboratories (14,29,36,52). The wear rate of conventional polyethylene has been shown to increase with increasing dilution of the serum used for lubrication (52). Consequently, the hip simulator wear results for highly cross-linked polyethylene acetabular liners are mostly reported in conjunction with the wear rate for a control group of conventional polyethylene acetabular liners tested under identical conditions.

The hip simulator tests are carried out at a frequency in the range of 1 to 2 Hz, with the articular pair immersed in 37°C to 40°C bovine serum. The studies are run for at least 2 to 5 million cycles, some for as long as 30 million cycles, with gravimetric and/or volumetric assessment of wear at regular intervals of 1 million cycles typically. The bovine serum used in the lubrication is replaced at these intervals as well. The particulate debris can be isolated from the used bovine serum for particle size and shape analysis.

The long-term performance of polyethylene components can be compromised due to chemical changes that may occur on the shelf and in vivo, such as oxidation of conventional polyethylene secondary to gamma sterilization. Hence, it is important to investigate the wear behavior of polyethylene following preconditioning of the acetabular liners with accelerated aging. Two main methods of accelerated aging, 3 to 5 weeks of storage at 80°C in air or 2 weeks of storage in 5 atm of pure O_2 pressure at 70°C, have been developed and adapted as standards (48,50). The hip simulator testing of preconditioned acetabular liners is typically carried out to investigate the device fatigue behavior of the type of polyethylene that is intended to be used.

Hip Simulator Testing with Clean Lubrication

Comprehensive analysis of the wear behavior of radiation cross-linked polyethylenes has been carried out by a number of research groups (14,29–31,34,36). We investigated the wear behavior of electron beam–irradiated (100 kGy) and melted acetabular liners in comparison with that of conventional acetabular liners using simulated normal gait in a Boston Hip Simulator (36). The highly cross-linked liners were machined from a UHMWPE stock that was electron beam irradiated to 100 kGy and melted. These liners were ethylene oxide steril-

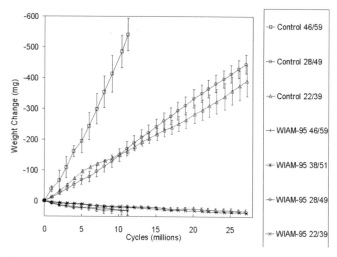

Figure 18-7 The average weight change of conventional (control) and highly cross-linked acetabular liners as tested on a Boston Hip Simulator. The highly cross-linked liners (WIAM-95) were electron beam irradiated to about 100 kGy and subsequently melted. The inner/outer diameter of the liners are indicated in the legend. (Reproduced with permission from Muratoglu OK, et al. Larger diameter femoral heads used in conjunction with a highly cross-linked ultra-high molecular weight polyethylene: a new concept. *J Arthroplasty.* 2001;16(8 suppl):24–30.)

ized. The conventional liners were machined from a UHMWPE stock and gamma sterilized in nitrogen. The hip simulator test was carried out to 20 million cycles and showed a wear rate of 14 ± 2 and 17 ± 1 mg per million cycles for conventional polyethylene liners that were tested with femoral head sizes of 22 and 28 mm, respectively (Fig. 18-7). The highly cross-linked polyethylene liners of both sizes showed no detectable weight loss during 20 million cycles.

There was a slight increase in the weight of the highly cross-linked acetabular liners due to fluid absorption from the bovine serum. We corrected the weight loss from wear by subtracting the weight gain that occurred in load-soak components that were only loaded but not subjected to motion. However, there are limitations to this correction because the liners, which are subjected to both motion and load, absorb slightly more fluid than their load-soak counterparts (5). As a result, the correction for fluid absorption by using the load-soak data as the correction factor leads to a slight underestimation of the actual weight loss. In instances in which there is no, or undetectable, weight loss in the motion cups, this differential increase in fluid absorption leads to a net increase in weight, as was the case with the highly cross-linked polyethylene liners in the study under discussion.

The weight loss data indicated no detectable wear in the highly cross-linked polyethylene liners. The optical analysis of the articular surfaces of the tested liners supported this finding. Visually the wear surfaces of the control liners were highly polished, even after only 5 million cycles of simulated gait, similar to wear surfaces of retrieved acetabular liners (25); such polishing is an indication of wear. No machining marks remained on the articular surfaces of the conventional polyethylene liners, also indicating substantial wear. In contrast, the highly cross-linked liners still retained the original machining marks on the articulating surfaces, which were visible at 5 million cycles but were slightly obscured after 20 million cycles due to heavy scratching. Though few scratches were noted at every million-cycle interval, the amount of scratching in the highly cross-linked motion liners progressively increased throughout the wear test period. Similar kinds of scratching also occurred with the control motion liners as well, but the wear process prevented the accumulation of the scratches and led to the highly polished appearance of the articulating surfaces of these control liners, with a few random scratches.

In the above study, the amount of linear penetration of the femoral heads into the load-soak liners was determined using a coordinate measuring machine (CMM) prior to the study and at the completion of each million cycles. Since the load-soak liners were not subjected to articulation, the penetration measured by the CMM method primarily represented creep. The total amount of creep measured in the load-soak liners of both materials was nearly the same. At 20 million cycles, the cumulative linear penetration in the load-soak liners was 0.10 ± 0.01 and 0.11 ± 0.01 mm with 28-mm inner diameter highly cross-linked liners and conventional liners ($p = 0.06$), respectively, and 0.15 ± 0.01 and 0.12 ± 0.01 mm with 22-mm inner diameter highly cross-linked liners and conventional liners ($p = 0.06$), respectively.

In another comprehensive study, McKellop et al. studied the wear rate of acetabular liners fabricated from gamma-irradiated UHMWPE stock as a function of radiation dose level between 33 and 500 kGy (29). The polyethylene stock material was irradiated with gamma radiation and subsequently melted to eliminate the residual free radicals. The liners were machined from the irradiated and melted polyethylene stock and sterilized with ethylene oxide gas. The testing was carried out on a Biaxial Rocking Hip Simulator for 3 million cycles at a frequency of 1 Hz in undiluted bovine serum. The study showed a marked decrease in wear rate with increasing radiation dose level, corroborating the findings of Muratoglu et al. (38). At doses exceeding 200 kGy, the acetabular liners showed a net weight gain even after correction by the loaded soak controls. These highly cross-linked liners also showed the presence of machining marks on the articular surfaces.

These investigations showed a marked increase in the wear resistance of polyethylene following irradiation and melting. The early investigations were carried out under ideal conditions of clean serum and polished femoral components, conditions that may not always be present in vivo. The following section reviews the effect of counterface roughness and the presence of third-body particles on the wear behavior of highly cross-linked and conventional polyethylenes.

The Effect of Counterface Roughness and Third-Body Particles on the Wear of Highly Cross-Linked Polyethylene

Another wear mechanism in vivo involves the presence of third-body particles, such as bone cement particles, which could increase the roughness of the counterface and accelerate the wear of the polyethylene acetabular liner. In several in vitro hip simulator studies in which the lubricating bovine serum was supplemented with third-body particles (e.g., barium sulphate containing bone cement particles), results for artificially roughened femoral heads and in vivo roughened explanted femoral heads were reported (8,31). These studies provide convincing evidence that the wear rate of cross-linked polyethylene is notably lower than that of conventional polyethylene under such adverse conditions.

McKellop et al. investigated the wear resistance of conventional and highly cross-linked polyethylene liners before and after accelerated aging and with femoral components with three degrees of roughness (31). The conventional liners were gas plasma sterilized. The highly cross-linked liners were fabricated from 50-kGy gamma-irradiated and melted polyethylene stock and were gas plasma sterilized. Three different roughness levels were achieved in the femoral heads used in the study: polished, roughened with 800 grit compound, and roughened with 320 grit compound. The wear test was performed on a Biaxial Rocking Hip Simulator at 1 Hz in undiluted bovine serum with gravimetric assessment of wear at intervals of 0.5 million cycles. The cross-linked liners were tested in unaged and aged forms; accelerated aging was achieved by maintaining the liners at 70°C in oxygen at 5 atm for 2 weeks. For the first 10 million cycles, the wear test was carried out with polished femoral heads, and the wear rates of the aged and unaged cross-linked polyethylene liners were lower than that of the conventional liners. Also, the wear rates of the aged and unaged cross-linked liners against both moderately and extremely roughened femoral heads were lower than those of the conventional liners. The wear rates of the cross-linked liners in the aged and unaged forms were comparable for all three roughness levels. This study demonstrated that wear reduction achieved by radiation cross-linking and melting persists even under aggressive conditions of accelerated aging and rough counterfaces.

The approach of using scratched or roughened metal countersurfaces (8,31) does not replicate the complex interaction of third-body particles entering and leaving the articular interface between a metal femoral head and a softer counterface. It is important to simulate this complex interaction to better understand the potential effects of third-body particles on the wear of polyethylene liners. One such study was carried out by Bragdon et al., who investigated the wear behavior of electron beam cross-linked and melted polyethylene acetabular liners articulating against 28-mm cobalt–chrome femoral heads in the presence of third-body particulate debris (8). The wear tests were performed in a Boston Hip Simulator, and conventional polyethylene (gamma in nitrogen) liners served as the control group. The highly cross-linked liners were sterilized with ethylene oxide gas. Two different types of third-body particles were chosen to represent severe and mild abrasive wear: Aluminum oxide particles with a mean particle size of 1 μm simulated severe abrasive wear conditions, and bone cement particles were used to investigate the effect of mild abrasive wear conditions. The latter were prepared by pulverizing prepolymerized bone cement powder containing barium sulfate in a freezer mill filled with liquid nitrogen. The powder was then sieved to obtain a population of particles about 30 μm in size. A concentration of 0.15 milligrams of particles per cubic centimeter of serum was used in that study. The hip simulator test was carried out to a total of 5 million cycles of simulated gait at a rate of 2 Hz.

During testing the third-body particles scratched the femoral heads. The heads were dull in appearance after testing with aluminum oxide particles and mildly scratched after testing with bone cement particles. In the presence of aluminum oxide particles, the incremental wear rates of conventional

UHMWPE averaged as high as 149 ± 116 mg per million cycles, compared with 37 ± 38 mg for the highly cross-linked components. With bone cement particles, the conventional UHMWPE components had an average incremental wear rate of 19 ± 5 mg per million cycles, whereas the wear rate of the highly cross-linked UHMWPE components was 0.5 ± 0.7 mg per million cycles. This study complemented the findings of McKellop et al. (31), demonstrating that the wear reduction of highly cross-linked polyethylene acetabular liners persists even under the adverse conditions of third-body particles.

CROSS-LINKED POLYETHYLENE AND EFFECT OF LARGE FEMORAL HEADS ON WEAR

An added benefit of cross-linked polyethylenes is the opportunity to use larger femoral head sizes. Until recently, the femoral head sizes used in total hip replacement implants were limited by the extent of wear of polyethylene. There is clinical evidence of increased volumetric wear (27) and increased risk for osteolysis (18) associated with larger femoral head diameters and conventional polyethylene. As a result, the most common femoral head diameters used are between 22 and 32 mm, the latter producing the maximum volumetric wear. However, there are a number of advantages to be gained from using femoral heads of larger diameter in total hip replacement surgery. These include greater range of motion, enhanced activities of daily living, greater intrinsic stability of the implant, reduced incidence of subluxation, reduced incidence of dislocation, less frequent impingement of the femoral neck on the polyethylene, and consequently reduced transfer of additional stress to the component–bone interface. In addition, the greater range of motion available is more accommodating to the inherent errors that occur in acetabular placement (i.e., an increased margin of safety if an error is made in shell placement) (21–23).

We reported on the in vitro evidence supporting the effectiveness of using nonstandard, more nearly normal femoral head sizes in metal–on–cross-linked polyethylene total hip replacement in terms of reduced wear (34). In that study, we used conventional polyethylene (gamma in nitrogen) acetabular liners and 100-kGy–irradiated and melted acetabular liners. The latter were ethylene oxide sterilized. The wear testing of the acetabular liners was carried for 11 million cycles on a Boston Hip Simulator with undiluted bovine serum as the lubricant. The conventional liners were tested with 46-mm femoral heads, and the highly cross-linked liners were tested with 28-, 38-, and 46-mm femoral heads. The polyethylene liner thickness was kept at 3 mm to determine the wear performance under worst-case dimensions. The wear as a function of simulated gait cycles is shown in Figure 18-7. The wear rate of the 46-mm conventional liners was 0.51 ± 0.04 mg per million cycles. The highly cross-linked polyethylene liners showed no detectable weight loss. Even though the weight change in the motion liners was corrected for fluid absorption using loaded soak controls, the highly cross-linked liners still showed a net weight gain. This is due to the specific increase in fluid uptake that occurs when motion is present along with loading and that therefore is not fully accounted for by the fluid uptake of the load soak control, as described earlier in this chapter (5). In addition, the machining marks present at the onset of testing persisted throughout the 11 million cycles with all three groups of highly cross-linked liners. The conventional polyethylene liners had a highly polished appearance, indicating the progression of wear as early as 0.5 million cycles.

The potential for reduced wear with larger femoral heads when the acetabular liner is fabricated from a highly cross-linked polyethylene increases the possibility of improving the range of motion, allowing increased activities of daily living, reducing impingement, reducing subluxation, reducing dislocation, improving treatment, preventing recurrent dislocation, and achieving greater forgiveness in positioning the acetabular component.

ANALYSIS OF EXPLANTED HIGHLY CROSS-LINKED ACETABULAR LINERS

The in vitro hip simulator wear studies demonstrating the improved wear resistance achieved with contemporary approaches for cross-linking of polyethylene have been discussed in detail (14,29–31,34,36). The highly cross-linked polyethylene acetabular liners have been in worldwide clinical use since 1998. A number of revisions have been reported for sepsis, recurrent dislocation secondary to implant malpositioning, and acetabular shell loosening with various types of highly cross-linked UHMWPEs (37). These early retrievals provide a unique opportunity to evaluate the effects of in vivo service on contemporary highly cross-linked UHMWPE components.

We reported on our observations with 16 highly cross-linked and melted and 19 conventional polyethylene acetabular components retrieved at revision surgery after an average in vivo duration of 6 months (37). The highly cross-linked group showed machining marks from the original manufacturing process in some areas and extensive scratching and some polishing of the articulating surfaces. The conventional group showed greater loss of machining marks, scratching, and polishing. The scratches observed on the articulating surfaces of the highly cross-linked explants could have been due to either wear resulting in loss of material or plastic deformation of the surface without loss of material. In order to separate the effects of wear and plastic deformation, we used polyethylene's "shape memory" property, which is triggered by melting: Any plastic deformation that does not lead to removal of polyethylene can be reversed by heating the material to above the melt temperature. Therefore, the shape memory property can be used to determine if the early in vivo changes in surface morphology are due to plastic deformation or to wear (material loss). In cases in which the surface damage results from actual removal of material (e.g., through wear), melting to trigger shape memory cannot restore the original surface morphology. If the surface damage is due to plastic deformation, the melt recovery can restore the original surface morphology.

Melt recovery experiments have consistently shown the disappearance of surface scratches and the restoration of the original machining marks in the highly cross-linked explants. An example is shown in Figure 18-8. In the conventional group, few of the scratches were eliminated, and only limited restoration of the machining marks was apparent. These ex vivo

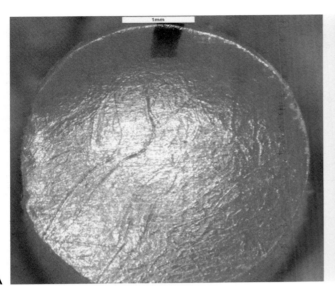
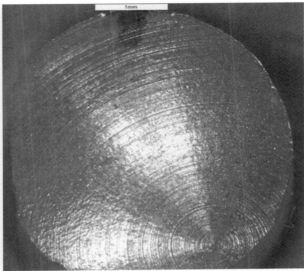

Figure 18-8 **A:** Typical surface morphology of an explanted highly cross-linked UHMWPE liner after 3 months in vivo before melting, showing such extensive scratching in the superior aspect of the articulating surface that machining marks are no longer obvious. **B:** After melting, there is near full recovery of the original machining marks. (Reproduced with permission from Muratoglu OK, et al. Surface analysis of early retrieved acetabular polyethylene liners: a comparison of standard and highly crosslinked polyethylenes. *J Arthroplasty.* 2004;19:68–77.)

observations confirmed that radiation cross-linking increases the wear resistance of polyethylene.

Highly cross-linked polyethylenes were developed not only for improved wear resistance but also for improved oxidation resistance. As discussed above, radiation cross-linking generates residual free radicals, which are the precursors to oxidative embrittlement in irradiated polyethylene. Manufacturers of highly cross-linked polyethylenes have adopted different methods of reducing the free radicals in irradiated polyethylene. One method is to use postirradiation melting followed by inert (nonradiation) sterilization techniques, such as use of ethylene oxide or gas plasma (Durasul, Longevity, Marathon). This method leads to undetectable levels of residual free radicals in the implantable device, hence improved oxidation resistance (36). An alternative method is to heat the irradiated polyethylene below the melting point (thermal annealing), which eliminates some but not all of the residual free radicals. Components manufactured with postirradiation annealing are typically gamma sterilized in nitrogen (e.g., Crossfire), introducing more residual free radicals into the polyethylene. The presence of residual free radicals with the latter method of annealing poses an instability problem, which could lead to deleterious chemical changes such as increased oxidation and crystallinity.

The adverse effects of residual free radicals became more apparent with the recent report from our laboratory comparing the oxidation levels measured in surgically explanted highly cross-linked polyethylenes of both melted and annealed types. In that study, we had a total of 9 irradiated, annealed, and gamma-sterilized acetabular liners and 18 irradiated and melted polyethylene components (11 acetabular and 5 tibial inserts). The oxidation levels and crystallinity of the explants were quantified using infrared microscopy and differential scanning calorimetry. The highly cross-

linked polyethylene components with residual free radicals (irradiated and annealed) oxidized in vivo, whereas those that had been melted after irradiation—and hence had no detectable residual free radicals—did not oxidize. Three of the irradiated and annealed components showed markedly elevated oxidation and crystallinity above the baseline values after in vivo service of less than 3 years, while none of the irradiated and melted components showed detectable oxidation or increase in crystallinity after in vivo durations up to 3 years.

One of the irradiated and annealed retrievals (33 months in vivo) had a subsurface "white band" (Fig. 18-9) that is characteristic of severe oxidative embrittlement previously observed in traditional components gamma sterilized in air (51). The other highly oxidized irradiated and annealed retrieval (18 months in vivo) had oxidation levels previously seen with traditional gamma-sterilized-in-air components after approximately 5 years in vivo. The subsurface oxidation peak in the highly oxidized retrieval (33 months in vivo) coincided with the "white band" shown in Figure 18-9. The shelf-stored irradiated and annealed component was kept in its original nitrogen package until the time of the study, and it only showed mild oxidation near the surface, with no detectable oxidation beyond 1.0 mm beneath the surface. In contrast, the retrieved highly oxidized component was oxidized even in the bulk region.

The elevated levels of oxidation and crystallinity measured in retrieved highly cross-linked polyethylene components that had been annealed after irradiation and contained residual free radicals are of great concern. These chemical changes could adversely affect device performance in the long term. Therefore, methods that improve long-term oxidation resistance of irradiated polyethylene should be used to avoid such undesirable outcomes.

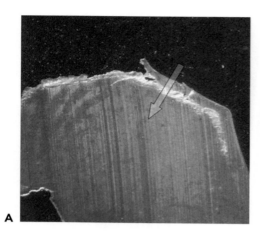

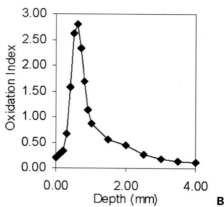

Figure 18-9 A: An irradiated and annealed polyethylene acetabular liner that was surgically removed after 33 months in vivo. Note the subsurface "white band," an indication of embrittlement. **B:** The embrittled region coincided with the subsurface oxidation peak. The in vivo oxidation of this polyethylene was due to the presence of residual free radicals; therefore, melting after irradiation to eliminate the free radicals or another method to stabilize the free radicals is essential.

SUMMARY

The technology of radiation cross-linking and melting is expected to reduce the incidence of revision surgery. More and more, total hip and knee patients include not only the elderly (>75 years) but also the young and the more active, increasing the demand for polyethylene components with low wear. The significance of the new highly cross-linked polyethylenes will be felt most in a decrease in mortality and morbidity, better patient outcomes, the long-term successful surgical treatment of young and active patients, and a potential decrease in health care costs.

Highly cross-linked polyethylenes have been in clinical use since 1998 in total hips and since 2000 in total knees. Several short-term in vivo radiographic follow-up studies (up to 3–4 years) showed a marked reduction in the femoral head penetration with highly cross-linked polyethylenes versus conventional polyethylenes (16,28,39). In addition, the analysis of explanted acetabular liners showed improved wear resistance with cross-linking (37). The in vivo observations (16,28,37,39) corroborate the findings from in vitro hip simulator tests (29–31,34,36).

REFERENCES

1. Atkinson JR, Cicek RZ. Silane crosslinked polyethylene for prosthetic applications, I: certain physical and mechanical properties related to the nature of the material. *Biomaterials.* 1983;4:267–275.
2. Atkinson JR, Cicek RZ. Silane crosslinked polyethylene for prosthetic applications, II: creep and wear behavior and a preliminary molding test. *Biomaterials.* 1984;5:326–335.
3. Atkinson JR, Dowling JM, Cicek RZ. Materials for internal prostheses: the present position and possible future developments. *Biomaterials.* 1980;1:89–96.
4. Blanchet TA, Peterson SL, Rosenberg KD. Serum lubricant absorption by UHMWPE orthopaedic bearing implants. *J Tribol.* (ASME Trans) 2001.
5. Bragdon C, O'Conner DO, Weinberg EA, et al. The effect of load plus motion versus load alone on fluid imbibition into UHMWPE. Paper presented at the 25th Annual Meeting of the Society for Biomaterials; Providence, RI; April 28-May 2, 1999.
6. Bragdon CR, O'Conner DO, Lowenstein JD, et al. The importance of multidirectional motion on the wear of polyethylene. *Proc Inst Mech Eng.* 1995;210:157–165.
7. Bragdon CR, O'Conner DO, Lowenstein JD, et al. A new pin-on-disk wear testing method for simulating wear of polyethylene on cobalt-chrome alloy in total hip arthroplasty. *J Arthroplasty.* 2001;16:658–665.
8. Bragdon CR, Jasty M, Muratoglu OK, et al. Third-body wear of highly cross-linked polyethylene in a hip simulator. *J Arthroplasty.* 2003;18:553–561.
9. Charlesby A. Cross-linking of polythene by pile radiation. *Proc R Soc Lond.* 1952;A215:187–215.
10. Charnley J. The long-term results of low-friction arthroplasty of the hip performed as a primary intervention. *J Bone Joint Surg.* 1972;54B:61–76.
11. Charnley J. Total hip replacement by low-friction arthroplasty. *Clin Orthop.* 1970;72:7–21.
12. Charnley J, Cupic Z. The nine and ten year results of the low-friction arthroplasty of the hip. *Clin Orthop.* 1973;No. 95:9–25.
13. Collier JP, Sperling DK, Currier JH, et al. Impact of gamma sterilization on clinical performance of polyethylene in the knee. *J Arthroplasty.* 1996;11:377–389.
14. Crowninshield R, Laurent MP, Yao JQ, et al. Cross-linking to improve THR wear performance. *Hip Int.* 2002;12:103–107.
15. de Boer J, Pennings A. Crosslinking of ultra-high molecular weight polyethylene in the melt by means of 2.5-dimethyl-2.5-bis(tert-butyldioxy)-3-hexyne, II: crystallization behaviour and mechanical properties. *Polymer.* 1982;23:1944–1952.
16. Digas G, Karrholm J, Malchau H, et al. RSA evaluation of wear of conventional versus highly cross-linked polyethylene acetabular components in vivo. Paper presented at the 49th Annual Meeting of the Orthopaedic Research Society; New Orleans, LA; Feb 2-5, 2003.
17. Edidin AA, Pruitt L, Jewett CW, et al. Plasticity-induced damage layer is a precursor to wear in radiation-cross-linked UHMWPE acetabular components for total hip replacement: ultra-high-molecular-weight polyethylene. *J Arthroplasty.* 1999;14:616–627.
18. Frankel A, Balderston RA, Booth RE, et al. Radiographic demarcation of the acetabular bone-cement interface: the effect of femoral head size. *J Arthroplasty.* 1990;5(suppl):1–3.
19. Goldring SR, Schiller AL, Roelk M, et al. The synovial-like membrane at the bone-cement interface in loose total hip replacements and its proposed role in bone lysis. *J Bone Joint Surg [Am].* 1983;65:575–584.
20. Goldring S, Jasty M, Paiement G. Tissue response to bulk and particulate biopolymers in a rabbit wound chamber model. *Orthop Trans.* 1986;11:288.
21. Jaramaz B, Nikou C, DiGioia AM. Effect of combined acetabular/femoral implant version on hip range of motion. *Transactions of 45th Annual Meeting of the Orthopedic Research Society.* 1999;24:926.
22. Jaramaz B, Nikou C, DiGioia AM. Effect of cup orientation and neck length in range of motion simulation. *Transactions of 43rd Annual Meeting of the Orthopedic Research Society.* 1997;22:286.
23. Jaramaz B, Nikou C, DiGioia AM. Sensitivity of impingement limits to error in cup placement. *Transactions of 44th Annual Meeting of the Orthopedic Research Society.* 1998;402.

24. Jasty M, Floyd WE, Schiller AL, et al. Localized osteolysis in stable, non-septic total hip replacement. *J Bone Joint Surg.* 1986;68A: 912–919.

25. Jasty MJ, Goetz DD, Lee KR, et al. Wear of polyethylene acetabular components in total hip arthroplasty: an analysis of 128 components retrieved at autopsy or revision operation. *J Bone Joint Surg.* 1997;79A:349–358.

26. Liao Y-S, Benya P, McKellop H. Effect of protein lubrication on the wear properties of materials for prosthetic joints. *J Biomed Mater Res.* 1999;48:465–473.

27. Livermore J, Ilstrup D, Morrey B. Effect of femoral head size on wear of the polyethylene acetabular component. *J Bone Joint Surg.* 1990;72A:518–528.

28. Martell JM, Incavo SJ. Clinical performance of a highly crosslinked polyethylene at two years in total hip arthroplasty: a randomized prospective trial. Paper present at the 49th Annual Meeting of the Orthopaedic Research Society; New Orleans, LA; Feb 2-5, 2003.

29. McKellop H, Shen FW, Lu B, et al. Development of an extremely wear resistant ultra-high molecular weight polyethylene for total hip replacements. *J Orthop Res.* 1999;17:157–167.

30. McKellop H, Shen FW, Lu B, et al. Effect of sterilization method and other modifications on the wear resistance of acetabular cups made of ultra-high molecular weight polyethylene: a hip-simulator study. *J Bone Joint Surg.* 2000;82A:1708–1725.

31. McKellop H, Shen FW, DiMaio W, et al. Wear of gamma-crosslinked polyethylene acetabular cups against roughened femoral balls. *Clin Orthop Relat Res.* 1999;No. 369:73–82.

32. Muratoglu OK, Merrill EW, Bragdon CR, et al. Effect of radiation, heat, and aging on in vitro wear resistance of polyethylene. *Clin Orthop Relat Res.* 2003;No. 417:253–262.

33. Muratoglu OK, O'Conner DO, Bragdon CR, et al. Gradient crosslinking of UHMWPE using irradiation in molten state for total joint arthroplasty. *Biomaterials.* 2001;23:717–724.

34. Muratoglu OK, Bragdon CR, O'Conner DO, et al. Larger diameter femoral heads used in conjunction with a highly cross-linked ultra-high molecular weight polyethylene: a new concept. *J Arthroplasty.* 2001;16(8 suppl):24–30.

35. Muratoglu OK, et al. Long term stability of radiation and peroxide cross-linked UHMWPE. Paper presented at the 23rd Annual Meeting of the Society for Biomaterials; New Orleans, LA; April 30-May 4, 1997.

36. Muratoglu OK, Bragdon CR, O'Connor DO, et al. A novel method of crosslinking UHMWPE to improve wear, reduce oxidation and retain mechanical properties. *J Arthroplasty.* 2001;16:149–160.

37. Muratoglu OK, Bragdon CR, O'Conner DO, et al. Surface analysis of early retrieved acetabular polyethylene liners: a comparison of standard and highly crosslinked polyethylenes. *J Arthroplasty.* 2004;19:68–77.

38. Muratoglu OK, Bragdon CR, O'Conner DO, et al. Unified wear model for highly crosslinked ultra-high molecular weight polyethylenes (UHMWPE). *Biomaterials.* 1999;20:1463–1470.

39. Nivbrant B, et al. In vivo wear and migration of high cross linked poly cups: a RSA study. Paper presented at the 49th Annual Meeting of the Orthopaedic Research Society; New Orleans, LA; 2003.

40. Ramamurti BS, Estok DM, Jasty M, et al. Analysis of the kinematics of different hip simulators used to study wear of candidate materials for the articulation of total hip arthroplasties. *J Orthop Res.* 1998;16:365–369.

41. Ramamurti B, Balaji S, Bragdon CR, et al. Loci of movement of selected points on the femoral head during normal gait: three-dimensional computer simulation. *J Arthroplasty.* 1996;11:845–852.

42. Saikko V. Effect of lubricant protein concentration on the wear of ultra-high molecular weight polyethylene sliding against a CoCr counterface. *J Tribol.* 2003;125:638–642.

43. Saikko V, Ahlroos T. Phospholipids as boundary lubricants in wear tests of prosthetic joint materials. *Wear.* 1997;207:86–91.

44. Saikko V, Ahlroos T. Type of motion and lubricant in wear simulation of polyethylene acetabular cup. *J Eng Med.* 1999;213:301–310.

45. Saikko V, Calonius O, Keranen J. Effect of counterface roughness on the wear of conventional and crosslinked ultrahigh molecular weight polyethylene studied with a multi-directional motion pin-on-pin device. *J Biomed Mater Res.* 2001;57:504–512.

46. Saikko V, Calonius O, Keranen J. Effect of slide track shape on the wear of ultra-high molecular weight polyethylene in a pin-on-disk wear simulation of total hip prosthesis. *J Biomed Mater Res.* 2004;69B:141–148.

47. Saikko V, Calonius O, Keranen J. Wear of conventional and cross-linked ultra-high-molecular-weight polyethylene acetabular cups against polished and roughened CoCr femoral heads in a biaxial hip simulator. *J Biomed Mater Res (Appl Biomater).* 2002;63:848–853.

48. Sanford W, Saum K. Accelerated oxidative aging testing of UHMWPE. *Trans Orthop Res Soc.* 1995;20:119.

49. Schmalzried T, Kwong LM, Jasty MJ, et al. The mechanism of loosening of cemented acetabular components in total hip arthroplasty: analysis of specimens retrieved at autopsy. *Clin Orthop.* 1992;No. 274:60–78.

50. Sun D, Stark C, J Dumbleton J. Development of an accelerated aging method for evaluation of long-term irradiation effects on UHMWPE implants. Paper presented at meeting of the American Chemical Society, Division of Polymer Chemistry; Washington, DC; Aug 21-24, 1994.

51. Sutula L, Collier JP, Saum KA, et al. The Otto Aufranc Award. Impact of gamma sterilization on clinical performance of polyethylene in the hip. *Clin Orthop.* 1995;No. (319):28–40.

52. Wang A, Essner A, Polineni VK, et al. Lubrication and wear of UHMWPE in total joint replacements. *Tribol Int.* 1998;31:17–33.

53. Wang A, Stark C, Dumbleton JH. Mechanistic and morphological origins of ultra-high molecular weight polyethylene wear debris in total joint replacement prostheses. [see comments]. *J Eng Med.* 1996;210:141–155.

54. Willert HG, Semlitsch M. Tissue reactions to plastic and metallic wear products of joint endoprostheses. *Clin Orthop.* 1996; No.333:4–14.

55. Willert H, Bertram H, Buchhorn G. Osteolysis in alloarthroplasty of the hip: the role of bone cement fragmentation. *Clin Orthop.* 1990;No. 258:108–121.

56. Willert HG, Bertram H, Buchhorn GH. Osteolysis in alloarthroplasty of the hip: the role of ultra-high molecular weight polyethylene wear particles. *Clin Orthop.* 1990;No. 258:95–107.

Clinical Wear Assessment

19

John M. Martell

Wear has been a major consideration in total hip arthroplasty since its introduction by Sir John Charnley in the late 1950s. Charnley's original prosthetic design attempted to limit wear by utilizing a 22.225-mm femoral bearing coupled with the low-friction material Teflon. Unfortunately, Teflon did not have adequate wear resistance, and the debris generated elicited an intense inflammatory reaction in the periprosthetic tissues. Sir John Charnley's subsequent designs used more durable ultrahigh molecular weight polyethylene as a bearing counterface (10). While less reactive to the tissues than Teflon debris, ultrahigh molecular weight polyethylene debris elicits an inflammatory response resulting in periprosthetic osteolysis and subsequent prosthetic loosening (11–13). In today's contemporary designs, particulate-mediated osteolysis and loosening are the primary factors limiting the long-term survival of implants (11,18,23).

Modifications to the design of the original Charnley low-friction arthroplasty prosthesis have been shown to influence the polyethylene wear rate. These changes include the material chosen for the articular surface (cobalt-chrome, titanium, ceramic) (3), the size of the bearing (22.225 mm, 26 mm, 28 mm, 32 mm) (31), the thickness of the polyethylene (1,15,30), and the propensity for debris generation (bead shedding and third-body wear from nonarticular surfaces and fretting of modular junctions) (21,25). Many of these design changes had an adverse effect on wear performance of the implants. While catastrophic failure is easily detected on radiographs, it is more difficult to appreciate the short-term effects

that design changes have on the polyethylene wear rate in vivo. While materials testing is a valuable tool for predicting the wear performance of new implant designs, tools for the clinical assessment of wear in patients are also critical. Hip simulators represent our best attempt at re-creating the mechanical environment of a total hip in vivo, yet only recently have simulator wear rate predictions been validated with clinically observed wear rates (33).

Early attempts to correlate clinical and radiographic outcomes with polyethylene wear rates yielded variable results (13,44). Studies with long-term data (more than 8 to 10 years), demonstrated significant correlations between clinical variables and measured wear rates (3,20,31). While useful for the assessment of long-term data, manual techniques of polyethylene wear measurement lack the precision and accuracy to assess the impact of design changes on wear performance using short-term data (14). Traditional manual techniques of measuring wear, including the methods of Charnley, Dorr, and Livermore, are accurate in experienced hands, but lack the precision necessary to assess wear rates in the short-term. It is important to understand the precision and accuracy of measurement techniques used to assess wear, particularly in the era of cross-linked polyethylene with predicted wear rates greater than 60 μm per year.

ASSESSMENT OF WEAR MEASUREMENT TECHNIQUES

The performance of a measurement instrument can be assessed in terms of precision and bias. Precision is the closeness of agreement between measurements taken under similar conditions while bias is the consistent or systematic difference between a set of measurements and an accepted reference value (3). Methods for the calculation of precision and accuracy are complex and depend on the experimental design use for data collection. A detailed discussion of these methods is

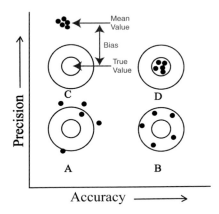

Figure 19-1 Instrument A has low accuracy and low precision while B has high accuracy (mean value = true value) but low precision. C demonstrates high precision with poor accuracy, and D is both accurate and precise. Instrument A is unusable, while instrument B can yield useful data if sample size is adequate and follow-up is sufficient. Instrument C is precise but inaccurate and contains systematic error (bias). If the bias of the instrument can be corrected through calibration, the instrument may yield acceptable data.

beyond the scope of this chapter; however, examples of methods for experimental designs often used in orthopaedics are given below. Both precision and bias are fundamental determinants of an instrument's accuracy. The relationship between precision, bias, and accuracy is demonstrated in Figure 19-1 and Table 19-1.

Bias

Bias is the consistent or systematic difference between a set of measurements and an accepted reference value.

Precision

Precision is the closeness of agreement between repeated independent test results obtained under stipulated conditions. When making 30 or more measurements of the same value using the same instrument, the ASTM standard practice E177-90a recommends that precision for the instrument at the measured value be expressed using a 95% level of confidence as shown in Equation 19-1a (2).

$$Precision\ (ASTM)_{>30\ measurements} = \pm 1.96 * S \quad (19\text{-}1a)$$

where: S = Standard deviation of the measurement series
When less then 30 observations exist in the series it is more appropriate to use Eq. 19-1b.

$$Precision\ (ASTM)_{<30\ measurements} = \pm t_{n-1} * \sqrt{2} * S \quad (19\text{-}1b)$$

where: S = Standard deviation of the measurement series
n = The number of observations in the series
When assessing the precision between two separate instruments (or separate observers), Bland and Altman advocate using the 95% confidence interval of the standard error to estimate the precision of agreement between measurement pairs obtained by different methods or different observers (Eq. 19-2) (6).

$$Precision\ (Pairs) = \pm t_{n-1} * \sqrt{2} * S_{diff} \quad (19\text{-}2)$$

where: S_{diff} = Standard deviation of the difference between measurement pairs
n = The number of observations in the series

Accuracy

Accuracy is the closeness of a measurement to the true value. A standard method of reporting accuracy has not been well established in the literature for clinical wear assessment. The ASTM standard recommends reporting bias and precision rather than accuracy (2). Published wear studies report on the accuracy of their polyethylene wear measurements in a variety of ways, making direct comparisons of accuracy between published techniques difficult. However, when the raw measurement data is given, the root mean square error (RMSE) may be calculated (Eq. 19-3).

$$RMSE = \sqrt{\frac{1}{n} \sum_{i=1}^{n} (x_i - T)^2} \quad (19\text{-}3)$$

where x = individual measurement
T = true value for measurement
Accuracy may also be reported as the standard error (SE) (Eq. 19-4).

$$Accuracy = \pm(SE) = \pm \frac{S_{dif}}{\sqrt{n}} \quad (19\text{-}4)$$

where S_{dif} = Standard deviation (measured value – true value)
n = Total number of observations

Repeatability

Repeatability may be reported as the precision within and between observers or as the repeatability coefficient as defined by Bland and Altman. The *repeatability coefficient* (RC) is defined as two times the standard deviation of the difference between two measurements taken under the same conditions (Eq. 19-5). Repeatability can be calculated for the same observer (intraobserver repeatability), or between different observers (interobserver repeatability) (5,6).

$$RC = \pm 2S_{dif} \quad (19\text{-}5)$$

where S_{dif} is the standard deviation (measured value – true value).

Standard Components of Variance Analysis

This approach uses analysis of variance to determine the percent variation contributed by each component of the measurement system. The percent measurement variation introduced by the measuring instrument, by the individual measuring the wear, and by variations in patient use are calculated (40). Ideally, in a good measurement system, the variation introduced by the instrument and the observer is less than the variation observed in the wear values as a result of patient clinical factors. While this technique yields detailed information on sources of potential error, a full analysis is time-consuming and requires multiple observations per observer and multiple observers.

TABLE 19-1

SAMPLE DATA FOR VALIDATION OF WEAR

Actual Wear (Microns)	Measured Wear1 (Microns)	Measured Wear2 (Microns)	Meas. 1-Actual	Meas. 2-Actual	Meas.1 - Meas.2 (Microns)
100	81	78.0	−19.0	−22.0	3
100	94	85.0	−6.0	−15.0	9
100	119	106.0	4.5	6.0	13
100	107	90.0	7.0	−10.0	17
100	110	140.0	10.0	40.0	−30
100	100	109.0	0.0	9.0	−9
100	115	98.0	15.0	−2.0	17
100	104	110.0	4.0	10.0	−6
100	95	88.0	−5.0	−12.0	7
100	111	100.0	11.0	0.0	11
100	100	95.0	0.0	−5.0	5
100	99	99.0	−1.0	−1.0	0
100	95	98.0	−5.0	−2.0	−3
Std dev	10.21	15.28	8.95	15.28	12.81
Precision (ASTM) <30 measurements			27.59	47.12	
Precision (ASTM) measurement pairs					7.75
Accuracy$_{(100)}$ RMSE	8.68	14.69			
Accuracy$_{(100)}$ (SE)	2.48	4.24			
RC (meas.1 vs meas.2)					25.62
n =	13.00				
t (df = 12) 95% two tailed =	2.18				
mean difference			1.19	−0.31	

This technique contains little bias (mean difference from standard = +1.19 and − 0.31 microns), reasonable precision and acceptable accuracy. The two measurement series have good precision to each other (± 7.75 microns), with 95% limits of agreement of 25.62 microns. Note that the method of reporting accuracy impacts the reported values.

Classifications of Wear Measurement Techniques

Published polyethylene wear studies differ with respect to the technique by which the measurements are made, the method by which they calculate wear, and the manner in which wear is reported.

Weight Bearing

The potential advantage of weight bearing is the assurance that the femoral bearing is in contact with the polyethylene of the acetabular component when the x-ray is acquired. Investigators have reported weight bearing to have both a significant and an insignificant (34,35) effect on wear measurements. Smith et al. showed significantly more wear with standing than with supine x-rays (39). Recently Digas et al. found a 50% difference between highly cross-linked and conventional polyethylene with standing, but not with supine, radiosterio-

metric analysis (RSA) studies. In this series the non-weight-bearing films were taken at 1 week postoperatively, while weight-bearing films were taken from 3 months on (16), making it difficult to attribute the difference observed entirely to weight bearing. In a prospective direct comparison of standing versus supine anteroposterior (AP) pelvis films, Moore et al. found no statistically significant difference in the wear measured with standing radiographs (35). Other investigators have shown that load bearing has no reproducible effect on the position of the femoral head in the acetabular component (34). Currently, there is no consensus on the importance of obtaining standing radiographs for wear studies.

Techniques of Analysis

Each measurement method can be classified as either a manual or a computer-assisted technique. Computer-assisted techniques may be further classified as those using edge detection and those that do not.

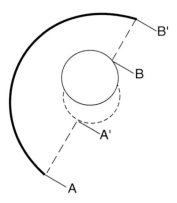

Figure 19-2 Wear is calculated by measuring A-A′ and subtracting its value from B-B′. This two-dimensional method requires only one follow-up radiograph, but detects only the component of wear directed toward the margin of the acetabular component (B′).

Method of Analysis

The method for calculating wear can be classified into four types: uniradiographic, which is based on analysis of one follow-up radiograph (Fig. 19-2); duoradiographic, which compares two radiographs to determine the maximum change in polyethylene thickness (Fig. 19-3); the dual circle method, which calculates wear based on the change in position of the femoral head center relative to the acetabular center on serial radiographs (Fig. 19-4); and the three-dimensional coordinate system (RSA).

Type of Wear Reported

Finally, the manner in which wear may be reported includes two-dimensional linear wear, three-dimensional linear wear, and volumetric wear. Two-dimensional linear wear assessment involves measuring only AP pelvis films and does not detect wear out of the AP plane. Three-dimensional linear wear measurements require an AP and lateral pelvis film for each time

point analyzed. While three-dimensional techniques detect 5% to 10% more wear than two-dimensional techniques, analysis of the lateral pelvis radiograph is often difficult, resulting in a drop in precision for three-dimensional analysis (26,32,42). Increased acetabular anteversion is the only clinical variable that has been significantly related to the likelihood of high out-of-plane wear. While significantly correlated ($p = 0.02$), the correlation coefficient is low and not useful for predicting those cases requiring three-dimensional analysis (32).

Volumetric wear may be calculated given the magnitude of two- or three-dimensional linear wear, the femoral head size, and the direction of the wear path with respect to the face of the cup (β angle). Historically, several published series have estimated volumetric wear assuming a β angle of 90°. With this assumption, the formula for calculation of volumetric wear becomes the volume of a cylinder (Fig. 19-5) (Eq. 19-6).

$$\text{Area of Cylinder} = \pi r^2 d, \qquad (19\text{-}6)$$

where r is the radius of the femoral head, and d is the linear wear. This method of reporting volumetric wear is less accurate than other published equations which take into account the direction of the wear path (27,29). Figure 19-6 demonstrates a case with equal linear wear in two different directions (β angles of zero and 90°). In this case the wear path with a β angle of 90° has two times greater volumetric wear than the wear path with a β angle of zero (parallel to the face of the cup). Additionally, close inspection of acetabular retrievals has demonstrated multiple wear paths, which cannot be accounted for when calculating volumetric wear from serial radiographs. When multiple wear paths are present, calculation of volumetric wear will underestimate the actual amount of volumetric wear present (45).

Uniradiographic Measurement Technique

Wear is determined by measuring the distance from the superior aspect of the femoral head to the superior acetabular rim (B-B′), and subtracting the distance from the inferior aspect of the femoral head to the inferior acetabular rim (A-A′). While this technique has the advantage of requiring only one follow-up

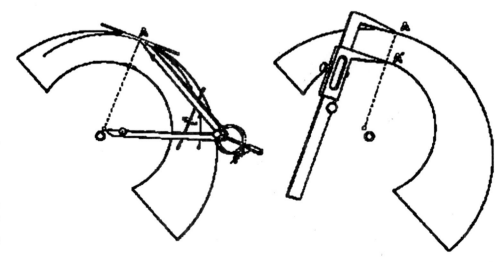

Figure 19-3 Duoradiographic measurement technique. The direction from the center of the femoral head (O) to the thinnest portion of the polyethylene is found at final follow-up (O-A). The distance from the edge of the head to the margin of the cup (A-A′) is measured along this line and subtracted from the measured polyethylene thickness along the same line on the initial radiograph. (From *J Bone Joint Surg.*, with permission.)

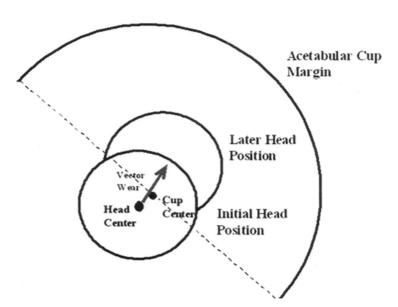

Figure 19-4   The dual circle technique. Motion of the femoral head center (A), with respect to the acetabular center (C), is followed on serial radiographs. This technique does not assume the femoral head center and acetabular centers are identical initially.

radiograph, its disadvantage is that wear directed away from the superior edge of the cup B′ is not well detected (Fig. 19-2).

Duoradiographic Measurement Technique

The direction from the center of the femoral head (O) to the thinnest portion of the polyethylene is found at final follow-up (O-A). The distance from the edge of the head to the margin of the cup (A-A′) is measured along this line and subtracted from the measured polyethylene thickness along the same line on the initial radiograph. This technique assumes

the femoral head center begins at the acetabular center. In offset polyethylene liner designs this is an invalid assumption, leading to errors in the magnitude and direction of wear detected (Fig. 19-3).

Dual Circle Technique

This method of determining wear follows the motion of the femoral head center (A), with respect to the acetabular center (C) on serial radiographs. While more versatile than the uni- and duoradiographic techniques, the precision and accuracy of this technique are dependent on the ability of the observer to find the center of the femoral head and the acetabular shell on serial radiographs. Computer-assisted techniques overcome this potential limitation by using edge detection and image analysis to reproducibly find the center of the femoral head and acetabular shell (Fig. 19-4).

Templating Technique

Templating is the most easily performed of all the wear analysis techniques. Magnified templates provided by the implant manufacturer show the thickness of the acetabular metal shell, allowing the remaining polyethylene thickness to be measured (Fig. 19-7). This assists in surgical decision-making regarding the timing of revision for polyethylene liner exchange (37).

Radiosteriometric Analysis

RSA is a computer-assisted three-dimensional technique based on two 40° radiographs of the patient while lying over a cage that allows calibration of the three-dimensional space around the patient. This technique follows the position of multiple tantalum markers fixed to the prosthesis and implanted in the bone at the time of surgery. This technique has high precision and accuracy in published implant migration studies (7,43),

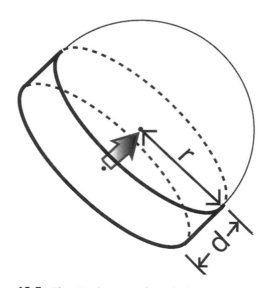

Figure 19-5   The simplest case for calculating volumetric wear occurs when the direction of wear *(large arrow)* is directly into the center of the cup (β angle of 90°). In this case, the volumetric wear is given by Equation 19-4 and equals the area of a cylinder with radius *r* and a height equal to the amount of wear *d*.

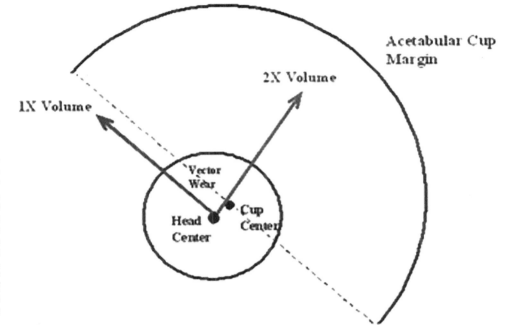

Figure 19-6 This figure demonstrates the effect that wear direction has on the volume of wear debris generated. In this case, identical linear wear results in a twofold difference in volumetric wear. When the wear path follows an angle of 90° (perpendicular to the cup face), volumetric wear is equal to the area of a cylinder (Eq. 19-4) (Fig. 19-5). When the wear path is directed toward the rim of the cup (β angle = 0), volumetric wear is equal to one half the area of a cylinder.

and recent work indicates a similarly high precision and accuracy for polyethylene wear determination (9). Wear is calculated directly from changes in the three-dimensional coordinates of the femoral head center (Fig. 19-8).

QUALITY CONTROL FOR X-RAY TECHNIQUE

Regardless of the wear-analysis techniques utilized, the quality of the radiographs has a direct impact on the precision of the data collected. The following criteria should be met before

analyzing an x-ray for wear. The entire acetabular component should be visible in each radiograph. AP pelvis radiographic projections should be comparable based on the appearance of the obturator foramen (symmetry). Additionally, for those techniques that cannot correct for beam position, the acetabulum should be located in approximately the same position on the radiograph for all examinations (Fig. 19-9). For lateral pelvis radiographs, the femoral bearing should appear round, indicating that the x-ray plate was correctly positioned perpendicular to the path of the x-ray beam. Failure to do so results in an oval appearance of the femoral head and introduces errors that are unacceptable for three-dimensional analysis (Fig. 19-10).

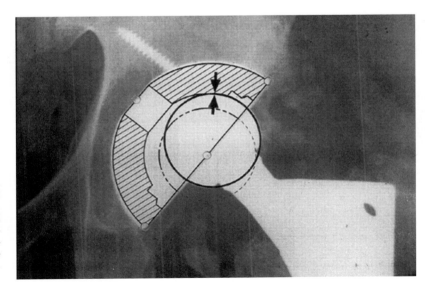

Figure 19-7 The templating technique depends upon magnified templates of the acetabular shell design, which includes the thickness of the metal. The template is superimposed on the femoral head and the distance to the inside edge of the acetabulum (*arrows*), representing the remaining polyethylene, is measured. In this case little polyethylene remains and revision for liner exchange is indicated. (From *J Bone Joint Surg.*, with permission.)

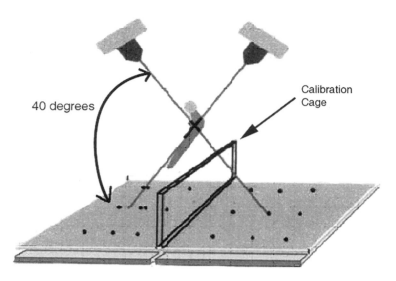

40 degrees

Calibration
Cage

Figure 19-8 RSA setup. The space surrounding the patient's implant is calibrated using a calibration cage containing tantalum markers. Analysis for wear is based upon two radiographs, each taken at 40° away from the horizontal plane. Motion of the femoral head in three-dimensional space with respect to markers on the acetabular component is reported as three-dimensional wear. (From Charles Bragdon, with permission.)

INTERPRETATION OF WEAR DATA

Once obtained, the manner in which wear is calculated and reported has an impact on the results. Therefore, it is important to understand the method used for calculating wear when attempting to compare results from different investigators. Wear data does not follow a Gaussian distribution (Fig. 19-11), and therefore, the statistical techniques used should be appropriate for nonparametric analysis (i.e., the Mann-Whitney test, not the student's t-test).

Bedding-in Analysis

Bedding-in consists of run-in wear, backside liner settling, and creep of the polyethylene. This phenomenon has been described by several authors and is generally limited to the first 18 months in the service life of an implant (17,36,41). The magnitude of the bedding-in effect can be estimated by the y intercept of the wear versus time curve for all data (41) (Fig. 19-12). Wear rates that include bedding-in will be higher than the true wear rates. Bedding-in is likely unique to each acetabular shell design and polyethylene locking mechanism. The duration of bedding-in can be assessed retrospectively based on the wear versus time curve. Prospectively, the bedding-in effect is complete when the wear rates stabilize and interval wear rates are not significantly different (Table 19-2) (32).

SUMMARY

There are many described techniques for the analysis of polyethylene wear in total hip arthroplasty. The precision and accuracy of these techniques vary (Table 19-3). Computer-based techniques with edge detection and image enhancement generally provide improved repeatability and precision compared to manual techniques. Nevertheless, quality control for radiographs in wear studies is critically important, since inadequate x-ray technique will often make wear analysis impossible by any means.

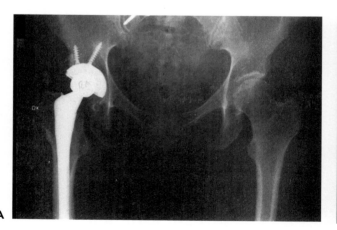

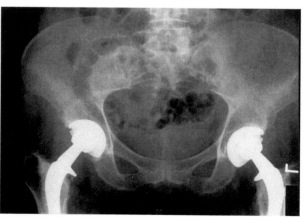

A   B

Figure 19-9 Unacceptable technique for the AP pelvis radiograph **(A)**, and correct technique **(B)**, with the iliac crest and the lesser trochanters both visible on the film.

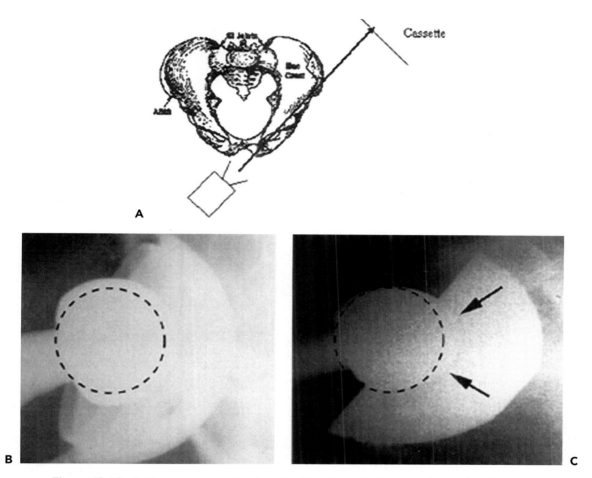

A

B   **C**

Figure 19-10   **A:** The correct setup for a lateral pelvis radiograph. The x-ray plate is placed perpendicular to the x-ray beam, which is parallel to the examination table and directed along the inguinal ligament (pubic tubercle to ASIS). **B:** Correct appearance of the lateral pelvis film, with a round femoral head. **C:** Unacceptable technique for the lateral pelvis film, with an oval-shaped femoral head *(arrows)*.

A standard method of reporting wear data is suggested. This includes reporting the duration and magnitude of bedding-in, along with the steady state (true wear rate). Steady-state wear has been reached when the yearly interval wear rates are no longer significantly different. The steady-state,

or true, wear rate is represented by the slope of the wear versus time plot with bedding-in excluded (Fig. 19-10). Reporting results in this fashion will allow more valuable comparisons of data reported by different investigators at multiple institutions.

Figure 19-11   A typical distribution of wear rates in a population of 85 patients, with normal curve superimposed. This distribution is skewed to the left with the median significantly smaller than the mean. High-wear outliers are contributing to the skewed distribution.

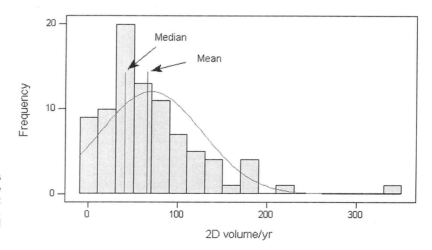

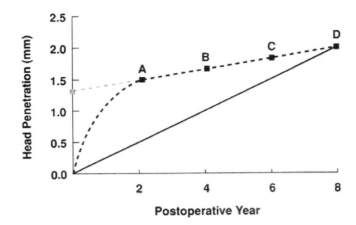

Figure 19-12 The apparent wear rate from time zero to point D, includes bedding-in and has a higher wear rate (slope), than the true steady-state wear rate (line A-D). The magnitude of the bedding in effect can be estimated by the y intercept of line A-D (1.4 mm). The true wear rate, in this example, can be estimated by the slope of the line fitting the data from 2 to 8 years. (From *J Bone Joint Surg.*, with permission.)

TABLE 19-2
COMPARISON OF LINEAR WEAR RATES BY YEARLY INTERVALS

Comparison Interval (years)	N	#1 Mean 2D Wear Rate (mm/year)	Standard Deviation	#2 Mean 2D Wear Rate (mm/year)	Standard Deviation	Paired t-test p value
1 to 2	53	0.327	0.238	0.200	0.132	0.000*
2 to 3	42	0.207	0.117	0.176	0.104	0.012*
3 to 4	34	0.192	0.100	0.180	0.199	0.323
4 to 5	34	0.164	0.078	0.155	0.065	0.420
5 to 6	36	0.162	0.091	0.155	0.090	0.242
6 to 7	29	0.174	0.105	0.068	0.099	0.218
7 to 8	16	0.141	0.071	0.136	0.078	0.500
8 to 9	17	0.138	0.079	0.143	0.070	0.348
9 to 10	13	0.157	0.064	0.152	0.073	0.395
10 to 11	7	0.158	0.065	0.160	0.057	0.735
11 to 12	2	0.156	0.099	0.150	0.071	0.856

A paired t-test comparing yearly wear rates demonstrated no significant difference in the two-dimensional wear rates after the third postoperative year. Completion of the bedding-in process is assumed by this time. (From *J Bone Joint Surg.*, with permission.)
*Significant difference at 95% level.

TABLE 19-3
CLASSIFICATION OF THE DIFFERENT PUBLISHED METHODS OF WEAR ANALYSIS

Wear Analysis	Method	Technique	Edge Detection	Wear Reported	Accuracy (mm)	Precision (mm)
Charnley (28)	Uniradiographic	Manual	N	2D	0.35	—
Dorr (19,37)	Uniradiographic	Manual	N	2D	0.4	1.96–3.05
Livermore (4,19,37)	Duoradiographic	Manual	N	2D	0.18	1.75–2.18
Maxima (22)	Duoradiographic	Computer	N	2D	0.50	0.01
Ebra (24)	Dual circle	Computer	N	2D	0.90	—
Engh Templatine (37)	Uniradiographic	Manual	N	2D	—	1.47
Engh	Dual circle	Manual	N	2D	—	—
Shaver (38)	Dual circle	Computer	Y	2D	0.076	0.018
Martell (8,19)	Dual circle	Computer	Y	2D, 3D, Vol.	0.060–0.1	0.040–0.67
Devane (15,19)	3D coordinate	Computer	Y	2D, 3D, Vol.	0.026–0.10	0.006–1.07
RSA (9)	3D coordinate	Computer	Y	2D, 3D	0.030–0.077	0.060

Precision and accuracy were calculated from data in each manuscript using Equations 1,2, and 4. Blank entries indicate the inability to calculate precision and accuracy with the data presented in the manuscript. 2D, two-dimensional; 3D, three-dimensional; Vol., volumetric.

REFERENCES

1. Astion DJ, Saluan P, Stulberg BN, et al. The porous-coated anatomic total hip prosthesis: failure of the metal-backed acetabular component. *J Bone Joint Surg Am.* 1996;78:755–766.
2. ASTM. *Practice E 177-90a.* West Conshohocken, PA: American Society for Testing and Materials; 2002.
3. Bankston AB, Faris PM, Keating EM, et al. Polyethylene wear in total hip arthroplasty in patient-matched groups. A comparison of stainless steel, cobalt chrome, and titanium-bearing surfaces. *J Arthroplasty.* 1993;8:315–322.
4. Bankston AB, Ritter MA, Keating EM, et al. Measurement of polyethylene thickness in total hip arthroplasty. A technique analysis. *J Arthroplasty.* 1994;9:533–538.
5. Bland JM, Altman DG. Comparing methods of measurement: why plotting difference against standard method is misleading. *Lancet.* 1995;346(8982):1085–1087.
6. Bland JM, Altman DG. Statistical methods for assessing agreement between two methods of clinical measurement. *Lancet.* 1986;1(8476):307–310.
7. Borlin N, Thien T, Karrholm J. The precision of radiostereometric measurements. Manual vs. digital measurements. *J Biomech.* 2002; 35:69–79.
8. Bragdon CR, Greene ME, Thanner J, et al. A five year clinical comparison of the measurement of femoral head penetration in THR using RSA and the Martell method. *Trans ORS.* 2004;29:181.
9. Bragdon CR, Yuan X, Perinchief R, et al. Precision and reproducibility of radiostereometric analysis (RSA) to determine polyethylene wear in a total hip replacement model. *Trans ORS.* 2001;47:1005.
10. Charnley J. *Low Friction Arthroplasty of the Hip: Theory and Practice.* New York: Springer-Verlag; 1978.
11. Charnley J. The long-term results of low-friction arthroplasty of the hip performed as a primary intervention. *J Bone Joint Surg Br.* 1972;54:61–76.
12. Charnley J. Total hip replacement by low-friction arthroplasty. *Clin Orthop.* 1970;72:7–21.
13. Charnley J, Halley DK. Rate of wear in total hip replacement. *Clin Orthop.* 1975;112:170–179.
14. Clarke JC, Black K, Rennie C, et al. Can wear in total hip arthroplasties be assessed from radiographs? *Clin Orthop.* 1976;121:126–142.
15. Devane PA, Horne JG. Assessment of polyethylene wear in total hip replacement. *Clin Orthop.* 1999;369:59–72.
16. Digas G, Karrholm J, Thanner J, et al. Highly cross-linked polyethylene in cemented THA: randomized study of 61 hips. *Clin Orthop.* 2003;417:126–138.
17. Dowd JE, Sychterz CJ, Young AM, et al. Characterization of long-term femoral-head-penetration rates. Association with and prediction of osteolysis. *J Bone Joint Surg Am.* 2000;82A:1102–1107.
18. Dumbleton JH, Manley MT, Edidin AA. A literature review of the association between wear rate and osteolysis in total hip arthroplasty. *J Arthroplasty.* 2002;17:649–661.
19. Ebramzadeh E, Sangiorgio SN, Lattuada F, et al. Accuracy of measurement of polyethylene wear with use of radiographs of total hip replacements. *J Bone Joint Surg Am.* 2003;85A:2378–2384.
20. Feller JA, Kay PR, Hodgkinson JP, et al. Activity and socket wear in the Charnley low-friction arthroplasty. *J Arthroplasty.* 1994;9:341–345.
21. Gilbert JL, Buckley CA, Jacobs JJ. In vivo corrosion of modular hip prosthesis components in mixed and similar metal combinations. The effect of crevice, stress, motion, and alloy coupling. *J Biomed Mater Res.* 1993;27:1533–1544.
22. Hardinge K, Porter ML, Jones PR, et al. Measurement of hip prostheses using image analysis. The maxima hip technique. *J Bone Joint Surg Br.* 1991;73:724–728.
23. Harris WH. The problem is osteolysis. *Clin Orthop.* 1995;311: 46–53.
24. Hendrich C, Bahlmann J, Eulert J. Migration of the uncemented Harris-Galante acetabular cup: results of the einbildroentgenanalyse (EBRA) method. *J Arthroplasty.* 1997;12:889–895.
25. Hop JD, Callaghan JJ, Olejniczak JP, et al. The Frank Stinchfield Award. Contribution of cable debris generation to accelerated polyethylene wear. *Clin Orthop.* 1997;344:20–32.
26. Hui AJ, McCalden RW, Martell JM, et al. Validation of two and three-dimensional radiographic techniques for measuring polyethylene wear after total hip arthroplasty. *J Bone Joint Surg Am.* 2003;85A:505–511.
27. Kabo JM, Gebhard JS, Loren G, et al. In vivo wear of polyethylene acetabular components. *J Bone Joint Surg Br.* 1993;75:254–258.
28. Kang JS, Park SR, Ebramzadeh E, et al. Measurement of polyethylene wear in total hip arthroplasty: accuracy versus ease of use. *Yonsei Med J.* 2003;44:473–478.
29. Kosak R, Antolic V, Pavlovcic V, et al. Polyethylene wear in total hip prostheses: the influence of direction of linear wear on volumetric wear determined from radiographic data. *Skeletal Radiol.* 2003;32:679–686.
30. Lee PC, Shih CH, Chen WJ, et al. Early polyethylene wear and osteolysis in cementless total hip arthroplasty: the influence of femoral head size and polyethylene thickness. *J Arthroplasty.* 1999;14:976–981.
31. Livermore J, Ilstrup D, Morrey B. Effect of femoral head size on wear of the polyethylene acetabular component. *J Bone Joint Surg Am.* 1990;72:518–528.
32. Martell JM, Berkson E, Berger R, et al. Comparison of two and three-dimensional computerized polyethylene wear analysis after total hip arthroplasty. *J Bone Joint Surg Am.* 2003;85:1111–1117.
33. Martell JM, Edidin A, Dumbleton J. Preclinical evaluation followed by randomized clinical study of a crosslinked polyethylene for total hip arthroplasty at two year follow-up. *Trans ORS.* 2001;26:163.
34. Martell JM, Leopold SS, Liu X. The effect of joint loading on acetabular wear measurement in total hip arthroplasty. *J Arthroplasty.* 2000;15:512–518.
35. Moore KD, Barrack RL, Sychterz CJ, et al. The effect of weight-bearing on the radiographic measurement of the position of the femoral head after total hip arthroplasty. *J Bone Joint Surg Am.* 2000;82:62–69.
36. Pedersen DR, Brown TD, Hillis SL, et al. Prediction of long-term polyethylene wear in total hip arthroplasty, based on early wear measurements made using digital image analysis. *J Orthop Res.* 1998;16:557–563.
37. .Pollock D, Sychterz CJ, Engh CA. A clinically practical method of manually assessing polyethylene liner thickness. *J Bone Joint Surg Am.* 2001;83:1803–1809.
38. Shaver SM, Brown TD, Hillis SL, et al. Digital edge-detection measurement of polyethylene wear after total hip arthroplasty. *J Bone Joint Surg Am.* 1997;79:690–700.
39. Smith SE, Harris WH. Total hip arthroplasty performed with insertion of the femoral component with cement and the acetabular component without cement. Ten to thirteen-year results. *J Bone Joint Surg Am.* 1997;79:1827–1833.
40. Snedecor GW, Cochran WG. In: Snedecor GW, Cochran WG, eds. The random effects model. *Statistical Methods.* Ames, IA: Iowa State University Press; 1980: 238–254.
41. Sychterz CJ, Engh CA Jr, Yang A, et al. Analysis of temporal wear patterns of porous-coated acetabular components: distinguishing between true wear and so-called bedding-in. *J Bone Joint Surg Am.* 1999;81:821–830.
42. Sychterz CJ, Yang AM, McAuley JP, et al. Two-dimensional versus three-dimensional radiographic measurements of polyethylene wear. *Clin Orthop.* 1999;365:117–123.
43. Valstar ER, Vrooman HA, Toksvig-Larsen S, et al. Digital automated RSA compared to manually operated RSA. *J Biomech.* 2000;33:1593–1599.
44. Woolson ST, Murphy MG. Wear of the polyethylene of Harris-Galante acetabular components inserted without cement. *J Bone Joint Surg Am.* 1995;77:1311–1314.
45. Yamaguchi M, Bauer TW, Hashimoto Y. Three-dimensional analysis of multiple wear vectors in retrieved acetabular cups. *J Bone Joint Surg Am.* 1997;79:1539–1544.

Bearing Surfaces

20

Mauricio Silva   Christian Heisel   Harry McKellop   Thomas P. Schmalzried

For the purpose of this chapter, the review and discussion of bearing surfaces will be limited to the femoral–acetabular articulation, the site of intended motion in a total hip arthroplasty: the surfaces of the ball and socket joint. The central issue is the wear of a bearing couple in vivo. Wear is the removal of material that results from relative motion between two opposed surfaces under load. While simple in concept, wear performance in vivo is a complex function of many factors including those related to the implanted components, variables in the surgical implantation procedure, and variables related to the patient.

MATERIAL PROPERTIES

Materials used in the manufacturing of femoral heads for metal-on-polyethylene (MOP) total hip replacement (THR) include the metal alloys, stainless steel (316L, F-56; Ortron-CFT; Chas. F. Thackray-DePuy International, Ltd., Leeds, U.K.), cobalt–chromium (F-75), and titanium alloy (6% aluminum, 4% vanadium; F-136) as well as ceramic materials, aluminum oxide, and zirconium oxide. Metal-on-metal (MOM) bearings have been cobalt–chromium on cobalt–chromium, while ceramic-on-ceramic (COC) bearings have been alumina on alumina.

Properties to consider when evaluating materials for bearings in THR include corrosion resistance, strength, ductility, hardness, and frictional characteristics (23) (Table 20-1). Friction is the resistance to movement between two surfaces in contact. Frictional characteristics are a result of material properties such as wettability (related to surface energy), manufacturing variables such as surface finish, and operating conditions such as lubrication. The degree of resistance is proportional to the load. The ratio between frictional force and load (friction/load) is the coefficient of friction, μ. The initial resistance to motion is the static coefficient of friction, μ_S. Once in motion, the resistance decreases to a dynamic coefficient of friction, μ_D. Because both chemical and mechanical interactions may occur, frictional forces depend on both the material composition and the roughness of the opposed surfaces. Lubricating conditions can change the nature of the interface between the moving surfaces and decrease friction. The coefficients of friction depend upon the nature and amount of lubricant present, as well as the speed of relative motion and the applied load.

SURFACE ROUGHNESS

A number of measurement parameters have been described for quantitative assessment of surface roughness (207). Conceptually, a contact or noncontact (laser) stylus scans the surface and makes an analog recording of the peaks and valleys over the specified length of the sample tracing. R_a is the arithmetic average of the absolute value of the measured profile height deviations as measured from the graphical center line (the line parallel to the general direction of the profile about which deviations are measured). R_a is the result of averaging a large number of data points and is relatively unaffected by occasional large deviations of the surface.

Other measurement parameters include R_q or the root mean square roughness. This is the root mean square value of the profile departures within the sampling length. This has been largely replaced by R_a. R_z is the average height difference between the highest peaks and lowest valleys of five sampling lengths. R_{max} is the largest of these and as such is sensitive to extreme values. R_p is the distance between the mean line of the profile and a line parallel to it that passes through the highest peak within the sampling length; R_p is sensitive to unusual peaks. R_{pm} is the

TABLE 20-1

COMPARISON OF PROPERTIES FOR BEARING SURFACE MATERIALS

	Stainless Steel	Cobalt Chromium	Ti-Al6, V4	Ceramics
Corrosion resistance	4	3	2	1
Modulus	3	2	4	1
Yield strength	2	1	2	3
Ductility	1	2	3	4
Hardness	3	2	4	1
Wettability	2	2	2	1

1, highest; 4, lowest.
Adapted from Black J. *Orthopaedic Biomaterials in Research and Practice*. Philadelphia: Churchill Livingstone; 1988.

average of the highest peak to mean line distance of five sampling lengths and is less affected by extreme values. R_m is the maximum profile valley depth, the distance between the lowest point on the profile and the mean line within the sampling length. Skewness is a measure of the asymmetry of the profile around the center line. A surface with a predominance of valleys will have negative skew, while a surface with a predominance of peaks will be positively skewed.

At this time it is not clear which parameters have the best correlation with in vivo wear performance. It seems logical that one should consider a number of parameters including those that describe the average deviation from the center line (R_a, R_z), those that describe peaks or asperities on the surface (R_p, R_{pm}), those that assess valleys or pores in the surface (R_m), and the symmetry of the profile (skewness). It should be kept in mind that these parameters are all derived from measurements of the surface tracing, and there may be significant correlations between parameters. A thorough surface roughness evaluation should include a visual comparison of the actual tracings and representative photomicrographs (scanning electron microscope) of the surface (Fig. 20-1).

Optical polishing techniques can achieve surfaces with peak heights as small as 0.005 μm (23). The surface roughness of currently available femoral heads ranges from an R_a of less than 0.03 μm to about 0.10 μm, and an R_{max} ranging from less than 0.10 to about 0.40 μm. The surface roughness of a femoral bearing can, however, change over time in vivo. The surface roughness of femoral heads retrieved after in vivo use is variable and can be several times higher than as manufactured, with R_a as high as 0.2 to 0.3 μm, a two- to threefold increase in the as-manufactured surface roughness (126,167,168). In the presence of hard third bodies, as can occur in vivo, surface abrasions (scratches) result in an increased surface roughness, and the wear rate of polyethylene (PE) can increase (81,168,184,277). Conversely, in "clean" operating conditions with little or no hard third bodies, such as in a laboratory wear simulator, motion against PE may result in polishing of the metal surface and a lower surface roughness (167). This suggests that a constant presence of hard third bodies, not a transient event, is necessary to maintain high femoral surface roughness. This also suggests that differences in the initial or as-manufactured surface roughness of a femoral head may not be as important in the long run as the in vivo operating conditions.

This mechanism for maintaining an increased surface roughness in vivo applies to all materials, but the susceptibility to scratching is a function of the hardness of the material. The decreased hardness of titanium alloy results in decreased abrasion resistance. Although the initial surface roughness of a titanium alloy femoral head may be equivalent to that of other bearing materials, there is greater potential for surface roughness to increase in vivo. In an environment with few or no hard third bodies, the wear performance of titanium alloy against PE can be comparable to the other metals (165,167,168), but the performance of titanium alloy against PE is affected to a greater degree by the presence of hard third bodies (168,184).

The abrasion resistance of cobalt–chromium alloy is considered superior to that of titanium alloy and stainless steel. Jasty et al. (126) studied the surface damage on 54 cobalt–chromium alloy femoral heads with in vivo service lives ranging from 8 months to 19 years. Forty-eight of the heads had some evidence of surface damage. The affected areas were usually discrete, measuring 1 to 20 mm^2 on the upper surface. Twenty-five of 31 (modular) heads (81%) from uncemented or hybrid hips and 11 of the 23 heads (48%) from cemented (nonmodular) hips showed surface damage involving more than 25% of the surface. Surface damage was more common, more extensive, and occurred after shorter periods of service in uncemented and in hybrid hips than in cemented hips. This suggests that the abrasive particles were mainly released from modular interfaces, metal backing, and/or porous coating.

Increased femoral head surface roughness may dramatically accelerate two-body abrasive wear of PE. Experimental studies indicate that a threefold increase in femoral roughness can cause at least a tenfold increase in the wear rate of PE (55,81). Specific increases in wear rate are dependent on the nature of the damage to the femoral head. Ceramics are harder and therefore more resistant to damage by third-body particles than metal counterfaces (54). For this reason, the increased hardness of ceramic materials is considered advantageous.

FRICTIONAL TORQUE

Charnley conducted an elaborate series of experiments to optimize the diameter of a metal on plastic bearing surface

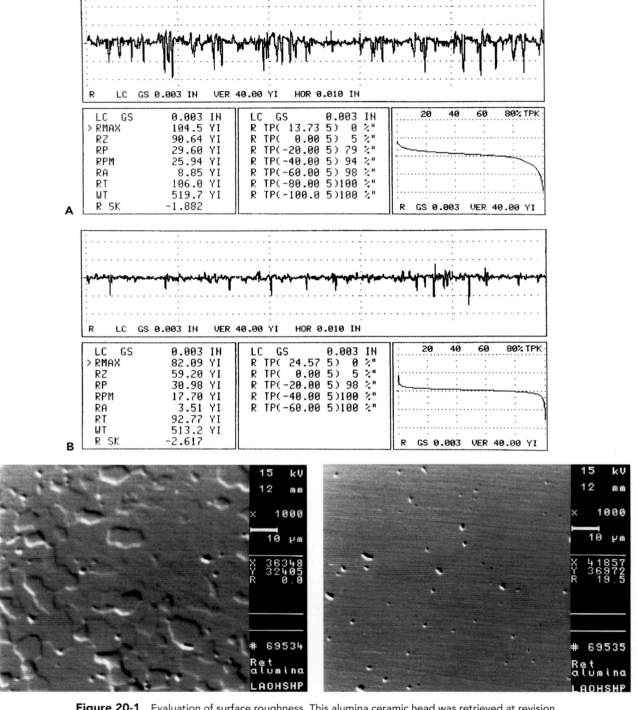

Figure 20-1 Evaluation of surface roughness. This alumina ceramic head was retrieved at revision surgery for rapid wear of PE and pelvic osteolysis after 39 months in situ. There was no grossly visible scratching, and the head appeared polished to the naked eye. **A:** Noncontact stylus (laser) profilometry of superior (weight bearing) portion of the head. **B:** Inferior (noncontact) portion of the same head. The superior portion obviously has higher surface roughness. Note the increase in deviations above, as well as below, the graphical center line resulting in increases in the measured parameters including R_a and R_{max} (which can be measured in micro-inches, as in this case, or in microns). The majority of the deviations and the largest deviations are below the center line (negative skew) suggesting loss of material with pores and "craters." **C:** Scanning electron photomicrograph (1000×) of the superior (weight bearing) portion of the head. **D:** Inferior (noncontact) portion of the same head. The inferior portion is considered to represent the original or as-manufactured surface. This visual comparison clearly illustrates differences in the two surfaces, presumably resulting from in vivo damage of the superior, weight bearing surface.

(40,43). The frictional torque of the Charnley prosthesis with a load of 890 N has been reported between 0.4 to 1.2 N m. Under similar conditions, the frictional torque of a 28-mm prosthesis, a 43-mm prosthesis, and a 51-mm prosthesis averaged 1.3, 2.7, and 3.2 N m, respectively (148). These values are 20 to 100 times smaller than the reported static torques to failure for cemented acetabular components (152). The coefficient of friction for the MOM bearing of the McKee–Farrar hip is roughly two to three times greater than that for the Charnley. The larger diameter of the McKee–Farrar (about 40 mm) amplifies this difference, and the result is a frictional torque that is up to 10 times greater than that in the Charnley (218). This value is still an order of magnitude less than the static torque-to-failure of an acutely implanted cemented acetabular component and lower than that reported for surface replacement components (152,218).

Contrary to theoretical considerations, frictional torque has not been demonstrated to be important in the initiation of aseptic loosening of either femoral or acetabular components (152,218). Accumulating evidence indicates that PE wear particles have a greater effect on the durability of implant fixation than frictional torque. From this perspective, the success of the Charnley low-friction arthroplasty is primarily a function of the low volumetric wear of the 22-mm bearing, not low frictional torque. Higher bearing surface friction and frictional torques can be tolerated if the release of wear particles to periprosthetic tissues is sufficiently low. Within the range of frictional torques generated by implants used to date, wear is a more important factor in survivorship than frictional torque. Large-diameter bearings can be successful if the wear rate is low. This is an important consideration as alternatives to PE bearings are being investigated.

The static and dynamic frictional torques of a bearing couple can be assessed with a pendulum comparator (40). In this device, the bearing couple is contained in a cell at the apex (fixed end) of pendulum. The cell is filled with lubricant such as dilute bovine serum, and a load is placed on the bearing through the cell. The free end of the pendulum is released, and the number of half-cycles is recorded until the pendulum stops. The number of swings to stopping decreases as ball diameter increases. A 41-mm McKee–Farrar demonstrated about one half the number of swings of a 32-mm MOP bearing. The 28-mm Metasul (Sulzer Medical Technology, Winterthur, Switzerland) MOM bearing has frictional torque characteristics similar to a 32-mm MOP bearing.

IN VIVO WEAR

The primary wear mechanisms are adhesion, abrasion, and fatigue. Adhesion involves bonding of the surfaces when they are pressed together under load. Sufficient relative motion results in material being pulled away from one or more surfaces, usually from the weaker material. Abrasion is a mechanical process, wherein asperities on the harder surface cut and plough through the softer surface, resulting in removal of material. When local stresses exceed the fatigue strength, that material then fails after a certain number of loading cycles, with release of material from the surface (210).

The conditions under which the prosthesis was functioning when the wear occurred have been termed the wear modes (164). Mode 1 wear results from the motion of two primary bearing surfaces one against each other, as intended. Mode 2 refers to the condition of a primary bearing surface moving against a secondary surface, which is not intended. Usually, this mode of wear occurs after excessive wear in mode 1. Mode 3 refers to the condition of the primary surfaces moving against each other, but with third-body particles interposed. In mode 3, the contaminant particles directly abrade one or both of the primary bearing surfaces. This is known as three-body abrasion or three-body wear. The primary bearing surfaces may be transiently or permanently roughened by this interaction, leading to a higher mode 1 wear rate. Mode 4 wear refers to two secondary (nonprimary) surfaces rubbing together. Examples of mode 4 wear include wear due to metal–cement or bone–cement interface motion or from relative motion of a porous coating, or other metallic surface, against bone (4,9,30,96,128,153); relative motion of the superior surface of a modular PE component against the metal support, so-called back-side wear (177,195,196); fretting between a metallic substrate and a fixation screw (80,141,198); and fretting and corrosion of modular taper connections and extra-articular sources (112,133,235). Particles produced by mode 4 wear can migrate to the primary bearing surfaces, inducing third-body wear (mode 3) (164).

Wear particles are a function of the type of wear (91,216). A smooth, highly polished femoral head wearing against PE in the absence of third bodies (as in a laboratory simulator) generates very small wear particles with comparatively little variation in size and shape. This intended or desired type of wear is the source of the numerous micron and submicron PE wear particles that have been associated with osteolysis and component loosening (164,215–217) (Fig. 20-2). The operating conditions in vivo are, however, variable, and analyses of retrieved components and periprosthetic tissues indicate that several types of wear which occur in vivo (91,164,184,216). Hard particles, such as bone or bone mineral, bone cement, metals, and ceramics, can affect the "baseline" wear by passing through the articulation, resulting in a transient three-body wear mechanism (215). The femoral head can be scratched by this interaction. Additionally or independently, hard particles may become embedded in the PE and act as an ongoing abrasive source. Increased femoral head surface roughness increases the rate of PE wear due to increased two-body abrasive wear (55,81,168,184,277). These types of wear generate particles that are larger and have more variability in size and morphology, but the relationship between the type of wear and the number of wear particles generated is not yet known.

The predominant type(s) of wear occurring from one hip to the next can be different. Further, in a specific hip there may be different types of wear occurring at different times during the service life. It seems logical that there would be more third bodies in the early postoperative period as a result of debris from the implantation procedure. There may then be a more "steady-state" level of third-body interactions, which is a function of the design and fixation of the implants. At any time, mechanical failure of some portion of the reconstruction may be a transient or continuous source of third bodies, resulting in transiently or constantly accelerated wear. A relatively "clean" joint will, therefore, be associated with a lower wear rate.

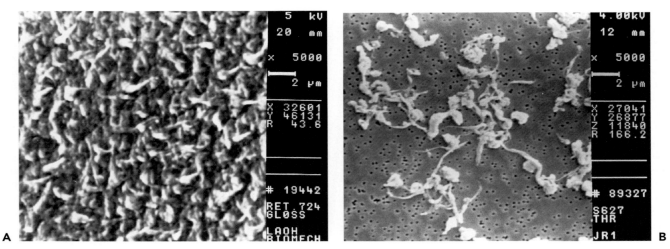

Figure 20-2   Polyethylene wear particles generated in vivo. **A:** Scanning electron photomicrograph (5000×) of the weight bearing region of a polyethylene acetabular component retrieved after in vivo use. This region appears smooth and glossy to the naked eye, having been "wear polished" in vivo with no gross evidence of surface damage. This visually bland region is the source of the numerous micron- and submicron-sized polyethylene wear particles. Note the "shag carpet" appearance with a nodular base and fibrillar strands. These submicroscopic features on the worn polyethylene surface have a high morphologic and dimensional correlation to the micron- and submicron-sized polyethylene particles retrieved from periprosthetic tissues. **B:** Scanning electron photomicrograph (5000×) of polyethylene wear particles retrieved from periprosthetic tissues.

ASSESSMENT OF IN VIVO WEAR

The clinical assessment of the performance of a bearing couple has traditionally been based on radiographic studies. In most MOP bearings, the wear of the metal ball is considered negligible. Using standard radiographs, the degree of the penetration of the femoral head into the socket is the linear wear of the bearing. Reference points are selected on the femoral and acetabular sides. The center of the femoral head is commonly employed, although the surface of the femoral head has also been used. Acetabular reference points include wire markers in PE components (42), the cement–prosthesis interface (144), and the implant–bone interface in cementless acetabular reconstructions (273). When penetration by the femoral head is studied radiographically, it is necessary to distinguish between true PE wear (removal of material) and other factors that contribute to the movement of the head, including creep (permanent plastic deformation of the PE liner) and bedding-in (settling-in of the PE liner into the metallic acetabular cup) (243). While creep depends on the material properties of the PE liner, bedding-in is a more complex phenomenon that involves not only the physical properties of the liner but also manufacturing characteristics of the modular acetabular system. Because creep and bedding-in decrease exponentially with time, it is now generally accepted that the majority of the deformation that occurs after the first 2 years or so is due to true wear (243,278).

The radiographic measurement method most commonly referenced is a variation of the duoradiographic technique described by Charnley and Halley (42) as reported by Livermore et al. (144). Using standard anteroposterior radiographs of the pelvis, an overlay template of concentric circles is used to simultaneously measure the diameter of the femoral

head on the radiograph (to assess the degree of radiographic magnification) and to identify the center of the femoral head. A compass is used to identify the shortest distance from the center of the femoral head to a point on the acetabular reference on the follow-up radiograph (Fig. 20-3). A measurement is then made between the same reference points on the initial postoperative radiograph. This method measures only wear which

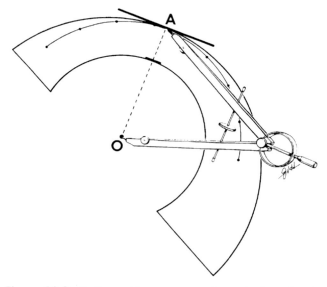

Figure 20-3   Radiographic assessment of wear in vivo using the technique of Livermore et al. (144). A compass is used to measure the shortest distance between the center point of the femoral head and the outer diameter of the acetabular component. The difference between this measurement on the most recent radiograph and the initial postoperative radiograph is a 2-D assessment of linear wear.

occurs in the plane of the radiograph and cannot detect any component of the wear vector which may occur out of the plane of the radiograph. After correcting for magnification, the difference in the measurement from the initial postoperative radiograph to the follow-up radiograph is the linear wear, which is conventionally expressed in millimeters. The linear wear rate is then calculated by dividing the linear wear by the time postimplantation. Linear wear rate is conventionally expressed as millimeters per year.

The accuracy of these methods is technique and observer dependent. Clarke et al. (46) found that repeated manual measurements of the femoral head diameter by clinicians varied by ±0.4 mm. Mathematical analysis of the duoradiographic technique revealed that the minimum error in such radiographic measurements was ±0.5 mm. The main sources of error were in deducing the position of the wear axis and the fundamental limitations of manual measurement. Griffith et al. (88) argued that when the wire marker of the acetabular component was aligned in the coronal plane, the duoradiographic technique provided consistent wear measurements to the nearest 0.5 mm, roughly half the error indicated by Clarke et al. The maximal single-observer measurement variation of the Livermore technique is reported to be 0.1 mm (144). An electronic digital caliper can measure to the nearest 0.05 mm, and the mean intraobserver error with this device is about 0.08 mm (273).

Volumetric wear is a measure of the amount of material removed from the bearing surfaces, and increased volumetric wear has been associated with component loosening and osteolysis (14,38,72,133,180,183,193,194,213,217). The association between volumetric wear and periprosthetic bone resorption appears to be related to the number of PE wear particles generated and released into the effective joint space (215). Assuming a 28-mm diameter bearing with a conservative linear wear rate of 0.05 mm/y (volumetric wear of about 30 mm^3) and wear particles equal in volume to a 10-μm-diameter sphere, then this wear volume would produce about 63 million particles. At one million steps per year, this translates to 63 wear particles per step. Such estimates are very sensitive to particle size. The number of particles produced by a given wear volume varies with the cube of the particle diameter. A single 10-μm spherical particle comprises the same volume as 8000 0.5-μm-diameter particles. If the typical wear particles are equal in volume to a 0.5-μm-diameter sphere, this results in 500 billion particles, which translates to 500,000 particles per step (164). Studies of wear particles retrieved from periprosthetic tissues and of worn PE surfaces are consistent with this latter estimate (164,229). Assuming constant wear particle size, increases in volumetric wear lead to increased numbers of PE wear particles. From a combined mechanical and biological perspective, optimization of in vivo wear requires not only a reduction of wear volume but a reduction in the generation of biologically active wear particles. A lower wear rate may not necessarily be preferred clinically if a higher number of biologically active wear particles is generated.

A calculation based on geometrical relationships has been used to estimate volumetric wear from the linear wear measurement. Assuming that the femoral head creates a roughly cylindrical wear track in the PE, the simple formula $v = \pi r^2 w$ has commonly been used to calculate volumetric wear, in which v is the volume change in the PE bearing, r is the radius of the femoral head, and w is the measured linear wear.

Again, assuming a negligible contribution due to creep in the long term, the wear of retrieved PE acetabular components has commonly been measured using variations of the "shadowgraph" technique (131,275). These techniques take a cast of the acetabular bearing surface and then uses the profile, or "shadow," of the cast to measure the wear track (Fig. 20-4). This method allows one to determine the angle of wear relative to the mouth of the component and to orient the cast along the true axis of wear. Thus the true wear vector (magnitude and direction) can be determined by this method. Although analysis of retrieved acetabular components indicates that the wear of PE components in vivo occurs frequently in one direction, multiple wear vectors have been found in 30% to 40% of retrieved implants (282,283). Impingement between the edge of the acetabular cup and the femoral component may be associated with multiple wear vectors (15,282,283).

A fluid displacement, or "volumetric," method has also been described to measure the wear of retrieved PE acetabular components (129). A femoral head of appropriate size is placed into the original articulating contour, and one measures the volume of fluid (oil) that is required to fill the remaining contour (the worn area). The interobserver variability is reportedly within ±5 mm^3, and the accuracy is reportedly within ±15 mm^3.

Kabo et al. (131) have compared linear wear measurements performed on retrieved acetabular components using a shadowgraph technique to those obtained by measurements made on standard clinical radiographs of the same hips. There was a close correlation between the two, although the radiographic measurements slightly underestimated the linear wear measured on the retrieved implants. This may, at least in part, be due to the fact that the wear vector is not consistently in the plane of the radiographs.

Computer-assisted wear measurement techniques have been developed (63,158). Based on selected points located on digitized radiographs, the computer-assisted vector wear analysis finds the circles that best fit the prosthetic femoral head and the acetabular component. When the centers of the acetabular component and the femoral head are found, the magnitude and direction of the femoral head vector displacement from the acetabular center can be calculated. Use of both anteroposterior and lateral projections allows construction of a three-dimensional (3-D) model. Comparison of serial radiographs gives both the magnitude and the direction of the femoral head displacement over time. Such computer-assisted techniques can reduce measurement variability due to difficulties related to single-reference point identification, angle of the radiographic beam, and patient positioning. A tenfold increase in the interobserver repeatability was observed when computer-assisted vector wear analysis were compared with the techniques of Livermore et al. for manual measurement of wear with the use of calipers or a digitizer (158).

Using a computer-assisted technique, average two-dimensional (2-D) linear wear rates between 0.15 and 0.24 mm/y have been reported (64,158). With the addition of anterior and posterior displacements, higher wear rates (average of 0.26 mm/y) were observed on 3-D analysis (64). However, the 2-D and 3-D wear measurements of the same hip have been

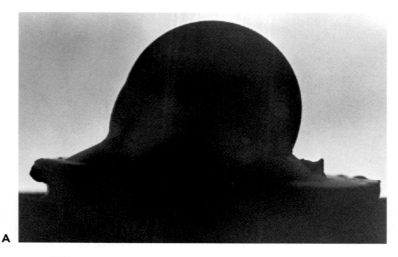

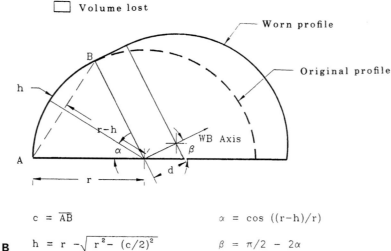

$$c = \overline{AB}$$

$$h = r - \sqrt{r^2 - (c/2)^2}$$

$$\alpha = \cos((r-h)/r)$$

$$\beta = \pi/2 - 2\alpha$$

B

Figure 20-4 Assessment of gross wear on retrieved polyethylene components. **A:** Cast of the worn, internal contour of the component. Note the double contour. The lower portion of a hemisphere (seen best on the left side) represents the original contour of the bearing, while the upper hemisphere is the path worn into the polyethylene by the femoral head. By analyzing this cast, the difference in the center points of the original contour and the wear path can be determined. **B:** Determination of the wear volume by the method of Kabo et al. (131). Volumetric wear is a portion of a cylinder dependent upon the depth and angle of wear (the wear vector).

shown to be highly correlated (115,159,247). In approximately 95% of cases, the 2-D and 3-D measurements of femoral head penetration are essentially equal; in 5% of hip replacements, there are differences between 2-D and 3-D wear assessments (159,247). These differences can be explained by the fact that, in these cases, the femoral head also moves in a direction that is perpendicular to the plane of the anteroposterior radiograph, creating a wear vector not detectable by a 2-D analysis (247). Acetabular anteversion, a factor associated with the amount of anterior translation of the femoral head, has a significant effect on the likelihood of such differences occurring (159). The repeatability of 2-D wear analysis has been shown to be four times better than that of the 3-D technique (159).

Because of the increased sensitivity of computer-assisted techniques in detecting small amounts of wear, measurements obtained with computer-assisted methods tend to be higher than wear measured with traditional methods. Using a zero wear model, Collier et al. (53) assessed the accuracy of the computer-assisted wear measurement methods described by Martell and Berdia (Hip Analysis Suite) (158) and Devane et al. (PolyWare) (63). Although no displacement of the head had occurred within the acetabular component, Hip Analysis Suite and PolyWare demonstrated mean head displacements of

0.27 mm (maximum of 0.65 mm) and 0.40 mm (maximum of 0.86 mm), respectively. The mean volumetric wear was 84 mm³ (maximum of 402 mm³) with the Hip Analysis Suite method and 126 mm³ (maximum of 498 mm³) with the PolyWare method. Hip Analysis Suite was more accurate than PolyWare for both linear and volumetric analysis ($p < 0.01$).

The wear of hard-on-hard bearing surfaces, such as MOM or COC, can be low enough to be unmeasurable on routine clinical radiographs. Further, the wear can also be too low to be measured on retrieved specimens using the shadowgraph technique (218). Consequently, computerized coordinate measuring machines have been employed to quantify the amount of wear. These devices can be used to assess the sphericity of bearing surfaces by comparing the measured dimensions in multiple planes to the best-fit circle. The deviations from sphericity measured by this technique include those due to the original manufacturing and changes in the surface due to wear. Since wear removes material, only positive deviations (elevations) of the cup profile or negative deviations (depressions) of the head profile (occurring in the load bearing area and/or with surface features consistent with systematic wear) are interpreted to be due to wear (166,218). The volume of wear can be calculated by integrating the depth of multiple individual wear points on the worn surface (166).

The stem provides an orientation reference for the location of wear on femoral heads. Such an orientation reference is not consistently present on acetabular components, although impingement wear can sometimes be used as a reference. Due to the nonspherical design of the acetabular bearing surface of several implants, this technique is less reliable for the measurement of acetabular wear.

CLINICAL STUDIES

There have been numerous studies on the in vivo wear of THRs. Table 20-2 summarizes some of this work. This collection is by no means complete. Rather, it is intended to provide some perspective and illustrate several general points. First, and most important, is that there are multiple variables that influence PE wear in vivo, and consequently PE wear rates are highly variable. If one looks not only at the average linear wear rates but also at the range of wear rates, all studies demonstrate substantial variability. In every study, regardless of the length of follow-up, there are a number of hips which have no radiographically measurable wear, and there are a few hips that demonstrate wear which is several times the average for that study. These large patient-to-patient variations in wear rate cannot be explained by differences in the wear resistance of the PE (264). This is not surprising considering the number of variables that contribute to wear in vivo, including those related to the patient, variables related to the hip reconstruction, and variables related to the technique of wear assessment.

Patient-related variables include age, gender, weight, general health, and the activity of the patient as it relates to the use of the hip prosthesis (214,221). Variables related to the hip reconstruction include the implanted materials (including but not limited to the PE-bearing material), design and manufacturing, and variables related to the surgical implantation procedure, including operative techniques, biomechanical considerations, and the initial as well as the long-term fixation of the implants. These variables are important from a wear perspective, as they can affect the loads and motions of the bearing, the lubrication, and the degree of three-body wear mechanisms. There is also variability due to differences in the method of wear assessment and the limitations of the measurement techniques, as discussed above. For these reasons, there are limitations on the strengths of comparisons made between different studies.

Clinical wear rates have traditionally been expressed using a denominator of time. This has been done as a matter of convenience, not accuracy. More appropriately, in vitro laboratory wear simulator studies have always used as a denominator the number of cycles. Similar to a set of automobile tires, the wear of a prosthetic hip is a function of use or the number of cycles and not a function of time in situ. The assumption made in clinical studies is that the activity of joint replacement patients, the actual use or number of cycles on the bearing, is about the same from patient to patient, or that any differences will "average out" over a large sample size. The limitations of this assumption must be recognized.

The walking activity of 111 total joint replacement patients has been studied using an electronic digital pedometer (221). These joint replacement patients were averaging about 0.9 million cycles for each lower extremity joint per year. This number is close to the average of 1.0 million cycles per year proposed by Seedhom et al. (225) based on their study of nine healthy (no prostheses) elderly people on vacation. The most important result, however, was not the average but the fact that there was a 45-fold difference in the range of gait cycles between the least active and the most active patient. The most active patient averaged 3.2 million cycles per year, about 3.6 times higher than average. These data indicate that individual differences in patient activity are a substantial source of variability. A 45-fold range in wear rates and high-end wear rates of more than 3.5 times the average wear rate can be accounted for by differences in patient activity. Age correlated with daily walking activity ($p = 0.048$) but with a high degree of variability (S.D. = 3040 steps per day). Patients less than 60 years old walked about 30% more on average than those 60 years of age or older ($p = 0.023$). Male patients walked about 30% more on average than the female patients ($p = 0.037$). Thus, variation in patient activity contributes to the variability in wear rates consistently seen in in vivo studies.

It is recognized that wear is function of use, not time (219). PE wear (linear penetration) in 37 hip replacements was assessed from digital images using a validated 2-D computer-assisted vector wear analysis. Patient activity was assessed with a pedometer, a step activity monitor, and a simple visual analog scale. This study demonstrated that wear was highly correlated to joint use.

Clinical wear studies to date have made retrospective comparisons of wear performance based on a specific variable, such as the type of PE, the size and material of the femoral head, the effect of metal backing, or the type of acetabular and/or femoral fixation. Because of the tremendous number of potentially confounding variables in such clinical studies, this fundamental limitation must be kept in mind. Further, great care should be taken in extrapolating the results to other reconstructions with that same generic variable. An example is the issue of metal backing. Cates et al. (38) have reported an increase in PE wear rate with one specific type of metal-backed cemented acetabular component compared to a cemented all-PE component. On the contrary, a different type of metal-backed acetabular component has been associated with lower PE wear rates in other cohorts (31,112). The issue cannot be as simple as the presence or absence of metal backing. Specific details of component design, materials, and manufacturing, as well as differences in patient populations, all must be carefully considered when evaluating PE wear rates in vivo.

The Charnley Low-Friction Arthroplasty

There have been more studies reported on the wear of the Charnley hip than any other type (31,41–43,73,88,112, 131,144,264,274–280). When considered in aggregate, these studies illustrate some features which may be general principles of wear for metal on ultrahigh molecular weight polyethylene (UHMWP) bearings in hip arthroplasty. There is variability not only in the range of wear rates for each study but also in the average wear rate for the numerous studies. The linear penetration rate is higher in the short term, then decreases to a lower level "steady state" which generally decreases slightly over time in situ (278). The increased penetration rate in the first year or two is thought to be due to creep and bedding-in. The bearing then settles into steady-state wear at a lower penetration rate which is a

TABLE 20-2
STUDIES OF WEAR RATES IN VIVO

Study	Acetabular Bearing	Femoral Head	Diameter (mm)	No. of Hips	Avg. Linear Wear Rate[a]	Range Linear Wear Rates[a]	Avg. Vol. Wear Rate[b] (Range)	Comments
Charnley et al. 1969 (43)	PTFE	SS	22	39	2.26		859	
Charnley and Cupic 1973 (41)	PE	SS	22	72	0.12		46	
Charnley and Halley 1975 (42)	PE	SS	22	72	0.15	0–0.6	57	
Griffith et al. 1978 (88)	PE	SS	22	493	0.07	0–0.24	27	
Wroblewski 1985 (275)	PE	SS	22	21	0.21	0–0.41	80	Radiographic
				21	0.19	0–0.52	72	Direct
Wroblewski 1986 (276)	PE	SS	22	103	0.10	0–0.43	36	15–21 year follow-up
Wroblewski et al. 1992 (277)	PE	SS	22	57	0.07	0.01–0.2	27	19–25 year follow-up
Wroblewski et al. 1996 (278)	XLP[c]	Alumina	22	19	0.06	0.024–0.32	22	Avg. 77 mo. follow-up
				14	0.23		87	First 18 months
				14	0.04		13	Avg. 91 mo. follow-up
				9	0.03		13	>8 yrs. follow-up
Livermore et al. 1990 (144)	PE	SS	22	227	0.13	0–0.39	49	
		SS	28	98	0.08	0–0.30	49	
		CoCr	32	60	0.10	0–0.32	80	
Isaac et al. 1992 (121)	PE	SS	22	87	0.21	<0.005–0.6	80	Direct
Schmalzried et al. 1992 (217)	PE			12	0.12	0.04–0.30	36	Autospy
Kabo et al. 1993 (131)	PE	SS	22	5	0.13		48	Direct
		CoCr	26	3	0.23		122	
			28	23	0.23		144	
		CoCr	32	9	0.21		172	
			36–54	20	0.38		314	
Cates et al. 1993 (38)	PE	Ti alloy	28	99	0.08	0–0.37	49	All-poly
		Ti alloy	28	134	0.11	0–0.31	68	MB
Hernandez et al. 1994 (106)	PE	Ti alloy	28	97	0.14	0–0.92	86	Hybrid hips
		Ti alloy	28	134	0.22	0–1.41	135	Cementless hips
Bankston et al. 1995 (12)	PE	SS	28	77	0.06		37	Patient matching
		CoCr	28	77	0.05		31	"
		Ti alloy	28	77	0.08		49	"
Callaghan et al. 1995 (31)	PE	SS	22	23	0.12		46	5 yr. machined
		SS	22	61	0.11		42	5 yr. molded
		CoCr	28	20	0.14		86	5 yr. molded
		CoCr	28	43	0.11		68	5 yr. molded MB
		CoCr	28	63	0.07		43	5 yr. machined hybrid
		CoCr	28	43	0.11		68	7–8 yr. molded MB
		SS	22	23	0.12		46	10 yr. machined
		SS	22	61	0.08		30	10 yr. molded
		CoCr	28	20	0.12		74	10 yr. molded
		SS	22	23	0.11		42	15 yr. machined
		SS	22	61	0.09		34	15 yr. molded
		SS	22	23	0.10		38	20–22 yr. machined
Nashed et al. 1995 (183)	PE	Ti Alloy		24	0.10			Cemented poly cup
		Ti Alloy		62	0.13			Cemented MB cup
		Ti Alloy		15	0.25			Cementless
		CoCr		74	0.17			Cementless
Bankston et al. 1995 (13)	PE	CoCr	28	54	0.05		31	Compression molded
		CoCr	28	54	0.11		68	Machined bar stock
Devane et al. 1995 (64)	PE	CoCr	26, 32	141	0.15			2-D computer
					0.26		79	3-D computer
Woolson and Murphy 1995 (273)	PE	CoCr	28	80	0.14	0–0.35	86	Cementless cups
Hop et al. 1997 (112)	PE	SS, CoCr	22, 28	181	0.086		52	Cable reattachment
		SS, CoCr	22, 28	189	0.074		46	Wire reattachment
Jasty et al. 1997 (129)	PE			22			35 (8–116)	Autopsy
				84			62 (8–256)	Cemented
				22			94 (12–284)	Cemented, MB
Eggli et al. 2002 (78)	PE	CoCr	22	49	0.11	SE (0.017)	41.5 (SE, 4.1)	
			32	40	0.15	SE (0.014)	120.3 (SE, 10.8)	

(continued)

TABLE 20-2
(continued)

Study	Acetabular Bearing	Femoral Head	Diameter (mm)	No. of Hips	Avg. Linear Wear Rate[a]	Range Linear Wear Rates[a]	Avg. Vol. Wear Rate[b] (Range)	Comments
Livingston et al. 1997 (145)	PE	CoCr	28	50	0.12			Avg. age 67.2 yrs.
	Hylamer	CoCr	28	26	0.13			Avg. age 66.5 yrs.
	Hylamer	CoCr	28	138	0.29			Avg. age 62.8 yrs.
	Hylamer	CoCr	28	20	0.29			Avg. age 47.7 yrs.
	Hylamer	Alumina	28	7	0.33			Avg. age 42.6 yrs.
Sychterz et al., 1998 (246)	PE		28, 32	84	0.22			Avg. age 54.2 yrs.
	Hylamer		28, 32	138	0.15			Avg. age 64.3 yrs.
Wroblewski et al. 2003 (279)	Hylamer	Zirconia	22.225	97	0.22	0.06–0.55		Radiographic
Ohashi et al. 1989 (187)	PE	CoCr	32	13	0.04		35	
		SS	28	106	0.04		26	
		Alumina	28	187	0.03		15	
Okumura et al. 1989 (188)	PE	SS	22		0.14		53	
		Alumina	28		0.08		49	
Sychterz et al. 1996 (245)	PE	CoCr, AlO2	32	26	0.07	0.02–0.18	245 (13–779)	Autopsy
Devane et al. 1997 (166)	PE	Ti Alloy	28	69	0.15			2-D cemented
					0.23		99	3-D cemented
	PE	Ti Alloy	28	70	0.25			2-D cementless
					0.36		155	3-D cementless
Shaver et al. 1997 (230)	PE	CoCr	28	43	0.15		47	2-D short-term
					0.09		27	2-D steady state
Sychterz et al. 1997 (242)	PE	CoCr	32	96	0.17	0.02–0.45	137 (16–362)	2-D computer
		Alumina	32	9	0.16			
Hernigou and Bahrami 2003 (107)	PE	Zirconia	28	40	0.41	0.25–0.57	171	12 years
	PE	Alumina	32	56	0.07	0.04–0.10	46	12 years
	PE	SS	28	20	0.13	0.07–0.19	53	12 years
	PE	SS	32	20	0.19	0.11–0.27	98	12 years
Heisel et al. 2004 (103)	XLP	CoCr-Ceramic	28	27			16	
		CoCr-Ceramic	32	7			22	
	PE	CoCr-Ceramic	28	2			70	
			32	22			89	
Schmalzried et al. 1996 (220)	CoCr	CoCr	28–41	5	4.20			McKee–Farrar (M-F)
McKellop et al. 1996 (166)	CoCr	CoCr		11	3.30		1.2 (0.12–2.6)	M-F fem. only
				2	5.20		2.3 (1.6, 3.0)	Ring fem. only
				6	5.90		3 (0.90–5.5)	Müller fem. only
Kothari et al. 1996 (136)	CoCr	CoCr	35, 41	22			0.5–8.5	M-F head and cup
Schmidt et al. 1996 (222)	CoCr	CoCr		17	6.60	0.1–28.0		M-F heads
				13	4.90	0.2–30.0		M-F cups
				10	2.00	0.7–6.2		Müller heads
				14	2.00	0.0–3.9		Müller cups
Willert et al. 1996 (267)	CoCr	CoCr		3	4.40	0.4–12.2	8.6 (0.66–22.36)	MF heads
				3	5.20	3.5–11.1		MF cups
				3	3.80	1.3–6.2	2.6 (0.22–5.98)	Müller heads
				3	4.40	1.5–7.9		Müller cups
Mittlemeier 1984 (178)	Alumina	Alumina			2.60			Cups
					5.50			Heads
Boutin et al. 1988 (27)	Alumina	Alumina			0.025			Theoretical potential
Walter 1992 (261)	Alumina	Alumina				0.025–5.0		

[a]mm/y for metal–plastic and microns per year for metal–metal and ceramic–ceramic.
[b]For radiographic studies, volumetric wear calculated from linear wear: $v = \pi r^2 w$.
[c]Cross-linked polyethylene.

result of a combination of factors. The wear rate is higher in patients less than 40 years of age at the time of surgery (0.20 mm/y), presumably due to the higher activity of these patients (234,274). The wear rate is low (0.02 mm/y) in cases where the surface of the femoral head is undamaged (277), and the wear rate is high (0.21 mm/) in hips with loose sockets (275).

Longitudinal studies of the Charnley hip with a ceramic head and cross-linked PE indicate an initial penetration rate of between 0.2 to 0.3 mm/y over a year to 18 months, which then slows to 0.022 mm/y (278). These features suggest caution when directly comparing results of studies with different lengths of follow-up. All other factors being equal, a shorter-term study will demonstrate a higher wear rate than a longer-term study. Further, in long-term studies, decreasing patient activity may also contribute to a decreasing wear rate over time.

Head Size

Volumetric wear rates can be calculated using the simple cylindrical formula $v = \pi r^2 w$, where, for any given amount of linear wear, the volumetric wear increases exponentially with increasing radius of the bearing. For a linear wear rate of 0.10 mm/y, the volumetric wear rate of a 22-mm head would be about 38 mm³/y, while the volumetric wear rate for a 32-mm head would be roughly doubled at 80-mm³/y. This has implications for the range of volumetric wear rates. A 22-mm bearing with a low linear wear rate of 0.05 mm/y would have a volumetric wear of about 19 mm³/y, while a high linear wear rate of 0.2 mm/y would have a volumetric wear of about 76 mm³/y. A 32-mm bearing with a low linear wear rate of 0.05 mm/y would have a volumetric wear of about 40 mm³/y, while a high linear wear rate of 0.2 mm/y would have a volumetric wear of about 161 mm³/y. For a given head size, volumetric wear increases linearly with depth of penetration, while the slope of the rate of increase increases with increasing head size (Fig 20-5). The range of volumetric wear rates (due to increases at the high end) will be therefore be substantially broader with larger head sizes.

In clinical studies, the linear wear rates associated with 32-mm heads have been equivalent to or greater than those with smaller head diameters (131,144). Even with equivalent linear wear rates, large-diameter heads yield significantly higher volumetric wear rates, which have been associated with bone resorption and component loosening (180,213,217).

Strictly from a wear perspective, 32-mm heads do not compare favorably to smaller-diameter heads.

As a further example of the effect of head size, because of their large diameters, surface replacements with PE components have volumetric wear rates that are 4 to 10 times higher than those of conventional total hips (131). It had been hoped that reduced PE stresses due to the larger contact area would result in reduced linear wear. This has not been the case. The linear wear rates of surface replacement components appear to be higher than those of smaller bearing couples. This may be due to a combination of factors including reduced PE thickness, higher patient activity levels, and/or increased femoral surface roughness (131). Within the range of contact areas for MOP prosthetic hip bearings (22 to 54 mm), it appears that the contact stresses and subsurface stresses of these highly conforming bearings are all sufficiently low such that any differences do not appreciably affect wear in vivo. It appears that the increased contact area and sliding distance of larger heads result in increased volumetric wear.

Based on their radiographic data, Livermore et al. (144) concluded that a prosthetic head of intermediate size, such as 28 mm, provided the best wear characteristics. In their study, the 28-mm bearings had a linear wear rate of 0.08 mm/y, which was significantly lower than that of the 22-mm (0.13 mm/y) and 32-mm (0.10 mm/y) bearings. The volumetric wear rates of the 28-mm and 22-mm components were the same. It is important to recognize that the conclusions of Livermore et al. were based on average linear wear values that were in the low end of the range of those reported for 28-mm bearings and in the middle to high end of the range of those reported for 22-mm bearings. This study compared different

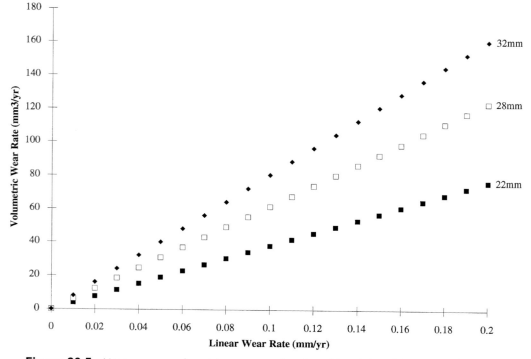

Figure 20-5 Linear versus volumetric wear as a function of head size. Given equivalent linear wear, volumetric wear increases as a function of head size. Using the simple formula for volumetric wear ($v = \pi r^2 w$), a linear wear rate of 0.1 mm/y with a 22-mm head produces a wear volume of 38 mm³/y, while the wear volume with a 32-mm head is roughly double at 80 mm³/y.

prosthetic designs from different manufacturers implanted by several surgeons, and unrecognized differences in these variables may have influenced their results.

The aggregate experience indicates that the linear wear rates of 28-mm and 22-mm bearings is generally not different by 0.05 mm/y, as was seen by Livermore et al. The aggregate experience indicates that the in vivo linear wear rates of 28-mm and 22-mm bearings are about the same (Table 20-2). Using similar measurement techniques, Callaghan et al. (31) studied the wear in five cohorts of total hips implanted by the same surgeon. The linear wear rate for the 22-mm components was comparable to that of 28-mm components. Again, there were differences in design and manufacturing that may have influenced the results. With roughly equivalent linear wear rates, the volumetric wear rate was significantly less for 22-mm components. In a further study by the same authors, in which the same acetabular and femoral components were used in 151 consecutive primary total hip arthroplasties, the wear rates obtained with 22-mm heads (105 hips) and 28-mm heads (46 hips) were compared. The long-term rate of penetration into the shell was 0.11 mm/y for the 22-mm heads and 0.17 mm/y for the 28-mm heads. However, the dislocation rate was significantly higher with the 22-mm heads (197).

The in vivo PE wear rate of cobalt–chrome femoral heads of 22 mm and 32 mm was compared in a prospective, randomized study by Eggli et al. (78), using a computer-assisted method. Although the mean linear wear rates were not significantly different (0.11 mm/y for the 22-mm heads vs. 0.15 mm/y for the 32-mm heads), the mean volumetric wear rates were significantly higher with the 32-mm heads (41.5 mm^3/y for the 22-mm heads vs. 120.3 mm^3/y for the 32-mm heads, $p<0.05$).

In clinical practice, when selecting the size of the bearing, one should consider the decreased risk of dislocation associated with larger head sizes. Strictly from a wear perspective, however, 22-mm-diameter MOP bearings are preferred.

Molded Versus Machined

Bankston et al. (13) reported a comparison of two groups of patients, one with compression-molded acetabular components and other components machined from stock bars. After patient matching, 54 patients were included in each group. Hips with a compression-molded PE acetabular component had an average linear wear rate of 0.05 mm/y, while hips with a PE component machined from bar stock had an average wear rate of 0.11 mm/y. While it is reasonable to question the effects of PE component manufacturing variables, the results of this study indicating a favorable effect of compression molding should be carefully interpreted in view of a number of other variables. This study compared two groups of patients implanted by two different surgeons at two different institutions with two different femoral components. Further, the base resins for the acetabular PE components were from two different manufacturers, and the components were made and sterilized by two different manufacturers. No difference in the wear rate of machined versus molded PE was seen in another study where the PE components were from the same manufacturer (31).

In a subsequent study, Ritter (203) reported the results of 549 cemented THRs in which a compression-molded acetabular component was used. In all cases, a cemented direct

compression–molded all-PE acetabular component, made from Hi-Fax 1900 resin, was utilized. The reported PE linear wear was between 0.05 and 0.06 mm/y.

Sterilization Methods

Over the last decade, clinical and laboratory research have revealed that sterilization methods can dramatically affect the in vivo performance of a PE component. Polyethylene components for total joint arthroplasty can be sterilized using gamma irradiation, gas plasma, or ethylene oxide. Gamma irradiation in an air environment was the industry standard since the early 1970s, using doses between 2.5 and 4 Mrad (1 megarad = 10^6 radiation absorbed dose = 10^4 gray), most commonly between 3.0 and 3.5 Mrad.

In addition to sterilization, gamma radiation breaks covalent bonds in the PE molecule. This produces free radicals, unpaired electrons from the broken covalent bonds, that can combine with oxygen (if present) during the irradiation process, during shelf-storage, and in vivo. Oxidation of the PE molecule is a chemical reaction that results in chain scission (fragmentation and shortening of the large polymer chains) and introduction of oxygen moieties into the polymer molecules (143). Such oxidation lowers the molecular weight of the polymer (which reduces its toughness), increases the density, and results in a reduction in fracture strength and elongation to break (51,169,204,240).

Peak levels of oxidation typically occur about 0.5 to 2 mm below the surface of a PE component, forming the so-called white bands seen on microtome sections of components sterilized by gamma radiation (240). As the degree of oxidation increases, so does the occurrence of fatigue cracking and delamination, as is observed in retrieved tibial components (19,50–52,268). Oxygen can diffuse into the components during shelf-storage and in vivo. Components with less than 1 year from the time of sterilization to the time of implantation exhibit lower in vivo oxidation and better in vivo performance than components with longer so-called shelf-life before implantation (58). In laboratory wear tests, PE that had been gamma irradiated in air and aged exhibited a higher wear rate than nonirradiated material (82). However, PE components that have been irradiated in air and tested within months exhibit lower wear rates than identical components that have not been irradiated, due to a favorable amount of cross-linking compared to the amount of oxidation.

Gamma irradiation in air has been abandoned as a sterilization method. Currently, two methods of sterilization are in use: nonradiation methods (gas plasma and ethylene oxide) and gamma irradiation using inert environments (without air). Nonradiation methods avoid the potential for high levels of oxidation, but no free radicals are created and there is no opportunity to produce cross-linking. Gamma irradiation in an oxygen-free environment still provides the benefits of cross-linking to the PE but prevents oxidation and its deleterious effects.

Ethylene oxide (EtO) is a known sterilizing agent that acts by altering the DNA structure in bacteria, spores, and viruses. Sterilization is accomplished by diffusion of EtO into the near-surface regions (139). The standard EtO sterilization process begins with a preconditioning period (at 46°C and 65% relative humidity) for 18 hours, followed by a 5-hour exposure to 100% EtO gas at 46°C and 0.04 MPa. An 18-hour forced air aeration period, at the same temperature, is required to allow diffusion of EtO out of UHMWPE (202).

Gas plasma is a surface sterilization method in which plasma, an ionized body of gas (i.e., peracetic acid, hydrogen peroxide), sterilizes surfaces by oxidizing biological organisms (29,52). Gas plasma sterilization is accomplished under dry, low-pressure, low-temperature conditions (52). The sterilization cycle with gas plasma takes between 1.2 and 4 hours, at temperatures lower than 50°C (139).

Hopper et al. (113) retrospectively analyzed the wear rates in a series of hips treated with conventional PE that had been sterilized with either gamma-in-air radiation (61 hips) or gas plasma (63 hips). The irradiated liners were stored with access to ambient oxygen for an average of 1 year prior to implantation. The PE liners that had been sterilized with gamma radiation in air had a significantly lower wear rate than those sterilized in gas–plasma (0.097 mm/y vs. 0.19 mm/y, $p < 0.001$), demonstrating the importance of cross-linking.

Components that have been sterilized by nonionizing methods such as EtO or gas plasma have no free radicals, thus there is no potential for oxidation either on the shelf or in the body. Ionizing radiation creates free radicals. If the components are radiated in an oxygen-free environment (such as in nitrogen) and stored in an oxygen-free environment (such as in a vacuum, barrier package), there is virtually no oxidation. However, the material contains free radicals that can react with oxygen, when present. If the barrier package is violated, ambient air will serve as a source of oxygen, and the free radicals will react over time. Once implanted, the component is exposed to dissolved oxygen in body fluids. Free radicals in the PE will react with the available oxygen over time. There is little data currently available on the relative rate of oxidation of PE in vivo. It appears that the rate of oxidation in vivo is lower than that in vitro, but there is debate as to how much lower. There is likely a multitude of factors that influence this process, including the resin type, the method of manufacturing, the number of available free radicals in the polymer, the degree of oxidation of the component at the time of implantation, and patient-related factors such as the characteristics of synovial fluid and the loads and motion patterns of the joint.

Cross-Linked Polyethylene

Cross-linking occurs when free radicals, located on the amorphous regions of PE molecules, react to form a covalent bond between adjacent PE molecules. Cross-linking can be accomplished using peroxide chemistry, variable-dose ionizing radiation, or electron beam irradiation. In other industries, cross-linking has long been recognized as a mechanism that improves the wear resistance of PE (87,171,172,191).

It is believed that cross-linking of the PE molecules resists intermolecular mobility, making it more resistant to deformation and wear in the plane perpendicular to the primary molecular axis. This has been demonstrated to dramatically reduce wear from crossing-path motion, as occurs in an acetabular cup (11,171). Wear simulator studies indicate that with optimal cross-linking the type of wear that occurs in acetabular cups can be reduced by greater than 95% (127,262). This effect has been seen even with larger (32-mm) head sizes (105).

Cross-linking has a detrimental effect on some fundamental material properties including yield strength, ultimate tensile strength, and elongation to break (171). The decrease in these properties is proportional to the degree of cross-linking. In general, oxidation and cross-linking are competing reactions. As cross-linking increases, oxidation decreases—and vice versa (161,172,232). For components that have been gamma irradiated in air, the relative amount of oxidation and cross-linking varies with depth from the surface of the component. This results in a corresponding variation in the wear resistance of the material as a function of depth from the surface (161,172,232).

Methods have been developed to produce components that have increased wear resistance due to cross-linking and do not oxidize on the shelf or in the body. Free radicals created in PE by ionizing radiation can be driven to a cross-linking reaction by heating the polymer to above the melting temperature (125°C to 135°C) (171). Components made from such "remelted" material have no residual free radicals, and thus there is no potential for subsequent oxidation when the component has been sterilized by EtO or gas plasma.

The manufacturing processes of the currently available products Marathon™ (DePuy), Longevity® (Zimmer), Durasul™ (Centerpulse), Crossfire™ (Stryker-Howmedica-Osteonics) and XLPE™ (Smith&Nephew) differ in dose and type of irradiation (gamma radiation or electron beam), thermal stabilization (remelting or annealing), machining, and final sterilization (163). For this reason, each material should be considered separately and the specific wear characteristics of each established through clinical studies.

Reoperation for any reason is the primary definition of failure of a THR. Unfortunately, this often requires a long follow-up period in order to demonstrate statistical and practical differences between implant systems. Shorter-term in vivo wear studies may help to predict long-term outcomes. Increased volumetric wear has been associated with component loosening and osteolysis (38,180,183,213,217). The association between volumetric wear and periprosthetic bone resorption appears to be related to the number and size of PE wear particles generated and released into the effective joint space (215). On this basis, a lower wear rate may not necessarily be clinically preferred if a higher number of biologically active wear particles are generated.

There are data available from clinical trials with small patient groups that show a reduction in wear rate associated with cross-linking (90,189,206,278). Martell et al. (160) evaluated 74 patients with a minimum follow-up of 2 years. Thirty-five patients received PE acetabular liners that had been gamma irradiated in air (historical standard), and 39 received a liner that was cross-linked with 3 Mrad of gamma irradiation in nitrogen and then heat annealed. Radiographs were analyzed with a computer-assisted technique (158). Hips with the historical standard PE had a mean volumetric wear rate of 94 (+78) mm^3/y compared to a mean of 54 (+70) mm^3/y in hips with the cross-linked PE ($p < 0.05$). The degree of clinical wear reduction associated with the intentionally cross-linked material was very similar to the degree of wear reduction seen in a hip wear simulator study comparing these same acetabular components (160). In another clinical study Martell and Incavo (161) compared 24 liners of highly cross-linked PE (Crossfire™; gamma irradiated to 7.5 Mrad, heat annealed at 120°C, sterilized with gamma irradiation at 2.5 to 3.5 Mrad while packaged in nitrogen) with 25 standard PE liners that were sterilized in the same manner. After 2 years follow-up the cross-linked PE showed a significant reduction in the linear wear of 53% (0.094 and 0.202 mm/y; $p = 0.008$).

Digas et al. (67) have prospectively compared a cemented, highly cross-linked PE acetabular component (Durasul™; electron beam radiation to 9.5 Mrad at 125°C, remelted at 150°C for 2 hours, sterilized with EtO) with a cemented PE component that had been sterilized with gamma irradiation in nitrogen. The in vivo wear, at a minimum follow-up of 2 years, was measured using radiostereometric analysis. The highly cross-linked acetabular cups showed 50% reduction in wear compared to the control group (0.06 and 0.13 mm, respectively).

Heisel et al. (103) measured linear and volumetric wear rates in 24 hips that received a conventional PE insert and 34 that received a cross-linked PE insert. In all these patients, activity was assessed by a computerized 2-D accelerometer. Patients with a conventional PE insert showed a mean linear wear rate of 0.13 mm/y and a mean volumetric wear rate of 87.6 mm³/y, while patients with a cross-linked PE insert showed a mean linear wear rate of 0.02 mm/y and a mean volumetric wear rate of 17.0 mm³/y. Wear in the group with cross-linked PE was 81% lower than that in the group with conventional PE ($p<0.00001$). Accounting for differences in patient activity, the adjusted wear rates per million cycles for a patient weight of 70 kg were 53 mm³/million cycles for conventional PE and 15 mm³/million cycles for cross-linked PE, a 72% reduction ($p = 0.0002$).

The increased wear resistance of cross-linked PE is fueling an increase in the use of larger-diameter heads. This trend is driving debates on the minimum thickness needed for a cross-linked PE component and the degree of increase in volumetric wear with larger head diameters.

Pulmonary Embolism Wear Particles

The number, shape, and size of PE wear particles is multifactorial: it is a function of the modes and mechanisms of wear that produce them, the stresses on the bearing surface, the motions, and the PE molecular orientation. Most of the PE wear particles produced in a prosthetic joint are micron to submicron in size and are produced in mode 1, in very large quantities, by well-functioning joints (164). The predominant wear mechanisms appear to involve microadhesion and microabrasion with the generation of many PE particles of less than 1 μm in length. The resultant wear damage is predominately burnishing and scratching (164).

Techniques have been developed to isolate and analyze wear particles generated in vivo by retrieving them from periprosthetic tissues (33,111,155,157,164,215,229). The concentration of debris particles from prosthetic joints is directly correlated to the duration of implantation (110) and can extend into the billions per gram of tissue (111,155,157,252). These data exist only for conventional PE so far because of the limited number of retrieved samples with cross-linked PE (211,212,216).

Significant differences in wear particles from cross-linked and non-cross-linked PE have been found in vitro. Cross-linked PE releases a relatively high number of submicron- and nanometer-sized PE particles and relatively fewer particles sev-

eral microns in dimension (79,118,119,201). These submicron particles induce a greater inflammatory response in vitro than do larger particles (79,118–120). Additionally, the cellular response is dependent on the shape of the particles; elongated particles generated a more severe inflammatory reaction than globular particles (284).

Illgen et al. (118) tried to correlate the volumetric wear to the biologic activity in vitro. They compared the wear of a cross-linked PE (Longevity®, e-beam irradiation to 9 Mrad, gas plasma sterilization) to a conventional PE (gamma-irradiated in nitrogen) measured in a hip simulator and afterward tested the biologic activity of the isolated particles in cell cultures. They found a reduced relative biologic activity for the cross-linked PE. As number, size, and shape of particles released by cross-linked PE liners depend on the material used (120), the mode of cross-linking (201), and patient-related wear factors (219), only clinical studies for each specific cross-linked PE can answer the question as to whether cross-linked PE offers a favorable benefit to risk ratio.

Head Material

Based on differences in material properties, there has been a natural tendency to compare the wear performance of various hip reconstructions based on the material composition of the femoral head. There have been concerns that the comparatively low hardness and poor abrasion resistance of titanium alloy could lead to increased wear rates in vivo. Similar to comparisons made based on other variables, the literature demonstrates wide variability in the average wear rates for PE against titanium alloy in vivo, ranging from 0.08 to 0.25 mm/y (Table 20-2).

Using matched groups with 77 patients per group, Bankston et al. (12) reported linear wear rates for 28-mm stainless steel, cobalt–chromium alloy, and titanium alloy femoral heads of 0.06, 0.05, and 0.08 mm/y, respectively. The authors' method of analysis did not indicate a difference at the 95% confidence interval, which led them to conclude that there was no difference in the wear rates. However, in clinical studies one should distinguish between a statistical difference and a practical difference (76). With longer follow-up, the 60% increase in PE wear rate of hips with titanium alloy heads compared to hips with cobalt–chromium alloy heads may lead to higher rates of osteolysis and component loosening.

Conversely, compared to cobalt–chromium alloys, ceramic materials have relatively high hardness and abrasion resistance. These materials can be highly polished and have better wettability and a lower coefficient of friction against PE. For these reasons, the wear rates of PE could theoretically be reduced with ceramic femoral heads. As is true of all other components in THRs, one should be aware of the tendency to compare and discuss ceramic heads in a generic fashion. Simply because one head is made of a ceramic material does not necessarily mean it will perform better than a cobalt–chromium product or similarly to another head made of ceramic material. Ultimately, total hip components are a product of a specific material, design, and manufacturing process. Our own retrieval analyses have demonstrated approximately threefold variability in the surface roughness of ceramic heads.

Ceramic materials used in the manufacturing of femoral heads are either aluminum oxide or zirconium oxide.

Furthermore, zirconia (ZrO_2) is available in two forms: (a) partially stabilized with yttria and (b) magnesia stabilized. Zirconia has a higher hardness and burst strength than alumina (Al_2O_3), but it is not thermostable. It can undergo phase transformation, probably due to its reduced heat conductivity (147,163). A practical effect of this material property is that zirconia femoral heads should not be sterilized in an autoclave. Usually yttrium oxide (Y_2O_3) is added to improve the material properties of zirconia. A new approach is the so-called zirconia-toughened aluminas (1–3). By mixing both materials, the composite achieves the high strength of zirconia and the thermal stability of alumina, although further studies have to evaluate the possible benefits of these composites.

Early clinical data on hip replacements using ceramic femoral heads articulating with PE came from either European or Japanese studies (49,187,188,223,277,288). The average wear rate of the hips with the ceramic head was always lower than those with the metal alloy head. However, the effect of potentially confounding variables, including age, weight, and type of components, was not addressed in these initial studies.

Subsequently, the performance of PE liners articulating with ceramic heads was compared to that of PE liners articulating with cobalt–chrome heads in two groups of patients that were matched on age, gender, weight, acetabular and femoral components, size of the head, manufacturer of the head, and surgical technique (244). The rate of wear of the ceramic-on-polyethylene (COP) group was slightly greater (0.09 mm/y) than that of the cobalt–chrome group (0.07 mm/y) ($p = 0.03$). The authors attributed these results to uncontrolled factors, such as third-body wear and levels of activity.

McKellop et al. (170) demonstrated in a hip simulator study that lower surface roughness reduces PE wear. Ceramic materials are much harder and can be polished to a lower surface roughness (made smoother) than metal heads. Alumina (Al_2O_3) or zirconia (ZrO_2) heads both have a high hardness and strength, which make them more difficult to scratch, and this can reduce abrasive wear (57,74,236).

Hernigou and Bahrami (107) studied the PE wear rates in 136 THRs where 28-mm zirconia heads ($n = 40$), 32-mm alumina heads ($n = 56$), 28 mm stainless steel heads ($n = 20$), or 32-mm stainless steel heads ($n = 20$) were utilized. The femoral implants and the type of PE were identical in all groups. At 5 years, the linear penetration rates were 0.043 mm/y for zirconia heads, 0.040 mm/y for alumina heads, 0.036 mm/y for 28-mm stainless steel heads, and 0.072 for 32-mm stainless steel heads. No significant differences were observed at this point, except for a significantly lower wear rate with zirconia heads as compared to 32-mm stainless steel heads. At 12 years, however, the mean linear wear penetration with zirconia heads (0.412 mm/y) was significantly higher than that with alumina heads (0.071 mm/y), 28-mm stainless steel heads (0.134 mm/y), and 32-mm stainless steel heads (0.192 mm/y). Similar results were observed for volumetric wear rates. The authors suggested that the increased wear observed with zirconia heads might be linked to a long-term degradation of the zirconia in vivo, associated with an altered roughness and roundness.

Hip simulator and clinical studies indicate that the wear of a COP bearing is at least equivalent to (21,65,134,244) or better

than that of a MOP bearing. Wear reduction of up to 50% has been reported (74,151,192,236,288).

Advances in the manufacturing of cobalt–chromium alloy heads achieved in recent years, which have improved sphericity and reduced surface roughness, could have theoretically resulted in lower PE wear rates. The magnitude of the reduction in PE wear provided by ceramic femoral heads, if any, also needs to be weighed against the magnitude of the increase in cost of the product.

Ceramics are brittle materials, creating the possibility of fracture of a ceramic head (32,45,108,116,137,176,178,179,186,271). A review of more than 500,000 current-generation alumina femoral heads indicates a fracture rate of 0.004% (4:100,000) (269). Even if the number of unreported cases is assumed to be three times higher (269), the fracture rate of ceramic heads is still much lower than that of femoral stems, which is around 0.27% (270:100,000) (102). Following a specific change in their manufacturing process in 1998, there was an increased rate of fracture of zirconia heads from one manufacturer (Prozyr®, SGCA Desmarquest, Vincennes Cedex, France, www.prozyr.com). It is important to recognize that the fracture risk of alumina or zirconia heads from other manufacturers was not affected by this occurrence.

With improvements in the manufacturing of ceramic materials, fracture of ceramic heads at this time is more often a function of design and manufacturing tolerances of morse taper junctions and not due to the ceramic material per se. Heavy patients and reconstructions with longer neck lengths (less contact area along the taper junction) and/or high offsets appear to be at increased risk. Theoretically, improvements in morse taper design and manufacturing can minimize or eliminate this problem.

Fixation

There are several studies which report on cementless acetabular fixation either with a cemented stem (hybrid hip) or cementless stem (Table 20-2). Callaghan et al. (31) reported an average linear wear rate of 0.07 mm/y for 63 hybrid hips with 28-mm cobalt–chromium alloy femoral heads. This group had the lowest linear wear rate of any of the five cohorts reported in that study. Hernandez et al. (106) reported an average linear wear rate of 0.14 mm per year for 97 hybrid hips with 28-mm titanium alloy femoral heads. Woolson and Murphy (273) reported an average linear wear rate of 0.14 mm/y for 58 hybrid hips and 22 cementless hips with 28-mm cobalt–chromium alloy femoral heads. Hernandez et al. (106) reported an average linear wear rate of 0.22 mm/y for 134 cementless hips with 28-mm titanium alloy femoral heads. Nashed et al. (183) reported an average linear wear rate of 0.25 mm/y for 15 cementless hips with titanium alloy femoral heads and an average linear wear rate of 0.17 mm/y for 74 cementless hips with cobalt–chromium alloy femoral heads.

The study of Callaghan et al. (31) suggests that the wear rate of cementless acetabular components can be equal to or perhaps better than that of cemented acetabular components. The studies of Hernandez et al. (106) and Nashed et al. (183), however, suggest that PE wear may be increased with cementless fixation. These results should be interpreted with caution because of the association with titanium alloy femoral heads. Similar to the proposal for cemented, metal-backed components, cementless acetabular and femoral components may differ in the amount of particles generated from the substrate, the porous coating, and the implant–bone interface. Such sources of hard third bodies could adversely affect PE wear. Recognizing the decreased abrasion resistance of titanium alloy, the performance of a bearing with this material would be affected to a greater degree by such a scenario.

Modularity

Modularity of the acetabular component has been identified as one of the variables that can affect PE wear. Initial studies by Callaghan et al. (31), Hernandez et al. (106), Nashed et al. (183), and Woolson and Murphy (273) that included hips with modular femoral heads, two-piece acetabular components, and/or screw fixation suggested this association.

The effects of acetabular liner modularity on PE wear and osteolysis were analyzed by Young and colleagues (286). A group of 41 hips treated with a nonmodular acetabular component was compared to a matched group of 41 hips treated with modular acetabular components, with mean follow-ups longer than 5 years. The nonmodular components demonstrated lower wear rates (0.11 versus 0.16 mm/y, $p = 0.22$), with 95% confidence intervals for the wear rates that were nearly half of those of the modular group (0.08 to 0.13 mm/y versus 0.11 to 0.20 mm/y, respectively). In addition, the nonmodular components were associated with lower rates of osteolysis (2% versus 22%, $p = 0.01$). Authors concluded that these results could be attributed to greater liner–shell conformity, greater liner thickness, and less liner–shell micromotion associated with nonmodular components.

Concern that wear particles and/or corrosion products from modular interfaces could migrate into the femoral–acetabular bearing and act as hard third bodies, adversely affecting wear performance, has been expressed (253). An example of the detrimental effects of hard third bodies, such as metallic debris, on the wear of PE is related to the use of cobalt–chromium cables for trochanteric reattachment. Compared to hips with monofilament wire reattachment, hips with cable reattachment had a higher rate of PE wear and acetabular component loosening (133).

METAL-ON-METAL BEARINGS

Aseptic loosening of early implants with a metal-on-metal (MOM) bearing was multifactorial and not uniformly due to the MOM bearings. As has been seen in hips which have MOP bearings, loosening of hips with MOM bearings occurred due to other factors such as suboptimal stem and/or cup design, manufacturing, or implantation technique (6,218,220,248,287). Many MOM implants lasted over two decades or are still functioning in patients who received the implant at a young age (218,220).

Materials and Design Considerations

The interplay of material(s), macrogeometry (diameter and clearance), microgeometry (surface topography), and lubrication influences the wear of MOM-bearing THRs to a far greater degree than MOP-bearing ones.

Alloys of cobalt (Co) and chromium (Cr) have been preferred for MOM bearings in THR because of their hardness. High chromium content provides good corrosion resistance. Carbon-rich compounds of Cr, Co, and molybdenum (Mo) are formed during manufacturing. These carbides, which are firmly adherent to the surrounding matrix, are approximately five times harder than the austenitic metallic phase of the matrix and are relatively brittle (222). The size and distribution of the carbides depends on the manufacturing process. Cast Co-Cr-Mo alloy (ASTM, F-75), which was used to manufacture the majority of first-generation MOM hips, has a relatively high carbon content of 0.2% to 0.3% and contains primarily Cr and Mo carbides, which result in asperities on the polished surface. The importance of dispersed carbides for wear resistance has been generally acknowledged (222).

The macrogeometry of a MOM bearing can be described in terms of the diameter(s) of the ball and the socket and the clearance of the resultant bearing couple. Clearance is the size of the gap between the surfaces at the equator of the bearing. For hemispherical bearings, clearance is a function of the difference in the diameters of the surfaces of the ball and socket. A ball and socket of exactly equal diameter mated together would have zero clearance and a maximal contact area for that size bearing. Contact area can be increased by increasing the size (diameter) of the bearing surfaces and/or by decreasing the clearance. Conversely, for a given diameter, increasing clearance decreases contact area. Contact stresses are a function of material properties and are inversely proportional to contact area. Clearance also influences lubrication, as the size of the gap has implications for the amount and type of lubrication. Smaller clearances encourage fluid film lubrication. Large clearances lead to a reduced contact area, loss of effective lubrication, and more rapid wear. However, too little clearance may lead to equatorial contact, very high frictional forces, high torque, and loosening of the implant (208). The limitations of current mass production manufacturing set the lower limit of clearance at about 20 μm. Wear rate, particularly during the initial run-in, increases rapidly with clearances above about 150 μm (39,166,173).

In addition to the contact area, another important variable is where the contact occurs. Given bearings of equivalent diameters, equatorial contact is associated with higher frictional torques than the same contact area in a more polar location. Equatorial bearing may have been a factor associated with failure of some early MOM THRs, and this is supported by retrieval studies (136). Consequently, relatively polar contact is preferred (136,166,218,260). Retrieval analyses of McKee–Farrar hips demonstrate variability in these parameters and likely represent an evolution of bearing surface design and manufacturing (136,218).

Lubrication

The lubricating fluid and conditions are important variables which influence friction and wear. The synovial fluid of normal, osteoarthritic, and rheumatoid joints has been characterized to some degree. The fluid is thixotropic; viscosity is a function of the shear strain rate, or velocity of motion, for practical purposes (208). Less is known about the fluid formed around total joint arthroplasties, but the composition and rheology are likely variable. A favorable film thickness to surface roughness ratio (lambda [λ] ratio) is desirable in order to maintain low friction between the articulating surfaces. This can be achieved by controlling the microtopography of the contacting surfaces and the elastic properties of the materials (208). Full-film lubrication completely separates the surfaces of a bearing. In this situation, the load is carried by the fluid, and wear of the bearings is minimal. Mixed-film lubrication partially separates the surfaces.

Mixed-film lubrication appears to be the operative mechanism in most MOM hip joints. For a given load and surface velocity, fluid film thickness is dependent on the properties of the fluid but can be influenced by the properties of the bearing materials, the macrogeometry of the bearing (which is a function of diameter and clearance), and the surface microtopography (surface finish) (208). Within the apparent contact area, the surfaces make actual contact only at the tips of asperities, and a lubricant film can influence wear significantly. As wear proceeds, the contact area at the asperity tips increases, and such "running-in" can produce a more favorable microgeometry for lubricant films to separate the surfaces and reduce wear (173).

Fluid-film lubrication is encouraged by making the femoral head as large as practically possible and the clearance as small as practically possible. For MOM bearings, in distinction from PE bearings, larger diameters can actually produce lower wear rates for similar manufacturing parameters (75,237).

Hip Simulator Tests

Medley et al. (173) described wear volumes ranging from 0.09 to 61 mm³ per million cycles and linear wear rates ranging from 1.3 to 100 μm per million cycles. In most tests, the wear rate decreased substantially after the first 0.1 to 0.5 million cycles. The authors suggest that lower wear was associated with larger effective radius (6 to 11 m) but there was a fair amount of scatter in the data. The poorest performance, however, was associated with a very high clearance of 630 μm.

The results of Chan et al. (39) showed that a higher wear occurred within the first million cycles, followed by a marked decrease in wear rate to lower, steady-state values. The total volumetric wear per million cycles was small, averaging 0.22 mm³/million cycles (range 0.05 to 0.85). An average wear rate of 0.40 mm³ per million cycles (range 0.02 to 1.9) was observed during the run-in period (first million cycles). Once the steady state was reached, an average wear rate of 0.08 mm³ per million cycles (range 0.03 to 0.21) was observed. With roughness held relatively constant, wear increased with increasing clearance ($R^2 = 0.65$, $p = 0.001$). Mass manufacturing control of tolerances below 20 μm is difficult, and the probability to match parts with an excessively tight fit would increase. Further, the bearing may deform during insertion or under load. The authors concluded that slightly larger clearances are necessary to increase the margin of safety.

Frictional Torque

The coefficient of friction for the MOM bearing of the McKee–Farrar hip is roughly two to three times greater than that for a MOP hip bearing. The larger diameter of the McKee–Farrar (about 40 mm) amplifies this difference, and

the result is a frictional torque that is up to ten times greater than that in the Charnley (218). This value is still an order of magnitude less than the static torque-to-failure of an acutely implanted cemented acetabular component and lower than that reported for MOP surface replacement components (8,40,43,77,148,257).

Contrary to theoretical considerations, frictional torque has not been demonstrated to be important in the initiation of aseptic loosening of either femoral or acetabular components. Accumulating evidence indicates that periprosthetic inflammation from PE wear particles has a greater effect on the durability of implant fixation than does frictional torque (8,77,148,257). From this perspective, the success of the Charnley low-friction arthroplasty is primarily a function of the low volumetric wear of the 22-mm-diameter bearing, not low frictional torque. Within the range of frictional torques generated by implants used to date, wear is a more important factor in survivorship than frictional torque. Large-diameter bearings can be successful if the wear rate is sufficiently low (152).

Retrieval Studies

Twenty-year performance has been reported of MOM hip articulations obtained at revision surgery after a mean implantation time of 21.3 years (218). The amount of wear was too small to be measured radiographically or by the shadowgraph technique. A computerized coordinate measuring machine was used to quantify the amount of wear by assessing the sphericity of bearing surfaces and comparing the measured dimensions in multiple planes to the best-fit circle. The worst-case estimate of combined femoral and acetabular linear wear was 4.2 μm/y—about 25 times less than that typically seen with PE.

Retrieval studies have shown average linear wear rates on the retrieved heads of about 0.004 mm/y, with an average volumetric wear rate of 1.5 mm³/y (136,166,222,267). The average linear wear rates on the cups are about 0.003 mm/y. The mean wear rate of the smaller-diameter McKee–Farrar balls is about twice that of the larger-diameter balls (1.4 vs. 0.7 mm³/y). This could be due to associated factors such as differences in clearance and/or effective radius, lubrication, or patient activity (166).

The wear rate of the MOM bearings decreases with time in situ. This is consistent with an initial conditioning phase or running-in: more rapid wear over the first 1 to 2 years, which is then followed by a lower steady-state wear rate (162,166,222,233).

Second-Generation MOM Bearings

In 1988 Müller and Weber reintroduced the MOM bearing under the brand name Metasul® (Centerpulse, Winterthur, Switzerland), a bearing that utilizes a carbide-containing, forged, Co-Cr-Mo alloy (Protasul-21WF) that reportedly has a clearance of 150 μm for the 28 mm articulation (181). With more than a decade of experience with second-generation MOM bearings, over 160,000 Metasul® bearings have been implanted, and this bearing technology has also been extended to large-diameter surface replacement components (7,259).

Clinical results of total hip systems with these bearings have generally been good (71,109,258,259,263). There are no reports of reoperations for a problem directly attributable to the MOM articulation. There has been no evidence of run-away wear, and few metal particles are seen in histologic sections (258,259,263). There have been, however, reoperations for infection, heterotopic ossification, instability, impingement, and aseptic loosening.

Impingement wear can be a source of metallosis, especially if a titanium alloy neck impinges on the Co-Cr acetabular articulation (117). For this reason, MOM articulations are more position sensitive than MOP joints. Larger-diameter bearings have a greater arc of motion, which decreases impingement risk.

Sieber et al. (233) reported on 118 Metasul components (65 heads and 53 cups) retrieved for dislocation (24%), loosening of the stem (17%), loosening of the cup (28%), and other reasons such as heterotopic ossification or infection (31%). None were revised for osteolysis. The mean time of implantation was 22 months (range 2 to 98 months). An update of this experience includes 297 retrieved head or cup components (281). The time between implantation and revision in this group ranged from 1 to 117 months with a similar distribution of indications (21% dislocation, 39% loosening of any component, 40% other reasons). The mean annual linear wear rate was found to decrease with the time from insertion, being between 25 and 35 μm/y for the running-in phase and reducing to a steady state of about 5 μm/y after the third year in both studies. The volumetric wear after the run-in period was estimated to be 0.3 mm^3/y, concluding that these MOM bearings have a volumetric wear rate more than 100 times lower than that of conventional PE bearings.

In clinical reports of hips with second-generation MOM bearings, with follow-up between 2.2 and 5 years, osteolysis is rare (109,258,259,263). Beaule et al., however, have reported a case of a well-fixed, cementless THR with a Metasul bearing with progressive diaphyseal osteolysis occurring within 2 years (18). There was minimal bearing surface wear and only small numbers of inflammatory cells in the tissues. Absent evidence of a foreign-body reaction, it was hypothesized that this was a case of osteolysis secondary to transmission of joint fluid pressure, rather than particulate-induced osteolysis (209).

Between 1991 and 1994, 74 Metasul bearings in the Weber cemented cup were implanted with a variety of femoral components. With up to 4 years follow-up (average 2.2), the clinical results were good to excellent and no hips had loosened. Twenty-seven of these patients had a contralateral metal on plastic bearing hip of similar design and none of these patients could detect a difference between the two hips (109). Complete clinical and radiographic data on 56 of these patients (56 hips), with follow-ups between 4 and 6.8 years (average 5.2 years) has also been reported (71). Good to excellent clinical results were found in 99% of cases. One patient required acetabular revision for loosening secondary to suboptimal cement technique. There were no loose or revised femoral components. There was no apparent osteolysis (71).

Metal–Metal Wear Particles

Wear particles from MOM bearings are nanometers in linear dimension, which is substantially smaller than PE wear particles

(68,69). Light microscopic analysis of tissue obtained from around MOM joints showed particles with variable and irregular shape (69). The size of metal particles reported by scanning electron microscopy studies ranges from 0.1 to 5 μm. The studies have suggested that large metallic particles observed with light microscopy were agglomerates of the smaller particles (69,95).

Transmission electron microscopy has demonstrated wear particles from Co-Cr-Mo bearings to be round to oval in shape with irregular boundaries. Most of the particles are smaller than 50 nm (range 6 nm to 1 μm) (68,234). Additional analysis of these retrieved wear particles indicates that the particles have several different elemental compositions. There are Co-Cr-Mo particles, but there is an even greater number of chromium oxide particles (35,37). It has been hypothesized that the Co-Cr-Mo particles are produced by the wear of the carbides on the bearing surfaces and the prosthesis matrix, and that the chromium oxide particles come from the passivation layer on the implant surface and possibly from oxidized chromium carbides (35,37).

There is little known about the rates of metallic particle production in vivo, lymphatic transport of metallic particles from the joint, and systemic dissemination (70,175). Utilizing information on volumetric wear rate and average particle size, it has been estimated that 6.7×10^{12} to 2.5×10^{14} metal particles are produced per year, which is 13 to 500 times the number of PE particles produced per year by a typical MOP joint (69). The aggregate surface area of these metal wear particles is substantial.

Biological Considerations

The large aggregate surface area of metal wear particles may have both local and systemic effects. Surface area has been identified as a variable affecting the macrophage response to particles (228). However, the local tissue reaction around MOM prosthesis, indicated by the number of histiocytes, is about one grade lower than that around MOP prostheses (69,70). A number of hypotheses have been proposed to explain this discrepancy (69). Since metal particles are considerably smaller than PE particles, histiocytes are able to store a larger number of metal particles, and therefore, the total number of histiocytes required to store the metal particles is lower. Very small particles may enter macrophages by pinocytosis instead of phagocytosis, which may alter the cellular response to the particles. It is also recognized that Co-Cr particles have greater potential for cytotoxicity than PE particles, and the cell may be incapable of the same inflammatory response. There may be a difference in the relative proportion of metal wear particles that are retained locally versus systemically distributed compared to PE wear particles. Dissolution of metal particles results in elevation of the cobalt and chromium ion concentrations in erythrocytes, serum, and urine (149).

In vitro studies have shown a dose–response effect with metal particles (100). Low to moderate concentrations of metal particles stimulate the release of cytokines, such as interleukin-1 (IL-1), interleukin-6 (IL-6), tumor necrosis factor-α, and prostaglandin E^2, that can lead to periprosthetic osteolysis and aseptic loosening (10,36,100,114,140,182,227). At higher concentrations, however, Co-Cr particles have been found to be cytotoxic (100,114,154,182,226,227), altering the phagocytic activity of macrophages and leading to cell death (36,100,200,227).

Although the volume of reactive periprosthetic inflammatory tissue associated with MOM bearings is less than with MOP, osteolysis can occur in hips with MOM bearings (18,218,220). The incidence of osteolysis associated with MOM bearings has not been well established but appears to be comparatively low (248,287).

Hypersensitivity

Due to the fact that all metals in a biological environment corrode (24,122), the ions released can combine with proteins and activate the immune system as antigens and elicit hypersensitivity responses (92). Nickel is the most common metal sensitizer in humans, followed by Co and Cr (17,85, 92,99,132). Because of the elevated level of Co and Cr ions in patients with a MOM bearing, there may be an increased risk of developing hypersensitivity. Aggregate worldwide experience with second-generation MOM bearings indicates that the incidence of hypersensitivity is approximately 2 per 10,000.

Implant-related hypersensitivity reactions are generally delayed cell-mediated responses (92,104,138). Delayed-type hypersensitivity is characterized by antigen activation of sensitized T lymphocytes that releases cytokines, resulting in a recruitment and activation of macrophages (92). Several case reports have associated the use of orthopedic implants with the appearance of immunogenic reactions (16,52,93, 174,205,250). Recently, some groups described specific histological changes in the tissues around revised MOM prostheses (5,62,265,266). They found lymphocytic infiltrations in the subsurface layer of the lining tissues, which were either diffuse or aggregated around small postcapillary vessels. The tissues of the MOM patients also showed significant ulcerations of the pseudosynovial surface compared to a group of metal-on-plastic patients. Interestingly, all these changes were less obvious in tissue retrieved from McKee–Farrar or loose cemented curved Co-Cr stems compared to modern MOM bearings (265). There seems to be no correlation between the amount of metal debris and the occurrence or extent of the immunological reaction (62). These immunological reactions are described with the term "aseptic lymphocytic vasculitis-associated lesions" (62). The clinical relevance of these findings is not clear yet, because only a small number of patients with MOM bearings had to be revised so far, and only a fraction of the revised cases show these histological changes.

Historically, testing for delayed-type hypersensitivity has been done in vivo by skin testing and in vitro by lymphocyte transformation testing and leukocyte migration inhibition testing. There are, however, many concerns about the applicability of skin test to the study of immune responses to implants. Unlike the typical acute dermal exposure to the antigen that occurs with the patch testing, it takes weeks to months of constant exposure prior to reports of dermal reactions to orthopaedic implants (92). Moreover, the diagnostic utility of patch testing could be affected by immunological tolerance, which could suppress dermal response to implants, or by impaired host immune response (92). In vitro delayed-type hypersensitivity testing remains an unpopular means of assessing metal hypersensitivity, mainly because of its labor-intensive characteristics and limited clinical results (92).

In patients with well-functioning implants, the prevalence of metal sensitivity is approximately 25%, which is roughly twice of that of the general population (92). The prevalence is approximately 60% among patients with a failed or poorly functioning implant. Because a malfunctioning or loose implant can generate metal particles, it is unclear whether metal hypersensitivity causes implant failure or vice versa (92). In either event, delayed type hypersensitivity should be considered when a patient with a well-fixed implant experiences chronic, aching pain with evidence of synovitis (an irritable range of motion) but has no objective evidence of infection. If a modular MOM bearing is being considered, the use of substrates without Co-Cr (e.g., titanium) will allow revision of only the bearings in cases were hypersensitivity develops.

Serum and Urine Ions

It is important to recognize that in modern THR prostheses there may be several sources of metal particle and ion generation. Systemic dissemination of soluble and particulate corrosion products from modular junctions has been described, including the presence of metallic particles in the lymph nodes, liver, and spleen (10,125,231,254,255).

In control subjects (no metallic implants) the levels of serum and urine Co and Cr are undetectable, or nearly undetectable (125).

For patients with clinically well-functioning hips with a MOP bearing, 36 months following surgery, the average serum Co level was 0.27 parts per billion (ppb) (range 0.15 to 1.59). The average serum Cr level was 0.18 ppb (range 0.015 to 1.46), and the average urine Cr level was 0.28 ppb (range 0.008 to 1.77). In these apparently well-functioning hips, the ion levels were 1 to 5 times higher than controls (124).

In modular total hips with a MOP bearing, with no or mild corrosion at the modular head and neck junction, serum and urine levels of Co averaged 0.94 ppb (range <0.54 to 1.65) and 0.92 ppb (range <0.3 to 1.14), respectively, and urine Cr levels averaged 1.0 ppb (range 0.54 to 1.92). With moderate or severe corrosion at the modular head and neck junction, the serum and urine levels of Co averaged 1.06 ppb (range 0.8 to 1.4) and 0.87 ppb (range <0.3 to 1.3), respectively, and the average urine Cr levels were 1.59 ppb (range 0.6 to 3.0) (125).

The levels of metal ions in serum and urine are further elevated in patients with MOM bearings (28,142,149). It appears that the ion levels are higher in the short term and decrease over time. This is consistent with a conditioning phase or running-in of the bearing. In resurfacing prostheses with an average bearing diameter of 48 mm (38 to 52 mm) and a minimum follow-up of 12 months, the average serum Co level was 1.8 ppb (range 0.6 to 4.3) and the average serum and urine Cr levels were 1.07 ppb (range 0.35 to 2.75) and 2.21 ppb (range 0.43 to 7.17), respectively (123).

The ion levels in subjects with Co-Cr alloy MOM THRs that had been in situ for an average of 24 years have been reported (123). The average serum Co level was 0.9 ppb (range <0.3 to 2.0). The average serum Cr level was 1.28 ppb (range 0.21 to 2.56), and the average urine Cr level was 1.22 ppb (range 0.26 to 2.59) (123).

The longer-term serum and urine ion levels produced by MOM bearings are not much higher than those produced by the modular junctions of femoral components. Unfortunately, the toxicological importance of these trace metal elevations has not been established, and available data do not answer questions regarding the risks of ion hypersensitivity, toxicity, and carcinogenesis (87,123,175,256). Since wear of a MOM bearing cannot generally be measured on a radiograph, serum and urine metal ion concentrations may be useful indicators of patient activity and the tribological performance of these bearings.

The distribution and histological effects of wear particles from a McKee–Farrar THR with an in vivo use of nearly 30 years has been described. Clinically, the implant was functioning well. Serum and urine levels of chromium and serum levels of cobalt, obtained 25 years after implantation and while the patient was healthy and active, were found to be 1.02 ppb, 0.51 ppb, and 0.66 ppb, respectively. Sections from multiple samples of the lymph nodes, spleen, liver, and kidney were examined with light microscopy. This tissue analysis did not reveal any evidence of end-organ damage or accumulation of metal particles. It appears that a patient with normal renal function is capable of clearing cobalt and chromium ions from his or her system (34).

Erythrocyte and urine metal analysis (cobalt, chromium, and titanium) was performed in 41 patients that have undergone modular THR in whom the only difference was the type of insert received: either metal or PE (149). Patients were followed for an average of 3.2 years (2.2 to 3.9 years). For patients that received a MOM articulation, the median erythrocyte cobalt, chromium, and titanium levels were 1.10 ppb (0.66 to 2.43), 2.5 ppb (1.18 to 3.13), and 1.80 ppb (1.15 to 2.75), respectively, and the median urine cobalt, chromium, and titanium levels were 14.73 ppb (5.29 to 28.78), 4.53 ppb (2.8 to 9.22), and 0.39 ppb (0.27 to 0.66), respectively, measured at a median of 2 years of follow-up. For patients that received a MOP articulation, the median erythrocyte cobalt, chromium, and titanium levels were 0.17 ppb (0.12 to 0.23), 1.30 ppb (1.00 to 1.83), and 1.50 ppb (1.15 to 2.08), respectively, and the median urine cobalt, chromium, and titanium levels were 0.29 ppb (0.2 to 0.37), 0.30 ppb (0.21 to 0.44), and 0.38 ppb (0.30 to 0.45), respectively, measured at a median of 2 years follow-up. Compared to patients receiving a MOP articulation, erythrocyte and urine levels of cobalt and chromium were significantly higher in patients receiving a MOM articulation (146). With such a modular acetabular bearing, the significance of such ion elevations has not been determined. Potential additional sources of ions include the acetabular morse taper connection.

The serum cobalt concentration was measured during the first 5 years after modular total hip arthroplasty in 100 patients that randomly received either a MOM articulation (50 patients) or a COP articulation (50 patients) (28). The median postoperative serum concentration in patients with a MOM bearing increased over the first year after the implantation, reaching its maximum level between the sixth and twelfth postoperative months (1 μg/L). After the first year, the serum cobalt concentrations remained relatively constant up to the fifth year, with levels between 0.55 and 0.75 μg/L. Serum cobalt concentrations on the COP group were below the detection limits at all time points.

Cancer Risk

Co and Cr wear particles have been shown to induce carcinoma in animal models (83,101), giving rise to the concern that such alloys could have the same effect in human tissues if present in sufficient amounts for a sufficient length of time.

The first well-documented case of cancer associated with total joint replacement was in a patient who developed a malignant fibrous histiocytoma 3.5 years after a MOM THR performed in December 1969 (241). There have been, at least, 24 additional cases reported in the English literature of malignancy occurring in association with a total hip or knee prostheses (249). Of the 25 reported cases of cancer following a total joint replacement, 21 involved sarcomas (249).

The risk of cancer after MOM THR has been assessed specifically in only one epidemiological study (256). In that study, the relative risk of cancer was reported to be 0.95 (95% confidence interval, 0.8 to 1.1), suggesting that there is no apparent increased risk of cancer development after MOM total hip arthroplasty. In addition, the risk of sarcoma after MOM THR was found to be 0.00 (95% confidence interval, 0.0 to 6.6) (256). However, the same study found the relative risk of hematopoietic cancer to be 1.59 (95% confidence interval, 0.8 to 2.8) following MOM THR and 3.77 (95% confidence interval, 0.9 to 17.6) for leukemia when MOM implants were compared with MOP implants. The confidence intervals are very broad for these data and encompass unity, indicating that the risk is statistically neither increased nor decreased. From an epidemiological perspective, these data are limited because of the small number of patients (579) who underwent MOM THR. Furthermore, the majority of patients in these reports have less than 10 years of follow-up. The latency of known carcinogens, such as tobacco, asbestos, and ionizing radiation, is several decades. Longer follow-up of large patient groups is needed to better assess the risk of cancer with any implant system (249). Since the goal of more wear resistant bearings is to reduce the need for reoperation, theoretical risks should be weighed against the risks of revision THR. In the Medicare population, the 90-day mortality following revision THR is 2.6%, which is significantly and substantially higher than that of primary total hip and directly related to the revision procedure (150). Rigorous long-term studies are needed to assess the relative risk to benefit ratios for total hip bearings.

CERAMIC-ON-CERAMIC BEARINGS

Ceramic bearings, made of alumina, have demonstrated the lowest in vivo wear rates to date of any bearing combination (27,47). The same principles of friction and lubrication reported for MOM bearings apply to ceramic-on-ceramic (COC) bearings. However, ceramics have two important properties that make them an outstanding material regarding friction and wear. Ceramics are hydrophilic, permitting a better wettability of the surface. This ensures that the synovial fluid-film is uniformly distributed over the whole bearing surface area. Secondly, ceramic has a greater hardness than metal and can be polished to a much lower surface roughness. Although the better wettability results in a slightly thinner fluid-film than with MOM bearings it is compensated by the reduced size of the asperities on the surface. Overall, this results in a favorable higher λ ratio and in a reduced coefficient of friction. This bearing combination is the most likely to achieve true fluid-film lubrication (44). However, because of the hardness of ceramics, the wear characteristics are sensitive to design, manufacturing, and implantation variables. Rapid wear has also been observed, generally associated with suboptimal positioning of the implants (45,271).

COC bearings currently in clinical use are made of alumina. Developments in the production process (sintering) have improved the quality of the material (20). Modern alumina ceramics have a low porosity, low grain size, high density, and high purity. Thus, hardness, fracture toughness, and burst strength increased (20,22,224). There are also in vitro tests that utilize zirconia and alumina/zirconia composites in order to improve wear characteristics (1–3), but these mixed oxides need further investigations before clinical trials can be conducted.

The United States experience with COC was initially limited to the Autophor/Xenophor prostheses, which were conceived and introduced in Europe by Mittlemeier (178,179). The clinical results with the Autophor were generally less satisfactory than those with established MOP designs, and COC implants were never widely used in the United States (151). Results from the past (mostly from Europe) showed survival rates of 75–84% after 10 years (22,186,271) and 68% after 20 years (94). In the patients aged 50 years and younger the survivorship rates were 84% after 10 years, 80% after 15 years (182), and 61% after 20 years (94).

Similar to the interpretation of MOM bearings based on the clinical performance of the McKee–Farrar prosthesis (218), perception of the performance of the COC bearing has been complicated by the fact that both the cementless femoral stem and the nonarticular portion of the cementless Autophor acetabular component had features that are now recognized as suboptimal (45). Follow-up studies show very low in vivo wear rates (94,130,199), but failures occurred as a result of inferior implant design and fixation technique (25,224). The current generation of COC bearings is frequently being utilized with implant systems that have demonstrated long-term successful fixation and excellent clinical results with a MOP bearing.

Two prospective, randomized multicenter trials are being performed in the United States with more than 300 patients enrolled in each study. Garino (84) reported the experience with the Transcend™ system (Wright Medical Technology), which was implanted with a modular cementless acetabular component in 333 cases, with either a cemented or cementless stem. With follow-up of 18 to 36 months (mean 22 months), 98.8% of the implants are still in situ. The second trial utilizes the ABC-System (Stryker–Howmedica–Osteonics), which was implanted in 349 cases (59,61). D'Antonio et al. (59) reported the most recent results of the six participating surgeons with the highest number of enrolled patients. This subgroup consists of 207 patients with 222 hips with a mean follow-up of 48 months. Five patients have been revised, with 97.7% of the implants in place. As an additional nonrandomized study arm, the Trident®-System (Stryker–Howmedica–Osteonics) was included in this multicenter study with 209 patients enrolled. One hundred seventy-five patients in the Trident® group have a minimum of 2 years follow-up with a revision rate of 1.4% (three revisions) (60).

One potential complication with these implants, which a surgeon should recognize, is liner chipping during insertion. This happened in 3 (1%) cases in the Transcend™ group and in 9 (2.6%) cases (162) in the ABC study group. The Trident® bearing has a metal-backed ceramic insert with an elevated titanium liner rim, and no intraoperative liner chipping has been reported in this group (59).

Performance of the ceramic bearing does appear to be sensitive to implant position. Hips with a lateral opening less than 30° or greater than 55° and/or a high neck-shaft angle (greater than about 140°) are at risk for neck–socket impingement and/or high wear as a result of stress concentration in the very stiff ceramic material (261).

Including the original study groups and additional implantations, at this time 1361 ceramic inserts have been implanted in these studies, and there have been no failures due to the bearing (59,84). No fractures of the implanted liners or ceramic heads have been reported. Fracture of a current-generation ceramic head happens with an incidence of 4 in 100,000 (269). It is too early to make a comparable statement about the acetabular inserts, as more data with a higher number of implants are needed. Results from the multicenter studies are encouraging with no liner fractures reported to date.

Microseparation and Wear Particles

Ceramic materials may have better biocompatibility than metal alloys (44), but the relative size, shape, number, reactivity, and local versus systemic distribution of the respective wear particles have not been fully determined.

Hatton et al. (98) investigated the tissues from ten noncemented COC THRs undergoing revision surgery. The tissues from the femoral and acetabular regions demonstrated the presence of intracellular particle agglomerates and mixed pathology, with areas that had no obvious pathology and areas that were relatively rich in macrophages, and over half of the tissues had in the region of 60% of necrosis. A bimodal size range of ceramic wear debris was observed, with particles as small as 5 to 90 nm (mean 24 nm) and as large as 0.05 to 3.2 μm (mean 0.43 μm). The authors suggested that the two types of ceramic wear debris are generated by two different wear mechanisms in vivo, with very small wear particles being generated under normal articulating conditions and larger particles being generated under microseparation conditions.

After total hip arthroplasty, the femoral head and the acetabular insert can separate up to 2 mm during the swing phase of a normal gait cycle (135). When a load is applied at heel strike in the stance phase, the femoral head moves vertically to relocate in the cup. With the geometry of a typical COC prosthesis, separations of only 2 mm will allow the femoral head to contact the rim acetabular liner, resulting in changes in the wear performance of the bearing couple (stripe wear) (239). Experimental studies have introduced microseparation into the swing phase of the hip joint simulator cycle, reproducing clinically relevant wear debris, wear mechanisms, and wear rates (185) and allowing varying degrees of joint laxity to be investigated.

The wear debris generated in vitro from COC articulations under normal and microseparation conditions has been characterized by Tipper et al. (251) with the use of transmission electron microscopy. Under standard simulation conditions, only nanometer-sized wear particles, ranging from 2 to 27.5 nm, were observed. When microseparation of the prosthetic components was introduced into the simulation, a bimodal distribution of wear particle sizes was observed, including nanometer-sized particles (1 to 35 nm), as well as micrometer-sized (0.02 to 1 μm) particles. The authors suggested that these larger particles originate from the wear stripe and were produced by the transgranular fracture of the ceramic.

This is especially important for COC designs, where microseparation conditions have resulted in wear rates up to 1.84 mm^3/million cycles, as compared to <0.1 mm^3/million cycles under normal conditions (239,251). Similar hip simulator test results were observed by Manaka et al. (156), who also compared the results of the hip simulator test with those obtained from retrieved components. The stripes from the simulator were narrower than short-term retrievals and much narrower than some long-term retrievals, suggesting that the variety of motions possible in the in vivo situation are not completely reproduced by the hip simulator.

Ceramic debris may not be bio-inert as initially assumed, because osteolysis has been described in some patients with a COC bearing (272,285). Some studies describe inflammatory and cytotoxic reactions on the cellular level, but the relationship to material, size, and particle number remains uncertain (86,97,98,146). It seems that there is less inflammatory reaction compared to MOM or MOP bearings in well-functioning prostheses (26). Ion toxicity is not an issue with ceramics because of their high corrosion resistance (26).

It is hoped that improvements in the manufacturing of ceramics and ceramic components will minimize or eliminate mechanical problems such as fracture and accelerated wear. It is also anticipated that "modern" COC bearings will be developed and marketed in the United States with established femoral components. Improved acetabular component fixation is needed and ceramic bearings will likely be combined with porous ingrowth fixation.

CONCLUSION

Cross-linked polyethylene, MOM, and COC bearings have all demonstrated lower in vivo wear rates than conventional metal-on-plastic couples. The degree of wear reduction is promising, but it may not directly translate into greater longevity of a THR for all patients. Continued close follow-up is needed to demonstrate a favorable benefit to risk ratio by reducing the number of revision surgeries. The use of any of these bearings has specific benefits and risks that should be considered on a patient-by-patient basis.

REFERENCES

1. Affatato S, Goldoni M, Testoni M, et al. Mixed oxides prosthetic ceramic ball heads. Part 3: Effect of the ZrO_2 fraction on the wear of ceramic on ceramic hip joint prostheses. A long-term in vitro wear study. *Biomaterials.* 2001;22:717–723.
2. Affatato S, Testoni M, Cacciari GL, et al. Mixed oxides prosthetic ceramic ball heads. Part 1: Effect of the ZrO_2 fraction on the wear of ceramic on polythylene joints. *Biomaterials.* 1999;20:971–975.
3. Affatato S, Testoni M, Cacciari GL, et al. Mixed-oxides prosthetic ceramic ball heads. Part 2: Effect of the ZrO_2 fraction on the wear of ceramic on ceramic joints. *Biomaterials.* 1999;20: 1925–1929.
4. Agins HJ, Alcock NW, Bansal M, et al. Metallic wear in failed titanium-alloy total hip replacements. A histological and quantitative analysis. *J Bone Joint Surg Am.* 1988;70A:347–356.
5. Al-Saffar N. Early clinical failure of total joint replacement in association with follicular proliferation of B-lymphocytes: a report of two cases. *J Bone Joint Surg Am.* 2002;84A: 2270–2273.
6. Amstutz HC, Campbell PA, McKellop H, et al. Metal on metal total hip replacement workshop consensus document. *Clin Orthop Relat Res.* 1996;329S:297–303.
7. Amstutz HC, Grigoris P. Metal on metal bearings in hip arthroplasty. *Clin Orthop Relat Res.* 1996;329(suppl):S11–S34.
8. Andersson GBJ, Freeman MAR, Swanson SAV. Loosening of the cemented acetabular cup in total hip replacement. *J Bone Joint Surg Br.* 1972;54B:590–599.
9. Anthony PP, Gie GA, Howie CR, et al. Localized endosteal bone lysis in relation to the femoral components of cemented total hip arthroplasties. *J Bone Joint Surg Br.* 1990;72B: 971–979.
10. Archibeck MJ, Jacobs JJ, Black J. Alternate bearing surfaces in total joint arthroplasty: biologic considerations. *Clin Orthop Relat Res.* 2000;379:12–21.
11. Baker DA, Hastings RS, Pruitt L. Study of fatigue resistance of chemical and radiation crosslinked medical grade ultrahigh molecular weight polyethylene. *J Biomed Mater Res.* 1999;46: 573–581.
12. Bankston AB, Cates H, Ritter MA, et al. Polyethylene wear in total hip arthroplasty. *Clin Orthop Relat Res.* 1995;317:7–13.
13. Bankston AB, Keating EM, Ranawat C, et al. Comparison of polyethylene wear in machined versus molded polyethylene. *Clin Orthop Relat Res.* 1995;317:37–43.
14. Barrack RL, Castro FP Jr, Szuszczewicz ES, et al. Analysis of retrieved uncemented porous-coated acetabular components in patients with and without pelvic osteolysis. *Orthopedics.* 2002;25:1373–1378.
15. Barrack RL, Schmalzried TP. Impingement and rim wear associated with early osteolysis after a total hip replacement : a case report. *J Bone Joint Surg Am.* 2002;84A:1218–1220.
16. Barranco VP, Soloman H. Eczematous dermatitis from nickel. *JAMA.* 1972;220:1244.
17. Basketter DA, Briatico-Vangosa G, Kaestner W, et al. Nickel, cobalt and chromium in consumer products: a role in allergic contact dermatitis? *Contact Dermatitis.* 1993;28:15–25.
18. Beaule PE, Campbell P, Mirra J, et al. Osteolysis in a cementless, second generation metal-on-metal hip replacement. *Clin Orthop Relat Res.* 2001;386:159–165.
19. Bell CJ, Walker PS, Abeysundera MR, et al. Effect of oxidation on delamination of ultrahigh-molecular-weight polyethylene tibial components. *J Arthroplasty.* 1998;13:280–290.
20. Bierbaum BE, Nairus J, Kuesis D, et al. Ceramic-on-ceramic bearings in total hip arthroplasty. *Clin Orthop Relat Res.* 2002;405: 158–163.
21. Bigsby RJ, Hardaker CS, Fisher J. Wear of ultra-high molecular weight polyethylene acetabular cups in a physiological hip joint simulator in the anatomical position using bovine serum as a lubricant. *Proc Inst Mech Eng H.* 1997;211:265–269.
22. Bizot P, Banallec L, Sedel L, et al. Alumina-on-alumina total hip prostheses in patients 40 years of age or younger. *Clin Orthop Relat Res.* 2000;379:68–76.
23. Black J. *Orthopaedic Biomaterials in Research and Practice.* Philadephia: Churchill Livingstone; 1988.
24. Black J. Systemic effects of biomaterials. *Biomaterials.* 1984;5: 11–18.
25. Boehler M, Plenk H Jr, Salzer M. Alumina ceramic bearings for hip endoprostheses: the Austrian experiences. *Clin Orthop Relat Res.* 2000;379:85–93.
26. Bos I, Willmann G. Morphologic characteristics of periprosthetic tissues from hip prostheses with ceramic-ceramic couples: a comparative histologic investigation of 18 revision and 30 autopsy cases. *Acta Orthop Scand.* 2001;72: 335–342.
27. Boutin P, Christel P, Dorlot JM, et al. The use of dense alumina-alumina ceramic combination in total hip replacement. *J Biomed Mater Res.* 1988;22:1203–1232.

28. Brodner W, Bitzan P, Meisinger V, et al. Serum cobalt levels after metal-on-metal total hip arthroplasty. *J Bone Joint Surg Am.* 2003;85A:2168–2173.

29. Bruck SD, Mueller EP. Radiation sterilization of polymeric implant materials. *J Biomed Mater Res.* 1988;22:133–144.

30. Burke DW, O'Connor DO, Zalenski EB, et al. Micromotion of cemented and uncemented femoral components. *J Bone Joint Surg Br.* 1991;73B:33–37.

31. Callaghan JJ, Pedersen DR, Olejniczak JP, et al. Radiographic measurement of wear in 5 cohorts of patients observed for 5 to 22 years. *Clin Orthop Relat Res.* 1995;317:14–18.

32. Callaway GH, Flynn W, Ranawat CS, et al. Fracture of the femoral head after ceramic-on-polyethylene total hip arthroplasty. *J Arthroplasty.* 1995;10:855–859.

33. Campbell PA, Ma S, Yeom B, et al. Isolation of predominantly submicron-sized UHMWPE wear particles from periprosthetic tissues. *J Biomed Mater Res.* 1995;29:127–131.

34. Campbell P, Urban RM, Catelas I, et al. Autopsy analysis thirty years following metal-on-metal total hip replacement. *J Bone Joint Surg Am.* 2003;85A:2218–2222.

35. Catelas I, Bobyn JD, Medley JB, et al. Size, shape, and composition of wear particles from metal-metal hip simulator testing: effects of alloy and number of loading cycles. *J Biomed Mater Res.* 2003;67A:312–327.

36. Catelas I, Campbell P, Dorey F, et al. Relationship between cytokines and metal particles in metal-metal THA's. Presented at: Orthopaedic Research Society Annual Meeting; 2001.

37. Catelas I, Campbell P, Medley JB, et al. Quantitative and compositional analysis of particles from metal-metal THRs. Presented at: European Society for Biomaterials 25th Anniversary Conference; 2001; London.

38. Cates HE, Faris PM, Keating EM, et al. Polyethylene wear in cemented metal-backed acetabular cups. *J Bone Joint Surg Br.* 1993;75B:249–253.

39. Chan FW, Bobyn JD, Medley JB, et al. Wear and lubrication of metal-on-metal hip implants. *Clin Orthop Relat Res.* 1999;369:10–24.

40. Charnley J. *Low Friction Arthroplasty of the Hip: Theory and Practice.* Berlin: Springer-Verlag; 1979.

41. Charnley J, Cupic Z. The nine and ten year results of the low-friction arthroplasty of the hip. *Clin Orthop Relat Res.* 1973;95:9–25.

42. Charnley J, Halley DK. Rate of wear in total hip replacement. *Clin Orthop Relat Res.* 1975;112:170–179.

43. Charnley J, Kamangar A, Longfield MD. The optimum size of prosthetic heads in relation to the wear of plastic sockets in total replacement of the hip. *Med Biol Eng.* 1969;7:31–39.

44. Christel PS. Biocompatibility of surgical-grade dense polycrystalline alumina. *Clin Orthop Relat Res.* 1992;282:10–18.

45. Clarke IC. Role of ceramic implants. Design and clinical success with total hip prosthetic ceramic-to-ceramic bearings. *Clin Orthop Relat Res.* 1992;282:19–30.

46. Clarke IC, Black K, Rennie C, et al. Can wear in total hip arthroplasties be assessed from radiographs? *Clin Orthop Relat Res.* 1976;121:126–142.

47. Clarke IC, Good V, Williams P, et al. Ultra-low wear rates for rigid-on-rigid bearings in total hip replacements. *Proc Inst Mech Eng H.* 2000;214:331–347.

48. Clarke IC, Gustafson A. Clinical and hip simulator comparisons of ceramic-on-polyethylene and metal-on-polyethylene wear. *Clin Orthop Relat Res.* 2000;379:34–40.

49. Clarke IC, Kabo JM. Wear in total hip replacement. In: *Hip Arthroplasty.* New York: Churchhill Livingstone; 1991:535–549.

50. Collier JP, Mayor MB, McNamara JL, et al. Analysis of the failure of 122 polyethylene inserts from uncemented tibial knee components. *Clin Orthop Relat Res.* 1991;273:232–242.

51. Collier JP, Sperling DK, Currier JH, et al. Impact of gamma sterilization on clinical performance of polyethylene in the knee. *J Arthroplasty.* 1996;11:377–389.

52. Collier JP, Sutula LC, Currier BH, et al. Overview of polyethylene as a bearing material: Comparison of sterilization methods. *Clin Orthop Relat Res.* 1996;333:76–86.

53. Collier MB, Kraay MJ, Rimnac CM, et al. Evaluation of contemporary software methods used to quantify polyethylene wear

54. Cooper JR, Dowson D, Fisher J. Ceramic bearing surfaces in artificial joints: resistance to third body damage. *J Med Eng Technol.* 1991;15:63–67.

55. Cooper JR, Dowson D, Fisher J. The effect of transfer film and surface roughness on the wear of lubricated ultrahigh molecular weight polyethylene. *Clin Mater.* 1993;14:295–302.

56. Cramers M, Lucht U. Metal sensitivity in patients treated for tibial fractures with plates of stainless steel. *Acta Orthop Scand.* 1977;48:245–249.

57. Cuckler JM, Bearcroft J, Asgian CM. Femoral head technologies to reduce polyethylene wear in total hip arthroplasty. *Clin Orthop Relat Res.* 1995;317:57–63.

58. Currier BH, Currier JH, Collier JP, et al. Shelf life and in vivo duration. Impacts on performance of tibial bearings. *Clin Orthop Relat Res.* 1997;342:111–122.

59. D'Antonio J, Capello W. Alumina ceramic bearings for total hip arthroplasty. *Semin Arthroplasty.* 2003;in press:

60. D'Antonio J, Capello W, Manley M, et al. Alumina/alumina ceramic bearings in THA. Presented at: Hip Society Meeting; 3–7 September 2002; Rochester, MN.

61. D'Antonio J, Capello W, Manley M, et al. New experience with alumina-on-alumina ceramic bearings for total hip arthroplasty. *J Arthroplasty.* 2002;17:390–397.

62. Davies A, Willert H, Campbell P, et al. Metal-on-metal bearing surfaces may lead to higher inflammation. Presented at: 70th Annual Meeting of the American Academy of Orthopaedic Surgeons; 2003.

63. Devane PA, Bourne RB, Rorabeck CH, et al. Measurement of polyethylene wear in metal-backed acetabular cups. I. Three-dimensional technique. *Clin Orthop Relat Res.* 1995;319:303–316.

64. Devane PA, Bourne RB, Rorabeck CH, et al. Measurement of polyethylene wear in metal-backed acetabular cups. II. Clinical application. *Clin Orthop Relat Res.* 1995;319:317–326.

65. Devane PA, Horne JG. Assessment of polyethylene wear in total hip replacement. *Clin Orthop Relat Res.* 1999;369:59–72.

66. Devane PA, Robinson EJ, Bourne RB, et al. Measurement of polyethylene wear in acetabular components inserted with and without cement. A randomized trial. *J Bone Joint Surg Am.* 1997;79A:682–689.

67. Digas G, Karrholm J, Thanner J, et al. Highly cross-linked polyethylene in cemented THA: randomized study of 61 hips. *Clin Orthop Relat Res.* 2003;417:126–138.

68. Doorn PF, Campbell PA, Amstutz HC. Metal versus polyethylene wear particles in total hip replacements. A review. *Clin Orthop Relat Res.* 1996;329(suppl):S206–S216.

69. Doorn PF, Campbell PA, Worrall J, et al. Metal wear particle characterization from metal on metal total hip replacements: transmission electron microscopy study of periprosthetic tissues and isolated particles. *J Biomed Mater Res.* 1998;42:103–111.

70. Doorn PF, Mirra JM, Campbell PA, et al. Tissue reaction to metal on metal total hip prostheses. *Clin Orthop Relat Res.* 1996;329(suppl):S187–S205.

71. Dorr LD, Wan Z, Longjohn DB, et al. Total hip arthroplasty with use of the Metasul metal-on-metal articulation. Four to seven-year results. *J Bone Joint Surg Am.* 2000;82A:789–798.

72. Dowd JE, Sychterz CJ, Young AM, et al. Characterization of long-term femoral-head-penetration rates. Association with and prediction of osteolysis. *J Bone Joint Surg Am.* 2000;82A:1102–1107.

73. Dowling JM, Atkinson JR, Dowson D, et al. The characteristics of acetabular cups worn in the human body. *J Bone Joint Surg Br.* 1978;60B:375–382.

74. Dowson D. A comparative study of the performance of metallic and ceramic femoral head components in total replacement hip joints. *Wear.* 1995;190:171–183.

75. Dowson D. New joints for the millennium: wear control in total replacement hip joints [abstract]. *Proc Inst Mech Eng H.* 2001;215:335.

76. Ebramzadeh E, McKellop H, Dorey F, et al. Challenging the validity of conclusions based on P-values alone: a critique of contemporary clinical research design and methods. *Instr Course Lect.* 1994;43:587–600.

77. Eftekhar NS, Pawluk RJ. Role of surgical preparation in acetabular cup fixation. In: *The Hip. Proceedings of the Eighth Open*

Scientific Meeting of the Hip Society. St. Louis: Mosby; 1980: 308–328.

78. Eggli S, z'Brun S, Gerber C, et al. Comparison of polyethylene wear with femoral heads of 22 mm and 32 mm. A prospective, randomised study. *J Bone Joint Surg Br.* 2002;84:447–451.

79. Endo M, Tipper JL, Barton DC, et al. Comparison of wear, wear debris and functional biological activity of moderately crosslinked and non-crosslinked polyethylenes in hip prostheses. *Proc Inst Mech Eng H.* 2002;216:111–122.

80. Engh GA, Dwyer KA, Hanes CK. Polyethylene wear of metal-backed tibial components in total and unicompartmental knee prostheses. *J Bone Joint Surg Br.* 1992;74B:9–17.

81. Fisher J. Surface damage to femoral head prostheses. *J Bone Joint Surg Br.* 1994;76B:852.

82. Fisher J, Chan KL, Hailey JL, et al. Preliminary study of the effect of aging following irradiation on the wear of ultrahigh-molecular-weight polyethylene. *J Arthroplasty.* 1995;10:689–692.

83. Freeman MA, Swanson SA, Heath JC. Study of the wear particles produced from cobalt-chromium-molybdenum-manganese total joint replacement prostheses. *Ann Rheumatic Dis.* 1969; 28(suppl):29.

84. Garino JP. Modern ceramic-on-ceramic total hip systems in the United States: early results. *Clin Orthop Relat Res.* 2000;379: 41–47.

85. Gawkrodger DJ. Nickel sensitivity and the implantation of orthopaedic prostheses. *Contact Dermatitis.* 1993;28:257–259.

86. Germain MA, Hatton A, Williams S, et al. Comparison of the cytotoxicity of clinically relevant cobalt-chromium and alumina ceramic wear particles in vitro. *Biomaterials.* 2003;24: 469–479.

87. Gillespie WJ, Henry DA, O'Connell DL, et al. Development of hematopoietic cancers after implantation of total joint replacement. *Clin Orthop Relat Res.* 1996;329(suppl):S290–S296.

88. Griffith MJ, Seidenstein MK, Williams D, et al. Socket wear in Charnley low friction arthroplasty of the hip. *Clin Orthop Relat Res.* 1978;137:37–47.

89. Grobbelaar CJ, du Plessis TA, Marais F. The radiation improvement of polyethylene prostheses. A preliminary study. *J Bone Joint Surg Br.* 1978;60B:370–374.

90. Grobbelaar CJ, Weber FA, Spirakis A, et al. Clinical experience with gamma irradiation-crosslinked polyethylene. A 14 to 20 year follow-up report. *S Afr Bone Joint Surg.* 1999;9:140–147.

91. Guttmann D, Schmalzried TP, Kabo JM, et al. Characterization of back-side wear in modular polyethylene liners. *Orthop Trans.* 1994;18:418.

92. Hallab N, Merritt K, Jacobs JJ. Metal sensitivity in patients with orthopaedic implants. *J Bone Joint Surg Am.* 2001;83A:428–436.

93. Halpin DS. An unusual reaction in muscle in association with Vitallium plate: a report of possible metal hypersensitivity. *J Bone Joint Surg Br.* 1975;57B:451–453.

94. Hamadouche M, Boutin P, Daussange J, et al. Alumina-on-alumina total hip arthroplasty: a minimum 18.5-year follow-up study. *J Bone Joint Surg Am.* 2002;84A:69–77.

95. Hanlon J, Ozuna R, Shortkroff S, et al. Analysis of metallic wear debris retrieved at revision arthroplsty. Presented at: Implant Retrieval Symposium of the Society for Biomaterials; 1992; St Charles, IL.

96. Harris WH, Schiller AL, Scholler JM, et al. Extensive localized bone resorption in the femur following total hip replacement. *J Bone Joint Surg Am.* 1976;58A:612–618.

97. Hatton A, Nevelos JE, Matthews JB, et al. Effects of clinically relevant alumina ceramic wear particles on TNF-alpha production by human peripheral blood mononuclear phagocytes. *Biomaterials.* 2003;24:1193–1204.

98. Hatton A, Nevelos JE, Nevelos AA, et al. Alumina-alumina artificial hip joints. Part I: A histological analysis and characterisation of wear debris by laser capture microdissection of tissues retrieved at revision. *Biomaterials.* 2002;23:3429–3440.

99. Haudrechy P, Foussereau J, Mantout B, et al. Nickel release from nickel-plated metals and stainless steels. *Contact Dermatitis.* 1994;31:249–255.

100. Haynes DR, Boyle SJ, Rogers SD, et al. Variation in cytokines induced by particles from different prosthetic materials. *Clin Orthop Relat Res.* 1998;352:223–230.

101. Heath JC, Freeman MA, Swanson SA. Carcinogenic properties of wear particles from prostheses made in cobalt-chromium alloy. *Lancet.* 1971;1:564–566.

102. Heck D, Partridge CM, Reuben JD, et al. Prosthetic component failures in hip arthroplasty surgery. *J Arthroplasty.* 1995;10: 575–580.

103. Heisel C, Silva M, dela Rosa MA, et al. Short-term in vivo wear of cross-linked polyethylene. *J Bone Joint Surg Am.* 2004;86A: 748–751.

104. Hensten-Pettersen A. Allergy and hypersensitivity. In: Morrey BF, ed. *Biological, Material, and Mechanical Considerations of Joint Replacements.* New York: Raven Press; 1993:353–360.

105. Hermida JC, Bergula A, Chen P, et al. Comparison of the wear rates of twenty-eight and thirty-two-millimeter femoral heads on cross-linked polyethylene acetabular cups in a wear simulator. *J Bone Joint Surg Am.* 2003;85A:2325–2331.

106. Hernandez JR, Keating EM, Faris PM, et al. Polyethylene wear in uncemented acetabular components. *J Bone Joint Surg Br.* 1994;76B:263–266.

107. Hernigou P, Bahrami T. Zirconia and alumina ceramics in comparison with stainless-steel heads. Polyethylene wear after a minimum ten-year follow-up. *J Bone Joint Surg Br.* 2003;85:504–509.

108. Higuchi F, Shiba N, Inoue A, et al. Fracture of an alumina ceramic head in total hip arthroplasty. *J Arthroplasty.* 1995;10:851–854.

109. Hilton KR, Dorr LD, Wan Z, et al. Contemporary total hip replacement with metal on metal articulation. *Clin Orthop Relat Res.* 1996;329(suppl):S99–S105.

110. Hirakawa K, Bauer TW, Stulberg BN, et al. Characterization of debris adjacent to failed knee implants of 3 different designs. *Clin Orthop Relat Res.* 1996;331:151–158.

111. Hirakawa K, Bauer TW, Stulberg BN, et al. Comparison and quantitation of wear debris of failed total hip and total knee arthroplasty. *J Biomed Mater Res.* 1996;31:257–263.

112. Hop JD, Callaghan JJ, Olejniczak JP, et al. Contribution of cable debris generation to accelerated polyethylene wear. *Clin Orthop Relat Res.* 1997;344:20–32.

113. Hopper RH Jr, Young AM, Orishimo KF, et al. Effect of terminal sterilization with gas plasma or gamma radiation on wear of polyethylene liners. *J Bone Joint Surg Am.* 2003;85A:464–468.

114. Howie DW, Rogers SD, McGee MA, et al. Biologic effects of cobalt chrome in cell and animal models. *Clin Orthop Relat Res.* 1996;329(suppl):S217–S232.

115. Hui AJ, McCalden RW, Martell JM, et al. Validation of two and three-dimensional radiographic techniques for measuring polyethylene wear after total hip arthroplasty. *J Bone Joint Surg Am.* 2003;85A:505–511.

116. Hummer CD, Rothman RH, Hozack WJ. Catastrophic failure of modular zirconia-ceramic femoral head components after total hip arthroplasty. *J Arthroplasty.* 1995;10:848–850.

117. Iida H, Kaneda E, Takada H, et al. Metallosis due to impingement between the socket and the femoral neck in a metal-on-metal bearing total hip prosthesis. A case report. *J Bone Joint Surg Am.* 1999;81A:400–403.

118. Illgen RL, Laurent MP, Watanuki M, et al. Highly crosslinked versus conventional polyethylene particles: an in vitro comparison of biologic activities. *Trans Orthop Res Soc.* 2003;28:poster 1438. Available at: http://www.ors.org/Transactions/49/1438.PDF. Accessed 9 November 2005.

119. Ingram JH, Fisher J, Stone M, et al. Effect of crosslinking on biological activity of UHMWPE wear debris. *Trans Orthop Res Soc.* 2003;28:poster 1439. Available at: http://www.ors.org/Transactions/49/1438.PDF. Accessed 9 November 2005.

120. Ingram J, Matthews JB, Tipper J, et al. Comparison of the biological activity of grade GUR 1120 and GUR 415HP UHMWPE wear debris. *Biomed Mater Eng.* 2002;12:177–188.

121. Isaac J, Wroblewski BM, Atkinson JR, et al. A tribological study of retrieved hip prostheses. *Clin Orthop Relat Res.* 1992;276: 115–125.

122. Jacobs JJ, Gilbert JL, Urban RM. Corrosion of metallic implants. In: Stauffer RN, ed. *Advances in Operative Orthopaedics.* St. Louis: Mosby; 1994:279–319.

123. Jacobs JJ, Skipor AK, Doorn PF, et al. Cobalt and chromium concentrations in patients with metal on metal total hip replacements. *Clin Orthop Relat Res.* 1996;329(suppl):S256–S263.

124. Jacobs JJ, Skipor AK, Patterson LM, et al. Metal release in patients who have had a primary total hip arthroplasty. A prospective, controlled, longitudinal study. *J Bone Joint Surg Am.* 1998;80:1447–1458.

125. Jacobs JJ, Urban RM, Gilbert JL, et al. Local and distant products from modularity. *Clin Orthop Relat Res.* 1995;319:94–105.

126. Jasty M, Bragdon CR, Lee K, et al. Surface damage to cobalt-chrome femoral head prostheses. *J Bone Joint Surg Br.* 1994;76B:73–77.

127. Jasty M, Bragdon CR, O'Connor DO, et al. Marker improvement in the wear resistance of a new form of UHMWPE in a physiologic hip simulator. *Trans Soc Biomater.* 1997;20:157.

128. Jasty MJ, Floyd WE, Schiller AL, et al. Localized osteolysis in stable, non-septic total hip replacement. *J Bone Joint Surg Am.* 1986;68A:912–919.

129. Jasty M, Goetz DD, Bragdon CR, et al. Wear of polyethylene acetabular components in total hip arthroplasty. An analysis of one hundred and twenty-eight components retrieved at autopsy or revision operations. *J Bone Joint Surg Am.* 1997;79A:349–358.

130. Jazrawi LM, Bogner E, Della Valle CJ, et al. Wear rates of ceramic-on-ceramic bearing surfaces in total hip implants: a 12-year follow-up study. *J Arthroplasty.* 1999;14:781–787.

131. Kabo JM, Gebhard JS, Loren G, et al. In vivo wear of polyethylene acetabular components. *J Bone Joint Surg Br.* 1993;75B:254–258.

132. Kanerva L, Sipilainen-Malm T, Estlander T, et al. Nickel release from metals, and a case of allergic contact dermatitis from stainless steel. *Contact Dermatitis.* 1994;31:299–303.

133. Kelley SS, Johnston RC. Debris from cobalt-chrome cable may cause acetabular loosening. *Clin Orthop Relat Res.* 1992;285:140–146.

134. Kim YH, Kim JS, Cho SH. A comparison of polyethylene wear in hips with cobalt-chrome or zirconia heads. A prospective, randomised study. *J Bone Joint Surg Br.* 2001;83B:742–750.

135. Komistek RD, Dennis DA, Ochoa JA, et al. In vivo comparison of hip separation after metal-on-metal or metal-on-polyethylene total hip arthroplasty. *J Bone Joint Surg Am.* 2002;84A:1836–1841.

136. Kothari M, Bartel DL, Booker JF. Surface geometry of retrieved McKee-Farrar total hip replacements. *Clin Orthop Relat Res.* 1996;329(suppl):S141–S147.

137. Krikler S, Schatzker J. Ceramic head failure. *J Arthroplasty.* 1995;10:860–862.

138. Kuby J. *Immunology.* New York: WH Freeman; 1994.

139. Kurtz SM, Muratoglu OK, Evans M, et al. Advances in the processing, sterilization, and crosslinking of ultra-high molecular weight polyethylene for total joint arthroplasty. *Biomaterials.* 1999;20:1659–1688.

140. Lee SH, Brennan FR, Jacobs JJ, et al. Human monocyte/macrophage response to cobalt-chromium corrosion products and titanium particles in patients with total joint replacements. *J Orthop Res.* 1997;15:40–49.

141. Lewis PL, Rorabeck CH, Bourne RB. Screw osteolysis after cementless total knee replacement. *Clin Orthop Relat Res.* 1995;321:173–177.

142. Lhotka C, Szekeres T, Steffan I, et al. Four-year study of cobalt and chromium blood levels in patients managed with two different metal-on-metal total hip replacements. *J Orthop Res.* 2003;21:189–195.

143. Li S, Burstein AH. Ultra-high molecular weight polyethylene. The material and its use in total joint implants. *J Bone Joint Surg Am.* 1994;76A:1080–1090.

144. Livermore J, Ilstrup D, Morrey B. Effect of femoral head size on wear of the polyethylene acetabular component. *J Bone Joint Surg Am.* 1990;72A:518–528.

145. Livingston BJ, Chmell MJ, Spector M, et al. Complications of total hip arthroplasty associated with the use of an acetabular component with a Hylamer liner. *J Bone Joint Surg Am.* 1997;79A:1529–1538.

146. Lohmann CH, Dean DD, Koster G, et al. Ceramic and PMMA particles differentially affect osteoblast phenotype. *Biomaterials.* 2002;23:1855–1863.

147. Lu Z, McKellop H. Frictional heating of bearing materials tested in a hip joint wear simulator. *Proc Inst Mech Eng H.* 1997;211:101–108.

148. Ma SM, Kabo JM, Amstutz HC. Frictional torque in surface and conventional hip replacement. *J Bone Joint Surg Am.* 1983;65A:366–370.

149. MacDonald SJ, McCalden RW, Chess DG, et al. Metal-on-metal versus polyethylene in hip arthroplasty: a randomized clinical trial. *Clin Orthop Relat Res.* 2003;406:282–296.

150. Mahomed NN, Barrett JA, Katz JN, et al. Rates and outcomes of primary and revision total hip replacement in the United States medicare population. *J Bone Joint Surg Am.* 2003;85A:27–32.

151. Mahoney OM, Dimon JH. Unsatisfactory results with a ceramic total hip prosthesis. *J Bone Joint Surg Am.* 1990;72A:663–671.

152. Mai MT, Schmalzried TP, Dorey FJ, et al. The contribution of frictional torque to loosening at the cement-bone interface in Tharies hip replacements. *J Bone Joint Surg Am.* 1996;78A:505–511.

153. Maloney WJ, Jasty M, Rosenberg A, et al. Bone lysis in well-fixed cemented femoral components. *J Bone Joint Surg Br.* 1990;72B:966–970.

154. Maloney WJ, Smith RL, Castro F, et al. Fibroblast response to metallic debris in vitro. Enzyme induction cell proliferation, and toxicity. *J Bone Joint Surg Am.* 1993;75A:835–844.

155. Maloney WJ, Smith RL, Schmalzried TP, et al. Isolation and characterization of wear particles generated in patients who have had failure of a hip arthroplasty without cement. *J Bone Joint Surg Am.* 1995;77A:1301–1310.

156. Manaka M, Clarke IC, Yamamoto K, et al. Stripe wear rates in alumina THR: comparison of microseparation simulator study with retrieved implants. *J Biomed Mater Res.* 2004;69B: 149–157.

157. Margevicius KJ, Bauer TW, McMahon JT, et al. Isolation and characterization of debris in membranes around total joint prostheses. *J Bone Joint Surg Am.* 1994;76A:1664–1675.

158. Martell JM, Berdia S. Determination of polyethylene wear in total hip replacements with use of digital radiographs. *J Bone Joint Surg Am.* 1997;79A:1635–1641.

159. Martell JM, Berkson E, Berger R, et al. Comparison of two and three-dimensional computerized polyethylene wear analysis after total hip arthroplasty. *J Bone Joint Surg Am.* 2003;85A:1111–1117.

160. Martell JM, Edidin A, Dumbleton J. Preclinical evaluation followed by randomized clinical study of crosslinked polyethylene for total hip arthroplasty at two years follow-up. Presented at: 47th Orthopaedic Research Society Annual Meeting; 2001.

161. Martell JM, Incavo SJ. Clinical perfromance of a highly crosslinked polyethylene at two years in total hip arthroplasty: a randomized prospective trial. *Trans Orthop Res Soc.* 2003;28: poster 1431. Available at: http://www.ors.org/Transactions/ 49/1431.PDF. Accessed 9 November 2005.

162. McCalden RW, Howie DW, Ward L, et al. Observation on the long-term wear behaviour of retrieved McKee-Farrar total hip replacement implants. *Trans Orthop Res Soc.* 1995;20:242.

163. McKellop HA. Bearing surfaces in total hip replacements: state of the art and future developments. *Instruc Course Lect.* 2001;50:165–179.

164. McKellop HA, Campbell PA, Park SH, et al. The origin of submicron polyethylene wear debris in total hip arthroplasty. *Clin Orthop Relat Res.* 1995;311:3–20.

165. McKellop H, Hosseinian A, Burgoyne K, et al. Polyethylene wear against titanium alloy compared to stainless steel and cobalt-chromium alloys. In: Anderson JM, ed. *Proceedings of the Second World Congress on Biomaterials.* Mt Laurel, NJ: Society for Biomaterials; 1984:313.

166. McKellop H, Park SH, Chiesa R, et al. In vivo wear of three types of metal on metal hip prostheses during two decades of use. *Clin Orthop Relat Res.* 1996;329S:128–140.

167. McKellop H, Rostlund T, Ebramzadeh E, et al. Wear of titanium 6-4 alloy in laboratory tests and in retrieved human joint replacements. In: Brown SA, Lemons JE, eds. *Medical Applications of Titanium and Its Alloys: The Material and Biological Issues.* STP 1272. West Conshohocken, PA: American Society for Testing and Materials; 1996.

168. McKellop HA, Sarmiento A, Schwinn CP, et al. In vivo wear of titanium-alloy hip prostheses. *J Bone Joint Surg Am.* 1990;72A:512–517.

169. McKellop HA, Shen FW, Campbell P, et al. Effect of molecular weight, calcium stearate, and sterilization methods on the wear

of ultra high molecular weight polyethylene acetabular cups in a hip joint simulator. *J Orthop Res.* 1999;17:329–339.

170. McKellop H, Shen FW, DiMaio W, et al. Wear of gamma-crosslinked polyethylene acetabular cups against roughened femoral balls. *Clin Orthop Relat Res.* 1999;369:73–82.

171. McKellop H, Shen FW, Lu B, et al. Development of an extremely wear-resistant ultra high molecular weight polyethylene for total hip replacements. *J Orthop Res.* 1999;17:157–167.

172. McKellop H, Shen FW, Lu B, et al. Effect of sterilization method and other modifications on the wear resistance of acetabular cups made of ultra-high molecular weight polyethylene. A hip-simulator study. *J Bone Joint Surg Am.* 2000;82A:1708–1725.

173. Medley JB, Chan FW, Krygier JJ, et al. Comparison of alloys and designs in a hip simulator study of metal on metal implants. *Clin Orthop Relat Res.* 1996;329(suppl):S148–S159.

174. Merle C, Vigan M, Devred D, et al. Generalized eczema from vitallium osteosynthesis material. *Contact Dermatitis.* 1992;27:257–258.

175. Merritt K, Brown SA. Distribution of cobalt chromium wear and corrosion products and biologic reactions. *Clin Orthop Relat Res.* 1996;329(suppl):S233–S243.

176. Michaud RJ, Rashad SY. Spontaneous fracture of the ceramic ball in a ceramic-polyethylene total hip arthroplasty. *J Arthroplasty.* 1995;10:863–867.

177. Mikulak SA, Mahoney OM, dela Rosa MA, et al. Loosening and osteolysis with the press-fit condylar posterior-cruciate-substituting total knee replacement. *J Bone Joint Surg Am.* 2001;83A:398–403.

178. Mittelmeier H. Eight years of clinical experience with self-locking ceramic hip prosthesis "Autophor." *J Bone Joint Surg Br.* 1984;66B:300.

179. Mittelmeier H, Heisel J. Sixteen-years' experience with ceramic hip prostheses. *Clin Orthop Relat Res.* 1992;282:64–72.

180. Morrey BF, Ilstrup D. Size of the femoral head and acetabular revision in total hip-replacement arthroplasty. *J Bone Joint Surg Am.* 1989;71A:50–55.

181. Müller ME. The benefits of metal-on-metal total hip replacements. *Clin Orthop Relat Res.* 1995;311:54–59.

182. Nakashima Y, Sun DH, Trindade MC, et al. Induction of macrophage C-C chemokine expression by titanium alloy and bone cement particles. *J Bone Joint Surg Br.* 1999;81B:155–162.

183. Nashed RS, Becker DA, Gustilo RB. Are cementless acetabular components the cause of excess wear and osteolysis in total hip arthroplasty? *Clin Orthop Relat Res.* 1995;317:19–28.

184. Nasser S, Campbell PA, Kilgus D, et al. Cementless total joint arthroplasty prostheses with titanium-alloy articular surfaces. A human retrieval analysis. *Clin Orthop Relat Res.* 1990;261:171–185.

185. Nevelos J, Ingham E, Doyle C, et al. Microseparation of the centers of alumina-alumina artificial hip joints during simulator testing produces clinically relevant wear rates and patterns. *J Arthroplasty.* 2000;15:793–795.

186. Nizard RS, Sedel L, Christel P, et al. Ten-year survivorship of cemented ceramic-ceramic total hip prosthesis. *Clin Orthop Relat Res.* 1992;282:53–63.

187. Ohashi T, Inoue S, Kajikawa K. The clinical wear rate of acetabular component accompanied with alumina ceramic head. In: Oonishi H, Aoli H, Sawai K, eds. *Bioceramics.* St. Louis: Ishiyaku EuroAmerica; 1989:278.

188. Okumura H, Yamamuro T, Kumar T. Socket wear in total hip prosthesis with alumina ceramic head. In: Oonishi H, Aoki H, Sawai K, eds. *Biomedics: Proceedings First International Symposium on Biceramics.* Tokyo: Ishiyaku EuroAmerica; 1989:258.

189. Oonishi H, Kadoya Y, Masuda S. Gamma-irradiated cross-linked polyethylene in total hip replacements: analysis of retrieved sockets after long-term implantation. *J Biomed Mater Res.* 2001;58:167–171.

190. Oonishi H, Takayaka Y, Clarke IC, et al. Comparative wear studies of 28-mm ceramic and stainless steel total hip joints over 2 to 7 year period. *J Long-Term Med Implants.* 1992;2:37–47.

191. Oonishi H, Takayama Y, Tsuji E. Improvement of polyethylene by irradiation in artificial joints. *Radiat Phys Chem.* 1992;39:495–504.

192. Oonishi H, Wakitani S, Murata N, et al. Clinical experience with ceramics in total hip replacement. *Clin Orthop Relat Res.* 2000;379:77–84.

193. Oparaugo PC, Clarke IC, Malchau H, et al. Correlation of wear debris-induced osteolysis and revision with volumetric wear-rates of polyethylene: a survey of 8 reports in the literature. *Acta Orthop Scand.* 2001;72:22–28.

194. Orishimo KF, Claus AM, Sychterz CJ, et al. Relationship between polyethylene wear and osteolysis in hips with a second-generation porous-coated cementless cup after seven years of follow-up. *J Bone Joint Surg Am.* 2003;85A:1095–1099.

195. Parks NL, Engh GA, Dwyer KA, et al. Micromotion of modular tibial components in total knee arthroplasty. *Orthop Trans.* 1994;18:611.

196. Parks NL, Engh GA, Topoleski LD, et al. Modular tibial insert micromotion. A concern with contemporary knee implants. *Clin Orthop Relat Res.* 1998;356:10–15.

197. Pedersen DR, Callaghan JJ, Johnston TL, et al. Comparison of femoral head penetration rates between cementless acetabular components with 22-mm and 28-mm heads. *J Arthroplasty.* 2001;16:111–115.

198. Peters PC Jr, Engh GA, Dwyer KA, et al. Osteolysis after total knee arthroplasty without cement. *J Bone Joint Surg Br.* 1992;74B:864–876.

199. Prudhommeaux F, Hamadouche M, Nevelos J, et al. Wear of alumina-on-alumina total hip arthroplasties at a mean 11-year followup. *Clin Orthop Relat Res.* 2000;379:113–122.

200. Rae T. A study on the effects of particulate metals of orthopaedic interest on murine macrophages in vitro. *J Bone Joint Surg Br.* 1975;57B:444–450.

201. Ries MD, Scott ML, Jani S. Relationship between gravimetric wear and particle generation in hip simulators: conventional compared with cross-linked polyethylene. *J Bone Joint Surg Am.* 2001;83A(suppl 2):116–122.

202. Ries MD, Weaver K, Beals N. Safety and efficacy of ethylene oxide sterilized polyethylene in total knee arthroplasty. *Clin Orthop Relat Res.* 1996;331:159–163.

203. Ritter MA. Direct compression molded polyethylene for total hip and knee replacements. *Clin Orthop Relat Res.* 2001;393:94–100.

204. Rose RM, Crugnola A, Ries M, et al. On the origins of high in vivo wear rates in polyethylene components of total joint prostheses. *Clin Orthop Relat Res.* 1979;145:277–286.

205. Rostoker G, Robin J, Binet O, et al. Dermatitis due to orthopaedic implants. A review of the literature and report of three cases. *J Bone Joint Surg Am.* 1987;69A:1408–1412.

206. Sakoda H, Voice AM, McEwen HM, et al. A comparison of the wear and physical properties of silane cross-linked polyethylene and ultra-high molecular weight polyethylene. *J Arthroplasty.* 2001;16:1018–1023.

207. Sander M. *A Practical Guide to the Assessment of Surface Texture.* Göttingen: Feinpruf GmbH; 1991.

208. Schey JA. Systems view of optimizing metal on metal bearings. *Clin Orthop Relat Res.* 1996;329(suppl):S115–S127.

209. Schmalzried TP, Akizuki KH, Fedenko AN, et al. The role of access of joint fluid to bone in periarticular osteolysis. A report of four cases. *J Bone Joint Surg Am.* 1997;79A:447–452.

210. Schmalzried TP, Callaghan JJ. Wear in total hip and knee replacements. *J Bone Joint Surg Am.* 1999;81A:115–136.

211. Schmalzried TP, Campbell P. Isolation and characterization of debris in membranes around total joint prostheses [letter; comment]. *J Bone Joint Surg Am.* 1995;77A:1625–1626.

212. Schmalzried TP, Campbell P, Schmitt AK, et al. Shapes and dimensional characteristics of polyethylene wear particles generated in vivo by total knee replacements compared to total hip replacements. *J Biomed Mater Res.* 1997;38:203–210.

213. Schmalzried TP, Guttmann D, Grecula M, et al. The relationship between the design, position, and articular wear of acetabular components inserted without cement and the development of pelvic osteolysis. *J Bone Joint Surg Am.* 1994;76A: 677–688.

214. Schmalzried TP, Huk OL. Patient factors and wear in total hip arthroplasty. *Clin Orthop Relat Res.* 2004;418:94–97.

215. Schmalzried TP, Jasty M, Harris WH. Periprosthetic bone loss in total hip arthroplasty. Polyethylene wear debris and the concept of the effective joint space. *J Bone Joint Surg Am.* 1992;74A:849–863.

216. Schmalzried TP, Jasty M, Rosenberg A, et al. Polyethylene wear debris and tissue reactions in knee as compared to hip replacement prostheses. *J Appl Biomater.* 1994;5:185–190.

217. Schmalzried TP, Kwong LM, Jasty M, et al. The mechanism of loosening of cemented acetabular components in total hip arthroplasty. Analysis of specimens retrieved at autopsy. *Clin Orthop Relat Res.* 1992;274:60–78.

218. Schmalzried TP, Peters PC, Maurer BT, et al. Long-duration metal-on-metal total hip arthroplasties with low wear of the articulating surfaces. *J Arthroplasty.* 1996;11:322–331.

219. Schmalzried TP, Shepherd EF, Dorey FJ, et al. Wear is a function of use, not time. *Clin Orthop Relat Res.* 2000;381:36–46.

220. Schmalzried TP, Szuszczewicz ES, Akizuki KH, et al. Factors correlating with long term survival of McKee-Farrar total hip prostheses. *Clin Orthop Relat Res.* 1996;329(suppl):S48–S59.

221. Schmalzried TP, Szuszczewicz ES, Northfield MR, et al. Quantitative assessment of walking activity after total hip or knee replacement. *J Bone Joint Surg Am.* 1998;80A:54–59.

222. Schmidt M, Weber H, Schon R. Cobalt chromium molybdenum metal combination for modular hip prostheses. *Clin Orthop Relat Res.* 1996;329(suppl):S35–S47.

223. Schuller HM, Marti RK. Ten-year socket wear in 66 hip arthroplasties. Ceramic versus metal heads. *Acta Orthop Scand.* 1990;61:240–243.

224. Sedel L. Evolution of alumina-on-alumina implants: a review. *Clin Orthop Relat Res.* 2000;379:48–54.

225. Seedhom BB, Dowson D, Wright V. Wear of solid phase formed high density polyethylene in relation to the life of artificial hips and knees. *Wear.* 1973;24:35–51.

226. Shanbhag AS, Jacobs JJ, Black J, et al. Effects of particles on fibroblast proliferation and bone resorption in vitro. *Clin Orthop Relat Res.* 1997;342:205–217.

227. Shanbhag AS, Jacobs JJ, Black J, et al. Human monocyte response to particulate biomaterials generated in vivo and in vitro. *J Orthop Res.* 1995;13:792–801.

228. Shanbhag AS, Jacobs JJ, Black J, et al. Macrophage/particle interactions: effect of size, composition and surface area. *J Biomed Mater Res.* 1994;28:81–90.

229. Shanbhag AS, Jacobs JJ, Glant TT, et al. Composition and morphology of wear debris in failed uncemented total hip replacement. *J Bone Joint Surg Br.* 1994;76B:60–67.

230. Shaver SM, Brown TD, Hillis SL, et al. Digital edge-detection measurement of polyethylene wear after total hip arthroplasty. *J Bone Joint Surg Am.* 1997;79A:690–700.

231. Shea KG, Lundeen GA, Bloebaum RD, et al. Lymphoreticular dissemination of metal particles after primary joint replacements. *Clin Orthop Relat Res.* 1997;338:219–226.

232. Shen FW, McKellop HA. Interaction of oxidation and crosslinking in gamma-irradiated ultrahigh molecular-weight polyethylene. *J Biomed Mater Res.* 2002;61:430–439.

233. Sieber HP, Rieker CB, Kottig P. Analysis of 118 second-generation metal-on-metal retrieved hip implants. *J Bone Joint Surg Br.* 1999;81B:46–50.

234. Silva M, Shepherd EF, Jackson WO, et al. Average patient walking activity approaches 2 million cycles per year: pedometers underrecord walking activity. *J Arthroplasty.* 2002;17: 693–697.

235. Silverton CD, Jacobs JJ, Rosenberg AG, et al. Complications of a cable grip system. *J Arthroplasty.* 1996;11:400–404.

236. Skinner HB. Ceramic bearing surfaces. *Clin Orthop Relat Res.* 1999;369:83–91.

237. Smith SL, Dowson D, Goldsmith AAJ. The effect of diametral clearances, motion and loading cycles upon lubrication of metal-on-metal hip replacements. *Proc Inst Mech Eng C.* 2001;215:1–5.

238. Soh EW, Blunn GW, Wait ME, et al. Size and shape of metal particles from metal-on-metal total hip replacements. *Trans Orthop Res Soc.* 1996;21:462.

239. Stewart TD, Tipper JL, Insley G, et al. Severe wear and fracture of zirconia heads against alumina inserts in hip simulator studies with microseparation. *J Arthroplasty.* 2003;18:726–734.

240. Sutula LC, Collier JP, Saum KA, et al. Impact of gamma sterilization on clinical performance of polyethylene in the hip. *Clin Orthop Relat Res.* 1995;319:28–40.

241. Swann M. Malignant soft-tissue tumour at the site of a total hip replacement. *J Bone Joint Surg Br.* 1984;66B:629–631.

242. Sychterz CJ, Engh CA Jr, Shah N, et al. Radiographic evaluation of penetration by the femoral head into the polyethylene liner over time. *J Bone Joint Surg Am.* 1997;79A:1040–1046.

243. Sychterz CJ, Engh CA Jr, Yang A, et al. Analysis of temporal wear patterns of porous-coated acetabular components: distinguishing between true wear and so-called bedding-in. *J Bone Joint Surg Am.* 1999;81:821–830.

244. Sychterz CJ, Engh CAJ, Young AM, et al. Comparison of in vivo wear between polyethylene liners articulating with ceramic and cobalt-chrome femoral heads. *J Bone Joint Surg Br.* 2000;82B: 948–951.

245. Sychterz CJ, Moon KH, Hashimoto Y, et al. Wear of polyethylene cups in total hip arthroplasty. A study of specimens retrived post mortem. *J Bone Joint Surg Am.* 1996;78A:1193–1200.

246. Sychterz CJ, Shah N, Engh CA. Examination of wear in Duraloc acetabular components: two- to five-year evaluation of Hylamer and Enduron liners. *J Arthroplasty.* 1998;13:508–514.

247. Sychterz CJ, Yang AM, McAuley JP, et al. Two-dimensional versus three-dimensional radiographic measurements of polyethylene wear. *Clin Orthop Relat Res.* 1999;365:117–123.

248. Szuszczewicz ES, Schmalzried TP, Petersen TD. Progressive bilateral pelvic osteolysis in a patient with McKee-Farrar metal-metal total hip prostheses. *J Arthroplasty.* 1997;12:819–824.

249. Tharani R, Dorey FJ, Schmalzried TP. The risk of cancer following total hip or knee arthroplasty. *J Bone Joint Surg Am.* 2001;83A:774–780.

250. Thomas RH, Rademaker M, Goddard NJ, et al. Severe eczema of the hands due to an orthopaedic plate made of Vitallium. *BMJ (Clin Res Ed).* 1987;294:106–107.

251. Tipper JL, Hatton A, Nevelos JE, et al. Alumina-alumina artificial hip joints. Part II: Characterisation of the wear debris from in vitro hip joint simulations. *Biomaterials.* 2002;23:3441–3448.

252. Tipper JL, Ingham E, Hailey JL, et al. Quantitative comparison of polyethylene wear debris, wear rate and head damage in retrieved hip prostheses. *Trans Orthop Res Soc.* 1997;22:355.

253. Urban RM, Jacobs JJ, Gilbert JL, et al. Migration of corrosion products from modular hip prostheses. Particle microanalysis and histopathological findings. *J Bone Joint Surg Am.* 1994;76A: 1345–1359.

254. Urban RM, Jacobs JJ, Tomlinson MJ, et al. Dissemination of wear particles to the liver, spleen, and abdominal lymph nodes of patients with hip or knee replacement. *J Bone Joint Surg Am.* 2000;82A:457–476.

255. Urban RM, Jacobs JJ, Tomlinson MJ, et al. Particles of metal alloys and their corrosion products in the liver, spleen and para-aortic lymph nodes of patients with total hip replacement prostheses. *Trans Orthop Res Soc.* 1995;20:241.

256. Visuri T, Pukkala E, Paavolainen P, et al. Cancer risk after metal on metal and polyethylene on metal total hip arthroplasty. *Clin Orthop Relat Res.* 1996;329(suppl):S280–S289.

257. Volz RG, Wilson RJ. Factors affecting the mechanical stability of the cemented acetabular component in total hip replacement. *J Bone Joint Surg Am.* 1977;59A:501–504.

258. Wagner M, Wagner H. Medium-term results of a modern metal-on-metal system in total hip replacement. *Clin Orthop Relat Res.* 2000;379:123–133.

259. Wagner M, Wagner H. Preliminary results of uncemented metal on metal stemmed and resurfacing hip replacement arthroplasty. *Clin Orthop Relat Res.* 1996;329(suppl):S78–S88.

260. Walker PS, Gold BL. The tribology (friction, lubrication and wear) of all-metal artificial hip joints. *Wear.* 1971;17:285–299.

261. Walter A. On the material and the tribology of alumina-alumina couplings for hip joint prostheses. *Clin Orthop Relat Res.* 1992; 282:31–46.

262. Wang A, Essner A, Polineni VK, et al. Wear mechanisms and wear testing of ultra-high molecular weight polyethylene in total joint replacements. In: *Polyethylene Wear in Orthopaedic Implants Workshop.* Mt Laurel, NJ: Society for Biomaterials; 1997:4–18.

263. Weber BG. Experience with the Metasul total hip bearing system. *Clin Orthop Relat Res.* 1996;329(suppl):S69–S77.

264. Weightman B, Swanson SAV, Isaac GH, et al. Polyethylene wear from retrieved acetabular cups. *J Bone Joint Surg Br.* 1991;73B: 806–810.

265. Willert H, Buchorn G, Fayyazi A, et al. Histopathological changes around metal/metal joints indicate delayed type hypersensitivity. Primary results of 14 cases. *Osteologie.* 2000;9: 2–16.

266. Willert HG, Buchorn GH, Fayyazi A, et al. Histopathological changes in tissues surrounding metal/metal joints: signs of delayed type hypersensitivity (DTH)? In: Rieker C, Oberholzer S, Wyss U, eds. *World Tribology Forum in Arthroplasty*. Bern: Hans Huber; 2001:147–166.

267. Willert HG, Buchhorn GH, Gobel D, et al. Wear behavior and histopathology of classic cemented metal on metal hip endoprostheses. *Clin Orthop Relat Res*. 1996;329(suppl):S160–S186.

268. Williams IR, Mayor MB, Collier JP. The impact of sterilization method on wear in knee arthroplasty. *Clin Orthop Relat Res*. 1998;356:170–180.

269. Willmann G. Ceramic femoral head retrieval data. *Clin Orthop Relat Res*. 2000;379:22–28.

270. Wilson JN, Scales JT. Loosening of total hip replacements with cement fixation. Clinical findings and laboratory studies. *Clin Orthop Relat Res*. 1970;72:145–160.

271. Winter M, Griss P, Scheller G, et al. Ten- to 14-year results of a ceramic hip prosthesis. *Clin Orthop Relat Res*. 1992;282:73–80.

272. Wirganowicz PZ, Thomas BJ. Massive osteolysis after ceramic on ceramic total hip arthroplasty. A case report. *Clin Orthop Relat Res*. 1997;338:100–104.

273. Woolson ST, Murphy MG. Wear of the polyethylene of Harris-Galante acetabular components inserted without cement. *J Bone Joint Surg Am*. 1995;77A:1311–1314.

274. Wroblewski BM. Charnley low friction arthroplasty in patients under the age of 40 years. In: Sevastik J, Goldie I, eds. *The Young Patient with Degenerative Hip Disease*. Stockholm: Almquvist and Wiksell; 1985:197–201.

275. Wroblewski BM. Direction and rate of socket wear in Charnley low-friction arthroplasty. *J Bone Joint Surg Br*. 1985;67B:757–761.

276. Wroblewski BM. 15–21-year results of the Charnley low-friction arthroplasty. *Clin Orthop Relat Res*. 1986;211:30–35.

277. Wroblewski BM, McCullagh PJ, Siney PD. Quality of the surface finish of the head of the femoral component and the wear rate of the socket in long-term results of the Charnley low-friction arthroplasty. *Proc Inst Mech Eng H*. 1992;206:181–183.

278. Wroblewski BM, Siney PD, Dowson D, et al. Prospective clinical and joint simulator studies of a new total hip arthroplasty using alumina ceramic heads and cross-linked polyethylene cups. *J Bone Joint Surg Br*. 1996;78B:280–285.

279. Wroblewski BM, Siney PD, Fleming PA. Wear of enhanced ultra-high molecular-weight polyethylene (Hylamer) in combination with a 22.225 mm diameter zirconia femoral head. *J Bone Joint Surg Br*. 2003;85B:376–379.

280. Wroblewski BM, Taylor GW, Siney P. Charnley low-friction arthroplasty: 19- to 25-year results. *Orthopedics*. 1992;15:421–424.

281. Wyss U, Rieker C. Metal-on-metal hip articulation. Presented at: 32nd Annual Course, Advances in Hip and Knee Arthroplasty; 2002.

282. Yamaguchi M, Bauer TW, Hashimoto Y. Three-dimensional analysis of multiple wear vectors in retrieved acetabular cups. *J Bone Joint Surg Am*. 1997;79A:1539–1544.

283. Yamaguchi M, Hashimoto Y, Akisue T, et al. Polyethylene wear vector in vivo: a three-dimensional analysis using retrieved acetabular components and radiographs. *J Orthop Res*. 1999;17:695–702.

284. Yang SY, Ren W, Park Y, et al. Diverse cellular and apoptotic responses to variant shapes of UHMWPE particles in a murine model of inflammation. *Biomaterials*. 2002;23:3535–3543.

285. Yoon TR, Rowe SM, Jung ST, et al. Osteolysis in association with a total hip arthroplasty with ceramic bearing surfaces. *J Bone Joint Surg Am*. 1998;80A:1459–1468.

286. Young AM, Sychterz CJ, Hopper RHJ, et al. Effect of acetabular modularity on polyethylene wear and osteolysis in total hip arthroplasty. *J Bone Joint Surg Am*. 2002;84A:58–63.

287. Zahiri CA, Schmalzried TP, Ebramzadeh E, et al. Lessons learned from loosening of the McKee-Farrar metal-on-metal total hip replacement. *J Arthroplasty*. 1999;14:326–332.

288. Zichner LP, Willert HG. Comparison of alumina-polyethylene and metal-polyethylene in clinical trials. *Clin Orthop Relat Res*. 1992;282:86–94.

Particle Debris

21

Harlan Levine   *W. Timothy Ballard*
Arun Shanbhag   *Joshua J. Jacobs*

The generation of particulate debris is a central focus of attention in the arthroplasty literature. The biologic response to wear debris is currently heralded as the single most important factor limiting the long-term durability of contemporary total hip and total knee replacement arthroplasty (31,41,103).

This chapter provides an historical perspective on wear debris in total joint replacements; summarizes current understanding of the mechanisms of particle generation, methods of particle analysis, and recognized types of particles; and concludes with a discussion of the impact of these data on prosthetic design.

HISTORY

The vast majority of early total hip arthroplasty failures were a result of infection (20). Fortunately, modern aseptic techniques, in conjunction with prophylactic perioperative antibiotics, have led to a drastic reduction in the incidence of postoperative infection. Subsequently, the durability of total hip arthroplasty has been primarily limited by aseptic loosening. Aseptic failures of cemented arthroplasties were at one time thought to result from a biologic reaction to the cement, and the term "cement disease" was coined (61). This was among many factors that stimulated the development of cementless prostheses; however, reports of periprosthetic bone resorption around cementless implants led to the realization that particle debris from a variety of sources in the prosthetic joint, regardless of the presence or absence of cement, can stimulate osteolysis (10,11,57,59,70,72,73,100,104,116,124).

Whereas studies of the ramifications of particle debris have been a focus of research only in the last 1 to 2 decades, wear, corrosion, and the generation of particle debris have been recognized since the 1950s. The precursors of modern total hip prostheses were metal femoral and acetabular components. The early Stanmore design utilized a cobalt-chromium-molybdenum (Co-Cr-Mo) implant with a horseshoe-shaped acetabular component designed to approximate the native acetabular articular surface. This design feature was credited with the production of abundant metallic wear debris and was replaced with a hemispherical cup with a continuous concave surface (34). The McKee-Farar prosthesis, another early cobalt-chromium (Co-Cr) design, combined a femoral component with a spherical head and a metal acetabular component in order to provide a low-friction articulation. Nonetheless, this all-metal device likewise produced a great deal of metallic debris under certain circumstances (34).

Charnley, after his investigations into animal joint lubrication, proposed the use of a boundary between the articulating ball and socket to reduce friction between the surfaces (21). Charnley then revolutionized total hip prosthetic design with his description of low-friction arthroplasty (20). He applied the principles of low frictional torque in developing a prosthesis with a small, 22-mm head that articulated with a thick polytetrafluoroethylene (Teflon) cup. Teflon was later abandoned because of excessive wear and adverse soft-tissue reaction to this particulate wear debris (22,23,25). Other polymers have subsequently been tried as articular surfaces, including polyacetal, high-density polyethylene, and polyesters, but because of high rates of clinical failure they have been abandoned in favor of the ultra high molecular weight polyethylene (UHMWPE) used in contemporary prostheses (68,78,121).

GENERATION OF PARTICLES

Particles may be generated from joint replacement components by two distinct processes: corrosion and wear. Corrosion refers to electrochemical dissolution of a metal. Some authors consider oxidative degradation of polymeric substances a form of corrosion as well. Wear, defined as removal of material as a consequence of relative motion between two abutting surfaces, may occur by a variety of mechanisms, including abrasion, adhesion, and fatigue, and results in the generation of wear particles. Wear modes refer to the conditions under which prosthetic components function when wear occurs and have been categorized into four types. Mode 1 wear is the wear that results from two primary bearing surfaces articulating against each other as designed. Mode 2 wear is wear that results from a primary bearing articulating with a unintended surface (e.g., metal femoral head with metal acetabular shell after catastrophic liner failure). Mode 3 wear is wear that results from the interposition of a third body between two primary articular surfaces. This leads to the abrasion of one or both of the articular surfaces, which then may cause an increase in Mode 1 wear. Mode 4 wear is the wear that results from motion between two surfaces where motion was not intended (e.g., backside polyethylene wear, head–taper junction fretting, and acetabular shell–screw junction fretting). The wear particles from Mode 4 wear can migrate into the joint to create Mode 3 wear, which can then increase Mode 1 wear (103).

Abrasive wear occurs when two surfaces with microscopic irregularities, or asperities, slide past one another while in intimate contact. The interaction generates particles, generally from the softer of the two substances. Abrasion is further enhanced when a third body is present, effectively creating surfaces with greater surface area and greater irregularities. Particles generated from the articulating surfaces themselves may act as third bodies and interact with the bearing surfaces. This mechanism is thought to explain the high rate of wear seen with non-ion-implanted titanium, which, relative to stainless steel and Co-Cr, has been shown to have limited resistance to abrasive wear (35,79).

Adhesive wear occurs when two opposing materials bond under contact load. Actual transfer of material from one surface to the other may occur, forming so-called transfer films. With the reinitiation of motion between the surfaces, particles may be broken free from one or both surfaces. These new particles then further contribute to wear via an abrasive mechanism.

Fretting refers to small cyclic motions, typically less than 100 µm, of one surface relative to another (J. L. Gilbert, personal communication, 1996). Fatigue wear results from the initiation, propagation, and coalescence of subsurface cracks, with resultant release of particles.

The discussion of wear would not be complete without some mention of friction. Frictional force is proportional to the coefficient of friction for the contact surfaces and the normal component of the contact force between the articulating surfaces. Frictional forces may be dramatically altered by the interposition of lubricants between the two articulating surfaces. The lambda ratio (λ) refers to the ratio of fluid-film thickness to the surfaces roughness. Lambda values greater than 3 imply that the fluid-film thickness is greater then the height of asperities on the articular surface and represent fluid-film lubrication. Lambda values between 1 and 3 represent mixed film lubrication, and values less then 1 represent boundary lubrication. As gamma values increase, friction and therefore wear decrease (44).

Synovial fluid and various other lubricants, however, are viscoelastic; that is, their material properties vary according to the velocity at which they are loaded. Hence, the determination of friction in the setting of a total joint articulation is complicated. Although wear and the coefficient of friction have not been directly correlated (35,102), the nature of the lubricant likely influences the generation of wear debris. The variability between lubricants and their impact on wear is critically important when comparing data from different in vitro wear models.

Particles may also be generated by corrosion (54). This may occur by precipitation of metal ions with anions present in body fluids or by grain egression as a consequence of intergranular corrosion (38). Corrosion and wear may be synergistic. Wear effectively produces an expanded surface area for electrochemical reactions and thus may lead to the acceleration of corrosion. In addition, fretting can disrupt the passivating oxide films that protect cobalt- and titanium-based alloys from corrosion, dramatically accelerating the corrosion rate (54).

Fretting corrosion of modular implants has been recognized as an important source of particles (Fig. 21-1). The modularity of femoral implants allows the mixing of various metals, as in the common case where a Co-Cr prosthetic head and neck is combined with a titanium alloy stem. The occurrence and significance of mixed-metal corrosion in this setting are controversial. Levine and Staehle (67) reported an increased rate of corrosion when Co-Cr-Mo was coupled with titanium-aluminum-vanadium (Ti6Al4V) versus when it was coupled with itself or stainless steel. Co-Cr-Mo has also been reported to incite a more significant capsular response in dogs when coupled with Ti6Al4V compared with same-metal couples (96). On the other hand, electrochemical analyses of mixed-metal couples suggest no potential problems with couples of cobalt alloy and titanium alloy. Electrochemical open-circuit-potential measurement and potentiostatic passive film-corrosion measurement suggest that Co-Cr alloy and stainless steel couples are unstable whereas Co-Cr alloy and titanium couples are stable (35). In addition, studies of several modular prostheses in which both the head and the stem are composed of Co-Cr-Mo have demonstrated significant crevice corrosion (38,77,117). In fact, one study reported less corrosion of Ti6Al4V when coupled with Co-Cr-Mo than when it was coupled with itself (13).

ANALYSIS OF PARTICLES

Specimens for particle analysis are derived from one of several sources: revision surgery, autopsy (90,118), prostheses in joint simulators (83,98), and nonprosthetic configurations of a material (107). For the purpose of comparing data, it is vital to consider not only the source of the test material but the testing environment as well, including the type of lubricant used during testing (if any) and the magnitude and frequency of applied loads.

Wear debris evaluation begins with optical observation. Evaluation with the unaided eye provides subjective data on gross wear, fracture, large debris, and macroscopic tissue characterization. Limited information may be gained with the use of a low-power dissecting microscope. Further characterization of the surface may be accomplished by measuring surface roughness with an instrument such as the Rotary Talysurf,

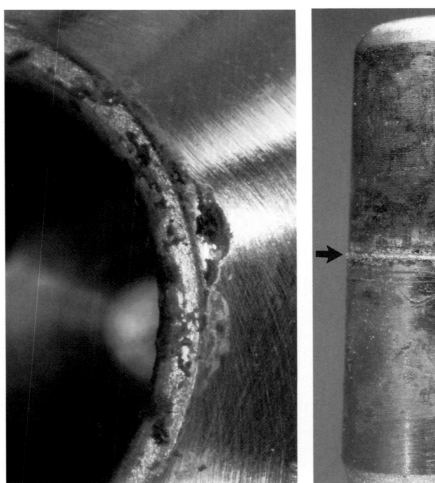
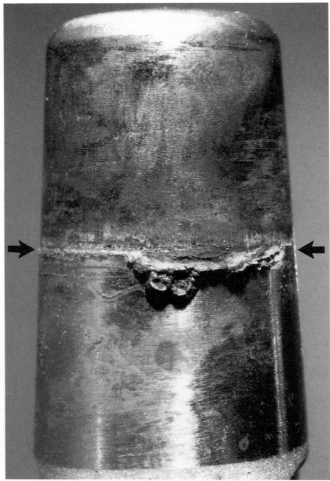

Figure 21-1 **A:** Dark green, glassy chromium-orthophosphate-hydrate–rich corrosion products deposited around the rim of the bore of a cobalt-chromium alloy head that was coupled with a titanium alloy stem (7×). **B:** Chromium-orthophosphate-hydrate–rich corrosion products circumscribing the neck of the prosthesis just distal to the head–neck junction (*arrows*) of a cobalt-chromium alloy femoral component (5×). (Reproduced with permission from Urban RM, Jacobs JJ, Gilbert JL, et al. Migration of corrosion products from modular hip prostheses. *J Bone Joint Surg.* 1994;76A:1345–1359.)

which permits measurements of roughness of 0.001 μm. Roughness standards have been established for orthopedic implant manufacturers, with an international standard of 0.05 mm set by the International Standards Organization for the surface finish and geometry of metallic components (53). The standard attained in practice for Charnley femoral heads is 0.025 mm (53).

Particles from tissue samples may be further examined microscopically, either within the tissue or after isolation from the tissue. For light microscopy, tissues can be processed routinely with formalin fixatives and paraffin embedding prior to sectioning and staining (Fig. 21-2). Polarized light techniques are particularly useful for visualization of UHMWPE (Fig. 21-3). Evaluation using these techniques is limited by artifacts introduced during processing and sectioning as well as by the fact that certain clearing agents used during paraffin processing, such as xylene, dissolve polymethylmethacrylate (PMMA) bone (19,121). Moreover, it has become increasingly apparent that the majority of particles are smaller than the limits of res-

olution for light microscopy (74,75,110). Oil red O, a common lipid stain, will also stain UHMWPE particles, but it is not as specific for their identification as oil immersion and polarized light (105).

Alternatively, tissues may be digested and particles isolated prior to evaluation. Although this further avoids some of the potential artifacts mentioned, it may introduce others. Nonetheless, these techniques permit the utilization of other analytic evaluation methodologies, such as scanning electron microscopy (SEM) and Fourier transform infrared spectroscopy. Metallic debris may be easily isolated from tissues with commercially available reagents and subsequent centrifugation (18,75,108). UHMWPE, however, is sensitive to certain reagents, and it is less dense than water, making it difficult to isolate by routine processing and centrifugation. Residue from papain, a proteolytic enzyme, tends to dry around UHMWPE and metal particles, making them difficult to accurately identify and measure (18). Soluene (Packard Chemical, IL, a solution of toluene and ammonium hydroxide,

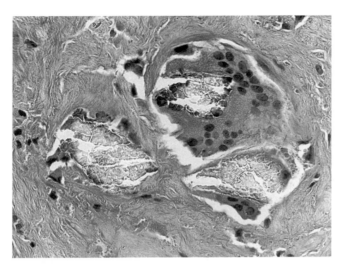

Figure 21-2 Light micrograph of foreign-body giant cells surrounding 50- to 70-μm chromium-orthophosphate-hydrate–rich particles in an area of marked fibrosis in the pseudocapsule (500×). (Reproduced with permission from Urban RM, Jacobs JJ, Gilbert JL, et al. Migration of corrosion products from modular hip prostheses. *J Bone Joint Surg.* 1994;76A:1345–1359.)

is particularly corrosive and therefore is not appropriate for certain filtration procedures. In addition, Soluene and hydroxide preparations may cause clumping of metal and UHMWPE debris. Campbell et al. (18) reported that this effect could be significantly overcome by extensive hot water washes and ultrasonication, but this is time consuming and results in loss of some of the product. Campbell et al. (19) subsequently refined the technique by performing density gradient ultracentrifugation of the digested tissues with a variable sucrose gradient. This technique has successfully yielded uncontaminated UHMWPE particles. Shanbhag et al. (110) used potassium hydroxide as a digestive agent, followed by extensive washing of the particles in distilled water. Using high-speed centrifugation in 95% ethyl alcohol, they essentially eliminated the loss of fine particles. They also routinely ultrsonicated the debris to prevent clumping and facilitate particle washing. Then by incorporating a hexane and ethyl alcohol separation technique, they were able to separate the UHMWPE particles from the remaining debris, permitting their more detailed evaluation. Alternatively, nitric acid digestion has been shown to eliminate calcium phosphate and hemosiderin contaminants while not altering the size or morphology of UHMWPE or metal particles (75).

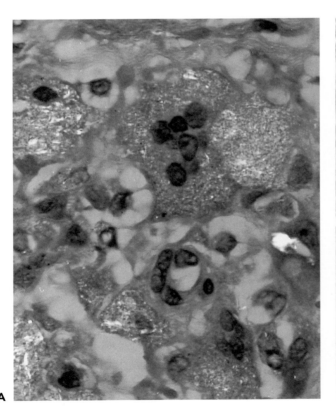

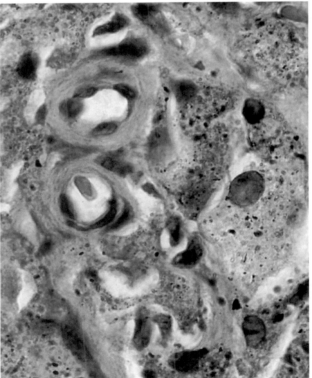

A   B

Figure 21-3 Photomicrograph of periprosthetic interfacial tissue removed from a failed cementless **(A)** and a failed cemented **(B)** total hip arthroplasty (50×). Numerous submicron birefringent particles, most likely polyethylene, are demonstrated by polarized light in A. Numerous dark metallic intracellular particles are also well visualized with nonpolarized light in B. (Reproduced with permission from Glant TT, Jacobs JJ, Mikecz K, et al. Particulate-induced, prostaglandin- and cytokine-mediated bone resorption in an experimental system and in failed joint replacements. *Am J Ther.* 1996;3:27–41.)

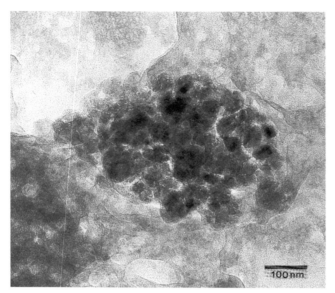

Figure 21-4 Transmission electron micrograph of intracellular particles aggregated within a histiocyte of an osteolytic lesion (100,000×). (Reproduced with permission from Urban RM, Jacobs JJ, Gilbert JL, et al. Migration of corrosion products from modular hip prostheses. *J Bone Joint Surg.* 1994;76A:1345–1359.)

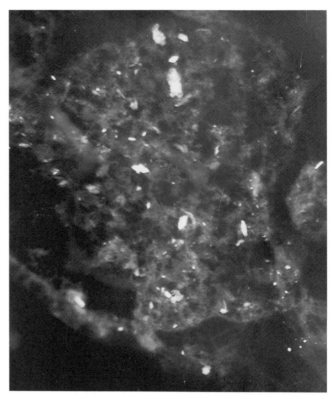

Figure 21-5 Back-scattered electron micrograph showing intracellular cobalt alloy particles 0.2 to 2.5 μm in size (20,000×). (Reproduced with permission from Jacobs JJ, Urban RM, Wall J, et al. Unusual foreign-body reaction to a failed total knee replacement: simulation of a sarcoma clinically and a sarcoid histologically. *J Bone Joint Surg.* 1995;77A:444–451.)

Particles may be identified and measured by several techniques. Transmission electron microscopy (TEM) allows qualitative visualization of intra- and extracellular particles (Fig. 21-4). Various computer-assisted image analyzers provide assistance in determining the two-dimensional measurements of a particular particle. However, it is difficult to measure particles with TEM because of the thinness of the sections, which are generally less than 0.1 mm. SEM overcomes some of these limitations (Fig. 21-5). Electronic sizing of isolated particles may also be accomplished with the use of laser scatter and electrozone techniques. Unfortunately, the accuracy of these measures has been recently called into question. Bobyn et al. (7) reported variable results not only when comparing the results of different methods used on the same solution but also when comparing the results of the same methods performed with different pieces of equipment.

Qualitative identification of particles requires different instruments. Whereas electron microscopy provides data on the morphology of particles, it does not by itself permit identification of their constituents. Fourier transform infrared spectroscopy, energy-dispersive x-ray spectroscopy, electron diffraction, and differential scanning calorimetry provide useful qualitative data for establishing the elemental identity of various particles (19,55,75,110).

No longer is particle analysis confined to periprosthetic tissue samples. Studies have shown sizable concentrations of metallic debris from primary total joint arthroplasties not only in regional lymph nodes, which drain prosthetic joints directly, but also in distant axillary lymph nodes (111). Furthermore, particles from less than 1 mm to greater than 7 mm in size of Co-Cr, stainless steel, commercially pure titanium, and Ti6Al4V alloy have been discovered in histiocytes from hepatic, splenic, and lymphatic tissues retrieved at autopsy from joint arthroplasty patients (119). Particles were

observed more frequently in association with multiple implants, revision total hip arthroplasty, long-duration primary arthroplasties, and periprosthetic wires or cables.

TYPES OF PARTICLES

Current data suggest that tissues adjacent to a failed joint prosthesis contain billions of particles per gram of tissue (74,75). A wide variety of particle types have been retrieved from periprosthetic tissues at the time of autopsy or revision, as well as from joint simulators. In general, these particles types may be classified as metallic, polymeric, and ceramic.

The majority of reports on periprosthetic metal debris pertain to Co-Cr and titanium (15,29). Metallic particles are characteristically gray to black, and although they may appear weakly birefringent under polarized microscopy, the appearance of birefringence is an optical artifact because the particles are actually opaque (102). Savio et al. (102) reported that metal particles are generally smaller than polymer particles but larger than ceramic particles. Submicrometer metallic particles have been described as globular or irregularly shaped as well as elongated with sharp corners (74,102). Larger Co-Cr particles, in the 1- to 5-μm size range, have been described more often as needle, rod, or splinter shaped (24,33,85,102). Even larger Co-Cr particles, from 5 μm to over 1 mm, have been described as irregularly shaped or globular. These particles tend to be extracellular and may actually represent aggregates or clusters of smaller particles (8,29,60,82).

The majority of titanium particles likewise range from under a micrometer to less than 5 μm in size (1,15,29,89,101) and have been described as blackish-gray material and fine powder (102). Occasional titanium particles from 5 μm up to 1 mm in size have been reported (6,29,82,110). A study by Maloney et al. (74) found the mean size of metallic particles to be 0.7 μm, and they suggested that previously reported techniques (using 4 M potassium hydroxide) may have caused dissolution of these smaller particles, leading to an underestimation of their mass.

The most common polymer particles encountered in association with joint prostheses are PMMA and UHMWPE particles. It has been suggested that their similarly birefringent appearance under polarized light may lead to confusion (102); however, PMMA, unlike UHMWPE, is normally not birefringent.

There are several potential sources of PMMA particles, including intraoperative debris, fatigue failure of cement, and fretting of bone–cement and prosthesis–cement interfaces. In addition, unconsolidated or poorly mixed PMMA may release 25- to 35-μm "prepolymerized spheres" (102). As mentioned in the previous section, certain elements of tissue processing for light microscopy dissolve PMMA, and therefore it may be represented by histologic voids, ranging from less than 1 μm (2) to greater than 1 mm in size (102). The particles or voids are irregularly shaped and have been described as multifaceted or resembling slivers of glass (14). Barium sulfate or zirconium oxide, which have been added to most PMMA since the 1970s to permit visualization of the cement on radiographs, has been reported in tissue voids left by PMMA (5,46,86,75,121).

UHMWPE debris is translucent and strongly birefringent under polarized light microscopy. The particles from the femoral area of aseptically loose femoral components are predominantly spherical or globular in shape, ranging from 0.1 to 1 μm, with a mean of 0.5 μm. Over 90% of these particles are less than 1 μm in size (18,74,75,110). The spherical particles are also associated with fibrillar attachments, either singly or forming aggregates of fine particles (45,48). The fibrils ranged from 0.3 to 1.0 μm wide to 10 to 25 μm in length (27,110). Debris over 100 μm in length have been described as large shards, shredded fibers, and flattened UHMWPE rolled in the articulation and resembling cigars (32,46,110).

UHMWPE debris is also detected in the empty screw holes of metal-backed acetabular components (73). UHMWPE in such locations behind stable components is also reported to be in the form of essentially spherical particles and aggregates of finer particles with fibrillar attachments (106). Despite the morphologic similarity, these UHMWPE particles are marginally larger than particles around femoral components. This distinction in the size of the particles at the two sites is important because several investigators have demonstrated that there is a relationship between particle size and bioreactivity, with phagocytosable debris much more bioreactive.

There has been great recent interest in the use of highly cross-linked UHMWPE in total joint arthroplasty as a means of decreasing the wear rates of the polyethylene bearing surfaces. It is known that the mechanical properties of UHMWPE are directly related to its molecular weight, crystalline ultra-

sturcture, chemical structure, and thermal history (64). The increased intramolecular cross-links of highly cross-linked UHMWPE are thought to better resist deformation and wear. In hip simulator studies, highly cross-linked polyethylene has shown up to 95% less wear than conventional UHMWPE (58,81) Using radiographic analysis to compare the wear rates of highly cross-linked polyethylene with those of conventional polyethylene, Martell et al. (75) demonstrated a reduction in the two- and three-dimensional wear rates of 42% and 50%, respectively. Muratoglu et al. (88), in a retrieval study, proposed that the early surface damage of acetabular liners is the result of plastic deformation in highly cross-linked polyethylene whereas it is more likely secondary to loss of material in conventional UHMWPE.

While early data indicate that highly cross-linked polyethylene may have better wear characteristics than conventional UHMWPE, there is a paucity of data demonstrating the in vivo effects of the wear particles from highly cross-linked polyethylene bearing surfaces. Studies show that the wear particles from highly cross-linked polyethylene are smaller (often in the submicrometer and nanometer range) than those from conventional UHMWPE (30,49,50,92). Controversy exists regarding the ability of these submicrometer particles to generate the inflammatory response that ultimately results in osteolysis. Green et al. (39) showed that smaller polyethylene particles (0.24 mm vs. 0.45 mm) generated less bone resorption in a cell culture study. Similarly, Illgen et al. (49) demonstrated in a cell culture study that the wear products of highly cross-linked polyethylene have a biologic reactivity similar to that of the wear products of conventional UHMWPE. However, other authors have found that submicrometer particles may induce a greater inflammatory response than smaller particles (30,49–51).

It is well known that particle morphology can strongly influence biological response. Yang et al. (125) demonstrated that elongated particles of UHMWPE were more biologically active than globular particles. The short-term data for highly cross-linked polyethylene is encouraging, but longer term clinical follow-up is necessary before any definitive conclusions can be formed regarding its ability to perform as a durable bearing surface while minimizing the generation of wear particles and the ensuing biologic response resulting in osteolysis.

A resurgence of interest in ceramic articulating surfaces has been driven by various reports of their excellent wear characteristics (28,97,99). Still, ceramic wear debris is reported, and particles are most commonly 1 to 5 μm in size (91). In a study of tissue retrieved at the time of revision, Hatton et al. (43) found a bimodal distribution of sizes of ceramic wear debris. Using SEM (low resolution), ceramic particles between 0.05 and 3.2 μm were found. Using TEM (high resolution), particles between 5 and 90 nm were visualized. It was theorized that the larger particles were generated from microseparation and impaction of the ceramic surfaces and that the smaller particles were generated from normal articulation of the bearing surfaces.

While often thought of as inert, ceramic wear debris may be able to generate a biologic response that leads to osteolysis (122,126), and recent studies have shown that ceramic particles can incite inflammatory and cytotoxic effects (36,42). Hatton et al. (42) demonstrated that tissues from around ceramic–ceramic hips had areas rich in macrophages, large amounts of neutrophils and lymphocytes, and areas with up to 60% necrosis/necrobiosis. The control group, tissue from Charnley metal-on-poly hips, showed the presence of giant cells and a dense macrophage infiltrate, but there was less than 30% necrosis/necrobiosis. There were significantly more neutrophils in the ceramic–ceramic tissues and significantly more macrophages and giant cells in the metal-on-poly group.

In certain clinical settings, relatively large numbers of particles of corrosion products have also been identified. Chromium-orthophosphate-hydrate–rich particles were noted at the modular prosthetic head–neck junction, in the UHMWPE liner, and in the pseudocapsule around the prosthesis (56,117,120). In fact, in certain cases, chromium orthophosphate was second only to UHMWPE in number of intracellular particles found in periprosthetic tissues. The vast majority of chromium orthophosphate particles are less than 5 μm, and they are described as noncrystalline, translucent, and colorless (117).

In addition to particles arising from the prosthesis or cement, certain anomalous particles have also been described. Silica has been reported in interfacial membranes, most likely a remnant of the catalyst used in UHMWPE manufacturing or a remnant of the sandblasting of metal prosthetic components (57,110). These are likely sources of trace amounts of aluminum as well. Furthermore, iron- and nickel-containing particles (stainless steel) were likely contaminants from surgical instruments. Calcium- and phosphorous-rich particles were noted and, judging from the ratio of their concentrations, were probably from bone mineral. Thus, bone particles are also present in the periprosthetic milieu. Although these anomalous particles may constitute only a small percentage of the overall particle burden, they may be important because of their propensity to act as third bodies, thereby increasing UHMWPE wear.

DESIGN CONSIDERATIONS

Although all components of the total hip prosthetic construct are susceptible to wear, the vast majority of particles recovered from membranes around contemporary prostheses are composed of UHMWPE (110). The design features affecting UHMWPE wear are currently a primary engineering focus. Increased rate of penetration of the femoral head into the UHMWPE has been correlated with increased rim wear of the acetabular component and with decreased survivorship of the prosthesis (53). The wear characteristics of UHMWPE have been shown to vary according to the age of the implant (94), the mode of sterilization (9,93–95), the method of implant fabrication (4), the thickness of the UHMWPE, and the presence or absence of a metal backing for the acetabular component (4). In study groups matched for age, weight, gender, and length of follow-up, machined UHMWPE was shown by Bankston et al. (4) to be associated with significantly greater wear than compression-molded UHMWPE.

The use of gamma radiation for sterilization of UHMWPE has been shown to result in increased cross-linking as well as scission of polymer chains, with resultant changes in crystallinity and water absorption (94,112). Rose et al. (95) subsequently demonstrated increased UHMWPE wear following

20-Mrad doses of gamma irradiation in air, whereas no significant differences were noted between unirradiated material and specimens irradiated with 2.5 Mrad, a dose commonly used for sterilization. Furthermore, the density of UHMWPE increases with time after gamma ray sterilization (9,93,94), and the changes in density are more pronounced at the surface than deeper in the substance, according to in vitro (93) and in vivo analyses (9). The increased density at the articulating surface appears to further increase stiffness and decrease ductility, thereby increasing contact stress and accelerating wear (94). However, gamma irradiation in inert gas environments, such as argon, may actually be associated with decreased wear by virtue of increasing cross-linking while minimizing oxidation (40,113).

Like the surface finish of the UHMWPE, the surface roughness of the femoral head may affect the rate of prosthetic wear. Nonetheless, irregularity of the surface finish of the prosthetic femoral head has not been directly correlated with increased UHMWPE wear or particle generation.

Cement and corrosion particles have access to the joint and have been found implanted in the UHMWPE (3,52,53,117). Increased wear has been associated with such implanted debris (52). Wroblewski et al. (123) performed detailed analyses of the articular surface of the UHMWPE and femoral head of hips revised for aseptic loosening of the femoral prosthesis with minimal UHMWPE penetration (average, 0.022 mm per year) radiographically and found excellent surface finish on the femoral head. In addition, minimal particulate implantation into the UHMWPE had occurred.

The optimal prosthetic femoral head diameter is controversial. Müller introduced a prosthesis with a 32-mm head, intended to provide increased hip stability and decreased UHMWPE wear (87). Livermore et al. (69) later reported greater volumetric wear with 32-mm heads than with 22- or 28-mm heads and reported the highest linear wear rate with 22-mm heads. Following this report, many surgeons turned to 28-mm heads. However, recent 20-year reports of excellent clinical results with the 22.25-mm head Charnley prosthesis further complicated the issue (16), which remains controversial.

The use of modular heads in total hip implants affords the surgeon flexibility in choosing head diameter and neck length while minimizing hospital inventory. Cyclic loading of this interface has been shown to yield abundant metallic particles in the range of sizes shown to be biologically active (7,26). In addition, fretting and crevice corrosion at this interface have been reported (37,54,71,77,80,115). These particles are important for two reasons. First, they may contribute to accelerated UHMWPE wear via third-body abrasion. Second, they may themselves contribute to macrophage stimulation and osteoclastic bone resorption (56,65).

Choice of materials is of utmost importance. Stainless steel has been generally abandoned in the United States for use hip prostheses and replaced with Co-Cr and titanium alloys. Despite easy machinability and low tissue reactivity, pure titanium is not a good choice for articulating surfaces because it is prone to fretting and has poor abrasion resistance. The wear properties, however, are greatly improved when titanium is anodized or ion-implanted (13,48).

In the 1970s, ceramic hip prostheses were introduced. Ceramic femoral heads possess excellent scratch resistance and therefore are capable of providing and maintaining an extremely smooth articulating surface. Hip joint simulator studies have demonstrated very encouraging wear characteristics for ceramic compared with metallic prostheses (28,97,99). Ceramic heads retrieved at revision and examined by SEM appear to maintain their smoothness and sphericity (114). Despite the potential benefits of improved wear characteristics, concern has arisen regarding catastrophic failure of these devices in vivo (17,45,62,84). Zirconia ceramic is a recently introduced alternative to alumina ceramic: it boasts decreased susceptibility to fracture while maintaining excellent wear characteristics. Unfortunately, fractures of zirconia have also been reported (47). Further, improvements in long-term clinical survivorship have not been demonstrated. In addition, the recent withdrawal of zirconia heads from the marketplace due to poor performance associated with a processing alteration has diminished enthusiasm for this material.

CONCLUSION

Recent data have contributed significantly to our understanding of the tribology of materials, the generation of periprosthetic particle debris, and the tissue response to particles. Advanced techniques of tissue digestion and high-resolution microscopy and spectroscopy have led to an increased appreciation for periprosthetic wear debris. The true volume of wear debris went unrecognized prior to the innovations of the past decade.

Whereas UHMWPE is the predominant particle type in the majority of joint replacement arthroplasties, large volumes of PMMA, bone, metals, and other species have been noted in certain clinical settings. Recent studies have focused on the size and quantity of particles. However, current data suggest that biologic responses are dictated not only by particle size but also by particle composition and surface properties (109). Future research should therefore be directed not only at particle sizing and quantification but also at determining the elemental composition, the surface morphology, and the nature of the organic surface deposits that these particles display. In vitro and in vivo animal experimentation requires the fabrication and procurement of particles similar to those produced by implants using techniques such as those developed by Leigh et al. (66), Buchhorn et al. (12), and Shanbhag et al. (107).

Many structural and material choices in prosthetic design reflect the data discussed herein. At our present level of understanding, particle debris is a key factor limiting the longevity of total hip arthroplasty and will therefore be the focus of many future research endeavors.

REFERENCES

1. Agins JH, Alcock NW, Bansal M, et al. Metallic wear in failed titanium-alloy total hip replacements. *J Bone Joint Surg.* 1988;70A: 347–356.
2. Anthony PP, Gie GA, Howie CR, et al. Localized endosteal bone lysis in relation to the femoral components of cemented total hip arthroplasties. *J Bone Joint Surg.* 1990;72B:971–979.
3. Atkinson JR, Dowson D, Isaac GH, et al. Laboratory wear tests and clinical observations of the penetration of femoral heads into acetabular cups in total replacement hip joints, II: explanted Charnley sockets after 2–16 years in vivo and determination of wear factors. *Wear.* 1985;104:225–244.
4. Bankston AB, Cates H, Ritter MA, et al. Polyethylene wear in total hip arthroplasty. *Clin Orthop.* 1995;317:7–13.
5. Betts F, Wright T, Slavati EA, et al. Cobalt-alloy metal debris in periarticular tissues from total hip revision arthroplasties: metal contents and associated histologic finding. *Clin Orthop.* 1992;276:75–82.
6. Black J, Sherk H, Bonini J, et al. Metallosis associated with a stable titanium-alloy femoral component in total hip replacement. *J Bone Joint Surg.* 1990;72A:126–130.
7. Bobyn JD, Tanzer M, Kryugier JJ, et al. Concerns with modularity in total hip arthroplasty. *Clin Orthop.* 1994;298:27–36.
8. Bos I, Johannisson R, Lohrs U, et al. Comparative investigations of regional lymph nodes and pseudocapsules after implantation of joint endoprostheses. *Pathol Res Pract.* 1990;186:707–716.
9. Bostrom MP, Bennett AP, Rimnac CM, et al. The natural history of ultra high molecular weight polyethylene. *Clin Orthop.* 1994;309:20–28.
10. Brown IW, Ring PA. Osteolytic changes in the upper femoral shaft following porous-coated hip replacement. *J Bone Joint Surg.* 1985;67B:218–221.
11. Buchert PK, Vaughn BK, Mallory TH, et al. Excessive metal release due to loosening and fretting of sintered particles on porous-coated hip replacement. *J Bone Joint Surg.* 1986;68A: 606–609.
12. Buchhorn GH, Willert HG, Semlitsch M, et al. Preparation, characterization, and animal testing for biocompatibility of metal particles of iron-, cobalt-, and titanium-based implant alloys. In: St. John KR, ed. *Particulate Debris from Medical Implants: Mechanisms of Formation and Biological Consequences.* Philadelphia: American Society for Testing and Materials; 1992: 177–188. ASTM Special Technical Publication 1144.
13. Budinski GK. Tribological properties of titanium alloys. *Wear.* 1991;151:203–217.
14. Bullough PG. Tissue reaction to wear debris generated from total hip replacements. In: *The Hip.* St. Louis: Mosby; 1973:80–91.
15. Bullough PG, DiCarlo EF, Hansraj KK, et al. Pathologic studies of total joint replacement. *Orthop Clin North Am.* 1988;19:611–625.
16. Callaghan JJ, Pederson DR, Olejniczak JP, et al. Radiographic measurement of wearing: 5 cohorts of patients observed for 5 to 22 years. *Clin Orthop.* 1995;317:14–18.
17. Callaway GH, Flynn W, Ranawat CS, et al. Fracture of the femoral head after ceramic-on-polyethylene total hip arthroplasty. *J Arthroplasty.* 1995;10:855–859.
18. Campbell P, Ma S, Schmalzried TP, et al. Technical note: tissue digestion for wear debris particle isolation. *J Biomed Mater Res.* 1994;28:523–526.
19. Campbell P, Ma S, Yeom B, et al. Isolation of predominantly submicron-sized UHMWPE wear particles from periprosthetic tissues. *J Biomed Mater Res.* 1995;29:127–131.
20. Charnley J. Arthroplasty of the hip. A new operation. *Lancet.* 1961;1:1129.
21. Charnley J. The lubrication of animal joints in relation to surgical reconstruction by arthroplasty. *Ann Rheum Dis.* 1960;19:10–19.
22. Charnley J. Stainless steel for femoral hip prostheses in combination with a high density polythene socket. *J Bone Joint Surg.* 1971;53B:342–343.
23. Charnley J. Tissue reactions to polytetrafluoroethylene. *Lancet.* 1963;2:1379.
24. Charosky CB, Bullough PG, Wilson PD. Total hip replacement failures: a histological evaluation. *J Bone Joint Surg.* 1973;55A:49–58.
25. Clarke IC, Kabo JM. Wear in total hip replacement. In: Amstutz HA, ed. *Hip Arthroplasty.* New York: Churchill Livingstone; 1991:535–553.
26. Cook SD, Barrack RL, Baffes GC, et al. Wear and corrosion of modular interfaces in total hip replacements. *Clin Orthop.* 1994;298:80–88.
27. Dannenmaier WC, Haynes DW, Nelson CL. Granulomatous reaction and cystic bony destruction associated with high wear rate in a total knee prosthesis. *Clin Orthop.* 1985;198:224–230.
28. Derbyshire B, Fisher J, Dowson D, et al. Comparative study of the wear of UHMWPE with zirconia ceramic and stainless steel femoral heads in artificial hip joints. *Med Eng Phys.* 1994;16: 229–236.
29. Dorr LD, Bloebaum R, Emmanual J, et al. Histologic, biochemical, and ion analysis of tissue and fluids retrieved during total hip arthroplasty. *Clin Orthop.* 1990;261:82–95.

30. Endo M, Tipper JL, Barton DC, et al. Comparison of wear, wear debris and functional biological activity of moderately crosslinked and non-crosslinked polyethylenes in hip prostheses. *Proc Inst Mech Eng [H].* 2002;216:111–122.

31. Engh CA Jr, Claus AM, Hopper RH Jr, et al. Long-term results using the anatomic medullary locking hip prosthesis. *Clin Orthop.* 2001;No. 393:137–146.

32. Evans CH, Mears DC. The wear particles of synovial fluid: their ferrographic analysis and pathophysiological significance. *Bull Prosthet Res.* 1981;18:13–26.

33. Evans EM, Freeman MAR, Miller AJ, et al. Metal sensitivity as a cause of bone necrosis and loosening of the prosthesis in total joint replacement. *J Bone Joint Surg.* 1974;56B:626–642.

34. Fielding JW, Stillwell WT. The evolution of total hip arthroplasty. In: Stillwell, Chandler, eds. *The Art of Total Hip Arthroplasty.* Orlando: 1987:1.

35. Galante JO, Rostoker W. Wear in total hip prostheses. *Acta Orthop Scand.* 1973;145(suppl):6–46.

36. Germain MA, Hatton A, Williams S, et al. Comparison of the cytotoxicity of clinically relevant cobalt-chromium and alumina ceramic wear particles in vitro. *Biomaterials.* 2003;24: 469–479.

37. Gilbert JL, Buckley CA, Jacobs JJ. In vivo corrosion of modular hip prosthesis components in mixed and similar metal combinations: the effect of crevice, stress, motion, and alloy coupling. *J Biomed Mater Res.* 1993;27(12):1533–1544.

38. Gilbert JL, Buckley CA, Jacobs JJ, et al. Intergranular corrosion–fatigue failure of cobalt-alloy femoral stems: a failure analysis of two implants. *J Bone Joint Surg.* 1994;76A:110–121.

39. Green TR, Fisher J, Matthews JB, et al. Effect of size and dose on bone resorption activity of macrophages by in vitro clinically relevant ultra high molecular weight polyethylene particles. *J Biomed Mater Res.* 2000;53:490–497.

40. Hamilton J, Schmidt M, Greer K. Improved wear of UHMWPE using a vacuum sterilization process. *Trans Orthop Res Soc.* 1996;21:20.

41. Hartley WT, McAuley JP, Culpepper WJ, et al. Osteonecrosis of the femoral head treated with cementless total hip arthroplasty. *J Bone Joint Surg.* 2000;82A:1408–1413.

42. Hatton A, Nevelos JE, Matthews JB, et al. Effects of clinically relevant alumina ceramic wear particles on TNF-alpha production by human peripheral blood mononuclear phagocytes. *Biomaterials.* 2003;24:1193–1204.

43. Hatton A, Nevelos JE, Nevelos AA, et al. Alumina-alumina artificial hip joints, I: a histological analysis and characterisation of wear debris by laser capture microdissection of tissues retrieved at revision. *Biomaterials.* 2002;23:3429–3440.

44. Heisel C, Silva M, Schmalzried TP. Bearing surface options for total hip replacement in young patients *J Bone Joint Surg.* 2003;85A:1366–1379.

45. Higuchi F, Shiba N, Inoue A, et al. Fracture of an alumina ceramic head in total hip arthroplasty. *J Arthroplasty.* 1995;10:851–854.

46. Howie DW, Cornish BL, Vernon-Roberts B. Resurfacing hip arthroplasty: classification of loosening and the role of prosthesis wear particles. *Clin Orthop.* 1990;255:144–159.

47. Hummer CD, Rothman RH, Hozack WJ. Catastrophic failure of modular zirconia-ceramic femoral head components after total hip arthroplasty. *J Arthroplasty.* 1995;10:848–850.

48. Hutchings R, Oliver WC. A study of the improved wear performance of nitrogen-implanted Ti-6Al-4V. *Wear.* 1983;92:143–153.

49. Illgen RL, Laurent MP, Watanuki M, et al. Highly crosslinked vs. conventional polyethylene particles: an in vitro comparison of biologic activities. *Trans Orthop Res Soc.* 2003;28:1438.

50. Ingram JH, Fisher J, Stone M, et al. Effect of crosslinking on biological activity of UHMWPE wear debris. *Trans Orthop Res Soc.* 2003;28:1439.

51. Ingram J, Matthews JB, Tipper J, et al. Comparison of the biological activity of grade GUR 1120 and GUR 415HP UHMWPE wear debris. *Biomed Mater Eng.* 2002;12:177–88.

52. Isaac GH, Atkinson JR, Dowson D, et al. The role of cement in the long term performance and premature failure of the Charnley low-friction arthroplasties. *Eng Med.* 1986;15:19–22.

53. Isaac GH, Wroblewski BM, Atkinson JR, et al. A tribological study of retrieved hip prostheses. *Clin Orthop.* 1992;276:115–125.

54. Jacobs JJ, Gilbert JL, Urban RM. Corrosion of metallic implants. In: Stauffer RN, ed. *Advances in Operative Orthopaedics.* Vol. 2. St. Louis: Mosby; 1994:279–319.

55. Jacobs JJ, Shanbhag A, Glant TT, et al. Wear debris in total joint replacements. *J Am Acad Orthop Surg.* 1994;2:212–220.

56. Jacobs JJ, Urban RM, Otterness I, et al. Biological activity of particulate chromium-phosphate corrosion products. *Trans Soc Biomater.* 1995;18:398.

57. Jacobs JJ, Urban RM, Schajowicz F, et al. Particulate-associated endosteal osteolysis in titanium-base alloy cementless total hip replacement. In: St. John KR, ed. Particulate debris from medical implants: mechanisms of formation and biological consequences. Philadelphia: American Society for Testing and Materials; 1992:52–60. ASTM Special Technical Publication 1144.

58. Jasty M, Bragdon C, O'Connor DO, et al. Marked improvement in the wear resistance of a new form of UHMWPE in a physiologic hip simulator. *Trans Soc Biomater.* 1997;20:157.

59. Jasty MJ, Floyd WE III, Schiller AL, et al. Localized osteolysis in stable, non-septic total hip replacement. *J Bone Joint Surg.* 1986;68A:912–919.

60. Johanson NA, Bullough PG, Wilson PD, et al. The microscopic anatomy of the bone-cement interface in failed total hip arthroplasties. *Clin Orthop.* 1987;No. 218:123–135.

61. Jones LC, Hungerford DS. Cement disease. *Clin Orthop.* 1987;225:192–206.

62. Krikler S, Schatzker J. Ceramic head failure. *J Arthroplasty.* 1995;10:860–862.

63. Kummer FJ, Rose RM. Corrosion of titanium/cobalt-alloy couples. *J Bone Joint Surg.* 1983;65A:1125–1126.

64. Kurtz SM, Muratoglu OK, Evans M, et al. Advances in the processing, sterilization, and crosslinking of ultra-high molecular weight polyethylene for total joint arthroplasty. *Biomaterials.* 1999;20:1659–1688.

65. Lee SH, Brennan FR, Jacobs JJ, et al. Human monocyte/macrophage response to cobalt-chromium corrosion products and titanium particles in patients with total joint replacements. *J Orthop Res.* 1997;15:40–49.

66. Leigh HD, Taylor P, Swaney A, et al. Research and development report: production of fine particulate ultra high molecular weight poly(ethylene) for biological response studies. *J Appl Biomater.* 1992;3:77–80.

67. Levine DL, Staehle RW. Crevice corrosion in orthopaedic implant metals. *J Biomed Mater. Res.* 1977;11:553–561.

68. Li SL, Burstein AH. Current concepts review. Ultra-high molecular weight polyethylene: the material and its use in total joint implants. *J Bone Joint Surg.* 1994;76A:1080–1090.

69. Livermore J, Ilstrup D, Morrey B. Effect of femoral head size on wear of the polyethylene acetabular component. *J Bone Joint Surg.* 1990;72A:518–523.

70. Lombardi AV, Mallory TH, Vaughn BK, et al. Aseptic loosening in total hip arthroplasty secondary to osteolysis induced by wear debris from titanium-alloy modular femoral heads. *J Bone Joint Surg.* 1989;71A:1337–1342.

71. Lucas LC, Buchanan RA, Lemons JE. Investigations on the galvanic corrosion of multi-alloy total hip prostheses. *J Biomed Mater Res.* 1981;15:731.

72. Maloney WJ, Jasty M, Harris WH, et al. Endosteal erosion in associate with stable uncemented femoral components. *J Bone Joint Surg.* 1990;72A:1025–1034.

73. Maloney WJ, Peters P, Engh C, et al. Osteolysis of the pelvis in association with acetabular replacement without cement. *J Bone Joint Surg.* 1993;75A:1627–1635.

74. Maloney WJ, Smith RL, Schmalzried TP, et al. Isolation and characterization of wear particles generated in patients who have had failure of a hip arthroplasty without cement. *J Bone Joint Surg.* 1995;77A:1301–1310.

75. Margevicius KJ, Bauer TW, McMahon JT, et al. Isolation and characterization of debris in membranes around total joint prostheses. *J Bone Joint Surg.* 1994;76A:1664–1675.

76. Martell JM, Verner JJ, Incavo SJ. Clinical performance of a highly cross-linked polyethylene at two years in total hip arthroplasty: a randomized prospective trial. *J Arthroplasty.* 2003;18[7 Suppl 1]:55–59.

77. Mathieson EB, Lindgren JU, Blomgren GGA, et al. Corrosion of modular hip prostheses. *J Bone Joint Surg.* 1991;73B:569–575.

78. Mathiesen EB, Lindgren U, Reinhold FP, et al. Wear of the acetabular socket: comparison of polyacetal and polyethylene. *Acta Orthop Scand.* 1986;57:193–196.

79. McKellop H, Kirkpatrick J, Markolf K, et al. Abrasive wear to Ti-6Al-4V prostheses by acrylic cement particles. *Trans Orthop Res Soc.* 1980;5:96.

80. McKellop HA, Sarmiento A, Brien W, et al. Interface corrosion of a modular head total hip prosthesis. *J Arthroplasty.* 1992;7:291–294.

81. McKellop H, Shen FW, Lu B, et al. Development of an extremely wear-resistant ultra high molecular weight polyethylene for total hip replacements. *J Orthop Res.* 1999;17:157–167.

82. Mears DC, Hanley EN, Rutkowski R, et al. Ferrographic analysis of wear particles in arthroplastic joints. *J Biomed Mater Res.* 1978;12:867–875.

83. Mejia LC, Brierley TJ. A hip wear simulator for the evaluation of biomaterials in hip arthroplasty components. *Biomed Mater Eng.* 1994;4:259–271.

84. Michaud RJ, Rashad SY. Spontaneous fracture of the ceramic ball in a ceramic-polyethylene total hip arthroplasty. *J Arthroplasty.* 1995;10:863–867.

85. Mirra JM, Amstutz HC, Matos M, et al. The pathology of the joint tissues and its clinical relevance in prosthesis failure. *Clin Orthop.* 1976;No. 117:221–240.

86. Mirra JM, Marder RA, Amstutz HC. The pathology of failed total joint arthroplasty. *Clin Orthop.* 1982;No. 170:175–183.

87. Müller ME. Total hip prostheses. *Clin Orthop.* 1970;72:46.

88. Muratoglu OK, Greenbaum ES, Bragdon CR, et al. Surface analysis of early retrieved acetabular polyethylene liners: a comparison of conventional and highly crosslinked polyethylenes. *J Arthroplasty.* 2004;19:68–77.

89. Nasser S, Campbell PA, Kilgus D, et al. Cementless total joint arthroplasty prostheses with titanium-alloy articular surfaces: a human retrieval analysis. *Clin Orthop.* 1990;261:171–185.

90. Pidhorz LE, Urban RM, Jacobs JJ, et al. A quantitative study of bone and soft tissues in cementless porous-coated acetabular components retrieved at autopsy. *J Arthroplasty.* 1993;8:213–225.

91. Pizzoferrato A, Stea S, Sudanese A, et al. Morphometric and microanalytical analyses of alumna wear particles in hip prostheses. *Biomaterials.* 1993;14:583–587.

92. Ries MD, Scott ML, Jani S. Relationship between gravimetric wear and particle generation in hip simulators: conventional compared with cross-linked polyethylene. *J Bone Joint Surg.* 2001;83A[Suppl 2]:116–122.

93. Rimnac CM, Klein RW, Betts F, et al. Post-irradiation aging of ultra-high molecular weight polyethylene. *J Bone Joint Surg.* 1994;76A:1052–1056.

94. Roe RJ, Grood ES, Shastri R, et al. Effect of radiation sterilization and aging on ultra high molecular weight polyethylene. *J Biomed Mater Rel Res.* 1981;15:209–230.

95. Rose RM, Goldfarb EV, Ellis E, et al. Radiation sterilization and the wear rate of polyethylene. *J Orthop Res.* 1984;2:393–400.

96. Rostoker W, Galante JO, Lereim P. Evaluation of couple/crevice corrosion by prosthetic alloys under in vivo conditions. *J Biomed Mater Res.* 1978;12:823–829.

97. Saikko VO. Wear of polyethylene acetabular cups against alumina femoral heads: 5 prostheses compared in a hip simulator of 35 million waling cycles. *Acta Orthop Scand.* 1993;64:507–512.

98. Saikko V, Paavolainen P, Kleimola M, et al. A five-station hip joint simulator for wear rate studies. *Proc Inst Mech Eng.* 1992;206:195–200.

99. Saikko VO, Paavolainen PO, Slatis P. Wear of the polyethylene acetabular cup: metallic and ceramic heads compared in a hip simulator. *Acta Orthop Scand.* 1993;64:391–402.

100. Santavirta S, Hoikka V, Eskola A, et al. Aggressive granulomatous lesions in cementless total hip arthroplasty. *J Bone Joint Surg.* 1990;72B:980–984.

101. Santavirta S, Konttinen YT, Hoikka V, et al. Immunopathological response to loose cementless acetabular components. *J Bone Joint Surg.* 1991;73B:38–42.

102. Savio JA, Overcamp LM, Black J. Size and shape of biomaterial wear debris. *Clin Mater.* 1994;15:101–147.

103. Schmalzried TP, Callaghan JJ. Wear in total hip and knee replacements. *J Bone Joint Surg.* 1999;81A;115–136.

104. Schmalzried TP, Jasty M, Harris WH. Periprosthetic bone loss in total hip arthroplasty. Polyethylene wear debris and the concept of the effective joint space. *J Bone Joint Surg.* 1992;74A:849–863.

105. Schmalzried TP, Jasty M, Rosenberg A, et al. Histologic identification of polyethylene wear debris using oil red O stain. *J Appl Biomater.* 1993;4:119–125.

106. Shanbhag AS, Bailey HO, Eror NG, et al. Characterization and comparison of UHMWPE wear debris retrieved from total hip and total knee arthroplasties. *Trans Orthop Res Soc.* 1996; 21:467.

107. Shanbhag AS, Hasselman CT, Rubash HE. Technique for generating submicrometer ultrahigh molecular weight polyethylene particles. *J Orthop Res.* 1996;14:1000–1004.

108. Shanbhag AS, Jacobs JJ, Black J, et al. Human monocyte response to particulate biomaterials generated in vivo and in vitro. *J Orthop Res.* 1995;13:792–801.

109. Shanbhag AS, Jacobs JJ, Black J, et al. Macrophage/particle interactions: effect of size, composition and surface area. *J Biomed Mater Res.* 1994;28:81–90.

110. Shanbhag AS, Jacobs JJ, Glant TT, et al. Composition and morphology of wear debris in failed uncemented total hip replacement. *J Bone Joint Surg.* 1994;76B:60–67.

111. Shea KG, Lundeen G, Zou L. Systemic dissemination of metal particulate to the lymphoreticular system in primary total arthroplasty. Presented at the meeting of the American Association of Orthopaedic Surgeons; Atlanta; 1996.

112. Shen C, Dumbleton JR. The friction and wear behavior of irradiated very high molecular weight polyethylene. *Wear.* 1974;30:349–364.

113. Sommerich R, Flynn T, Schmidt M, et al. The effects of sterilization on contact area and wear rate of UHMWPE. *Trans Orthop Res Soc.* 1996;21:486.

114. Sugano N, Nishii T, Nakata K, et al. Polyethylene sockets and alumina ceramic heads in cemented total hip arthroplasty: a ten-year study. *J Bone Joint Surg.* 1995;77B:548–536.

115. Svensson O, Mathiesen EB, Reinholt FB, et al. Formation of a fulminant soft-tissue pseudotumor after uncemented hip arthroplasty. *J Bone Joint Surg.* 1988;70A:1238.

116. Tanzer M, Maloney WJ, Jasty M, et al. The progression of femoral cortical osteolysis in association with total hip arthroplasty without cement. *J Bone Joint Surg.* 1992;74A:404–410.

117. Urban RM, Jacobs JJ, Gilbert JL, et al. Migration of corrosion products from modular hip prostheses. *J Bone Joint Surg.* 1994;76A:1345–1359.

118. Urban RM, Jacobs JJ, Sumner DR, et al. The bone-implant interface in femoral stems with noncircumferential porous coating in specimens retrieved at autopsy. *J Bone Joint Surg.* 1996;78A:1068–1081.

119. Urban RM, Jacobs JJ, Tomlinson MJ, et al. Dissemination of wear particles to the liver, spleen and abdominal lymph nodes of patients with hip or knee replacement. *J Bone Joint Surg.* 2000;82A:457–477.

120. Urban RM, Jacobs JJ, Tomlinson MJ, et al. Migration of corrosion products from the modular head junction to the polyethylene bearing surface and interface membranes of hip prostheses. In: Galante JO, Rosenberg AG, Callaghan JJ, eds. Total Hip Revision Surgery. New York: Raven Press; 1995:61–71.

121. Willert HG, Semlitsch M. Tissue reactions to plastic and metallic wear products of joint endoprostheses. In: Geschwind N, Debrunner HU, eds. Total Hip Prosthesis. Baltimore: Williams & Wilkins; 1976:205–239.

122. Wirganowicz PZ, Thomas BJ. Massive osteolysis after ceramic on ceramic total hip arthroplasty: a case report. *Clin Orthop.* 1997;338:100–104.

123. Wroblewski BM, McCullagh PJ, Siney PD. The quality of the surface finish of the head of the femoral component and the wear rate of the socket in long-term results of the Charnley low-friction arthroplasty. *Proc Inst Mech Eng.* 1992;206:181–183.

124. Xenos JS, Hopkinson WJ, Callaghan JJ, et al. Osteolysis around an uncemented cobalt chrome total hip arthroplasty. *Clin Orthop.* 1995;317:29–36.

125. Yang SY, Ren W, Park Y, et al. Diverse cellular and apoptotic responses to variant shapes of UHMWPE particles in a murine model of inflammation. *Biomaterials.* 2002;23:3535–3543.

126. Yoon TR, Rowe SM, Jung ST, et al. Osteolysis in association with a total hip arthroplasty with ceramic bearing surfaces. *J Bone Joint Surg.* 1998;80A:1459–1468.

Biological Response to Wear Debris: Cellular Interactions Causing Osteolysis

Arun S. Shanbhag   *Manish K. Sethi*   *Harry E. Rubash*

Total joint replacements (TJRs) have experienced a steady stream of advances and innovations since their introduction more than half a century ago. Improvements in surgical techniques, prevention of infection, selection of materials, optimization of manufacturing techniques, and refined methods of fixation have resulted in a TJR procedure that is one of the most cost effective means of relieving pain and restoring joint mobility and function (9). The vast majority of patients receiving joint replacements will enjoy more than 20 years of pain-free functional outcome, but this success has also increased societal expectations. Increasing numbers of joint replacements are being performed in younger patients, who need the components to last a longer life span, and live an active lifestyle, placing higher demands on components,

which results in higher rates of failure (112). Looking forward, the survivorship of TJR in a young and active cohort will present the locus of our challenges. Recent advances in improving wear resistance of materials have resulted in implants that are more durable. But compromised material properties, together with a longer patient life span, point to a more realistic, delayed appearance of osteolysis. Additionally, we already have a conventional ultra-high molecular weight polyethylene (UHMWPE) implant patient base of more than 5 million who are at a higher risk for implant failure. There is thus a need to understand the biological mechanisms by which joint replacements fail. The opportunities from such investigations include the development of technologies to detect bone loss early, and medical therapies to treat and prevent osteolysis.

A common mode of implant failure is associated with a localized granulomatous reaction resulting in resorption of the bone, which compromises bony anchors stabilizing the implant and leads to a painfully loose implant. In the absence of bacterial infection, this is termed "aseptic loosening" or "osteolysis." In the absence of medical management alternatives, revision surgery is required to débride the site and insert new components.

The underlying etiology of aseptic loosening has been explored for more than 3 decades, and several mechanisms have been proposed as causative of aseptic loosening. A wear-mediated biological phenomenon is the leading pathway causing periprosthetic bone resorption. The 1994 NIH Consensus Statement (111) and its year 2000 update (66) both emphasized the role of UHMWPE wear debris as a major cause of osteolysis and aseptic loosening. Additional contributory factors include mechanical conditions such as high fluid pressure and implant instability leading to increased relative bone resorption.

Mechanical perturbations at the implant interface can synergize the effect of particles, and it appears that a smaller dose of debris can initiate bone resorption when accompanied by interfacial micromotion. An adaptive immune response to implant materials, including specific patient responses, cannot be ignored in the biological cascade leading to osteolysis. In this chapter, we concisely discuss the important mechanisms and pathways leading to peri-implant bone loss and provide a roadmap for investigations aimed at therapeutic advances.

HISTORICAL PERSPECTIVE ON OSTEOLYSIS

Charnley recognized loosening in total hip replacements (THR) in the 1960s when the poly-tetrafluoroethylene (PTFE) acetabular components he used required revision within 3 years (13–16). Histopathological analyses of tissues retrieved during revision surgery demonstrated the presence of particulate debris surrounded by foreign body giant cells forming a "caseating granulomata and sterile pus." In order to prove that particulate PTFE debris caused the granulomas, Charnley implanted finely divided PTFE subcutaneously in his thigh and after 3 months could palpate the larger nodules (15). These findings provided Charnley with the rationale to switch to a more wear resistant polyethylene for the articulating surface, used to this day with minor modifications (126).

Willert and Semlitsch extensively analyzed histopathological sections from around failed joint replacements and proposed that aseptic loosening of implants was caused by excessive wear debris generated from the polyethylene liner. The retrieved periprosthetic tissues contained sheets of macrophages laden with various types of particulate wear debris in a fibrous stroma, intermingled with multinucleated giant cells encapsulating larger debris (Figs. 22-1 and 22-2) (101,102,164,168). According to Willert's hypothesis, wear debris generated at the articulating surface would routinely be cleared from the joint space by macrophage phagocytosis and transported via the lymphatic system (164,168). If the amount of wear debris generated exceeded the clearance capacity of the local vasculature,

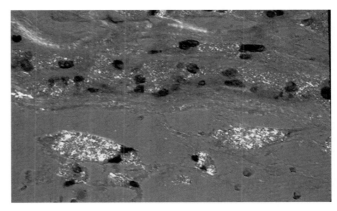

Figure 22-1 Histology of clinical peri-implant interfacial tissue under polarized light. Note macrophages laden with internalized birefringent polyethylene particles. Nuclei appear squished to the right edge of the cell. Birefringence is also observed in other cells in the collagenous tissue. (Micrograph was kindly provided by Prof. Joshua J Jacobs, Rush Medical University, Chicago, IL.) See Color Plate.

debris would be retained locally within the macrophages, stimulating them and leading to the formation of a periprosthetic granuloma (164,168). As the amount of wear debris increases, granulomas initiated in the joint capsule would advance distally into the cement–bone interface, sacrificing bone–implant anchors and resulting in component loosening (164).

Although the original observations of Willert and Semlitsch were made with cemented components, a similar process is believed to occur in uncemented implants (72,89,124,165,166). By carefully studying the tissues around failed components, Willert and Semlitsch further suggested that the "whole environment" of the joint participated in clearing prosthetic wear debris (164). Schmalzried et al. elaborated by pointing out that joint fluid can carry wear debris from the articulation to all fluid accessible areas (124). The pattern of debris migration and deposition would determine whether the debris would be linearly dispersed along the component, or accumulated in discrete pockets, leading to their characteristic focal lytic appearances (124). Implant design

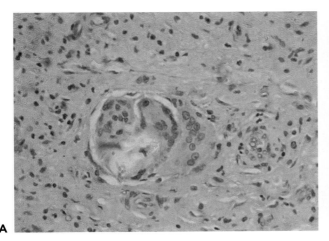
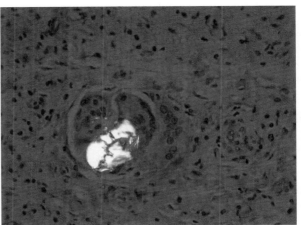

A   **B**

Figure 22-2 Histology of clinical peri-implant interfacial tissue under normal incident **(A)** and polarized light **(B)**. In each figure, a foreign body giant cell has encapsulated a larger fragment of birefringent polyethylene and isolated it from the surrounding tissue. Note the numerous nuclei in the giant cell. See Color Plate.

features such as surface smoothness and provision of surface texture, and porosities to encourage bone ingrowth all play critical roles in determining the pattern of wear debris migration and accumulation as well as the subsequent radiographic manifestation of lesions (7,124,130). As an aside, although we recognize that osteolysis and aseptic loosening have different radiographic manifestations, for the purposes of this discussion we neglect the distinction and focus on the similar underlying biological mechanisms.

Investigations of clinical materials during autopsies have confirmed the local clearance aspects of wear debris. Through the use of histopathology and electron microscopy, wear debris was identified at remote sites such as the lungs, kidneys, liver, spleen, and lymph nodes of patients with well-functioning joint replacements (50,54,69,156). In many of these cases, despite the presence of wear debris and an associated inflammatory response, there was no discernible radiographic finding of osteolysis, suggesting a threshold or a dose effect of wear debris.

BRIEF NOTE ON THE MAGNITUDE OF WEAR IN PATIENTS

Although more exhaustive discussions of wear in joint replacements occur in other chapters in this book, we take this opportunity to cast the magnitude of wear perhaps in a slightly more illuminating light. The amount of wear of the acetabular liner depends in part on the distance that the surface of the femoral head slides against it. Each walking step produces an excursion of about 2 cm between the hard metal femoral head and the UHMWPE liner. Estimating 1 million paces of the hip in a year of normal activities and a 28-mm diameter head, some 2463 m^2 of material surfaces move against each other (138). This is approximately the area of seven basketball courts. Imagine dragging your sneakers across the entire surface of a basketball court times seven in one year! Moreover, given an average range of motion of 90°, the femoral head annually travels a linear distance of approximately 14 miles within the acetabular cup. This area and distance helps us to conceptualize the magnitude of the articulating surfaces susceptible to wear in TJR, and marvel at the already phenomenal success in limiting wear in patients. Clinically, then, osteolysis appears to be directly related to wear of the UHMWPE liner (6,23,24). The direct relationship between polyethylene wear and degree of osteolysis is well supported by radiographic measurements in patients (31).

ANALYSES OF CLINICAL TISSUES

Biochemical analyses of clinical materials harvested during revision surgery, have provided the foundations for studying the pathogenesis of osteolysis. By placing retrieved tissues in organ culture, investigators identified the mediators released by cells in the peri-implant region, which in turn provided insight into the microenvironment at the bone–implant interface. Goldring et al. used organ culture techniques to demonstrate that peri-implant membranous tissues were capable of producing biological mediators such as collagenase and prostaglandin E_2 (PGE_2) that had the capacity to stimulate

osteoclasts to resorb bone (42). This important finding demonstrated that the interfacing fibrous membrane was not a mere tissue appendage but participated actively in the biological process leading to implant loosening. Since then, numerous investigators have shown that this interfacial tissue is capable of secreting a variety of mediators; enzymes; prostaglandins; potent proinflammatory cytokines such as interleukins (IL-1α, IL-1β, and IL-6); tumor necrosis factor-α (TNF-α); and growth factors such as platelet-derived growth factor (PDGF) (29,44,74,132). Matrix-degrading enzymes such as gelatinase, stromelysins, and various matrix metalloproteinases, including MMP-1, MMP-9, MMP-10, MMP-12, and MMP-13, are also released (79,113,146,147), as well as chemokines that recruit inflammatory cells to the site, such as monocyte chemoattractant proteins (MCP-1), monocyte inflammatory proteins MIP-1α and MIP-1β, and IL-8. This array of chemokines, growth factors, proinflammatory and anti-inflammatory cytokines, and mediators indicate the potent ability of periprosthetic tissues to not only recruit but also stimulate cells capable of propelling osteoclastic bone resorption and fibrous tissue formation (17,29,42,43,74,132).

Immunohistochemistry and in situ hybridization have pinpointed gene expression for these cytokines in the peri-implant tissues, confirming their localized synthesis and release. Potent free radicals such as nitric oxide are induced in the granulomatous tissues, confirming their participation in the osteolytic cascade (114,163). Importantly, while a variety of cell types are present at the bone–implant interface, including fibroblasts, lymphocytes, eosinophils, and basophils, inflammatory mediators are specifically transcribed and secreted by macrophages with phagocytized wear debris (47,73), highlighting their central role in causing osteolysis.

In a recent review, Jacobs et al. summarized why it is difficult to draw further insight from studies of peri-implant tissues (70). The authors highlighted the lack of relevant controls, the potential for laboratory artifacts given the variations in techniques, the large scatter due to biological variability, and the tendency for over simplification of an essentially complex interaction that involves mediators, receptors, inhibitors, and synergistic interactions (70).

CHARACTERISTICS OF WEAR DEBRIS ASSOCIATED WITH OSTEOLYSIS

In an earlier chapter, we comprehensively discussed the composition and characteristics of wear debris found around TJRs. Here we briefly highlight the common types of wear debris, particularly from the perspective of understanding their biological response.

Wear detritus around TJRs can arise from several sources. The predominant debris identified in osteolytic tissues (representing 70–95% of the debris burden) is particulate UHMWPE from the articulating surfaces (1,35,92,128,137). UHMWPE debris present around failed total hip, total knee, as well as total shoulder components has been retrieved and analyzed (11,58,75,87,92,93,128,129,137). These particles are predominantly spheroids 0.1 to 2.0 μm in size. Fibrils interconnecting the spheroids and forming larger aggregates are also present (Fig. 22-3) (11,92,137). Wear also occurs on the convex, nonarticulating surface of the UHMWPE acetabular

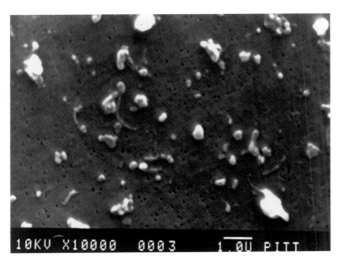

Figure 22-3 Scanning electron microscopy (SEM) micrograph of UHMWPE particles retrieved from around the femoral component of patients with aseptically loose total hip replacements. Note the spherical morphology of the debris, with occasional fibrillar attachments. Scale bar is 1 μm.

liner due to liner motion against the metal backing and abrasion of the UHMWPE at the rim of the screw holes (28,65,127). Unoccupied filled screw holes in the metal backing are repositories of debris generated at the back surface, as well as debris that has migrated from the articulating surfaces (65,129,162). Such UHMWPE particles are generally larger than those present around the femoral components (Figs. 22-4 and 22-5) (127,129). Unfilled screw holes provide wear debris access to the area behind the ingrowth cup, resulting in pelvic osteolysis observed during clinical follow-up (90) and in autopsy retrievals (155). Metal screws that provide initial shell stability can abrade the liner, resulting in larger shards and fibrils; and their fretting wear can also generate metallic debris.

The newest generation of cross-linked UHMWPE (XLPE) exhibits a dramatic decrease in wear in laboratory hip simulator studies (96,107). The size distribution of XLPE debris extracted from hip simulators is similar to that from conventional UHMWPE (118,123,139). The particles from both are approximately 0.2 μm, much smaller than the debris reported from clinical retrievals (92,93,137). XLPE debris is also characterized by a striking absence of fibrils (118,139). Using in vitro models, Fisher et al. demonstrated that XLPE debris is more inflammatory to macrophages and stimulates higher levels of inflammatory mediators (33). Huddleston et al. recently reported that human macrophages are particularly stimulated by XLPE debris and release more than 2 to 4 times the level of inflammatory mediators incited by conventional polyethylene debris (64). Clearly, this is an emerging area of concern and needs to be fully investigated.

Metallic debris represents a small fraction of the debris burden in UHMWPE articulations and typically results from abrasion of the stem against bone or cement (92,137). An important source of metallic debris in THR is at the modular femoral head and neck junction. The "Morse taper"–head connection is conducive to fretting wear and further introduces a crevice for subsequent generation of corrosion products (21,38,98). These corrosion products can be fragments of component oxides in various combinations, including chromium orthophosphate, which has been identified in interfacial tissues (71,88). Fretting is an important source of metal debris, particularly in multimodular components used to customize prostheses. Silicates and stainless steel particles are found in small amounts in clinical tissues and are possible contaminants from drilling and reaming tools (137). Unusually, silicates and other similar debris may be introduced on the surface of the component as a consequence of their polishing and lapping treatments during manufacture (97,117). Although the smaller fraction of these metallic particles would suggest they play a minor role, such debris elicit particularly aggressive cellular responses and may participate in initiating and/or instigating an inflammatory process that would otherwise be subclinical (40,52,70,71,134,135). Of particular

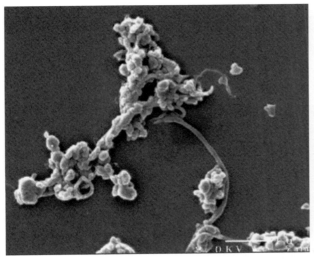

A

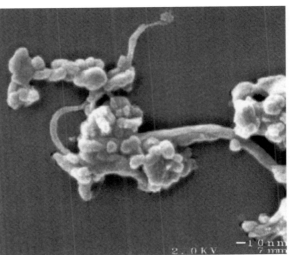

B

Figure 22-4 SEM micrographs of UHMWPE particles retrieved from around the acetabular component of patients with aseptically loose total hip replacements. Note that the majority of debris appears as aggregates of fine spherical debris and fibrils. Scale bars are 5 μm **(A)** and 10 μm **(B)**.

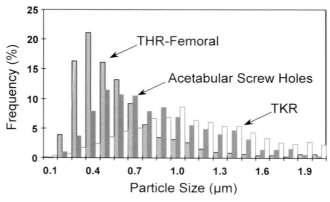

Figure 22-5 Size distribution of UHMWPE wear debris extracted from clinical cases of failed total joint replacements. Debris from around the femoral components of total hip replacements (THR-Femoral) are finer than debris from the acetabular screw holes, which are in turn finer than UHMWPE debris from around failed total knee replacements (TKR). It is this size discrepancy that is believed to result in the higher macrophage stimulation in THR and the consequent higher rates of osteolysis. The lower failure rates of TKR are believed to be due to the larger size of the UHMWPE debris, which consequently is less stimulatory to macrophages. (Data adapted from Shanbhag AS, Jacobs JJ, Glant TT, et al. Composition and morphology of wear debris in failed uncemented total hip replacement. *J Bone Joint Surg [Br]*. 1994;76:60–67. Shanbhag AS, Bailey HO, Hwang DS, et al. Quantitative analysis of ultrahigh molecular weight polyethylene (UHMWPE) wear debris associated with total knee replacements. *J Biomed Mater Res.* 2000;53:100–110.)

concern is the potential for such harder debris to drive between the head and UHMWPE articulating surfaces, where it can lead to third-body wear, accelerating UHMWPE debris generation.

Given that the periprosthetic tissues contain many types and sizes of particulate debris, it is not possible to ascertain which of the debris species is primarily involved in initiating the granulomatous reaction. In vitro and in vivo models are required to determine and confirm the incriminating particle species as well as identify the sequence of events leading to implant loosening.

MACROPHAGES IMPEL OSTEOLYSIS

In Vitro Macrophage–Particle Interactions

Based on histopathological analyses of clinical specimens, various cell types involved in the chronic inflammatory process and their spatial relationships have been well established. The presence of macrophages and multinucleated foreign body giant cells with internalized debris in the periprosthetic granuloma and bony erosions is universally reported (20,89,101,102,167,168). Macrophages are sentinels of the immune response, primary cells at any site of inflammation and, along with short-lived neutrophils, key participants in innate immunity. With their abilities to degrade protein and process and present antigen, macrophages orchestrate the recruitment and activity of B-lymphocytes and T-lymphocytes and coordinate the adaptive immune response (106,143). Macrophages also mount an aggressive response to debris and secrete mediators associated with osteoclast recruitment, proliferation, differentiation, and maturation (76,80,85). This concerted and continuous biological process disrupts the homeostatic balance between osteoclasts and osteoblasts, degrades the bone–implant anchors, and eventually leads to implant loosening. A schematic of the pathophysiology associated with wear debris–mediated osteolysis is presented in Figure 22-6.

Macrophages cultured with wear debris in vitro thus provide a well-developed and clinically relevant model for dissecting

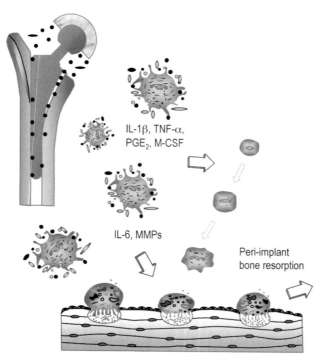

IL-1β, TNF-α, PGE₂, M-CSF

IL-6, MMPs

Peri-implant bone resorption

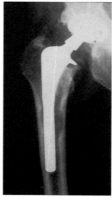

Figure 22-6 Schematic representation of the pathophysiology of wear debris–mediated osteolysis.

the sequence of events occurring at the bone–implant interface. They permit studying different variables individually, without interactions from confounding factors. The primary goal of an in vitro cell–particle interaction is to determine if particles can stimulate macrophages and other cells to release inflammatory mediators and if the resulting inflammation is capable of initiating bone resorption.

Although there are advantages to using transformed or immortalized macrophage cell lines, it is clinically more pertinent to use primary cells and their inherent variability to develop relevant models. Since macrophages in interfacial membranes are believed to be derived from circulating mononuclear cells, peripheral blood monocytes are the target cells of choice for studying and reproducing macrophage–particle interactions (68,83,84,95,133,134).

Early studies on macrophage–particle interactions focused on the toxicity of different particles. Co, Ni, and Co-Cr alloy particles in phagocytosable sizes decreased phagocytic ability and damaged cell membranes extensively, leading to cell death, whereas Ti alloy particles were less deleterious (37,115,116). Both poly-methylmethacrylate (PMMA) and UHMWPE caused varying levels of cell death, though far less than metal particles (60–62). Shanbhag et al. demonstrated that cell death increased with increasing dose of challenging particles (134,135). Macrophages cultured with Ti particles for 24 hours were barely affected by particle concentrations representing one tenth the surface area of cells, whereas increasing the particle concentration 10-fold resulted in approximately a 50% decrease in cellular synthesis. A 100-fold increase in the particle concentration, which then represented 10 times the surface area of cells, nearly abolished DNA synthesis. This cytotoxic effect is also dependent on the composition of the debris, as polystyrene particles at comparable concentrations had a smaller cytoxic effect (135). Particle toxicity directly impacts cellular ability to secrete mediators. Haynes et al. demonstrated that Co-Cr alloy particles caused extensive macrophage death within hours and did not elicit synthesis and secretion of high levels of inflammatory mediators (52). Ti alloy particles, however, were less toxic, and the resulting cell death occurred nearly 24 hours later, providing sufficient opportunity for macrophages to synthesize and secrete copious amounts of inflammatory mediators (52).

Mathews et al. compared the human macrophage response to a range of sizes of UHMWPE particles and reported that finer particles elicit higher levels of cytokines such as IL-1β and IL-6 and granulocyte-macrophage colony-stimulating factor (GM-CSF) (95). Fine PMMA particles also stimulated macrophages to release IL-1β, IL-6, PGE$_2$, and the enzyme hexosaminidase (49). Larger debris particles on the other hand were not stimulatory (49). Response is related not only to size; Human macrophages also discerned minor elemental differences between two similar clinically used Ti-based alloy: TiAlV and TiAlNb, and released higher cytokine levels with TiAlV particles (120). To account for varying densities of metallic and polymeric particles, Shanbhag et al. normalized for surface area of debris and demonstrated that metallic debris consisting of TiAlV (Fig. 22-7) and CpTi particles, for example, was the most stimulatory in eliciting a variety of inflammatory mediators, including PGE$_2$, IL-1α, IL-1β, and IL-6 (133,134). UHMWPE wear debris, either retrieved from patients with failed THRs or fabricated in the laboratory in clinically similar sizes, was less stimulatory than metal particles but significantly more stimulatory than nonstimulated cells (Fig. 22-8) (133,134). Nakashima et al. documented that macrophage phagocytosis of wear debris may not be necessary and that surface recognition may suffice to elicit high levels of TNF-α and IL-6 (110). Cytokine release follows intracellular signaling pathways and includes the translocation of transcription factor NF-κB, an intermediary for TNF-α gene expression (110). Inflammatory macrophages also release chemokines, which are essential for recruiting new as well as precursor cells to the site of perturbation (84,109).

Inflammatory cytokines, enzymes, and mediators play an important role in stimulating bone resorption, especially IL-1, TNF-α, and PGE$_2$, WWch are potent stimulators of osteoclasts. These cytokines act in an autocrine and paracrine manner, recruit other cells to the site, and elicit additional cytokine release. Osteoclast precursors are also recruited, differentiate to maturation, and their stimulation is facilitated. Matrix metalloproteinases (MMPs) degrade organic matrix, whereas osteoclasts dissolve the mineral component of bone. That cells do indeed follow these steps is evidenced by osteoclastic bone resorption in ^{45}Ca-labeled murine calvaria placed in organ culture with supernatants from macrophage particle cultures (Fig. 22-9) (39,40,53,63,133,136). Even when wear debris alone is surgically placed over the calvaria, the resident and recruited macrophage response initiates an inflammatory cascade resulting in bone resorption (125).

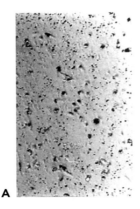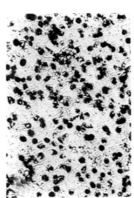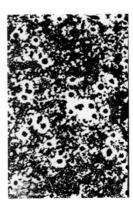

Figure 22-7 Human peripheral blood macrophages cultured for 24 hours with TiAlV particles dosed at 0.1 × the surface area of the macrophages (**A**), 1 × the surface area (**B**), and 10 × the surface area (**C**).

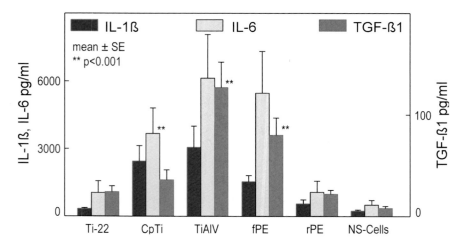

Figure 22-8 Levels of mediators released by human macrophages stimulated with various types of debris. Human macrophages were dosed with debris representing 10 × the surface area of cells and cultured for 24 hours. The spent conditioned medium was analyzed for various proinflammatory mediators with the ability to stimulate bone resorption. Macrophages also release the growth factor TGF-β1, which directs fibroblast proliferation and formation of the fibrous interfacial tissue. Ti-22, Titanium 22 μm; CpTi, commercially pure titanium; TiAlV, Ti-Al-V alloy; fPE, fabricated polyethylene; rPE, retrieved polyethylene; NS, nonstimulated control cells. (Data adapted from Shanbhag AS, Jacobs JJ, Black J, et al. Human monocyte response to particulate biomaterials generated in vivo and in vitro. *J Orthop Res.* 1995;13:792–801.)

Anti-Inflammatory Component of Macrophage Action

Complementing the exhaustively studied catabolic sequelae of macrophage interaction, an anti-inflammatory healing response is also evident. Vascular endothelial growth factor (VEGF) expression in tissues has been reported, along with its copious secretion in macrophages stimulated by particles in vitro (103). Moreover, macrophages release growth factors such as TGF-β$_1$ and stimulate fibroblast proliferation (133). IL-1 is also a key fibrogenic factor (27,32,94,104). The angiogenic role of VEGF, in concert with the fibrogenic role of TGF-β$_1$ and IL-1, suggests that macrophages engage in formation of the fibrovascular interfacial tissue as a healing response to particle-mediated inflammation. This healing aspect is ongoing in the peri-implant region. While bone is resorbed, intervening spaces are refilled by a vascularized interfacial tissue (25,26,133,148).

Modulation of Fibroblasts

In the periprosthetic milieu, fibroblasts primarily lead to scar tissue, encapsulating the inflammation (26). The very presence of fibrous tissue at the bone–implant interface prevents bone ingrowth because the tissues occupy the space where bone might have grown. Therefore, fibroplasia at the interface compromises the extent of ingrown bone, prevents stable fixation, and makes implants more susceptible to loosening. Fibroblasts are facultative phagocytes and are directly stimulated by wear debris to release enzymes potently able to degrade the organic components of bone (58,91,174). Thus, fibroblasts associated with interfacial tissue play an important role in the biological cascade leading to osteolysis.

Maloney et al. studied fibroblast–particle interactions and found a correlation between fibroblast proliferation and particle toxicity (91). When bovine synovial fibroblasts were cultured with Ti particles, phagocytosis was accompanied by membrane

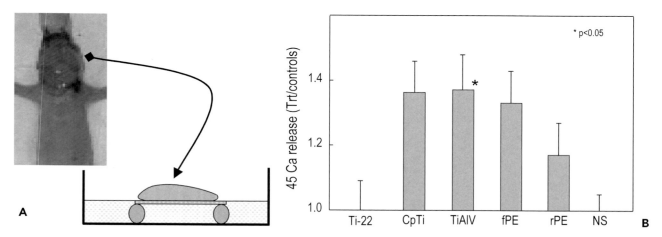

Figure 22-9 A: Calvaria were harvested from 5-day old, ^{45}Ca-labeled mice and placed in organ culture. Media was supplemented with spent conditioned media from human macrophages cultured with various types of particulate debris. Macrophages when stimulated with particles release a variety of mediators that lead to bone resorption in the murine calvaria. B: ^{45}Ca release from calvaria is representative of the bone resorptive capacity of the particle-stimulated macrophages. Ti-22, titanium 22 μm; CpTi, commercially pure Titanium; TiAlV, Ti-Al-V alloy; fPE, fabricated polyethylene; rPE, retrieved polyethylene; NS, nonstimulated control cells.

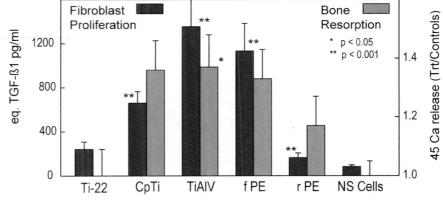

Figure 22-10 Fibroblast proliferation and bone resorption effected by human macrophages cultured with various particulate wear debris. Spent conditioned medium from macrophage–particle cultures was supplemented in fibroblast cultures or cultured with dissected, prelabeled newborn murine calvaria.

ruffling and filopodial extension. Conversely, when exposed to cobalt particles, fibroblasts underwent cytoplasmic shrinking and crenation, features associated with cell death (91). A succeeding study by Yao et al. demonstrated that fibroblasts stimulated by metallic debris produced elevated levels of bone-resorbing enzymes such as collagenase, stromelysin, and metalloproteinases (174). In conjunction with these findings, Shanbhag et al. revealed that particle-free conditioned medium collected from monocytes challenged with wear debris, stimulated fibroblast proliferation (Fig. 22-10) (133). Cellular mediators present in conditioned medium such as IL-1 and TGF-β_1 induce fibrosis, even if levels are insufficient to cause bone resorption (133). Therefore, the deleterious consequences of acute fibrosis at the bone–implant interface may have a synergistic role in osteolysis and aseptic loosening: fibrous tissue impedes initial bone ingrowth, and bone resorption is additionally stimulated by fibroblast-secreted mediators.

Wear Debris Effects on Osteoblasts

In normal physiology, osteoclastic bone *resorption* is balanced by osteoblastic bone *formation* (157). Osteoblastic activity is particularly crucial at the bone–implant interface. If the rate of bone formation is compromised, the "system" cannot compensate for pathologic bone loss consequent to debris-mediated inflammation. This is exactly what happens in vitro when particles are cultured with osteoblasts.

Investigators noted that MG-63 human cell activity was adversely affected by UHMWPE or Ti debris in a dose-dependent manner (22,173). Debris stimulated osteoblast proliferation but also PGE_2 production, and consequently cellular differentiation and extracellular matrix synthesis was inhibited (22). Similarly, Vermes et al. demonstrated that particle phagocytosis by osteoblasts stimulates the secretion of IL-6, which initiates osteoblast differentiation, but bone formation is also suppressed, as type-I collagen synthesis is inhibited (160,161).

Thus the presence of wear debris has a threefold effect: (a) osteoclast differentiation and activation are stimulated by particles through the release of IL-1, IL-6, TNF-α, and other inflammatory mediators; (b) these same mediators repress osteoblast function and synthesis of matrix; and (c) fibroblast activity is stimulated.

As a consequence, bone resorbed by the osteoclastic activity is replaced not by similar mineralized tissue but by fibrous tissue, resulting in the loss of bony anchors and implant fixation.

Animal Models for Developing Wear-Mediated Osteolysis

Animal models serve multiple purposes. Earlier models were developed to demonstrate the inflammatory potential of particles in vivo and confirm that wear debris introduction was sufficient to lead to peri-implant bone loss. Recently, smaller animals have been used, and research with these models has focused on interfering with specific aspects of the biochemical pathway leading to osteolysis.

Howie et al. studied the inflammatory reaction to particulate high-density polyethylene around a non-weight-bearing bone cement plug in a rat model (56,57). Animals receiving a bone cement plug and no wear debris had a complete shell of new bone surrounding the cement plug, 2 weeks after implantation. Repeated injections of polyethylene particles in the knee resulted in the formation of fibrous tissue containing macrophages, giant cells, and particles, which in turn led to the radiographically evident bone resorption around the plugs. Goodman et al. utilized a rabbit tibial-defect model and demonstrated that introduction of particulate PMMA debris too can lead to a florid fibrohistiocytic and giant cell reaction similar to that observed around loose clinical components (44–46).

Larger animals offer the opportunity to perform a partial or THR, as well as introduce wear debris. In an earlier canine model, a femoral component was placed in an overreamed dog femur, along with PMMA particles. At 4 months postoperative, radiolucent lines characteristic of implant loosening were observed at the bone–cement interface (144). Turner et al. also developed loosening in a canine model of cemented THR by overreaming the femur at the time of surgery and fixing the prosthesis with an admixture of blood, bone debris, and doughy cement (150). At 11 months, the animals developed radiographic signs of loosening together with the characteristic granulomatous reaction (150).

Dowd et al. developed a canine model for uncemented THR (30) and investigated the contribution of different types of wear debris: Ti alloy, Co-Cr alloy, or high-density polyethylene. A stable fiber-metal–coated TiAlV femoral component articu-

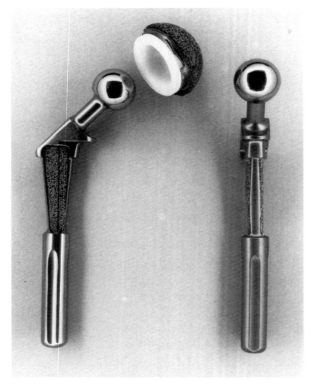

Figure 22-11 TiAlV femoral component with a CpTi fiber–metal mesh recessed by 2 mm. During implantation, wear debris is placed in the resulting gap. The nonmodular head articulates with a UHMWPE liner with a fiber-metal–backed acetabular shell.

lated against an UHMWPE acetabular liner with a fiber-metal–backed metal shell (Fig. 22-11). During the surgical procedure, particulate debris was introduced into a 2-mm proximal gap contiguous with the porous coating. A 12-week postoperative duration resulted in a granuloma laden with fibroblasts, macrophages, and foreign body giant cells, with phagocytosed wear debris (30). In organ culture, these tissues released high levels of inflammatory cytokines, mediators, and enzymes such as IL-1, PGE$_2$, collagenase, and gelatinase (30). The striking similarity of the canine membrane histology and

biochemistry, to those around clinically loosened components makes such a model potentially valuable in understanding the factors involved in aseptic loosening (Fig. 22-12). By using clinically relevant UHMWPE debris and extending the duration to 24 weeks postimplantation, researchers found radiolucencies had developed around the implant that were strikingly similar to the endosteal scalloping in clinical cases of failed THR (51,131) (Fig. 22-13). When placed in organ culture, the granulomatous tissues released elevated PGE$_2$ levels (51,131). These studies confirm conclusively that wear debris in the peri-implant region has the potential to cause osteolysis.

ROLE OF OSTEOBLASTS IN OSTEOCLAST DIFFERENTIATION

Three interrelated regulators of osteoclast differentiation and maturation have recently been identified (67,70,169). RANKL (receptor activator of NFκB ligand) is expressed by marrow stromal cells and is critical for osteoclast differentiation; it is referred to as an osteoclast differentiation factor. It is part of the TNF-α superfamily with the acronym TRANCE (TNF-α–related activation-induced cytokine) (151,152,175). Mice lacking RANKL have clear defects in osteoclastogenesis and develop osteopetrosis (176). Osteoprotegerin (OPG) is a stromal cell–secreted glycoprotein, is a member of the TNF-receptor family of proteins, and can block osteoclast differentiation from precursor cells in a dose-dependent manner (8,10,105,140). OPG acts as a decoy protein binding to RANKL and prevents interaction with its receptor, in turn impeding osteoclastogenesis (80,140,153). Mice lacking OPG develop severe osteoporosis and brittle bones (77,78,100,176). RANK (receptor for activation of NFκB), the receptor for RANKL, is expressed on the surface of osteoclast precursors and also has similarities to the TNF family (3,82,108). RANK–RANKL interactions are essential for inducing osteoclastogenesis and stimulate osteoclast activity (108). Studies using knockout mice underscore the importance of this interaction, and neither protein by itself can separately induce osteoclast maturation and bone resorption (82,169).

The identification of these three important regulators of osteoclastogenesis (RANK, RANKL, and OPG) provides

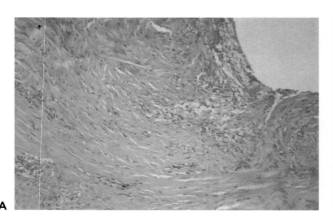
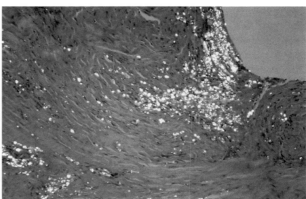

A   **B**

Figure 22-12 Histology of peri-implant granulomatous tissue from a canine uncemented total hip replacement (12 weeks) under normal incident **(A)** and polarized light **(B)**. Birefringent polyethylene debris are dispersed within the tissues. See Color Plate.

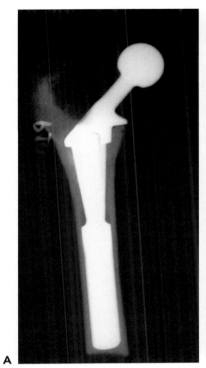
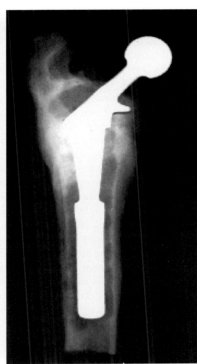

Figure 22-13 Contact femoral radiographs from canines at the end of 24 weeks. **A:** In control animals, no wear debris was introduced and no osteolysis was observed. **B:** In canines with introduced UHMWPE debris, marked endosteal scalloping was observed all around the implant.

unique opportunities to determine the specific role of various cytokines in the biochemical pathway leading to osteoclast-mediated bone resorption. The close association of these signalling molecules to TNF-α appeared to indicate a direct correlation between TNF-α and bone resorption. Experimental studies supported this thesis when very low concentrations of TNF-α were able to stimulate osteoclast activation and potentiate the effect of RANKL (36). In mice with NFκB knockout, a transcription factor associated with TNF-α, osteoclastogenesis was prevented (169). TNF-α also prevents osteoclast apoptosis and appears to prolong the survival of osteoclasts (81). Such targeted investigations have lead to TNF-α being considered "atop the inflammatory pyramid" driving bone resorption.

OPPORTUNITIES FOR THERAPEUTIC MANAGEMENT OF OSTEOLYSIS

With cytokines playing a critical role in bone resorption, there has been a rush to identify the primary mediator responsible for bone resorption. The thinking goes that blocking this key mediator could lead to blocking the entire inflammatory cascade, and thus prevent bone resorption. Early attempts were made to modulate inflammation using nonsteroidal anti-inflammatory drugs (NSAIDS), including cox-2 inhibitors. Although these efforts were of limited utility, they highlighted the complexity of the system. For example, indomethacin could be used to effectively block PGE_2, but it only inhibited a portion of the bone resorption in [45]Ca-labeled murine calvaria (39,40), indicating multiple mediators acting in concert.

Anti-TNF Therapies

The identification of the three osteoclast regulators described earlier (RANK, RANKL, and OPG) and their critical association with bone resorption has focused attention on TNF-α as the cytokine most responsible for encouraging osteolysis, which it does through the facilitation and augmentation of osteoclast differentiation as well as activation of pre-existing osteoclasts (67). Experimental studies also supported this hypothesis. Algan et al. reported that anti-TNF-α antibody was able to significantly inhibit bone resorption by supernatants from particle-stimulated macrophages (2).

The importance of TNF-α was also supported by elegant in vivo work using knockout mice and carefully designed anti-TNF compounds. Schwarz et al. persuasively demonstrated that Ti particles introduced on the calvaria of mice provoked severe inflammation associated with TNF-α and caused bone resorption (125). In mice with a p55 TNF receptor knockout, the inflammation and ensuing bone resorption was suppressed (125). Using a soluble protein based on the p75 TNF receptor (Etanercept, Immunex, Seattle, WA), Childs et al. revealed that Ti-induced calvarial bone resorption could be completely blocked, demonstrating the drug's ability to *prevent* osteolysis (19). When the drug was administered 5 days after Ti implantation and with inflammation already established, further osteolysis was prevented, indicating its potential for *treating* osteolysis (19). Further solidifying the role of TNF-α at the apex of the wear-mediated osteolytic cascade, gene delivery of the soluble inhibitor of TNF-α prevented associated inflammation and bone resorption (18,145).

These encouraging findings led to the development of a clinical trial to evaluate the efficacy of Etanercept in treating established osteolysis in clinical patients (67,141). Twenty patients were recruited into the study and randomized to receive Etanercept or placebo. Progression of the osteolytic lesion was determined using volumetric Cat Scan and associated algorithms to develop 3-D volume data. At the end of the 1-year clinical trial, the Etanercept treatment did not affect the size of the lesion. There was an actual increase in osteolytic volume in both patient groups. Measures of urine N-telopeptides and functional assessment also failed to demonstrate treatment efficacy (141). The authors suggest that a larger number of patients would have been required to determine the efficacy of this drug. Rather it appears that patients have a highly evolved inflammatory cascade with multiple redundant and compensatory pathways. It is more likely that, instead of a single mediator, a panel of inflammatory cytokines together impel the inflammation, leading to osteolysis along parallel paths that converge at the osteoclast. Presciently, Horowitz et al. reported on the inadequacy of inhibiting TNF-α using an innovative culture model (59). In a co-culture with adherent macrophages and particles, mouse calvaria was supported on a mesh in the same well (59). In this system, while neutralizing antibodies completely inhibited TNF-α, it could not prevent PGE_2 release, nor completely block bone resorption as measured by ^{45}Ca release (59).

Bisphosphonate Therapies

In the study by Horowitz et al., pamidronate (a bisphosphonate) was the only drug capable of inhibiting osteoclasts and prevented bone resorption (59). This assessment was shared by Shanbhag et al. as well. In a canine model of uncemented THR, they evaluated the effect of oral bisphosphonate (alendronate, Merck, Rahway, NJ) in preventing osteolysis stimulated by submicron UHMWPE particles (131). To kindle the inflammatory cascade around uncemented components, submicron UHMWPE and/or metallic wear debris was introduced around the femoral components intraoperatively. At 24 weeks after surgery, endosteal scalloping and radiolucencies were observed surrounding the implants in untreated canines, consistent with aseptic loosening. In canines treated with oral alendronate, the osteoclast-mediated bone loss was completely inhibited (Fig. 22-14). Yet the underlying inflammation to wear debris still smoldered. Radiographs showcased excellent bone–implant interface, but the thin interfacing tissue was laden with macrophages and phagocytosed wear debris and released high levels of inflammatory mediators (Figs. 22-15 and 22-16) (51,131). Thus it appears, that in treated animals, even though the macrophages were stimulated by the wear debris to initiate the inflammatory cascade, bisphosphonate treatment prevented the end effector cells (osteoclasts) from excavating the surrounding bone (131). This finding is consistent with the literature indicating that bisphosphonates act as specific inhibitors of osteoclast-mediated bone resorption with no known anti-inflammatory effects (Fig. 22-17) (59,119).

These findings were confirmed in a rat model of osteolysis in which a UHMWPE plug was placed in the rat proximal tibia and high-density polyethylene was injected intra-articularly. Infusing alendronate around the implant successfully prevented the peri-implant bone loss observed in control animals (99). In separate rats, osteolysis was allowed to develop for 10 weeks postsurgery, and alendronate was infused for a subsequent 6 weeks. At the end of the treatment phase, bone volumes around the implants were preserved and even recovered to near nontreated levels (99). Thadani et al. observed similar results (149). Reaping the benefits of the newer, more potent bisphosphonate zoledronate (Zometa,

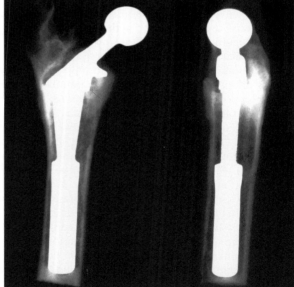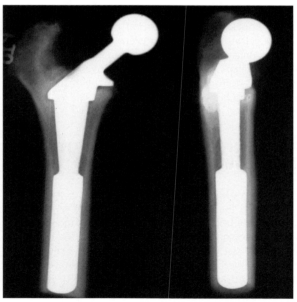

A,B   C,D

Figure 22-14 Contact femoral radiographs from canines untreated (**A** and **B**) and treated (**C** and **D**) with oral alendronate. Canines underwent uncemented total hip replacement. Particulate debris (UHWMPE, Co-Cr, and TiAlV) was introduced intraoperatively. Treated canines received daily oral alendronate therapy starting at week 1. After 24 weeks, peri-implant bone resorption was inhibited in treated animals.

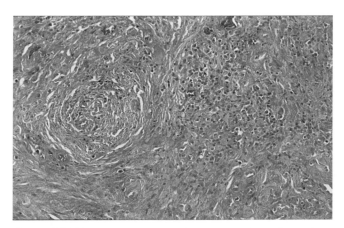

Figure 22-15 Light micrograph of an interfacial membrane from a canine with an uncemented total hip replacement and submicron UHMWPE debris introduced around the implant intraoperatively. Tissues were harvested and analyzed at the end of the 24-week study. Note the significant macrophage infiltrate with intracellular and extracellular wear debris present (magnification, 100×). See Color Plate.

Novartis, Basel, Switzerland), von Knoch et al. demonstrated in a mouse model that a single subcutaneous dose protects against particle-induced inflammation for 14 days. These studies establish in animal models at least, that bisphosphonate treatment can inhibit osteoclast-mediated osteolysis around joint replacements.

In clinical settings, the results have been less optimistic. Lyons et al. studied the effect of alendronate therapy in patients who demonstrated aseptic loosening and who were awaiting revision surgery in the United Kingdom (86). In this patient cohort, a 6-month oral treatment conferred no advantage and did not alter the need for revision surgery (86).

A randomized multicenter clinical trial was also undertaken to evaluate the effect of alendronate on the radiographic progression of osteolytic lesions. Two dosing regimens were considered: an osteoporosis dose (10 mg/d) and a Paget's disease dose (35 mg/d). Patients with femoral osteolysis post-THR ($n = 123$) were randomized to various treatment regimens, radiographs were digitized, and osteolytic lesions measured (121). After an 18-month study period, neither of the two alendronate doses had an effect on lesion size. The lack of treatment effect might have been due to the lower sensitivity of radiographs in detecting subtle changes in lesion size (121). CT scans might have performed better. Based on clinical trials, it is apparent that dosing of bisphosphonates, as well as sensitive methods to evaluate treatment efficacy, need to be developed.

Preventing Stress Shielding

Clinical evidence suggests that bisphosphonates may be effective in preventing the diffuse bone loss associated with stress shielding (48). Particularly around THRs, the insertion of a stiff metal implant alters the loading pattern of the surrounding bone. Body weight is transferred along the implant to the femoral diaphysis, bypassing the proximal femur. During the first 3 months after insertion of the implant, bone mineral density (BMD) decreases by 3% to 14% in all Gruen zones around the implant (159). Most of the decrease occurs within the first year, bottoming out at about a 23% loss from the preoperative level in the calcar region (Gruen zone 7). In subsequent years, further decreases generally do not occur, and a slight restoration may be seen (159). The artificially induced osteopenia may compromise implant stability if allowed to progress.

In a sheep femoral hemiarthroplasty model, intravenous infusion of zoledronate initiated 1 month preoperatively and continued monthly reduced calcar bone resorption and prevented the destructive effects of stress shielding over 4 months postimplantation (48). In a clinical trial in patients with uncemented THR, Venesmaa et al. reported a similarly positive finding (158). A 6-month treatment of oral alendronate was effective in preventing bone loss associated with stress shielding. In untreated patients, BMD in the proximal femur decreased by 17%, which was abrogated in alendronate-treated patients, resulting in a 0.9% decrease compared with preoperative levels (158). Similarly, Lyons et al. reported slight increases in BMD compared with placebo controls in primary THR recipients receiving alendronate (86). Soininvaara et al. demonstrated the protective effect of alendronate treatment in patients with total knee replacements (TKRs) (142). In

Figure 22-16 Mediators released by interfacial tissues harvested from canines at the end of a 24-week study. Canines underwent uncemented total hip replacement. Particulate debris—UHWMPE, TiAlV, Co-Cr, or a mix of particles (UHMWPE:TiAlV:Co-Cr = 90:5:5)—was introduced intraoperatively. Some canines (mix + Rx) received daily oral alendronate therapy starting at week 1. At sacrifice, peri-implant tissues were harvested and placed in organ culture, and the spent conditioned medium was assayed for prostaglandin E_2 and interleukin-1 using bioassays. Bisphosphonate therapy did not affect macrophages stimulated and releasing inflammatory, but the osteoclastic bone resorption was completely blocked, as can be seen in figure 22-14.

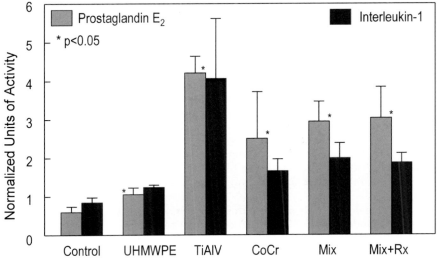

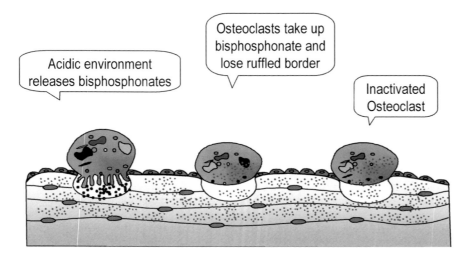

Figure 22-17 Mechanism of bisphosphonate action. Bisphosphonates are bound to the hydroxyapatite mineral. Osteoclasts attempting bone resorption create a localized acidic environment that releases the bisphosphonates and enters the osteoclast. Within the cell, bisphosphonates interfere with the mevalonate pathway, leading to many cellular changes, including loss of ruffled border and possible apoptosis.

patients receiving alendronate (10 mg/d), along with a calcium supplement (500 mg), distal femoral BMD was maintained at presurgical levels. In patients receiving only the calcium supplement, significant bone loss occurred over the 1-year duration of the study. These studies highlight the beneficial effects of bisphosphonate therapy in maintaining improved bone quality in patients with joint replacements and possibly improving their long-term durability.

Improving Implant Stability

The long-term success of uncemented TJR is critically dependent on the initial biological fixation being stable. Most of the initial implant migration occurs within 6 months postsurgery, at which time the implant stabilizes. If implant migration continues past 1 year, then loosening is imminent (122). In a clinical trial of patients with TKR followed for more than 10 years, Ryd et al. confirmed that all cases of implant loosening were associated with continuous migration of tibial components (122). The concern with bisphosphonate use to prevent bone resorption in the immediate postoperative period is that crucial fracture healing is also taking place. Hindering osteoclastic activity might retard bone remodeling and mineralization, and negatively impact the long-term stability of components. Hilding et al. demonstrated in a double-blinded clinical trial that perioperative treatment of oral clodronate was effective in reducing tibial component migration in cemented TKR (55). Patients were dosed with oral clodronate starting 3 months before surgery, and treatment continued till 6 months after surgery. Component migration was assessed using RSA at 6 months and 1 year postoperative. Not only did bisphosphonate treatment stabilize the implants (rotation and translation were significantly reduced), but it also protected the components from migration at the 1-year point as well. The authors explained that bisphosphonates protect the necrotic bone layer under the tibial components, which otherwise would have been replaced by a fibrous tissue interface, resulting in inadequate fixation and consequent implant motion (55).

Astrand and Aspenberg explored this hypothesis further in an animal model of bone necrosis. They demonstrated that a higher clinical dose of systemic alendronate effectively shuts down resorption of necrotic bone, which then provides a scaffold for new osteoid deposition (5). They speculated that since bisphosphonates prevent the detrimental effects of necrotic bone revascularization, the drug could be used in treating osteonecrosis. Resorption of the necrotic bone would be reduced until sufficient new bone has formed, preventing structural collapse of the femoral head (5). Such protective effects could potentially be used to prevent resorption of structural bone autografts and allografts by simply soaking the grafts for 10 minutes in a bisphosphonate solution before implantation (4). Clinical studies exploring these hypotheses are yet to be conducted.

Other Therapeutic Opportunities

In the past decade, the concept of delivering genes to a target site for their therapeutic effects has become popular. Ulrich-Vinther et al. investigated the effects of a single intramuscular injection of an adenoviral vector coexpressing OPG in the murine calvaria model of particle-induced osteolysis and showed a complete inhibition of osteolysis (154). Goater et al. reported on the potential of ex vivo transfected synoviocytes in inhibiting Ti-stimulated bone resorption in a murine model (41). Gene therapy for OPG was also effective in protecting against UHMWPE-induced osteoclastogenic cytokine release and bone calcium release in a murine air-pouch model (170).

Blocking the effect of IL-1 using gene therapy for IL-receptor antagonist protein (IRAP) was also effective in blocking release of UHMWPE-induced inflammatory cytokines (171,172). Adenoviral IL-10 also appears to have anti-inflammatory properties. Introducing and coexpressing a viral IL-10 gene in fibroblastlike synoviocytes inhibited the release of Ti-mediated TNF-α and IL-1 and subsequent osteoclastogenesis (12).

FUTURE DIRECTIONS

Wear debris causes osteolysis. Any and all developments to reduce the wear debris burden will extend the durability of joint replacements.

The development of alternate bearing materials has been the focus of vigorous activity. Specifically, cross-linked

UHMWPE has the potential to significantly improve the longevity of joint replacements. XLPE liners reduce generated debris by up to 90%, but the debris from these liners is biologically more inflammatory to macrophages than conventional UHMWPE (33,64). Consequently, an aggressive vigilance program to replace liners at the first signs of wear or osteolysis would be required. Particularly from a public health perspective, further studies investigating the biology of XLPE debris are sorely needed.

Clinical attempts to block inflammatory mediators using therapeutic agents have thus far been unsuccessful. This is particularly surprising coming on the heels of several studies demonstrating persuasive results in animals, particularly in models with sophisticated "gene–knock-out" mice. Yet the clinical response in humans to these same therapeutic molecules is underwhelming. What then do these studies imply about the role of small animal models? Despite minimal genetic differences between species, the importance of innumerable compensatory mechanisms and redundant inflammatory pathways in the human system cannot be overstated. In addition, with variable bioavailability and species-specific pharmacokinetic parameters, a safe therapeutic window may not be achievable for this application in patients. These trials also suggest that, rather than a single mediator driving inflammatory bone resorption, a panel of mediators with complex interrelationships likely share the burden of impelling wear debris–mediated osteolysis in patients. Any therapeutic endeavors would have to be correspondingly complex. Blocking maturation of osteoclasts by overexpressing OPG appears to be a promising approach, considering that, more than the particle-mediated inflammation, it would directly cap available RANKL and prevent the rise of new osteoclasts.

Certainly gene therapy provides exciting possibilities for the future. Although investigators have demonstrated dramatic results in small animals, clinical reality may intrude on this optimism. Delivery of genes using a viral vector remains unresolved and controversial. Will patients accept the introduction of an adenoviral vector to treat an essentially nonlethal or non-life-threatening pathologic process around their joint replacement? This might seem doubtful given that the surgical alternative is a routinely performed revision whose risks are currently quantifiable and whose outcomes are more predictable. In the hands of an experienced master surgeon, the complications of revision surgery are not much greater than those of a primary joint replacement and more acceptable than the potential toxicity and long-term consequences of proposed experimental agents. What then would compel a patient and treating physician to take on the unknown risks associated with repeated gene delivery using viral vectors or other carriers? For surgeons to clinically use gene therapy for osteolysis, it must first be widely accepted as a treatment for other "quality-of-life" diseases. Only then might patients accept this over other alternatives.

Bisphosphonates still appear to hold promise, primarily because many older recipients of joint replacements likely present signs of subclinical osteoporosis. Bisphosphonates are widely used in patients, and their safety, reliability, and efficacy in inhibiting bone resorption are well documented in long-term clinical studies. To be effective in treating osteolysis, bisphosphonates may need to be administered at the very onset of osteolysis, which is undetectable using currently accepted sur-

veillance methods. If the lesion is still small, is asymptomatic, and does not compromise implant stability, there may be an opportunity for attempting bisphosphonates. Bisphosphonates do not appear to be terribly effective when the lytic lesion is rapidly expanding, the implant is already loose, or loosening is imminent. Clinical trials also indicate that effective dosing of bisphosphonates for prevention and management of osteolysis in joint replacement patients has still not been determined.

To match the sophistication of current therapeutic modalities, there is a corresponding need for sensitive methods to track the efficacy of treatments. Clinical studies have highlighted the limitations of x-rays and CT scans. Importantly, efforts need to be directed at means to detect bone resorption much earlier—before it compromises implant stability and requires drastic revision surgery. Developments in functional genomics have sadly not yet impacted joint replacement and osteolysis studies. The slower development of end user–friendly data mining tools has likely contributed to this lack of progress. Yet, a combination of gene expression profiling and protein chip investigations offers the best hope for well-designed nonsurgical interventions.

Developers of treatments will also need to address the costs of new treatments, particularly in an increasingly cost-conscious social environment. Compare Etanercept, which costs nearly $10,000 for an annual treatment, with the surgical cost of $31,000 for revision surgery (34). Gene therapy costs are still undetermined.

SUMMARY

In this interdisciplinary arena, where multiple specialization and skill sets intersect, advances in joint replacement have been truly phenomenal. A joint replacement lasting more than 20 years appears to be a reality. If that is not enough, new materials are still being developed, implant designs are being refined, surgical skills are being honed, and operative times shaved thin. Blood loss has been squeezed, and complications are predictable. Postoperative rehabilitation procedures have been optimized, patients are weight bearing earlier, and they are attaining greater range of motion. These wide-ranging but coordinated contributions have advanced the entire field, improving the final outcome for the patient. For total joint replacements to become a *routine* procedure is itself a marvel and attests to the efforts of all who toil in this field.

REFERENCES

1. Abb J, Zander H, Abb H, et al. Association of human leucocyte low responsiveness to inducers of interferon alpha with HLA-DR2. *Immunology.* 1983;49:239–244.
2. Algan SM, Purdon M, Horowitz SM. Role of tumor necrosis factor alpha in particulate-induced bone resorption. *J Orthop Res.* 1996; 14:30–35.
3. Anderson DM, Maraskovsky E, Billingsley WL, et al. A homologue of the TNF receptor and its ligand enhance T-cell growth and dendritic-cell function. *Nature.* 1997;390(6656):175–179.
4. Aspenberg P, Astrand J. Bone allografts pretreated with a bisphosphonate are not resorbed. *Acta Orthop Scand.* 2002;73:20–23.
5. Astrand J, Aspenberg P. Systemic alendronate prevents resorption of necrotic bone during revascularization: a bone chamber study in rats. *BMC Musculoskelet Disord.* 2002;3(1):19.
6. Berger RA, Jacobs JJ, Quigley LR, et al. Primary cementless acetabular reconstruction in patients younger than 50 years old: 7- to 11-year results. *Clin Orthop.* 1997;344:216–226.

7. Bobyn JD, Jacobs JJ, Tanzer M, et al. The susceptibility of smooth implant surfaces to periimplant fibrosis and migration of polyethylene wear debris. *Clin Orthop.* 1995;311:21–39.

8. Boyle WJ, Simonet WS, Lacey DL. Osteoclast differentiation and activation. *Nature.* 2003;423(6937):337–342.

9. Bozic KJ, Rosenberg AG, Huckman RS, et al. Economic evaluation in orthopaedics. *J Bone Joint Surg [Am].* 2003;85A:129–142.

10. Bucay N, Sarosi I, Dunstan CR, et al. Osteoprotegerin-deficient mice develop early onset osteoporosis and arterial calcification. *Genes Dev.* 1998;12:1260–1268.

11. Campbell P, Ma S, Yeom B, et al. Isolation of predominantly submicron-sized UHMWPE wear particles from periprosthetic tissues. *J Biomed Mater Res.* 1995;29:127–131.

12. Carmody EE, Schwarz EM, Puzas JE, et al. Viral interleukin-10 gene inhibition of inflammation, osteoclastogenesis, and bone resorption in response to titanium particles. *Arthritis Rheum.* 2002;46:1298–1308.

13. Charnley J. Anchorage of the femoral head prosthesis to the shaft of the femur. *J Bone Joint Surg.* 1960;42B:28–30.

14. Charnley J. Tissue reaction to implanted plastics. In: Charnley J, ed. Acrylic Cement in Orthopedic Surgery. Edinburgh: E&S Livingstone; 1970:1–9.

15. Charnley J. Tissue reactions to polytetrafluorethylene [Letter to the editor]. *Lancet.* 1963;1963:1379.

16. Charnley J, Follacci FM, Hammond BT. The long-term reaction of bone to self-curing acrylic cement. *J Bone Joint Surg.* 1968;50B: 822–829.

17. Chiba J, Rubash HE, Kim KJ, et al. The characterization of cytokines in the interface tissue obtained from failed cementless total hip arthroplasty with and without femoral osteolysis. *Clin Orthop.* 1994;300:304–312.

18. Childs LM, Goater JJ, O'Keefe RJ, et al. Effect of anti-tumor necrosis factor-alpha gene therapy on wear debris-induced osteolysis. *J Bone Joint Surg [Am].* 2001;83A:1789–1797.

19. Childs LM, Goater JJ, O'Keefe RJ, et al. Efficacy of etanercept for wear debris-induced osteolysis. *J Bone Miner Res.* 2001;16:338–347.

20. Coleman DL, King RN, Andrade JD. The foreign body reaction: a chronic inflammatory response. *J Biomed Mater Res.* 1974;8: 199–211.

21. Collier JP, Surprenant VA, Jensen RE, et al. Corrosion between the components of modular femoral hip prostheses. *J Bone Joint Surg [Br].* 1992;74:511–517.

22. Dean DD, Schwartz Z, Liu Y, et al. The effect of ultra-high molecular weight polyethylene wear debris on MG63 osteosarcoma cells in vitro. *J Bone Joint Surg [Am].* 1999;81:452–461.

23. Devane PA, Bourne RB, Rorabeck CH, et al. Measurement of polyethylene wear in metal-backed acetabular cups, I: three-dimensional technique. *Clin Orthop Relat Res.* 1995;319: 303–316.

24. Devane PA, Bourne RB, Rorabeck CH, et al. Measurement of polyethylene wear in metal-backed acetabular cups, II: clinical application. *Clin Orthop Relat Res.* 1995;319:317–326.

25. Diegelmann RF, Cohen IK, Kaplan AM. Effect of macrophages on fibroblast DNA synthesis and proliferation. *Proc Soc Exp Biol Med.* 1982;169:445–451.

26. Diegelmann RF, Cohen IK, Kaplan AM. The role of macrophages in wound repair: a review. *Plast Reconstr Surg.* 1981;68:107–113.

27. Dinarello CA. Interleukin-1. *Rev Inf Dis.* 1984;6:51–95.

28. Doehring TC, Saigal S, Shanbhag AS, et al. Micromotion of acetabular liners: measurements comparing the effectiveness of locking mechanisms. *Trans Orthop Res Soc.* 1996;21:427.

29. Dorr LD, Bloebaum R, Emmanual J, et al. Histologic, biochemical, and ion analysis of tissue and fluids retrieved during total hip arthroplasty. *Clin Orthop Relat Res.* 1990;261:82–95.

30. Dowd JE, Schwendeman LJ, Macaulay W, et al. Aseptic loosening in uncemented total hip arthroplasty in a canine model. *Clin Orthop.* 1995;319:106–121.

31. Dowd JE, Sychterz CJ, Young AM, et al. Characterization of long-term femoral-head–penetration rates: association with and prediction of osteolysis. *J Bone Joint Surg [Am].* 2000;82A:1102–1107.

32. Dower SK, Call SM, Gillis S, et al. Similarity between the interleukin 1 receptors on a murine T-lymphoma cell line and on a murine fibroblast cell line. *Proc Natl Acad Sci USA.* 1986;83: 1060–1064.

33. Fisher J, McEwen HM, Tipper JL, et al. Wear, debris, and biologic activity of cross-linked polyethylene in the knee: benefits and potential concerns. *Clin Orthop Relat Res.* 2004;428:114–119.

34. Frankowski JJ, Watkins-Castillo S. *Primary Total Knee and Hip Arthroplasty Projections for the US Population to the Year 2030.* Rosemont, IL: American Academy of Orthopaedic Surgeons; 2002.

35. Friedman RJ, Black J, Galante JO, et al. Current concepts in orthopaedic biomaterials and implant fixation. *Instr Course Lect.* 1994;43:233–255.

36. Fuller K, Murphy C, Kirstein B, et al. TNF-alpha potently activates osteoclasts, through a direct action independent of and strongly synergistic with RANKL. *Endocrinology.* 2002;143:1108–1118.

37. Garrett R, Wilksch J, Vernon-Roberts B. Effects of cobalt-chrome alloy wear particles on the morphology, viability and phagocytic activity of murine macrophages in vitro. *Aust J Exp Biol Med Sci.* 1983;61:355–369.

38. Gilbert JL, Buckley CA, Jacobs JJ. In vivo corrosion of modular hip prosthesis components in mixed and similar metal combinations: the effect of crevice, stress, motion, and alloy coupling. *J Biomed Mater Res.* 1993;27:1533–1544.

39. Glant TT, Jacobs JJ. Response of three murine macrophage populations to particulate debris: bone resorption in organ cultures. *J Orthop Res.* 1994;12:720–731.

40. Glant TT, Jacobs JJ, Molnar G, et al. Bone resorption activity of particulate-stimulated macrophages. *J Bone Miner Res.* 1993;8: 1071–1079.

41. Goater JJ, O'Keefe RJ, Rosier RN, et al. Efficacy of ex vivo OPG gene therapy in preventing wear debris induced osteolysis. *J Orthop Res.* 2002;20:169–173.

42. Goldring SR, Schiller AL, Roelke M, et al. The synovial-like membrane at the bone-cement interface in loose total hip replacements and its proposed role in bone lysis. *J Bone Joint Surg [Am].* 1983;65:575–584.

43. Goodman SB, Chin RC. Prostaglandin E2 levels in the membrane surrounding bulk and particulate polymethylmethacrylate in the rabbit tibia: a preliminary study. *Clin Orthop.* 1990; 257:305–309.

44. Goodman SB, Chin RC, Chiou SS, et al. A clinical-pathologic-biochemical study of the membrane surrounding loosened and nonloosened total hip arthroplasties. *Clin Orthop.* 1989;244: 182–187.

45. Goodman SB, Fornasier VL, Kei J. The effects of bulk versus particulate polymethylmethacrylate on bone. *Clin Orthop.* 1988;232: 255–262.

46. Goodman SB, Fornasier VL, Kei J. The effects of bulk versus particulate ultra-high-molecular-weight polyethylene on bone. *J Arthroplasty.* 1988;3(suppl):S41–S46.

47. Goodman SB, Knoblich G, O'Connor M, et al. Heterogeneity in cellular and cytokine profiles from multiple samples of tissue surrounding revised hip prostheses. *J Biomed Mater Res.* 1996;31: 421–428.

48. Goodship AE, Lawes TJ, Green J, et al. The use of bisphosphonates to inhibit mechanically related bone loss in aseptic loosening of hip prostheses. *Trans Orthop Res Soc.* 1998;23:2.

49. Gonzalez O, Smith RL, Goodman SB. Effect of size, concentration, surface area, and volume of polymethylmethacrylate particles on human macrophages in vitro. *J Biomed Mater Res.* 1996;30: 463–473.

50. Gray MH, Talbert ML, Talbert WM, et al. Changes seen in lymph nodes draining the sites of large joint prostheses. *Am J Surg Path.* 1989;13:1050–1056.

51. Hasselman CT, Shanbhag AS, Kovach C, et al. Osteolysis and aseptic loosening in a canine uncemented total hip arthroplasty (THA) model. *Trans Orthop Res Soc.* 1997;22:22.

52. Haynes DR, Rogers SD, Hay S, et al. The differences in toxicity and release of bone-resorbing mediators induced by titanium and cobalt-chromium-alloy wear particles. *J Bone Joint Surg [Am].* 1993;75(6):825–834.

53. Herman JH, Sowder WG, Anderson D, et al. Polymethylmethacrylate-induced release of bone-resorbing factors. *J Bone Joint Surg.* 1989;71A:1530–1541.

54. Hicks DG, Judkins AR, Sickel JZ, et al. Granular histiocytes of pelvic lymph nodes following total hip arthroplasty: the presence of wear debris, cytokine production, and immunologi-

cally activated macrophages. *J Bone Joint Surg.* 1996;78A: 482–496.

55. Hilding M, Ryd L, Toksvig-Larsen S, et al. Clodronate prevents prosthetic migration: a randomized radiostereometric study of 50 total knee patients. *Acta Orthop Scand.* 2000;71:553–557.

56. Howie DW, Vernon-Roberts B. The synovial response to intraarticular cobalt-chrome wear particles. *Clin Orthop.* 1988;232: 244–254.

57. Howie DW, Vernon-Roberts B, Oakeshott R, et al. A rat model of resorption of bone at the cement-bone interface in the presence of polyethylene wear particles. *J Bone Joint Surg.* 1988;70A: 257–263.

58. Horikoshi M, Dowd J, Maloney WJ, et al. Activation of human fibroblasts and macrophages by particulate wear debris from failed total hip and total knee arthroplasty. *Trans Orthop Res Soc.* 1994;19:199.

59. Horowitz SM, Algan SA, Purdon MA. Pharmacologic inhibition of particulate-induced bone resorption. *J Biomed Mater Res.* 1996;31:91–96.

60. Horowitz SM, Doty SB, Lane JM, et al. Studies of the mechanism by which the mechanical failure of polymethylmethacrylate leads to bone resorption. *J Bone Joint Surg.* 1993;75A: 802–813.

61. Horowitz SM, Frondoza CG, Lennox DW. Effects of polymethylmethacrylate exposure upon macrophages. *J Orthop Res.* 1988;6:827–832.

62. Horowitz SM, Gautsch TL, Frondoza CG, et al. Macrophage exposure to polymethyl methacrylate leads to mediator release and injury. *J Orthop Res.* 1991;9:406–413.

63. Horowitz SM, Gonzales JB. Effects of polyethylene on macrophages. *J Biomed Mater Res.* 1997;15:50–56.

64. Huddleston JI, Hayata K, Kawashima M, et al. Human macrophage response to highly cross-linked UHMWPE debris. *Trans Orthop Res Soc.* 2006;31:700.

65. Huk OL, Bansal M, Betts F, et al. Polyethylene and metal debris generated by non-articulating surfaces of modular acetabular components. *J Bone Joint Surg.* 1994;76B:568–574.

66. *Implant Wear in Total Joint Replacement.* Rosemont, IL: American Academy of Orthopaedic Surgeons; 2001.

67. Ingham E, Fisher J. The role of macrophages in osteolysis of total joint replacement. *Biomaterials.* 2005;26:1271–1286.

68. Ingham E, Green TR, Stone MH, et al. Production of TNF-alpha and bone resorbing activity by macrophages in response to different types of bone cement particles. *Biomaterials.* 2000;21:1005–1013.

69. Jacobs JJ, Patterson LM, Skipor AK, et al. Postmortem retrieval of total joint replacement components. *J Biomed Mater Res.* 1999; 48:385–391.

70. Jacobs JJ, Roebuck KA, Archibeck M, et al. Osteolysis: basic science. *Clin Orthop.* 2001;393:71–77.

71. Jacobs JJ, Urban RM, Gilbert JL, et al. Local and distant products from modularity. *Clin Orthop.* 1995;319:94–105.

72. Jacobs JJ, Urban RM, Schajowicz F, et al. Particulate-associated endosteal osteolysis in titanium-base alloy cementless total hip replacement. In: St John KR, ed. *Particulate Debris from Medical Implants: Mechanisms of Formation and Biological Consequences.* Philadelphia: American Society for Testing and Materials; 1992: 52–60. ASTM Special Technical Publication no. 1144.

73. Jiranek WA, Machado M, Jasty M, et al. Production of cytokines around loosened cemented acetabular components: analysis with immunohistochemical techniques and in situ hybridization. *J Bone Joint Surg [Am].* 1993;75:863–879.

74. Kim KJ, Rubash HE, Wilson SC, et al. A histologic and biochemical comparison of the interface tissues in cementless and cemented hip prostheses. *Clin Orthop.* 1993;287:142–152.

75. Klimkiewicz JJ, Iannotti JP, Rubash HE, et al. Aseptic loosening of the humeral component in total shoulder arthroplasty. *J Shoulder Elbow Surg.* 1998;7:422–426.

76. Kobayashi K, Takahashi N, Jimi E, et al. Tumor necrosis factor alpha stimulates osteoclast differentiation by a mechanism independent of the ODF/RANKL-RANK interaction. *J Exp Med.* 2000;191:275–286.

77. Kong YY, Feige U, Sarosi I, et al. Activated T cells regulate bone loss and joint destruction in adjuvant arthritis through osteoprotegerin ligand. *Nature.* 1999;402(6759):304–309.

78. Kong YY, Yoshida H, Sarosi I, et al. OPGL is a key regulator of osteoclastogenesis, lymphocyte development and lymph-node organogenesis. *Nature.* 1999;397(6717):315–323.

79. Konttinen YT, Ainola M, Valleala H, et al. Analysis of 16 different matrix metalloproteinases (MMP-1 to MMP-20) in the synovial membrane: different profiles in trauma and rheumatoid arthritis. *Ann Rheum Dis.* 1999;58:691–697.

80. Lacey DL, Timms E, Tan HL, et al. Osteoprotegerin ligand is a cytokine that regulates osteoclast differentiation and activation. *Cell.* 1998;93:165–176.

81. Lee SE, Chung WJ, Kwak HB, et al. Tumor necrosis factor-alpha supports the survival of osteoclasts through the activation of Akt and ERK. *J Biol Chem.* 2001;276:49343–49349.

82. Li J, Sarosi I, Yan XQ, et al. RANK is the intrinsic hematopoietic cell surface receptor that controls osteoclastogenesis and regulation of bone mass and calcium metabolism. *Proc Natl Acad Sci USA.* 2000;97:1566–1571.

83. Lind M, Trindade MC, Nakashima Y, et al. Chemotaxis and activation of particle-challenged human monocytes in response to monocyte migration inhibitory factor and C-C chemokines. *J Biomed Mater Res.* 1999;48:246–250.

84. Lind M, Trindade MC, Schurman DJ, et al. Monocyte migration inhibitory factor synthesis and gene expression in particle-activated macrophages. *Cytokine.* 2000;12(7):909–913.

85. Lum L, Wong BR, Josien R, et al. Evidence for a role of a tumor necrosis factor-a (TNF-a)-converting enzyme-like protease in shedding of TRANCE, a TNF family member involved in osteoclastogenesis and dendritic cell survival. *J Biol Chem.* 1999;274: 13613–13618.

86. Lyons AR, Owen JE, Freedholm DA, et al. Effect of alendronate on periprosthetic bone mass. Transactions of the 10th Combined Meeting of the Orthopaedic Associations of the English Speaking World; Auckland, New Zealand; February 1–6,1998:209.

87. Mabrey JD, Afsar-Keshmiri A, McClung GA, et al. Comparison of UHMWPE particles in synovial fluid and tissues from failed THA. *J Biomed Mater Res.* 2001;58:196–202.

88. Maloney WJ, Herzwurm P, Paprosky W, et al. Treatment of pelvic osteolysis associated with a stable acetabular component inserted without cement as part of a total hip replacement. *J Bone Joint Surg [Am].* 1997;79:1628–1634.

89. Maloney WJ, Jasty M, Harris WH, et al. Endosteal erosion in association with stable uncemented femoral components. *J Bone Joint Surg [Am].* 1990;72:1025–1034.

90. Maloney WJ, Smith RL. Periprosthetic osteolysis in total hip arthroplasty: the role of particulate wear debris. *Instr Course Lect.* 1996;45:171–182.

91. Maloney WJ, Smith RL, Castro F, et al. Fibroblast response to metallic debris in vitro: enzyme induction cell proliferation, and toxicity. *J Bone Joint Surg [Am].* 1993;75:835–844.

92. Maloney WJ, Smith RL, Schmalzried TP, et al. Isolation and characterization of wear particles generated in patients who have had failure of a hip arthroplasty without cement. *J Bone Joint Surg [Am].* 1995;77:1301–1310.

93. Margevicius KJ, Bauer TW, McMahon JT, et al. Isolation and characterization of debris in membranes around total joint prostheses. *J Bone Joint Surg.* 1994;76A:1664–1675.

94. Martin M, Resch K. Interleukin 1: more than a mediator between leukocytes. *TIBS.* 1988;9:171–177.

95. Matthews JB, Besong AA, Green TR, et al. Evaluation of the response of primary human peripheral blood mononuclear phagocytes to challenge with in vitro generated clinically relevant UHMWPE particles of known size and dose. *J Biomed Mater Res.* 2000;52:296–307.

96. McKellop H, Shen FW, Lu B, et al. Development of an extremely wear-resistant ultra high molecular weight polyethylene for total hip replacements. *J Orthop Res.* 1999;17:157–167.

97. Merchant KK, Rohr WL, Lintner WP, et al. Orthopaedic implant surface debris. *Trans Orthop Res Soc.* 1995;20:164.

98. Mevellec C, Burleigh TD, Shanbhag AS. Corrosion in modular femoral hip prostheses: a study of 22 retrieved implants. Proceedings of the 15th Southern Biomedical Engineering Conference; Dayton, OH; March 29–31, 1996:3–4.

99. Millett PJ, Allen MJ, Bostrom MP. Effects of alendronate on particle-induced osteolysis in a rat model. *J Bone Joint Surg [Am].* 2002;84A:236–249.

100. Min H, Morony S, Sarosi I, et al. Osteoprotegerin reverses osteoporosis by inhibiting endosteal osteoclasts and prevents vascular calcification by blocking a process resembling osteoclastogenesis. *J Exp Med.* 2000;192:463–474.

101. Mirra JM, Amstutz HC, Matos M, et al. The pathology of the joint tissues and its clinical relevance in prosthesis failure. *Clin Orthop.* 1976;117:221–240.

102. Mirra JM, Marder RA, Amstutz HC. The pathology of failed total joint arthroplasty. *Clin Orthop.* 1982;170:175–183.

103. Miyanishi K, Trindade MC, Ma T, et al. Periprosthetic osteolysis: induction of vascular endothelial growth factor from human monocyte/macrophages by orthopaedic biomaterial particles. *J Bone Miner Res.* 2003;18:1573–1583.

104. Mizel SB. Production and quantitation of lymphocyte-activating factor (interleukin 1). In: Herscowitz HB, Holden HT, Bellanti JA, et al., eds. *Manual of Macrophage Methodology: Collection, Characterization, and Function.* New York: Marcel Dekker; 1981: 407–416.

105. Morinaga T, Nakagawa N, Yasuda H, et al. Cloning and characterization of the gene encoding human osteoprotegerin/osteoclastogenesis-inhibitory factor. *Eur J Biochem.* 1998;254:685–691.

106. Morrissette N, Gold E, Aderem A. The macrophage: a cell for all seasons. *Trends Cell Biol.* 1999;9:199–201.

107. Muratoglu OK, Bragdon CR, O'Connor DO, et al. A novel method of cross-linking ultra-high-molecular-weight polyethylene to improve wear, reduce oxidation, and retain mechanical properties. Recipient of the 1999 HAP Paul Award. *J Arthroplasty.* 2001;16:149–160.

108. Nakagawa N, Kinosaki M, Yamaguchi K, et al. RANK is the essential signaling receptor for osteoclast differentiation factor in osteoclastogenesis. *Biochem Biophys Res Commun.* 1998;253:395–400.

109. Nakashima Y, Sun DH, Trindade MC, et al. Induction of macrophage C-C chemokine expression by titanium alloy and bone cement particles. *J Bone Joint Surg [Br].* 1999;81:155–162.

110. Nakashima Y, Sun DH, Trindade MC, et al. Signaling pathways for tumor necrosis factor-alpha and interleukin-6 expression in human macrophages exposed to titanium-alloy particulate debris in vitro. *J Bone Joint Surg [Am].* 1999;81:603–615.

111. National Institutes of Health. *Total Hip Replacement.* Bethesda, MD, National Institutes of Health; 1994. NIH Consensus Statement.

112. Older J. Charnley low-friction arthroplasty: a worldwide retrospective review at 15 to 20 years. *J Arthroplasty.* 2002;17:675–680.

113. Pap T, Pap G, Hummel KM, et al. Membrane-type-1 matrix metalloproteinase is abundantly expressed in fibroblasts and osteoclasts at the bone-implant interface of aseptically loosened joint arthroplasties in situ. *J Rheumatol.* 1999;26:166–169.

114. Puskas BL, Menke NE, Huie P, et al. Expression of nitric oxide, peroxynitrite, and apoptosis in loose total hip replacements. *J Biomed Mater Res.* 2003;66A:541–549.

115. Rae T. The biological response to titanium and titanium-aluminum-vanadium alloy particles, I: tissue culture studies. *Biomaterials.* 1986;7:30–36.

116. Rae T. A study on the effects of particulate metals of orthopaedic interest on murine macrophages in vitro. *J Bone Joint Surg.* 1975; 57B:444–450.

117. Ricci JL, Kummer FJ, Alexander H, et al. Technical note: embedded particulate contaminants in textured metal implant surfaces. *J Appl Biomater.* 1992;3:225–230.

118. Ries MD, Scott ML, Jani S. Relationship between gravimetric wear and particle generation in hip simulators: conventional compared with cross-linked polyethylene. *J Bone Joint Surg [Am].* 2001;83A[Suppl 2, Pt 2]:116–122.

119. Rodan GA, Fleisch HA. Bisphosphonates: mechanisms of action. *J Clin Invest.* 1996;97:2692–2696.

120. Rogers SD, Howie DW, Graves SE, et al. In vitro human monocyte response to wear particles of titanium alloy containing vanadium or niobium. *J Bone Joint Surg [Br].* 1997;79:311–315.

121. Rubash HE, Dorr LD, Jacobs JJ, et al. Does alendronate inhibit the progression of periprosthetic osteolysis? *Trans Orthop Res Soc.* 2004;29:1888.

122. Ryd L, Albrektsson BE, Carlsson L, et al. Roentgen stereophotogrammetric analysis as a predictor of mechanical loosening of knee prostheses. *J Bone Joint Surg [Br].* 1995;77:377–383.

123. Saikko V, Calonius O, Keranen J. Wear of conventional and cross-linked ultra-high-molecular-weight polyethylene acetabular cups against polished and roughened CoCr femoral heads in a biaxial hip simulator. *J Biomed Mater Res.* 2002;63:848–853.

124. Schmalzried TP, Jasty M, Harris WH. Periprosthetic bone loss in total hip arthroplasty: polyethylene wear debris and the concept of the effective joint space. *J Bone Joint Surg [Am].* 1992;74: 849–863.

125. Schwarz EM, Lu AP, Goater JJ, et al. Tumor necrosis factor-alpha/nuclear transcription factor-kappaB signaling in periprosthetic osteolysis. *J Orthop Res.* 2000;18:472–480.

126. Shanbhag AS. What experimental approaches (tissue retrieval, in vivo, in vitro, etc) have been used to investigate the biologic effects of particles? In: Wright TM, Goodman SB, eds. *Implant Wear in Total Joint Replacements.* Rosemont, IL: American Academy of Orthopaedic Surgeons, 2001:114–123.

127. Shanbhag AS, Bailey HO, Eror NG, et al. Characterization and comparison of UHMWPE wear debris retrieved from total hip and total knee arthroplasties. *Trans Orthop Res Soc.* 1996;21:467.

128. Shanbhag AS, Bailey HO, Hwang DS, et al. Quantitative analysis of ultrahigh molecular weight polyethylene (UHMWPE) wear debris associated with total knee replacements. *J Biomed Mater Res.* 2000;53:100–110.

129. Shanbhag AS, Bailey HO, Hwang DS, et al. Chemical and morphological characterization of wear debris associated with acetabular screw holes. *Trans Soc Biomater.* 1995;18:325.

130. Shanbhag AS, Hasselman CT, Jacobs JJ, et al. Biologic response to wear debris. In: Callaghan JJ, Rosenberg AG, Rubash HE, eds. *The Adult Hip.* Philadelphia: Lippincott-Raven Publishers; 1998: 279–288.

131. Shanbhag AS, Hasselman CT, Rubash HE. The John Charnley Award. Inhibition of wear debris mediated osteolysis in a canine total hip arthroplasty model. *Clin Orthop.* 1997;344:33–43.

132. Shanbhag AS, Jacobs JJ, Black J, et al. Cellular mediators secreted by interfacial membranes obtained at revision total hip arthroplasty. *J Arthroplasty.* 1995;10:498–506.

133. Shanbhag AS, Jacobs JJ, Black J, et al. Effects of particles on fibroblast proliferation and bone resorption in vitro. *Clin Orthop.* 1997;342:205–217.

134. Shanbhag AS, Jacobs JJ, Black J, et al. Human monocyte response to particulate biomaterials generated in vivo and in vitro. *J Orthop Res.* 1995;13:792–801.

135. Shanbhag AS, Jacobs JJ, Black J, et al. Macrophage/particle interactions: effect of size, composition and surface area. *J Biomed Mater Res.* 1994;28:81–90.

136. Shanbhag AS, Jacobs JJ, Black J, et al. Pro- and anti-inflammatory mediators secreted from infacial membranes obtained at revision total hip arthroplasty. In: Buchorn GH, Willert HG, eds. *The Implant/Bone Interface.* Gottingen: Hogrefe and Huber; 1997.

137. Shanbhag AS, Jacobs JJ, Glant TT, et al. Composition and morphology of wear debris in failed uncemented total hip replacement. *J Bone Joint Surg [Br].* 1994;76:60–67.

138. Shanbhag AS, Rubash HE. Wear: the basis of particle disease in total hip arthroplasty. *Tech Orthop.* 1994;8:269–274.

139. Shanbhag AS, Vai CW, Qureshi SA, et al. Characteristics of cross-linked UHMWPE wear debris. *Trans Orthop Res Soc.* 2001;26:2.

140. Simonet WS, Lacey DL, Dunstan CR, et al. Osteoprotegerin: a novel secreted protein involved in the regulation of bone density. *Cell.* 1997;89:309–319.

141. Smith SE, Harris WH. Total hip arthroplasty performed with insertion of the femoral component with cement and the acetabular component without cement: ten- to thirteen-year results. *J Bone Joint Surg.* 1997;79:1827–1833.

142. Soininvaara TA, Jurvelin JS, Miettinen HJ, et al. Effect of alendronate on periprosthetic bone loss after total knee arthroplasty: a one-year, randomized, controlled trial of 19 patients. *Calcif Tissue Int.* 2002;71:472–477.

143. Solbach W, Moll H, Rollinghoff M. Lymphocytes play the music but the macrophage calls the tune. *Immunol Today.* 1991; 12:4–6.

144. Spector M, Shortkroff S, Hsu HP, et al. Tissue changes around loose prostheses: a canine model to investigate the effects of an antiinflammatory agent. *Clin Orthop.* 1990;261:140–152.

145. Sud S, Yang SY, Evans CH, et al. Effects of cytokine gene therapy on particulate-induced inflammation in the murine air pouch. *Inflammation.* 2001;25:361–372.

146. Takagi M, Santavirta S, Ida H, et al. Matrix metalloproteinases and tissue inhibitors of metalloproteinases in loose artificial hip joints. *Clin Orthop.* 1998;352:35–45.

147. Takei I, Takagi M, Santavirta S, et al. Messenger ribonucleic acid expression of 16 matrix metalloproteinases in bone–implant interface tissues of loose artificial hip joints. *J Biomed Mater Res.* 2000;52:613–620.

148. Takemura R, Werb Z. Secretory products of macrophages and their physiological functions. *Am J Physiol.* 1984;246(1 Pt 1):C1–9.

149. Thadani PJ, Waxman B, Sladek E, et al. Inhibition of particulate debris-induced osteolysis by alendronate in a rat model. *Orthopedics.* 2002;25:59–63.

150. Turner TM, Urban RM, Sumner DR, et al. Revision, without cement, of aseptically loose, cemented total hip prostheses. *J Bone Joint Surg.* 1993;75A:845–862.

151. Udagawa N, Takahashi N, Akatsu T, et al. Origin of osteoclasts: mature monocytes and macrophages are capable of differentiating into osteoblasts under a suitable microenvironment prepared by bone marrow–derived stromal cells. *Proc Natl Acad Sci U S A.* 1990;87:7260–7264.

152. Udagawa N, Takahashi N, Jimi E, et al. Osteoblasts/stromal cells stimulate osteoclast activation through expression of osteoclast differentiation factor/RANKL but not macrophage colony-stimulating factor: receptor activator of NF-kappa B ligand. *Bone.* 1999;25:517–523.

153. Udagawa N, Takahashi N, Yasuda H, et al. Osteoprotegerin produced by osteoblasts is an important regulator in osteoclast development and function. *Endocrinology.* 2000;141:3478–3484.

154. Ulrich-Vinther M, Carmody EE, Goater JJ, et al. Recombinant adeno-associated virus-mediated osteoprotegerin gene therapy inhibits wear debris-induced osteolysis. *J Bone Joint Surg [Am].* 2002;84A:1405–1412.

155. Urban RM, Jacobs JJ, Sapienza CI, et al. Interface tissues and modes of particulate debris infiltration in 25 cementless acetabular components retrieved at autopsy. *Trans Orthop Res Soc.* 1996; 21:45.

156. Urban RM, Jacobs JJ, Tomlinson MJ, et al. Dissemination of wear particles to the liver, spleen, and abdominal lymph nodes of patients with hip or knee replacement. *J Bone Joint Surg [Am].* 2000;82:457–476.

157. Vaes G. Cellular biology and biochemical mechanism of bone resorption: a review of recent developments on the formation, activation, and mode of action of osteoclasts. *Clin Orthop.* 1988; 231:239–271.

158. Venesmaa PK, Kroger HP, Miettinen HJ, et al. Alendronate reduces periprosthetic bone loss after uncemented primary total hip arthroplasty: a prospective randomized study. *J Bone Miner Res.* 2001;16:2126–2131.

159. Venesmaa PK, Kroger HP, Miettinen HJ, et al. Monitoring of periprosthetic BMD after uncemented total hip arthroplasty with dual-energy x-ray absorptiometry: a 3-year follow-up study. *J Bone Miner Res.* 2001;16:1056–1061.

160. Vermes C, Chandrasekaran R, Jacobs JJ, et al. The effects of particulate wear debris, cytokines, and growth factors on the functions of MG-63 osteoblasts. *J Bone Joint Surg [Am].* 2001;83A:201–211.

161. Vermes C, Roebuck KA, Chandrasekaran R, et al. Particulate wear debris activates protein tyrosine kinases and nuclear factor kappaB, which down-regulates type I collagen synthesis in human osteoblasts. *J Bone Miner Res.* 2000;15:1756–1765.

162. von Knoch F, Jaquiery C, Kowalsky M, et al. Effects of bisphosphonates on proliferation and osteoblast differentiation of human bone marrow stromal cells. *Biomaterials.* In press.

163. Watkins SC, Macaulay W, Turner D, et al. Identification of inducible nitric oxide synthase in human macrophages surrounding loosened hip prostheses. *Am J Pathol.* 1997;150:1199–1206.

164. Willert HG. Reactions of the articular capsule to wear products of artificial joint prostheses. *J Biomed Mater Res.* 1977;11:157–164.

165. Willert HG, Bertram H, Buchhorn GH. Osteolysis in alloarthroplasty of the hip: the role of one cement fragmentation. *Clin Orthop Relat Res.* 1990;258:108–121.

166. Willert HG, Bertram H, Buchhorn GH. Osteolysis in alloarthroplasty of the hip: the role of ultra-high molecular weight polyethylene wear particles. *Clin Orthop Relat Res.* 1990;258:95–107.

167. Willert HG, Ludwig J, Semlitsch M. Reaction of bone to methacrylate after hip arthroplasty: a long-term gross, light microscopic, and scanning electron microscopic study. *J Bone Joint Surg [Am].* 1974;56:1368–1382.

168. Willert HG, Semlitsch M. Tissue reactions to plastic and metallic wear products of joint endoprostheses. In: Gschwend N, Debrunner HU, eds. *Total Hip Prosthesis.* Baltimore: Williams & Wilkins; 1976:205–239.

169. Wooley PH, Schwarz EM. Aseptic loosening. *Gene Ther.* 2004;11: 402–407.

170. Yang SY, Mayton L, Wu B, et al. Adeno-associated virus-mediated osteoprotegerin gene transfer protects against particulate polyethylene-induced osteolysis in a murine model. *Arthritis Rheum.* 2002;46:2514–2523.

171. Yang S, Wu B, Mayton L, et al. IL-1Ra and vIL-10 gene transfer using retroviral vectors ameliorates particle-associated inflammation in the murine air pouch model. *Inflamm Res.* 2002;51: 342–350.

172. Yang SY, Wu B, Mayton L, et al. Protective effects of IL-1Ra or vIL-10 gene transfer on a murine model of wear debris-induced osteolysis. *Gene Ther.* 2004;11:483–491.

173. Yao J, Cs-Szabo G, Jacobs JJ, et al. Suppression of osteoblast function by titanium particles. *J Bone Joint Surg [Am].* 1997;79:107–112.

174. Yao J, Glant TT, Lark MW, et al. The potential role of fibroblasts in periprosthetic osteolysis: fibroblast response to titanium particles. *J Bone Miner Res.* 1995;10:1417–1427.

175. Yasuda H, Shima N, Nakagawa N, et al. A novel molecular mechanism modulating osteoclast differentiation and function. *Bone.* 1999;25:109–113.

176. Yasuda H, Shima N, Nakagawa N, et al. Osteoclast differentiation factor is a ligand for osteoprotegerin/osteoclastogenesis-inhibitory factor and is identical to TRANCE/RANKL. *Proc Natl Acad Sci USA.* 1998;95:3597–3602.

Autografts

Victor M. Goldberg   *Jean Welter*

23

Reconstructing a hip that has significant bone loss from arthritic problems or from failed total hip arthroplasty is a challenge for the orthopedic surgeon. Although there are myriad materials for reconstructing the bone lost after failed hip arthroplasty, the biologic approach, using either autogenous or allogeneic bone, is an important technique. Autogenous bone has been shown to be superior to allogeneic bone in its ability to regenerate bone (15,16,37,44). Because of limited autogenous supply and potential significant donor-site morbidity, however, the use of allograft and bone substitute has increased in the past decade (1,15,21,38,43).

The biologic activity of a graft is a synergy between its inherent biology and its ability to induce the surrounding host tissue to provide the osteoprogenitor stem cells that will ultimately become osteogenic tissue (31,39,40). Although this biologic activity of a graft in its surrounding host bed is critical to its incorporation, the mechanical environment is also important (4,23,27). Instability at the graft–host junction will usually result in graft failure and resorption. Further, there is a strong and important interaction between the biologic aspects of bone grafts and the clinical circumstances (36). The soft tissue usually present after a failed total hip arthroplasty is typically fibrotic and poorly vascularized and provides an inferior support for bone graft incorporation.

Because of the complex interaction between the biologic activity of the bone graft, the mechanical environment, and the host environment, it is important for the surgeon to understand each of these in order to choose the graft material that will result in a successful reconstruction.

It may be useful to define some of the terms frequently used in the context of bone grafts. The term "bone graft" refers to transplanted bone and can thus apply to *autografts* (tissue transferred from one anatomic site to another in the same individual), *allografts* (a graft between genetically dissimilar individuals of the same species), or *xenografts*: (tissue transplanted across species barriers). Some authors prefer the use of "graft" for living tissue and use "implant" for all others. "Bone graft substitute" generally refers to man-made substances and naturally occurring substances that have been processed.

Bone grafts can be further classified according to their composition (*cortical, corticocancellous, cancellous*), their anatomical site of origin, or the state of their blood supply (*nonvascularized, revascularized*). Allografts are described based on preservation method (*fresh, freeze-dried*) or other processing steps (*demineralized, irradiated*). As these factors affect the properties of the material, they influence the proper choice of material for a particular clinical situation.

Although there is an increasing demand for allograft bone, there is an important role for autogenous bone in reconstructing the bone-deficient hip. This chapter reviews bone graft function, the biologic events of incorporation of cancellous and cortical autogenous bone grafts, and general clinical principles. Alternative biosynthetics are discussed briefly.

BONE GRAFT FUNCTION

The biologic activity of bone grafts is the result of two functions, osteogenesis and mechanical support (14,15,31,36). *Osteogenesis* is the formation of new bone by viable cells in the graft or by invading cells from the surrounding host tissue. Fresh autogenous bone grafts have been shown to provide cells that survive transplantation, that are nourished by diffusion, and that synthesize early new bone (15,42). However, only about 10% of the graft cells in nonvascularized cancellous bone survive to participate in bone formation. Ultimately, these cells will become necrotic, and the graft will be repopulated by osteoprogenitor cells from the host. A graft of cancellous bone, because of its large surface area, has a greater propensity than cortical bone for forming active new bone. The process of activating and recruiting host osteoprogenitor cells to migrate into the graft area and then to differentiate into osteoblasts is called *osteoinduction* (31,39,40). This biologic process is a complex series of events that results in the recruitment of mesenchymal stem cells from the surrounding host tissues. Osteoinduction is modulated by the bone morphogenic proteins and cytokines present in both autografts and processed allografts (31).

Osteoconduction is the term for the graft function that provides the three-dimensional structure for the ingrowth of host capillaries, perivascular tissue, and osteoprogenitor cells from the recipient bed into the graft (13,15). This osteoconduction function is provided not only by both autografts and allografts but also by such biomaterials as ceramic. Physical characteristics of the graft, including porosity, pore size, pore connectivity, and three-dimensional architecture, affect its osteoconductive activity. The final and critical function of bone grafts is to give mechanical support (13,15). Cortical grafts may provide some mechanical support initially. Ultimately, mechanical support is the result of remodeling of the original graft under the influence of the host's mechanical demands (25).

THE BIOLOGY OF BONE GRAFTS

In 1914, Phemister noted,

> When a defect in the course of a long bone is filled by a transplant, nature is confronted with three tasks to perform, namely:
> I. The preservation of nutrition and re-establishment of circulation of the transplant.
> II. The union of the ends of the transplant with the ends of the fragments.
> III. The transformation of the transplant into a duplicate of the normal bone whose place it fills.

These principles are still central to bone graft physiology.

The biologic events of bone graft incorporation make up a prolonged process that, for a cancellous graft, usually results in the complete resorption and replacement of the graft by host bone (39). Cortical autografts, in contrast, may never be completely resorbed. They usually remain an admixture of graft bone and host bone (3,6,17). Because of this prolonged remodeling activity of the graft, it is difficult to define the endpoint of incorporation. The process can be considered functional, however, when the graft can withstand the normal loads of the activities of daily living. To understand and evaluate the incorporation of bone grafts, researchers have used radiographic, histologic, scintigraphic, and biomechanical methods. It is the histologic process of incorporation, however, that best reflects the biologic events of this process (13–15,39).

Bone graft incorporation is a sequence of interrelated phases that use all these bone graft functions (13,15,39). The initial inflammatory response results in the early migration of inflammatory cells and fibroblasts. Early on the graft is surrounded by a hematoma. Entrapped platelets degranulate, releasing growth factors such as platelet-derived growth factor (PDGF) and TGF-β1. Because their vascular supply has been interrupted, most cells within the graft die within the first

days. Osteoinduction occurs rapidly and consists of chemotaxis, mitosis, and differentiation of the osteoprogenitor cells. During the first week, chondroid material is seen, and very rapidly, by day 10, osteoblasts are present. This osteoinductive potential is mediated by a family of peptides known as osteogenins (31). These osteogenins, present in demineralized bone matrix, are destroyed by treatment with alkaloid proteases and mercaptoethanol (15). Osteoconduction proceeds in large cortical autografts for many years and results in the resorption of the original graft tissue and replacement with new host bone. This remodeling is a response to weight bearing. Its success depends on a balance between revascularization and osteogenesis in response to applied loads. Bone graft incorporation is a dynamic continuum of the intrinsic biologic activity of the bone graft, the perigraft environment, and the host–graft mechanical interactions.

BIOLOGY OF CANCELLOUS AUTOGRAFTS

Cancellous grafts are composed of porous, highly cellular trabecular bone and are used to stimulate and enhance bone healing. In terms of clinical outcome, cancellous autografts remain the "gold" standard against which all other grafting procedures are judged. Cancellous autografts are the only commonly used grafts that provide osteogenesis; they provide osteoconduction and osteoinduction as well. Owing to their open structure and large surface area, the incorporation of these grafts is the quickest; complete turnover and integration with the host site can be completed as early as 6 to 12 months postoperatively (13).

Initially in incorporation, hemorrhage and inflammation are seen. The surface osteophytes survive by diffusion, and new bone is rapidly identified as immature woven trabeculae synthesized on the graft bone (13). The revascularization of a cancellous graft in the first few days after implantation precedes the ingrowth of new osteoprogenitor cells as well as osteoclasts. Even during the early phases of incorporation, graft resorption occurs with formation. The graft-derived low-molecular-weight peptides called bone morphogenic protein (BMP), active during the first weeks after transplantation, induce the perigraft host osteoprogenitor cells to migrate into the graft tissue (40).

The later phase of incorporation of cancellous autograft is characterized by osteoconduction that proceeds rapidly with new capillary ingrowth. The osteoprogenitor cells divide rapidly and differentiate into osteoblasts that line the dead trabeculae and deposit seams of osteoid around the core of dead bone. This osteoid results in increased radiographic bone density, increased width of individual trabeculae, and increased mechanical strength. The remodeling and complete replacement of the nonviable graft bone is explained by Wolff's law (25). This remodeling ultimately produces a construct with the biomechanical properties able to withstand the normal loads of daily activity. Marrow tissue, which reforms in the later phase of incorporation, continues to provide the osteogenic precursor cells for bone graft remodeling. Cancellous autografts are usually resorbed completely and replaced by viable new host bone within a year after the process has begun (Fig. 23-1).

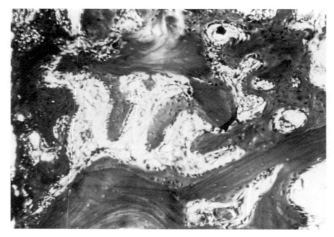

Figure 23-1   Fresh cancellous autograft completely replaced by new bone 1 year after transplantation.

BIOLOGY OF CORTICAL BONE GRAFTS

Cortical grafts are composed of relatively nonporous lamellar bone. They are used primarily to provide immediate mechanical support for a major bony defect. Cortical autograft incorporation proceeds in a manner similar to cancellous autograft incorporation but at a much slower pace (3,6,17,33). Because of the density of cortical bone, however, a cortical graft has a decreased rate of revascularization and remodeling. Central to the process of any graft incorporation is the vascular penetration of the graft by host tissue. This vascular ingrowth into the Volkmann and haversian canals of a cortical graft must await the osteoclastic resorption of bone. The slower revascularization usually results in cortical bone becoming more radiolucent and significantly weaker than normal bone. This decrease in strength may last for months to years after transplantation, depending on the graft size and the implantation site.

The uncoupling of bone resorption and bone formation is a result of the differential activity of osteoblasts and osteoclasts (14). Osteoclasts can resorb bone at a rate of 50 μm per day, whereas osteoblasts can synthesize new bone tissue at a rate of only 1 μm of bone per day (14). This uncoupling may cause cortical bone grafts to fail even under the best circumstances.

After cortical transplantation, new bone tissue is seen in the first month; however, even at 1 year, cortical autografts remain an admixture of necrotic donor bone and viable new host tissue (Fig. 23-2). The remodeling of these grafts in response to the mechanical stimuli is a prolonged process similar to that for normal skeletal bone; it involves the osteonal system rather than interstitial lamellae. Ultimately, the graft may be remodeled both spatially and temporally and may become identical with the surrounding host tissue. The complete incorporation of a cortical graft depends a great deal on the mechanical stability of the graft and its capacity to be mechanically stressed.

VASCULARIZED CORTICAL AUTOGRAFTS

Although there is infrequent use of vascularized cortical autografts to reconstruct deficient bone for total hip arthro-

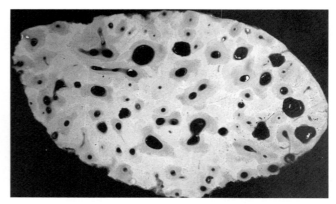

Figure 23-2   Fresh cortical autograft 1 year after transplantation, demonstrating a mixture of necrotic donor bone and viable host tissue.

plasty, they are used to some extent to reconstruct the hip after tumor excision or trauma. The biology of this autograft differs significantly from that of nonvascularized tissue and should be understood for completeness. Vascularized cortical autograft is provided with an immediate blood supply and suffers only transient ischemia (3,11,12,17,33). Over 90% of the donor osteocytes survive the transplantation episode (Fig. 23-3). The graft–host interface heals rapidly, and the normal uncoupling of bone resorption and formation is usually not seen. Thus, the vascularized cortical graft will usually not be weakened by resorption. In this regard, the graft may provide load-bearing characteristics early in the incorporation. Further, the vascularized cortical autograft is incorporated independent of the host bed and thus may function in biologically deficient host environments. These grafts are also clinically useful when segments of host tissue loss are larger than 6 cm. Like nonvascularized autografts, however, vascularized autografts must be supported with appropriate internal or external fixation until the graft–host interface heals and the segmental graft hypertrophies in response to the mechanical loading at its new site. Drawbacks are the even more limited supply of suitable donor sites, an increase in donor site morbidity due to the

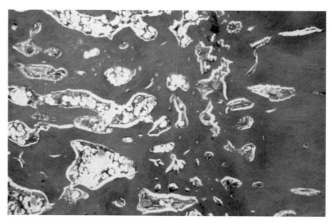

Figure 23-3   Cross section of vascularized fibular autograft at 6 months, with viable bone maintaining structure (stained with hematoxylin and eosin, 5×).

extensive dissection of the vascular pedicle and muscle cuff, and the increased technical difficulty of the microvascular anastomosis.

BONE-GRAFTING COMPLICATIONS

Besides donor site morbidity, bone-grafting procedures are affected by three major complications. Fractures primarily affect cortical grafts and may occur because the graft was inadequately sized for the host bone. The remodeling process described above weakens cortical grafts, predisposing them to late fracturing. Nonunions may be caused by inadequate stabilization or, in the case of allografts, by immunological rejection. Graft infections, although they can often be treated or prevented by antibiotics, may require graft removal (35). Finally, massive graft resorption may occur (usually, in the case of allografts, because of immunological rejection).

BONE GRAFT SUBSTITUTES

Although autogenous cancellous bone is the gold standard for bone-grafting material, it has a number of disadvantages, as has been discussed. Allogeneic bone is an alternative; however, its disadvantages include immunologic incompatibility, an increased risk of infection, slow and incomplete incorporation, and the risk of viral transmission (35,38). Because of these disadvantages, a myriad of biosynthetic bone graft substitutes are presently under investigation, and some are already in clinical use (Table 23-1) (2,9,21,22,26,30,39). These materials may be useful as osteoconductive matrices or as osteoinductive proteins, with or without osteoprogenitor mesenchymal stem cells. The major osteoconductive matrices that are presently being investigated and are in clinical use to some extent include collagen, ceramic, and degradable matrices (1,19,21,26,28). These bone graft substitutes are generally porous structures that, when implanted into bone, serve as a structural template for host-derived new bone formation. Some types may, at least transiently, provide some structural support.

Osteoconductive materials usually serve as a passive scaffold for the host vascular and cellular responses. The implant stimulates the attachment and migration of vascular and osteogenic cells within the graft material. Osteoconductive materials increase the probability that the entire gap or void space will become filled with host bone. They also serve as a placeholder or spacer that blocks the ingress of soft tissues into the gap. The porosity, pore size, pore connectivity, and three-dimensional architecture, as well as the chemical composition and surface structure of the implant, all affect osteoconduction. Pore sizes of 100 to 500 μm, with lateral interconnections of 100 μm or greater, seem to be ideal (1).

Collagen is the major constituent of demineralized bone matrix, and it is the material around which mineralization occurs. Collagen fibers appear to serve as a nucleation site for the deposition of mineral by interacting with noncollagenous matrix proteins to promote hydroxyapatite crystal deposition. Animal studies indicate that collagen alone lacks osteogenic capacity but that it provides an osteoconductive substratum (26,39). In this regard, studies by Werntz et al. (26,41) suggested that fibrillar collagen was an effective material when

combined with bone marrow to heal large segmental defects in rats. However, in the absence of bone marrow, collagen alone was significantly inferior to autologous cancellous bone in supporting the healing of these defects. Rubash et al. (20,24; H. E. Rubash, personal communication) have published a series of studies on the ingrowth and formation of bone in defects on an uncemented fiber–metal total hip replacement model in dogs. The data from this series demonstrate that defect healing is enhanced by grafting material. At 6 weeks, ingrowth into defects containing the collagen-hydroxyapatite-tricalcium phosphate (collagen-HA/TCP) bone mixture was maximal, compared with ingrowth in control animals after 12 or 24 weeks. In addition, their model of autogenous bone grafting, initially slow to provide ingrowth, promoted significant ingrowth into defect sites at 24 weeks, and the ingrowth was comparable to ingrowth into the implant at sites away from the osseous defects. The studies by Rubash et al. support the grafting of bone defects in revision total joint arthroplasty and reaffirm the importance of the osteoconductive potential of HA/TCP as a graft material.

Calcium phosphate biomaterials (ceramics) provide a high degree of biocompatibility and the matrix for osteoconduction to occur. There are a number of different ceramics composed of hydroxyapatite or tricalcium phosphate, or both (1,21,22,30). These materials are prepared as porous implants and can be supplemented for clinical use with solubilized fibrillar collagen and bone marrow. Since hydroxyapatite and tricalcium phosphate have differing rates of resorption and porosity, a mixture of the two appears to provide an improved clinically applicable material. Studies using a defined rat femoral defect model showed a significantly higher regeneration of the defect using a ceramic with a 60% HA and 40% TCP composition combined with soluble fibrillar collagen and bone marrow (8,9,26). This combination was highly effective in repairing the large femoral segmental defects in this rat model, as shown by radiologic, histologic, and biomechanical methods. When ceramics are in a block form, little inflammation is seen; however, small granules of calcium phosphates may invoke a foreign-body giant cell reaction.

There are a number of ceramics presently being utilized in clinical studies (2,21,22). These include tricalcium phosphate materials that are synthesized as particulates, are biodegradable, and are used for repair of contained bone defects. Other bioceramics consist of combinations of tricalcium phosphate, hydroxyapatite, and/or calcium sulfate, and they have generally been approved for use in repairing these same contained bone defects. Injectable calcium phosphates have been developed that may be useful for restoring non-weight-bearing osseous defects but have little application in the repair of segmental bone loss (21). Although bioceramics are attractive as materials because of their biocompatibility, their ability to support osteoconduction, and their possible role as a stimulator of osteogenesis, their major drawback is that they are brittle and have low impact and fracture resistance. Another problem with calcium phosphate materials is that their biodegradation and incorporation are unpredictable. However, these materials do offer a potentially important alternative to autogenous and allogeneic bone grafts.

The isolation of an osteoinductive factor by Marshall Urist in 1978 (39) opened an entirely different approach to the treatment of bone loss. When used as bone graft substitutes,

TABLE 23-1

BONE SUBSTITUTES (UNITED STATES)

Product and Description	Company
Anorganic	
Bio-Oss: bovine hydroxyapatite (HA)	Osteohealth, Shirley, NJ
OsteoGraft: human HA	Ceramed, Lakewood, CO
Comments: These products are particulates; they do not biodegrade; primary role would be as space fillers in non-load-bearing craniofacial sites. They probably should be augmented with autograft.	
Collagen, factors (growth factors)	
Grafton: Gelatinized demineralized bone matrix	Osteotech, Shrewsbury, NJ
Demineralized bank bone preparations	Numerous sources
Comments: These products are manufactured as particulates (although bank bone preparations can be in block formats) and have varying degrees of biologic activity. They are biodegradable and probably should be augmented with autograft; particulates have been used mostly in non-load-bearing craniofacial sites.	
Ceramics	
Synthograft: TCP	Johnson and Johnson, Somerville, NJ
Augmen: TCP	Miter, Worthington, OH
Orthograft: TCP	DuPuy, Warsaw, IN
Comments: These products are particulates and biodegradable and should be used in non-stress-bearing areas such as periodontal defects.	
Hapset: TCP + calcium sulfate	Lifecore Biomedical, Chaska, MN
Comments: This product is prepared as a paste for insertion into dental extraction sites. It is questionable whether extraction sites, which ordinarily regenerate new bone, require treatment.	
OsteoGen: Synthetic HA	Impladent, Holliswood, NY
ProOsteon: Coralline-derived HA	Interpore International, Irvine, CA
Comments: These products are particulates and nonbiodegradable and should be used in non-stress-bearing areas such as periodontal defects. ProOsteon has been Food and Drug Administration (FDA)-approved for use in metaphyseal defects.	
Collagraft: HA (65%) + TCP (35%), combined with 95% type I bovine collagen and 5% type III	Zimmer, Warsaw, IN
Comments: This product is supplied in strips, and the manufacturer suggests that for best results autogenous blood should be added. Application sites recommended are spinal fusions and bone cystic cavities. The collagen and TCP should be biodegradable with time.	
Healos	
Comments: Healos is a similar resorbably product based on a porous, open cell matrix formed from corss-linked collagen fibers coated with resorbable hydroxyapatite.	Orquest, Mountain View, CA
Perioglas: a bioglass	U.S. Biomaterials, Alachua, FL
BioGran: a bioactive glass	Orthovita, Malvern, PA
Comments: These are particulate materials with dentoalveolar applications in non-stress-bearing sites. The products are nonbiodegradable or slowly biodegradable.	
Calcium sulfate (plaster of paris)	
Comments: Calcium sulfate was first used as a resorbable bone graft substitute in the 19th century and remains in use today. It is a hemihydrate prepared by heating gypsum. Calcium sulphate is used as pellets or in injectable form. It is useful in antibiotic-laden form for the treatment of infected defect sites. It offers little mechanical support and dissolves relatively rapidly (30–60 days) in vivo.	*OsteoSet, Wright Medical Technology, Arlington, TN* *Wright Medical Technology;* *BonePlast, Interpore Cross, Irving, CA*
Injectable calcium phosphates	
Bone Source: tetracalcium phosphate + dicalcium phosphate dihydrate	Leibinger, Dallas, TX
Norian SRS: Monocalcium phosphate monohydrate + α-tricalcium phosphate + calcium carbonate + sodium phosphate	Norian Corp., Cupertino, CA
True Bone: various calcium phosphates	Etex Corp., Cambridge, MA
Comments: These materials may be useful for restoring non-weight-bearing osseous defects, such as cystic cavities; with suitable porosity and biodegradability, delivery of vulnerary molecules may be possible.	
Polymers, nonbiodegradable	
HTR-PMI: Calcium-layered polymethylmethacrylate + hydroxyethylmethacrylate	Lorenz, Jacksonville, FL
Comments: A granular product used to repair periodontal defects and cranioplasties; not suitable for weightbearing structures.	

osteoinductive agents are intended to induce and promote differentiation of undifferentiated mesenchymal stem cells to osteogenic cells. Compounds with known osteoinductive properties include bone marrow, TGF-β, the bone morphogenetic proteins (BMPs), the FGFs, the insulinlike growth factors (IGFs), and PDGF. Bone morphogenic protein has been shown to be a major osteoinductive protein, and along with other growth factors, it has become a central focus of recent research activities (31,42).

Bone marrow has been used directly to stimulate bone formation in bone defects and nonunions. Autogenous bone marrow can be harvested through a minute incision using a large-bore cannula with minimal morbidity. For nonunion, the marrow can be injected percutaneously into the site. Its efficacy is based on the presence of pluripotent mesenchymal stem cells in the marrow. These cells, however, are quite rare (0.001% or less of the nucleated cells) and become significantly rarer among the debilitated or aged patient populations most likely to require such adjuvant therapy. Thus, it may be advantageous to attempt to enrich or culture-expand these cells before reimplantation. Bone marrow can also be used as an adjuvant to augment bone grafts or bone substitutes (24).

Another major source of these growth factors can be found in demineralized bone matrix (DBM) (9,26). DBM is prepared from pulverized cortical bone by extracting the internal phase with a 0.5 N hydrochloric acid solution. The demineralization unmasks acid-resistant BMPs and other growth factors that remain in the matrix. BMPs promote bone formation by inducing the differentiation of mesenchymal cells to chondroblasts, which deposit a chondroid extra cellular matrix. This subsequently undergoes endochondral ossification. Studies have demonstrated the capability of demineralized bone matrix to repair a rat femoral defect model (9). It appears that the demineralization process enhances the osteoinductive activity and further improves the access of surrounding osteoprogenitor cells to these proteins. Demineralized bone may be made from either autologous or allogeneic material. The one clinically approved material available is a gelatinized, demineralized bone matrix from allogeneic material (21). These demineralized products are usually particulate but can be made in other formats, are biodegradable, and are generally well tolerated by the host, since antigenic determinants have been significantly modified. These materials are useful for enhancing bone repair in non-load-bearing defects but do require well-vascularized sites for activity.

Growth factors can be also enriched from the patient's blood at the time of surgery or can be obtained as highly purified or recombinant proteins. In the future, gene therapy may allow the delivery to the graft site of genetically modified cells that will act as growth factor factories. Besides the BMPs discussed above, numerous other growth factors have osteoinductive capacity. Some of these are still in the experimental stages; some are commercial products. For example, protein-derived growth factors had a stimulatory effect on fracture healing in a rabbit osteotomy model, and basic fibroblast growth factor (bFGF) is produced in bone during the early phase of fracture healing. It has an anabolic and mitogenic effect on osteoblasts and their precursors. Mixtures of bone-derived growth factors are also undergoing clinical trials, either alone or as adjuvants with DBM or ceramics. Ossigel

(Orquest, Mountain View, CA) is an injectable matrix that combines hyaluronic acid and bFGF. It is intended to promote fracture union and is currently under clinical evaluation in Europe (19). In the Autologous Growth Factors (AGF) (Interpore Cross International Inc, Irvine, CA) approach, a proprietary gel is enriched with the buffy coat of the patient's blood and is placed at the fracture site. The gel is thus enriched with growth factors, especially TGF-β and PDGF (19).

BMPs are members of the expanding TGF-β superfamily of growth factors. BMPs have been cloned and sequenced and are available as highly purified recombinant proteins. The most extensively studied BMPs are OP-1/BMP-7 and BMP-2.

OP-1 Implant (Stryker Corporation, Kalamazoo, MI) contains rhOP-1 and a bovine collagen carrier that has FDA approval. It is intended as an autograft alternative in refractory nonunions. It is reconstituted from a lyophilized powder and then implanted as a paste.

In Fuse (Medtronic-Somafor-Danek, Minneapolis, MN) is a new material containing rhBMP-2 collagen sponge carrier and is approved for spine fusions. In clinical studies, rhBMP-2 bone graft substitutes combined with titanium interbody fusion cages for lumbar spinal fusion demonstrated osteoinduction (28).

Other nonbiologic bone graft substitutes have an advantage over biological materials in that the physical properties (mechanics, surface chemistry, porosity, connectivity, etc.) can be controlled during manufacture.

Polymers such as polylactic acid-based and polyglycolic acid-based polymers have a long history as resorbable surgical suture materials. They have also been used as resorbable fracture fixation implants. PolyGraft BGS (Osteobiologics Inc, San Antonio, TX) is a porous polylactide-coglycolide, calcium sulfate, and polyglycolide fiber composite approved by the FDA to fill bony structure. The PolyGraft product family includes granules and preformed cubes, blocks, and cylinders (21).

It is clear that future technology for bone regeneration will focus on newer approaches, such as gene therapy, tissue engineering, and molecules that can be easily manufactured, to provide a combination of both osteoconduction and osteoinduction. At the present time, these bone substitutes are useful for nonstructural applications; however, newer materials will be available in the future that may have applicability as substitutes for large structural defects.

Gene therapy still has a certain science fiction aura, but animal studies suggest that it will eventually become clinically useful. In gene therapy, genetic information in the form of DNA (or occasionally RNA) is transferred to cells to alter their gene expression patterns for therapeutic purposes. The alteration can be positive; that is, the cell expresses or overexpresses proteins encoded by the gene (e.g., cytokines or growth factors beneficial to the repair process). The alteration can also be negative; that is, the genetic information is designed to inhibit or down-regulate the expression of endogenous genes.

An advantage to this approach is that it can easily be used in conjunction with most any of the grafts or graft substitutes discussed above. The genetic material can be injected directly at the site of interest, as naked DNA, as a complex designed to facilitate entry into the cells, or in a viral (adenoviral or retroviral) vector. It is possible to target the expression of the gene product, for example, by using regulatory sequences that function only in selected cell types. Alternatively, the patient's own cells can be harvested, culture expanded, genetically modified, and then reimplanted.

An issue with this approach is controlling the duration of the expression of the gene product at the target site. In most cases, a short-term, reversible, localized therapeutic effect is desired, and usually achieved. However, the possibility of creating stable transformants with long-term expression of the gene product exists, as does the possibility of inadvertent malignant transformation of the modified cells (7,29).

Tissue engineering is the result of the confluence of biological, physical, and engineering sciences (18,29). The goal of tissue engineering is to create living biological analogs of tissues in vitro for subsequent implantation. This can be as simple as culture-expanding progenitor cells from various sources (bone marrow, fat, peripheral blood) for reimplantation or can involve extensive in vitro bioreactor culture in combination with specialized scaffolds and cytokines or growth factors. Although tissue engineering is currently the focus of much academic and industry research, there are no actual commercial products for use as bone graft substitutes at this time. Limited clinical trials are underway in the Netherlands for one cell–scaffold composite product as an adjunct in hip revision surgery (VivescOs, IsoTis, Bilthoven, The Netherlands). A major tissue-engineering–related problem is that bone is a vascular tissue. Thus, the successful tissue engineering of large bone implants will have to address the formation of a built-in microvascular system in vitro, still a major challenge.

GENERAL CLINICAL PRINCIPLES OF BONE GRAFTING

To achieve a successful bone grafting procedure, the clinician must choose a bone graft that is appropriate for the specific biologic and mechanical environment into which it will be placed. Thus the clinical situation will usually dictate the source and type of bone graft to be used (4,36). The size and type of pelvic or femoral bone loss will determine whether autogenous tissue has an application. For example, well-contained small defects of the pelvis may be reconstructed with morselized cancellous autografts. In contrast, large uncontained segmental defects of the proximal femur usually require massive processed cortical and cancellous allografts (5,23).

The clinical outcome of any bone-grafting procedure depends on the local and systemic conditions of the recipient (27,36). The preparation of the host bed is critical and requires excision of fibrous scar tissue, treatment of infection, an adequate blood supply, and satisfactory soft-tissue coverage. To select the appropriate bone graft, the surgeon must understand the clinical indication for the graft. Important questions are: What is the primary functional requirement of the bone graft? Is it osteogenesis or immediate structural support? Further, secure fixation of a bone graft to the host bone is critical to ensure a successfully incorporated graft (27).

The major sources of autogenous bone are the ilium, fibula, and tibia (14). The ribs are also a useful source of cortical bone. The outer table of the iliac crest is the site most frequently used when both cancellous bone and cortical bone are required. The anterior ilium just proximal to the anterior superior spine is a useful source of cortical and cancellous bone for reconstructing contained and smaller uncontained segmental defects. Precautions must be taken to protect the inner pelvic wall and to prevent excessive bleeding. The anterior medial tibia is useful for full-thickness cortical grafts that provide osteogenesis, osteoconduction, and structural support. The disadvantage of using the tibia as a donor is the need to protect the tibia to prevent fractures and longer rehabilitation. The fibular midshaft and proximal fibula are excellent donor sites for cylindrical cortical bone to be used to reconstruct segmental defects and to support contained cystic bone losses of the pelvis or femur.

Good sources of cancellous and corticocancellous bone graft are the proximal head and neck of the femur, useful for reconstructing deficient bone during primary total hip replacement. After the soft-tissue attachments and remaining cartilage are removed, the femoral head and neck can be used as a bulk corticocancellous graft or can be morselized to fill cavities in the ilium or proximal femur.

The technique of using cancellous grafts usually requires the formation of chips or morselized particles. Particle size is critical, because particles less than 75 to 125 μm are rapidly resorbed and do not participate in effective osteogenesis. These grafts must be contained by surrounding bony tissue or by other techniques.

The removed femoral head and neck are effective sources of corticocancellous bone. The femoral head may be used as a bulk graft to reconstruct segmental defects (Fig 23-4). The long-term outcome of grafts of this nature, however, remains in doubt (10). Recent reports suggest that the autogenous femoral heads do survive and incorporate into the host. They appear to provide a source of restoring bone stock (23,34). If this autogenous bone graft is used to reconstruct segmental defects, excellent fixation of the graft to the host tissue is of central importance (27). Cancellous screws or bolts usually give adequate fixation. Cages may be necessary to support the bone graft. To be effective, the graft should be oriented along the stress lines of the pelvis if possible, although this is still somewhat controversial (34). These grafts, however, suffer from the normal biologic processes of incorporation. The invasion of host blood vessels results in the resorption of the bulk graft, and if concomitant bone formation is not maintained, the structural integrity of the autograft will be undermined, and a clinical failure will result. Because of the controversy in the literature about using bulk cancellous autografts, the use of morselized cancellous bone has become more widespread (4,23). Cancellous bone grafts—because of their large surface area, effective revascularization, and rapid osteogenesis and osteoinduction—are excellent for filling contained defects. Figure 23-5 illustrates the use of morselized cancellous autograft to reconstruct a contained acetabular bone defect. The soft-tissue lining must be removed to bleeding host bed and the cavity packed with cancellous bone.

Cortical bone grafts can provide support and osteoconduction. They are typically used as single or dual onlay grafts to reconstruct segmental defects or to contain cystic defects. However, because of the usual need in these clinical circumstances for large grafts, autografts (which would typically be taken from the tibia and fibula) are less useful, so in most circumstances allogeneic bone must be available. The clinical experience with cortical autografts parallels our experimental

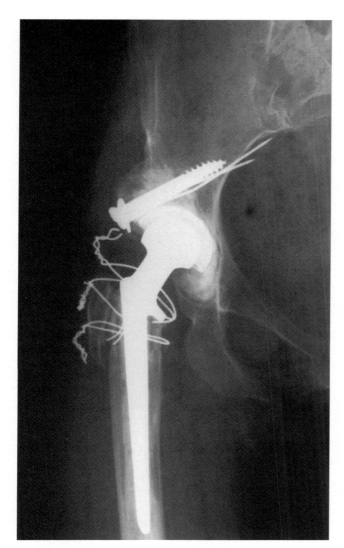

Figure 23-4 Fresh morselized cancellous autograft has been used to reconstruct this contained pelvic bone loss.

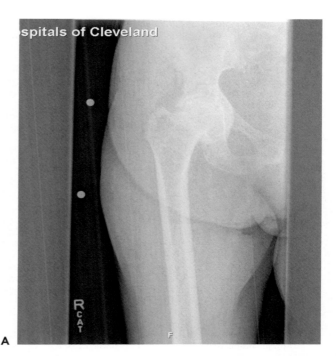

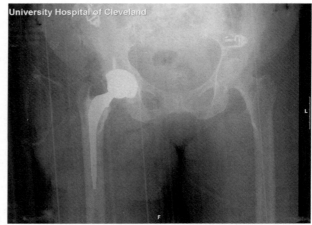

Figure 23-5 Anterior posterior radiograph of an 84-year-old patient with significant protrusio acetabulim. The contained central acetabular defect was reconstructed using morselized autograft.

observations (4,27). It is important to provide intrinsic and stable graft–host fixation and satisfactory soft-tissue coverage. The graft must be protected from full weight bearing for a prolonged period of time, because fatigue fractures are often seen from 6 months to 3 years after surgery. When appropriately used with stable internal fixation, the graft does incorporate, it unites to the host tissue, and it hypertrophies.

CONCLUSION

A good clinical outcome for bone grafting in primary and revision total hip arthroplasty requires that the clinician understand the biologic and mechanical environment into which the graft will be placed. This understanding, coupled with an appreciation of the cellular and molecular interaction of the bone graft with its host, will provide reproducible techniques for reconstituting bone loss in primary and revision total hip arthroplasty and after tumor excision or trauma. Surgically preparing an excellent host bed, providing

an adequate blood supply, and selecting appropriate bone graft material for the clinical demand will enable the graft to biologically and functionally incorporate into the host and provide the ultimate load-bearing function required for a successful clinical outcome.

REFERENCES

1. Bucholtz RW. Nonallograft osteoconductive bone graft substitutes. *Clin Orthop Relat Res.* 2002;No. 395:44–52.
2. Cornell CN, Lane JM, Chapman M, et al. Multicenter trial of Collagraft as bone graft substitute. *J Orthop Trauma.* 1991;5:1–8.
3. Dell PC, Burchardt H, Glowczewski FP Jr. A roentgenographic, biomechanical, and histological evaluation of vascularized and non-vascularized segmental fibular canine autografts. *J Bone Joint Surg.* 1985;67A:105–112.

4. Emerson RH Jr. Bone grafts. In: Callaghan JJ, Dennis DA, Paprosky WG, et al., eds. *Orthopaedic Knowledge Update: Hip and Knee Reconstruction*. Rosemont, IL: American Academy of Orthopaedic Surgeons; 1995:49–56.

5. Emerson RH Jr, Malinin TI, Cuellar AD, et al. Cortical strut allografts in the reconstruction of the femur in revision total hip arthroplasty: a basic science and clinical study. *Clin Orthop.* 1992;285:35–44.

6. Enneking WF, Burchardt H, Puhl JJ, et al. Physical and biological aspects of repair in dog cortical-bone transplants. *J Bone Joint Surg.* 1975;57A:237–252.

7. Gamradt SC, Liebernman JR. Genetic modification of stem cells to enhance bone repair. *Ann Biomed Eng.* 2004;32:136–147.

8. Gebhart M, Lane JM, Rose K, et al. Effect of demineralized bone matrix (DBM) and bone marrow (BM) on bone defect repair. *Orthop Trans.* 1985;9:258–259.

9. Gepstein R, Weiss RE, Hakllel T. Bridging large defects in bone by demineralized bone matrix in the form of powder: a radiographic, histological, and radioisotope-uptake study in rats. *J Bone Joint Surg.* 1987;69A:984–992.

10. Gerber SD, Harris WH. Femoral head autografting to augment acetabular deficiency in patients requiring total hip replacement: a minimum five-year and an average seven-year follow-up study. *J Bone Joint Surg.* 1986;68A:1241–1248.

11. Goldberg VM, Shaffer JW, Field G, et al. Biology of vascularized bone grafts. *Orthop Clin North Am.* 1987;18:197–205.

12. Goldberg VM, Shaffer JW, Stevenson S, et al. Biology of vascularized bone grafts. In: Friedlaender GE, Goldberg VM, eds. *Bone and Cartilage Allografts*. Park Ridge, IL: American Academy of Orthopaedic Surgeons; 1991:13–26.

13. Goldberg VM, Stevenson S. Natural history of autografts and allografts. *Clin Orthop.* 1987;225:7–16.

14. Goldberg VM, Stevenson S. Bone transplantation. In: Evarts CM, ed. *Surgery of the Musculoskeletal System*. New York: Churchill Livingstone; 1989:115–150.

15. Goldberg VM, Stevenson S. The biology of bone grafts. *Semin Arthroplasty.* 1996;7:12–17.

16. Goldberg VM, Stevenson S, Shaffer JW. Biology of autografts and allografts. In: Friedlaender GE, Goldberg VM, eds. *Bone and Cartilage Allografts*. Park Ridge, IL: American Academy of Orthopaedic Surgeons, 1991:3–12.

17. Goldberg VM, Stevenson S, Shaffer JW, et al. Biological and physical properties of autogenous vascularized fibular grafts in dogs. *J Bone Joint Surg.* 1990;72A:801–810.

18. Goldberg VM. Selection of bone grafts for revision total hip arthroplasty. *Clin Orthop Relat Res.* 2000;381:68–76.

19. Greenwald AS, Boden SD, Goldberg VM, et al. Bone-graft substitutes: facts, fictions and applications. *J Bone Joint Surg.* 2001;83[Supp 2]:98–103.

20. Greis PE, Kang JD, Silvaggio V, et al. A long-term study on defect filling and bone ingrowth using a canine fiber metal total hip model. *Clin Orthop.* 1992;274:47–59.

21. Hollinger JO, Brekke J, Gruskin E, et al. Role of bone substitutes. *Clin Orthop.* 1996;324:55–65.

22. Holmes RE, Bucholz RW, Mooney V. Porous hydroxyapatite as a bone-graft substitute in metaphyseal defects: a histometric study. *J Bone Joint Surg.* 1986;68A:904–911.

23. Huo MH, Friedlaender GE, Salvati EA. Bone graft and total hip arthroplasty: a review. *J Arthroplasty.* 1992;7:109–120.

24. Kang JD, McKernan DJ, Kruger, M, et al. Ingrowth and formation of bone in defects in an uncemented fiber-metal total hip-replacement model in dogs. *J Bone Joint Surg.* 1991;73A:93–104.

25. Kushner A. Evaluation of Wolff's law of bone formation. *J Bone Joint Surg.* 1940;22:589–596.

26. Lane JM, Cornell CN, Werntz JR, et al. Clinical applications of biosynthetics. In: Friedlaender GE, Goldberg VM, eds. *Bone and Cartilage Allografts*. Park Ridge, IL: American Academy of Orthopaedic Surgeons, 1991;279–294.

27. Lin KY, Bartlett SP, Yaremchuk MJ, et al. The effect of rigid fixation on the survival of onlay bone grafts: an experimental study. *Plast Reconstr Surg.* 1990;86:449–456.

28. Ludwig SC, Boden SD. Osteoinductive bone graft substitutes for spinal fusion: a basic science summary. *Orthop Clin North Am.* 1999;30:635–645.

29. Mauney JR, Blumberg J, Pirun M, et al. Osteogenic differentiation of human bone marrow stromal cells on partially demineralized bone scaffolds in vitro. *Tissue Eng.* 2004;10:81–92.

30. Ohgushi H, Okumura M, Tamai S, et al. Marrow induced osteogenesis in porous hydroxyapatite and tricalcium phosphate: a comparative histomorphometric study of ectopic bone formation. *J Biomed Mater Res.* 1990;24:1563–1570.

31. Reddi AH, Wientroub S, Muthukumaran N. Biologic principles of bone induction. *Orthop Clin North Am.* 1987;189:207–212.

32. Sanches-Sotelo J, Berry DJ, Trousale RT, et al. Surgical treatment of developmental dysplasia of the hip in adults, II: arthroplasty options. *J Am Acad Orthop Surg.* 2002;10:334–344.

33. Shaffer JW, Field GA, Goldberg VM, et al. Fate of vascularized and nonvascularized autografts. *Clin Orthop.* 1985;197:32–43.

34. Stans AA, Pagnano MW, Shaughnessy WJ, et al. Results of total hip arthroplasty for Crowe type III developmental hip dysplasia. *Clin Orthop.* 1998;348:149–157.

35. Stevenson S. Experimental issues in histocompatibility of bone grafts. In: Friedlaender GE, Goldberg VM, eds. *Bone and Cartilage Allografts*. Park Ridge, IL: American Academy of Orthopaedic Surgeons; 1991:45–54.

36. Stevenson S, Emery SE, Goldberg VM. Factors affecting bone graft incorporation. *Clin Orthop.* 1996;323:66–74.

37. Stevenson S, Li XQ, Davy DT, et al. Critical biological determinants of nonvascularized cortical bone graft incorporation: quantifying a complex process and structure. *J Bone Joint Surg.* 1997;79A:1–16.

38. Tomford WW, Mankin HJ, Friedlaender GE, et al. Methods of banking bone and cartilage for allograft transplantation. *Orthop Clin North Am.* 1987;18:241–247.

39. Urist MR. Bone transplants and implants. In: Urist MR, ed. *Fundamental and Clinical Bone Physiology*. Philadelphia: JB Lippincott; 1980:331–368.

40. Urist MR, Silverman BF, Büring K, et al. The bone induction principle. *Clin Orthop* 1967;53:243–283.

41. Werntz JR, Lane JM, Piez C, et al. The repair of segmental bone defects with collagen and marrow. *Orthop Trans* 1986;10:262.

42. Wozney JM, Rosen V, Celeste AJ, et al. Novel regulators of bone formation: molecular clones and activities. *Science.* 1988;242:1528–1534.

43. Younger EM, Chapman MW. Morbidity at bone graft donor sites. *J Orthop Trauma.* 1989;3:192–195.

44. Zeiss IM, Nisbet NW, Heslop BF. Studies on transference of bone, II: vascularization of autologous and homologous implants of cortical bone in rats. *Br J Exp Pathol.* 1960;41:345–363.

Allografts

D. Luis Muscolo   *Miguel A. Ayerza*
Victor M. Goldberg

24

The use of massive bone allografts for reconstruction of large defects dates back to the beginning of this century (105). Parrish (140), Volkov (180), Ottolenghi (136), and Nilsonne (132) in the 1960s and 1970s, and, more recently, Mankin et al. (110,111,114), reported clinical results of allografts used to replace bone and joint loss in tumors.

Recent long-term studies of allograft replacement after bone tumor resections rated 73% of all allografts and 77% of reconstructions utilizing both an allograft and a prosthesis as either excellent or good (112). There is also a report on a small series of femur allografts with good function and radiographic scores that were followed for at least 24 years (128).

Bone allografts were first used mainly for reconstructions after excision of tumors, often in patients with poor function and life expectancy. However, the use of allografts has been expanded to include bone deficiencies caused by severe trauma, congenital abnormalities, and, more frequently, extensive resorptions of bone secondary to nonseptic loose components of failed joint arthroplasties.

Among the advantages of utilizing bone allografts rather than autografts are that the amount of allograft is unlimited and there is not the inconvenience of donor site morbidity. Allografts also provide mechanical quality for major defects such as pelvic column or proximal femur losses (69,70). In addition, osteochondral grafts are not available from autologous sources for large defects. Host ligaments and muscles can be reattached to the allografts. Healing then restores joint stability and function. Also, if healing at the host–donor junction occurs when using allograft–prosthesis composites, load sharing with normal translation of forces between the prosthetic implant and the host bone is observed.

The disadvantages of using bone allografts include potential disease transmission and an unpredictable incidence of infections, fractures, resorptions, and host–donor junction complications. Additionally, allografts are replaced by host bone slowly and unpredictably, perhaps the basis of fractures and failure. Because of the immunological rejection that is seen with fresh bone allografts, these grafts are processed by either freezing or freeze-drying and by irradiation. The grafts are obviously not viable but do provide osteoconduction and/or osteoinduction functions. Processing the grafts is convenient for storage, reduces immunogenicity, and may reduce the risk of disease transmission.

In revision total hip replacements, the acetabulum or the femur is frequently structurally deficient as a result of stress shielding, wear particle osteolysis, fractures, or perforations. Each revision may involve some additional loss of bone. Conventional attempts to manage these deficiencies include recementing techniques, resection arthroplasty, arthrodesis, augmentation with bone autografts, and tumor or custom implants (77,83,120). Bone stock may also be reconstituted with bone allografts. Several authors have reported the use of nonstructural or massive segmental allografts to salvage severe bone loss associated with failed total hip arthroplasties (33,39,41,53,57,67,71,82,137,148,176).

Particulate morselized bone allografts are often used to repair contained acetabular or femur defects at revision surgery (39,51,53,119), and evidence of biologic incorporation and bone stock restoration has been reported

(9,55,74,78,84,153,158). Recent studies have reported the histological outcome of impaction allografting of the proximal femur for revision total hip arthroplasty. The retrieved specimens showed zones of differentiation similar to those reported for massive allografts. There were areas of dead bone surrounded by zones of partially revascularized, viable cancellous bone (5).

Cortical strut allografts have been used to restore continuity to a defective cortex in revision total hip arthroplasties (4,41,82,83,137). The histologic and mechanical response to strut grafts in animals has been well documented (41). Cortical strut grafts predictably unite to the host femur and remodel, mature, and augment the host bone structure (82). Clinical success with this type of allograft has been reported to be as high as 96% (74,82).

Structural acetabular allografts are often used when multiple revisions of the acetabulum have led to severe loss of bone stock. Original studies on the use of structural acetabular allografts have not been encouraging, finding a failure rate of 30% at 2 years, 32% at 6, and 47% at 10 years, with an unacceptably high migration of components into allografts (87,92,98, 139,181,182). However, other studies have reported lower failure rates (40,50,66,138,139,164,173). It has been suggested that the use of a stronger allograft rigidly fixed against the host ilium markedly improves results (139). In addition, a structural allograft used to provide support for an acetabular component seems likely to be very effective if the graft involves less than 50% of the acetabulum or if it supports greater loads (50). Information regarding biologic incorporation of these reconstructions is scarce; however, one study showed evidence of revascularization of allografts 6 months after surgery (77,155,159). There are some data to indicate that at the time of re-revision the acetabular bone stock was sufficient to support an uncemented socket, suggesting some bone restoration was achieved (2,101). Hemipelvic allografts are mainly indicated for reconstructions after tumor resections. High complication rates have been reported with this technique (1,66,79,99).

The use of proximal femoral structural allografts in revision total hip arthroplasty has been increasing (11,68,74, 80,81,93,117). The use of proximal femoral allografts in conjunction with prostheses has replaced the initial use of massive whole-joint hip osteoarticular allografts because of the failures caused by cartilage necrosis and subchondral bone collapse (58,120). One report showed that proximal femoral allografts used to restore uncontained circumferential defects of multiple revised total hip arthroplasties had a success rate of 85% at an average follow-up of 5 years (68). Similarly, femoral allograft composites implanted after tumor resections showed a survival rate of 76% at 10 years (186). This type of reconstruction has also been reported as a valid option for treating a deficient femoral bone in a revision of a hip arthroplasty that had failed as a result of infection (7).

The main complications of allografts in revision total hip arthroplasty are infection, fracture, resorption, and nonunion (116). Understanding the biology of incorporation and immune responses to these bioimplants is crucial for predicting, preventing, and treating these complications.

Treating severe bone loss with a safe and predictable organic material has definite advantages over the use of synthetic implants. Bone allografting safety depends on banking procedures, but predictability is related to biologic events between the host and the graft. Bone grafts stimulate in the host a series of partially known phenomena that lead to progressive incorporation and, through biomechanical loading, adaptive remodeling. Bone allografts also trigger an immune response that may have a definite impact on the final outcome. Surgeons involved with this type of reconstructive procedure should consider this biologic sequence when selecting a bone graft so that expectations of the clinical result will be reasonable.

BIOLOGIC PRINCIPLES OF GRAFT INCORPORATION

Bone graft incorporation is a process that involves the host and the graft and ends with the remodeling of the transplanted tissue in response to biomechanical loading. How rapidly the graft will be incorporated depends on the type of graft; its size, structure, and fixation; the vascularity of the host bed; and the graft's genetic compatibility with the receptor. The physiologic events include inflammation and hemorrhage, osteogenesis, osteoconduction, osteoinduction, and, finally, remodeling. The previous chapter presents the basic physiology of bone graft incorporation. The difference between autografts and allografts is emphasized in this chapter.

Inflammation and Hemorrhage. This initial event in fresh allografts is similar to the event in autografts, except an immune response is seen early and usually results in the rapid resorption of the graft. There is almost no new viable bone produced.

Osteogenesis. Although most osteocytes will die, some osteoblasts and osteoclasts can survive in fresh or vascularized autografts. However, usually within the first 10 to 14 days the donor cells are killed by the immune response of the host when a fresh allograft is used. The function of new bone formation seen in processed allografts is a result of their ability to provide a passive scaffold (osteoconduction) or bone morphogenic proteins (osteoinduction).

Osteoconduction. Through the process of osteoconduction, the bone graft supports the growth of sprouting capillaries, perivascular tissues, and osteoprogenitor cells from the host into the three-dimensional structure of the graft. Bone, other biologic materials, and nonbiologic materials share this ability to provide a framework for ingrowth of these tissues (146). Osteoconduction does not require live cells. Nonetheless, it provides the appropriate surface to support the vascularization, growth, and remodeling of bone (32,38). Processed allografts retain this function.

Osteoinduction. The ability of extracellular bone matrix to trigger donor mesenchymal pluripotential progenitor cells to transform into chondrocytes and osteoblasts, forming new bone, is called osteoinduction (143). The differentiation of these cells is modulated by low-molecular-weight peptides collectively known as "bone morphogenetic proteins" (BMPs). The majority of these BMPs belong to the transforming growth factor-β (TGF-β) superfamily of proteins (38). Most BMPs, including BMP_2 to BMP_7, induce bone in similar ways, but specific molecular activities result in various amounts of new cartilage or bone formation (183).

Urist showed that the implantation of demineralized bone at extraskeletal sites induced cartilage and bone formation through the process of osteoinduction (29,144,177). Osteoinduction does not require live cells, it is most effective with demineralized bone, it is active not only in autografts but also in modified preserved allografts, and it is destroyed by autoclaving (29).

Remodeling. Allografts incorporate more slowly and incompletely than autografts (62). Particulate allografts are usually resorbed and replaced by new host bone, but structural corticocancellous allografts may never be completely remodeled, retaining areas of graft necrotic bone along with the viable host new bone.

The initial revascularization rate, the biomechanical load-sharing between the graft and the host, and donor–recipient tissue matching greatly influence the final remodeling and the capacity of large segmental allografts to perform as supporting structures.

VASCULARIZED ALLOGRAFTS

Vascularized bone allografts potentially offer more biologic and mechanical advantages than nonvascularized bone allografts (61,123). *En bloc* whole joint transplantation avoids the potential complications of anatomic donor–recipient mismatching, joint instability, and articular cartilage deterioration that may occur with hemiarticular, nonvascularized allografts. Also, in segmental, structural, nonarticular allografts, if a vascular bed can be maintained, graft viability can be preserved by osteogenesis from transplanted cells without going into resorption and revascularization from the host, reducing allograft fracture, nonunion, and resorption rates.

Unfortunately, immunologic rejection of osteocytes and vascular endothelium may occur as early as 3 days postoperatively when animal vascularized bone allografts are used (63). Although changes caused by rejection could be prevented by immune suppression with cyclosporine (63), adverse effects at the required doses make it difficult to administer this drug after skeletal, nonvital-organ transplantation (126). Advances in the capacity to induce recipient immune tolerance or in tissue matching with the donor are needed before vascularized bone allografts can be clinically applied.

IMMUNOLOGY OF BONE ALLOGRAFTS

Efforts to elucidate the immune response that occurs in reaction to bone allografts date back to the early 1950s (10,22,23,27,43,85,91). However, it is only recent information related to the immunogenicity of transplanted tissues that has stimulated their potential use as bone substitutes.

The immune response generated by transplanted tissue is considered to be one of the main causes of failure of bone allografts, and evidence that frozen bone is also immunogenic has been reported (45). By using different immunologic assays and vascularized, fresh, and frozen osteoarticular allografts in animals, sensitization against donor antigens has been demonstrated (12,13,30,46,48,90,102,103,147,160,161). The major histocompatibility complex (MHC) is a chromosome region of overwhelming importance in determining the

fate of allografts. Class I antigens and class II antigens, which are encoded by genes from the MHC, are both capable of activating T cells. Abundant experimental, clinical, and genetic evidence indicates that the human leukocyte antigen (HLA) chromosomal complex is the major determinant of histocompatibility in humans (2). Rats grafted with allogeneic bone (totally mismatched) showed a stronger response than those receiving semiallogeneic (partially mismatched) bone allografts (60,89,130), suggesting that the response that generates fresh bone allografts is directly related to the MHC.

Stevenson et al. (163) placed fresh and frozen osteochondral allografts orthotopically in the major weight-bearing bone of a genetically controlled group of dogs to reproduce in vivo mechanical stresses, and they radiographically and histologically evaluated the results. Their data suggest that disparities between histocompatibility antigens modulate the incorporation of bone into massive osteochondral allografts. The effect of histocompatibility matching, assessed histologically and radiologically after orthotopic bone transplantation in mice and dogs, also has been reported (17,18,75). The degree of bone healing in donor–recipient combinations differing at the MHC was weaker than for syngeneic controls (76).

These animal studies, along with reports of anti-HLA antibodies against freeze-dried (47) and frozen bone allografts (145,171), support the need for clinical trials of histocompatibility-typed bone allografts in humans (70,114,129).

IMMUNOGENICITY OF HUMAN BONE ALLOGRAFTS

Muscolo et al. (127) performed HLA histocompatibility studies between donor and recipient in patients receiving frozen bone allografts, including a cross-match test against the donor (and a panel of healthy control lymphocytes), and the HLA phenotypes (class I and class II) of the donor and recipient. This group of patients was radiographically evaluated using the proposed Musculoskeletal Tumor Society scoring system at an average follow-up of 55 months (42).

In an attempt to evaluate histologic evidence of immune response against the transplant, material was obtained from transplants in a group of patients by punch, by open biopsy, or from a surgical specimen. The mean radiographic score for this group of patients was 72%. All patients with a negative cross-match test with the potential donor received the transplant regardless of the matching for the HLA antigens. The group with zero donor–recipient antigen matches had a mean radiographic score of 67%. The group with one HLA-A antigen match had a mean radiographic score of 71%. The group with one HLA-B antigen match had a mean radiographic score of 83%. Finally, the group in which the donor and recipient shared more than one antigen had a mean radiographic score of 76%. The differences between these four groups were not statistically significant (Fig. 24-1). The comparison between the patients with zero donor–recipient antigen matches (with a mean radiographic score of 67%) and the group of patients with at least one antigen match (and a mean radiographic score of 75%) was not statistically significant.

Histologic features of immune rejection in solid organ transplantations are well established. Infiltration of the allograft

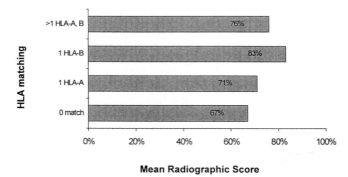

Figure 24-1 Fresh-frozen bone allografts, HLA class I antigen-matched with the donor, and radiographic score.

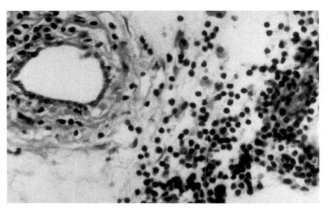

Figure 24-3 Photomicrograph of the specimen in Figure 24-2, obtained at higher magnification. Note an intense perivascular round cell infiltration and histologic features of vasculitis (hematoxylin and eosin, 350×). See Color Plate.

CORRELATION OF HLA MATCHING WITH ACCEPTANCE AND REJECTION

with lymphocytes and macrophages usually is associated with perivascular cellular infiltration and arterial vasculitis, defined as intramural inflammatory cell infiltration altering the vascular wall (156,166). A fibroproliferative process involving endothelial and mesenchymal cells also has been described (3). Histology has been accepted as the reference method for diagnosis of immune rejection. Also, it has been reported that graft survival and biopsy histology support the concept that donor matching for HLA will diminish rejection and increase the success of cardiac transplantation (187). Histologic material obtained from the authors' study was evaluated in relation to the radiographic score. Infiltration of round cells and the presence of vascular lesions (defined as vasculitis with swelling of endothelial cells or proliferative changes in the vessels) were observed in some patients (Figs. 24-2 and 24-3). This group of patients showed a mean radiographic score of 37%, whereas the group of patients without round cell infiltration showed a mean radiographic score of 62% (Fig. 24-4). The comparison between these two groups was statistically significant, suggesting that the immune response generated by frozen bone allografts might be related to low radiographic performance. Those allografts showing lymphocyte infiltration or vascular lesions scored radiographically lower than those that did not.

The human MHC is defined by three HLA class I loci that encode the A, B, and C specificities (2). The loci in the HLA class II, or D, region are now usually divided into four subregions, DR, DQ, DO, and DP (1690). The expression of class I antigens had been defined in most if not all nucleated cells and is dependent on regulatory factors, the most important being interferon. The class II antigens have a more restricted tissue distribution.

The importance of HLA matching to graft survival of organs such as the kidney, heart, lung, pancreas, and liver has been studied extensively (134). The transplant results for HLA-identical transplants from living, related donors are unsurpassed, and it is well accepted that kidneys from living, related donors are associated with better survival than cadaver kidneys (118). Controversy, however, persists regarding the impact of HLA A, B, and DR donor–recipient matching on cadaverous donor renal allograft survival (95). Data from larger registries indicate

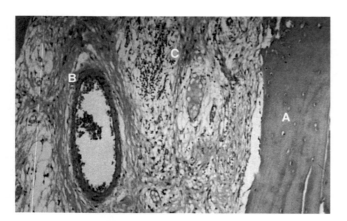

Figure 24-2 Human fresh-frozen cancellous bone allograft. Photomicrograph showing a bone marrow space lined by viable bone trabeculae (A). Note perivascular fibrosis (B) and round cell infiltration (C) (hematoxylin and eosin, 150×). See Color Plate.

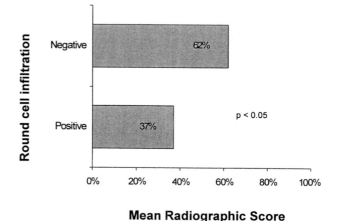

Figure 24-4 Fresh-frozen bone allograft round cell infiltration and radiographic score.

a significant benefit in graft survival for recipients of well-matched grafts (56,134,135,150); however, other single-center reports do not reflect this same benefit (95,118).

A significant benefit from transplanting cadaveric kidneys with the best matches (zero mismatched or six antigens matched) has been reported (118). However, data show that matching does not significantly affect graft survival except in the case of six-antigen-match kidneys (65). Furthermore, the zero-mismatched or six-mismatched recipients made up less than 8% of the total population studied, with 92% of the patients having one to five mismatches and not showing any significant difference in graft survival (65). But in a recent collaborative transplant study, a positive correlation of HLA matching in kidney and heart transplantation was obtained, even in cyclosporin-treated patients (134). Results from the previously presented authors' studies of musculoskeletal transplants showed a higher radiographic score for the groups of patients with one or more HLA class I antigen matches between donor and recipient than for the group with no matches. However, differences between the groups were not statistically significant.

One should also consider the extensive polymorphism of the HLA system when analyzing these latter results. At present, there are at least 25 allelic specificities defined by alloantisera in the HLA-A locus, 50 in the HLA-B locus, and 14 in the HLA-DR subregion. In addition, this study did not utilize the results of tissue typing in a preoperative manner to select recipients. As previously stated, all patients who had a negative cross-match with a potential donor had the transplantation regardless of the results of tissue matching. Thus, few patients had more than one antigen match with the donor, which is very different from the necessary three or four antigen matches for class I HLA antigens that are needed to obtain beneficial results when performing kidney or heart allografts (134). The effect of HLA matching and graft survival may also be obscured by the fact that subgroups exist for both class I and class II antigens. These are relatively new subdivisions of the previously identified antigens and are not yet defined by conventional serologic techniques (118). HLA matching is based on the premise that the transplantation antigens are the same as those that elicit an antibody response, but allograft rejection is essentially a cellular phenomenon. It is becoming clear that T cells and antibodies recognize different MHC products, and serologic definition of HLA, therefore, will not predict exact T cell–mediated alloreactivity (122).

Traditionally, HLA matching has been performed by counting the number of mismatched antigens. There are two antigens each in the A, B, and DR loci. However, molecular analysis of HLA specificities demonstrates that the number of antigens mismatched is not clearly correlated with the number of amino acids mismatched. If antibodies are directed against specific amino acids, it would be necessary to count all the amino acid differences (165,167). Therefore, scientists have attempted to cut the HLA molecule into peptides of different lengths and then match the transplants for the peptides (165). It has been reported that for kidney allografts, matching the peptides of the HLA A and B loci is associated with graft outcome and that this matching method may be more effective for transplants (165). An alternative explanation of the HLA matching effect might be that some mismatches are more immunocompetent than others. Allografts

with highly immunocompetent mismatches would be rejected early (56).

Major histocompatibility complex molecules contain a peptide-binding groove (8). Recent findings indicate that peptides normally occupy this site (122) and that the primary biologic role of HLA is to carry peptides to T cells. Allo-MHC molecules present in allografted tissues are recognized as complexes of allo-MHC plus peptides and not only as alloantigens (37,100). Different tissues express different peptides, and it might be inadequate to try to assess immunity against bone cells using donor blood lymphocytes, because T cells recognize MHC plus peptides (184). The role then of MHC molecules is to select peptides from inside the cell and to present them at the cell surface, where MHC peptide complexes can be recognized by T lymphocytes (174,184).

PATHWAYS OF IMMUNE RECOGNITION

Large frozen bone allografts are atypical nonviable transplants, and antigens are slowly released from dead cells over a long period of time (162). There are two routes for alloimmunization. First, there is the direct pathway, in which T cells recognize intact allo-MHC with a binding peptide on the surface of the donor antigen-presenting cell (APC). Second, there is the indirect pathway, in which T cells recognize processed alloantigen that has been shed from the graft and taken up by the recipient APC. These endogenous peptides may be derived from minor histocompatibility or tissue-specific antigens (37,100,184). Frozen bone allograft should sensitize the host through the indirect pathway, because it does not provide a viable APC (Fig. 24-5).

T cells primed by the direct pathway play a dominant role in acute early allograft rejection, whereas T cells primed by the indirect pathway may play the dominant role in chronic rejection (151,152). There is evidence also that the indirect pathway of alloantigen recognition is related to tolerance induction of nonviable grafts (25). Studies performed with corneal (72) and cultured pancreatic cell allografts (25,26) in which donor

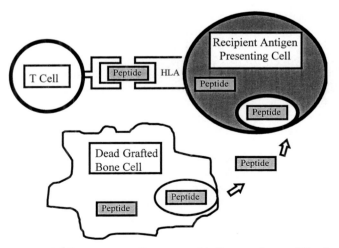

Figure 24-5 Schematic illustration of indirect pathway of T cell recognition of bone allografts. T cell, recipient T cell; peptide, minor histocompatibility or tissue-specific antigen; HLA, human leukocyte antigen.

APC were eliminated suggest that indirect presentation of graft antigens by host APC may be involved in the generation of regulatory T cells that in turn interfere with the generation of the graft-specific T cell response in vivo, thereby generating immunologic tolerance (25,26). This recent information applied to frozen bone allografts as nonviable tissues with no APC may support the idea that they either generate a chronic type of rejection or might be able to induce an immune tolerant state in the recipient. This may explain the difficulties inherent in correlating donor–recipient HLA mismatches with frozen bone allograft performance as well as explain the reported failures to correlate anti-HLA antibodies with the clinical status of the allografts (171). However, one recent long-term study assessing survival of massive frozen osteoarticular allografts suggested that matching for MHC class II antigens had an effect on graft survival (49,114).

With our present knowledge regarding the immunobiology of processed nonviable grafts, it seems rational either to explore ways to induce clinical immune tolerance in the recipient or to tissue-match for HLA and bone tissue–specific antigens. A multicenter trial using large tissue banks would provide the basis of an important clinical study. Clinical application of viable, vascularized bone allografts may need prospective tissue matching or new advances in immune modulation of acute rejection of organ transplants.

BIOMECHANICAL PROPERTIES OF PRESERVED FORMS OF BONE ALLOGRAFTS

In clinical practice, the most commonly used grafts are fresh-frozen or freeze-dried preserved allografts that have been irradiated or autoclaved (170). To plan a reconstructive procedure, it is important to understand the effects of these different conservation methods on the strength of the allografts.

Published reports reveal that fresh-frozen allografts have biomechanical properties that are similar to those of fresh allografts (21,97,141,154). Although optimal length and storage temperature have not been determined, it seems that bone grafts may be stored several years at –70°C to –80°C without significant deterioration of biologic or biomechanical properties.

Comparisons of biomechanical behavior between animal fresh-frozen and freeze-dried bone allografts have been reported (14,15,20,142). Data from these studies suggest that freeze-drying has a deleterious effect on the torsional and bending strength but not on the capacity to resist compressive forces. The biological properties of osteoconduction and osteoinduction are generally preserved. In one study, magnified examination of the freeze-dried specimens showed longitudinal microscopic cracks after the specimens were rehydrated (142). These defects were not observed in any of the frozen specimens, so it is unlikely that they were initiated during the freezing stage of the freeze-drying process. In another study, the effect of rehydration on freeze-dried human femora and tibiae matched pairs was analyzed (24). The authors concluded that this stage of the freeze-drying process may adversely affect graft strength and stiffness. Defects seemed to have originated during the drying stage.

These changes may have a significant impact on clinical practice, depending on how the graft material is used. When

graft is morselized for filling a cystic defect, mechanical strength might be irrelevant. On the other hand, when segmental or structural grafts are subjected to significant torsional loads, frozen bone would be biomechanically better than freeze-dried bone.

To decrease the risk of infectious disease transmission, different sterilization techniques, such as irradiation and ethylene oxide treatment, may be used. The biomechanical consequences of these procedures have been studied (97,157,175). Irradiation effect is controversial and seems to be dose specific. Below 3 Mrad, there appears to be little difference in the biomechanical properties of the tested specimens, but above this level a significant change in the breaking strength has been observed. This effect is magnified if the allograft is freeze-dried as well as irradiated (175). Results from a study of machined femora that were tested by applying three-point bending, compression, and torsion forces showed a significant reduction in the bending strength with 3.0-Mrad irradiation of freeze-dried bone but no change in compression or torsion strength (97). The screw pullout strength of bone allografts with different forms of preservation has been analyzed (157). Irradiated and ethylene oxide–treated specimens did not differ significantly from controls; the only specimen treatment that required significantly less force for screw pullout was freeze-drying. It is questionable whether this method of processing should be used for structural allograft reconstructions in which screw fixation is mandatory.

The effect of different conservation methods on the strength of bone allografts should be considered so that the reconstructive procedure will adequately account for the type and amount of load that the graft will require. When grafted segments are subject to significant torsional loads, a frozen bone would be better biomechanically than a freeze-dried bone. In situations that do not result in significant loading of the graft, or when compression forces are the primary concern, frozen and freeze-dried allografts are both biomechanically acceptable.

In an effort to improve the incorporation of these processed cortical allografts without compromising their biomechanical properties, new methodologies have been developed. Perforation of the graft increases the available surface area for ingrowth and ongrowth of new bone (34,104). Additionally, it provides easier access to the intramedullary canal. Several studies have demonstrated that perforated grafts indeed have more new bone ingrowth than similar nonperforated grafts (34,104). These grafts are also more porous in the 6 months following surgery because of the increased area availability to osteoclasts for bone resorption. This method may also help revascularization of the allografts by providing channels for ingrowth of host blood vessels. However, the overall repair process is not that different from standard cortical grafts. Perforation of the graft has raised some concern in the past about the possibility of stress rises at the perforation sites. (16,19). Studies have shown, however, that the strength of the bone immediately following drilling is not diminished significantly in either compression or bending (18,34). There is a decrease in the overall strength after 4 weeks, but this was associated with the increased porosity of the graft rather than with the drill holes. By 6 weeks after transplantation, the strength of the graft returned to that of the nonperforated grafts. Recent studies have combined partial demineralization with perforation of the graft and have demonstrated a positive effect on overall osteoinduction while preserving some of the biomechanical properties of the graft (104). Overall cortical allograft incorporation is a complex process that has significant variables that influence the ultimate incorporation and function of the graft.

MODES OF ALLOGRAFT FAILURE

The most common complications and causes of allograft clinical failures are infections, resorptions, fractures, and nonunions.

Infection

Infection rates correlate with the magnitude of the allograft reconstructive procedure. Extensive surgical exposures and adjuvant chemotherapeutic regimes are associated with infection rates as high as 14% (35,172). Another study showed no infections after allograft reconstructions for revision joint arthroplasty or for a tumor with no adjuvant therapy, but it showed a 13% infection rate in patients who had chemotherapy, radiotherapy, or both (86). The transfer of infections with grafts from bone banks does not seem to be a relevant factor if the bone banks follow appropriate guidelines (107). The dissimilarity between organisms grown from donor tissues and those grown from cultures of material from patients who had clinical infections suggests that contamination of the culture-negative allografts was probably not responsible for most clinical infections (172).

Small particulate bone allografts have a negligible clinical incidence of infection compared with large structural allografts (172). This observation might be related to prolonged surgery, problems with soft-tissue coverage and wound necrosis, the use of chemotherapy, or the big dead spaces generally observed in patients receiving a large allograft. However, differences in the biology of incorporation might be implicated. Particulate allografts are more rapidly revascularized and remodeled than structural allografts, which retain extensive necrotic areas for many years (44). These dead spaces are unreachable by antibiotics and unprotected by the bactericidal effect of the immune system.

The efficiency of sterilization of musculoskeletal tissue by irradiation depends on the biologic properties of allografts. In fact, the dose differential required for sterility and preservation of graft osteoinductive properties, for a normal rate of union between the donor and receptor, and for prevention of fractures is uncertain (36,86,125,178). It has been suggested that infection might be a subtle sign of allograft rejection (44,107). Nonunion and bone resorption rates are higher in infected allografts and both are potentially related to poor donor–receptor tissue matching.

Resorption

Partial resorption as a cause of clinical failures has been reported after acetabular and femoral structural allograft reconstructions (87,92,121,128), with rates as high as 36%. Graft resorption is frequently associated with, and may be the triggering factor for, nonunion (128), fracture (6), or infection (35,107,129,172).

Massive allograft resorption is a relatively infrequent but devastating complication. Late infections and allograft resorptions are the main factors that influence long-term results (114,128). Both have been related to a host immune response (88). Bone resorption is mediated by cytokine production by activated immune cells or activated osteoblasts and osteoclasts. The authors of this chapter have reported evidence that gross antigen mismatches between donor and recipient might generate massive resorption and collapse of an osteoarticular allograft (129).

Nonunion and Fracture

Nonunion rates at the allograft–host bone junction vary from 9% (110) to 23% (59), with most series reporting an incidence of 10% to 15% (4,58,113). One proposed modification to lower nonunion and fracture rates is to alter the osteotomy geometry to limit its motion and enhance healing (28). The mechanical and functional properties of transverse and step-cut osteotomies have been compared in an in vivo canine model (115). The step-cut osteotomy was associated with significantly greater structural stiffness than the transverse osteotomy. The dogs with the step-cut osteotomy also experienced significantly less weight bearing than the dogs with a transverse osteotomy. It was concluded that there is no advantage to altering the osteotomy configuration from the traditional transverse osteotomy.

The effects of internal fixation on the healing of large allografts have also been reported (124,179). In a sheep tibia allograft model, the union and incorporation of intercalary allografts after fixation with a locked intramedullary nail or a dynamic compression plate were not measurably different (124). Data from a recent human study (179) suggest that diaphyseal junctions healed slowly, by an average of 9 months after the operation, whereas metaphyseal junctions healed more rapidly, usually in less than 6 months. The authors recommended neutralization of forces across the junction with either a plate or an intramedullary nail, and they also reported no significant difference in the rate of union between the methods of fixation. However, the use of a plate was associated with a higher rate of allograft fracture. This association was also reported by other authors, who suggest that structural defects, such as screw holes, create a mechanical stress riser that fails with fatigue (168). It appears that fractures originate at the defect and extend into the unprotected segment of the graft. For this reason, the authors recommended the use of intramedullary fixation, which provides much longer allograft protection and avoids cortex defects (168).

Bone grafting to promote healing across gaps at the allograft–host junction has been proposed, but it has not been consistently successful (179). It is easy to obtain a stable fixation and some compression at the allograft–host junction with the use of a plate, but it is important to consider stress risers and their relationship to allograft fractures. Although intramedullary nails may avoid screw holes, small gaps and unstable allograft–host junctions are commonly seen. Interlocking nailing may provide control of rotation when adequate bone is available. However, placement of the locking screws in the allograft may increase the risk of fracture. For this reason, methylmethacrylate has been used in some patients to augment intramedullary fixation and to avoid allograft screw holes (168). Although no adverse effect on healing was identified in these patients, future surgery, such as joint replacement, would be more difficult after this technique has been used.

Published reports suggest that fractures generally occur approximately 24 months after the implantation of the graft (6,185), and most have occurred by 4 years. It has been suggested that resorption through rapid revascularization might lead to mechanical weakness and fracture of the graft (6,52,121). However, intraoperative evidence obtained at the time of surgical treatment of fractured allografts suggests the opposite (168): areas of poor revascularization occurred at the fracture site, and new bone was formed only by the reparative process. It is not clear if rapid revascularization triggers bone resorption, possibly through immune recognition of foreign antigens, or if lack of revascularization and stress risers created at time of implantation are responsible for mechanical failure.

More retrieval analyses of fractured and nonfractured specimens, along with histologic markers of immune responses, are needed to clarify this issue.

HUMAN BONE ALLOGRAFTS: CLINICAL HISTOLOGIC AND RETRIEVAL STUDIES

There are a number of long-term clinical studies reporting the outcome of bone allografts used for reconstruction after tumor excision or as an adjunct in revision total hip arthroplasty. One recent study of 893 allografts reported that 75% demonstrated an excellent or good result and did not fail because of tumor problems (114). Intercalary grafts had the best outcome, alloarthrodeses the worst. Most of the graft failures occurred in the first 3 years, and after 5 years the allografts appeared to reach a stable condition.

Allograft use for revision total hip arthroplasty has become common because of the increasing number of failures caused by osteolytic bone loss resulting from wear particles. Cancellous allografts to treat bone defects in acetabular revision have been used for the last 2 decades, with controversial but yet effective outcomes (Fig. 24-6). The grafts have been used to reconstruct contained defects, with success reported as high as 85% at 12 years after surgery (158). Complete graft incorporation has been demonstrated in autopsy retrievals or punch biopsy up to 7 years after the graft procedures. By contrast, bulk allografts used to reconstruct larger segmental acetabular defects have had less than ideal outcomes (108). Failure of the allograft with resorption and acetabular loosening has been reported to be 60% at 10 years. Most of these failures may be due to fatigue fractures of the graft occurring when more than 50% of the socket support is provided by the graft.

Revision femoral reconstruction usually requires allografting, either segmental or cavitary, because of the large defect size. Morselized frozen allograft impacted into the medullary canal with a cemented stem has been reported by Gie et al. to have generally satisfactory short-term outcomes (54). Although, as noted earlier in this chapter, revascularization and remodeling to viable new bone occurs, the long-term assessment remains unknown. Onlay cortical strut allografts

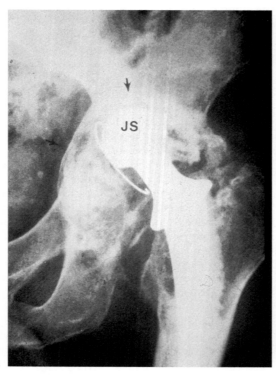
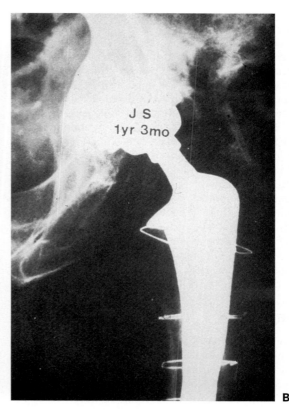

A **B**

Figure 24-6 **A:** AP radiograph demonstrating a failed acetabular component. **B:** AP radiograph of one and a half year postop bone grafting showing excellent incorporation of cancellous morselized allograft.

are useful for treating a femur with a cortical defect. Clinical and radiographic outcomes are consistently satisfactory, with success rates as high as 99% at intermediate time points (54). As shown radiographically, these grafts usually remodel by rounding their ends and demonstrate adaptive changes as a response to the loads on the host femur. Massive bulk femoral allografts used with a long-stem femoral component provide an approach to the reconstruction of major proximal femoral bone loss. Although the functional clinical results at intermediate and longer-term follow-up have varied, with reoperation rates reported to be 10% to 41%, the frozen allografts usually are preserved, with minimal resorption and union at the host–allograft junction observed in 90% of the patients (117).

Extensive histologic observations of allografts related to incorporation rates or resorption under different circumstances in experimental animals have been reported. Although these experiments have been extremely valuable for furthering general understanding of the different incorporation rates of various types of bone grafts used in various genetic circumstances, information from human allograft specimens is sparse.

Clinical and histologic data from patients with small failed fresh osteochondral allografts have been reported (133). Material from the excised grafts showed evidence of viable hyaline cartilage–producing matrix. The degree of replacement of the graft by host bone as a result of creeping substitution was variable but increased with time. Grafts retrieved after more than 44 months had complete bony replacement. In a second study by the same group (31), using autoradiography of sections labeled with radioactive precursors of ribonucleic acid synthesis, viability of articular cartilage in biopsies of small fresh osteochondral grafts was found. The viability of cartilage might be related to its ability to survive without a blood supply and to avoid exposure to the immune system (109). However, a study of retrieved osteochondral allografts in a canine model showed viability of chondrocytes only when the subchondral plate was intact and no pannus covered the articular surface. All but one of the fresh antigen-mismatched allografts had a marked lymphoplasmacytic and fibrous pannus across the articular surface, mononuclear cells in intertrabecular spaces, and little new bone formation (161).

Postmortem retrieval analysis of morselized, particulate, frozen bone allograft after cancellous impaction grafting in the femur (106) and in acetabular reconstructions (84) has also been reported (5) (Fig. 24-7). Although only four cases were studied, progression of graft incorporation was seen to be related to the length of time the graft had been in situ. An allograft retrieved 83 months after transplantation showed trabeculae enveloped by new host bone rimmed by normal osteoblasts. These few cases suggest that morselized, particulate allografts that are placed in an acetabular or femoral defect and are not intended to bear a substantial load become incorporated.

The natural history of bone allografts is difficult to define through these studies, because most specimens are obtained from transplants that failed as a result of infection, resorption, or fracture. Those excised for nongraft-related complications such as tumor recurrence may be indicative of a properly functioning graft. Histologic analyses of limited biopsies obtained from human processed massive allografts have been reported (64,129,149). In one study (64), only two cases were reported

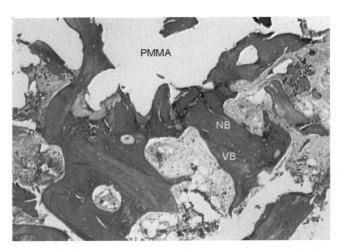

Figure 24-7 Histology image of an autopsy retrieval after impaction grafting demonstrating labeled spaces that had been occupied by cement. Inside is PMMA, then a layer of varying thickness composed of impacted graft. See Color Plate.

from what the authors considered to be functioning grafts because the materials were obtained during reoperations for minor complications. Little resorption–apposition was present, and then predominantly in subperiosteal areas. Inflammatory infiltration was seldom found. Another study reported biopsies of cartilage and subchondral bone from half-joint knee allografts up to 8 years after grafting with deep-frozen allogeneic grafts (149). A slow substitution of grafted bone and cartilage was found to begin at 12 months.

The authors of this chapter studied biopsies obtained from fresh-frozen massive allografts followed for 9 to 18 months (129). Both revascularization and new bone formation were studied in the periosteal, cortical, or medullary transplant areas. Revascularization and new bone formation seem to be correlated; if the graft was revascularized, the event was almost always followed by good new bone formation (Figs. 24-8 to 24-10).

Isolated cases of retrieved specimens after amputation for tumor recurrence or graft collapse (94,96,140) and a series of four allografts, two of which were not infected and were studied more than 3 months after transplantation, have been reported (125). Host bone growth into donor bone at the graft–host interface and extensive areas of necrotic bone with no clear evidence of an immune response were found.

Another histologic analysis of four retrieved fresh-frozen massive osteoarticular allografts obtained 1 to 25 years after transplantation has been reported (129,131). Although extensive areas remained necrotic, periosteal, cortical, and medullary revascularization and new bone formation were found. All specimens showed histologic union between donor and recipient, but in one specimen retrieved after 27 months because of graft resorption, there was strong evidence of an immune response (129). The specimen obtained after 25 years in situ was a hip osteoarticular graft in which articular fibrocartilage and areas of bone remodeling with necrotic and newly formed bone were found (128).

The most extensive study of retrieved allografts was reported by Enneking and Mindell (44), who included a series of 16 retrieved specimens. Their basic findings were strong

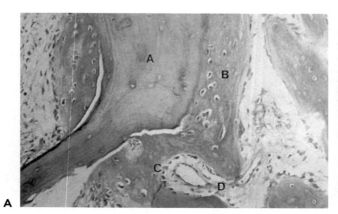

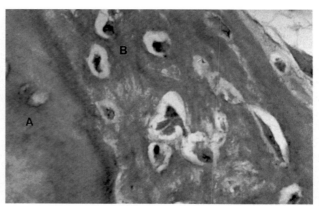

Figure 24-8   Human fresh-frozen cancellous bone allograft. **A:** Low-magnification photomicrograph showing a large complete necrotic cancellous trabeculum (A) lined by newly formed bone (B). Another area shows bone remodeling with active osteoblasts and osteoclasts (C). The marrow is well vascularized (D) (hematoxylin and eosin, 150×). **B:** Higher-magnification photomicrograph of the same area, showing a necrotic trabeculum with dead osteocytes (A) and viable osteocytes on a newly formed trabeculum (B) (hematoxylin and eosin, 400×). See Color Plate.

attachment between soft tissues and allograft surface, the ability of fractured grafts to heal, routine union at the donor–recipient site, and necrotic articular cartilage with remarkably good architecture even after 5 years. No radiographic or histologic evidence of allograft resorption about the cement or loosening in composite allografts was found. The authors' observations support these findings (Figs. 24-11 and 24-12). Although a slow and incomplete repair, apparently based mainly on osteoconduction (not osteoinduction), was the norm, both rapid resorption and advanced bone repair appeared possible. No histocompatibility studies between donor and recipient were done, and no signs of acute immune rejection were found. However, two allografts were retrieved because of a supposed rejection, possibly caused by loose fibrovascular tissue with some chronic inflammatory cells that resulted in the expression of a low-grade, indolent immune response to antigens present in the graft. Additional studies of retrieved allografts with different fixation and processing techniques, including tissue typing for donor and recipient, are needed to clarify the role of each variable in the clinical outcome of allografts.

SUMMARY

The surgeon, when considering graft options for reconstruction in revision total hip replacement, should evaluate the amount of bone loss, the load requirements, and the biologic and biomechanical properties of available grafts. At the time of implantation, processed bone allografts are nonviable structures. Biologic events induce a progressive incorporation of the graft but also a possible immune response against foreign antigens. Because of their lack of viable cells, allografts prompt either an indolent, chronic type of rejection or an immunologic state of tolerance in the host. When particulate, morselized bone allografts are used to repair contained defects, mechanical strength might be irrelevant. On the other hand, when segmental or structural grafts are indicated, the effect of different preservation methods on bone allograft strength should be considered. Risk of infectious disease is decreased with different sterilization techniques, but these techniques have potential biomechanical effects.

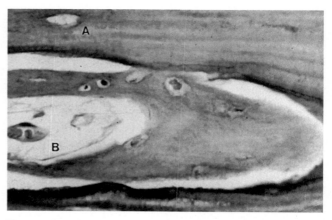

Figure 24-9   Human fresh-frozen cancellous bone allograft. Photomicrograph shows a necrotic bone trabeculum (A) with active osteoclastic resorption (B) (hematoxylin and eosin, 300×). See Color Plate.

Figure 24-10   Human fresh-frozen cortical bone allograft. Photomicrograph shows a necrotic haversian canal (A) with central capillary revascularization and new bone formation (B) (hematoxylin and eosin, 350×). See Color Plate.

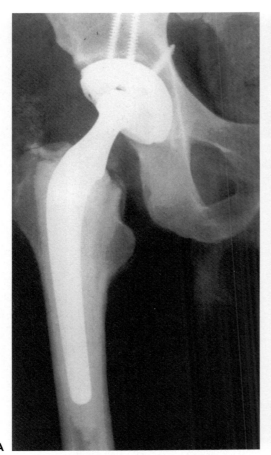

A

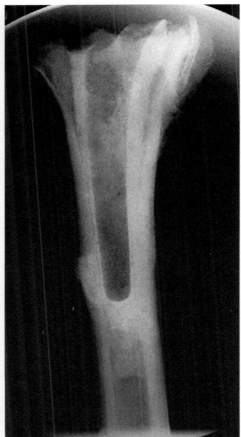

B

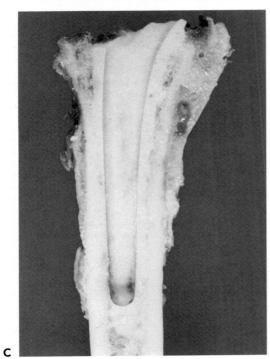

C

Figure 24-11 Fresh-frozen hip allograft composite. **A:** AP radiograph of a total femur allograft with a proximal total hip prosthesis, made 34 months after insertion. **B:** Cut-surface anteroposterior radiograph of the dissected specimen retrieved at 35 months because of local tumor recurrence. **C:** Photograph of the same cut surface showing no evidence of resorption of the allograft about the cement or loosening. See Color Plate.

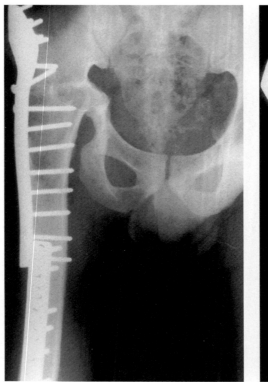
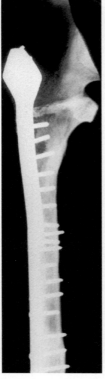
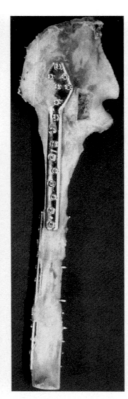
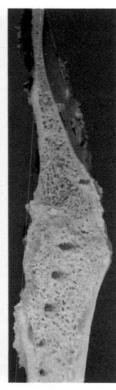

A,B   C,D

Figure 24-12 Fresh-frozen intercalary allograft. **A:** AP radiograph of a hip arthrodesis with an intercalary allograft made 20 months after insertion. **B:** AP radiograph of the dissected specimen retrieved at 23 months because of a local tumor recurrence, showing cancellous (proximal) and cortical (distal) unions. **C:** Photograph of the same specimen showing both osteotomies. **D:** Photograph of the cut surface of the proximal osteotomy, showing cancellous union. See Color Plate.

Future advances will include ways to preserve allograft viability and the development of cellular and molecular biologic techniques for enhanced graft incorporation. Procedures to modulate the immune response or to ensure tissue-specific matching of donor and recipient also need to be developed.

REFERENCES

1. Aho AJ, Ekfors T, Dean PB, et al. Incorporation and clinical results of large allografts of the extremities and pelvis. *Clin Orthop.* 1994;No. 307:200–213.
2. Albrechtsen D, Moen T, Thorsby E. HLA matching in clinical transplantation. *Transplant Proc* 1983;15:1120–1123.
3. Al-Dossari GA, Jessurun J, Bolman RM III, et al. Pathogenesis of obliterative bronchiolitis: possible roles of platelet-derived growth factor and basic fibroblast growth factor. *Transplantation.* 1995;59:143–145.
4. Allan DG, Lavoie GJ, McDonal S, et al. Proximal femoral allografts in revision hip arthroplasty. *J Bone Joint Surg.* 1991; 73B:235–240.
5. Bauer, TW, Muschler GF. Bone graft materials. *Clin Orthop.* 2000; No. 371:10–27.
6. Berry BH, Lord CF, Gebhardt MC, et al. Fractures of allografts. *J Bone Joint Surg.* 1990;72A:825–833.
7. Berry DJ, Chandler HP, Reilly DT. The use of bone allografts in two-stage reconstruction after failure of hip replacements due to infection. *J Bone Joint Surg.* 1991;73A:1460–1468.
8. Bjorkman PJ, Saper MA, Samraovi B, et al. The foreign antigen binding site and T cell recognition regions of class I histocompatibility antigen. *Nature.* 1987;329:512–518.
9. Blackley HR, Davis AM, Hutchison CR, et al. Proximal femoral allografts for reconstruction of bone stock in revision arthroplasty of the hip: a nine to fifteen-year follow-up. *J Bone Joint Surg.* 2001;83:346-354.
10. Bonfiglio M, Jeter WS, Smith CL. The immune concept: its relation to bone transplantation. *Ann N Y Acad Sci.* 1955;59:417–433.
11. Borja FJ, Mnaymneh W. Bone allografts in salvage of difficult hip arthroplasties. *Clin Orthop.* 1985;197:123–130.
12. Bos GD, Goldberg VM, Powell AE, et al. The effect of histocompatibility matching on canine frozen bone allografts. *J Bone Joint Surg.* 1983;65A:89–96.
13. Bos GD, Goldberg VM, Zika JM, et al. Immune responses of rats to frozen bone allografts. *J Bone Joint Surg.* 1983;65A:239–246.
14. Bright R, Burchard H. The biomechanical properties of preserved bone grafts. In: Friedlander G, Mankin H, Sell K, eds. *Bone Allografts: Current State of the Art.* Boston: Little, Brown; 1983: 223–232.
15. Bright R, Burstein A. Material properties of preserved cortical bone. *Trans Orthop Res Soc.* 1968;3:210.
16. Brooks D. Burstein A, Frankel V. The biomechanics of torsional fractures: the stress concentration effect of a drill hole. *J Bone Joint Surg.* 1970;52A:507–514.
17. Burchardt H. The biology of bone graft repair. *Clin Orthop.* 1983;No. 174:28–42.
18. Burchardt H, Glowczewskie FP, Enneking WF. Allogeneic segmental fibular transplants in azathioprine-immunosuppressed dogs. *J Bone Joint Surg.* 1977;59A:881–894.
19. Burstein A, Currey J, Frankel VH, et al. Bone strength: the effect of screw holes. *J Bone Joint Surg.* 1972, 54A:1143–1156.
20. Burstein A, Frankel V. A standard test for laboratory animal bone. *J Biomech.* 1971;4:155–158.
21. Burwell RG. The fate of freeze dried bone allografts. *Transplant Proc.* 1976;8(suppl):95.

22. Burwell RG. Studies in the transplantation of bone: the immune responses of lymph nodes draining second-set homografts of fresh cancellous bone. *J Bone Joint Surg.* 1962;44B:688–710.

23. Chalmers J. Transplantation immunity in bone homografting. *J Bone Joint Surg.* 1959;41B:160–179.

24. Conrad EU, Ericksen DP, Tencer AF, et al. The effects of freeze-drying and rehydratation on cancellous bone. *Clin Orthop.* 1993;290:279.

25. Coulombe M, Gill RG. Tolerance induction to cultured islet allografts: characterization of the tolerant state. *Transplantation.* 1994;57:1195–1200.

26. Coulombe M, Gill RG. Tolerance induction to cultured islet allografts: the status of antidonor reactivity in tolerant animals. *Transplantation.* 1994;57:1201–1207.

27. Curtiss PH Jr, Wilson PD. A comparison of the healing of homogeneous bone and autogenous fresh bone grafts with and without administration of cortisone. *Surg Gynec Obstet.* 1953;96:155–161.

28. Czitrom AA. Allograft reconstruction after tumor surgery in the appendicular skeleton. In: Czitron AA, Gross AE, eds. *Allografts in Orthopaedic Practice.* Baltimore: Williams & Wilkins; 1992:83–119.

29. Czitron AA. Biology of bone grafting and principles of bone banking. In: Weinstein SL, ed. *The Pedriatic Spine.* New York: Raven Press; 1994:1285–1298.

30. Czitrom AA, Axelrod T, Fernandes B. Antigen presenting cells and bone allotransplantation. *Clin Orthop.* 1985;197:27–31.

31. Czitrom A, Keating S, Gross AE. The viability of articular cartilage in fresh osteochondral allografts after clinical transplantation. *J Bone Joint Surg.* 1990;72A;574–581.

32. Damien CJ, Parsons JR. Bone graft and bone graft substitutes: a review of current technology and applications. *J Appl Biomater.* 1991;2:187–208.

33. Delloye C, Simon P, Nyssen-Behets C, et al. Perforations of cortical bone allografts improved their incorporation. *Clin Orthop.* 2002;396:240–247.

34. DeWae H, Chen F, Su E, et al. Use of structural bone graft with cementless acetabular cups in total hip arthroplasty. *J Arthroplasty.* 2003;18:23–28.

35. Dick HM, Strauch RJ. Infection of massive bone allografts. *Clin Orthop.* 1994;306;46–53.

36. Dziedzic-Goclawska A, Ostrowski K, Stachowicz W, et al. Effect of radiation sterilization on the osteoinductive properties and the rate of remodeling of bone implants preserved by lyophilization and deep-freezing. *Clin Orthop.* 1991;272:30–37.

37. Eckels D. Alloreactivity: allogeneic presentation of endogenous peptides or direct recognition of MHC polimorphism. *Tissue Antigens.* 1990;35:49–55.

38. Einhorn TA. Current concept review. Enhancement of fracture healing. *J Bone Joint Surg.* 1995;77A:940–956.

39. Elting JJ, Zicat BA, Mikhail WEM, et al. Impaction grafting: preliminary report of a new method for exchange femoral arthroplasty. *Orthopaedics.* 1995;18:107–112.

40. Emerson RH, Head WC, Berklacich FM, et al. Noncemented acetabular revision arthroplasty using allograft bone. *Clin Orthop.* 1989;249:30–42.

41. Emerson RH, Malinin TI, Cuellar AD, et al. Cortical strut allografts in the reconstruction of the femur in revision total hip arthroplasty: a basic science and clinical study. *Clin Orthop.* 1992;285:35–43.

42. Enneking WF. Discussion of the functional evaluation system. In: Enneking WF, ed. *Limb Salvage in Musculoskeletal Oncology.* New York: Churchill Livingstone; 1987:622–623.

43. Enneking WF. Histological investigation of bone transplants in immunological prepared animals. *J Bone Joint Surg.* 1957;39A:597–615.

44. Enneking WF, Mindell ER. Observations on massive retrieved human allografts. *J Bone Joint Surg.* 1991;73A:1123–1142.

45. Friedlaender GE. The antigenicity of preserved allografts. *Transplant Proc.* 1976;8[Suppl 1]:195–200.

46. Friedlaender GE. Bone allografts: the biological consequences of immunological events. *J Bone Joint Surg.* 1991;73A:1119–1122.

47. Friedlaender GE, Horowitz MC. Immune responses to osteochondral allografts: nature and significance. *Orthopaedics.* 1992;15:1171–1175.

48. Friedlaender GE, Strong DM, Sell KW. Studies on the antigenicity of bone: donor-specific anti-HLA antibodies in human recipients of freeze-dried allografts. *J Bone Joint Surg.* 1984;66A:107–112.

49. Friedlaender G, Strong DM, Tomford WW, et al. Long term followup of patients with osteochondral allografts: a correlation between immunologic rsponses and clinical outcome. *Orthop Clin North Am.* 1999;30:583–590.

50. Garbuz D, Morsi E, Gross AE. Revision of the acetabular component of a total hip arthroplasty with a massive structural allograft: study with a minimum five-year follow-up. *J Bone Joint Surg.* 1996;78A:693–697.

51. Gates HS, McCollum DE, Poletti SC, et al. Bone grafting in total hip arthroplasty for protrusio acetabulum. *J Bone Joint Surg.* 1990;72A:248–251.

52. Gebhardt M, Roth YF, Mankin HJ. Osteoarticular allografts for reconstruction in the proximal part of the humerus after excision of a musculoskeletal tumor. *J Bone Joint Surg.* 1990;72A:334–345.

53. Gie GA, Linder L, Ling RSM, et al. Impacted cancellous allografts and cement for revision total hip arthroplasty. *J Bone Joint Surg.* 1993;75B:14–21.

54. Gie GA, Timperley AJ, Lamberton TD: Femoral revision: impaction bone grafting and cement. In: Lieberman J, Berry D, eds. *Advanced Reconstruction Hip.* American Academy of Orthopaedic Surgeons; 439–448.

55. Gieson EB, Lamerigts NM, Verdonschot N, et al. Mechanical characteristics of impacted morcellised bone grafts used in revision of total hip arthroplasty. *J Bone Joint Surg.* 1999;81B:1052–1057.

56. Gilks WR, Gore SM, Bradley BA. Renal transplant rejection: transient immunodominance of HLA mismatches. *Transplantation.* 1990;50:141–146.

57. Gill TJ, Sledge JB, Muller ME. The management of severe acetabular bone loss using structural allograft and acetabular reinforcement devices. *J Arthroplasty.* 2000;15:1–7.

58. Gitelis S, Heligman D, Quill G, et al. The use of large allografts for tumor reconstruction and salvage of the failed total hip arthroplasty. *Clin Orthop.* 1988;231:62–70.

59. Gitelis S, Piasecki P. Allograft prosthetic composite arthroplasty for osteosarcoma and other aggressive bone tumors. *Clin Orthop.* 1991;270:197.

60. Goldberg VM, Bos GD, Heiple KG, et al. Improved acceptance of frozen bone allografts in genetically mismatched dogs by immunosuppression. *J Bone Joint Surg.* 1984;66A:937–950.

61. Goldberg VM, Bos G, Powell A, et al. The effect of histocompatibility matching on canine frozen bone allografts. *J Bone Joint Surg.* 1983;65A:89–96.

62. Goldberg VM, Stevenson S, Shaffer JW. Biology of autografts and allografts. In: Friedlander GE, Goldberg VM, eds. *Bone and Cartilage Allografts.* Park Ridge, IL: American Academy of Orthopaedic Surgeons; 1989:3–12.

63. Gornet MF, Randolph MA, Schofield BH, et al. Immunologic and ultrastructural changes during early rejection of vascularized bone allografts. *Plast Reconstr Surg.* 1991;88:860–868.

64. Gouin F, Passuti N, Verriele V, et al. Histological features of large bone allografts. *J Bone Joint Surg.* 1996;78B:38–41.

65. Greenstein SM, Schechner RS, Louis P, et al. Evidence that zero antigen-matches cyclosporine-treated renal transplant recipients have graft survival equal to that of matched recipients: reevaluation of points. *Transplantation.* 1990;49:332–336.

66. Gross AE, Allan DG, Catre M, et al. Bone grafts in hip replacement surgery: the pelvic side. *Orthop Clin North Am.* 1993;24:679–695.

67. Gross AE, Allan DG, Leitch KK, et al. Proximal femoral allografts for reconstruction of bone stock in revision arthroplasty of the hip. *Instruct Course Lect.* 1996;45:143–147.

68. Gross AE, Allen G, Lavoie G. Revision arthroplasty using allograft bone. *Instr Course Lect.* 1993;45:363–380.

69. Gross AE, Garbuz DG, Morsi ES. Acetabular allografts for restoration of bone stock in revision arthroplasty of the hip. *Instruct Course Lect.* 1996;45:135–142.

70. Gross AE, Hutchison CR, Alexeeff M, et al. Proximal femoral allografts for reconstruction of bone stock in revision arthroplasty of the hip. *Clin Orthop.* 1995;319:151–158.

71. Gross AE, Lavoie MV, McDermott P, et al. The use of allograft bone in revision of total hip arthroplasty. *Clin Orthop.* 1985;No. 197:115–122.

72. Guymer RH, Mandel TE. A comparison of corneal, pancreas, and skin grafts in mice. *Transplantation.* 1994;57:1251–1262.

73. Haddah FS, Garbuz DS, Masri BA, et al. Structural proximal femoral allografts for failed total hip arthroplasty (THA): a minimum review of five years. *J Bone Joint Surg.* 2000;82:830–836.

74. Halliday BR, English HW, Timperley AJ, et al. Femoral impaction grafting with cement in revision total hip replacement: evolution of the technique and results. *J Bone Joint Surg.* 2003;6B:809–817.

75. Halloran PF, Lee EH, Ziv I, et al. Orthotopic bone transplantation in mice: studies of the alloantibody response. *Transplantation.* 1979;27:420–426.

76. Halloran PF, Ziv I, Lee EH, et al. Orthotopic bone transplantation in mice: technique and assessment of healing. *Transplantation.* 1979;27:414–419.

77. Hamadouche M, Mathieu M, Meunier A, et al. Histological findings in a proximal femoral allograft ten years following revision total hip arthroplasty: a case report. *J Bone Joint Surg.* 2002;84A:269–273.

78. Hamadouche M, Oakes DA, Berry DJ. Bone grafting for total joint arthroplasty. In: Lieberman J, Friedlaender G, eds. *Bone Regeneration and Repair.* Totowa, NJ: Humana Press; 2005:263–289.

79. Harrington KD. The use of hemipelvic allografts or autoclaved grafts for reconstruction after wide resections of malignant tumors of the pelvis. *J Bone Joint Surg.* 1992;74A:331–341.

80. Harris WH. Revision surgery for failed, nonseptic total hip arthroplasty: the femoral side. *Clin Orthop.* 1982;No. 170:8–20.

81. Head WC, Berklacich FM, Malinin TI, et al. Proximal femoral allografts in revision total hip arthroplasty. *Clin Orthop.* 1987; No. 225:22–36.

82. Head WC, Emerson RH, Malinin TI. Freeze-dried cortical strut allografts for femoral reconstruction in revision hip replacement surgery. *Instruc Course Lect.* 1996;45:131–134.

83. Head WC, Wagner RA, Emerson RH, et al. Restoration of femoral bone stock in revision total hip arthroplasty. *Orthop Clin North Am.* 1993;24:697–703.

84. Heekin RD, Engh CA, Vinh T. Morselized allograft in acetabular reconstruction: a postmortem retrieval analysis. *Clin Orthop.* 1995;No. 319:184–190.

85. Herndon CH, Chase SW. The fate of massive autogenous and homogenous bone grafts including articular surfaces. *Surg Gynec Obstet.* 1954;98:273–290.

86. Hernigou P, Delepine G, Goutallier D, et al. Massive allografts sterilised by irradiation: clinical results. *J Bone Joint Surg.* 1993; 75B:904–913.

87. Hooten JP, Engh CA Jr, Engh CA. Failure of structural acetabular allografts in cementless revision hip arthroplasty *J Bone Joint Surg.* 1994;76B:419–422.

88. Horowitz MC, Friedlander GE. The immune response to bone grafts. In: Friedlander GE, Goldberg VM, eds. *Bone and Cartilage Allografts.* Park Ridge, IL: American Academy of Orthopaedic Surgeons; 1989:85–101.

89. Horowitz MC, Friedlaender GE. Induction of specific T-cell responsiveness to allogeneic bone. *J Bone Joint Surg.* 1991;73A:1157–1168.

90. Horowitz MC, Friedlaender GE, Qian HY. T cell activation and the immune response to bone allografts. *Trans Orthop Res Soc.* 1994;19:180.

91. Inclan A. The use of preserved bone graft in orthopaedic surgery. *J Bone Joint Surg.* 1942;24:81–96.

92. Jasty MJ, Harris WH. Total hip reconstruction using frozen femoral head allografts in patients with acetabular bone loss. *Orthop Clin North Am.* 1987;18:291–299.

93. Jofe MH, Gebhardt MC, Tomford WW, et al. Reconstruction for defects of the proximal part of the femur using allograft arthroplasty. *J Bone Joint Surg.* 1988;70A:507–516.

94. Kandel RA, Pritzker KP, Langer F, et al. The pathologic features of massive osseous grafts. *Hum Pathol.* 1984;15:141–146.

95. Kerman RH, Kimball PM, Lindholm A, et al. Influence of HLA matching on rejections and short- and long-term primary cadaveric allograft survival. *Transplantation.* 1993;56:1242–1247.

96. Kocialkowski A, Wallace WA, Harvey L. Fate of frozen intercalary allograft at one year after implantation with adjuvant chemotherapy treatment. *Clin Orthop.* 1991;No. 272:146–151.

97. Komender A. Influence of preservation on some mechanical properties of human harvesian bone. *Mater Med Pol.* 1976;8:13.

98. Kwong LM, Jasty M, Harris WH. High failure rate of bulk femoral head allografts in total hip acetabular reconstructions at 10 years. *J Arthroplasty.* 1993;8:341–346.

99. Langlais F, Vielpeau C. Allografts of the hemipelvis after tumour resection: technical aspects of four cases. *J Bone Joint Surg.* 1989; 71B:58–62.

100. Lechler RI, Lombardi G, Batchelor JR, et al. The molecular basis of alloreactivity. *Immunol Today.* 1990;11:83–88.

101. Lee BP, Cabanela M, Wallrichs S. et al. Bone-graft augmentation for acetabular deficiencies in total hip arthroplasty: results of long-term follow-up evaluation. *J Arthroplasty.* 1997;12;503–510.

102. Lee WP, Pan YC, Randolph MA, et al. Cell-mediated and humoral responses to the components of vascularized limb allografts. *Trans Orthop Res Soc* 1988;13:63.

103. Lee WP, Yaremchuk MJ, Pan YC, et al. Relative antigenicity of components of a vascularized limb allograft. *Plast Reconstr Surg.* 1991;87:401–411.

104. Lewandronski KW, Tomford WW, Schomacker KT, et al. Improved osteoinduction of cortical bone allografts: a study of the effects of laser perforation and partial demineralization *J Orthop Res.* 1997;15:748–756.

105. Lexer E. Joint transplantations and arthroplasty. *Surg Gynec Obstet.* 1925;40:728–809.

106. Ling RSM, Timperley AJ, Linder L. Histology of cancellous impaction grafting in the femur. *J Bone Joint Surg.* 1993;75B:693–696.

107. Lord F, Gebhardt MC, Tomford WW, et al. Infection in bone allografts. *J Bone Joint Surg.* 1988;70A:369–375.

108. MacDonald SJ, Mehin R. Acetabular revision: structural grafts. In: Lieberman J, Berry D, eds. *Advanced Reconstruction Hip.* Chicago: American Academy of Orthopaedic Surgeons; 2005:335–342.

109. Malinin TI, Mnaymneh W, Lo HK, et al. Cryopreservation of articular cartilage. *Clin Orthop.* 1994;No. 303:18–32.

110. Mankin HJ, Doppelt S, Tomford W. Clinical experience with allograft implantation: the first ten years. *Clin Orthop.* 1983;No. 174:69.

111. Mankin HJ, Folgeson FS, Thrasher AZ, et al. Massive resection and allograft transplantation in the treatment of malignant bone tumors. *N Engl J Med.* 1976;294:1247–1255.

112. Mankin HJ, Gebhardt MC, Jennings CL, et al. Long-term results of allograft replacement in the management of bone tumors. *Clin Orthop.* 1996;No. 324:86–97.

113. Mankin HJ, Gebhardt MC, Springfield DS. The clinical use of frozen cadaveric allografts in the management of bone tumors. In: Friedlander GE, Goldberg VM, eds. *Bone and Cartilage Allografts.* Park Ridge, IL: American Academy of Orthopaedic Surgeons; 1991:247–253.

114. Mankin HJ, Hornicek FJ, Gebhardt MC, et al. Bone allograft transplantation. In: Lieberman JR, Friedlaender GE, eds. *Bone Regeneration and Repair: Biology and Clinical Applications.* Totowa NJ: Humana Press; 2005:241–261.

115. Markel MD, Wood SA, Bogdanske JJ, et al. Comparison of allograft/endoprosthetic composites with a step-cut or transverse osteotomy configuration. *J Orthop Res.* 1995;13:639–641.

116. Martin WR, Sutherland CJ. Complications of proximal femoral allografts in revision total hip arthroplasty. *Clin Orthop.* 1995;No. 295:161–167.

117. Masri BA, Duncan CP. Femoral revision: allograft prosthetic composite. In: Lieberman J, Berry D, eds. *Advanced Reconstruction Hip.* Chicago: American Academy of Orthopaedic Surgeons; 2005:449–458.

118. Matas AJ, Frey DJ, Gillingham KJ, et al. The impact of HLA matching on graft survival and on sensitization after a failed transplant: evidence that failure of poorly matched renal transplants does not result in increased sensitization. *Transplantation.* 1990;50:599–607.

119. McCollum DE, Nunley JA, Harrelson JM. Bone grafting in total hip replacement for acetabular protusion. *J Bone Joint Surg.* 1980;62A:1065–1073.

120. McGann W, Mankin HJ, Harris WH. Massive allografting for severe failed total hip replacement. *J Bone Joint Surg.* 1986;68A:4–12.

121. Mnaymneh W, Malinin TI, Lackman RD, et al. Massive distal femoral osteoarticular allografts after resection of bone tumors. *Clin Orthop.* 1994;303:103–115.

122. Möller E. Advances in and future of tissue typing. *Transplant Proc.* 1991;23:63–66.

123. Moran CG, McGrory BJ, Bronk JT, et al. Reperfusion injury in vascularized bone allografts. *J Orthop Res.* 1995;13:368–374.

124. Muir P, Johnson KA. Tibial intercalary allograft incorporation: comparison of fixation with locked intramedullary nail and dynamic compression plate. *J Orthop Res.* 1995;13:132–137.

125. Munting E, Wilmart JF, Wijne A, et al. Effect of sterilization on osteoinduction: comparison of five methods in demineralized rat bone. *Acta Orthop Scand.* 1988;59:34–38.

126. Muramatsu K, Doi K, Kawai S. Vascularized allogeneic joint, muscle, and peripheral nerve transplantation. *Clin Orthop.* 1995; 320:194–204.

127. Muscolo DL, Ayerza MA, Calabrese ME, et al. HLA matching, radiographic score, and histologic findings in massive bone allografts. *Clin Orthop.* 1996;326:115–126.

128. Muscolo DL, Ayerza MA, Calabrese ME, et al. Long term performance of massive allografts. In: Galante JO, Rosenberg AG, Callaghan JJ, eds. *Total Hip Revision Surgery.* New York: Raven Press; 1995:445–460.

129. Muscolo DL, Caletti E, Schajowicz F, et al. Tissue-typing in human massive allograft of frozen bone. *J Bone Joint Surg.* 1987; 69A:583–595.

130. Muscolo DL, Kawai S, Ray RD. Cellular and humoral immune response analysis of bone allografted rats. *J Bone Joint Surg.* 1976;58A:826–832.

131. Muscolo DL, Petracchi LJ, Ayerza MA, et al. Massive femoral allografts followed for 22 to 36 years. *J Bone Joint Surg.* 1992; 74B:887–892.

132. Nilsonne U. Homologous joint-transplantation in man. *Acta Orthop Scand.* 1969;40:429–447.

133. Oakeshott RD, Farine I, Pritzker KPH, et al. A clinical and histological analysis of failed fresh osteocondral allografts. *Clin Orthop.* 1988;233:283–294.

134. Opelz G. Collaborative transplant study: 10 year report. *Transplant Proc.* 1992;24:2342–2355.

135. Opelz G. The role of HLA matching and blood transfusions in the cyclosporine era. *Transplant Proc.* 1989;221:609–612.

136. Ottolenghi CE. Massive osteo and osteoarticular bone grafts: technique and results of 62 cases. *Clin Orthop.* 1972;87:156–164.

137. Pak JH, Paprosky WG, Jablonsky WS, et al. Femoral strut allografts in cementless revision total hip arthroplasty. *Clin Orthop.* 1993;295:172–178.

138. Paprosky WG, Bradford MS, Jablonsky WS. Acetabular reconstruction with massive acetabular allografts. *Instruct Course Lect.* 1996;45:149–159.

139. Paprosky WG, Magnus RE. Principles of bone grafting in revision total hip arthroplasty: acetabular technique. *Clin Orthop.* 1994;298:147–155.

140. Parrish FF. Allograft replacement of all or part of the end of a long bone following excision of a tumor. *J Bone Joint Surg.* 1973;55A:1–22.

141. Pelker RP, Friedlander GE, Markham TC. Biomechanical properties of bone allografts. *Clin Orthop.* 1983;174:54–57.

142. Pelker RP, Friedlander GE, Marham TC, et al. Effects of freezing and freeze-dryng on the biomechanical properties of rat bone. *J Orthop Res.* 1984;1:405–411.

143. Reddi AH, Wientroub S, Muthukumaran N. Biologic principles of bone induction. *Orthop Clin North Am.* 1987;18:207–212.

144. Riley EH, Lane JM, Urist MR, et al. Bone morphogenetic protein-2: biology and applications. *Clin Orthop.* 1996;324:39–46.

145. Rodrigo JJ, Fuller TC, Mankin HJ. Cytotoxic antibodies in patients with bone and cartilage allografts. *Trans Orthop Res Soc.* 1976;1:131.

146. Rodrigo JJ, Prolo DJ. Allografts. In: Chapman M, ed. *Operative Orthopaedics.* Philadelphia: Lippincott; 1988:911–928.

147. Rodrigo JJ, Schnaser AM, Reynolds HM Jr, et al. Inhibition of the immune response to experimental fresh osteoarticular allografts. *Clin Orthop.* 1989;243:235–253.

148. Saleh KJ, Jaroszynski G, Woodgate I, et al. Revision total hip arthroplasty with the use of structural acetabular allograft and reconstruction ring. *J Arthroplasty.* 2000;15:951–958.

149. Salenius P, Holmstron T, Koskinen EV, et al. Histological changes in clinical half-joint allograft replacements. *Acta Orthop Scand.* 1982;53:295–299.

150. Sanfilippo F, Goeken N, Niblack G, et al. The effect of first cadaver renal transplant HLA A, B match on sensitization levels and transplant rates following graft failure. *Transplantation.* 1987;43:240–244.

151. Sayeg MH, Perico N, Gallon L, et al. Mechanisms of acquired thymic unresponsiveness to renal allografts. *Transplantation.* 1994;58:125–132.

152. Sayeg MH, Watschinger B, Carpenter CB. Mechanisms of T cell recognition of alloantigen. *Transplantation.* 1994;57:1295–1302.

153. Schreurs BW, Bolder SBT, Gardeniers JWM, et al. Acetabular revision with impacted morselized bone grafting and cemented cup: a 15 to 20 year follow-up of 62 revision arthroplasties. *J Bone Joint Surg.* 2004;86B:492–497.

154. Sedlin E. A rheologic model for cortical bone. *Acta Orthop Scand.* 1965;36(suppl):83.

155. Shih CH, Chen CH, Tsai MF, et al. Incorporation of allograft for acetabular reconstruction: single photon emission CT in 21 hip arthroplasties followed for 2.5–5 years. *Acta Orthop Scand.* 1994; 65:589–594.

156. Sibley RK. Pathology and immunopathology of solid organ graft rejection. *Transplant Proc.* 1989;21:14–17.

157. Simonian PT, Conrad EU, Chapman JR, et al. Effect of sterilization and storage treatments on screw pullout strength in human allograft bone. *Clin Orthop.* 1994;302:290–296.

158. Sloof T, Buma P, Schreurs B, et al. Acetabular and femoral reconstruction with impacted graft and cement. *Clin Orthop.* 1996;324: 108–115.

159. Somers JFA, Timperley AJ, Norton M, et al. Block allografts in revision total hip arthroplasty. *J Arthroplasty.* 2002;17:562–568.

160. Stevenson S. The immune response to osteochondral allografts in dogs. *J Bone Joint Surg.* 1987;69A:573–581.

161. Stevenson S, Dannucci GA, Sharkey NA, et al. The fate of articular cartilage after transplantation of fresh and cryopreserved tissue: antigen-matched and mismatched osteochondral allografts in dogs. *J Bone Joint Surg.* 1989;71A:1297–1307.

162. Stevenson S, Horowitz M. Current concepts review. The response to bone allografts. *J Bone Joint Surg.* 1992;74A:939–947.

163. Stevenson S, Li XQ, Martin B. The fate of cancellous and cortical bone after transplantation of fresh and frozen tissue: antigen-matched and mismatched osteochondral allografts in dogs. *J Bone Joint Surg.* 1991;73A:1143–1156.

164. Stiehl JB. Acetabular allograft reconstruction in total hip arthroplasty, I: current concepts in biomechanics. *Orthop Rev.* 1991;20: 339–341.

165. Takemoto S, Terasaki PI. HLA peptide matching. *Transplant Proc.* 1991;23:2039–2042.

166. Tamura F, Vogelsang GB, Reitz BA, et al. Combination thalidomide and cyclosporine for cardiac allograft rejection: comparison with combination methylprednisolone and cyclosporine. *Transplantation.* 1990;49:20–25.

167. Terasaki PI, Takemoto S, Park MS, et al. Molecular HLA matching. *Transplant Proc.* 1991;23:365–367.

168. Thompson RC, Pickvance EA, Garry D. Fractures in large-segment allografts. *J Bone Joint Surg.* 1993;75A:1663–1673.

169. Thorsby E. Structure and function of HLA molecules. *Transplant Proc.* 1987;19:29–35.

170. Tomford WW, Mankin HJ, Friedlander GE, et al. Methods of banking bone and cartilage for allograft transplantation. *Orthop Clin North Am.* 1987;18:241–248.

171. Tomford W, Springfield D, Mankin H, et al. The immunology of large frozen bone allograft transplantation in humans: antibody and T lymphocyte responses and their effects on results. *Trans Orthop Res Soc.* 1994;19:184.

172. Tomford WW, Thongphasuk J, Mankin HJ, et al. Frozen musculoskeletal allografts. *J Bone Joint Surg.* 1990;72A:1137–1143.

173. Trancik TM, Stulberg BN, Wilde AH, et al. Allograft reconstruction of the acetabulum during revision total hip arthroplasty:

clinical, radiographic and scintigraphic assessment of the results. *J Bone Joint Surg.* 1986;68A:527–533.

174. Tremblay N, Fontaine P, Perreault C. T lymphocyte responses to multiple minor histocompatibility antigens generate both self-major histocompatibility complex-restricted and cross-reactive cytotoxic T lymphocytes. *Transplantation.* 1994;58:59–67.

175. Triantafyllou N, Sotiropoulos E, Triantafyllou J. The mechanical properties of lyophilized and irradiated bone grafts. *Acta Orthop Belg.* 1975;41:35.

176. Tyer HDD, Huckstep RL, Stalley PD. Intraluminal allograft restoration of the upper femur in failed total hip arthroplasty. *Clin Orthop.* 1987;224:26–32.

177. Urist MR. Bone formation by autoinduction. *Science.* 1965;150:893–899.

178. Urist MR, Hernandez A. Excitation transfer in bone: deleterious effects of cobalt 60 radiation sterilization of bank bone. *Arch Surg* 1974;109:486–493.

179. Vander Griend RA. The effect of internal fixation on the healing of large allografts. *J Bone Joint Surg.* 1994;76A:657–663.

180. Volkov M. Allotransplantation of joints. *J Bone Joint Surg.* 1970;52B:49–53.

181. Whiteside LA, Pollack FH. Failure of suport allografts. *J Arthroplasty.* 1992;7:271.

182. Wilson MG, Nikpoor N, Aliabadi P, et al. The fate of acetabular allografts after bipolar revision arthroplasty of the hip: a radiographic review. *J Bone Joint Surg.* 1989;71A:1469–1479.

183. Wozney JM, Rosen V. Bone morphogenetic proteins and their gene expresion. In: Noda M, ed. *Cellular and Molecular Biology of Bone.* San Diego: Academic Press; 1993:131–167.

184. Yamamoto S, Ito T, Nakata S, et al. The rejection mechanism of rat pancreaticoduodenal allografts with a class I MHC disparity. *Transplantation.* 1994;57:1217–1222.

185. Zehr RJ, Enneking WF, Heare T, et al. Fractures in large structural allografts. In: Brown KLB, ed. *Complications of Limb Salvage.* Montreal: 1991;3–8. International Symposium on Limb Salvage.

186. Zehr RJ, Enneking WF, Scarborough MT. Allograft–prosthesis composite versus megaprosthesis in proximal femoral reconstruction. *Clin Orthop.* 1996;322:207–223.

187. Zerbe TR, Arena VC, Kormos RL, et al. Histocompatibility and other risk factors for histological rejection of human cardiac allografts during the first three months following transplantation. *Transplantation.* 1991;52:485–490.

The Role of Bone Graft Substitutes in Total Hip Arthroplasty

25

Wellington K. Hsu   *Jay R. Lieberman*

Despite excellent clinical results after primary total hip arthroplasty, wear debris-generated periprosthetic osteolysis is the leading cause for revision total hip arthroplasty procedures. Osteolysis, which is generated by macrophages initiating an inflammatory response, leads to loss of bone stock around implants and can result in loosening of the prosthetic components (31). Multiple classification systems exist that characterize periprosthetic osteolytic defects. Paprosky et al. (81,82) published two useful classification systems for acetabular and femoral bone loss that can facilitate preoperative planning. Acetabular bone defects are categorized according to the extent and location of bone loss and the component migration (Table 25-1) (29,48). Osteolytic defects can also be categorized as either cavitary or segmental deficiencies, which aids in the choice of bone-graft (29,48). Cavitary defects, which do not affect the structural integrity of bone, are predominately treated with particulate grafts, while segmental defects may require structural grafts to provide mechanical support.

The stability of the prosthetic component is the critical element that dictates the choice of treatment strategies. There is a risk of underlying structural damage when either a well-fixed porous-coated acetabular socket or a cementless or cemented femoral stem is removed. Furthermore, there is no guarantee that a new component will have equal or better ingrowth than a previously ingrown prosthesis. Thus, many surgeons treat osteolytic lesions around well-fixed cementless acetabular components with a strategy that involves a liner exchange, retention of the acetabular cup, and débridement and grafting of osteolytic lesions. Similarly, lesions in the greater trochanteric region have also been treated with débridement and bone-grafting, with retention of a well-fixed cementless femoral stem. Maloney et al. (70) evaluated the treatment of pelvic osteolysis in a total of 68 patients with either acetabular revision and bone-grafting (type I) or component retention, liner exchange, and bone-grafting of the lesion (type II). In this study, 40 patients were treated with revision and bone-grafting, while 28 underwent a type II procedure. At a mean follow-up of 3.5 years, all acetabular cups were stable, and the osteolytic lesion on plain radiographs decreased in size regardless of treatment, although it was not possible to determine if the bone-graft actually became incorporated into the host bone (6,70).

The successful treatment of any bone repair problem requires recognition of biologic processes associated with bone healing. Four critical elements influence bone repair. First, an osteoinductive signal that can recruit or stimulate the differentiation of osteoprogenitor cells into osteoblasts is required. Second, responding cells that can respond to an osteoinductive signal must be either present at the bone defect site or supplied by the surgeon. Third, an osteoconductive matrix providing a three-dimensional scaffold for new bone formation is necessary. Finally, an adequate vascular supply is

TABLE 25-1

PAPROSKY CLASSIFICATION OF ACETABULAR BONE DEFICIENCY IN REVISION TOTAL HIP REPLACEMENT

Type	Description
1	Minimal lysis or component migration
2A	Superior–medial migration <2 cm
2B	Superolateral migration <2 cm
3A	Migration >2 cm, ischial lysis present
3B	Same as 3A with disruption of the Kohler line, indicative of profound medial loss; pelvic dissociation may be present

Reproduced from Paprosky WG, Perona PG, Lawrence JM. Acetabular defect classification and surgical reconstruction in revision arthroplasty: a 6-year follow-up evaluation. *J Arthroplasty.* 1994;9:33–44.

critical for the early migration of progenitor cells, osteoclasts, and other inflammatory agents into the repair site. Before treatment is implemented, the orthopedic surgeon must initially assess the inherent biologic potential of the bone repair site and then select a bone-graft strategy based on this information.

In the assessment of an osteolytic defect, there are multiple elements that must be evaluated. Is the component stable or will revision of the component be necessary? If the component is to be retained, how will the osteolytic lesion be treated? When should surgical intervention occur? If removal of the component is necessary, will a structural or nonstructural bone-graft be required? What prosthesis should be used for the revision procedure? And finally, what is the best biologic agent to use to manage the bone loss?

The appropriate selection of bone-graft substitutes in revision hip surgery remains controversial. The fate of bone-grafts after implantation has not been well studied, and consequently the extent of their incorporation into host bone to provide structural integrity and future bone stock remains unclear. Furthermore, at the present time, there is no clinically relevant animal model that approximates the rigorous biologic environment surrounding revision hip surgery. Therefore, there is no consensus among arthroplasty surgeons regarding the choice of appropriate bone-graft agent, the timing of the surgical intervention, and outcome measures.

New radiologic methods that can quantify the amount of periprosthetic osteolysis have been developed, including volumetric CT scanning, which can quantitate the volume of osteolytic defects (68). Novel three-dimensional imaging can offer accurate assessments of bone loss surrounding implants. Although still in its infancy, this technology allows surgeons to longitudinally assess the size of osteolytic lesions and may aid in the evaluation of the efficacy of different treatment strategies for revision THA.

The purpose of this chapter is to review the available preclinical and clinical data regarding the treatment of osteolytic defects using a variety of bone-graft substitutes. The results of structural allografts are not reviewed in this chapter.

AUTOGRAFTS

Autogenous bone-graft remains the gold standard for bone-grafting for orthopedic procedures because it alone offers three of the four necessary components for bone repair: osteoinductive signals from associated growth factors, osteogenic cells, and an osteoconductive matrix. A number of animal models have provided insight into the incorporation of cancellous grafts into host bone (45). Histological and biomechanical evidence indicates that autogenous cancellous graft offers incorporation into host bone in 6 to 12 months. Two distinct phases have been described in the incorporative process: an early phase characterized by active bone resorption and formation, and a late phase identified by creeping substitution (95). By 1 year after surgery, complete remodeling and incorporation of the graft is seen (95).

Autogenous cortical graft, which provides excellent structural support but limited osteoinductive capability, is used mainly for segmental bone defects in orthopedic surgery. Cortical bone demonstrates a significantly slower rate of revascularization and incorporation in animal models than does cancellous bone-graft (9,15,16,44). Resorption occurs via osteoclastic activity, which is seen after 6 weeks (30). Autografts then lose their initial strength until revascularization has taken place. Their clinical use in revision THA is currently limited.

The use of autologous bone-graft in the setting of revision THA typically presents a number of concerns for the arthroplasty surgeon. The elderly patient population presents clinical problems such as osteoporosis, poor bone stock, and the surgical risks of increased operative time. Furthermore, structural compromise of the donor site, overall increased morbidity, and supply–demand discrepancies often make the use of autogenous bone unattractive for revision THA. Reamed cancellous bone obtained from the preparation of an acetabular component is also a source of autograft bone. Although the best indications for autograft bone are for small, cavitary defects behind stable implants, they are not routinely used.

ALLOGRAFTS

Allograft bone offers advantages over autogenous bone-graft in that there is an abundant supply of graft material, and the morbidity associated with autograft harvest is subsequently eliminated. Allografts are either preserved through frozen or freeze-dried processes or offered as fresh specimens. Fresh samples elicit a vigorous immune response and are thus predominantly used for tumor reconstruction or joint resurfacing. The process of freeze-drying decreases antigenicity, reducing the host's cell-mediated immune response and leading to increased graft incorporation (10,17). However, freeze-drying also decreases osteogenic activity and hinders host vascular invasion. This loss of osteoinductive capabilities leads to a higher incidence of nonunion and delayed union than occurs with autografts (45). Furthermore, resorption of cancellous allograft proceeds at a slower rate than with autogenous graft, leaving necrotic tissue at the surgical site for longer time periods. Necrotic allograft bone has been reported at the site of implantation even years after surgery (44,91). The risk of disease transmission from musculoskeletal tissue donors also exists with the use of allografts, but this risk has been found to be low. New standards in screening donor tissue enforced by the American Association of Tissue Banks have reduced the risk of HIV disease transmission to no greater than 1 in 1.5 million (39). In the past 5 years, no cases of HIV transmission have been reported in more than 2 million cases in which allograft bone was used (87).

Allograft bone has been used extensively to treat bone loss associated with the revision of acetabular and femoral components. Cancellous bone-graft is commonly used to treat cavitary defects in the acetabulum and lytic lesions around well-fixed acetabular components. Other uses of particulate graft are seen in conjunction with reconstruction cages, impaction grafting with cement, and the bone-grafting of osteolytic defects around the greater trochanteric region (18,62).

The incorporation rates of allograft bone have not been well delineated. Radiographic appearance is currently the most common method used to assess allograft incorporation into host bone, which often does not correlate with histologic incorporation. Using these methods of evaluation, one study reported a 95% rate of radiographic incorporation into cementless acetabular revisions at a mean follow-up of 7 years (34). However, the use of high-resolution imaging studies may offer better detection methods for the orthopedic surgeon. The earliest evidence of incorporation of cancellous allograft bone was identified by single photon emission CT scan at 13 months in both primary and revision total hip arthroplasty (90). Another study using bone scintigraphy every 6 months revealed that uptake around the bone-grafting site became normal only 2 years after the procedure (58).

Histologic evaluations of cancellous allografts used during revision THA have been obtained from biopsies during revision procedures and postmortem specimens. In a postmortem retrieval study, specimens from three patients representing separate time points after revision acetabular arthroplasty with a noncemented cup and cancellous fresh-frozen allograft were histologically examined (49). At 18 months after revision procedure, allograft fragments were well visualized among osteoclasts and a myxofibrous stroma. At 53 months, allograft bone was still visible but less distinguishable from adjacent host bone. Finally, at 83 months, the graft had almost completely incorporated, as allograft material was only visible using high-power microscopy (49).

Other studies of histologic specimens from revision THA with acetabular impaction grafting at the time of reoperation confirm delayed incorporation of allograft bone (99). Twenty-four hip biopsy specimens from 20 different patients retrieved up to 15 years after impaction grafting of morselized cancellous bone chips for primary and revision cemented acetabular reconstructions were examined. Fresh-frozen femoral head allografts (revision hips) and autograft femoral heads (primary hips) were prepared using either a rongeur, bone mill, or both. New bone formation was reported as early as 3 months after the procedure, and remodeling lamellar bone was noted at 15 months (99). Specimens obtained 8 to 30 months after surgery all revealed newly formed trabecular bone, with fewer allograft remnants and greater cortical bone than earlier sections. Nearly 90% of the bone-graft was incorporated in specimens obtained after a follow-up of 10 years or longer (99). A variable amount of bone-graft remained unincorporated even at long-term follow-up.

Although it is not known why full graft incorporation does not occur, it is likely influenced by the extent of the bone loss, the biologic potential of the host bone, the biomechanical stresses on the particulate graft, and the local immune response to the allograft bone. Studies have shown that cartilage fragments not removed at the time of surgery did not incorporate at long-term follow-up (99). This demonstrates that thorough débridement and removal of cartilage and fibrous tissue are necessary for optimal graft incorporation. Although evidence suggests that the technique of impaction bone-grafting with large morselized bone chips can restore bone stock during revision total hip arthroplasty, the results cannot be generalized to either the treatment of osteolytic defects associated with cementless acetabular revision components or the bone-grafting of osteolytic lesions around well-fixed cementless components.

In femoral component revisions, allograft bone is used for femoral impaction bone-grafts with cement fixation (41) and the grafting of large lytic lesions in the greater trochanter. Although the use of impaction grafting with cancellous allograft to augment femoral defects has been described (40,41), recent interest has been directed toward the potential advantages of using cortical morselized allograft. Biomechanical and clinical studies have compared the outcomes in patients who received either impacted cortical or cancellous morselized allograft with revision femoral components (56,57). In a retrospective study, the clinical outcomes in 50 patients (25 treated with morselized graft derived from cortical bone and 25 treated with morselized graft derived from cancellous bone) after a mean of 5.2 years follow-up were compared. Significantly better results in terms of clinical outcome, pain, and radiographic stem subsidence were reported when revision femoral stems were reconstructed with impacted morselized cortical allograft than with cancellous bone-graft (56). The authors concluded that cortical allograft offers enhanced early implant stability that limits micromotion and stem subsidence between the graft and the implant, leading to improved clinical outcomes (56).

Analysis of postmortem femoral specimens after impaction grafting supports the incorporation of morselized allograft into host bone. Histologic examination of retrieved femurs $3^1/_2$ years after impaction grafting showed three distinct areas of graft incorporation: an inner zone containing necrotic bone with evidence of creeping substitution, a middle zone with viable cancellous bone, and an outer zone filled with remodeled cortical bone (66). However, despite excellent histologic and radiographic results, stem subsidence has been reported with the use of this technique (33). Long-term evaluation of morselized allograft in femoral components is needed.

These studies indicate that despite early evidence of allograft incorporation on plain radiographs, residual bone-graft is still likely to be present histologically. This finding identifies the major concern regarding exclusive use of allograft bone in revision procedures. Allograft cancellous chips are frequently used to bone-graft contained cavitary defects or osteolytic lesions around well-fixed implants. Although these grafts appear to be incorporated on plain radiographs, it remains unclear if these grafts actually incorporate and restore host bone stock (38). We are particularly concerned about the ability of this material to incorporate when it is used alone to treat osteolytic lesions around well-fixed components. There appears to be little chance for this type of graft to incorporate when it is implanted through the screw holes in the cup. In this setting, the granulomatous tissue cannot be completely removed, and the remaining tissue prevents the graft material from contacting host bone. Furthermore, it is not clear if the host bone has the biologic potential to incorporate the allograft bone even when the bone-graft is placed through a trapdoor in the ilium. Further study is required to define role of allograft bone in revision hip arthroplasty.

DEMINERALIZED BONE MATRIX

Demineralized bone matrix (DBM) is created through the acid extraction of the mineralized phase of bone. The preparation of DBM was originally characterized by Urist et al. (96,97) and then modified by Reddi and Huggins (85). Allogeneic bone is crushed to a particle size of 74 to 420 μm, followed by demineralization in 0.5N HCL mEq/g for 3 hours (35). Methods of processing follow the same initial steps; however, additives and refining techniques differ depending on the source and company involved. Commercial preparations also use different carriers, such as glycerol, hyaluronic acid, gelatin, and calcium sulfate powder. There are few comparative studies that evaluate the different DBM preparations available (83).

DBMs have been found to have rich osteoconductive capabilities but questionable osteoinductive capabilities. DBMs have been shown to induce rapid revascularization and serve as an excellent osteoconductive scaffold (35). Much of their biologic activity is attributed to growth factors and proteins that are contained in the extracellular matrix and survive various processing methods. However, the osteoinductive capacity of DBM is dependent not only on the original donor but also on the different commercial sterilization and handling methods. Sterilization by ethylene oxide and use of gamma irradiation, for example, have been found to significantly reduce osteoinductivity (1,74).

Despite their wide use and variable processing methods, DBMs have been tested in few animal models and laboratory studies. DBMs, like allograft bone, are not subject to the rigorous testing of the FDA because they are classified as minimally manipulated tissue for transplantation. Recent studies have demonstrated the variability of these preparations in inducing osteogenic activity in an intramuscular animal model (89), a rat femoral defect (79), and a rat spine fusion model (83). In the rat femoral defect model, only 8 of 48 specimens healed at 12 weeks when treated with two different DBMs with either a hyaluronic acid or glycerol carrier (79). The authors concluded that when used alone, DBMs have excellent osteoconductive capabilities but minimal osteoinductive potential in bone healing. In a separate study using a rat spine fusion model, widely variable osteoinductive potential was demonstrated using different commercially available DBM preparations (83). This wide variability of biologic activity of DBMs is likely influenced not only by the carrier but also by the demineralization and sterilization methods (83).

DBMs have been used successfully as bone-graft extenders to promote spinal fusion and the healing of long bone nonunions (4,36,52,54). Recent studies have also combined the use of autologous bone marrow and DBM in promoting bone repair (21,92). In revision THA, DBMs have been utilized as bone-graft substitutes in the treatment of small, contained cavitary defects (35,43). They may also be routinely used in the future as bone-graft extenders in association with autologous bone marrow cells obtained from aspiration or cancellous grafts.

There is a need for further study of the influence of donor age and sex, processing, and the biologic activity of DBMs (47). Both the lack of FDA oversight and the wide variety of graft donors contribute to the variability in outcome from the use of DBM. Furthermore, different preparations are combined with different carriers, and these influence the osteoconductive activity of the DBMs. Since the DBMs do not all have the same biologic potential, the optimal product for each clinical situation needs to be determined. It is yet unknown if DBMs are associated with the restoration of host bone stock when used to treat an osteolytic defect. To date, no studies have analyzed the capability of DBMs to integrate into an in vivo environment. Evidence of histologic and radiographic incorporation rates after long-term follow-up is needed.

CERAMICS

Ceramic carriers are derived from a process called sintering, which uses high temperatures to extract individual crystals that fuse together at crystal grain boundaries (35). The osteoconductive matrices used in conjunction with these carriers are composed of hydroxyapatite, tricalcium phosphate, and/or calcium sulfate (13). Commercial calcium phosphate materials are produced with pore diameters between 200 and 500 μm, approximating the structure of human trabecular bone (51). Klawitter et al. concluded that the size and interconnectivity of the pores of an implant are important in allowing bony ingrowth and blood vessels to integrate within the carrier (55). However, other investigators have indicated that the degree of interconnectivity porosity (12% to 80%) and pore size (range, <1 μm to 1500 μm) do not inhibit bone formation (67).

Ceramics possess a number of attractive qualities as a biologic substitute in orthopedic surgery. Ceramics have been found to be safe, osteoconductive, and compatible with biologically active cells such as autologous bone marrow (35). Furthermore, these carriers provide compression resistance, which is advantageous in certain orthopedic procedures. For example, interporous hydroxyapatite was directly compared with autograft in a randomized series of 40 tibial plateau fractures requiring metaphyseal bone-grafting after internal fixation. The authors concluded that both groups exhibited satisfactory and comparable radiographic, histologic, and clinical results (14).

Calcium–collagen graft, which is composed of hydroxyapatite, tricalcium phosphate, and both type I and III collagen, has been used clinically to augment fracture healing in acute long-bone fractures (19). When compared with autologous bone-graft, there were no differences between the two groups in terms of union rate or outcome measures (19). Tricalcium phosphate is another porous ceramic that undergoes partial conversion to hydroxyapatite once it is metabolized in the body (39). However, because it is resorbed faster than hydroxyapatite and has a more unpredictable biodegradation profile, tricalcium phosphate is rarely used in the clinical setting (50).

TABLE 25-2

CALCIUM-BASED BONE–GRAFT SUBSTITUTES CLEARED FOR MARKETING IN THE UNITED STATES

Product	Company	Type	FDA-Approved Uses
Collagraft	Zimmer	Bovine collagen, hydroxyapatite, and tricalcium phosphate; available in granular and strip forms	Traumatic bone defects less than 30 cc
Pro Osteon	Interpore Cross	Coralline hydroxyapatite granules and blocks; 200, 500, and R forms	Traumatic metaphyseal defects of long bones
Osteoset	Wright Medical Technology	Calcium sulfate pellets	All bone defects
Vitoss	Orthovita	Ultraporous beta-tricalcium phosphate	Bone defects of the spine, extremities, and pelvis
SRS	Norian	Calcium phosphate (carbonated apatite) injectable cement	None

Reproduced from Finkemeier CG. Bone-grafting and bone-graft substitutes. *J Bone Joint Surg.* 2002;84A: 454–464.

Although ceramics can be used to treat bone defects secondary to osteolysis, these carriers do have limitations. Interporous hydroxyapatite has brittle handling properties and minimal tensile strength. The ceramic must be rigidly fixed to the surrounding tissue to protect it from shear and torsional stresses (39). Furthermore, its use in diaphyseal defects is limited since restoration of bending strength increases only to less than 10% of that of cortical bone (13). The resorption characteristics of ceramics also vary depending on the preparation. Newer commercial fabrications may display more rapid resorption in vivo, thereby permitting more complete bone remodeling (13). Finally, when used alone, calcium phosphate carriers do not provide osteogenic activity.

The clinical utility of ceramics in the realm of revision THA has yet to be studied. A number of calcium-based bone-graft substitutes have been approved for marketing in the United States (Table 25-2). Pro Osteon (hyaluronic acid block), Osteoset (calcium sulfate), and Vitoss (tricalcium phosphate) are FDA approved for use in treating non-weight-bearing bone defects in the extremities and pelvis (3), but none of these materials has been rigorously evaluated in revision THA. Calcium sulfate graft material has been used primarily as an osteoconductive filler and resorbs as newly formed bone remodels. Clinical uses in pellet form have been reported in non-weight-bearing areas in revision hip and knee arthroplasties (5). Although radiographic incorporation was noted, histologic data were not available to confirm incorporation. Ceramics can be used to treat cavitary defects; however, the material must be used carefully because if the particles migrate into the joint space, they can induce third-body wear. Adverse inflammatory reactions have also been reported (60). Both preclinical studies in animals and clinical trials are necessary to evaluate the potential efficacy of calcium phosphate ceramics in revision THA.

An injectable inorganic calcium phosphate has been used to augment fracture healing in humans. The malleable substance hardens within minutes, forming a structure of low crystallinity and grain size similar to the mineral phase of bone (46). After 12 hours, an osteoconductive apatite of high compressive strength of 55 Mpa is formed that is eventually replaced by host bone (23). Clinical uses have been reported in distal radius (53,59) and hip fractures (46), but no studies have been performed in revision THA.

AUTOLOGOUS CELLS

Autologous human bone marrow cells provide osteogenic capability through the action of secreted cytokines and growth factors. Bone marrow contains osteoprogenitor cells and growth factors that actively recruit host mesenchymal stem cells to undergo osteoblastic differentiation. Recent research has reported the ability of bone marrow to stimulate bone formation (102). In vitro expansion of mesenchymal stem cells with a ceramic carrier composed of hydroxyapatite and beta-tricalcium phosphate ceramic in canines promoted superior healing of a critical-sized femoral defect compared with autologous bone marrow alone (12).

Autologous cells provide significant osteoinductive capabilities through osteogenic cells; however, when used alone, they lack localized structural support. For this reason, the combination of bone-graft substitutes and autologous marrow has been assessed in tibial nonunions, bone cysts, and comminuted fractures associated with bone loss (22,65,80,92). The goal is to combine the osteogenic activity of bone marrow cells with the osteoconductive capability of the demineralized bone matrix. Autologous cells, with or without matrix, have also been used to treat nonunions of carpal bones, tibia, femur, and humerus (35).

Bone marrow cells are easily accessible through aspiration from the posterior iliac wing, and a recent study has recommended the harvest of smaller volumes (2 cc) of bone marrow in order to obtain a higher concentration of osteoblast progenitor cells (76). Muschler et al. reported the use of a selective cell attachment technique that allows mesenchymal stem cells to be concentrated from bone marrow aspirates (78). When combined with cancellous bone matrix, the enriched cellular composite graft obtained using this method induced a greater spine fusion mass volume in a canine model than cancellous bone matrix alone (78).

Early evidence in animals supports further investigation into the use of autologous bone marrow with an osteoconductive carrier in revision THA. With the addition of a suitable carrier, the combination offers three of the four necessary elements for bone repair: osteogenic bioactive factors, responding cells, and a matrix to encourage ingrowth of host capillaries. Together, the use of autologous cells with a carrier offers components for bone repair similar to factors provided by autogenous bonegraft. This technique also avoids complications associated with bone-graft harvesting and may reduce the risk of infection. However, there are concerns about the potential variability in human bone marrow cellularity as well as an age-related decline in progenitor cells (77). Although the benefits of bonegrafting with autologous cells are supported by a strong theoretical basis and success in animal models, further studies into the use of autologous cells combined with a suitable carrier as a bone-graft substitute during revision THA are needed.

GROWTH FACTORS

The discovery of bone morphogenetic proteins (BMPs) by Urist in 1965 (94) has led to a diverse area of research dedicated to the identification and characterization of osteoinductive growth factors. Members of the TGF-β superfamily, BMPs have been proposed for a number of applications in orthopedic surgery (104). Recombinant BMP-2 and BMP-7 (or osteogenic protein-1) have been evaluated in numerous preclinical models, and successful healing in long bone defects has been reported (24,25,28,103,104). Similar findings have been demonstrated in spinal arthrodesis models in animals (6,72,86,101). In fact, FDA approval has been granted for the use of rh-BMP-2 to enhance anterior spinal fusion (8) and for the use of rh-OP-1 to treat fresh tibia fractures and recalcitrant long bone nonunions (37,71). Human clinical trials evaluating the efficacy of rh-BMP in treating open tibia fractures, distraction osteogenesis, and osteonecrosis of the hip are underway (98).

Both rh-BMP-2 and rh-OP-1 induce bone formation in humans, but there are valid concerns regarding the large doses of BMP required to produce an adequate biologic response. Although milligram doses are necessary to achieve bony union in clinical trials, BMP in human bone is measured in nanogram amounts. It has been hypothesized that the collagen carriers presently being used are inefficient delivery vehicles (32).

BMPs have been assessed in several different animal models related to revision total hip arthroplasty, including osteolytic defects around well-fixed implants and the incorporation of femoral strut allografts. There is interest in the potential use of recombinant growth factors to heal large osteolytic bone defects, since such defects are a common problem in the setting of revision THA. In six canines, bilateral 8 mm × 5 mm acetabular defects (Fig. 25-1) were created adjacent to cementless

press-fit components (2). Each defect was either left empty or treated with an OP-1 device composed of 3.5 mg rh-OP-1/g type I collagen or allograft bone. Bone healing within the defect was then evaluated radiographically and histologically 6 weeks after surgery (2). The periprosthetic defects treated with rh-OP-1 exhibited greater bone healing than control groups, with bone density and trabecular pattern similar to those of intact acetabulum (Fig. 25-2).

Rh-BMP-2 placed in an αBSM carrier (calcium phosphate) was used in a separate canine model to assess bone ingrowth into an acetabular component (11). Special reamers were used to create a 1-mm defect between the acetabular dome and component in a total of 15 dogs. Then 240 μg of rh-BMP-2 was applied to the backside of the cup. The dogs were assessed

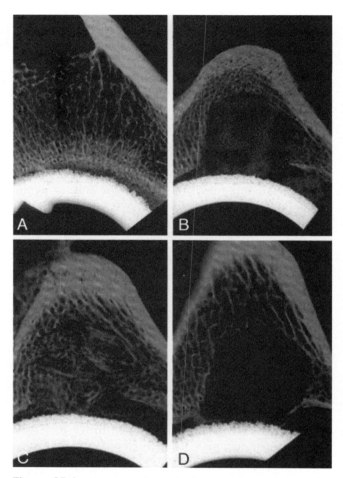

Figure 25-1 Contact radiographs from representative acetabular defect areas 6 weeks after total hip replacement in canines are shown (magnification, 1×). **A:** The radiograph of an acetabulum with no defect shows the cancellous bone structure and the contact between bone and the porous-coated implant. **B:** The radiograph of a defect treated with rh-OP-1 shows defect filling with new trabecular bone and gap filling and substantial new bone contact with the porous-coated surface of the acetabular component. **C:** The radiograph of a defect grafted with allograft bone shows some defect filling; however, only limited new bone contact with the porous surface is seen. **D:** Very little new bone was observed filling the empty defect, with little bone contact with the porous surface at 6 weeks postoperative. (Adapted from Barrack RL, Cook SD, Patron LP, et al. Induction of bone ingrowth from acetabular defects to a porous surface with OP-1. *Clin Orthop.* 2003;417:41–49.)

stringent biologic environment than these models offer. Second, in these models, the growth factors were used in young healthy animals with otherwise excellent bone stock, as opposed to the weaker, sclerotic bone often seen in revision THA. Finally, the bone defects were created at the time of the surgical procedure so that wear debris-associated cytokines were not present prior to the implantation of the acetabular component. There is a need for an animal model that accurately simulates the biological environment both of a loose acetabular component and osteolysis associated with well-fixed acetabular implants.

Strut allografts offer mechanical support and are used with internal fixation in revision THA for periprosthetic fractures and cases with proximal femoral bone loss. The grafts help reconstitute and stabilize existing cortical bone and offer immediate structural support. However, the incorporation of these cortical allografts is typically slow. Enhancing the incorporation and healing of strut allografts would lead to earlier weight bearing, faster recovery times, and possibly improved clinical outcomes.

Cook et al. recently reported the successful use of rh-OP-1 to augment onlay allograft strut healing to the femur in a canine model (26). After undergoing bilateral cortical strut graft procedures, 14 dogs each had one femur treated with an allograft strut that was coated with 1.25 mg of rh-OP-1. Results from this study demonstrated markedly improved radiographic and histologic healing of onlay allografts with use of rh-OP-1 at all time points (26). Rh-OP-1–treated animals also experienced significantly greater graft–host incorporation than the controls, as well as abundant new bone formation adjacent to the allograft (26). However, a major limitation of the study was that the strut grafts were secured to a normal femur and not used to stabilize one with a bone defect.

In a separate canine model, a 2.5-cm proximal femoral bone defect created adjacent to a cementless femoral prosthesis at the time of total hip arthroplasty was used to test the ability of recombinant protein to restore lost bone stock in 16 dogs (75). A femoral prosthesis impregnated with rh-BMP-2 with a biodegradable synthetic polymer at different concentrations along the proximal medial part of the stem was then implanted at the time of surgery and examined by plain radiographs and histologic specimens. Twelve weeks after implantation, new bone formation was seen in all groups treated with rh-BMP-2, with reconstitution of the medial defect in the high-dose recombinant protein groups (500 µg and 1000 µg) (75). The authors concluded that the use of rhBMP-2 with this delivery system could potentially restore bone stock during revision surgery without a bone-grafting procedure (75).

Additional studies indicate that recombinant growth factors may improve incorporation at allograft–host bone junctions. In a canine segmental femoral defect model in 21 dogs, local treatment with a 0.92-mg dose of rh-BMP-2 on an absorbable collagen sponge applied to a cortical allograft–host bone junction resulted in denser bone structure and better bone formation than was found in junctions treated with autogenous graft and collagen sponge alone at the 14-week time point (84,104). These authors concluded that rh-BMP-2 had a greater impact on the recruitment of osteoprogenitor cells and subsequent osteoblastic differentiation than autogenous bone-graft (104).

Results from early clinical studies using rh-OP-1 in revision THA have been reported (27). In four different human cases,

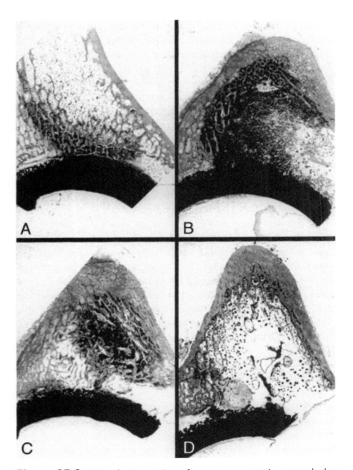

Figure 25-2 Histologic sections from representative acetabular defect areas 6 weeks after total hip replacement in canines are shown (stain, basic fuchsin and toluidine blue; magnification, 1×). **A:** A histologic section through an acetabulum with no defect shows the normal trabecular bony structure. **B:** The rh-OP-1–treated defects had significantly more new bone formation compared with unfilled defects and a trend toward restoration of the normal trabecular patterns. **C:** New bone and allograft bone were present and difficult to distinguish in the histologic section through a defect treated with allograft bone. Some bony contact with the porous-coated implant was observed. **D:** Little filling and ingrowth with bone in the empty acetabular defects were seen. (Adapted from Barrack RL, Cook SD, Patron LP, et al. Induction of bone ingrowth from acetabular defects to a porous surface with OP-1. *Clin Orthop.* 2003;417:41–49.)

in three groups (rh-BMP-2 and αBSM carrier, carrier alone, or untreated control) in this study. Radiographic and histologic examination 12 weeks after implantation demonstrated that rh-BMP-2 in the αBSM carrier induced bridging bone formation up to the underlying porous coating (11). Scanning electron micrographs of the five animals in the rh-BMP-2/αBSM group revealed new trabecular bone with a thickness close to that of the surrounding host bone. The authors concluded that the use of recombinant BMP-2 with an αBSM carrier could result in improved implant fixation. Although this canine model simulated a primary total hip arthroplasty, rh-BMP-2 may also be useful for enhancing ingrowth in revision THA.

These results are promising, but the animal models used in these studies have inherent limitations. First, the conditions surrounding a human revision THA may harbor a far more rh-OP-1 was used as an adjuvant with proximal femoral allo-graft, bulk femoral head allograft, cortical strut allograft, or morselized allograft in the treatment of osteolytic defects during revision THA. The authors reported greater and more rapid bone formation and enhanced graft incorporation in each case in which rh-OP-1 was used than occurred with allograft alone (27). However, no histologic analysis was available in this study. The findings in these studies involving canines and humans show promise with respect to the future use of recombinant growth factors in the treatment of bone defects associated with revision THA.

As stated previously, the critical issue associated with the use of recombinant BMP is that large doses are required to induce an adequate osteoinductive response. Since collagen carriers have not been shown to be efficient delivery vehicles, new ones need to be developed to enhance the release of BMP at the site of bone repair. Furthermore, the identification of appropriate carriers for different clinical scenarios is essential in order to reduce both the dose and cost of recombinant proteins. BMPs are also quite expensive, and they may not be cost-effective for the treatment of revision THA patients. As a result, any use of BMPs to treat osteolytic defects would be off-label in the United States at this time. However, BMP-2 and BMP-7 are osteoinductive, and continued research directed toward optimizing the use of these recombinant growth factors is worthwhile, since they have the biologic potential to obviate the need for autogenous bone-grafting and to enhance the ingrowth of cementless components.

GENE THERAPY AND TISSUE ENGINEERING

Tissue engineering remains an attractive potential option for revision THA because of its ability to closely approximate the biology of autologous bone-graft. Strategies utilizing the combination of bone-graft substitutes, recombinant proteins, and/or gene transfer strategies could offer additional options for revision THA.

Gene therapy involves the in vitro transfer of genetic material to cells to stimulate in vivo expression of a targeted protein. Gene therapy systems are composed of the DNA sequence; a vector, such as a virus, to mobilize the genetic material in question; and target cells to express the protein. The main advantage of such a system is the continuous local production of growth factors, as opposed to a single treatment dose of protein that may get rapidly degraded. This difference may prove to be critical in a stringent biological environment when sustained growth factor production is required for osseous repair.

A number of animal studies have demonstrated the efficacy of gene therapy in healing long bone defects (61,63,64) and spinal fusion in animals (7,100). Bone marrow cells transduced with an adenoviral vector containing the BMP-2 gene have been successful in healing long bone defects in a rat critical-sized femoral defect model (63). When compared with treatment with rh-BMP-2, no difference in defect strength was observed on biomechanical testing; however, histomorphometric analysis revealed that use of ex vivo gene therapy resulted in significantly denser trabecular bone. Similar results have been found in a rat posterolateral spine fusion model (101).

RANKL, a growth factor that directly stimulates osteoclastic resorption of bone, has been proposed to be a critical factor in the development of osteolysis. One recent study has used gene therapy in a mouse calvarial model to inhibit this factor. An ex vivo gene therapy system was used to transduce fibroblastlike synoviocytes with the coding sequence for a natural RANKL antagonist protein, osteoprotegerin (OPG) (42). The small amount of OPG produced by these transduced cells was found to be effective in blocking osteoclastogenesis induced by titanium wear particles, in comparison with cells transduced with a lacZ control gene (42). Successful inhibition of wear debris–induced osteolysis was also attained with a single intramuscular injection of a recombinant adeno-associated viral vector expressing OPG (93).

These studies show promise for the potential clinical uses of gene therapy. However, since these are elective procedures, patient safety is essential. In the arena of revision THA, the prospects of structural allograft incorporation or the regeneration of osseous defects could be greatly improved with the sustained delivery of proteins that enhance bone production. Moreover, in the future, prostheses could be developed that deliver growth factors, cytokines, or antibiotics locally, thus enhancing bone ingrowth or the treatment of infections.

CLINICAL APPLICATIONS

A number of questions regarding the treatment of osteolysis around both loose and well-fixed implants need to be answered. When a revision of an acetabular component is being performed, what is the best biologic agent to use to reconstitute bone stock? When osteolytic lesions are identified around well-fixed components, when is the best time to intervene? At the time of polyethylene liner exchange, should osteolytic lesions be grafted? Do small lesions have healing potential of their own or is there a "critical window" when intervention is crucial? If a bone-grafting procedure is to be performed, what surgical technique offers the greatest opportunity for graft incorporation? Is a trapdoor in the ilium necessary to débride the lesion and facilitate packing of a biologic substance? Would this type of approach affect long-term cup stability? What material should be used when bone-grafting these lesions? The current literature lacks definitive evidence to help arthroplasty surgeons make these important decisions.

Any proposed treatment must consider the biologic factors necessary for adequate bone repair: the supply of osteoinductive factors, responding cells, an osteoconductive matrix to support bone formation, and an adequate vascular supply. Since small cavitary lesions do not compromise structural integrity, nonstructural bone-graft substitutes may be used. On the femoral side, strut allografts are often necessary for larger, uncontained defects in weight-bearing regions.

Contained cavitary defects are often encountered at the time of a revision of a loose acetabular component. The treatment options are dependent on the size, location, and structural integrity of the bone defect. In patients with cavitary defects that are surrounded by well-vascularized and otherwise healthy bone, a number of biologic agents are available for use. For example, DBM, allograft chips, and ceramic carriers each provide an osteoconductive matrix for bone repair. Although there are data suggesting that allografts do lead to bone incorporation over time (58,90), long-term study of the efficacy of all bone-graft substitutes is necessary.

In general, when there is an osteolytic defect around a well-fixed acetabular component, the cup is usually left in place and a polyethylene liner exchange is performed. It has not been established when the best time is to intervene in these cases. It must be remembered that radiographs often underestimate the size of these lesions. Judet views can often be helpful when evaluating these patients. In a recent study, Mehin et al. recommended that when osteolysis involves 50% of the shell circumference on the anteroposterior or lateral views, polyethylene liner exchange and bone-grafting are recommended to prevent loss of fixation of the shell (73). However, surgical intervention may be necessary earlier, depending on the extent of polyethylene wear and the location of the osteolytic lesion. It is essential that surgeons clearly convey to patients the importance of close follow-up when managing polyethylene wear and/or osteolysis with nonoperative treatment.

The quality of bone surrounding an osteolytic defect is often quite variable. Some surgeons have not grafted these lesions at the time of the liner exchange out of concern that the graft may not incorporate because the area is not stressed. However, we believe that these lesions should be thoroughly débrided and grafted in the hope that some bone will incorporate and be available for future revision procedures. In addition, if the area is not grafted, wear debris will accumulate over time, which could lead to further loss of bone stock.

Bone-grafting is often performed through the screw holes in the cup, through a trapdoor in the ilium, or through lytic lesions when they are at the periphery of the component. At this time it has not yet been definitively established which approach is best. One important advantage of bone-grafting through the holes in the back of the cup is that there is no risk of destabilizing the acetabular component. However, this approach makes it extremely difficult to completely débride all of the granulomatous tissue in the lytic lesion and adequately pack the bone-graft. The debris found associated with osteolysis may actually prevent graft incorporation (70). An alternative approach that allows better visualization and access to defects behind acetabular components is to use access channels that may have already been formed or to create a bone window, or trapdoor, in the ilium. However, since cementless acetabular components are stabilized by discrete pseudopods of bone, these areas of bone ingrowth must not be disrupted when creating a bone window adjacent to the cup. In general, the senior author (Lieberman) will make a trapdoor in the ilium unless there is a major risk of destabilizing the well-fixed acetabular component. The lytic lesion must be thoroughly débrided of all granulomatous tissue. Recently, using this technique, we have started supplementing bone-graft substitutes with autologous bone marrow harvest in the hopes of enhancing graft incorporation. Between 30 and 70 cc of bone marrow can be easily harvested from the iliac crest. This strategy enables us to supply osteogenic cells, responding cells, and an osteoconductive matrix to the osteolytic lesion.

The advent of three-dimensional CT scans has led to a major advance in the ability to characterize osteolytic defects surrounding THA. Volumetric analysis allows accurate quantification of osteolysis, and the senior author's experience suggests that it could become useful in determining the need

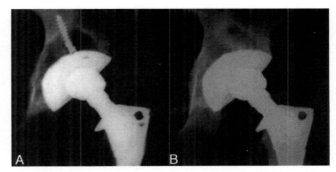

Figure 25-3   **A:** A preoperative plain AP radiograph shows an osteolytic lesion superior to cementless acetabular component. Treatment of this lesion was performed through existing screw holes with packing of allograft bone chips around a stable component. **B:** A plain radiograph taken 3 years after surgical intervention shows apparent incorporation of the allograft chips. *Clin Orthop* 2003;417:183–194.

for revision THA in some patients. A preoperative radiograph is shown depicting the typical appearance of an osteolytic lesion above an otherwise stable acetabular component (Fig. 25-3A). Cancellous allograft chips were then inserted through the screw holes of the acetabular cup, which was retained. A plain radiograph taken 3 years postoperatively suggests graft incorporation and healing of the osteolytic lesion (Fig. 25-3B). Figure 25-4 demonstrates the high-resolution images from three-dimensional reconstructions of an artifact-suppressed CT scan (VirtualScopics, Inc., Rochester, NY) performed 3 years postoperatively. Since this technology has the ability to differentiate between host bone, residual allograft, and osteolytic lesions (68), the images indicate that there is incomplete graft incorporation and that a portion of the osteolytic lesion remains untreated. The CT scan reveals the limitation of grafting an osteolytic lesion through holes in the acetabular cup.

Preclinical studies have used rh-BMP-2 (11) and rh-OP-1 (26) in primary THA animal models to treat acetabular and femoral bone defects and augment the healing of femoral strut grafts. These results have been promising, with radiographic and histologic evidence of bridging bone formation to a porous ingrowth surface (11,75). Although further study is required in a more rigorous model truly simulating a revision THA in order to determine its cost-effectiveness, the use of recombinant proteins for the augmentation of revision procedures remains promising.

DISCUSSION

Revision THA often presents a number of difficulties, including osteolytic bone defects, poor biological environment, and compromised bone stock. Generators of particulate wear debris lead to implant loosening, which remains the leading cause of component failure. Bone-graft and bone-graft substitutes are vital to a joint surgeon's armamentarium in dealing with issues of bone loss, prosthetic stability, and clinical outcome. Available data for these substances vary widely, and careful evaluation is necessary to identify the appropriate use of various bone-graft agents.

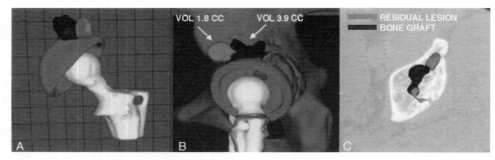

Figure 25-4   An AP **(A)** and lateral **(B)** view of three-dimensional reconstructions of an artifact-suppressed CT scan (VirtualScopics, Inc. Rochester, NY) from the same patient shown in Figure 25-3A,B. Color imaging allows differentiation between the host bone, the allograft, and the residual osteolytic lesion. Volumetric measurements are shown (B) for each section. A two-dimensional axial CT scan **(C)** identifies the corresponding region of the ilium superior to the acetabular component. The images suggest that the residual osteolytic lesion remains despite bone-grafting through the screw holes. Further research is required to delineate the clinical significance of such a lesion. *Clinical Orthop* 2003;417:183–194. See Color Plate.

Several limitations exist in the clinical and basic science data for bone-graft agents. First, animal models that are used to simulate circumstances surrounding human revision THA fall short in critical areas. Periprosthetic defects used to challenge biologic substitutes are created in healthy, bleeding bone, in contrast to the variable quality seen in clinical situations. Second, few randomized clinical trials have been used to compare the efficacy of different treatments. Third, routine radiographic imaging does not accurately characterize host incorporation of bone-graft in humans. Plain radiographic signs of incorporation often misrepresent the progress of graft incorporation histologically.

Recent studies have reported the use of volumetric computerized tomography as an outcome measure in the assessment of periprosthetic osteolysis (20,88). Claus et al. created various sized osteolytic lesions around bilateral total hip replacements in human cadavers and tested the accuracy of three-dimensional computed tomographic (3DCT) scans in determining volume and location (20). Although osteolysis in the ilium and acetabular rim was more easily identified than that in the ischium and pubis, 81% of all lesions were correctly identified by 3DCT scan. The authors concluded that computed tomography imaging analysis is a more powerful and accurate tool than plain radiography for the assessment of pelvic osteolysis (20).

Because it can reliably quantify the size of osteolytic lesions, three-dimensional imaging offers a comprehensive perspective on an osteolytic lesion that is beyond the capability of plain radiography and may be quite useful in certain patients. Although this technology may enable surgeons to evaluate the efficacy of various bone-graft substitutes in clinical and preclinical trials, it probably should not be used on a routine basis at this time because of the cost of these studies.

Bone loss in revision THA is a difficult problem in terms of treatment, longitudinal follow-up, and clinical outcome. Not only do revision THA patients often exhibit poor bone repair potential, but graft substitute incorporation rates also have not been well studied. Novel treatment strategies and imaging technology may soon provide the arthroplasty surgeon with significantly more options for dealing with this clinical problem.

Currently established treatment options, including the use of allograft or autograft bone, may soon be supplemented with recombinant growth factors or products from cell-based therapies, which may enhance their osteoinductive potential. Although cost-effectiveness must be assessed, novel biologic substitutes may be used to enhance bone repair in more stringent biologic environments. In making these critical decisions, surgeons must assess the host biologic environment and ensure that the four elements critical for promoting bone repair are present: bioactive factors, responding cells, matrix, and an adequate vascular supply. At the present time, the senior author combines bone marrow aspirates with bone-graft substitutes when treating osteolytic lesions. Further study into the efficacy of bone-graft substitutes will hopefully lead to improved clinical outcomes in the treatment of revision THA.

REFERENCES

1. Aspenberg P, Johnsson E, Thorngren KG. Dose-dependent reduction of bone inductive properties by ethylene oxide. *J Bone Joint Surg.* 1990;72B:1036–1037.
2. Barrack RL, Cook SD, Patron LP, et al. Induction of bone ingrowth from acetabular defects to a porous surface with OP-1. *Clin Orthop.* 2003;417:41–49.
3. Bauer TW, Smith ST. Bioactive materials in orthopaedic surgery: overview and regulatory considerations. *Clin Orthop.* 2002;395: 11–22.
4. Berven S, Tay BK, Kleinstueck FS, et al. Clinical applications of bone-graft substitutes in spine surgery: consideration of mineralized and demineralized preparations and growth factor supplementation. *Eur Spine J.* 2001;10[Suppl 2]:S169–177.
5. Blaha JD. Calcium sulfate bone-void filler. *Orthopedics.* 1998;21:1017–1019.
6. Boden SD, Martin GJ Jr, Horton WC, et al. Laparoscopic anterior spinal arthrodesis with rhBMP-2 in a titanium interbody threaded cage. *J Spinal Disord.* 1998;11:95–101.
7. Boden SD, Titus L, Hair G, et al. Lumbar spine fusion by local gene therapy with a cDNA encoding a novel osteoinductive protein (LMP-1). *Spine.* 1998;23:2486–2492.
8. Boden SD, Zdeblick TA, Sandhu HS, et al. The use of rhBMP-2 in interbody fusion cages: definitive evidence of osteoinduction in humans: a preliminary report. *Spine.* 2000;25:376–381.
9. Bonfiglio M. Repair of bone-transplant fractures. *J Bone Joint Surg.* 1958;40A:446–455; discussion 455–456.
10. Bos GD, Goldberg VM, Zika JM, et al. Immune responses of rats to frozen bone allografts. *J Bone Joint Surg.* 1983;65A:239–246.

11. Bragdon CR, Doherty AM, Rubash HE, et al. The efficacy of BMP-2 to induce bone ingrowth in a total hip replacement model. *Clin Orthop.* 2003;417: 50–61.

12. Bruder SP, Kraus KH, Goldberg Vm, et al. The effect of implants loaded with autologous mesenchymal stem cells on the healing of canine segmental bone defects. *J Bone Joint Surg.* 1998;80A: 985–996.

13. Bucholz RW. Nonallograft osteoconductive bone-graft substitutes. *Clin Orthop.* 2002;395:44–52.

14. Bucholz RW, Carlton A, Holmes R. Interporous hydroxyapatite as a bone-graft substitute in tibial plateau fractures. *Clin Orthop.* 1989;240:53–62.

15. Burchardt H. The biology of bone-graft repair. *Clin Orthop.* 1983;174:28–42.

16. Burchardt H, Jones H, Glowczewski F, et al. Freeze-dried allogeneic segmental cortical-bone-grafts in dogs. *J Bone Joint Surg.* 1978;60A:1082–1090.

17. Burwell RG. Studies in the transplantation of bone, V: the capacity of fresh and treated homografts of bone to evoke transplantation immunity. *J Bone Joint Surg.* 1963;45B:386–401.

18. Cabanela ME, Trousdale RT, Berry DJ. Impacted cancellous graft plus cement in hip revision. *Clin Orthop.* 2003;417: 175–182.

19. Chapman MW, Bucholz R, Cornell C. Treatment of acute fractures with a collagen-calcium phosphate graft material: a randomized clinical trial. *J Bone Joint Surg.* 1997;79A:495–502.

20. Claus AM, Totterman SM, Sychterz CJ, et al. Computed tomography to assess pelvic lysis after total hip replacement. *Clin Orthop.* 2004;422:167–174.

21. Connolly JF. Injectable bone marrow preparations to stimulate osteogenic repair. *Clin Orthop.* 1995;313:8–18.

22. Connolly JF, Guse R, Tiedeman J, et al. Autologous marrow injection as a substitute for operative grafting of tibial nonunions. *Clin Orthop.* 1991;266:259–270.

23. Constantz BR, Ison IC, Fulmer MT, et al. Skeletal repair by in situ formation of the mineral phase of bone. *Science.* 1995;267(5205): 1796–1799.

24. Cook SD, Baffes GC, Wolfe MW, et al. The effect of recombinant human osteogenic protein-1 on healing of large segmental bone defects. *J Bone Joint Surg.* 1994;76A:827–838.

25. Cook SD, Baffes GC, Wolfe MW, et al. Recombinant human bone morphogenetic protein-7 induces healing in a canine long-bone segmental defect model. *Clin Orthop.* 1994;301:302–312.

26. Cook SD, Barrack RL, Santman M, et al. The Otto Aufranc Award. Strut allograft healing to the femur with recombinant human osteogenic protein-1. *Clin Orthop.* 2000;381:47–57.

27. Cook SD, Barrack RL, Shimmin A, et al. The use of osteogenic protein-1 in reconstructive surgery of the hip. *J Arthroplasty.* 2001;16[8 Suppl 1]:88–94.

28. Cook SD, Wolfe MW, Salkeld SL, et al. Effect of recombinant human osteogenic protein-1 on healing of segmental defects in non-human primates. *J Bone Joint Surg.* 1995;77A:734–750.

29. D'Antonio JA, Capello WN, Borden LS, et al. Classification and management of acetabular abnormalities in total hip arthroplasty. *Clin Orthop.* 1989;243:126–137.

30. Dell PC, Burchardt H, Glowczewski FP Jr. A roentgenographic, biomechanical, and histological evaluation of vascularized and non-vascularized segmental fibular canine autografts. *J Bone Joint Surg.* 1985;67A:105–112.

31. Dunbar MJ, Blackley HR, Bourne RB. Osteolysis of the femur: principles of management. *Instr Course Lect.* 2001;50:197–209.

32. Einhorn TA. Clinical applications of recombinant human BMPs: early experience and future development. *J Bone Joint Surg.* 2003;85A[Suppl 3]:82–88.

33. Emerson RH Jr, Head WC, Berklacich FM, et al. Noncemented acetabular revision arthroplasty using allograft bone. *Clin Orthop.* 1989;249:30–43.

34. Etienne G, Bezwada HP, Hungerford DS, et al. The incorporation of morselized bone-grafts in cementless acetabular revisions. *Clin Orthop.* 2004;428: 241–246.

35. Finkemeier CG. Bone-grafting and bone-graft substitutes. *J Bone Joint Surg.* 2002;84A:454–464.

36. Frenkel SR, Moskovich R, Spivak J, et al. Demineralized bone matrix: enhancement of spinal fusion. *Spine.* 1993;18:1634–1639.

37. Friedlaender GE, et al. Osteogenic protein-1 (bone morphogenetic protein-7) in the treatment of tibial nonunions. *J Bone Joint Surg.* 2001;83A[Suppl 1, Pt 2]:S151–158.

38. Gamradt SC, Lieberman JR. Bone-graft for revision hip arthroplasty: biology and future applications. *Clin Orthop.* 2003;417: 183–194.

39. Gazdag AR, Lane JM, Glaser D, et al. Alternatives to autogenous bone-graft: efficacy and indications. *J Am Acad Orthop Surg.* 1995;3:1–8.

40. Gie GA, Linder L, Ling RS, et al. Contained morselized allograft in revision total hip arthroplasty: surgical technique. *Orthop Clin North Am.* 1993;24:717–725.

41. Gie GA, Linder L, Ling RS, et al. Impacted cancellous allografts and cement for revision total hip arthroplasty. *J Bone Joint Surg.* 1993;75B:14–21.

42. Goater JJ, O'Keefe RJ, Rosier RN, et al. Efficacy of ex vivo OPG gene therapy in preventing wear debris induced osteolysis. *J Orthop Res.* 2002;20: 169–173.

43. Goldberg VM. Selection of bone-grafts for revision total hip arthroplasty. *Clin Orthop.* 2000;381:68–76.

44. Goldberg VM, Stevenson S. The biology of bone-grafts. *Semin Arthroplasty.* 1996;12–17.

45. Goldberg VM, Stevenson S. Natural history of autografts and allografts. *Clin Orthop.* 1987;225:7–16.

46. Goodman SB, Bauer TW, Carter D, et al. Norian SRS cement augmentation in hip fracture treatment: laboratory and initial clinical results. *Clin Orthop.* 1998;348:42–50.

47. Greenwald AS, Boden SD, Goldberg VM, et al. Bone-graft substitutes: facts, fictions, and applications. *J Bone Joint Surg.* 2001;83A [Suppl 2, Pt 2]:98–103.

48. Haddad FS, Masri BA, Garbuz DS, et al. Femoral bone loss in total hip arthroplasty: classification and preoperative planning. *Instr Course Lect.* 2000;49:83–96.

49. Heekin RD, Engh CA, Vinh T. Morselized allograft in acetabular reconstruction: a postmortem retrieval analysis. *Clin Orthop.* 1995;319:184–190.

50. Hollinger JO, Brekke J, Gruskin E, et al. Role of bone substitutes. *Clin Orthop.* 1996;324:55–65.

51. Jarcho M. Calcium phosphate ceramics as hard tissue prosthetics. *Clin Orthop.* 1981;157:259–278.

52. Johnson EE, Urist MR, Finerman GA. Resistant nonunions and partial or complete segmental defects of long bones: treatment with implants of a composite of human bone morphogenetic protein (BMP) and autolyzed, antigen-extracted, allogeneic (AAA) bone. *Clin Orthop.* 1992;277:229–237.

53. Jupiter JB, Winters S, Sigman S, et al. Repair of five distal radius fractures with an investigational cancellous bone cement: a preliminary report. *J Orthop Trauma.* 1997;11:110–116.

54. Kakiuchi M, Hosoya T, Takaoka K, et al. Human bone matrix gelatin as a clinical alloimplant: a retrospective review of 160 cases. *Int Orthop.* 1985;9:181–188.

55. Klawitter JJ, Bagwell JG, Weinstein AM, et al. An evaluation of bone growth into porous high density polyethylene. *J Biomed Mater Res.* 1976;10:311–323.

56. Kligman M, Con V, Roffman M. Cortical and cancellous morselized allograft in revision total hip replacement. *Clin Orthop.* 2002;401:139–148.

57. Kligman M, Rotem A, Roffman M. Cancellous and cortical morselized allograft in revision total hip replacement: a biomechanical study of implant stability. *J Biomech.* 2003;36: 797–802.

58. Kondo K, Nagaya I. Bone incorporation of frozen femoral head allograft in revision total hip replacement. *Nippon Seikeigeka Gakkai Zasshi.* 1993;67:408–416.

59. Kopylov P, Runnqvist K, Jonsson K, et al. Norian SRS versus external fixation in redisplaced distal radial fractures: a randomized study in 40 patients. *Acta Orthop Scand.* 1999;70:1–5.

60. Lee GH, Khoury JG, Bell JE, et al. Adverse reactions to OsteoSet bone-graft substitute: the incidence in a consecutive series. *Iowa Orthop J.* 2002;22:35–38.

61. Lee JY, MUsgrave D, Pelinkovic D, et al. Effect of bone morphogenetic protein-2-expressing muscle-derived cells on healing of critical-sized bone defects in mice. *J Bone Joint Surg.* 2001;83A:1032–1039.

62. Leopold SS, Jacobs JJ, Rosenberg AG. Cancellous allograft in revision total hip arthroplasty: a clinical review. *Clin Orthop.* 2000;371:86–97.

63. Lieberman JR, Daluiski A, Stevenson S, et al. The effect of regional gene therapy with bone morphogenetic protein-2-producing bone-marrow cells on the repair of segmental femoral defects in rats. *J Bone Joint Surg.* 1999;81A:905–917.

64. Lieberman JR, Le LQ, Wu L, et al. Regional gene therapy with a BMP-2-producing murine stromal cell line induces heterotopic and orthotopic bone formation in rodents. *J Orthop Res.* 1998;16:330–339.

65. Lindholm TS, Urist MR. A quantitative analysis of new bone formation by induction in compositive grafts of bone marrow and bone matrix. *Clin Orthop.* 1980;150:288–300.

66. Ling RS, Timperley AJ, Linder L. Histology of cancellous impaction grafting in the femur: a case report. *J Bone Joint Surg.* 1993;75B:693–696.

67. Liu DM. Influence of porous microarchitecture on the in vitro dissolution and biological behavior of porous calcium phosphate ceramics. *Mater Sci Forum.* 1997;250:183–208.

68. Looney RJ, Boyd A, Totterman S, et al. Volumetric computerized tomography as a measurement of periprosthetic acetabular osteolysis and its correlation with wear. *Arthritis Res.* 2002;4:59–63.

69. Maloney WJ, Herzwurm P, Paprosky W, et al. Treatment of pelvic osteolysis associated with a stable acetabular component inserted without cement as part of a total hip replacement. *J Bone Joint Surg.* 1997;79A:1628–1634.

70. Maloney WJ, Paprosky W, Engh CA, et al. Surgical treatment of pelvic osteolysis. *Clin Orthop.* 2001;393:78–84.

71. Maniscalco P, Gambera D, Bertone C, et al. Healing of fresh tibial fractures with OP-1: a preliminary report. *Acta Biomed Ateneo Parmense.* 2002;73:27–33.

72. Martin GJ Jr, Boden SD, Marone MA, et al. Posterolateral intertransverse process spinal arthrodesis with rhBMP-2 in a nonhuman primate: important lessons learned regarding dose, carrier, and safety. *J Spinal Disord.* 1999;12:179–186.

73. Mehin R, Yuan X, Haydon C, et al. Retroacetabular osteolysis: when to operate? *Clin Orthop.* 2004;428:247–255.

74. Munting E, Wilmart JF, Wijne A, et al. Effect of sterilization on osteoinduction: comparison of five methods in demineralized rat bone. *Acta Orthop Scand.* 1988;59:34–38.

75. Murakami N, Saito N, Takahashi J, et al. Repair of a proximal femoral bone defect in dogs using a porous surfaced prosthesis in combination with recombinant BMP-2 and a synthetic polymer carrier. *Biomaterials.* 2003;24:2153–2159.

76. Muschler GF, Boehm C, Easley K. Aspiration to obtain osteoblast progenitor cells from human bone marrow: the influence of aspiration volume. *J Bone Joint Surg.* 1997;79A:1699–1709.

77. Muschler GF, Nitto H, Boehm CA, et al. Age- and gender-related changes in the cellularity of human bone marrow and the prevalence of osteoblastic progenitors. *J Orthop Res.* 2001;19:117–125.

78. Muschler GF, Nitto H, Matsukura Y, et al. Spine fusion using cell matrix composites enriched in bone marrow-derived cells. *Clin Orthop.* 2003;407:102–118.

79. Oakes DA, Lee CC, Lieberman JR. An evaluation of human demineralized bone matrices in a rat femoral defect model. *Clin Orthop.* 2003;413:281–290.

80. Ohgushi H, Goldberg VM, Caplan AI. Repair of bone defects with marrow cells and porous ceramic: experiments in rats. *Acta Orthop Scand.* 1989;60:334–339.

81. Paprosky WG, Burnett RS. Assessment and classification of bone stock deficiency in revision total hip arthroplasty. *Am J Orthop.* 2002;31:459–464.

82. Paprosky WG, Perona PG, Lawrence JM. Acetabular defect classification and surgical reconstruction in revision arthroplasty: a 6-year follow-up evaluation. *J Arthroplasty.* 1994;9:33–44.

83. Peterson B, Zhang J, Iglesias R, et al. Osteoinductivity of commercially available demineralized bone matrix: preparations in a spine fusion model. *J Bone Joint Surg.* 2004;86A:2243–2250.

84. Pluhar GE, Manley PA, Heiner JPJRV, et al. The effect of recombinant human bone morphogenetic protein-2 on femoral reconstruction with an intercalary allograft in a dog model. *J Orthop Res.* 2001;19:308–317.

85. Reddi AH, Huggins C. Biochemical sequences in the transformation of normal fibroblasts in adolescent rats. *Proc Natl Acad Sci U S A.* 1972;69:1601–1605.

86. Sandhu HS, Kanim LE, Toth JM, et al. Experimental spinal fusion with recombinant human bone morphogenetic protein-2 without decortication of osseous elements. *Spine.* 1997;22:1171–1180.

87. Sandhu HS, Khan SN, Suh DY, et al. Demineralized bone matrix, bone morphogenetic proteins, and animal models of spine fusion: an overview. *Eur Spine J.* 2001;10[Suppl 2]:S122–131.

88. Schwarz EM, Campbell D, Totterman S, et al. Use of volumetric computerized tomography as a primary outcome measure to evaluate drug efficacy in the prevention of peri-prosthetic osteolysis: a 1-year clinical pilot of etanercept vs. placebo. *J Orthop Res.* 2003;21:1049–1055.

89. Schwartz Z, Mellonig JT, Carnes DL, et al. Ability of commercial demineralized freeze-dried bone allograft to induce new bone formation. *J Periodontol.* 1996;67:918–926.

90. Shih CH, Chen CH, Tsai MF, et al. Incorporation of allograft for acetabular reconstruction: single photon emission CT in 21 hip arthroplasties followed for 2.5–5 years. *Acta Orthop Scand.* 1994;65: 589–594.

91. Stevenson S. Biology of bone-grafts. *Orthop Clin North Am.* 1999;30:543–552.

92. Tiedeman JJ, Garvin KL, Kile TA, et al. The role of a composite, demineralized bone matrix and bone marrow in the treatment of osseous defects. *Orthopedics.* 1995;18:1153–1158.

93. Ulrich-Vinther M, Carmody EE, Goater JJ, et al. Recombinant adeno-associated virus-mediated osteoprotegerin gene therapy inhibits wear debris-induced osteolysis. *J Bone Joint Surg.* 2002;84A:1405–1412.

94. Urist MR. Bone: formation by autoinduction. *Science.* 1965;150(698):893–899.

95. Urist MR. Bone transplants and implants. In: Urist MR, ed. *Fundamental and Clinical Bone Physiology.* Philadelphia: JB Lippincott; 1980:331–368.

96. Urist MR, Dawson E. Intertransverse process fusion with the aid of chemosterilized autolyzed antigen-extracted allogeneic (AAA) bone. *Clin Orthop.* 1981;154:97–113.

97. Urist MR, Silverman BF, Buring K, et al. The bone induction principle. *Clin Orthop.* 1967;53:243–283.

98. Valentin-Opran A, Wozney J, Csimma C, et al. Clinical evaluation of recombinant human bone morphogenetic protein-2. *Clin Orthop.* 2002;395:110–120.

99. van der Donk S, Buma P, Slooff TJ, et al. Incorporation of morselized bone-grafts: a study of 24 acetabular biopsy specimens. *Clin Orthop.* 2002;396:131–141.

100. Viggeswarapu M, Boden SD, Liu Y, et al. Adenoviral delivery of LIM mineralization protein-1 induces new-bone formation in vitro and in vivo. *J Bone Joint Surg.* 2001;83A:364–376.

101. Wang JC, Kanim LE, Yoo S, et al. Effect of regional gene therapy with bone morphogenetic protein-2-producing bone marrow cells on spinal fusion in rats. *J Bone Joint Surg.* 2003;85A:905–911.

102. Whang PG, Lieberman, JR Clinical issues in the development of cellular systems for use as bone-graft substitutes. In: Laurencin CT, ed. *Bone-Graft Substitutes: A Multidisciplinary Approach.* West Conshohocken, PA: American Society for Testing and Materials International; 2003:142–164.

103. Yasko AW, Lane JM, Fellinger EJ, et al. The healing of segmental bone defects, induced by recombinant human bone morphogenetic protein (rhBMP-2): a radiographic, histological, and biomechanical study in rats. *J Bone Joint Surg.* 1992;74A:659–670.

104. Zabka AG, pluhar GE, Edwards RB, et al. Histomorphometric description of allograft bone remodeling and union in a canine segmental femoral defect model: a comparison of rhBMP-2, cancellous bone-graft, and absorbable collagen sponge. *J Orthop Res.* 2001;19: 318–327.

CLINICAL SCIENCE

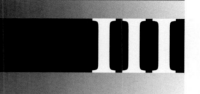

History and Physical Exam

26

Steven A. Purvis   Seth S. Leopold

A thorough history and physical exam remains as important as ever in the evaluation of patients with hip pain. Although magnetic resonance imaging and hip arthroscopy permit identification of pathoanatomy with greater precision than was possible before the adoption of those techniques, most adult hip diagnoses still may be made using a combination of skillful questioning, careful examination, and plain radiographs.

The principal goals of an effective history and physical examination are as follows:

■ Consideration of life-threatening or limb-threatening diagnoses, such as malignancy, vascular pathology, acute infection, and severe or progressive neurological conditions
■ Determination of whether the source of the patient complaint is nonorthopedic, orthopedic but para-articular or extra-articular in origin, or intra-articular
■ Creation of a manageable differential diagnosis, to which further workup, including diagnostic imaging, can be applied

THE HISTORY

Chief Complaint

The chief complaint is the essential first element of an effective history, and it sets the tone for the rest of a well-obtained problem-based history. Ideally, the surgeon will begin the interview with a suitable open-ended question that will put the patient at ease and allow that individual to introduce the problem in his or her own words. Time pressure frequently leads to physicians interrupting their patients after only a few seconds. This common but unfortunate approach can keep the surgeon from learning what specifically the patient seeks from the encounter or from getting a sense for the emotional state of the patient; hurrying the encounter at this early stage may have the unintended effect of actually making the visit less efficient.

Most adults seeking care for hip-related problems do so because of pain. Less commonly, stiffness or gait disturbances prompt these evaluations. Although the chief complaint will tend to move the interview in a particular direction—for example, a young patient presenting to an urgent care center with 12 hours of severe groin pain and fever in contrast to an older patient presenting with 6 months of gradually worsening groin pain and decreased tolerance to activities requiring weight bearing—it remains important to maintain a wide "search image" for all reasonable possibilities at this early point in the interview. The former patient is likely to have septic arthritis but could easily be experiencing a first presentation of inflammatory arthritis; the latter patient is most likely to have osteoarthritis of the hip, but more ominous conditions such as malignancy will need to be excluded during the remainder of the history and physical examination as well as through the use of appropriate diagnostic testing.

History of Present Illness

This portion of the interview permits the patient to better describe the important symptoms mentioned in the chief complaint and allows a skilled examiner to elicit information that may not be volunteered as relevant but that nonetheless can help narrow the differential diagnosis.

If pain is the presenting symptom, it is important to determine its characteristics, including severity, location, duration, association with particular activities (such as weight bearing, sitting, or twisting), ameliorating and exacerbating factors, interference with daily activities, and radiation, either from the lumbar spine or down the lower extremity. Having patients rate pain on a visual-analog or Likert scale is helpful during the initial history as one measure of the impact of the problem on the patient's lifestyle as well as for later use in gauging the response to treatments. Pain that is severe, unrelenting, rapidly worsening, or associated with neurological fallout and/or constitutional symptoms mandates prompt (sometimes emergent) evaluation to exclude certain time-sensitive diagnoses, such as joint sepsis, acute osteomyelitis, malignancy with impending pathological fracture, and spinal cord compression.

The location of pain from intra-articular hip conditions varies but broadly falls into one of three patterns: groin pain, thigh pain, and buttock pain. These patterns are attributable to Hilton's law, which states that each major nerve that crosses a joint sends sensory fibers to that joint; fibers from the three important nerves that cross the hip—the obturator, femoral, and sciatic nerves—account for the groin, thigh, and buttock pain patterns, respectively. They also account for some of the patterns of pain from nonorthopedic sources that can masquerade as hip pathology, such as groin pain from ovarian cysts.

Stiffness is another area of importance to patients, who frequently will state that they can no longer reach shoes or socks because the hip will not allow comfortable positioning. Patients often are told they are limping even before they become aware of it; a painful limp that is most prominent during the first few steps after prolonged sitting (so-called start-up pain or "gelling") is common in osteoarthritis, but persistently abnormal gait patterns can occur with any painful condition around the hip. In the section on physical examination, further details about gait assessment are provided.

More remote elements of the history of present illness may be important, as well. Childhood illnesses or conditions such as slipped capital femoral epiphysis (SCFE), Legg–Calvé–Perthes disease, developmental dysplasia of the hip, prior joint infections, or early-onset inflammatory arthritides, including juvenile rheumatoid arthritis, are common causes of hip problems in the adult population and need to be identified in the history. Trauma, whether remote or recent, is also an important etiology of adult hip arthritis. Risk factors for osteonecrosis of the femoral head, including the use of exogenous glucocorticoids like prednisone, excessive alcohol consumption, personal or family history of hypercoagulable states, and certain occupational exposures such as extreme barotrauma, are worth specifically covering in patients with hip pain of unknown etiology.

Previous surgery on the hip, though properly considered in its own section of a formal history and physical, is perhaps more conveniently gathered during the history of present illness. It is important to get as much information as is practical about prior surgical exposures and the specific manufacturer and type of implants that may be in place at this time, although these details are sometimes obscure to the patient.

Although the present review cannot cover all presentations of all hip diagnoses, the following section outlines the typical elements of the history of present illness as they often appear in several common conditions.

Intra-articular Conditions

Osteoarthritis
This disease is classically associated with more advanced age but is being seen and treated more frequently in younger patients, sometimes as a result of prior trauma. Patients most often complain of pain with activities, walking, or simply trying to put on their shoes and socks. Stiffness and decreased range of motion, along with crepitation and changes in gait, are also frequent complaints in this group of patients. Radiographic characteristics include asymmetric joint space narrowing, sclerosis, subchondral cysts, and periarticular osteophytes. Osteoarthritis is the primary diagnosis in an overwhelming majority of hip arthroplasties.

Inflammatory Arthritis
This large category includes rheumatoid arthritis, systemic lupus erythematosus, psoriatic arthritis, ankylosing spondylitis, and literally dozens of other inflammatory, crystal-related, and autoimmune arthropathies. These patients will often present with symptoms of inflammation in more than one joint, which may be acute in nature and necessitate ruling out an infectious process as the first step in the workup. They also may have stiffness, which may be worst in the morning and then improve through the day. Multiple joint involvement is important to document, as this may have significant impact on both the patient and therapeutic decision-making (both medical and surgical). Radiographic changes include symmetric joint space narrowing, cysts, osteopenia, and sometimes periarticular spurring.

Infectious Arthritis
Pyogenic arthritis of the hip is a true orthopedic emergency, requiring prompt workup and (often) surgical treatment. Patients often appear acutely ill, have severe joint pain that is worse with motion or weight bearing, and have constitutional symptoms like fever, chills, and malaise. Failure to diagnose infectious arthritis in a timely manner can lead to catastrophic results.

Osteonecrosis of the Femoral Head
Often called avascular necrosis or AVN, this condition affects approximately 500,000 people in the United States. Patients are commonly diagnosed in their 30s or 40s; making the diagnosis early requires a high degree of suspicion on the part of the physician. Common risk factors include hypercoagulable states, exogenous corticosteroid intake, alcohol abuse, high-dose irradiation, sickle cell disease, and Caisson's disease (barotrauma), among many others. More than 40% of patients who have osteonecrosis have no clear risk factors, and in fact this disease may be multifactorial in etiology. Patients describe a deep throbbing or sharp pain that is worsened with activity but frequently present even at rest or with minimal motion of the hip. Radiographic findings, though classic in appearance with sclerosis, subchondral collapse, and fragmentation, are usually not present early in the disease process. If avascular necrosis is suspected, obtaining an MRI has become the standard of care as well as the most reliable test to make the diagnosis, as an MRI provides more useful anatomic information regarding the location and extent of the lesion than is possible with scintigraphy (bone scan). Since over 50% of patients with this condition have bilateral involvement at some point in the disease course, it is reasonable to obtain an MRI of the whole pelvis (both hips) at the time of the screening evaluation. Also, since as many as 15% of patients with osteonecrosis of the femoral head will have other joint

involvement, it is important to inquire about symptoms in the ankles, knees, and shoulders, which are the most common other sites. This diagnosis accounts for nearly 10% of hip arthroplasties performed in the United States.

Femoroacetabular Impingement

This diagnosis has relatively recently become recognized as a cause of premature degenerative arthritis of the hip. The pathoanatomy involves abnormal contact between the anterior femoral neck and the acetabular rim, causing damage to the labrum and articular surfaces. Most often seen in young active persons, these patients describe pain that can be exacerbated by athletic activities, walking, or prolonged sitting. This diagnosis is best made by correlating history, physical findings, and radiographs; on physical exam, the most useful maneuver is the impingement sign, also called the flexion–adduction–internal rotation (FADIR) test (3,5). With the patient supine, the examiner brings the hip passively into flexion, internal rotation, and adduction across the midline; from this position, if the test is positive, further passive internal rotation will reproduce the patient's hip pain. As mentioned, further diagnostic imaging, including plain radiographs perhaps as well as an MRI, help to show diagnostic changes associated with this condition.

Labral Pathology

Pain from labral pathology may mimic other types of hip pain and may be aggravated by increased activity levels, particularly those that involve twisting and flexing. Labral pathology is most often diagnosed in younger patients with a history of hip dysplasia. If symptoms persist for long periods, this diagnosis can be difficult to distinguish from femoroacetabular impingement. Plain radiographs may reveal subtle dysplasia, and an MRI with intra-articular contrast can confirm the diagnosis, allowing proper treatment planning (6).

Transient Osteoporosis of the Hip

Transient osteoporosis of the hip (TOH) is a painful but self-limiting condition that is often confused with osteonecrosis of the femoral head. It has two demographic peaks, one in men in the 6th and 7th decades of life and another in women in the third trimester of pregnancy. TOH causes unilateral acute hip pain of insidious onset. The pain is generally worse with activity and decreases with rest. There is typically no history of antecedent trauma, but most patients can remember when the pain started. Decreases in range of motion may or may not be found. Radiographs reveal osteoporosis starting at about 2 months after the onset of symptoms, which resolves on serial films, usually within 6 to 9 months. On MRIs, there are diffuse signal changes suggestive of marrow edema, involving the head and neck of the femur down to the intertrochanteric line; MRI findings are present before changes are noted on plain films. In contrast, findings in hips with AVN are localized to signal changes in the femoral head, usually in the subchondral area (4).

Malignancy

Though rare as a primary diagnosis when evaluating patients with hip pain, this diagnosis should not be forgotten. Intracapsular tumors, bone lesions (primary or metastatic), and soft-tissue tumors (chondral or synovial) can be causes of hip pain. Extracapsular tumors can also cause hip pain by either direct compression or invasion into the hip, as well as cause referred pain from more distant tumor processes.

Para-articular Conditions

Trochanteric Bursitis

This is a common cause of pain in the adult hip. Symptoms are mechanical in nature and are easily reproduced with palpation along the lateral aspect of the greater trochanter. Symptoms often include pain that can radiate locally, burning, and difficulty lying on the affected hip at night. Treatment rarely requires more than conservative therapy.

Spinal Stenosis

In patients presenting for hip pain that do not have classic physical findings of hip disease, spinal stenosis is a diagnosis that should be investigated. Patients are usually in the same age group; describe insidious onset of pain (usually worse with walking or extension of the lumbar spine), paresthesias, and "giving way"; rarely have the dermatomal pain pattern often seen with a herniated disc; and often describe the pain as being relieved with flexion of the lower lumbar spine. Workup includes radiographic images as well as CT scan.

Snapping Hip and Piriformis Syndrome

In the "snapping" hip, the patient complains that certain ranges of motion cause a pop or snap, usually in the anterior hip. The examiner can often reproduce the snap and palpate it during the exam. Diagnosis sometimes can be confirmed with iliopsoas bursography. Piriformis syndrome causes a pain and or burning usually described in the buttock area along the course of the piriformis tendon. The sciatic nerve may be locally irritated as it courses under the tendon.

Iliotibial Band Friction Syndrome

This condition typically is seen in more active patients, usually younger runners, who complain of pain in the lateral distal femur that can radiate and is activity related. Ober's test (described later in this chapter) is helpful in making the diagnosis.

Nonorthopedic Conditions around the Hip

A high index of suspicion in the face of an atypical history and physical exam can lead the clinician to local pathologies around the hip. Pyelonephritis, ovarian cysts, hernias, and fibromyalgia with atypical pain patterns are diagnoses that can lead a patient presenting to the orthopedist's office.

Past Medical History

A thorough medical history is important, not only because of the occasional chronic illness that can manifest with hip symptoms (such as sickle cell anemia and osteonecrosis of the femoral head), but because awareness of medical comorbidities have profound implications for surgical decision-making and perioperative management. While most hip surgeons will engage medical consultants prior to surgery when significant comorbid conditions are present, it is worth being aware of the common medical issues that bear most heavily on surgical outcomes. One commonly used systematic approach to this problem was recently outlined by Eagle et al. (2).

TABLE 26-1

ACTIVITY ENERGY REQUIREMENT ESTIMATES (METS)

1 MET	Self-care: feed, dress, toilet
	Ambulation in the house
	1–2 blocks community ambulation 2–3 mph
	Light housework
4 METs	Flight of stairs
	Community ambulation at 4 mph
	Run short distances
	Golf, bowling, dancing
10 METs	Strenuous sports, swimming, singles tennis, skiing, basketball

Adapted from Eagle KA, Brundage BH, Chaitman BR, et al. Guidelines to perioperative cardiovascular evaluation of noncardiac surgery. *Circulation.* 1996;93;1278–1317. Report of the American College of Cardiology/American Heart Association Task Force on Practical Guidelines.

TABLE 26-2

RISK PROFILE, BY TYPE OF SURGERY

High risk
- Major emergency surgery (increased risk if elderly)
- Aortic or other major vascular surgery
- Prolonged surgeries with expected large fluid shifts

Intermediate risk
- Carotid endarterectomy
- Major head/neck surgery
- Intraperitoneal, intrathoracic, and prostate surgery
- Major open orthopedic surgery (including arthroplasty)

Low risk
- Endoscopic surgery
- Arthroscopic surgery
- Superficial procedures

Adapted from Eagle KA, Brundage BH, Chaitman BR, et al. Guidelines to perioperative cardiovascular evaluation of noncardiac surgery. *Circulation.* 1996;93;1278–1317. Report of the American College of Cardiology/American Heart Association Task Force on Practical Guidelines.

This group's work suggests that perioperative cardiac risk in noncardiac surgery patients is closely related to several factors: the type of surgery and the hemodynamic effects specifically related to the procedure as well as the patient's cardiac functional capacity at baseline. Functional capacity can be expressed in metabolic equivalent levels (METs) and can indicate perioperative and long-term risks in surgical candidates. Patients unable to meet a 4 MET demand level (equivalent to climbing a flight of stairs) have a higher risk of perioperative cardiac conditions (Table 26-1). The task force also classified surgery-specific risks (Table 26-2), with emergency surgery being labeled high risk and many elective orthopedic procedures, including hip arthroplasty, being classified as intermediate risk (2).

Past Surgical History

As mentioned earlier, it is more convenient to gather information about prior operations on the affected hip(s) during the history of present illness. The more general past surgical history is useful for identifying otherwise overlooked medical comorbidities and systemic conditions. Sometimes, for example, patients who have had coronary artery bypass grafting, which may have cured angina for them, will not identify themselves as patients with significant coronary artery disease, as they consider themselves "cured." Responses to prior surgical treatments—whether of the hip, other joints, or other parts of the body—are sometimes predictive of postoperative response to future surgery and therefore may be helpful to obtain.

Social History

The social history provides important insight into the patient's treatment goals, available resources for postoperative recuperation, the demands the home environment might impose, and risk factors for poor surgical outcomes. Learning the type and intensity of patient's job demands is crucial for counseling about postoperative return to function and expected limitations. Awareness of whether the patient lives alone, whether the patient's home has stairs and where the available bedrooms are, and the proximity of the home to available care

(such as outpatient physical therapy for patients who live in more remote areas) play a role in the preoperative planning process. Social habits, such as excessive alcohol intake or illicit drug use, can predict noncompliance with aftercare and failure of arthroplasty because of traumatic dislocations and infections in intravenous drug users. Ongoing litigation and workers' compensation claims likewise are associated with failure in many types of elective orthopedic surgery, including lower-extremity reconstruction (7).

Family History and Review of Systems

These sections occasionally are helpful and are worth completing as part of an initial evaluation. Certain risk factors for osteonecrosis of the femoral head are heritable; for example, if a patient is diagnosed with a hypercoagulable state, family screening may be indicated. The review of systems will occasionally turn up constitutional complaints that can point toward or away from certain diagnoses (such as inflammatory arthritis or malignancy) and will more than occasionally identify uncontrolled or poorly managed medical comorbidities that need attention prior to elective surgical interventions.

THE PHYSICAL EXAMINATION

Gait

It is commonly stated that the physical examination begins when the patient walks into the exam room. A careful eye for gait abnormalities can provide valuable and occasionally diagnostic information before the surgeon even asks any questions. Four abnormal gait patterns commonly are seen in the hip clinic are described in this section.

Trendelenburg Gait

The Trendelenburg gait is seen in patients with abductor (gluteus medius) dysfunction, weakness, denervation, or transection; it is also known as "abductor lurch." Patients are noted to move their trunk and head over the affected hip just prior to the stance phase of gait to prevent falling to the unaffected side. This condition is nearly pathognomonic for intra-articular hip pathology, but it is not helpful for distinguishing one intra-articular cause from another.

Antalgic Gait
This gait is characterized by a shortened stance phase of the gait cycle. Any painful lower-extremity condition from hip to toes can cause it, but it commonly suggests the problem is other than the hip, as intra-articular hip pathology more typically will present with a Trendelenburg gait, if any gait abnormality is to be detected.

Circumduction
This pattern is most suggestive of limb-length inequality, particularly if there is also joint stiffness. In this gait pattern, the limb is rotated away from and then toward the body through the gait cycle to permit clearance of the long leg from the ground.

Steppage
This gait pattern requires a "high" step to clear the toes on the affected limb as a result of equinus deformity or foot drop. If the latter is present, the examining physician should seek an explanation from the patient. Etiologies include common peroneal and sciatic nerve palsies, L4-L5 nerve root pathology, and rarely myopathy (e.g., polio) or neuropathy.

Inspection: Posture, Leg Length, and Incisions

Patients with hip symptoms routinely should be disrobed and placed in a gown for a thorough orthopedic examination. Following examination of gait, it is worth having the patient stand for examination of posture from the front and from the side. From this inspection, the presence of spinal deformity, lower-extremity asymmetries or malalignments, and stigmata of systemic disease (such as the joint deformities of rheumatoid arthritis and the skin findings of psoriatic arthritis) can be identified.

Next, with the patient lying supine, an assessment of leg length should be made. So-called true leg length is determined by measuring from a fixed structure such as the anterior-superior iliac spine or the pubic symphysis to the medial malleolus and comparing that distance with the distance on the contralateral side. "Apparent" limb-length differences may be assessed by measuring from the umbilicus to the medial malleolus on each side; this is of fairly limited utility, and the patient's own perception of leg length has as much, if not more, clinical relevance.

Limb-length differences that are identified can be confirmed and the patient's perception of limb length assessed using leg-length blocks. It is also important to distinguish true leg-length differences from fixed pelvic obliquity. Inspection and palpation of the posterior superior iliac spines permit the examiner to do this; calibrated blocks further facilitate the process. Fixed pelvic obliquity will not be corrected with the calibrated blocks, and the examiner must then look at the lumbosacral spine as the most common etiology. Apparent pelvic obliquity that is corrected with the use of the blocks should lead the examiner back to a true leg-length discrepancy as the likely cause.

The final important element of inspection is examination of the hip(s) in question for prior incisions, wounds, and infectious signs such as draining sinuses.

Palpation

Palpation of bony landmarks about the pelvis and hips—including the iliac crests, anterior and posterior superior iliac spines, greater trochanters, and, if possible, the ischial tuberosities—should be done, as these are occasional trigger points in fibromyalgia patients or patients with tendonitis or enthesopathy. Provocative tests for certain para-articular pain sources, such as Ober's test for iliotibial band syndrome, can be performed now. With the patient lying on the table in a lateral decubitus position, the examiner abducts the leg while extending the hip to demonstrate tightness of the iliotibial band. While palpating the landmarks mentioned, it is necessary to document any areas of point tenderness as well as further evidence of pelvic obliquity.

Quick Tests for Intra-articular Pathology

One of the goals of the physical examination is to help distinguish intra-articular pathology from para-articular conditions and nonmusculoskeletal diagnoses. Several maneuvers offer presumptive evidence of an intra-articular hip condition; these maneuvers, perhaps with the exception of tests for femoroacetabular impingement, are not specific to particular conditions. It is worth noting that no physical exam maneuver is sufficiently sensitive or specific to malignancy, and imaging tests and appropriate tissue studies are required to make that diagnosis. Conversely, if a lesion is identified in the region of the hip on imaging, reasonable care should be used in manipulating the extremity on physical examination, and if the lesion poses a risk of pathological fracture, the patient should be advised to restrict weight bearing until appropriate treatment is arranged. Following are several tests that suggest intra-articular hip pathology:

Active Straight-Leg Raise
Telemetric studies demonstrate that a simple supine straight-leg raise of 6 inches generates a $1.8 \times$ body weight joint-reaction force across the hip joint (1). As a result, performing this maneuver often will trigger the familiar symptoms—whether groin pain, thigh pain, or buttock pain—if the symptoms are caused by intra-articular pathology. If the examiner adds slight manual resistance to the straight-leg raise, the test becomes more sensitive but less specific, as too much resistance might bother patients with low-back pain.

Passive Rotation and Flexion Contractures
Patients with intra-articular hip pathology frequently lose comfortable rotation before range of motion is affected in other planes. Many patients, in later stages of disease in fact go on to develop external rotation contractures. Passive internal rotation with the hip gently flexed will therefore reproduce the familiar hip symptoms in patients with intra-articular sources of pain. Asymmetric range of motion, particularly in rotation, also is suggestive of hip pathology.

Hip flexion contractures often are not diagnosed but can be severe and may have reconstructive implications. The presence of a flexion contracture is determined using the Thompson test. This maneuver involves having the patient extend both legs fully, then manually draw the asymptomatic (contralateral) hip to the chest and hold it tightly there using both arms. If the symptomatic hip remains flat on the table, no significant hip flexion contracture exists. Comparison can then be made with the opposite hip. If one of the hips has been replaced, this test should not be performed, as it requires taking the hip outside the safe motion range and risks dislocation.

Trendelenburg Test

This test is carried out with the examiner behind the standing patient. While observing the posterior superior iliac spine, the examiner asks the patient to stand on one leg. If abductor function is normal, the PSIS should remain level. If this does not occur, abductor dysfunction is confirmed.

Flexion–Adduction–Internal Rotation (Impingement) Test

Femoroacetabular impingement can be tested for by bringing the hip slowly to 90° of flexion, bringing it to adduction, and slowly internally rotating the femur; during this process it is possible to feel the position of anterior impingement (5). Likewise labral pathology can be elicited with a similar maneuver, the FADIR maneuver. Though the provocative tests for impingement and labral pathology are similar, these are in fact very different pathologies and difficult to distinguish on physical examination. Appropriate imaging studies often are diagnostic. Radiographs should include anteroposterior and lateral views, with the anteroposterior often appearing normal on viewing; the lateral view, however, will often show the classic osteophytes in the anterolateral neck. An MRI arthrogram should also be obtained to fully assess the labrum and the acetabular cartilage (3).

DISTAL NEUROCIRCULATORY EXAMINATION

While in common use, the terms "neurovascularly intact" or "NVI" have little information value. Invariably, should a patient's neurocirculatory status change following a proce-dure, having a more detailed description of the baseline status will be useful to the surgeon.

Important elements of the vascular examination include the presence and strength of peripheral pulses, skin temperature and color, and capillary refill. Significant abnormalities noted on this portion of the examination warrant preoperative workup and/or consultation.

Venous circulation is often overlooked on the baseline orthopedic examination. Findings suggestive of postthrombotic syndrome—including prominent varicosities, bluish discoloration of the feet or ankles, and venous stasis ulcers—should be evaluated before elective hip surgery using venous Doppler and duplex ultrasonography. Chronic deep-vein thrombosis is sometimes present in the age demographic of a typical reconstructive hip surgery practice, and awareness of this condition has implications for perioperative thromboprophylaxis.

Finally, the neurological status of the lower extremities should be assessed, with documentation of the motor function of muscles whose innervation may be in jeopardy during typical hip exposures, including the peroneal branch of the sciatic nerve (extensor hallucis longus and tibialis anterior muscle function) and the femoral nerve (quadriceps function). Deep tendon reflexes or their absence should be documented, as should any sensory changes. Abnormalities identified on physical examination should be evaluated prior to elective hip surgery.

REFERENCES

1. Davy DT, Kotzar GM, Brown RH, et al. Telemetric force measurements across the hip after arthroplasty: *J Bone Joint Surg [Am]*. 1980;70:45.
2. Eagle KA, Brundage BH, Chaitman BR, et al. Guidelines to perioperative cardiovascular evaluation of noncardiac surgery. *Circulation*. 1996;93;1278–1317. Report of the American College of Cardiology/American Heart Association Task Force on Practical Guidelines.
3. Ganz R, Parvizi J, Beck M, et al. Femoroacetabular impingement: a cause for osteoarthritis of the hip. *Clin Orthop Rel Res.* 2003;417; 112–120.
4. Guerra JJ, Steinberg M. Current concepts review: distinguishing transient osteoporosis from avascular necrosis of the hip. *J Bone Joint Surg [Am]*.1995;77:616–624.
5. MacDonald SJ, Garbuz D, Ganz R. Clinical evaluation of the symptomatic young adult hip. *Semin Arthroplasty*. 1997;8:3–9.
6. McCarthy JC, Noble PC, Schuck MR, et al. The role of labral lesions to development of early degenerative hip disease. *Clin Orthop Rel Res.* 2001;393:25–37.
7. Mont MA, Mayerson JA, Krackow KA, et al. Total knee arthroplasty in patients receiving workers' compensation. *J Bone Joint Surg [Am]*. 1998;80:1285–1290.

Radiographic Evaluation of the Hip

Derek R. Armfield   *Jeffrey D. Towers*

Radiography remains the primary diagnostic imaging tool for disease of the adult hip and serves as a crucial first step in a comprehensive imaging strategy. Unfortunately, it is all too common to witness diagnostic and therapeutic misadventures initiated by the results of advanced imaging studies interpreted in isolation, which are only resolved when a plain radiograph is carefully reviewed. It cannot be overemphasized that all other imaging modalities should be interpreted as complementary to the initial plain radiographs.

ROUTINE RADIOGRAPHY

Diagnostic Goals

It is critical that radiography of the hip be both performed and interpreted accurately so that reliable data are used in diagnosis and management. Defined goals for image quality and diagnosis, tailored to the clinical setting in which radiography is performed, aid in reducing the exposure of patients and staff to ionizing radiation from unnecessary or repeat examinations and provide for more efficient and cost-effective clinical practice.

The clinical setting defines the ordered differential diagnosis that must be satisfied by the radiographic examination. In the setting of acute trauma, fracture and dislocation (and their sequelae) are of foremost concern. In the setting of chronic mechanical pain, disorders of the hip articulation or associated myotendinous structures become paramount, and in the presentation of nonmechanical pain, neoplasm and infection are more highly considered. For surgical follow-up, evaluation of hardware or prosthetic position and fixation, status of bone healing, and complications of intervention are of greatest interest. Finally, the condition and habitus of the patient become important considerations in performing and interpreting radiographs, particularly in the setting of acute trauma and surgical follow-up. An imaging strategy should not only provide accurate diagnosis and staging of the primary disorder, but also screen for other differential considerations and associated pathology in an orderly progression based on the likelihood of pathology and the relative strengths of imaging modalities with respect to their costs.

Screening radiography is the primary imaging study of such a strategy, with supplemental radiographic views or complementary imaging studies obtained either to clarify findings from screening radiographs or to identify pathology that may be radiographically occult when the likelihood or significance of occult pathology warrants further imaging.

Equipment, Film Screens, Quality Assurance

Radiographs are commonly obtained in three settings: the hospital radiology department (commonly from the emergency department), the portable examination in the operating suite or recovery room, and examination in the outpatient setting. The widest variety of equipment and technique is encountered in the outpatient setting. A blinded review of film quality by Levin et al. involving examinations performed by radiologists and nonradiologists found great differences in quality among practitioners, with examinations performed under a radiologist's supervision to be of the highest quality. Orthopedists ranked significantly but only slightly behind, followed by a variety of physician subspecialists whose examinations were clearly inferior in quality. Nonphysicians (podiatrists, chiropractors, etc.) ranked last in film quality with the majority of studies performed by some groups being insufficient for diagnosis (80).

One reason for this difference in quality may be differences in radiographic equipment, particularly in the outpatient setting. The production of high-quality images begins with high-quality equipment appropriate for the demands of imaging various parts of the body. The radiographic image begins with the x-ray generator and tube, which in concert produce the x-ray beam consisting of electrons boiled from the surface of a tungsten filament. Metal collimators then cone the beam to suit the size and shape of the object to be studied, avoiding excessive exposure of the patient and scattered radiation. As the beam passes through the body, differential attenuation of the x-ray beam by various types of substances and tissues yields the levels of gray that provide image contrast. The beam then encounters metallic grids of various types that reduce scattered radiation after the beam leaves the body, further improving spatial resolution and contrast. Finally, there is the cassette, which when exposed to radiation produces visible light which in turn exposes the silver emulsion on the film with the image we recognize as the radiograph. High-voltage, three-phase generators are recommended for most radiographic examinations, particularly those involving larger body parts, like the hip, which require greater penetration and flux of x-ray photons. Lower-voltage, single-phase generators are often used in outpatient settings solely for distal extremity radiographs, which require much less generator performance but are inappropriate for examination of larger body parts. Some single-phase, fully rectified, high-frequency generators approach the performance of three-phase generators and may be used for larger body parts, eliminating the need for special power lines and siting restrictions (127).

The film–screen combination most commonly used for hip radiography is dual-emulsion regular speed with a dual-sided phosphorous screen cassette. Although greater detail and exposure latitude may be obtained from single-emulsion fine-grain film, the radiation exposure necessary for such film is much greater and is generally not considered to be worthwhile in the hip, where the benefit of added spatial resolution is minimal and the drawback of gonadal irradiation is of great concern. Several manufacturers market high-speed film, which reduces exposure in examination of the hip by using larger or planar silver granules in the film emulsion. The larger grain size reduces spatial resolution, and the benefit of reduced exposure must be weighed against this loss of diagnostic information.

Radiographic grids are metallic and polymer devices that are somewhat like a thin louvered shade and are constructed to align the metallic linear shades, commonly made of lead, with the plane of the x-ray beam, between the patient and the film cassette. The grid shades allow only those x-ray beams aligned with the grid to pass, blocking out scattered beams from the patient which greatly degrade image quality. Although the use of a grid slightly increases the radiation dose received by the patient, it is essential to high-quality radiography, particularly of large body parts such as the hip, which generate a great deal of scattered radiation (127).

PACS

Radiology departments, hospitals, and imaging centers are increasingly converting processes to filmless or digital-only work flow environment. This transformation process requires the incorporation of a picture archival computer system (PACS). Components of a PACS system include digital source images, computer network, database server, archival system, patient information database/security (radiology information systems), and end-user interfaces and workstations (120).

Cross sectional modalities such as computed tomography (CT) and magnetic resonance imaging (MRI) have digital output capabilities, but plain films are typically acquired via computed radiography (CR) or digital radiography (DR) equipment, although images could be digitized from conventional radiographs with a scanner. The major difference between CR and DR technologies is that CR requires user handling between x-ray exposure (i.e., handling a film cassette) and image acquisition (laser reading of x-ray information), whereas DR either directly or indirectly transforms x-ray data into a digital image without interval handling (120). This results in potentially faster acquisition and improved work flow, although DR is typically more expensive.

While there are many benefits for the orthopedist in a filmless work environment, including elimination of lost films, timeliness of image availability, and ability to view images remotely, many challenges remain in orthopedic workflow pertaining to the hip. Preoperative planning is variably available electronically and is often vendor limited. Printing images to accurate full size may pose challenges, and intraoperative image management is not fully optimized. Finally, full integration of electronic image delivery and patient information systems has not matured to provide a consistent outpatient-to-inpatient environment. Because of the complexity, many workflow and budgetary issues must be addressed prior to the implementation of a PACS system, as the transformation process can be expensive, time-consuming, and subject to user and clinician frustration. However, the benefits include improved efficiency, decreased costs, improved user convenience and satisfaction, and potentially improved diagnostic capabilities.

QUALITY ASSURANCE

A comprehensive quality assurance program is vital to any practitioner who performs radiographs, not only to ensure high standards of film quality but to ensure that radiation exposures are within acceptable standards. The process includes routine calibration and periodic inspection of radiography equipment, commonly as part of the manufacturer's service contract, and daily monitoring of film developers. Ongoing inspection of cassettes for defects or contaminants that result in artifacts, film exposure and positioning technique, and review of overall image quality are essential. Finally, blinded comparison of film interpretation between readers, with grading of interpretive variance in categories of significance related to patient care, completes the quality assurance process (127).

SAFETY ISSUES

Exposure to ionizing radiation entails minimal but very real risk, which can be segregated into somatic risk to the patient (or those otherwise exposed to radiation, including in utero offspring), and genetic risk to the human genome by gonadal irradiation. To an individual, the effect of radiation exposure increases in significance with greater total exposure, which may be cumulative over many years, and the individual's age. The younger the individual, the more significant the effect of exposure. Many factors, including natural background radiation, may influence how much radiation exposure would theoretically induce carcinogenesis or measurable genetic mutations in a population, and though there is considerable disagreement regarding the relative biological risk of radiation, guidelines exist for acceptable exposure for diagnostic purposes (48).

The unit used to express radiation exposure has traditionally been the roentgen (R); the radiation dose is the roentgen absorbed dose (rad); and the normalized dose, which accounts for modifiers of exposure, is the roentgen equivalent in humans (rem). The SI unit used to denote radiation dose is the gray (Gy), which is equivalent to 100 rad, and for normalized dose, the sievert (Sv), which is equivalent to 100 rem. The National Council on Radiation Protection and Measurements periodically issues recommendations on exposure allowances, which have progressively diminished over the past decades as more data regarding biological effects of radiation are available. Current maximal permissible doses are 1.5 rem/person/year for the general population and 5 rem/person/year for those in a profession in which exposure to radiation is necessary (43). Those professionals or workers who exceed this maximum permissible dose may be restricted in their use of and proximity to radiation devices. Workers routinely exposed to ionizing radiation are issued radiation badge monitors, which allow a cumulative record of exposure.

The underlying assumption of these guidelines is that all radiation is potentially harmful, and all reasonable steps to reduce exposure should be uniformly undertaken. For patients, these steps include prescreening women of childbearing age for the possibility that they may be pregnant (to avoid fetal exposure), appropriate shielding of genitals, and accurate examination performance to minimize repeat exposures. For personnel, monitoring of career exposure by dosimeters, shielding of the body and thyroid, and strict attention to fluoroscopic technique are of vital importance. Finally, the ordering physician may make the greatest impact in reducing patient and personnel exposure with judicious use of diagnostic fluoroscopy and radiography.

POSITIONING AND TECHNIQUE

The radiographic study of the hip most commonly consists of an anteroposterior (AP) and either a cross-table or externally rotated frog-leg lateral view (50). We also include an AP view of the pelvis in our screening examination of the hip to examine the sacrum, sacroiliac joints, pelvis, and contralateral hip. In the setting of atraumatic pain, the hip may be internally rotated for the AP radiograph, which accommodates femoral anteversion and brings the femoral neck into a plane perpendicular to the anteroposterior x-ray beam. For the lateral projection, the patient's hip is flexed and externally rotated with the x-ray beam directed anteroposteriorly (Figs. 27-1 and 27-2).

Bony landmarks are helpful for determining adequacy of the AP and lateral exposures. On the AP radiograph, the greater tuberosity and lesser tuberosity should be clearly defined. The greater tuberosity should not significantly overlap the femoral neck. The calcar femoris should be clearly visible, and there should be very little elliptical overlap between the anterior and posterior margins of the femoral head–neck junction. The most common error in AP radiography of the hip is that of allowing external rotation of the hip (Fig. 27-3). This results in overlap of the greater trochanter with the femoral neck and medially profiles the lesser tuberosity. At the level of the femoral head–neck junction, it results in lack of parallelism between the femoral head and x-ray beam with the posterior femoral head–neck junction projecting superior to the anterior femoral head–neck junction. This may occasionally be of some diagnostic concern, particularly where femoral head osteophytosis overlaps the subcapital region of the femoral neck in external rotation, simulating a sclerotic fracture line (see Fig. 27-32).

In the setting of trauma, the study is performed with as little manipulation of the patient's position as possible. For the AP radiograph, this may accomplished by rotating the entire patient to achieve a true AP of the hip. Similarly, the lateral radiograph is obtained by a cross-table lateral in which the contralateral hip is flexed, and the beam is directed laterally with caudocephalad angulation across the femoral neck. If after examination by this technique no fracture can be detected, a frog-leg lateral may be obtained depending on the likelihood of fracture by clinical examination (50).

SPECIAL VIEWS

Pelvis

Inlet and outlet views are generally employed in addition to the AP radiograph in evaluation of the bony pelvis (Fig. 27-4). The inlet view is obtained from an AP projection angled caudally approximately 40°. In this projection, the ring of the pelvis is optimally delineated. Fractures of the pubic rami and rotational malalignment of the pelvis are best assessed. The outlet projection is obtained again in the AP plane with cranial angulation of again approximately 40°. Vertical translation or malalignment of the pelvis is best demonstrated by this projection (137).

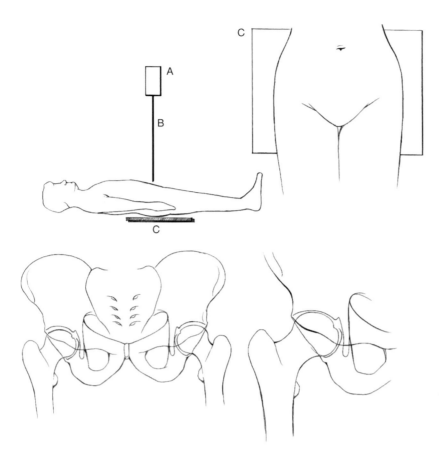

Figure 27-1 Technique for AP radiography of the pelvis and hip: x-ray tube (*A*), collimated x-ray beam (*B*), and film cassette (*C*). The exposure is centered between the umbilicus and pubis for the pelvic examination and centered over the ilioinguinal ligament for AP radiograph of the hip.

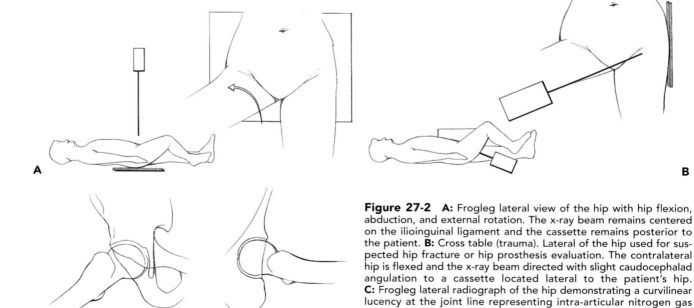

Figure 27-2 **A:** Frogleg lateral view of the hip with hip flexion, abduction, and external rotation. The x-ray beam remains centered on the ilioinguinal ligament and the cassette remains posterior to the patient. **B:** Cross table (trauma). Lateral of the hip used for suspected hip fracture or hip prosthesis evaluation. The contralateral hip is flexed and the x-ray beam directed with slight caudocephalad angulation to a cassette located lateral to the patient's hip. **C:** Frogleg lateral radiograph of the hip demonstrating a curvilinear lucency at the joint line representing intra-articular nitrogen gas (*arrow*) formed during intra-articular negative pressure from hip abduction and flexion.

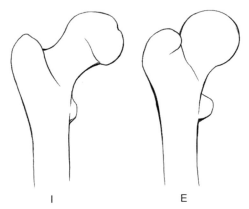

Figure 27-3 Line representation of internal and external AP radiographs of a hip. In internal rotation, the femoral neck is elongated and the lesser trochanter less pronounced. With external rotation, the greater trochanter overlaps the femoral neck to a greater extent and the lesser trochanter is more prominent in profile.

Acetabulum

The acetabulum is evaluated on the AP radiograph and, most commonly, with Judet method obliques when supplemental views are obtained. Judet obliques are obtained by rotating the patient approximately 45° from the supine position with the beam directed anteroposteriorly (Fig. 27-5A). Although one hip may be collimated in isolation, this view is commonly used to evaluate both acetabula simultaneously. The anterior oblique acetabulum has its anterior (iliopubic) column and posterior rim best delineated, while the posterior oblique best demonstrates the posterior (ilioischial) column and the anterior rim (Fig. 27-5B) (50).

Other views for evaluation of the acetabulum, including the false profile view, sitting AP, sitting lateral, and Chassard–Lapine semiaxial views have been used in the past (78). The information demonstrated by these views is now more reliably and accurately portrayed by computed tomography, and these views are rarely used in current practice.

Hip

A variety of special views of the hip have been described, primarily for evaluation of the weight-bearing surface in various positions (40). These include abduction/adduction AP views, weight-bearing acetabular oblique views, sitting AP and sitting lateral views (135). Traction radiography, used to outline the articular surfaces of the hip by forming nitrogen gas during joint distraction, has also been described for evaluation of the articular surface of the hip (89) (Fig. 27-6). These supplemental views are rarely used clinically, having been largely replaced by CT and MRI.

TOMOGRAPHY

The role for conventional tomography of the hip has progressively diminished with the advent of CT and MRI. The benefits of tomography primarily lie in its ability to directly image the hip in the coronal and sagittal plane, demonstrating the contour of the femoral head and neck. The relative drawbacks of the technique are its limited tissue contrast, artifacts from metallic hardware, radiation exposure, and cost as other techniques utilizing electronic display (CT and MRI) become more rapid and less expensive (35). The most common indication for hip tomography is the characterization of displaced femoral neck fractures. Tomography has traditionally been the method of choice for evaluation of complicated avascular necrosis in which characterization of the degree and extent of femoral head flattening may affect management. This role has largely been replaced by MRI, which can directly assess femoral head marrow, the subchondral plate, and the articular surface of the hip simultaneously (132). Although tomography may occasionally reveal fractures in a patient that are not seen by plain films, its role in evaluating radiographically occult acute fractures of the femoral neck has been replaced by MRI as well (114). This is particularly relevant to the patient with decreased bone mass (particularly the elderly) in whom fractures of the femoral neck are often both radiographically occult and not demonstrable by conventional tomography, but clearly evident at MRI examination (91).

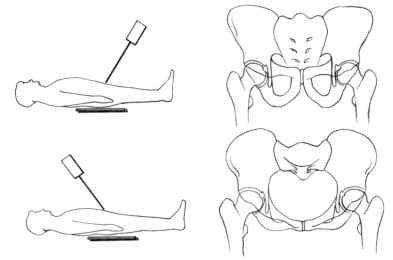

Figure 27-4 Outlet and inlet views of the pelvis. The outlet view (*top*) provides a projection parallel to the plane of the pelvic rim and perpendicular to the face of the sacrum. The sacrum appears elongated, the symphysis pubis overlies it, the obturator foramina are prominent, and the ischial tuberosities and ischiopubic synchondroses are well demonstrated. Vertical instability of the pelvis is best assessed on this view. Pelvic inlet view (*below*) parallel to the anterior sacral surface demonstrating the pelvic rim. Rotational instability of the pelvis is best examined with this projection.

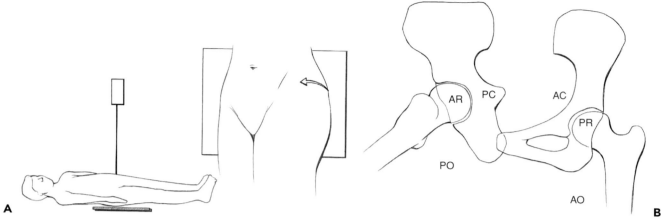

Figure 27-5 **A:** Judet oblique view of the hip (right posterior oblique, left anterior oblique). The patient is rotated with respect to the cassette and the cassette exposed through an anteroposterior approach. The opposite oblique (left posterior oblique, right anterior oblique) would be obtained by rotating the patient in the opposite direction. **B:** Linear representation of radiographic anatomy for Judet oblique (right posterior oblique, left posterior oblique). Note demonstration of contralateral column and acetabular rim anatomy. Posterior oblique (PO) demonstrates the posterior column and anterior rim, while the anterior oblique (AO) demonstrates the anterior column and posterior rim anatomy.

Tomography of the hip is best performed by complex polytomography rather than linear tomography, as greater spatial resolution and spatial separation is possible with greater complexity of tube and film cassette motion. The machinery required to perform polytomography accurately must be manufactured at very close tolerances to allow complex motion, while at the same time maintaining a very consistent and narrow (1 to 3 mm) plane of resolution. Increasingly, the cost of tomographic equipment and maintenance makes the examination less attractive from a cost standpoint. At our institution, the charges for single-plane tomography (coronal or sagittal only) exceeds that of CT of the hip. Two-plane tomography (coronal and sagittal) exceeds that of MRI examination. While some of this

increased cost is due to decreased utilization of tomography as CT and MRI are more heavily utilized, much of the increased cost of tomography lies with the diminishing number of tomography manufacturers, greater cost in service and repair of equipment, and greater cost in technologist time to perform the examination.

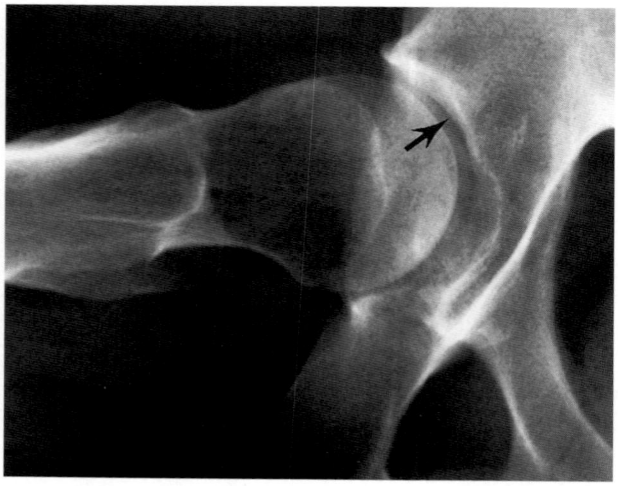

COMPUTED TOMOGRAPHY

Computed tomography is commonly used to evaluate the hip, both for primary disorders of the hip and for postoperative evaluation, particularly of prostheses (39,102,1134).

The most common use of CT in evaluating primary disorders of the hip is for the evaluation of trauma (Fig. 27-7). Depiction of pelvic/acetabular fractures and osseous sequelae of hip dislocation, and, importantly, detection of intra-articular osseous fragments are better performed by CT than by plain radiography or tomography. The greater tissue contrast of CT when compared with radiography and tomography allows detection of periarticular pathology related to trauma, including characterization of deep retroperitoneal hematomas and peripheral degloving injuries.

In the clinical setting of a neoplasm, the most common use of CT is characterization of calcifications seen by plain radiography. This may include tumor matrix within bone or characterization of soft tissue calcification or ossification. CT is rarely used in our institution for evaluation of arthritis, which is predominantly diagnosed by plain radiography. The use of finecut CT with multiplanar reconstruction algorithms has been described by several authors for evaluating hip pathology (94). Although touted as an alternative to planar tomography with advantages in speed, multiplanar display, and tissue contrast, this technique has not gained wide acceptance in clinical practice to date because the CT study must be carefully performed and reconstructed at the CT console. With recent advances in CT workstations and reconstruction software,

Figure 27-6 Frog-leg lateral radiograph of the hip demonstrating a curvilinear lucency at the joint line representing intra-articular nitrogen gas (*arrow*) formed during intra-articular negative pressure from hip abduction and flexion.

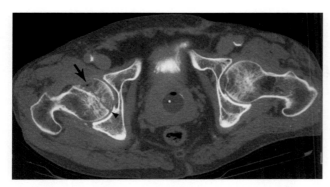

Figure 27-7 Transaxial CT of the hips showing a transchondral fracture of the right femoral head. Avulsive transchondral defect anteriorly (*arrow*) lies at the margin of a rotated transchondral fragment. Medial extent (*arrowhead*) shows involvement of the posterior margin of the fovea.

some expect that in the near future multiplanar CT will further replace tomography for most applications.

For evaluation of the prosthetic hip, CT offers several advantages over plain radiography and tomography. Some artifact is typically encountered from metallic prosthetic components, but this can be minimized by increasing the kilovolt potential (KvP) and milliampere (MaS) settings of the x-ray tube, which provides a more energetic beam and more photon flux for the x-ray detectors (see Fig. 27-9). While this more energetic photon profile may diminish soft tissue contrast, it does allow depiction of osseous structures adjacent to prosthetic components in the majority of cases. Titanium components are particularly well imaged by CT as their x-ray attenuation is much less than that of stainless steel and chromium alloys.

Examination of the prosthetic hip by CT directly demonstrates the axial relationships of components and is generally obtained in the clinical setting of recurrent prosthetic dislocation or chronic pain. Evaluation of component position, osseous integrity of bone stock, detection and characterization of intrapelvic cement, and detection of prosthetic loosening may take place (99,109).

Tilt (or abduction) of the acetabular component of total hip arthroplasty is evaluated on the AP scanogram, or scout view, in a fashion similar to that of plain radiography. The scanogram is a digital radiograph acquired by moving the patient through the bore of the scanner using the motorized

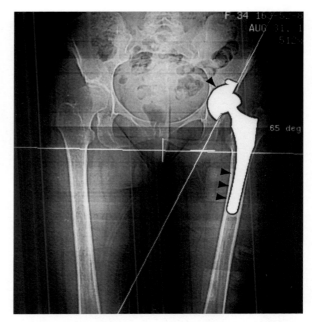

Figure 27-8 AP CT scanogram of the pelvis showing 65° abduction of left total hip arthroplasty relative to the interischial line. Prominent duct band about metallic total hip arthroplasty component represents a normal CT artifact (*arrowheads*).

table while the detectors and x-ray tube are held stationary. The acetabular angle is measured relative to a line drawn across the ischial tuberosities, normally 40° plus or minus 10° (Fig. 27-8). Acetabular version may be directly measured from an axial CT image obtained through the central portion of the acetabular prosthesis. Although it may be necessary to image the acetabular component at the superior margin of the metallic femoral head component to reduce scatter, this generally does not affect accuracy and is often unnecessary when higher KvP and MaS technique is used. Acetabular version is measured relative to perpendicular from a line drawn across the ischial spines, normally 10° plus or minus 5° (Fig. 27-9).

For patients presenting for revision of acetabular components of total hip arthroplasty, clinical diagnostic goals are determining the adequacy of bone stock of the anterior and posterior columns and localizing intrapelvic cement relative to pelvic vasculature. We use high-KvP, high-MaS technique

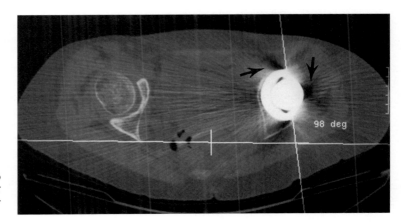

Figure 27-9 Transaxial CT examination of total hip arthroplasty showing 8° anteversion (from perpendicular to interischial spinous line). Note significant beam hardening artifact (*arrows*), but overall diagnostic study.

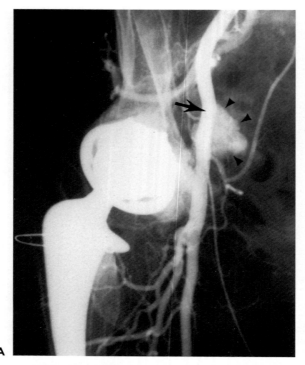

A

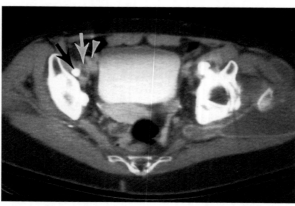

B

Figure 27-10   Preoperative evaluation for total hip arthroplasty revision. **A:** AP exposure during common iliac arteriography. The common iliac artery (*arrow*) overlies a large intrapelvic collection of cement (*arrowheads*). **B:** Noncontrast transaxial CT of the pelvis showing intrapelvic cement (*black arrow*), iliopsoas muscle (*white arrow*), and common iliac artery and vein (*arrowhead*). Since vascular anatomy showed no contact between major vasculature and intrapelvic cement and had little artifact, intravenous contrast was not used. Contact of vessels with cement or proximity within 1 cm is considered to be indicative of vasculature at risk for injury during revision.

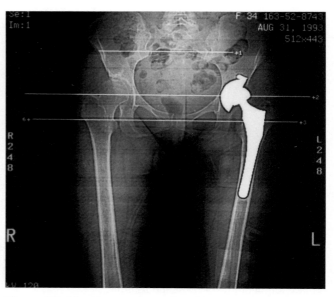

Figure 27-11   AP scanogram of total hip arthroplasty showing cuts through the center of the femoral head and widest portion of the femoral stem. A scan was also obtained through the femoral condyles.

with 3-mm collimation cuts taken at 5-mm intervals from approximately 3 cm above the acetabular cup through the symphysis pubis. Acetabular protrusio and osseous deficiency of the anterior column, posterior column, or both are reliably demonstrated by this technique. In our experience, localization of intrapelvic cement with respect to pelvic vasculature has generally not required intravenous contrast (102) (Fig. 27-10). Studies are monitored as they are performed, and, if the pelvic vasculature is well seen, contrast is not administered. If there is

difficulty visualizing the pelvic vasculature as it relates to intrapelvic cement, intravenous contrast is then administered to clarify their spatial relationship.

A dynamic CT examination of the prosthetic hip to detect axial loosening of the femoral component has been described, which we have modified for use in our clinical practice to evaluate patients with mechanical-type pain and equivocal radiographs (39,109). A preliminary AP scanogram is obtained, and axial images through the center of the femoral head, the widest portion of the femoral stem (prosthetic metaphysis), and the midfemoral condyles are obtained (Fig. 27-11). With a specially designed positioning boot, the leg is maximally internally and externally rotated, the end point being patient discomfort. CT images through the prosthetic femoral metaphysis and femoral condyles are then repeated. Measurement of prosthetic femoral metaphyseal anteversion is then made in the neutral, internal rotation, and external rotation positions and compared. Measurement error is considered to be <2° (Fig. 27-12). A discrepancy of measured anteversion >2° between any of the three positions is considered evidence of axial rotation of the femoral stem within the medullary canal of the femur (Fig. 27-13). When using these criteria, Fletcher found dynamic CT examination to be 91.6% sensitive and 90% specific with a positive predictive value of 91.6% in differentiating patients with loose components from those with documented stability (39). Reinus et al. used a similar technique using different femoral condylar landmarks and without using a positioning boot, reporting 67% sensitivity and 100% specificity for femoral component loosening (109). Their diminished sensitivity was from failure to diagnosis what they termed partial loosening, defined as intraoperative movement of a femoral stem with a torque wrench using force between 8.5 and 17 N m.

For the subgroup of patients with late femoral prosthetic pain and unequivocal plain radiographic evidence of loosening,

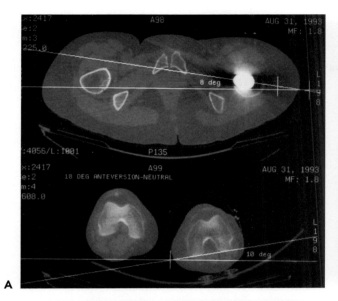

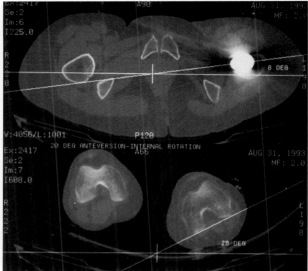

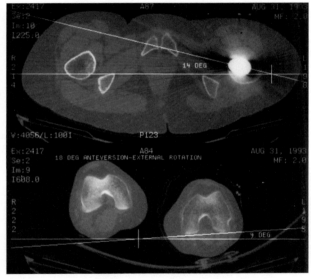

Figure 27-12 **A:** Transaxial images through the femoral component (*top*) and femoral condyles (*bottom*). The angle between the axis of the femoral component and the posterior intercondylar line represents the degree of version of the femoral component. In the neutral position, it measured 18°. **B:** With internal rotation, the angle between the femoral component and posterior condylar line of the femur measured 20°, within acceptable measurement error. **C:** With external rotation, femoral anteversion measures 18°, identical to neutral position.

there is likely no benefit in further imaging to determine femoral fixation. By contrast, the patient with equivocal radiographic evidence of loosening in the setting of pain often benefits from such an examination, in our experience. The alternative choices to detect prosthetic loosening are radionuclide imaging, which has mixed results in predicting loosening; hip arthrography, which carries a very small but real risk of introducing infection to a sterile prosthesis; and operative dislocation to evaluate fixation of the femoral component (1,4,7,70,95).

Multislice/Multidetector CT

The latest generation CT scanners are faster and provide greater detail than their predecessors. Known as multislice or multidetector scanners, they employ a larger detector segmented into smaller independent detectors instead of single x-ray detectors capturing information (4 to 64 detectors). This allows scanners to acquire data more quickly and with a thinner collimation so

that the volumetric data contains volume elements, or voxels, that are similar in size in *x*, *y*, and *z* dimensions. This process is known as an isotropic data set acquisition and allows reformatted images to be obtained in any plane of reformation with similar high spatial resolution (19).

Increased photon flux can help decrease metallic artifact, which is often a problem in imaging the postoperative hip. In general the amount of photon flux is limited by tube current. With multislice CT, low pitch setting can result in higher effective tube limits and increased photon flux, which can decrease metallic artifact and allow for better assessment of adjacent bone and soft tissues around metal (19) (Fig. 27-14). Conventional helical CT has been used to evaluate for acetabular osteolysis and periprosthetic bone and soft tissue changes suspicious for infection (21,28). Decreased artifact associated with multislice CT may allow for improved diagnoses.

One disadvantage of multislice CT is increased radiation dose, which mathematically has a small but real potential to induce cancer (41,66).This issue is particularly important in

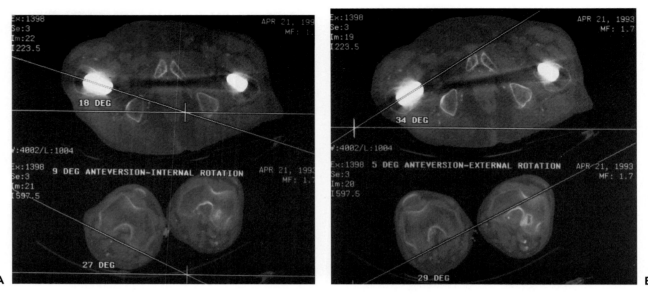

Figure 27-13 CT rotation study in patient with pain but no radiographic features of loosening. **A:** Nine degrees anteversion is measured between the femoral component and posterior condylar line in internal rotation. **B:** Five degrees anteversion is measured between the femoral stem and posterior intercondylar line during external rotation. This represents a significant discrepancy and indicates axial rotation of the femoral component within the femur during external rotation.

the pediatric population, where parameters for CT should be adjusted to prevent excessive radiation, as these patients have more radiosensitive tissue and a smaller body habitus which increases radiation dose (24). In the adult orthopaedic population this issue is less sensitive because of examination of hardware often involves extremities which are less radiosensitive.

However, pelvic and gonadal radiation does occur with CT examination of the hip, and excessive and inappropriate use should be avoided particularly in younger and smaller individuals. There should also be consideration for discussing these risks with patients by the ordering physician or radiologists, as patients are often uniformed (76). Another small

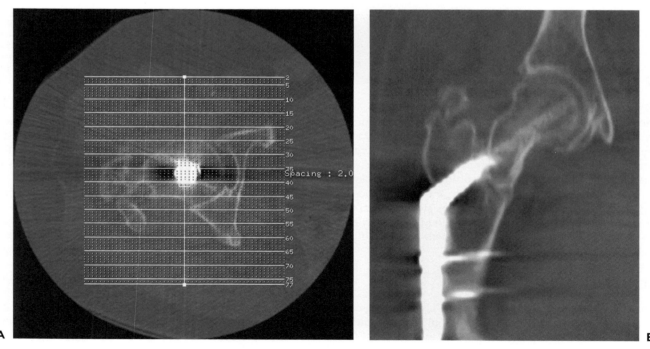

Figure 27-14 **A:** Scout image from multislice CT demonstrating coronal orientation of reformatted images in a patient with persistent pain after dynamic hip screw placement. **B:** Isotropic reformatted image demonstrates minimal artifact and persistent fracture line.

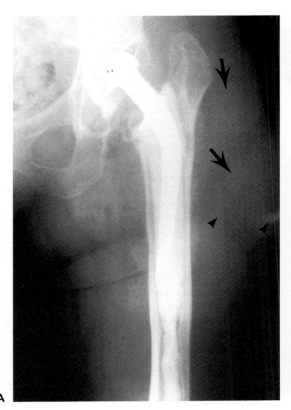 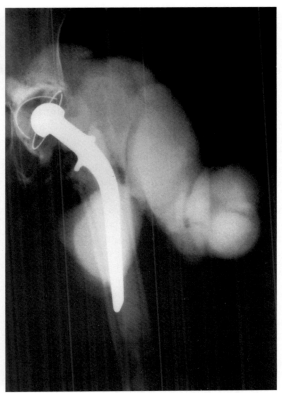

A   B

Figure 27-15 Arthrogram of infected total hip arthroplasty. **A:** Initial radiograph shows marked bone cement interface lucency about both the femoral and acetabular components with total hip arthroplasty. Note the lobulated soft tissue mass lateral to the femur (*arrows*) and cement debris within the lobulated mass (*arrowheads*). **B:** Postinjection arthrogram showing large sinus tract emanating from infected total hip arthroplasty corresponding to soft tissue mass seen in A.

disadvantage of multislice is the large volumetric data set that is created and must be interpreted and stored. Conventional axial interpretation methods of each image can be overwhelming, and 3D workstation analysis of data will be increasingly utilized as software and hardware constraints improve (119).

HIP ASPIRATION AND ARTHROGRAPHY

For the patient with acute, unilateral, atraumatic hip pain with normal radiographic findings, the clinical differential includes gout, pseudogout, and infection. Prompt aspiration of the hip for detection of infection is mandatory, either in the operating suite or in the radiology department (106).

Prior to aspiration, the common femoral artery is palpated and marked with a permanent marker. The skin is prepared with iodine soap (Betadine) and the area draped in a sterile fashion. Adherence of strict aseptic technique is mandatory to avoid introducing microorganisms through the skin, and it is imperative to avoid areas of abnormal skin during needle placement.

A variety of approaches have been described for fluoroscopic needle placement. All share a common goal of placing the needle at the femoral head–neck junction above the zona orbicularis, where joint fluid typically accumulates. We generally use an anterior approach in hip arthrography, with the

patient positioned supine, knee slightly flexed, and the hip held in internal rotation by sandbags applied to the leg and foot laterally. Under fluoroscopic examination, the skin is marked lateral to the femoral artery. Following skin preparation and draping, the needle is placed through the skin and, using sequential fluoroscopic images, is advanced toward the femoral head–neck junction along the lateral margin of the femoral head. Joint aspiration may be performed if fluid can be collected at this location. If no fluid is obtained, confirmation of needle position may be made by instillation of radiographic contrast. Although authors have previously reported bactericidal effects of radiographic contrast, it has been more recently shown that nonionic contrast agents show no bactericidal or bacteriostatic properties and that most ionic contrast agents display no significant bactericidal effects either (13). In the setting of suspected hip infection, we generally use nonionic contrast agents for confirmation of needle placement. After needle placement is confirmed, nonbacteriostatic saline is instilled and reaspirated, with the fluid submitted for gross, crystal, and chemical analysis as well as culture and Gram stain (Fig. 27-15).

For evaluation of the prosthetic hip, arthrography is used to detect infection (both with aspiration and by definition of sinus tracts) and has also been used to evaluate for prosthetic loosening.

In suspected prosthetic loosening, the arthrogram technique is modified (95,139). The patient is again positioned supine with the hip in internal rotation fixed by sandbags applied to the lateral aspect of the leg and foot. The femoral artery is again palpated and marked, and an anterolateral approach is used so that the radiopaque femoral head does not obscure needle position. The needle is directed toward a concave surface at the femoral head–neck junction of the component where fluid is likely to collect. Once the needle has been placed on the metallic component, aspiration is attempted. If fluid is obtained, it is submitted for analysis as above. Once this is accomplished, the position of the needle tip is confirmed with a very small injection of contrast, generally Renografin 60. Upon confirmation of needle position, a scout image of the entire component in the AP projection is obtained. A manual subtraction film may be made, or if digital subtraction equipment is available this may also be used. Progressive injection of 5-mL aliquots of contrast is made and serial exposures are obtained. Larger aliquots may be administered as the study progresses and the capacitance of the pseudocapsule is established. Subtraction technique with subsequent exposures may be used to outline contrast accumulation between bone and acrylic cement or the prosthesis. Following instillation of contrast, CT or conventional tomography may also be used to supplement the examination.

PERCUTANEOUS BONE BIOPSY

Biopsy of cancellous and cortical bone may be performed percutaneously with a variety of trephine needles. The study may be performed fluoroscopically or more commonly done under CT guidance. After preliminary examination, a route of needle placement is selected that avoids neurovascular structures. In the setting of suspected tumor, particularly sarcoma, consultation should be made with the orthopedic oncologist to define soft tissue planes to be crossed during the procedure, to be coordinated with potential resection surgery (111).

A skin mark is made over the appropriate entry site and the site is thoroughly prepared with iodine soap. The site is then draped with sterile towels. Using sequential CT images or fluoroscopic guidance, the needle guide and trocar are placed at the cortical surface. The trocar is then removed and replaced by the trephine needle, which is rotated and pushed through the bone cortex. Once the cortex has been traversed, the cortical plug is cleared and submitted for histopathologic examination. The trephine needle is then replaced into the defect in the cortex and advanced through the cancellous bone. On removal, the cancellous bone plug is expressed by a plunger inserted into the trephine needle. Marrow aspiration may be performed at the same time, either through the cortical hole with the trephine needle or following cancellous biopsy. By varying the approach through the cortical window, numerous cancellous biopsies may be obtained in a similar fashion.

PERCUTANEOUS SOFT TISSUE BIOPSY

Automated percutaneous biopsy guns are available in a variety of gauges and lengths for core biopsy of extraskeletal masses. Using similar technique as percutaneous biopsy, the site is localized and the automated biopsy gun is loaded and locked to prevent accidental discharge. The needle is then placed at the periphery of the lesion with a clear excursion through and across the lesion (generally about 2.5 cm). Care is taken to avoid neurovascular structures, both in placing the needle and in the expected excursion of the needle following discharge. The needle is then discharged through the lesion and removed to reveal the core biopsy. Detachable systems are available in which the outer guide of the needle may be maintained within the patient while the inner core biopsy needle is removed to reveal the biopsy specimen. Using this technique, repeated biopsies of the same lesion may be obtained from placement of a single needle. It is important to note that repositioning of the needle is mandatory upon each discharge since both the inner needle and outer guide move the same amount during each automated biopsy.

DIAGNOSTIC/THERAPEUTIC PELVIC INJECTIONS

Fluoroscopic- and CT-guided injections around the hip pelvis may be therapeutic and/or diagnostic and help differentiate between primary and referred hip pain. Target sites depend upon clinical scenario but often include sacroiliac joint, piriformis muscle/sciatic nerve, hamstring insertion, pubic symphysis, or iliopsoas bursa/tendon sheath (Fig. 27-16) (11,12,15,17,28,33,34,36,37,51,60,82,99,117,140). A 22-gauge spinal needle is typically advanced under image guidance using usual sterile conditions. Approximately 1 to 5 mL of anesthetic agent is then injected (1% preservative-free lidocaine or 0.5% bupivicaine), depending on size of anatomic target and body habitus, usually in combination with 40 to 80 mg of Depomedrol or appropriate steroid equivalent, depending upon the clinical situation. Some studies advocate use of botulinum toxin for piriformis injection (22,33,105). Selection of image guidance depends upon personal preference and availability of equipment; however, many referring physicians appreciate visualizing the precise needle localization with CT guidance.

RADIOGRAPHIC ANATOMY AND LANDMARKS

In the AP projection, the acetabular landmarks commonly used include the iliopubic or iliopectineal line delineating the anterior column, the ilioischial line denoting the posterior column, the teardrop outline at the inferior margin of the medial acetabular border, and the anterior and posterior acetabular rims. The anterior rim extends as a radiographic edge of greater radiopacity extending from the lateral acetabulum to the caudal base of the superior pubic ramus. The posterior rim extends from the lateral acetabulum to the lateral margin of the ischium. Finally, the medial edge of the horseshoe-shaped articular surface of the acetabulum can be seen well on the AP radiographic superiorly, ending at about the level of the fovea of the femoral head. The anterior and posterior caudomedial margins of the acetabular articular surface are commonly seen as curvilinear radiopacities just lateral to the teardrop (6) (Fig. 27-17).

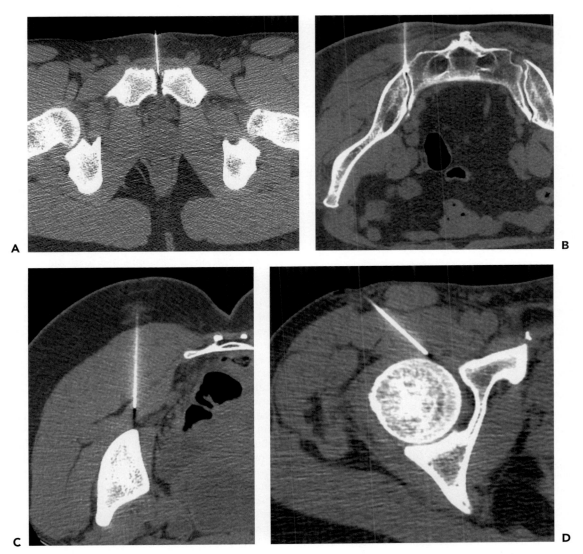

Figure 27-16 CT guided needle placements for pain in the following regions. **A:** Pubic symphsis. **B:** Sacroiliac joint. **C:** Piriformis. **D:** Iliopsoas bursa.

The femur has several radiographic anatomic features seen on the AP radiograph. The femoral head with its medial fovea capitas is seen in profile. The femoral head–neck junction is variable in appearance, particularly in the presence of circumferential osteophytosis. Anterolaterally, the head–neck junction contains a triangular area of irregular cortex which is contacted by the iliofemoral ligaments during hip extension. This area may have cystic foci within it, commonly referred to as synovial herniation pits and recently associated with femoroacetabular impingement (96,103) (Fig. 27-18). The femoral neck blends laterally into the greater trochanter and posteromedially into the lesser trochanter. The medial femoral neck is thicker than the lateral femoral neck and continues through the lesser trochanter as the calcar femoris, an area of intramedullary lamellar (compact) bone (118). Within the medullary space of the femoral head and femoral neck are several trabecular bands that are readily apparent on the AP radiograph. A group of these trabeculae arise from the medial femoral neck, extending proximally across the midportion of

the femoral head–neck junction to the superior central portion of the femoral head comprising the primary compressive trabecular band. A similar arcuate group of trabeculae forming the primary tensile group arise from the lateral femoral cortex and greater trochanter, extending across the lateral portion of the femoral neck, crossing the primary compressive trabecular group, to the medial femoral head. Secondary compressive and tensile trabecular groups and a greater trochanteric group are also present. Patterns of osteoporotic trabecular loss corresponding to these groups of trabeculae have been used as a method to grade the severity of osteoporosis by Singh and coworkers, who reported orderly loss of secondary and primary groups as osteoporosis progressed (45) (Fig. 27-19). This method of estimating osteoporosis has been supplanted by more accurate and reproducible direct measurement of bone mineralization by quantitative bone densitometers.

In the lateral projection, femoral version can be identified. The greater trochanter overlaps the femoral neck, and the lesser trochanter can be seen in profile posteriorly on a well-

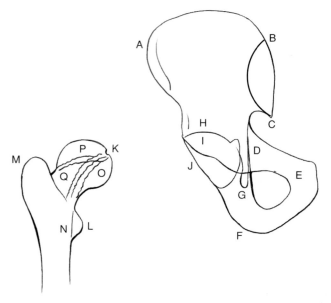

Figure 27-17   Line representations of AP radiographic anatomy of the hip. Anterior iliac crest (*A*). Posterior iliac crest (*B*). Iliopubic (iliopectineal) line (*C*). Ilioichial line (*D*). Pubis (*E*). Ischial tuberosity (*F*). Acetabular (teardrop) denoting the quadrilateral surface of the nonarticular medial acetabulum (*G*). Superior articular surface of the acetabulum (*H*). Note its termination just lateral to the quadrilateral surface. The caudal margin of the articular surface of the acetabulum is often curvilinear. Anterior acetabular rim (*I*). Posterior acetabular rim (*J*). These are recognizable radiographically as edges of density connecting from the superolateral acetabular margin to the caudal margin of the pubis and lateral margin of the ischium, respectively. Fovea of the femoral head (*K*). Lesser trochanter (*L*). Greater trochanter (*M*). Calcar femoris (*N*). Primary compressive group of trabeculae (*O*). Primary tensile group of trabeculae (*P*). Ward's triangle (*Q*), an area of relatively sparse trabeculation.

positioned lateral view. When performed as a frog-leg lateral, the acetabular anatomy is relatively unchanged in appearance. When obtained as a cross-table lateral, the radiograph outlines the caudal aspect of the ischial tuberosity and may demonstrate portions of the acetabular rim anteriorly and posteriorly, though it is rarely of clinical use in the native hip. Following total hip arthroplasty placement, the cross-table lateral may be more helpful in estimating acetabular version, generally using a perpendicular to the table as a reference (69).

Radiographic Measurements

Although measurement of anatomic landmarks is more commonly used in the interpretation of pediatric hip and pelvic radiographs, several are of use in examining the adult. The femoral neck–shaft angle is measured between the central axes or center lines of the femoral neck and shaft, generally accepted to be 125°, with a range of about 120° to 140° (71) (Fig. 27-20). The plate–shaft angle of the femoral neck is measured by a perpendicular to the physeal scar relative to the center line of the neck. It is commonly difficult to measure due to the curvature of the physeal remnant and is not commonly used. Femoral neck version is measured anatomically by comparison of the femoral neck center line to either the epicondylar axis of the distal femur or the condylar plane. It is generally accepted to be 14° anteverted from the femoral condylar

plane. Measurement of femoral version in vivo is difficult on standard radiographs due to variability in rotation of the femur and the necessity to compare the femoral neck axis to the shaft instead of the intercondylar plane. Standard radiographs may reveal gross abnormalities of version, and a seated AP view has been described to improve evaluation of version specifically, but CT provides ideal axial images of the hips and knees from which the femoral version can be reliably measured (59). When performed as a dedicated study for measurement purposes only, the cost of such an examination may rival plain radiography.

Acetabular protrusio is identified by constructing a line (of Kohler) from the medial border of the body of the ischium to the tangent of the medial border of the ilium (Fig. 27-21). Protrusion exists if the acetabulum passes medial to that line (71).

A number of measurements exist for the detection and characterization of developmental dysplasia of the hip. Most are used in infants and children, and many rely on radiographic landmarks present only in the immature skeleton. The acetabular angle, or index, is commonly used in infants and small children to identify acetabular dysplasia. It is measured as the angle between a line drawn between the triradiate cartilage of the acetabulae (Hilgenreiner's line) and a second line drawn from the triradiate cartilage to the lateral border of the acetabulum. A modified acetabular index is used for adults, in which the angle is measured between a line drawn between the caudal margins of the acetabular teardrops, and a second drawn between the teardrop and the lateral acetabulum (Fig. 27-22). The acetabular depth is measured by the longest perpendicular from the medial acetabulum to a line drawn between the teardrop and the lateral acetabular border. Shenton's line is occasionally helpful in evaluating the relationship of the femoral head and acetabulum of the adult hip, observed as the confluent arch made by the inferior border of the superior pubic ramus and the medial border of the femoral neck (Fig. 27-23).

A commonly accepted method of evaluating congruence of the hip in older children, which is occasionally used in adults, is by the center edge angle of Wiberg, modified by Massie and Howorth (90) (Fig. 27-23A). The measurement is made by drawing a line from the center of the femoral head to the lateral edge of the acetabulum, and measuring its incident angle from a second line drawn directly cephalocaudad from the center of the femoral head. The main advantage of the center edge angle as compared with other measurements of articular congruence is its relative independence from changes in hip position. The migration percentage index is also occasionally used to demonstrate hip incongruence, obtained by dividing the width of uncovered head by the width of the entire head multiplied by 100 (108).

Normal Variants

A variety of anatomic variants occur about the hip, particularly during skeletal development. Many are simply normally overlapping structures that during slight changes in position have an unexpected appearance, simulating pathology, whereas others represent accessory or vestigial structures. The etiology of these are generally unknown, and while most are incidental findings, some may be symptomatic. In general, most are of

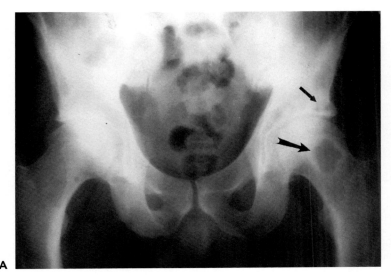

A

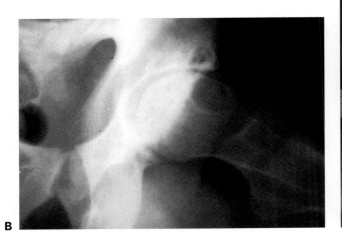

B

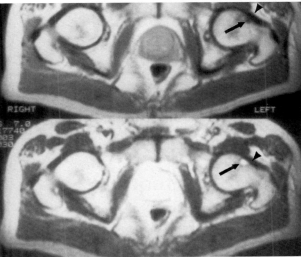

C

Figure 27-18 Synovial herniation pit. **A:** AP radiograph of the pelvis showing osteoarthritis of both hips with a subchondral (Ecker's) cyst in the superolateral acetabulum (*small arrow*). A large geographic mass overlies the femoral head–neck junction with sharply circumscribed, sclerotic borders. **B:** Frog-leg lateral view more clearly shows both the acetabular subchondral cyst and the anterior junctional location of the femoral mass. The location is typical for a synovial herniation pit, occurring at the "rough" zone of the femoral head/neck junction underlying the iliofemoral ligaments. Intrusion of synovium between undulations in the cortex is thought to give rise to these structures. **C:** Transaxial MRI in another patient with proton density weighting (*top*) and T2 weighting (*bottom*) showing proximity of synovial herniation pit (*arrows*) to iliofemoral ligaments (*arrowheads*) as well as fluid signal within herniation pit itself.

no significance other than in being mistaken for more serious abnormalities.

In the adult, the size and shape of the femoral head and fovea capitas vary, often appearing to represent flattening of the femoral head. The caudal margins of the acetabular articular surfaces may simulate lytic areas where they overlap the femoral head. The gluteal and inguinal skin folds may form curvilinear lucencies simulating fractures but can almost always be followed beyond the osseous cortex, allowing differentiation. Similarly, in the absence of a hip effusion, a vacuum may be created within the articulation, especially during abduction and external rotation. The resulting curvilinear lucencies may mimic fracture lines.

Variance in trabeculation of the femoral head at the borders of compressive and tensile trabecular groups may mimic a lytic mass in osteoporotic individuals, particularly in the lateral aspect of the femoral head (104). The appearance is exaggerated in the presence of a displaced subcapital fracture and may lead to the erroneous diagnosis of a pathologic fracture (Fig. 27-24). In the subtrochanteric femur and midilium of osteoporotic individuals, bizarre arrays of trabeculae termed *bone reinforcement*

bars are common and may be mistaken for chondroid tumor matrix or osteonecrosis. Bone islands or stenoses are foci of compact bone occurring within cancellous bone and appear radiographically as sclerotic foci of variable size, but usually less than 1 cm in diameter. They are of no clinical significance and occur in epiphyseal or metaphyseal areas predominantly (Fig. 27-25). They are generally ovoid, oriented parallel to surrounding trabeculae, with a spiculated border from the insertion of adjacent trabeculae. They may become large and lose characteristic features in the pelvis and may be mistaken for osteoblastic metastases, but bone scan is diagnostic, with no increased uptake of radionuclide (126). Familial conditions of cortical mosaicism exist, in which multiple bone islands (osteopoikilosis) or coalescent linear foci of sclerotic bone (osteopathia striata) may be seen, which should not be mistaken for metastatic disease (Fig. 27-26). A condition that may be symptomatic and is occasionally seen with these disorders is melorheostosis, in which endosteal curvilinear sclerotic bone is found and whose appearance has been likened to dripping candle wax (111).

Accessory ossification centers about the acetabulum (os acetabulae) are common and have a variety of appearances,

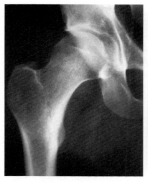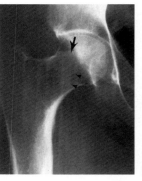

Figure 27-19 Variance in radiographic density of osseous structures of the hips. **A:** Normal individual with thick cortex of acetabular teardrop, superior pubic ramus, femoral neck, and sub-trochanteric femoral diaphysis. Note dense three-dimensional mesh of trabeculae throughout the femoral head. **B:** Osteoporotic individual with both cortical and trabecular bone loss. Note thin but sharply circumscribed cortex of acetabular teardrop, superior pubic ramus, and femoral neck. The subtrochanteric diaphysis is thinner than in patient A but is still relatively robust. Trabecular loss has resulted in prominence of the tensile band of trabeculae (*arrow*) and indistinctness of the primary compressive group (*arrowheads*).

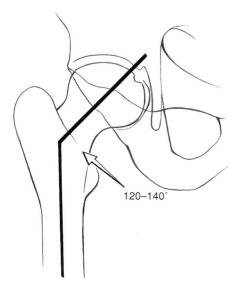

Figure 27-20 Neck shaft angle of the femur. The centroid of the femoral head and neck form the femoral line while the shaft of the subtrochanteric femur determines the shaft line. Values of less than 120 indicate varus while values greater than 140 indicate valgus.

ranging from punctate calcification and ossification within the acetabular labrum to large crescentic ossicles at the lateral acetabular margins. The latter should not be mistaken for acetabular rim fractures, as accessory ossicles have corticated margins at their junction with the acetabulum in contrast to the uncorticated margins of an acute fracture (Fig. 27-27).

RADIOGRAPHIC PATHOLOGY OF THE HIP

Accurate diagnosis of hip disease by interpretation of radiographs depends on several conditions being met. The radiograph must first demonstrate the abnormalities; the findings must be identified, characterized, and differentiated from artifacts and normal variants; and the significance of the findings must be determined. In short, the patient's intrinsic pathology must be recognized within the image. Fortunately, bone lends itself well to portraying its pathology by radiography, having high intrinsic radiographic contrast with nonosseous tissue and a dynamic crystalline architecture that reveals pathology by accommodating to its presence. To recognize radiographic pathology, one must first possess a familiarity with pathologic conditions affecting the hip, the manner in which musculoskeletal tissues respond to them, and where the process is most likely to occur.

The following discussion is intended to serve as a categorical review of common radiographic pathology rather than a

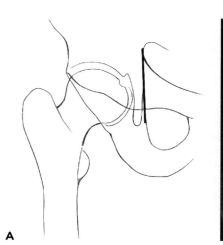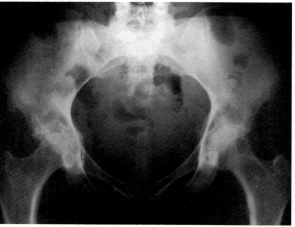

Figure 27-21 A: Kohler's ilioischial line. Protrusion of the femoral head medial to this line indicates acetabular protrusio. **B:** AP radiograph of the hip in a patient with longstanding rheumatoid arthritis showing axial migration of the right femoral head with early acetabular protrusio. Note diminutive appearance of femoral head from circumferential erosion.

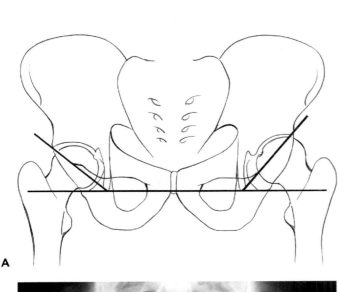

A

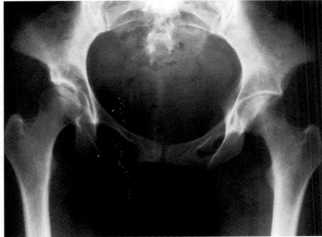

B

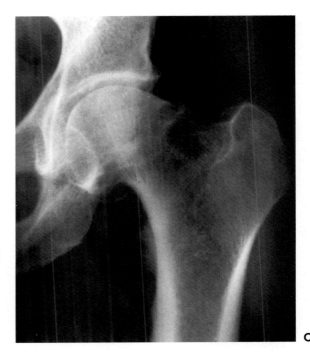

C

Figure 27-22 **A:** Modified acetabular index for adults using a line tangent to both acetabular teardrops. A line connecting the acetabular teardrop with the lateral acetabular margin defines the acetabular angle or index. Note an increased acetabular angle on the dysplastic left hip in contrast to the right. **B:** Developmental dysplasia of the hip with coxa valga and shallow acetabular index. Note thickened quadrilateral surface (superior teardrop) and diminished size of right hemipelvis. **C:** Adult presentation of slipped capital femoral epiphysis (SCFE). Deformity of femoral head may suggest developmental dysplasia, but varus rather than valgus deformity and normal appearance of teardrop indicate SCFE.

completely inclusive encyclopedic reference, with examples chosen to portray the typical radiographic appearance of common entities. As with the normal hip, the hip affected by disease has a variety of radiographic appearances for the same condition based on many factors, including the age and condition of the patient, the duration and severity of disease, and the nature of treatment.

Trauma

The two main sequelae of acute traumatic injury of the hip, fracture and dislocation, occur with differing frequency depending on the patient population to be considered. Hip dislocation occurs primarily in younger adults, generally in the setting of high-velocity motor vehicle accidents. The majority are posterior in direction, with the femoral head positioned superolateral to the acetabulum and the leg internally rotated

and adducted. Most occur when the knee is hit by the automobile dashboard, driving the femoral head posteriorly, and are commonly associated with posterior acetabular rim and column fractures. Anterior dislocations are less common, occurring from forced abduction and external rotation of the hip with the femoral head located inferomedially with the leg externally rotated and abducted (81). Associated fractures of the anterior rim of the acetabulum, greater trochanter, and femoral neck may be seen. In both, transchondral fractures of the femoral head may be observed (see Figs. 27-7 and 27-27). Following reduction, persistent widening of the hip on plain radiographs or persistent severe pain may suggest entrapped fracture fragments and warrant examination by CT, which is the study of choice to identify occult acetabular fractures and intra-articular bone fragments. Later complications of hip dislocation include degenerative joint disease, heterotopic ossification, and osteonecrosis, the latter of which is best examined by MRI.

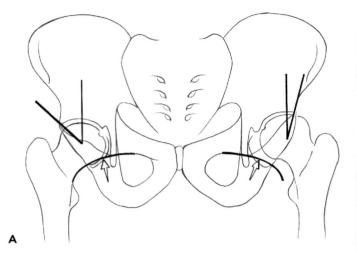

A

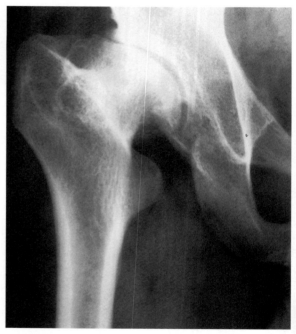

B

Figure 27-23 **A:** The center edge (CE) angle is obtained by establishing the centroid of the femoral head and comparing a line drawn from its vertical to the lateral acetabular margin. As lateral translation of the head progresses, the CE angle diminishes. Compare the normal architecture on the right with the dysplastic, laterally translocated hip on the left. Shenton's line, referring to confluence between the inferior border of the superior pubic ramus and the medial femoral neck, may also be used in advanced cases of hip incongruence from dysplasia or fracture. Contiguous curvilinear relationship is maintained on the right while lateral translocation on the left disrupts the normal relationship. **B:** Advanced developmental dysplasia of the hip. Note the femoral head deformity, shallow acetabular angle, and thickened quadrilateral surface with a triangular appearing teardrop. Shenton's line is grossly disrupted.

The elderly are affected to a greater extent by minor trauma from falls in which hip fracture is the major result and osteoporosis a major contributor. Acute fractures of the proximal femur may be of the femoral head (commonly in younger patients, associated with dislocation) or in subcapital, transcervical, basicervical, intertrochanteric, or subtrochanteric locations

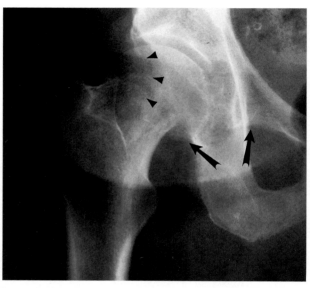

Figure 27-24 Pseudolytic lesion in patient with displaced subcapital fracture. Observe marked apparent demineralization in the superolateral margin of the femoral head. No pathologic process was found following hemiarthroplasty placement. Also note disruption of Shenton's line (*arrows*).

(Fig. 27-28). Classification schemes based on these common fracture locations as well a schemes based on other criteria exist. Avulsion fractures of the greater and lesser trochanter frequently occur, and it is important to recall that the traumatized patient complaining of a painful hip may have a fracture not sufficiently displaced to detect by plain film. It is now known that many fractures of the hip and pelvis are radiographically occult, particularly in the elderly and osteoporotic, and a strong clinical suspicion of fracture should warrant immediate examination by MRI (Figs. 27-29 and 27-30). The examination should include the symptomatic hip as well as the pelvis and contralateral hip,

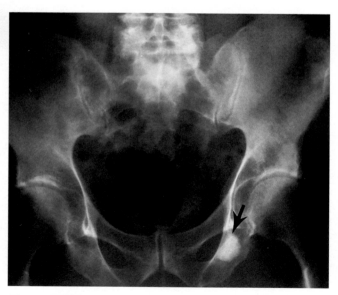

Figure 27-25 Bone island. An unusually large very radiodense lesion in the ischium. Because of its unusual size, this lesion was biopsied revealing enostosis (bone island).

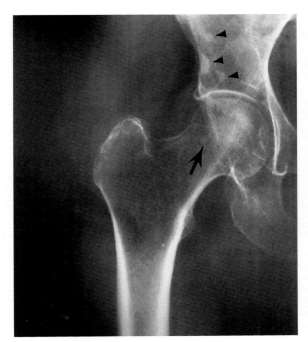

Figure 27-26 Osteopoikolosis. Numerous typical bone islands both at the femoral head–neck junction (*arrow*) and acetabulum. Note that the ellipsoid axis of the lesions are parallel to the trabeculae in which they exist.

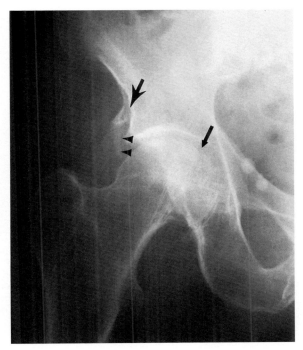

Figure 27-27 Displaced acetabular rim fractures simulating os acetabulum. The displacement, lack of circumferential cortication (*arrow*), and heterotopic ossification (*arrowheads*) differentiate this from os acetabulum. Note barely perceptible femoral head fracture clearly identifiable by CT.

as patients complaining of posttraumatic hip pain may have an occult fracture of the sacrum, ilium, pubis, or ischium (91) (Figs. 27-31 and 27-32). Contusions, hematomas, and muscle injuries that may mimic fracture clinically can also be identified and differentiated from more serious injuries by MRI. In our practice and in the radiology literature, MRI has proven valuable as a sensitive and, more importantly, specific tool to identify occult fracture and injuries that mimic fracture in patients presenting with signs and symptoms of hip fracture but negative or equivocal radiographs, allowing appropriate discharge from the emergency department or timely and appropriate treatment.

Stress fractures of the hip in the athlete and insufficiency fractures of the hip in the elderly are occasionally diagnosed by plain radiographs as linear areas of sclerosis, both in the femoral neck where they are generally subcapital in location and in the acetabulum in which the fractures are usually in the axial plane just above the superior articular surface. Frequently,

these fractures may be radiographically occult and the clinical suspicion indicates examination by MRI, which is again the study of choice for diagnosis in the patient with negative or equivocal radiographs (Fig. 27-33).

Pathologic fractures of the hip may be seen in association with infection, metastatic disease, primary neoplasm (benign or malignant), metabolic disease, or tumorlike disease such as Paget's disease of bone. In the setting of neoplasm, bone involved with more than 50% tumor is considered at risk for pathologic fracture, but there is not universal acceptance of this dictum or the manner in which circumferential extent is determined, and prophylactic treatment is often initiated based on a variety of criteria (Fig. 27-34).

Complications of fracture reduction and fixation include malunion, nonunion (atrophic and hypertrophic), degenerative

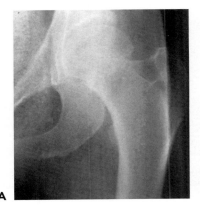
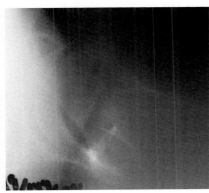

Figure 27-28 Subcapital fracture of the femoral neck. **A:** AP radiograph demonstrating substantial valgus displacement. **B:** Cross-table lateral view of the femoral neck showing posterior displacement of the femoral head.

A

B

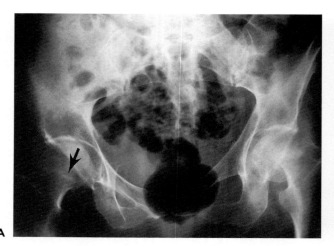
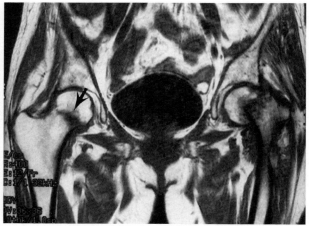

A   B

Figure 27-29 Traumatic and stress fractures. Patient with several months of hip pain bilaterally with acute left hip pain following a fall. **A:** AP radiograph of the pelvis showing a subcapital fracture of the left femoral head with varus angulation and advanced displacement. Note ill-defined sclerotic band at the subcapital region of the right femoral neck. **B:** Coronal T1-weighted MRI of both hips showing displaced subcapital fracture on the left and nondisplaced stress fracture of the left hip (*arrow*). The left femoral neck fracture likely represented displacement of an existing stress fracture during the patient's fall.

joint disease, osteonecrosis, para-articular heterotopic ossification, and infection in addition to mechanical complications of fixation hardware. Radiography is routinely used to monitor fracture healing and identify complications. The extent to which residual angulation, displacement, or foreshortening affects hip biomechanics after a fracture has healed defines malunion and varies with the type of fracture. The degree to which an individual patient is affected by residual malalignment varies considerably, and terms used to describe fracture alignment should reflect this. Terms most appropriate to describe fracture reduction include *anatomic reduction* in which no difference from the prefracture morphology can be detected, *near-anatomic reduction* in which the fragments are closely aligned to normal but are not

ideal, and *nonanatomic reduction* in which gross disturbance of alignment persists. Subjective qualifiers, such as good, satisfactory, or poor, do not describe reduction in terms of the anatomic ideal and may lead to false assessments of outcome.

Malposition of fixation components is the most common postoperative hardware complication and is evaluated by portable radiographs either intraoperatively or postoperatively at the time fracture reduction is assessed. It may be difficult to determine if hardware is intra-articular radiographically due to the three-dimensional curvature of the hip articulation, and if suspicion warrants, fluoroscopy may be used to obtain a view of the hardware and joint in profile (123). CT or plain tomography may identify the position of

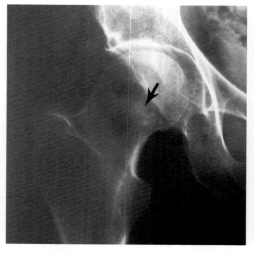
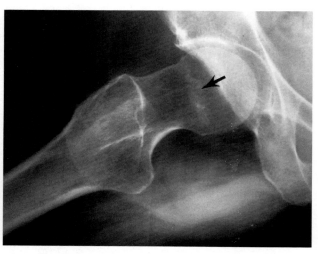

Figure 27-30 Stress fracture. Follow-up radiographs from previous patient. AP and frog-leg radiographs show a more clearly apparent sclerotic band across the subcapital portion of the femoral neck 6 weeks following the initial radiograph.

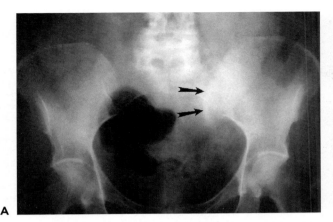

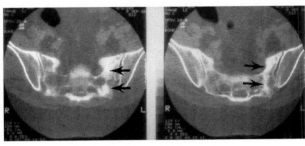

Figure 27-31 Sacral insufficiency fracture. **A:** AP radiograph showing asymmetric sclerosis overlying the left hemisacrum. **B:** Transaxial noncontrast CT scan of the sacrum showing typical sagittal plane distribution of linear sclerosis and sacral insufficiency fracture.

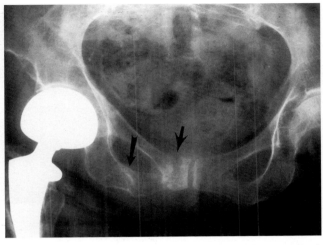

Figure 27-33 Insufficiency fracture of the pubis. Patient with hemiarthroplasty and right hip pain, without trauma. Osteosclerosis and cortical disruption of right parasymphyseal pubis (*short arrow*) and ischiopubic synchondrosis (*long arrow*) indicating insufficiency fracture.

hardware relative to the joint to greater advantage, if radiography or fluoroscopy are equivocal, and may be augmented by the use of intra-articular contrast.

Later complications of hardware include infection, loosening and motion of plates, backing out of screws, and fracture of hardware. Although bony reaction generally accompanies loss of fixation, change in the relative position of hardware may rarely be the only radiographic feature of loosening.

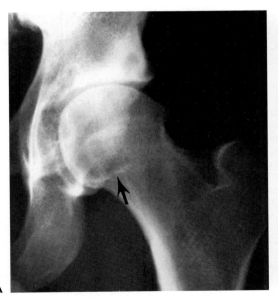

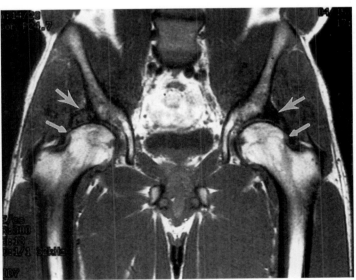

Figure 27-32 Stress fracture mimicked by osteophytes. **A:** Patient with known osteoarthritis of the hip with recent exacerbation of pain following activity. Observe a band of sclerosis traversing the medial subcapital region of the femoral neck. Although this is felt to represent circumferential osteophytosis, an MRI was obtained because of the patient's symptoms. **B:** Coronal T1-weighted MRI examination of both hips showing no evidence of a stress fracture of the femoral necks but marginal osteophytosis of the femoral heads (*small arrows*) and extensive acetabular sclerosis (*large arrows*).

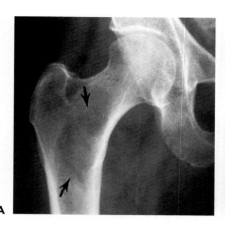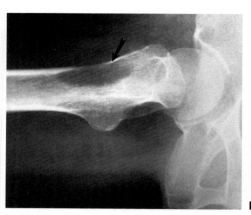

Figure 27-34 Metastatic breast carcinoma. **A:** AP radiograph showing barely perceptible area of lucency in the intertrochanteric region of the femur (*arrows*). **B:** Frog-leg lateral view showing anterior cortical destruction and moth eaten border. Although this lesion did not circumferentially involve more than 50% of the femoral intertrochanteric cortex, it was prophylactically instrumented.

Articular Disorders

The hip is commonly affected by arthropathy, with rare involvement by some entities such as gout, and frequent or even characteristic involvement by others. Joint narrowing is the characteristic finding of articular disease, representing cartilaginous destruction from any disorder that enzymatically, chemically, or mechanically destroys cartilage and is not specific for any one entity. The location of joint narrowing within the hip and subsequent migration of the femoral head toward the acetabulum differs between articular disorders and may provide evidence for specific entities (55). Conditions that affect the entire cartilage surface, such as inflammatory or infectious arthritis, result in diffuse cartilage loss and joint narrowing, with axial migration of parallel to the neck (Fig. 27-35). Disorders that narrow specific regions of the hip, such as

osteoarthritis, result in either superior or medial migration, with axial migration when both the superior and medial areas of the joint are affected to a similar extent (109). When they affect bone, articular disorders of the hip are recognized by their symmetric involvement of both the acetabulum and femoral head, as compared to extra-articular disorders that tend to involve one bone or the other primarily, with later involvement of the joint. Table 27-1 provides a summary of common disorders.

Osteoarthritis

Degenerative joint disease is the most common disorder of the hip, and while it was largely disregarded as a natural consequence of aging, recent interest by many investigators has contributed much to the understanding of this disease. Terminology for this condition may be confusing. The terms

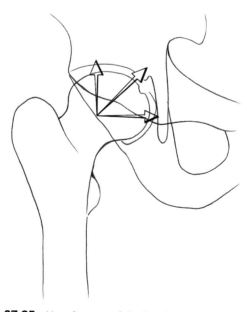

Figure 27-35 Line diagram of the hip showing superior, medial, and axial migration patterns in the femoral head. Superior and medial migration generally indicate asymmetric cartilage loss, usually degenerative. Axial migration (*central arrow*) generally indicates diffuse cartilage loss seen in inflammatory arthropathies.

TABLE 27-1

ARTICULAR DISORDERS AFFECTING THE ADULT HIP

Osteoarthritis
Primary or idiopathic
Secondary (degenerative joint disease)
Rheumatoid arthritis and juvenile chronic arthritis
The seronegative spondyloarthropathies
Psoriatic arthritis
Reiter's disease
Ankylosing spondylitis
Inflammatory bowel associated arthropathy
Connective tissue disease
Crystal arthropathies
Gout
CPPD
CHA
Miscellaneous disorders
Rapidly destructive hip disease
Chondrolysis
Pigmented villonodular synovitis
Synovial (osteo) chrondromatosis
Metabolic and endocrine disease
Nutritional disorders
Radiation chrondrosis and osteonecrosis
Osteoarthritis

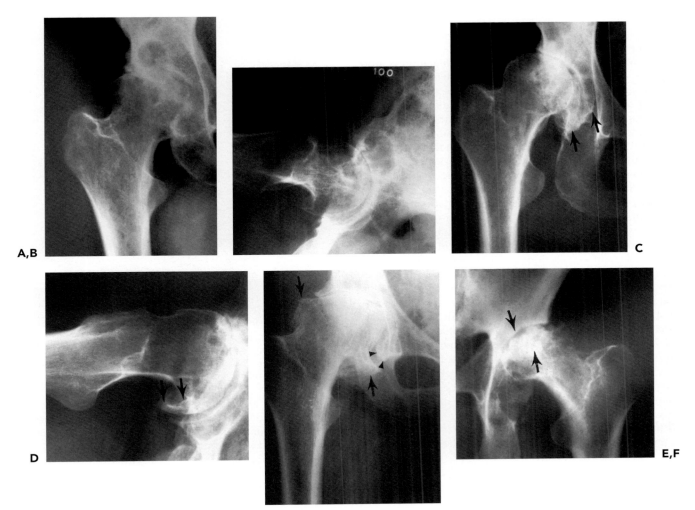

Figure 27-36 Radiographic features of degenerative osteoarthritis. **A:** Joint line narrowing (superior) with subchondral sclerosis and prominent subchondral cyst formation. Although there is flattening of the femoral head, the distribution of cystic changes cross the acetabular and femoral head surfaces indicate osteoarthritis rather than osteonecrosis as the primary disorder. **B:** Frog-leg lateral from A showing asymmetric joint loss anteriorly coinciding with subchondral cyst formation. **C:** Osteophytosis with secondary femoral head translocation. Dysplastic appearing acetabulum from advanced superior degenerative wear with prominent medial acetabular osteophyte (*arrows*) and advanced lateral translocation of the femoral head. **D:** Lateral radiograph from C showing large posteromedial femoral osteophyte (*arrow*) matching acetabular osteophyte from C. **E:** End-stage osteoarthritis with double teardrop appearance of medial osteophytosis (*arrowheads*) and large medial femoral head osteophyte (*arrow*) resulting in advanced lateral translocation and superior joint narrowing. **F:** Secondary degenerative arthrosis from primary inflammatory arthropathy in patient with previous septic arthritis. Although the primary process is erosive arthropathy, subchondral sclerosis and acetabular eburnation are prominent degenerative features (*arrows*).

osteoarthritis and *degenerative joint disease* are used synonymously in the United States. As the condition lacks inflammation typically denoted by the *-itis* suffix, some prefer to use the suffix *-osis* yielding the term *osteoarthrosis*.

Osteoarthritis may be classified by primary, or idiopathic, and secondary types, with the secondary types being the result of some other primary disorder. Although there is considerable disagreement regarding this classification, and careful review of primary osteoarthritis may reveal prior disorders leading to degenerative arthritis, evidence of a genetic predisposition to some types of osteoarthritis suggests that there may be some rationale for its use. Finally, any insult to the

joint may lead to secondary osteoarthritis in the hip. The primary insult can commonly be discerned radiographically and may be a source of some confusion in interpretation.

Osteoarthritis has several characteristic radiographic features which reflect the histopathology of the disease. Joint narrowing, osteophytosis, subchondral sclerosis, cyst formation, intra-articular bodies, and malalignment are findings that together or in groups are characteristic for the disease (47) (Fig. 27-36).

Joint narrowing follows cartilaginous destruction and is seen in any disorder that enzymatically, chemically, or mechanically destroys cartilage and is not specific for any one entity. In osteoarthritis, joint narrowing is mostly superior. Superolateral migration of the femoral head is more commonly seen in women and is usually asymmetric or unilateral, occurring in 15% to 50% of cases (110). Superomedial migration is more common in men and is usually bilateral, often occurring at a younger age, and is seen in 35% to 50% of cases. Medial migration is seen in 10% to 35% of cases and is commonly symmetric.

Osteophytosis is characteristic of osteoarthritis, representing osteochondral excrescences extending from the margins of the joint, termed *marginal osteophytes,* or from the subchondral plate at the center of the chondral surface, termed *central osteophytes.* In the hip, marginal osteophytosis may occur either laterally or medially about the fovea and medial acetabular rim, the latter occasionally associated with lamellar buttressing of the medial femoral neck (88). These medial marginal osteophytes have been implicated in the lateral translation of the femoral head thought to lead to incongruent contact of the hip articular surfaces, resulting in rapid superior joint narrowing (84,100). With severe osteoarthritis, subchondral cysts may be a very prominent feature, and collapse of the subchondral plate overlying cysts may occur. The final appearance may be difficult to distinguish from osteonecrosis with secondary osteoarthritis, and to further confound diagnosis, foci of osteonecrosis may be seen adjacent to osteoarthritic joints. The symmetry of femoral and acetabular involvement and the advanced nature of the degenerative changes with relatively minor collapse may be helpful clues to the diagnosis, and comparison with previous films is generally diagnostic.

Rheumatoid and Juvenile Chronic Arthritis

Hip involvement in rheumatoid arthritis is less common than peripheral small joint disease but when present is predominantly bilateral and symmetric, similar to the distribution of the disease throughout the remainder of the involved joints (30). Uniform cartilage loss is typical, with axial migration of the femoral head. Protusio acetabula is common in advanced cases, and the femoral head commonly becomes diminutive in advanced disease following recurrent longstanding inflammatory erosion (58) (Fig. 27-37). Osteoporosis is a common feature, and while secondary osteoarthritis may occur, it is unusual for it to predominate radiographically. Inflammatory synovial pannus may cause erosions of the femoral neck, though these are uncommon. Intraosseous subchondral cysts are common and may be quite large in size. While fibrous ankylosis of the joint may occur in end-stage disease, bony ankylosis is very unusual.

Juvenile chronic arthritis is a term used to include many inflammatory arthropathies that occur in childhood and adolescence, with features of adult forms of rheumatoid arthritis and seronegative spondyloarthropathies. Hip involvement is common, in contrast to adult rheumatoid arthritis, with patients typically presenting with end-stage erosive arthropathy as young adults, testament to years of inflammatory disease (3). Inflammation during skeletal development may lead to epiphyseal overgrowth and coxa valga, and bony ankylosis is a common feature of the disease (116).

In both juvenile and adult forms of rheumatoid disease, occipitocervical instability is common in patients with disease severe enough to consider surgery. Screening of the cervical spine by neutral, flexion, and extension lateral radiographs should be routinely performed preoperatively to identify

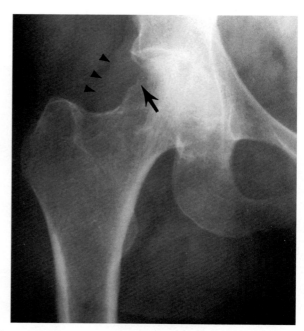

Figure 27-37 Rheumatoid arthritis. AP radiograph demonstrating axial migration of the femoral head from concentric diffuse cartilage loss. Superolateral marginal erosions (*arrow*) from overlying hypertrophic synovial pannus (*arrowhead*).

those at risk for neurologic injury during anesthesia. Basilar invagination, or cranial settling, refers to the tendency of the odontoid (and its surrounding pannus) to migrate cephalad toward the foramen magnum as ligaments become lax. In rheumatoid arthritis, the diagnosis is difficult due to concurrent erosions making identification of the odontoid tip difficult or impossible. Redlund has proposed a modified scheme for evaluating cranial settling in which distance from the C2 base is measured from McGregor's line, which eliminates variation due to odontoid erosion. Values <34 mm in men and 29 mm in women were considered evidence of vertical instability. Atlantoaxial instability is considered present when >3 mm is present between the anterior arch of C1 and the odontoid (107).

The Seronegative Spondyloarthropathies

Ankylosing spondylitis, enteropathic arthropathy, psoriatic arthritis, and Reiter's disease are inflammatory arthritides that affect the spine and appendicular skeleton to varying degrees, are not associated with production of rheumatoid factor, and occur in patients with HLA-B27 antigen expression. Radiographically, the hallmark of these disorders are enthesophytes, that is, osseous excrescences occurring at insertions of ligaments, tendons, or joint capsules (entheses) into bone. Sacroiliitis, characterized by erosions and sclerosis, is common and may help to differentiate subgroups.

Ankylosing spondylitis and its radiographic clone enteropathic arthropathy are typically bilateral in sacroiliac distribution and usually symmetric. Following inflammatory episodes and erosive arthropathy, ankylosis of the sacroiliac joints and spine is typical, with thin bridging enthesophytes, termed *syndesmophytes,* which are characteristic of the disorder. Hip and shoulder involvement generally lags behind spinal disease

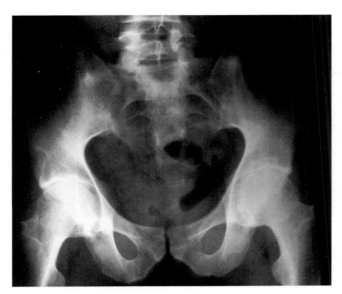

Figure 27-38 Ankylosing spondylitis. Symmetric axial narrowing of both hips associated with complete ankylosis of both SI joints. Symmetric hip and shoulder erosive arthropathy is characteristic of the disorder in its later stages.

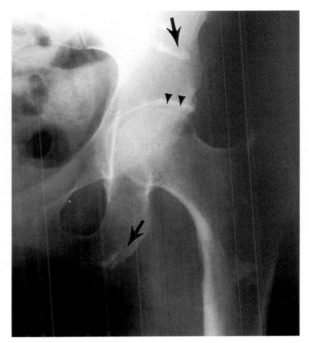

Figure 27-39 Calcium hydroxyapatite deposition and pyrophosphate arthropathy. Entheseal deposition of hydroxyapatite in the hamstring and rectus femoris musculature as well as linear chondrocalcinosis (*arrowhead*) of the hip.

radiographically and predominates over distal appendicular disease. Involvement of the hips is manifest by diffuse cartilage loss with axial migration, and bony ankylosis of the hips may occur in advanced disease. Discrete erosions, subchondral cysts, and sclerosis are not typical features of the disorder (31) (Fig. 27-38).

Reiter's disease and psoriatic arthritis rarely involve the hips, preferentially involving the peripheral joints, and typically have unilateral or asymmetric bilateral sacroiliitis. Spine involvement differs from ankylosing spondylitis by the absence of syndesmophytes and by the presence of curvilinear ossification crossing lateral to the disc, termed *paravertebral ossification*.

Crystal Arthropathies

Calcium hydroxyapatite (CHA), calcium pyrophosphate dihydrate (CPPD), and monosodium urate are the commonest of the many crystals that may precipitate in or around joints, causing arthropathies that often have distinctive radiographic features. Of these three, CPPD crystals most commonly affect the joint itself; CHA crystals may involve tendons about the hip and, less commonly, the articular components of the hip; and gout is rarely seen in and about the hip (111).

Terminology may be confusing in CPPD deposition disease. *Chondrocalcinosis* is a term indicating the radiologic or pathologic presence of CPPD crystals in hyaline or fibrocartilage, is not diagnostic of crystal arthropathy in and of itself and is frequently seen in osteoarthritis. *Pyrophosphate arthropathy* indicates arthropathy from CPPD crystal deposition, which most commonly appears as degenerative arthritis in a specific distribution in the patellofemoral, metacarpophalangeal, radiocarpal, and triscaphe joints. It may also have a destructive appearance similar to that of neuropathic disease. *Pseudogout* is the description of one of the clinical manifestations of the disease, in which acute inflammatory monoarthropathy mimics gout, but aspiration of the joint

reveals CPPD crystals. CPPD deposition disease may be seen in association with a variety of metabolic conditions (112).

The hip is commonly symptomatic in the disorder, and chondrocalcinosis is frequently present but is more difficult to see than in the knee. Osteoarthritic changes are mostly seen, usually of the superolateral portion of the joint. Subchondral cysts may be quite large, in contrast to osteoarthritis. Less commonly, diffuse joint destruction with axial narrowing and protrusio may be seen, and a neuropathic appearance is occasionally encountered.

Though periarticular calcification may occur with CPPD deposition disease, it more frequently is the result of CHA deposition. Appearing as discrete, globular, or faceted calcifications generally a few millimeters in diameter, as compared to the fine linear calcification from CPPD, CHA deposition about the hip most commonly involves the gluteal enthesis on the greater trochanter, the trochanteric bursae, and hamstring tendons in the posterior aspect of the ischial tuberosity (138) (Fig. 27-39). Gout rarely involves the hip, though some accounts associating it with osteonecrosis have been reported. These may reflect incidental precipitation of monosodium urate crystals within or around necrotic bone rather than a true association between the clinical disorders.

Miscellaneous Disorders

Rapidly destructive hip disease has been described as a condition of unknown etiology occurring in young adults with, as the name implies, rapid and unrelenting destruction of the joint within months or years (14). The diagnosis is one of exclusion, and rapid radiographic change is the only characteristic feature.

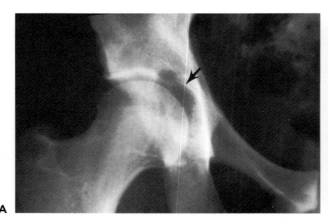

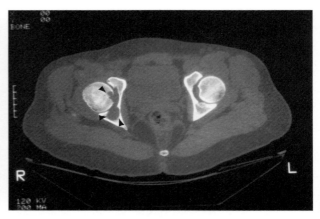

Figure 27-40 Pigmented villonodular synovitis. **A:** AP radiograph of the hip showing a geographic region of osteolysis in the acetabulum suspected to represent neoplasm. **B:** Noncontrast CT examination of the hip showing osteolysis of the posterior acetabulum and perifoveal femoral head (*arrowheads*) suggesting a synovial rather than osseous origin of the process. Pigmented villonodular synovitis was found at biopsy.

Chondrolysis accompanies joint pathology from trauma, radiation, infection, inflammatory and degenerative arthritis, and by disuse (93). Direct destruction may occur, or interference with hydrodynamic cartilage nutrition may play a role in certain conditions. Idiopathic chondrolysis is a condition with a predilection for the hip, mostly occurring in adolescent females, and presenting radiographically as concentric narrowing of the hip with osteoporosis, small subcortical erosions, and, occasionally, enlargement of the femoral head with degenerative changes seen later in the disease.

Pigmented villonodular synovitis (PVNS) and synovial osteochondromatosis are conditions in which well-defined erosions of the femoral neck may be seen in the presence of a normal joint space. PVNS only rarely calcifies, and osteochondromatosis may also lack calcification in which case some have termed it *synovial chondromatosis*. The conditions do not lead directly to cartilage loss, though in synovial osteochondromatosis, loose bodies may mechanically injure the joint. Plain film findings may be diagnostic, although MRI is generally useful to differentiate the disorders with susceptibility artifact seen in PVNS from hemosiderin deposition and discrete rice bodies seen in osteochondromatosis (Figs. 27-40 and 27-41).

Transient osteoporosis is a disorder in which radiographic demineralization of the femoral head and neck occurs spontaneously, after minor trauma or in pregnancy, with no articular abnormalities and resolves over months (62). The cause of the disorder is unknown, but some have speculated a relationship to reflex sympathetic dystrophy and to a condition seen by MRI termed *transient marrow edema* (5,57). No relationship to osteonecrosis has been established.

Radiation in doses used for therapy may result marrow necrosis in the adult, which in the hip most commonly affects the femoral head. Importantly, hip pain after radiation therapy often heralds insufficiency fractures, most commonly of the sacrum and pubis (85). When plain films are unrevealing, the history of pelvic or hip pain following radiation may warrant MRI examination, by which occult fracture and marrow necrosis are easily diagnosed (74).

Metabolic, endocrine, and nutritional disorders result in generalized osseous pathology. Osteoporosis is the most common and most important, being implicated in the majority of hip fractures in the elderly (45). Radiographic features of osteoporosis include cortical thinning, secondary and subsequent primary trabecular loss, and, finally, bone reinforcement lines. Diagnosis is made by quantitative mineral densitometry,

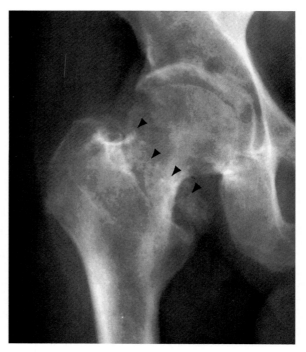

Figure 27-41 AP radiographic of the hip showing curvilinear cluster of calcifications and early degenerative arthrosis in primary synovial osteochondromatosis. The primary form is generally distinguished from the secondary form by the innumerable, small similarly sized intra-articular bodies that contrast the larger, disparate sized intra-articular body seen in secondary synovial osteochondromatosis.

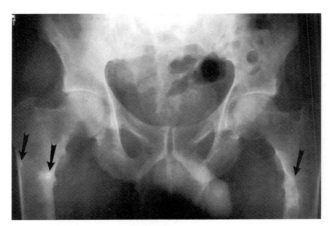

Figure 27-42 Osteomalacia. Bilateral subtrochanteric medial predominant femoral stress fractures with overall heterogeneous osseous mineralization and ill-defined trabeculae.

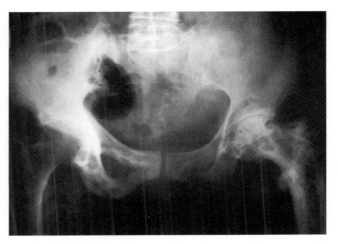

Figure 27-44 Mixed phase Paget disease of bone. AP radiograph of the pelvis showing dense sclerosis of the right innominate bone and sclerosis with areas of lysis in the left femur with varus deformity (Shepherd's crook deformity). In addition, diffuse bony enlargement is present.

most commonly dual-energy x-ray absorptiometry (DEXA). Insufficiency fractures are the predominant complication and are frequently radiographically occult. MRI or bone scan may diagnose these fractures not detectable on plain film with MRI having greater sensitivity and equal sensitivity in most studies.

Osteomalacia is an increasingly uncommon disorder that may have increased, normal, or, most commonly, diminished bone mass. Demineralization is evident radiographically but results in indistinct cortex and trabeculae, as abnormal ossification of bone matrix proceeds. Bowing deformities may occur in the femoral necks, and insufficiency fractures may occur, usually on the concave side of the deformity (Fig. 27-42). Bilateral insufficiency fractures suggest the disorder. In contrast to osteoporosis, in which patients are asymptomatic prior to fracture, osteomalacia may cause diffuse bone pain.

Involvement is generally appendicular rather than axial, as seen in osteoporosis.

Hyperparathyroidism may be seen either as a primary condition or, more commonly, in association with renal insufficiency. Hyperparathyroidism results in bone resorption, particularly in subligamentous locations, which may be prominent around the SI joints and may be accompanied by erosive arthropathy with sclerosis. Osteoclastomas may occur in primary and secondary disease, manifest as well-defined lytic masses. Since this disorder is now diagnosed and treated early in its course, fulminant radiographic findings are uncommon. The combination of secondary hyperparathyroidism and abnormal vitamin D metabolism seen in renal failure has been termed *renal osteodystrophy*. Radiographic features of osteomalacia, osteoporosis, and hyperparathyroidism may be seen in addition to bone and joint pathology related to dialysis (49). Metabolic disease may be seen in concert with osteonecrosis, most commonly in sickle-cell disease, and Gaucher's disease (Fig. 27-43). Paget's disease of bone is an idiopathic disorder affecting individuals over the age of 60, presenting as monostotic or polyostotic lesions beginning near epiphyseal remnants with contiguous spread throughout bone as lytic (early) mixed lytic and sclerotic, and sclerotic bone (late). Radiographs are generally diagnostic, and recognition is important to differentiate from malignancy (Fig. 27-44). Lytic phase Pagetic bone is extremely vascularized, which may pose a surgical hazard.

Avascular Necrosis

Radiography plays a critical role in the evaluation of ischemic necrosis of the femoral head. Radiographs are obtained on initial presentation and, if negative, MRI is usually obtained for diagnosis and differentiation from other disorders (25). Following diagnosis, plain films may be used to follow the osseous response to necrosis and the mechanical complications of osteochondral collapse and arthrosis. The staging system described by Steinberg is most commonly used for radiographic description (129) (Table 27-2). Utilizing radiography and scintigraphy (with the more recent addition of MRI), the

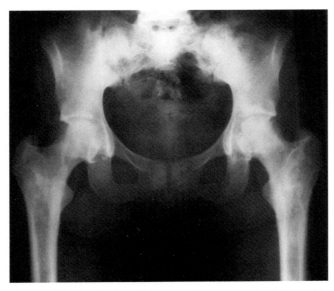

Figure 27-43 Sickle-cell disease. AP radiograph of the pelvis showing diffuse osteosclerosis with predeliction for the femoral heads (stage II avascular necrosis) and nonarticular cancellous bone (medullary necrosis).

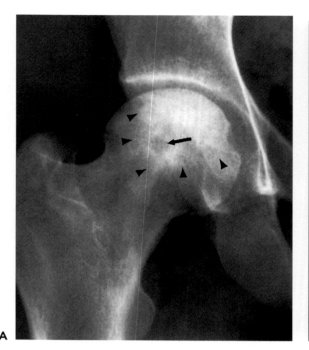
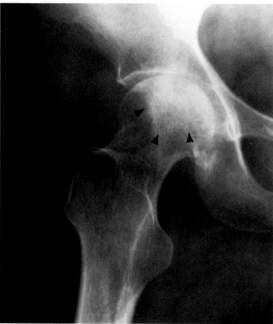

A

B

Figure 27-45 Avascular necrosis. **A:** AP radiograph of the hip demonstrating central lucency (*arrow*) and peripheral sclerosis (*arrowheads*) in Ficat stage II avascular necrosis. **B:** Frog-leg lateral view of the same patient again showing femoral head sclerosis.

TABLE 27-2
RADIOGRAPHIC STAGING OF FEMORAL HEAD AVASCULAR NECROSIS BY STEINBERG

Stage	Criteria
0	Normal x-ray, bone scan, and MRI
I	Normal x-ray, *abnormal* bone scan or MRI
II	Patchy sclerosis or lucency of femoral head
	A. Mild (<15%)
	B. Moderate (15%–30%)
	C. Severe (>30%)
III	Subchondral collapse (crescent sign)
	A. Mild (<15%)
	B. Moderate (15%–30%)
	C. Severe (>30%)
IV	Flattening of femoral head without joint narrowing
	A. Mild (<15%)
	B. Moderate (15%–30%)
	C. Severe (>30%)
V	Flattening of femoral head with joint narrowing or acetabular involvement
	A. Mild (<15% of surface and <2 mm depression)
	B. Moderate (15%–30% of surface or 2–4 mm depression)
	C. Severe (>30% of surface or >4 mm depression)
VI	Advanced degenerative arthrosis
	A. Mild
	B. Moderate
	C. Severe (determined as above, with estimate of acetabular involvement)

stages parallel the pathologic changes within the femoral head. The percent involvement of the head and appearance of the anterosuperior subchondral surface are helpful in predicting outcome.

Early in the disease, radiographs are normal as ischemia and necrosis affect cellular but not crystalline elements and are thus detectable by MRI as areas of excess free water and by scintigraphy as either diminished or increased uptake (132). Months later, the reactive response leads to hyperemia of surrounding bone sparing the necrotic focus (which has no blood supply), leading to diffuse osteoporosis with apparent radiographic sclerosis of the necrotic region (63). This pattern is not commonly detected, as the difference in bone density may be minimal on a macroscopic scale. As the reactive response continues, the hyperemic border of necrotic bone becomes fibrous and is in turn enveloped by hypertrophic bone, yielding the classic radiographic features of epiphyseal lucency with surrounding sclerosis (Fig. 27-45). Larger lesions may undergo transient elastic deflection of the cartilaginous surface overlying the necrotic segment, impacting the dead trabecular bone beneath. As the osteochondral surface regains its shape, a crescentic zone between it and the underlying trabeculae emerges and is recognized radiographically as a subchondral lucency known as the crescent sign (97) (Fig. 27-46). This important feature indicates mechanical failure of the necrotic and reactive bone and portends a poor outcome. With time, the osteochondral segment inevitably fails to spring back from its deflections and remains permanently flattened, or an entire segment of cartilage and underlying bone may collapse into the femoral head. The resulting incongruence of the hip leads to progressive degenerative arthrosis (Figs. 27-47 and 27-48).

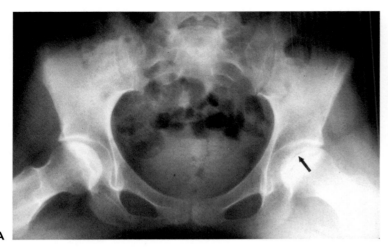
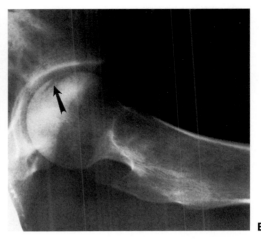

A   B

Figure 27-46   Crescent sign. **A:** Frog-leg view of both hips showing osteosclerosis and lucent crescent on the left, indicating transient osteochondral collapse with elastic recoil. **B:** Single lateral view of the left hip in the same patient more clearly delineating the subchondral crescent within the sclerotic femoral head caused by transient osteochondral collapse. This radiograph features the hallmark of Ficat stage III avascular necrosis indicating mechanical failure of the femoral head during the reparative phase of osteonecrosis.

Tomography may occasionally help to clarify the extent or depth of displacement in advanced osteonecrosis of the femoral head but has been largely supplanted by MRI, which when performed with newer dedicated coils and high-resolution technique is capable of multiplanar demonstration of collapse, cartilage degeneration, and evaluation of marrow. CT may be of help with thin collimation technique and multiplanar reconstruction, but the plane of section is not optimal to evaluate the superior weight-bearing surface of the femoral head, and further evaluation of this application may be needed.

Periarticular Disorders

The hip is not a common site for involvement for inflammatory enthesopathy, but mechanical greater trochanteric bursitis and iliopsoas bursitis are common conditions and are often radiographically occult (57,86,121,128,136). Upon occasion, calcium hydroxyapatite deposition may be seen in

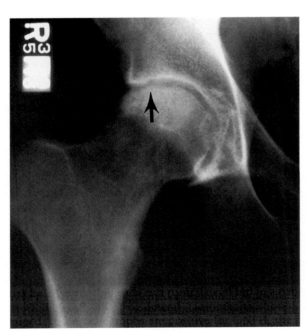

Figure 27-47   Fixed flattening of the superior weight-bearing femoral head. Although the joint space is relatively well preserved, the fixed incongruence of the femoral head in Stage IV disease inevitably leads to degenerative arthrosis.

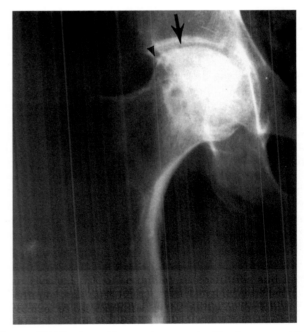

Figure 27-48   Stage V avascular necrosis. Fixed segmental flattening of the femoral head (*arrow*) with joint space loss medially and osteophytosis laterally (*arrowhead*).

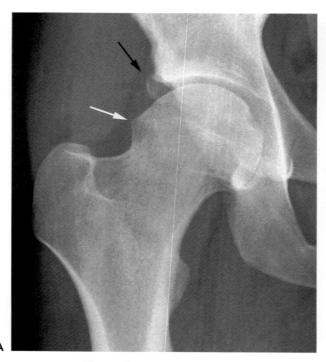
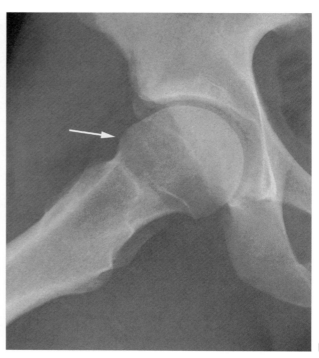

A   B

Figure 27-49   25-year-old male with AP view of the right hip showing loss of normal sphericity and loss of normal offset of the femoral head-neck junction due to presence of a bony excrescence (*white arrow*) **(A)**. A large periacetabular ossicle (*black arrow*) is noted that may be associated with underlying labral injury. Frogleg lateral view demonstrates loss of normal offset at the femoral head-neck junction **(B)**.

the iliopsoas enthesis at the lesser trochanter or about the greater trochanter, and rarely, inflammatory enthesophytes may be seen. Symptoms may precede radiographic identification of calcifications, and the diagnosis may be made by MRI examination (77). Finally, lumbar radiculopathy, inguinal hernia, and disorders of urinary and reproductive organs may mimic hip disorders and should be considered when intrinsic hip pathology is not apparent clinically or by imaging.

Femoroacetabular Impingement

Femoroacetabular impingement (FAI) is a recently recognized and important concept associated with labral injury and arthritis (8,9,10,42,68,72,75,79,83). The most common types have subtle but identifiable radiographic findings. FAI is categorized into two basic types: Type 1 and Type 2. Type 1, also known as cam type or pistol grip deformity, has a bony bump at the femoral head-neck junction, resulting in loss of normal offset. Type 2, or pincer type, result from over coverage of the acetabulum, usually anteriorly, related to subtle retroversion. Both types are predisposed to collision of the femoral head-neck junction with acetabular rim, causing resultant injury to the cartilage and intervening labrum, and thus, the term impingement. Hybrid combinations of both major types of FAI exist.

The radiographic appearance of Type 1 impingement demonstrates loss of normal offset of the femoral head-neck junction and loss of normal sphericity of the femoral head (Fig. 27-49). Radiographically, this finding is best see with a cross-table lateral view, but in some cases, can also be appreciated on an AP view or frogleg lateral view (Fig. 27-50). One

study has showed that femoral head-neck junction offset on a cross-table later view in asymptomatic patients measured more than 11.5 mm, but offset in symptomatic patients measured less than 7.2 mm (Fig. 27-50) (32). Type 1 FAI can also be identified with cross-sectional imaging, such as CT or MR arthrography, using oblique axial images parallel to the femoral neck and measuring an alpha angle (Fig. 27-51) (98).

Synovial herniation pits seen on plain film or cross-sectional imaging studies were often considered normal variants in the past, but are now suspicious markers for Type 1 FAI (Fig. 27-18) (79). Anecdotally, there may also be an association with Type 1 FAI and small periacetabular ossicles, which could be related to underlying labral tears.

Type 2 impingement is generally associated with acetabular retroversion. This is best seen on a well-centered AP view of the pelvis. Radiographically, the anterior acetabular rim, which appears as a thin line arising from the pubis to the lateral acetabulum, should not cross over the posterior acetabular rim extending from the ischium. This cross-over usually occurs superiorly, and it has been termed the cross-over sign (Fig. 27-52) (113). However, evaluation for this radiographic finding requires a well-centered view of the pelvis without significant pelvic tilt or rotation, so that the projectional appearance of the anterior acetabular rim, in relation to the posterior rim, is not altered (44,125). Cross-sectional imaging, such as CT or MR, can also detect retroversion, but one must analyze the superior aspect of the acetabulum and not the midportion (83).

The cause of FAI is unclear, but is likely multifactorial and related to subtle physeal growth injury and subsequent healing with minor anatomic deformity. It is, however, possible

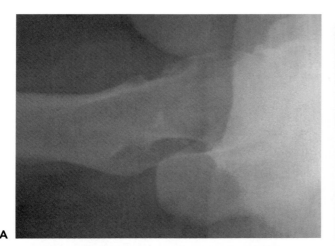

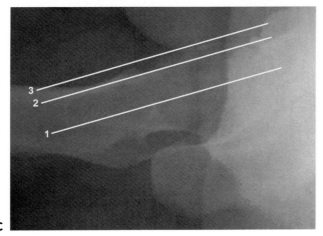

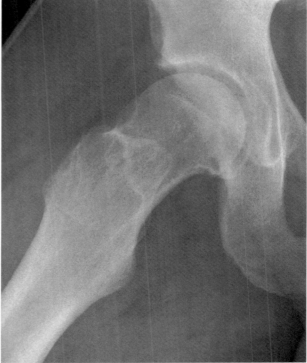

Figure 27-50 28-year-old male with clinical findings of FAI. Cross-table lateral view (**A**) clearly shows loss of femoral head-neck offset, which is less apparent on conventional frogleg lateral view (**B**). Quantitative evaluation of loss of offset on cross-table lateral view can be obtained by measuring the distances between lines drawn along the anterior femoral cortex (line 2) and the anterior aspect of the femoral head (line 3), which are parallel to a line along the center of the femoral neck (line 1) (**C**).

that an underlying soft issue injury (i.e., labral tear) or joint microinstability could predispose to a chronic bony reaction in response to altered biomechanics, reminiscent of Fairbanks, like changes of the knee.

Infection

Septic arthritis is best diagnosed by examination of joint fluid or aspirate in the acute presentation of atraumatic hip pain where radiographs are normal. If the process is not recognized and treated promptly, cartilage destruction is rapid and diffuse, leading to axial narrowing of the hip, often with osteoporosis, and ankylosis may be a late feature (20,27) (Fig. 27-53).

Osteomyelitis is a term that implies infection of medullary bone, usually with associated necrosis. Other conditions in skeletal infection include infectious periostitis, in which infection occurs at and between the periosteum and underlying cortex, and cortical osteitis, where infection has involved the intracortical haversian system. *Infectious osteitis* is a term used to indicate sterile inflammation of bone marrow associated with an adjacent infection or infected but viable bone. Osseous infection may occur from direct inoculation, often from open fractures, an adjacent infection such as decubitus ulcers, or hematogenously (111).

In the acute setting, radiographs may reveal only subtle permeative trabecular destruction as the process spreads, and MRI or scintigraphy (with bone-seeking agents and/or indium-labeled leukocytes) is diagnostic. Later, endosteal destruction, immature periostitis, and soft tissue masses may be noted with greater definition of bone loss (Fig. 27-54). MRI performed with administration of intravenous gadolinium-based contrast commonly differentiates viable from nonviable bone and soft tissue and may help in choosing between antibiotic therapy alone (viable enhancing tissue) or surgical excision of nonviable, nonenhancing tissue. Chronic osteomyelitis is characterized radiographically by the formation of sequestra of dead bone and infected debris and the involucrum of reactive sclerosis by the bone in an effort to contain the process. Examination by CT may define the extent and location of sequestra to better advantage and, due to its greater tissue contrast, is more commonly used than tomography.

Neoplasm

Virtually every neoplasm affecting the musculoskeletal system may involve the hip, and a review of each is beyond the scope of this chapter. Recognition of the radiographic features used in diagnosis and characterization of neoplasm are of greater importance and will be summarized.

Plain films are used to identify and characterize skeletal masses, CT is used to characterize mineralized matrix of masses, and MRI is used to both identify radiographically

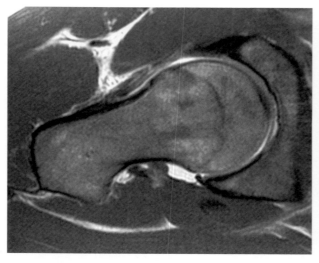

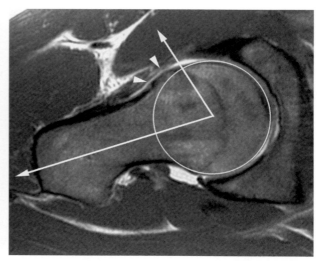

A

B

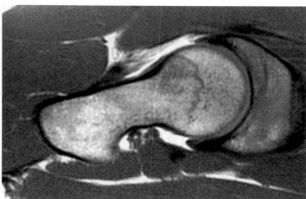

C

Figure 27-51 Oblique axial MR image of the right hip in same patient as Figure 27-49 showing loss of normal femoral head-neck offset consistent with cam impingement (A). Figure B illustrates measurement of the alpha angle. A ray parallel to the femoral neck, originating from the center of a best-fit circle of the femoral head, is drawn first. An additional ray is then drawn from the center of the femoral head to the point where the anterior cortex of the head-neck junction deviates from the circumference of the best-fit circle. Alpha angle values greater than 50 degrees suggest cam impingement (Type 1). In this case, the angle is greater than 80 degrees and arrowheads mark the bony excrescence, which contributes to impingement. Figure C demonstrates a different patient with normal appearance of the femoral head-neck offset on an oblique axial MR image parallel to the femoral neck.

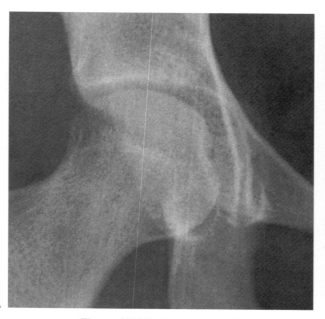

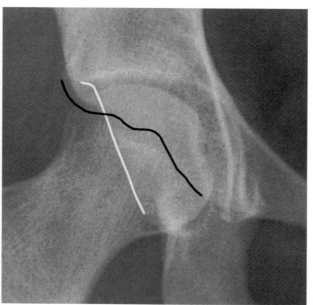

A

B

Figure 27-52 Same images of a well-centered AP view of the pelvis emphasizing the right hip with (A) and without (B) annotation shows cross over of the anterior acetabular rim (black line) with posterior rim (white line) involving the superior aspect of the acetabulum. This is known as the cross-over sign, which is indicative of subtle acetabular retroversion predisposing to pincer type impingement.

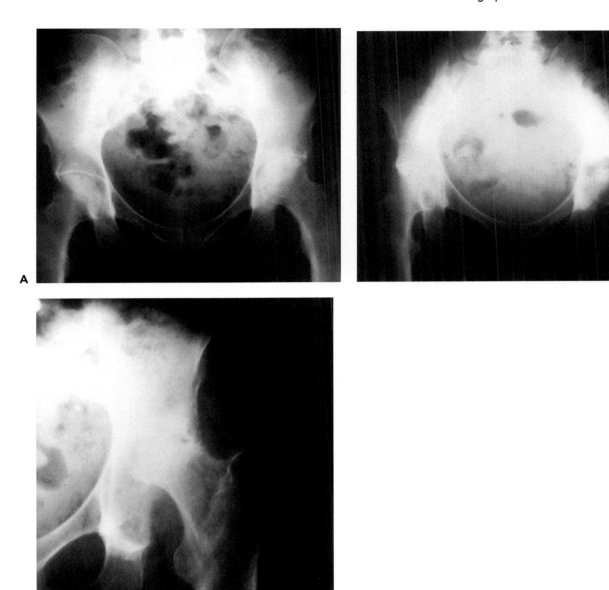

Figure 27-53 Septic arthritis. **A:** Initial radiograph showing early axial narrowing of the left hip thought to be due to inflammatory arthritis. **B:** AP radiograph of the pelvis 1 week following initial radiograph **(A)** showing rapid destruction of the hip. Aspiration yielded *Candida albicans*. **C:** Follow-up radiograph showing progressive destruction of the femoral head and acetabulum.

occult masses and locally stage extent of spread. CT and MRI do not generally differentiate benign from malignant disease to a greater extent than plain film. Scintigraphy is used to identify occult masses as well and may screen the entire body.

Masses may represent neoplasm, inflammation, or infection and so are referred to as aggressive or indolent radiographic processes, recognizing the overlap of pathology. Some are radiographically pathognomonic, but most share features with a limited host of other entities and may only be definitively diagnosed upon biopsy. Importantly, the biopsy must be interpreted in concert with imaging findings, as they are complementary and errors in diagnosis may come from histologic analysis in isolation.

Finally, the radiologic staging of the patient with primary skeletal neoplasm (sarcoma) must include local imaging prior to biopsy, plain films followed by MRI, and examination of the chest to evaluate for metastatic disease, which is best performed by CT (101).

Radiographic features used to distinguish indolent from aggressive processes reflect both the nature of the mass and the response of bone to it. Tumors may be osteolytic or

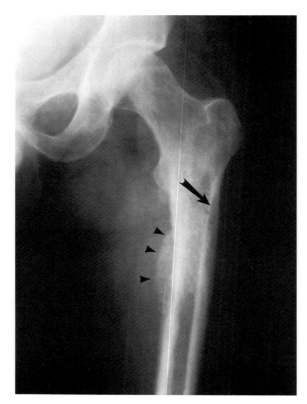

Figure 27-54 Osteomyelitis. Thirty-four-year-old laborer with rapid onset of leg pain and initially normal radiograph. Follow-up radiograph demonstrates medial periostitis and a diffuse permeative lesion throughout the subtrochanteric femur. Although initially felt to represent an aggressive round cell tumor, biopsy revealed gross pus. Radiographic distinction between acute suppurative osteomyelitis and aggressive neoplasm may be impossible and mandate biopsy.

osteoblastic or both. The transition between normal and abnormal bone is generally sharply defined in indolent processes, while broad and ill defined in aggressive processes. Well-defined lesions are termed *geographic*, intermediately defined lesions are termed *moth-eaten*, and poorly defined are termed *permeative* (73) (Fig. 27-55). *Margination* refers to the presence and type of border about the mass, including reactive sclerosis. *Location* within a bone includes the anatomic region (diaphysis, metaphysis, or epiphyseal equivalent) and cross-sectional location (central medulla, peripheral medulla, cortex, periosteum). *Matrix* refers to the substance of the mass itself and may be bland, having no radiographic features. Chondroid matrix has rings, arcs, and punctate foci of calcification and may be seen in certain benign and malignant cartilage tumors. Tumor bone, which may be cloudy or spiculated, indicates bone-forming tumors such as osteosarcoma or osteoblastoma. Distinguishing tumor bone from heterotopic bone may be difficult, but tumor bone is most immature at the periphery of the lesion, whereas heterotopic bone is most mature peripherally, and CT may help in characterization of such matrix. Periosteal response to a slow-growing lesion is generally thick and well defined, whereas aggressive lesions provoke thin, often layered periosteal responses that may appear as onion skin. If interrupted by the mass, the border of the layered periosteal response is termed a *Codman's triangle* and may be seen in infection and tumor. The most highly aggressive lesions may result in a sunburst array of spiculated subperiosteal new bone. An associated soft tissue mass may be seen with bony masses, more commonly in sarcomas and infection than in metastatic disease (84). Using these criteria and the patient's clinical history, one of three conclusions should be reached in every case. Either the mass is completely characteristic of benign disease and needs to be left alone or followed radiographically (Fig. 27-56), it is completely characteristic of aggressive disease and needs to be staged and biopsied, or it is a lesion lacking enough features to make a diagnosis, warranting supplemental studies, biopsy, or follow-up, depending on its most dominant features.

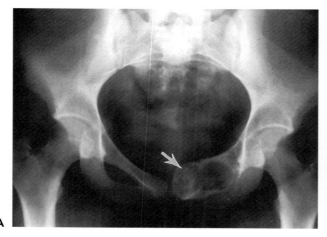

A

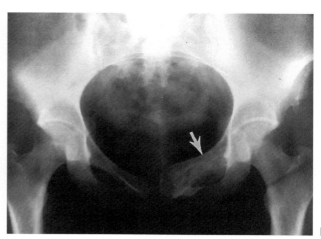

B

Figure 27-55 Aneurysmal bone cyst. **A:** Initial AP radiograph of the pelvis showing an expansile geographic lesion in the superior pubic ramus on the left. Apparent chondroid matrix in the perisymphyseal pubis raise the possibility of a chondroid tumor but the expansile well-demarcated borders are more consistent with either a unicameral bone cyst or aneurysmal bone cyst (found at biopsy). **B:** Follow-up radiograph following curettage showing sclerosis of the lesion with similar appearance to initial matrix morphology.

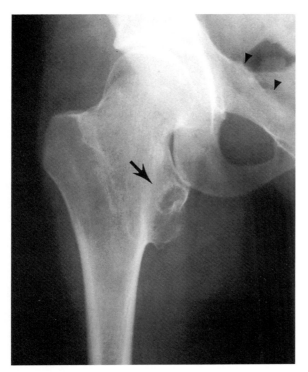

Figure 27-56 Multiple hereditory exostoses (diaphyseal aclasis). Large medial osteochondroma (exostosis) with endomedullary continuity of lesion (*arrow*), distinguishing it from juxtacortical lesions and heterotopic ossification. Note sessile exostoses along pubic ramus and intertrochanteric line (*arrowheads*). While there is a malignant potential for osteochondromas, the radiographic appearance of the primary lesions do not require other imaging, and the lesions can be followed clinically and with occasional radiographs.

The Prosthetic Hip

Complications of arthroplasty may occur from errors in positioning during surgery, infection, mechanical failure of prosthesis or bone, or by a biological response to wear material that in turn leads to mechanical failure of fixation (16). Plain films are almost always diagnostic, whereas CT has specific utility in evaluating prosthetic component position and in detection of early failure of femoral stem fixation (23).

Postoperatively, position of components, cement technique, and identification of fracture are of most importance, and portable films in the recovery suite are most commonly used. Once the patient's condition has stabilized, an AP and cross-table lateral views are obtained by standard technique, including all hardware and cement. Rarely, component failure or periprosthetic fracture may occur in the subacute setting, more often in revision and in osteoporosis (38) (Fig. 27-57).

Infection may be seen acutely, subacutely, or in late follow-up; commonly has no immediate radiographic features; and must be diagnosed on clinical suspicion and aspiration. Later features include pericement or periprosthetic bone destruction and mechanical loosening (130) (Fig. 27-58).

Dislocation may occur at any time postoperatively and is often the result of component malposition (56). AP and cross-table radiographs should demonstrate about 45° abduction and 10° anteversion of the acetabular component, and 15° anteversion of the femoral stem. Offset overlap on the AP projection may be seen with either anteversion or retroversion, although some have proposed that the degree of overlap between AP views of the hip and pelvis differs from different central beam alignment, allowing differentiation of anteversion and retroversion. We have not found this to be a reliable

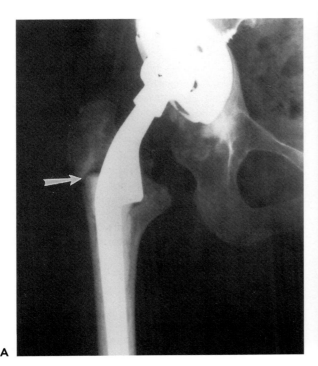

A

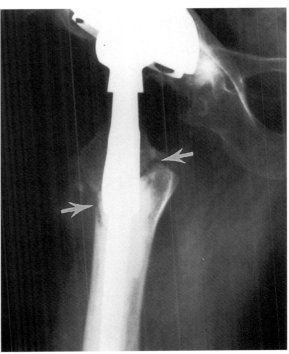

B

Figure 27-57 Periprosthetic fracture of the intertrochanteric femur. **A:** AP radiograph showing questionable lucency of the lateral cortex at the proximal margin of the femoral cement column in a patient with an atraumatic history. **B:** Frog-leg lateral view showing anterior and posterior cortical fracture of the greater trochanter.

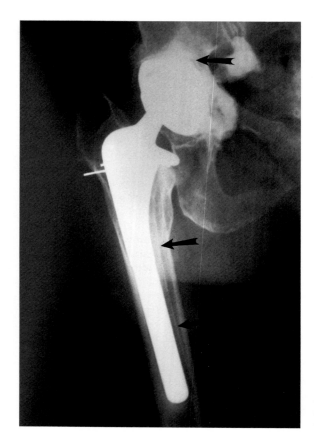

Figure 27-58 Infected total hip arthroplasty. Advanced periprosthetic lucency about the femoral stem and circumferential but modest bone cement interface lucency about acetabular component of total hip arthroplasty. Hip aspiration yielded *Staphylococcus aureus* despite the well-demarcated periprosthetic lucencies.

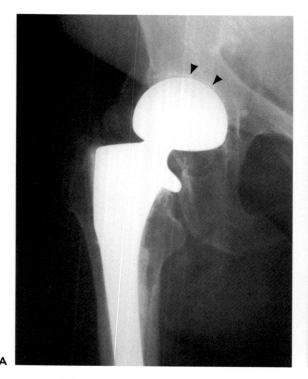

A

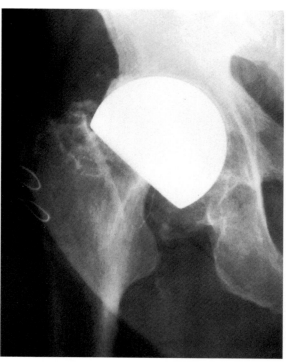

B

Figure 27-59 Chondrolysis. **A:** Hemiarthroplasty of the right hip showing focal medial narrowing of acetabular chondral surface in patient with early chondrolysis. **B:** Advanced chondrolysis circumferential acetabular narrowing in patient with femoral head hemiarthoplasty.

observation, and when plain radiography is unrevealing we perform a limited CT examination that directly demonstrates true acetabular and femoral version and tilt.

In long-term follow-up, several radiographic abnormalities may be seen about components, and comparison with recent and distant previous studies is of great help in detecting abnormalities. In the presence of a femoral hemiarthroplasty, the acetabular cartilage may degrade resulting in progressive narrowing or chondrolysis, which is often only seen in comparing previous to recent examinations (Fig. 27-59).

Complications of total hip arthroplasty femoral components tend to occur earlier than acetabular (54,87). Mechanical stem failure presents as fracture of the component, generally of the mid- to distal femoral stem and may be easily overlooked when other findings are present (52). Periprosthetic fractures in the chronic setting are usually posttraumatic, and at the level of the femoral stem tip.

Resorption of metaphyseal trabecular and cortical bone is common about femoral stems of hemi- or total arthroplasty and is the result of unloading of bone as load is transferred from femoral neck cortex, in the native state, to the femoral stem and subtrochanteric cortex in the presence of a femoral arthroplasty (18,61,87,115). Termed *stress shielding*, it generally is of no concern and should not be mistaken for a significant abnormality (Figs. 27-60 and 27-61).

The biological–nonbiological interface of an arthroplasty has been termed the *effective joint space* and may be apparent radiographically as a very thin lucent zone between either cement and bone or prosthesis and bone of both femoral and acetabular components (26,67). With time, wear particles may accumulate in recesses of this space and, if they are of a critical size, incite a reactive histiocytic response termed *membrane disease*, *particle disease*, or *aggressive osteolysis* from among others (46,53). Radiographically, scalloped lucent foci of variable size occur at the biological–nonbiological interface, with or without sclerotic margination (131). Comparison with previous films shows a progressive, unrelenting course, and in longstanding disease, mechanical loosening or fracture may occur (2).

Mechanical loosening of the femoral stem is apparent radiographically by several features (87,133). Motion of the component during examination from one position to another indicates loosening (86,93). Periprosthetic or bone–cement interface lucency does not indicate loosening in and of itself, and acceptable lucency differs in cemented and uncemented components (Fig. 27-62). In general, more than 2 mm of lucency is considered a cutoff in which loosening of a cemented prosthesis should be considered, but more important than the width of the lucency is the distribution. Diffuse, circumferential lucency or that which widens beyond a central

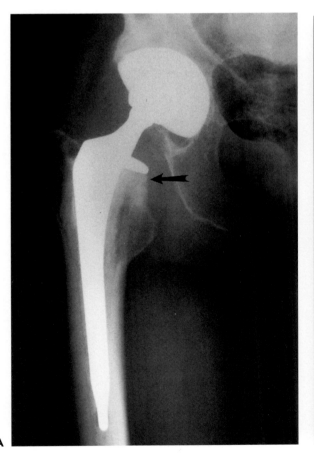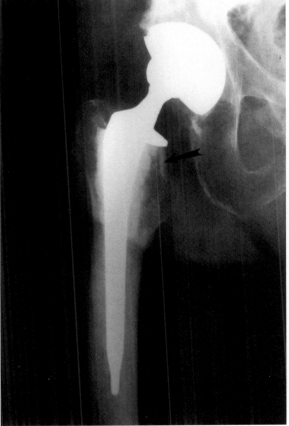

A   **B**

Figure 27-60 Stress shielding. **A:** Initial AP radiograph of the hip showing dense cortical bone of the remnant of the medial femoral neck. **B:** Subsequent AP radiograph showing advanced metaphyseal bone loss in the proximal femur, particularly in the medial femoral neck remnant with preservation of mineralization in the subtrochanteric diaphysis.

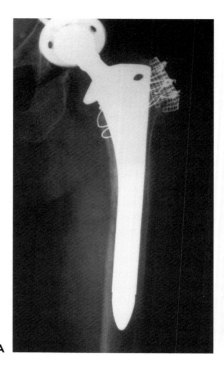

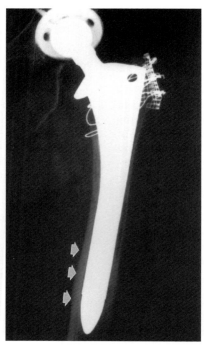

Figure 27-61 Cortical hypertrophy from load transfer. **A:** Revision total hip arthroplasty showing relatively uniform femoral cortex. **B:** Subsequent AP radiograph showing distal cortical hypertrophy from increased mechanical load at the femoral stem tip. Proximal bone loss is negligible.

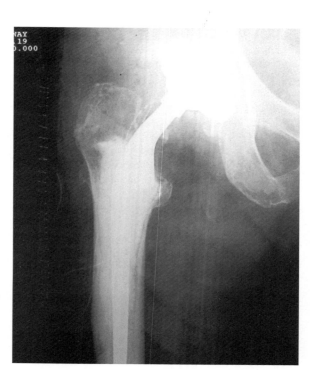

Figure 27-62 Bone cement interface lucency immediately following revision total hip arthroplasty. On follow-up examination, there was no significant change in its appearance despite its relative prominence medially and extensive length of involvement. Progressive change rather than absolute width of bone cement interface lucencies should be considered more indicative of osteolysis or mechanical loosening.

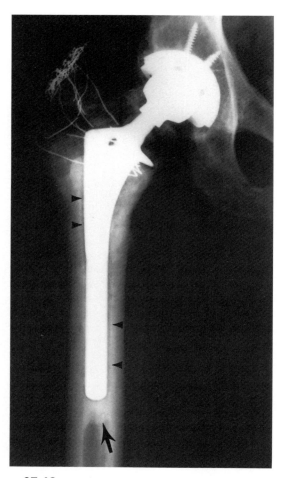

Figure 27-63 Mechanical loosening of uncemented femoral component of total hip arthroplasty. Observe circumferential periprosthetic lucency predominating inferomedially and superolaterally consistent with a mid stem fulcrum. Pronounced endomedullary pedestal which in isolation is generally not a significant radiographic finding (*arrow*).

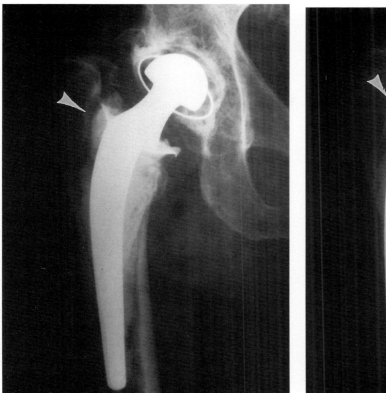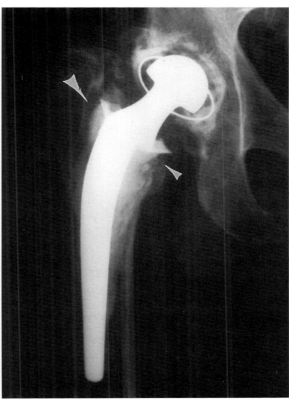

Figure 27-64 Acetabular and femoral component failure of total hip arthroplasty. **A:** AP radiograph of the hip showing asymmetry of the femoral head within the acetabular cup (asymmetric wear), advanced bone cement interface lucency about the medial acetabular component and femoral component varus. **B:** Progressive degeneration of superior acetabular polymethylmethacrylate and polyethylene. While no appreciable change in the bone cement interface lucency about the femoral stem can be seen, closer approximation of the femoral mesh with the lesser trochanter and progressive varus indicates subsidence and loss of fixation.

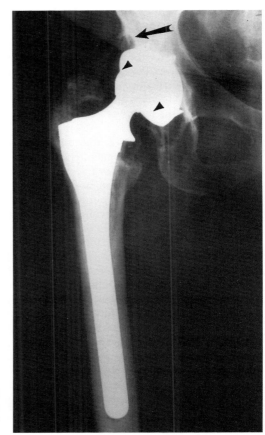

Figure 27-65 Asymmetric wear of acetabular component. The femoral head (outlined by *arrowheads*) lies asymmetrically within the acetabular cup indicating advanced polyethylene wear. Some early osteolysis is present, particularly at the superior margin of the acetabulum (*arrow*).

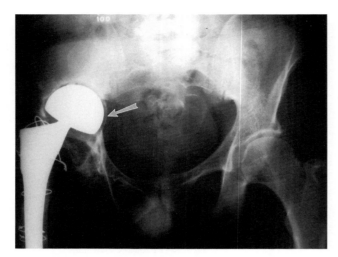

Figure 27-66 Advanced acetabular protrusio. Hemiarthroplasty of the right hip showing advanced cephaloaxial migration with marked thinning of the anterior and medial acetabulum.

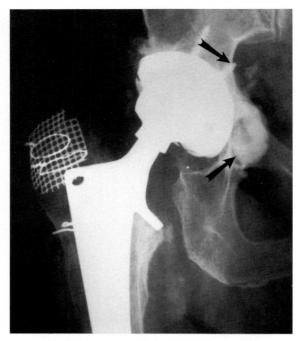

Figure 27-67 Intrapelvic cement and intrapelvic screw in revision total hip arthroplasty. Intrapelvic cement and screws increase the risk of major vascular trauma during revision surgery and may warrant CT examination to evaluate position of pelvic vasculature relative to screws and cement.

fulcrum is more suspicious than focal lucency. Some have termed this latter appearance the *windshield washer sign,* as the perilucency sclerosis is akin in shape to that of snow pushed to the edge of an automobile windshield. Most refer to the finding as toggling of the component about a fulcrum (Fig. 27-63). Interval change is critical in evaluation, as scattered linear lucencies about components are common. The most reliable indicator of loosening of a component is subsidence, or intrusion, which may be difficult if not impossible to detect without previous examinations and is often the only sign of mechanical loss of fixation (see Fig. 27-60). As mentioned earlier, dynamic CT examination may help in diagnosis of femoral lucency in which history and plain films are not definitive. Although arthrography has been traditionally used for detection of component loosening when plain radiographs are equivocal, opinion remains divided on criteria for performance, interpretation, and significance of conclusions drawn (87,95). Perhaps the most widely accepted use for arthrography in the setting of a painful arthroplasty is that of aspiration when infection is considered (115).

Acetabular component complications tend to occur later than femoral, though overall their frequencies are thought to be similar. The polyethylene liner of the acetabular component may wear asymmetrically, predominantly superiorly (Fig. 27-64). Any measurable difference in superolateral and anteromedial centralization of the femoral component with respect to the acetabular component indicates asymmetric wear (Fig. 27-65). With advanced wear, fragmentation and gross collapse of the polyethylene liner may occur and may be difficult to detect radiographically. Periprosthetic lucencies about acetabular components may be difficult to detect superiorly, as cephalad migration of the component occurs as well, and medial lucency or change in component position may be the only clue to loss of fixation and loosening (122) (Fig. 27-66). Protrusio may occur with either cemented or uncemented components. In evaluation of an arthroplasty for revision, careful examination of the anterior and posterior column and medial wall in planning acetabular augmentation and identification of intrapelvic cement or screws is of great importance (Fig. 27-67). When plain films show

intrapelvic cement, CT examination can define its position relative to pelvic vasculature. Intravenous administration of contrast may be necessary to define vessels on occasion.

REFERENCES

1. Alazraki N. Diagnosing prosthetic joint infection. *J Nucl Med.* 1990;31:1955–1957.
2. Amstutz HC, Campbell P, Kossovsky N, et al. Mechanism and clinical significance of wear debris-induced osteolysis. *Clin Orthop.* 1992;276:7–18.
3. Ansell BM, Unlu M. Hip involvement in juvenile chronic polyarthritis [abstract]. *Ann Rheum Dis.* 687–688.
4. Antti-Poika I, Josefsson G, Konttinen Y, et al.. Hip arthroplasty infection. *Acta Orthop Scand.* 1990;61:163–169.
5. Apel DM, Vince KG, Kingston S. Transient osteoporosis of the hip: a role for core decompression? *Orthopedics.* 1994;17:629–632.
6. Armbuster TG, Guerra J, Resnick D, et al. The adult hip: an anatomic study. *Radiology.* 1978;128:1–10.
7. Barrack RL, Tanzer M, Kattapuram SV, et al. The value of contrast arthrography in assessing loosening of symptomatic uncemented total hip components. *Skeletal Radiol.* 1994;23:37–41.
8. Beall DP, Sweet CF, Martin HD, et al. Imaging findings of femoroacetabular impingement syndrome. *Skeletal Radiol* 2005.
9. Beck M, Kalhor M, Leunig M, et al. Hip morphology influences the pattern of damage to the acetabular cartilage: femoroacetabular impingement as a cause of early osteoarthritis of the hip. *J Bone Joint Surg Br* 2005;87:1012–1018.
10. Beck M, Leunig M, Parvizi J, et al. Anterior femoroacetabular impingement: Part II. Midterm results of surgical treatment. *Clin Orthop Relat Res.* 2004;418:67–73.
11. Beck PV, Mahajan G, Wilsey BL, et al. Fluoroscopic and electromyographic guided injection of the piriformis muscle with botulinum toxin type B. *Pain Med.* 2002;3:179.
12. Benzon HT, Katz JA, Benzon HA, et al. Piriformis syndrome: anatomic considerations, a new injection technique, and a review of the literature. *Anesthesiology.* 2003;98:1442–1448.

13. Blake MP, Halasz SJ. Effect of X-ray contrast media on bacterial growth. *Australasian Radiol.* 1995;39:10–13.
14. Bock GW, Garcia A, Weisman MH, et al. Rapidly destructive hip disease: clinical and imaging abnormalities. *Radiology.* 1993;186: 461–466.
15. Braun J, Bollow M, Seyrekbasan F, et al. Computed tomography guided corticosteroid injection of the sacroiliac joint in patients with spondyloarthropathy with sacroiliitis: clinical outcome and followup by dynamic magnetic resonance imaging. *J Rheumatol.* 1996;23:659–664.
16. Brown CS, Knickerbocker WJ. Radiologic studies in the investigation of the causes of total hip replacement failure. *J Can Assoc Radiol.* 1973;24:245–253.
17. Brown JA, Braun MA, Namey TC. Pyriformis syndrome in a 10-year-old boy as a complication of operation with the patient in the sitting position. *Neurosurgery.* 1988;23:117–119.
18. Bryan JM, Sumner DR, Hurwitz DE, et al. Altered load history affects periprosthetic bone loss following cementless total hip arthroplasty. *J Orthop Res.* 1996;14:762–768.
19. Buckwalter KA, Rydberg J, Kopecky KK, et al. Musculoskeletal imaging with multislice CT. *AJR Am J Roentgenol.* 2001;176:979–986.
20. Bulmer JH. Septic arthritis of the hip in adults. *J Bone Joint Surg Br.* 1966;48:289–298.
21. Chiang PP, Burke DW, Freiberg AA, et al. Osteolysis of the pelvis: evaluation and treatment. *Clin Orthop.* 2003;417:164–174.
22. Childers MK, Wilson DJ, Gnatz SM, et al. Botulinum toxin type A use in piriformis muscle syndrome: a pilot study. *Am J Phys Med Rehabil.* 2002;81:751–759.
23. Clements RW, Nakayama HK. Radiographic methods in total hip arthroplasty. *Radiol Technol.* 1980;51:589–600.
24. Cody DD, Moxley DM, Krugh KT, et al. Strategies for formulating appropriate MDCT techniques when imaging the chest, abdomen, and pelvis in pediatric patients. *AJR Am J Roentgenol.* 2004;182:849–859.
25. Cohen JM, Hodges SC, Weinreb JC, et al. MR imaging of iliopsoas bursitis and concurrent avascular necrosis of the femoral head. *J Comput Assist Tomogr.* 1985;9:969–971.
26. Cook SD, Thomas KA, Haddad RJ. Histologic analysis of retrieved human porous-coated total joint components. *Clin Orthop.* 1988;234:90–101.
27. Curtiss PH, Klein L. Destruction of articular cartilage in septic arthritis. Part I: *J Bone Joint Surg Am.* 1973;45:797–886.
28. Cyteval C, Hamm V, Sarrabere MP, et al. Painful infection at the site of hip prosthesis: CT imaging. *Radiology.* 2002;224:477–483.
29. Dussault RG, Kaplan PA, Anderson MW. Fluoroscopy-guided sacroiliac joint injections. *Radiology.* 2000;214:273–277.
30. Duthie RB, Harris CM. A radiographic and clinical survey of the hip joint in sero-positive rheumatoid arthritis. *Acta Orthop Scand.* 1969;40:346–364.
31. Dwosh IL, Resnick D, Becker MA. Hip involvement in ankylosing spondylitis. *Arthritis Rheum.* 1976;19:683–692.
32. Eijer H, Leunig M, Mahomed N, et al. Cross-table lateral radiographs for screening of anterior femoral head-neck offset in patients with femoro-acetabular impingement. *Hip Int* 2001;11: 37–41.
33. Fanucci E, Masala S, Sodani G, et al. CT-guided injection of botulinic toxin for percutaneous therapy of piriformis muscle syndrome with preliminary MRI results about denervative process. *Eur Radiol.* 2001;11:2543–2548.
34. Fanucci E, Masala S, Squillaci E, et al. Pyriformis muscle syndrome: CT/MR findings in the percutaneous therapy with botulinic toxin. *Radiol Med Torino.* 2003;105:69–75.
35. Fishman EK, Magid D, Mandelbaum BR, et al. Multiplanar (MPR) imaging of the hip. *RadioGraphics.* 1986;6:7–54.
36. Fishman LM, Dombi GW, Michaelsen C, et al. Piriformis syndrome: diagnosis, treatment, and outcome—a 10-year study. *Arch Phys Med Rehabil.* 2002;83:295–301.
37. Fishman SM, Caneris OA, Bandman TB, et al. Injection of the piriformis muscle by fluoroscopic and electromyographic guidance. *Reg Anesth Pain Med.* 1998;23:554–559.
38. Fitzgerald RH, Brindley GW, Kavanagh BF. The uncemented total hip arthroplasty. *Clin Orthop.* 1988;235:61–66.
39. Fletcher F, Donaldson T, Wasielewski M, et al. A dynamic test for the diagnosis of loosened uncemented femoral components in total hip arthroplasty. Presented at: 23rd Annual Hip Course; 1993; Boston, MA.
40. Friedman L, Dubowitz B, Hurwitz J, et al. The 30° cephalad anteroposterior tilt view to stage avascular necrosis of the femoral head. *J Can Assoc Radiol.* 1988;39:213–215.
41. Frush DP. Review of radiation issues for computed tomography. *Semin Ultrasound CT MR.* 2004;25:17–24.
42. Ganz R, Parvizi J, Beck M, et al. Femoroacetabular impingement: a cause for osteoarthritis of the hip. *Clin Orthop Relat Res.* 2003; 417:112–120.
43. Gibbs SJ. Basic mechanism of radiation injury-somatic and genetic. In: American College of Radiology, ed. *Radiation Risk: A Primer.* Reston, VA: American College of Radiology; 1996:5–13.
44. Giori NJ, Trousdale RT. Acetabular retroversion is associated with osteoarthritis of the hip. *Clin Orthop Relat Res.* 2003:263–269.
45. Gluer CC, Cummings SR, Pressman A, et al. Prediction of hip fractures from pelvic radiographs: the study of osteoporotic fractures. *J Bone Min Res.* 1994;9:671–677.
46. Goetz DD, Smith EJ, Harris WH. The prevalence of femoral osteolysis associated with components inserted with or without cement in total hip replacements. *J Bone Joint Surg Am.* 1994;76: 1121–1129.
47. Gofton JP, Trueman GE. Studies in osteoarthritis of the hip. Part II. *Can Med Assoc J.* 1971;104:791–799.
48. Gray JE. Safety (risk) of diagnostic radiology exposures. In: American College of Radiology, ed. *Radiation Risk: A Primer.* Reston, VA: American College of Radiology; 1996:15–17.
49. Greenfield GB. Roentgen appearance of bone and soft tissue changes in chronic renal disease. *AJR Am J Roentgenol.* 1972; 116:749–757.
50. Greenspan A. *Orthopedic Radiology.* Philadelphia: JB Lippincott; 1988:5.2–5.18.
51. Gunaydin I, Pereira PL, Daikeler T, et al. Magnetic resonance imaging guided corticosteroid injection of the sacroiliac joints in patients with therapy resistant spondyloarthropathy: a pilot study. *J Rheumatol.* 2000;27:424–428.
52. Harris WH. The first 32 years of total hip arthroplasty. *Clin Orthop.* 1992;274:6–11.
53. Harris WH. The problem is osteolysis. *CORR.* 1995;311:46–53.
54. Harris WH, Sledge CB. Total hip and total knee replacement. *N Engl J Med.* 1990;323:725–731.
55. Hayward I, Bjorkengren AG, Pathria MN, et al. Patterns of femoral head migration in osteoarthritis of the hip: a reappraisal with CT and pathologic correlation. *Radiology.* 1988;166:857–860.
56. Hedlundh U, Ahnfelt L, Hybbinette CH, et al. Surgical experience related to dislocations after total hip arthroplasty. *J Bone Joint Surg Br.* 1996;78:206–209.
57. Helfgott SM. Unusual features of iliopsoas bursitis. *Arthritis Rheum.* 1988;31:1331–1333.
58. Hermodsson I. Roentgen appearances of arthritis of the hip. *Acta Radiol Diagn.* 1972;12:865–881.
59. Hernandez RJ, Tachdjian MO, Noznanski AK. CT determination of femoral torsion. *AJR Am J Roentgenol.* 1981;137:97–101.
60. Holt MA, Keene JS, Graf BK, et al. Treatment of osteitis pubis in athletes. Results of corticosteroid injections. *Am J Sports Med.* 1995;23:601–606.
61. Huiskes R. Stress shielding and bone resorption in total hip arthroplasty: clinical versus computer simulation studies. *Acta Orthop Belgica.* 1993;59(suppl 1):118–129.
62. Hunder GG, Kelly PJ. Roentgenologic transient osteoporosis of the hip. *Ann Intern Med.* 1968;68:539–552.
63. Hungerford, DS. Early diagnosis of ischemic necrosis of the femoral head. *Johns Hopkins Med J.* 1975;137:270
64. Ito K, Minka MA 2nd, Leunig M, et al. Femoroacetabular impingement and the cam-effect. A MRI-based quantitative anatomical study of the femoral head-neck offset. *J Bone Joint Surg Br.* 2001;83:171–176.
65. Jager M, Wild A, Westhoff B, et al. Femoroacetabular impingement caused by a femoral osseous head-neck bump deformity: clinical, radiological, and experimental results. *J Orthop Sci.* 2004;9:256–263.
66. Kalra MK, Prasad S, Saini S, et al. Clinical comparison of standard-dose and 50% reduced-dose abdominal CT: effect on image quality. *AJR Am J Roentgenol.* 2002;179:1101–1106.

67. Kaplan PA, Montesi SA, Jardon OM, et al. Bone-ingrowth hip prostheses in asymptomatic patients: radiographic features. *Radiology.* 1988;169:221–227.

68. Kassarjian A, Yoon LS, Belzile E, et al. Triad of MR arthrographic findings in patients with cam-type femoroacetabular impingement. *Radiol* 2005;236:588–592.

69. Kattapuram SV, Lodwick GS, Chandler H, et al. Porous-coated anatomic total hip prostheses: radiographic analysis and clinical correlation. *Radiology.* 1990;174:861–864.

70. Katz JF. Arthrography in Legg-Calvé-Perthes disease. *J Bone Joint Surg Am.* 1968;50:467–472.

71. Keats TE, Teeslink R, Diamond AE, et al. Normal axial relationships of the major joints. *Radiology.* 1966;87:904–907.

72. Klaue K, Durnin CW, Ganz R. The acetabular rim syndrome. A clinical presentation of dysplasia of the hip. *J Bone Joint Surg Br* 1991;73:423–429.

73. Kricun ME. Radiographic evaluation of solitary bone lesions. *Orthop Clin North Am.* 1983;14:39.

74. Kursunoglu-Brahme S, Cervilla V, Vint V, et al. Magnetic resonance appearance of sacral insufficiency fractures. *Skeletal Radiol.* 1990;19:489–493.

75. Lavigne M, Parvizi J, Beck M, et al. Anterior femoroacetabular impingement: Part I. Techniques of joint preserving surgery. *Clin Orthop Relat Res* 2004;418:61–66.

76. Lee CI, Haims AH, Monico EP, et al. Diagnostic CT scans: assessment of patient, physician, and radiologist awareness of radiation dose and possible risks. *Radiology.* 2004;231:393–398.

77. Lee JKD, Glazer HS. Psoas muscle disorders: MR imaging. *Radiology.* 1986;160:683–687.

78. Letournel E, Jutet R. Radiology of the normal acetabulum. In: *Fractures of the Acetabulum.* 2nd ed. New York: Springer-Verlag; 1993:29–31.

79. Leunig M, Beck M, Kalhor M, et al. Fibrocystic changes at anterosuperior femoral neck: prevalence in hips with femoroacetabular impingement. *Radiol* 2005;236:237–246.

80. Levin DC. The practice of radiology by nonradiologists: cost, quality and utilization issues. *AJR Am J Roentgenol.* 1994;162:513–518.

81. Levin PE, Browner BB. Dislocations and fractures of the hip. In: Steinberg M, ed. *The Hip and Its Disorders.* Philadelphia: WB Saunders; 1991:222–246.

82. Levine WN, Bergfeld JA, Tessendorf W, et al. Intramuscular corticosteroid injection for hamstring injuries. A 13-year experience in the National Football League. *Am J Sports Med.* 2000;28:297–300.

83. Li PL, Ganz R. Morphologic features of congenital acetabular dysplasia: one in six is retroverted. *Clin Orthop Relat Res* 2003:245–253.

84. Lodwick GS, Wilson AJ, Farrell C. Determining growth rates of focal lesions of bone from radiographs. *Radiology.* 1980;134:577.

85. Lundin B, Björkholm E, Lundell M, et al. Insufficiency fractures of the sacrum after radiotherapy for gynaecological malignancy. *Acta Oncol.* 1990;29:211–215.

86. Lyons CW, Berquist TH, Lyons JC, et al. Evaluation of radiographic findings in painful hip arthroplasties. *Clin Orthop.* 1985;195:239–251.

87. Manaster BJ. From the RSNA Refresher Courses. Total hip arthroplasty: radiographic evaluation. *RadioGraphics.* 1996;16:645–660.

88. Martel W, Braunstein EM. The diagnostic value of buttressing of the femoral neck. *Arthritis Rheum.* 1978;21:161–164.

89. Martel W, Poznanski AK, Kuhns LR. Further observations on the value of traction during roentgenography of the hip. *Invest Radiol.* 1971;6:1–8.

90. Massie WK, Howorth MB. Congenital dislocation of hip: method of grading results. *J Bone Joint Surg Am.* 1950;32:519–531.

91. May DA, Purins JC, Smith DK. MR imaging of occult traumatic fractures and muscular injuries of the hip and pelvis in elderly patients. *AJR Am J Roentgenol.* 1996;166:1075–1078.

92. Meachim G, Path MR, Hardinge K, et al. Methods for correlating pathological and radiological findings in osteoarthritis of the hip. *Br J Radiol.* 1972;45:670–676.

93. Moule NJ, Golding JSR. Idiopathic chondrolysis of the hip. *Clin Radiol.* 1974;25:247–251.

94. Mudge B, Riesett M, Magid D, et al. Multiplanar imaging of the hip: a systemic approach. *Radiol Technol.* 1988;59:307–311.

95. Mulcahy DM, Fenelon GC, McInerney DP. Aspiration arthrography of the hip joint. Its uses and limitations in revision hip surgery. *J Arthroplasty.* 1996;11:64–68.

96. Nokes SR, Volger JB, Spritzer CE, et al. Herniation pits of the femoral neck: appearance at MR imaging. *Radiology.* 1989;172:231–234.

97. Norman A, Bullough P. The radiolucent crescent line: an early diagnostic sign of avascular necrosis of the femoral head. *Bull Hosp Joint Dis.* 1963;24:99–104.

98. Notzli HP, Wyss TF, Stoecklin CH, et al. The contour of the femoral head-neck junction as a predictor for the risk of anterior impingement. *J Bone Joint Surg Br* 2002;84:556–560.

99. O'Connell MJ, Powell T, McCaffrey NM, et al. Symphyseal cleft injection in the diagnosis and treatment of osteitis pubis in athletes. *AJR Am J Roentgenol.* 2002;179:955–959.

100. Odenbring S, Berggren AM, Peil L. Roentgenographic assessment of the hip-knee-ankle axis in medial gonarthrosis. *Clin Orthop.* 1993;289:195–196.

101. Panicek DM, Gatsonis C. Rosenthal D. CT and MR imaging in the local staging of primary malignant musculoskeletal neoplasms: report of the Radiology and Diagnostic Oncology Group. *Radiology.* 1997;202:237–246.

102. Petrera P, Trakru S, Mehta S, et al. Revision total hip arthroplasty with a retroperitoneal approach to the iliac vessels. *J Arthroplasty.* 1996;11:704–708.

103. Pitt MJ, Graham AR, Shipman JH, et al. Herniation pit of the femoral neck. *AJR Am J Roentgenol.* 1982;138:1115.

104. Pope TL Jr. Pseudopathologic fracture of the femoral neck. *Skeletal Radiol.* 1981;7:129.

105. Porta M. A comparative trial of botulinum toxin type A and methylprednisolone for the treatment of myofascial pain syndrome and pain from chronic muscle spasm. *Pain.* 2000;85:101–105.

106. Razzano CD, Nelson CL, Wilde AH. Arthrography of the adult hip. *Clin Orthop.* 1974;99:86–94.

107. Redlund-Johnell I, Petterson H. Vertical dislocation of the C1 and C2 vertebrae in rheumatoid arthritis. *Acta Radiol Diagn.* 1984;25:133–141.

108. Reimer J. The stability of the hip in children. A radiological study of the results of muscle surgery in cerebral palsy. *Acta Orthop Scand Suppl.* 1980;184:1–100.

109. Reinus WR, Merkel KC, Gilden JJ, et al. Evaluation of femoral loosening by CT imaging. *AJR Am J Roentgenol.* 1996;166:1439–1442.

110. Resnick D. Patterns of migration of the femoral head in osteoarthritis of the hip. Roentgenophraphic-pathologic correlation and comparison with rheumatoid arthritis. *AJR Am J Roentgenol.* 1975;124:62–74.

111. Resnick D, Niwayama G, eds. *Diagnosis of Bone and Joint Disorders.* 2nd ed. Philadelphia: WB Saunders; 1988.

112. Resnick D, Niwayama G, Goergen TG. Clinical, radiographic and pathologic abnormalities in calcium pyrophosphate dihydrate deposition disease (CPPD): pseudogout. *Radiology.* 1977;122:1–15.

113. Reynolds D, Lucas J, Klaue K. Retroversion of the acetabulum. *J Bone Joint Surg Br* 1999;81:281–288.

114. Rizzo PF, Gould ES, Lyden JP, et al. Diagnosis of occult fractures about the hip. *J Bone Joint Surg Am.* 1993;75:395–401.

115. Roberts P, Walters AJ, McMinn DJW. Diagnosing infection in hip replacements. *J Bone Joint Surg Br.* 1992;74:265–269.

116. Rombouts JJ, Rombouts-Lindemans C. Involvement of the hip in juvenile rheumatoid arthritis. *Acta Rheum Scand.* 1971;17:248–267.

117. Rosenberg JM, Quint TJ, de Rosayro AM. Computerized tomographic localization of clinically-guided sacroiliac joint injections. *Clin J Pain.* 2000;16:18–21.

118. Rosenthal DI, Scott JA. Biomechanics important to interpret radiographs of the hips. *Skeletal Radiol.* 1983;9:185–188.

119. Rubin GD. 3-D imaging with MDCT. *Eur J Radiol.* 2003;45:S37–S41.

120. Samei E, Seibert JA, Andriole K, et al. AAPM/RSNA tutorial on equipment selection: PACS equipment overview: general guide-

lines for purchasing and acceptance testing of PACS equipment. *Radiographics*. 2004;24:313–334.

121. Schaberg JE, Harper MC, Allen WC. The snapping hip syndrome. *Am J Sports Med*. 1984;12:361–365.

122. Schmarlzried TP, Jasty M, Harris WH. Periprosthetic bone loss in total hip arthroplasty. *J Bone Joint Surg Am*. 1992;74:849–863.

123. Shaw JA. Preventing unrecognized pin penetration into the hip joint. *Orthop Rev*. 1984;13:142–152.

124. Siebenrock KA, Schoeniger R, Ganz R. Anterior femoro-acetabular impingement due to acetabular retroversion. Treatment with peri-acetabular osteotomy. *J Bone Joint Surg Am*. 2003;85A:278–286.

125. Seibenrock KA, Kalbermatten DF, Ganz R. Effect of pelvic tilt on acetabular retroversion: a study of pelves from cadavers. *Clin Orthop Relat Res* 2003:241–248.

126. Smith J. Giant bone islands. *Radiology*. 1973;107:35.

127. Sprawls P, ed. *Physical Principles of Medical Imaging*. Gaithersville, MD: Aspen Publishers; 1987.

128 Staple TW, Jung D, Mork A. Snapping tendon syndrome: hip tenography with fluoroscopic monitoring. *Radiology*. 1988;166: 873–874.

129. Steinberg ME, Steinberg DR. Avascular necrosis of the femoral head. In: Steinberg ME, ed. *The Hip and Its Disorders*. Philadelphia: WB Saunders; 1991:623–647.

130. Tigges S, Stiles RG, Roberson JR. Appearance of septic hip prostheses on plain radiographs. *AJR Am J Roentgenol*. 1994;163:377–380.

131. Tigges S, Stiles RG, Roberson JR. Complications of hip arthroplasty causing periprosthetic radiolucency on plain radiographs. *AJR Am J Roentgenol*. 1994;162:1387–1391.

132. Totty WG, Murphy WA, Ganz WI, et al. Magnetic resonance imaging of the normal and ischemic femoral head. *AJR Am J Roentgenol*. 1984;143:1273.

133. Vresilovic EJ, Hozack WJ, Rothman RH. Radiographic assessment of cementless femoral components. *J Arthroplasty*. 1994;9:137–141.

134. Wasielewski RC, Cooperstein LA, Kruger MP, et al. Acetabular anatomy and the transacetabular fixation of screws in total hip arthroplasty. *J Bone Joint Surg Am*. 1990;72:501–508.

135. Watkins GL, Moore TF. *Atypical Orthopedic Radiographic Procedures*. St. Louis: Mosby Year Book; 1993.

136. Weinreb JC, Cohen JC, Maravilla KR. Iliopsoas muscles: MR study of normal anatomy and disease. *Radiology*. 1985;156: 435–440.

137. Weissman BN, Sledge CB, eds. In: *Orthopedic Radiology*. Philadelphia PA: WB Saunders; 1986:335–495.

138 Wepfer JF, Reed JG, Cullen GM, et al. Calcific tendonitis of the gluteus maximus tendon (gluteus maximus tendonitis). *Skeletal Radiol*. 1983;9:198.

139. Willems D, Verhelst M, Van Odijk J, et al. Diagnostic value of arthrography in painful total hip replacements. *J Belge Radiol*. 1973;56:213–222.

140. Wist A. Treatment of symphysiolysis with hydrocortisone-procaine injections. *Ann Chir Gynaecol Fenn*. 1968;57:98–100.

Radionuclide Imaging

Robert H. Fitzgerald, Jr.   *Lawrence P. Davis*   *Dheeraj K. Rajan*

Nuclear medicine is a unique subspecialty in the field of diagnostic imaging. Unlike other imaging techniques, nuclear medicine techniques depend on the administration of radioactive materials to the patient and their subsequent external detection. The radioactive materials used have the same biological and chemical properties as their nonradioactive counterparts. This principle permits their use in monitoring a wide range of physiologic processes and aids in the diagnosis of a large number of specific disease entities.

COMPOSITION OF RADIOPHARMACEUTICALS

Nuclear medicine image production begins with the oral or intravenous administration of a radiotracer, often termed a *radiopharmaceutical*. The radiopharmaceutical is usually composed of two parts: a radionuclide and an organ-specific compound. The radionuclide is a radioactive isotope of a normally stable element that emits energy as it decays to a stable, lower energy, "ground" state. This decay process can be in a single step or multiple cascadelike steps that form a variety of intermediate unstable compounds before reaching a stable state. The emitted energy can be in the form of electromagnetic radiation such as γ rays or x-rays or in the form of particles such as positron, β, or α particles. The decay scheme, rate of decay, and types of energy emitted are all well established for each radionuclide used in clinical nuclear medicine.

Most common radionuclides used in nuclear medicine emit discrete photons of energy in the form of γ rays or x-rays. γ rays and x-rays have similar properties. The difference between them is that γ rays originate in the excited unstable atomic nucleus, and x-rays originate in the electron shell outside the nucleus. Both γ rays and x-rays lose some of their energy as they interact with atoms in the body. In soft tissue, half the photons are lost every 4 to 6 cm as they travel through the body. However, γ rays and x-rays are thought of as penetrating radiation because they can still penetrate the body and be detected externally.

Particles emitted during radioactive decay cannot penetrate out of the body and by themselves cannot be used for imaging. The α and β particles are thought of as ionizing radiation because they lose all their energy inside the body as a result of collisions with atoms and molecules. During these collisions, energy is transferred to orbital electrons resulting in ionization and excitation of these atoms. It is this ionization process that is responsible for the radiobiological effects of these particles. The α and β particles deliver most of their energy in soft tissue very close to their origin. The α particles have a range on the order of μm, whereas the β particles have a range usually less than 1 cm. Although not used in imaging, β particles can be used for radionuclide therapy. Two common examples of this are iodine-131 and strontium-89. Iodine-131, like nonradioactive iodine, is accumulated in the thyroid. Its β particle can be used to treat overactive thyroid glands, as well as functioning thyroid cancer and its distant metastases. Strontium-89 is an alkaline earth that can substitute for calcium in the calcium hydroxyapatite bone crystal. Its β particle is now routinely used to treat pain from diffuse bone metastases, commonly from prostate and breast carcinoma.

Positrons also release their energy through ionization. However, as a positron comes to rest, it combines with an electron. When this occurs, the positron and electron are annihilated and two 0.511-MeV γ photons are released, 180° apart. This unique phenomenon of annihilation radiation is the basis for positron emission tomography. Fluorine-18, nitrogen-13, oxygen-15, and carbon-11 are the most common positron emitters used in nuclear medicine.

If only a radionuclide is administered, it will often circulate in the blood pool without accumulating in the organ of interest. To accumulate a radionuclide in a specific organ, it must be tagged or labeled to a biologically active molecule, often termed an *organ-specific compound*. It is this organ-specific compound that determines where the radionuclide will accumulate and what organ can be imaged. Although this labeling process can occasionally be complex and take several hours to perform, as is the case with labeled white cells, it is more often a fairly simple process that can be accomplished in under 30 minutes. The vast majority of nuclear medicine procedures use the same radionuclides (technetium-99m, indium-111, gallium-67, thallium-201, and isotopes of iodine) because they are easily detected externally. Each nuclear medicine procedure, however, requires a different organ-specific compound.

NUCLEAR MEDICINE IMAGE CREATION

Once a radiopharmaceutical is prepared and administered to the patient, the distribution of its radioactivity must be externally detected and mapped in order to create an image. The most common detector used to produce nuclear medicine images is a gamma camera, first created by Hal Anger in 1957 (3). The basic principles of this equipment are still used today in the modern nuclear medicine department. When photons are emitted from the patient, they first encounter a collimator attached to the surface of the camera's detector. The purpose of the collimator is to define the field of view of the detector and the direction of travel of protons allowed to reach the detector. Collimators are most often made of lead foil with multiple holes. Primary photons with accurate positional information travel through these holes to the detector, whereas off-angled scattered photons are absorbed by the lead of the collimator. The photons next encounter the detector. All contemporary gamma cameras use a thallium-activated sodium iodide crystal as a detector. The crystals are big enough (usually more than 40 to 50 cm in diameter) to cover a large portion of the patient at any one time. When the sodium iodide crystal absorbs a τ or x-ray, it "scintillates" or emits light. Behind the crystal is an array of photomultiplier tubes. These tubes convert the light energy to an electric pulse and amplify it by approximately one million times. Multiple square or hexagonal photomultiplier tubes are attached to the sodium iodide crystal. The electric output of each individual photomultiplier tube is used to define the x and y coordinates of the photon interaction within the crystal and its appropriate position on the image created. The electric output of all the photomultiplier tubes is summed to create a "Z" pulse. The Z pulse is then subjected to pulse height analysis to determine whether it is in the desired energy range of a primary photon or represents interaction with a scattered photon and should be rejected.

The gamma camera allows formation of an image proportional to the intensity and distribution of radioactivity in the body. Images can be obtained over seconds in order to monitor rapidly changing events such as blood flow or, as is more often the case, over minutes to monitor more slowly changing physiologic events. In the past, gamma cameras had one detector. Today, multiheaded gamma cameras are becoming significantly more common. Dual-headed gamma cameras with two opposing detectors may become the equipment of choice in a modern nuclear medicine department because of increased patient throughput. There is a substantial time savings generated by imaging from the patient's front and back or, by moving the detectors, from both sides simultaneously. Triple-headed gamma cameras are most useful as dedicated equipment for brain and cardiac imaging.

Nuclear medicine images are most often planar images. Like a photograph, they are two-dimensional representations of the three-dimensional distribution of radioactivity in the organ of interest. These images are easier and less time-consuming to create and interpret. There is also significantly less detector quality assurance required. However, image quality can be degraded by background activity in the tissues in front of or behind the organ of interest. The pathology in the organ can also be obscured by normal surrounding organ activity.

In order to improve image quality and the sensitivity of lesion detection, a process called single-photon emission computed tomography (SPECT) was developed (27). This process can be used to obtain cross-sectional images of the distribution of the radioactivity in the body. The most common SPECT systems consist of one to three sodium iodide detectors mounted on a gantry. The detector heads rotate around the long axis of the patient and acquire data through 180° to 360° angular sampling at small (3° to 10°) angle increments. The data are collected at each angular position and then stored on a computer in a 64 × 64 or 128 × 128 matrix. Similar to CT, the images are mathematically reconstructed using a "back-projection" technique. The concept of back-projection is that each count in the raw data represents the cumulative activity from a line projecting through the object and perpendicular to the camera face. When all of the projection views from around the body are superimposed, an image is reconstructed. The images are then mathematically manipulated and filtered in order to enhance specific characteristics of the image, such as background subtraction, edge enhancement, and suppression of statistical noise (Fig. 28-1). The data can be reconstructed to form transverse, sagittal, or coronal images (Fig. 28-2). The SPECT process eliminates background activity surrounding the region of interest and can improve image quality. However, there is a tradeoff. The SPECT equipment is significantly more expensive than planar gamma cameras, an issue that will become increasingly more important with upcoming health care reform. The images are more time-consuming to computer process and interpret than planar images. Quality assurance of SPECT equipment is significantly more demanding than for planar equipment. The center of rotation is a measure of the alignment of the opposing detectors. Misalignment by more than one pixel may cause significant image degradation. Pixel size, detector uniformity, spatial resolution, and linearity must also be carefully calibrated.

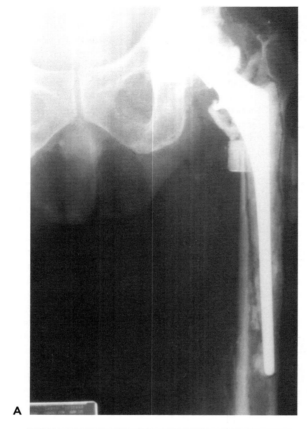

A

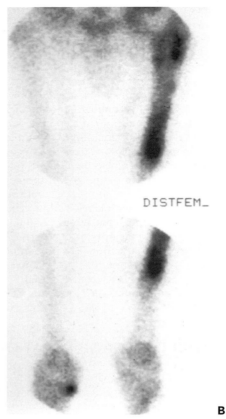

DISTFEM_

B

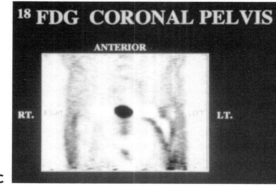

¹⁸ FDG CORONAL PELVIS

ANTERIOR

RT.   RIGHT   LEFT   LT.

C

Figure 28-1 A painful cemented total hip arthroplasty in a retired 79-year-old truck driver following revision total hip arthroplasty 2 years previously. **A:** Anteroposterior roentgenograph of a left total hip arthroplasty with subsidence of the femoral component that has a circumferential radiolucent line. There is erosion of the endosteal cortex laterally about the tip of the femoral component. **B:** Bone scan of the hips and femurs reveals intense uptake about the proximal and distal aspects of the femoral component. **C:** SPECT image of the pelvis demonstrates uptake about the femoral component consistent with an infection of the femoral component.

RISKS OF RADIOPHARMACEUTICALS

Adverse reactions associated with radiopharmaceuticals are much less common than with iodinated contrast media. The overall incidence of adverse reactions in the United States has been estimated as 1 to 6 reactions per 100,000 radiopharmaceutical administrations (59). These rare reactions are usually mild, consisting of nausea, dyspnea, bronchospasm, hypotension, itching, flushing, hives, chills, bradycardia, muscle cramps, and dizziness. More recently, there has been concern for the possibility of reactions due to the development of human antimouse antibodies (HAMA) after administration of murine-based radiolabeled monoclonal antibodies.

Because of the radiation burden to the patient associated with the administration of radiopharmaceuticals, nuclear medicine techniques should be used judiciously in all patients, but especially in the pediatric population. Different nomograms have been developed using such factors as age, weight, and body surface area to decrease the amount of radioactivity administered to children compared to the typical adult dose.

There are no true absolute contraindications to nuclear medicine imaging. Physicians should be concerned about the possibility of pregnancy in women of childbearing age. If necessary, a pregnancy test can be carried out before administration of a radiopharmaceutical. Pregnancy is not an absolute contraindication. The risks (of radiation) and benefits (of identifying the pathology) of such procedures must be fully understood by the referring physician, the patient, and the family. Breast-feeding poses unique problems. For technetium-99m-based

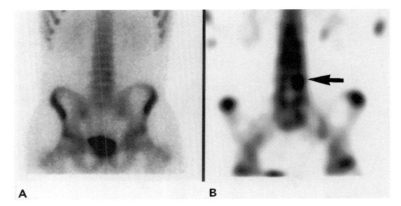

Figure 28-2 Anterior planar **(A)** and coronal SPECT **(B)** bone scan images from a 17-year-old boy with unexplained back pain. The planar image shows little if any abnormal tracer uptake. The SPECT image shows intense focal tracer uptake at L4 *(arrow)*.

radiopharmaceuticals, breast-feeding should be suspended for up to 12 hours. For isotopes of iodine breast-feeding must be terminated after the procedure in order to avoid exposure to the baby. The same may hold true after gallium-67 and thallium-201 imaging.

RADIONUCLIDE IMAGING OF THE MUSCULOSKELETAL SYSTEM: BONE SCINTIGRAPHY

Bone scintigraphy has been available for over 30 years and is one of the most commonly performed nuclear medicine procedures. Refined many times over the last three decades, numerous radiopharmaceuticals have been introduced during this time. Because the mineral portion of bone is calcium hydroxyapatite [$Ca_5(PO_4)_3(OH)$], and with the calcium and phosphorus in bone in equilibrium with the plasma, it would seem reasonable that radioisotopes of calcium and phosphorus would be ideal bone-imaging agents. Unfortunately, calcium-45 and phosphorus-32, common radioisotopes of calcium and phosphorus, are pure β emitters and do not emit a β ray. They have been employed for metabolic studies but are not useful for external imaging. Calcium-47, a γ-emitting radionuclide, was first used for external bone imaging in the early 1960s (11). Its high-energy (1.297 MeV) photons were poorly detected, and significant septal penetration in the collimator resulted in a very poor quality images. Its long physical half-life (4.5 days) and β decay produced a relatively high radiation dose to the patient.

All periodic table group IIA elements will substitute for calcium in the calcium hydroxyapatite crystal. A radioisotope of one of these group IIA elements, strontium-85, was the radionuclide of choice for bone scanning until the early 1970s (9,16). However, use of strontium-85 was limited by its higher than ideal τ photon energy (514 keV) and long half-life (65.1 days) resulting in a high radiation dose. Imaging was done 48 hours after injection to allow clearance of background activity and the radiotracer excreted in the gut. Strontium-85 was usually only used to image malignant conditions because of its high radiation burden. Strontium-87m was also an early bone-scanning agent, but its slow blood clearance and poor bone-to-soft-tissue ratio severely limited image quality. Strontium-89 is a commonly used radionuclide in current nuclear medicine practice. Because it is mainly a β emitter it is

not suitable for imaging. Its current role is in treatment of pain from diffuse bone metastases. It has an efficacy of approximately 80% in patients with bone metastases from prostate and breast cancer and significantly improves quality of life (15).

Fluorine-18 was introduced in the early 1960s as a bone-scanning agent because it will substitute for the OH group in the bone crystal (6). It has a rapid plasma clearance and high bone uptake, but did not become popular because of its expense, high photon energy peak (511 keV), and short half-life (109 minutes), which limited its availability.

In 1971, technetium-99m phosphates were first introduced as bone-scanning agents (64). The first phosphate compounds were pyrophosphates (P-O-P bonds) but were replaced by diphosphonates (P-C-P bonds) because of their more rapid blood clearance and higher bone-to-background ratio. One of these agents, technetium-99m methylene diphosphonate (MDP), continues as the standard for radionuclide bone imaging (65).

The major determinants of technetium-99m MDP uptake in bone is blood flow and metabolic bone activity. Bone scanning is very sensitive to blood flow (31). When blood flow is significantly decreased (such as in gangrene), abnormally increased uptake may not be seen despite superimposed bone pathology such as osteomyelitis. In the opposite extreme, a region of cellulitis with increased blood flow to the underlying bone may show increased bony uptake even without true bone pathology.

The metabolic activity of the bone is the major factor controlling tracer uptake. The tracer chemisorbs onto the surface of the hydroxyapatite bone crystal by substitution of the phosphate portion of the tracer for the inorganic phosphate in the bone crystal (28). Technetium-99m MDP accumulates in the perivascular fluid adjacent to the interface between uncalcified and calcified bone matrix. Newly developed bone mineral in regions of high metabolic activity, such as that seen in acute fracture, infection, or tumor, has the largest surface area exposed to the radiotracer, as well as the highest phosphate-to-calcium ratio. These factors account for the greater amount of tracer uptake in these regions. Areas of low metabolic activity, such as in osteoporotic bones, have less available surface area, a lower phosphate-to-calcium ratio, and less tracer uptake.

After intravenous administration, approximately 50% of the technetium-99m MDP absorbs onto the bone crystal. The

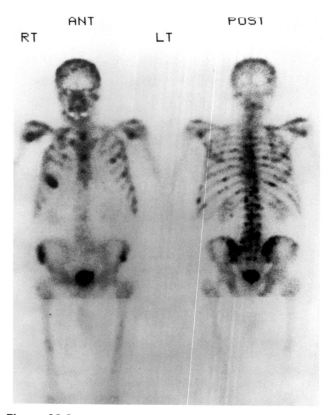

Figure 28-3 Anterior and posterior images from a total-body bone scan on a 88-year-old man with prostate cancer. Notice areas of increased tracer uptake throughout the skeleton including skull and distal femurs representing diffuse bone metastases.

infection, and arthritis can all demonstrate a similar scan appearance. Radiographs of those regions shown to be abnormal on bone scan often are required to differentiate between different types of pathology. In cases of suspected infection, other radionuclide studies such as leukocyte or gallium scans, in conjunction with the bone scan, are invaluable in making a more accurate diagnosis.

APPLICATIONS

Tumors

One of the most common indications for bone scintigraphy is in the evaluation of bone tumors. This procedure is of most benefit in the evaluation of metastatic bone disease, but it also plays a role in the assessment of primary bone tumors. Bone scanning is a rapid and cost-effective approach for assessing the entire skeletal system in a patient with possible bone metastases. Examining the entire skeletal system in these patients is important because approximately 20% of metastases occur in the more distal appendicular skeleton and skull (30) (Fig. 28-3). In some malignancies, such as renal or thyroid cancer, bone metastases are demonstrated as areas of decreased tracer uptake ("cold spots") instead of increased uptake ("hot spots") (Fig. 28-4). This is due to a large region of bone destruction without a surrounding reparative process.

Bone scintigraphy does have a role in the evaluation of primary bone tumors, both malignant and benign. Bone scans routinely show a region of intense uptake in the tumor. Other bones in the involved extremity also can show a mild

remainder of the activity is in the blood pool resulting in soft tissue background uptake. With time, this background activity is cleared by the kidneys into the bladder. Peak tracer uptake occurs in the bone by approximately 20 minutes. Imaging is often delayed for 2 to 4 hours postinjection in order to clear background activity and improve the bone to background ratio. Total-body or localized images can be obtained requiring about 30 to 60 minutes of imaging time. Images of a specific skeletal region of interest can be obtained over seconds at the time of tracer injection yielding dynamic images of blood flow. Images acquired minutes after injection show soft tissue uptake. In conjunction with the 2- to 4-hour delayed images, these images constitute a "three-phase bone scan." This technique can be of value in patients with suspected osteomyelitis.

Bone radiography is often the first imaging procedure performed in patients with symptoms of bone pathology. However, bone radiography usually requires approximately 40% to 50% bone destruction before a lesion can be identified. Bone scintigraphy, on the other hand, assesses bone physiology and is an extremely sensitive technique for the detection of bone abnormalities. Thus, lesions are detected significantly earlier on bone scans then on radiographs. However, although the technique has high sensitivity, it also has poor specificity. Regions of abnormal uptake can be seen in any area of increased bone turnover. Tumor, fracture,

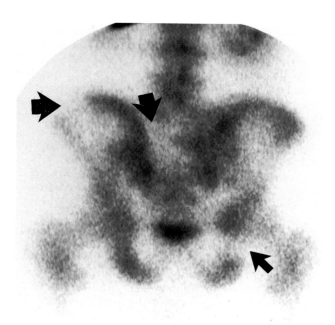

Figure 28-4 Posterior pelvis image from a bone scan in a patient with renal cell carcinoma. Notice areas of decreased tracer uptake (*arrows*) representing metastases to the sacrum, left ilium, and right ischium.

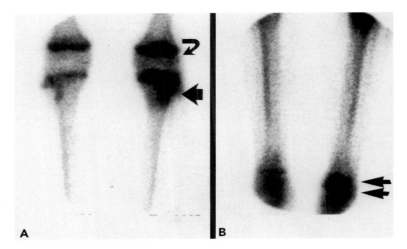

Figure 28-5 Anterior images of the knees **(A)** and shins **(B)** from a bone scan on a 15-year-old boy with an osteogenic sarcoma of the left proximal tibia. The primary lesion shows intense increased uptake (*straight arrow*). There is also an expanded pattern of increased uptake in the distal femur (*curved arrow*) and ankle (*double arrow*).

to moderate increase in uptake (Fig. 28-5). This expanded pattern of tracer uptake may be due to changes in blood flow or gait (8). Because of this phenomenon, bone scanning is not of value in determining local tumor extent. The role of bone scanning in these patients is to look for distant spread of disease. Multiple myeloma is the most common primary bone tumor in adults. It is primarily a lytic tumor without much reparative osteoblastic response. Bone scans in multiple myeloma are characteristically less sensitive then bone radiographs, and this disease is one of the few current indications for a radiographic skeletal survey.

Bone scintigraphy will show increased tracer uptake in many benign bone tumors such as nonossifying fibromas, enchondromas, osteochondromas, and large bone islands. However, the most dramatic abnormal uptake is in osteoid osteomas. Osteoid osteoma is one of the most common benign bone tumors in children and young adults. The tumor commonly occurs in the femur, tibia, and spine and classically presents with pain at night relieved by aspirin. The lesion is typically diagnosed with plain radiographs or CT. Bone scintigraphy is useful when an osteoid osteoma is suspected but radiographs are not diagnostic. Bone scans commonly demonstrate increased uptake in all phases of a three-phase

bone scan (5) (Fig. 28-6). Successful surgical removal of the lesion can be facilitated by localizing the nidus of the tumor with a preoperative or intraoperative bone scan.

Metabolic Bone Disease

Bone scintigraphy has not become a popular modality for the evaluation of metabolic bone disease. However, the technique could be of great value in demonstrating the extent of bone involvement and response to therapy in conditions such as Paget's disease, hyperparathyroidism, renal osteodystrophy, and osteomalacia. Paget's disease is a common disorder generally involving many bones, but in 20% of patients it is monostotic (19). Bone scintigraphy is extremely valuable in assessing the extent of disease because it can rapidly and sensitively evaluate the entire skeletal system (Fig. 28-7). With the advent of powerful bisphosphonates to treat Paget's disease, a new role of bone scintigraphy is to confirm remission. Bone scintigraphy may also be able to predict the need for further therapy (58).

Metabolic bone diseases such as renal osteodystrophy, osteomalacia, and primary hyperparathyroidism commonly demonstrate diffuse increased tracer uptake throughout the entire skeletal system (20). Finally, in patients with primary

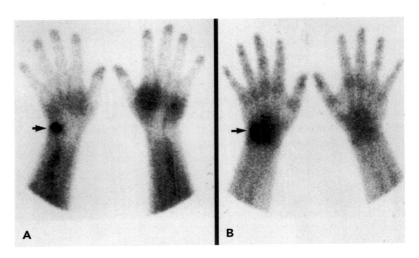

Figure 28-6 Blood pool **(A)** and 2-hour delay **(B)** bone scan images from a patient with an osteoid osteoma of the wrist. Notice intense tracer uptake (*arrow*) in the tumor on both phases of the exam.

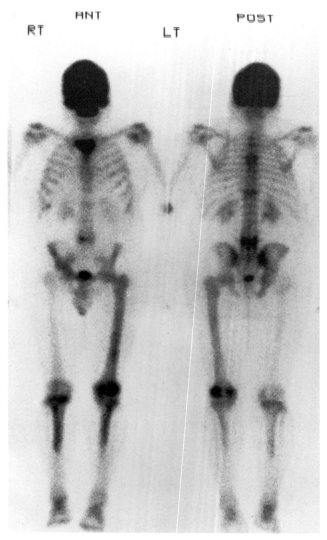

RT   ANT   LT   POST

Figure 28-7 Anterior and posterior total-body bone scan images from a 66-year-old man with Paget's disease. There is abnormal tracer uptake in the skull, sternum, spine, pelvis, left femur, and both tibias.

hyperparathyroidism and renal osteodystrophy, soft tissue uptake in the lungs and stomach can be seen (Fig. 28-8), whereas in patients with osteomalacia, pseudofractures can cause multiple areas of increased uptake (63).

Infection

Bone scintigraphy has had a longstanding role in the evaluation of patients with suspected musculoskeletal infection. The differentiation of patients with simple cellulitis from those with underlying osteomyelitis can be a difficult clinical problem. Three-phase bone scintigraphy has been shown to be extremely effective in differentiating bone infection from soft tissue infection. Bone scintigraphy can document osteomyelitis within 24 to 72 hours of onset of symptoms. The study is abnormal 10 to 14 days before there is enough bone loss to be identified on radiographs (22). In patients with cellulitis, the first two (blood flow and blood pool)

phases of the three-phase bone scan reveal minor to moderate but diffuse increased uptake involving the infected soft tissues. The delayed third (bone) phase of the scan may be normal or show mild diffuse increase uptake due to regional hyperemia caused by the cellulitis (Fig. 28-9). In patients with osteomyelitis, all three phases demonstrate significant abnormal tracer uptake. The uptake becomes more intense and more focal, localizing to the involved bone, when comparing the early to the late phases of the bone scan (Fig. 28-10). In adults and children who have normal bone radiographs and no underlying bone pathology that increases bone turnover, the bone scan has very high sensitivity and specificity for the diagnosis of osteomyelitis. In these patients, sensitivity has been estimated as 94% and specificity as 95% (60). The limitation of bone scintigraphy is in patients with underlying bone pathology that will increase bone metabolism. Bone scintigraphy is notoriously nonspecific for osteomyelitis in patients with previous bone trauma, bone surgery such as prosthetic joint replacements or amputations, decubitus ulcer infections, diabetic neurotrophic arthropathy, and paraplegia with extensive heterotrophic ossification. Bone scintigraphy will be positive in all of these conditions and by itself cannot accurately identify patients with superimposed osteomyelitis. In this patient population, the sensitivity of bone scintigraphy remains high, approximately 95%, but specificity drops significantly to approximately 33% (60). In these patients where bone scintigraphy is not specific, other nuclear medicine procedures such as gallium or leukocyte scintigraphy can be very helpful in making a more definitive diagnosis of osteomyelitis. This will be discussed later in this chapter.

Another limitation of bone scanning for the diagnosis of osteomyelitis may be in the neonate (40). Sensitivities as low

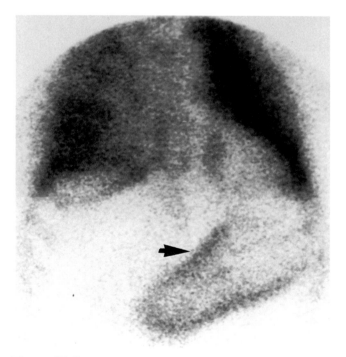

Figure 28-8 Anterior chest and abdomen image from a bone scan on a patient with renal osteodystrophy. Notice diffuse tracer uptake in the lungs and in the wall of the stomach (*arrow*).

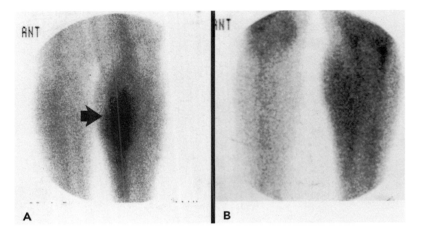

Figure 28-9 Anterior blood pool (**A**) and 3-hour delay (**B**) bone scan images of the shins from a patient with cellulitis on the left. Notice the increased activity on the blood pool image (*arrow*) which decreases in intensity on the delayed image.

as 30% have been reported in this patient population although recent studies revealed sensitivities of 87% (7). Osteomyelitis can also appear as regions of decreased activity in both adults and children (43). This appearance can be seen with osteomyelitis of the femur associated with septic arthritis of the hip (Fig. 28-11) and with osteomyelitis of the spine. Abscess formation in such enclosed spaces causes increased pressure and thrombosis of the blood supply. This leads to decreased blood flow and lack of tracer delivery to the region (69).

Evaluation of Bone Interventional Procedures

Scintigraphy is of value in assessing patients after skeletal interventional procedures. Vascularized bone grafts from the iliac crest, rib, or fibula are commonly used for reconstruction after bone resection. This technique may be used for hip reconstruction in femoral neck nonunion as well as in the treatment of osteonecrosis. Bone scintigraphy is helpful to confirm that the graft's blood supply is still patent. Vascular compromise may result in graft failure and lack of bony union. Well-vascularized grafts demonstrate normal or diffusely increased tracer uptake throughout the graft with focally increased uptake at the sites of resection, whereas poorly vascularized grafts demonstrate significantly decreased tracer uptake or a "cold" defect (46). Scans performed after 1 week postoperatively may give a false impression of graft viability due to new bone deposition on even nonvascularized grafts.

One of the most common indications for scintigraphy after a bony interventional procedure is the evaluation of the painful joint replacement. Hip and knee replacements are common procedures, with more than 120,000 of each performed in the United States annually (23,24). The most common cause of prosthesis pain is loosening. It is extremely important for patient management to differentiate painful prostheses that are loose from those that are infected. The rate of prosthesis infection is under 1% for primary hip replacements (23) and under 2% for primary knee replacements (24). This rate becomes significantly greater after surgical revision of the prosthesis.

Plain radiographs are usually the first imaging procedure used to assess a painful prosthesis. The classic findings of loosening are a radiolucent zone of 2 mm or wider at the cement–bone interface or a lucent zone at the prosthesis–cement interface (2) These findings, however, are not always seen in patients with loosening, and they cannot differentiate loosening from infection.

Bone scintigraphy is often the next imaging procedure used to evaluate a painful prosthesis. Increased tracer uptake can be seen surrounding a normal asymptomatic hip prosthesis for 12 to 24 months after surgery due to bone remodeling (68). Increased uptake can be seen in an asymptomatic knee prosthesis for up to 6 to 12 years postoperatively and is usually most intense around the tibial component (54). This normal uptake should decrease over time, but it limits the value of scintigraphy in differentiating normal from abnormal.

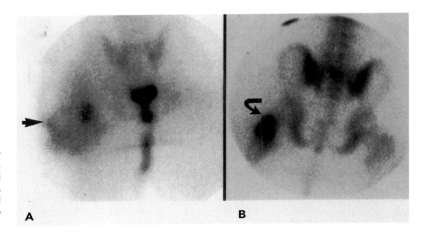

Figure 28-10 Posterior blood pool (**A**) and 3-hour delay (**B**) bone scan images of the pelvis from a patient with left hip cellulitis and superimposed osteomyelitis of the left greater trochanter. There is mild diffuse activity (*straight arrow*) on the blood pool image which becomes more intense and localizes to the bone (*curved arrow*) on the delayed image.

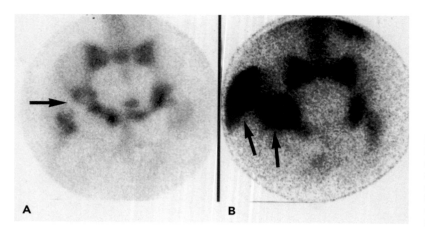

Figure 28-11 Posterior 3-hour delay bone scan **(A)** and leukocyte scan **(B)** images of the pelvis from a patient with left hip cellulitis, septic arthritis, and superimposed osteomyelitis. Notice the region of decreased tracer uptake on the bone scan in the left femoral head and neck (*arrow*). This corresponds to diffuse leukocyte uptake (*double arrows*) indicating significant infection.

The appearance of abnormal uptake surrounding a painful prosthesis has been used to help differentiate loosening from infection. A loose hip prosthesis commonly shows abnormal tracer uptake at the trochanters, prosthetic tip, and, if involved, the acetabulum (Fig. 28-12), whereas infection tends to show diffuse uptake surrounding the entire prosthesis (66) (Fig. 28-13). A loose knee prosthesis can demonstrate abnormal uptake most frequently at the tibial plateau, but infection can have a similar scan appearance (30). Although bone scintigraphy is very sensitive for diagnosing prosthetic infection, it is not specific and alone cannot reliably differentiate infection from loosening. Additional nuclear medicine procedures such as indium leukocyte scintigraphy can be used to make a more specific diagnosis. This topic will be discussed later in this chapter. However, bone scintigraphy can also be used to identify which patients might require eventual revision surgery. In a study by Miles et al., patients whose hip replacements showed increased activity at the lesser trochanter and prosthetic tip were less likely to have a spontaneous resolution of symptoms and more likely to need revision surgery (47).

Alterations of Blood Supply

Reflex Sympathetic Dystrophy

Reflex sympathetic dystrophy (RSD) occurs following injury to bone and/or soft tissue. The clinical diagnosis is based on diffuse pain associated with reduced function, stiffness of joints, and dystrophic changes of the skin and soft tissues.

Radiographically, the bones characteristically demonstrate patchy osteoporosis. However, sensitivity is 60% to 70% and normal exams are common (38). Three-phase bone scans have become widely accepted for establishing the diagnosis. RSD is thought to be secondary to sympathetic nervous system injury. This results in vascular dilatation, increased blood flow, and increased tracer delivery to the extremity of concern. The typical bone scan appearance is a generalized increased activity of the extremity with marked tracer accentuation in the periarticular regions on all three phases of the bone scan (Fig. 28-14). Delayed imaging has been found to be 94% to 100% sensitive in the diagnosis of RSD (25,44). Specificity is approximately 80%.

Radiation Therapy

Radiation therapy is the treatment of choice, both palliative and/or curative, for a number of malignancies. In the field of orthopedic oncology, radiation therapy is used for Ewing's sarcoma, osteosarcomas, chondrosarcomas, multiple myeloma, and a number of benign bone tumors. It is also used for therapy of metastatic bony disease.

The extent of radiation effects in tissue is influenced by the degree of injury to supporting structures, most notably the vascular system. Osteoblasts and osteoclasts are radiosensitive

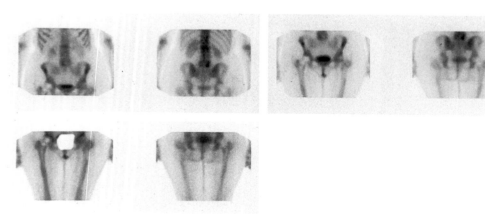

Figure 28-12 Bone scans of a painful total hip arthroplasty. There is discrete uptake about the acetabulum, greater trochanter, and tip of the femoral component seen with aseptic loosening.

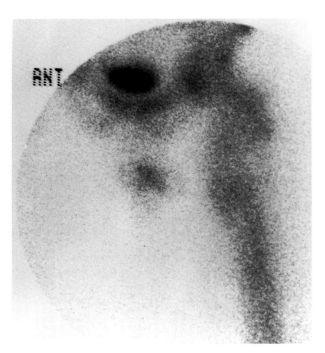

Figure 28-13 Anterior bone scan image of the left femur in a patient with a left hip prosthesis. Notice the diffuse increased tracer uptake surrounding the femur suggesting infection.

and die. Endarteritis with obliteration of the lumen leads to ischemia of the irradiated area (34). With no vascular supply to the irradiated region, imaging is compromised because of the inability to distribute tracer. On bone scintigraphy, these areas appear as regions of relative lack of tracer uptake (Fig. 28-15).

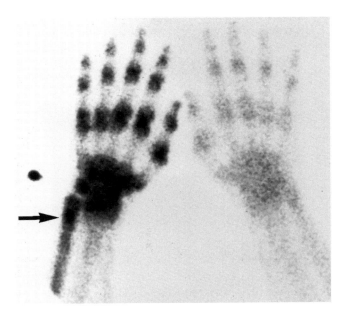

Figure 28-14 Three-hour delay bone scan image in a patient with a right forearm injury and right hand pain. There is abnormal increased uptake in all the joints of the right hand and wrist suggesting reflex sympathetic dystrophy. There is also increased uptake in the right ulna (*arrow*) due to the injury.

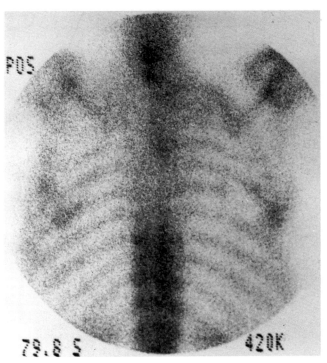

Figure 28-15 Posterior bone scan image of the chest in a patient who received radiation therapy for esophageal carcinoma. There is abnormally decreased tracer activity in the upper thoracic spine when compared to the rest of the spine due to the effect of the radiation on the bone.

Osteonecrosis

Osteonecrosis occurs when there is interruption of blood supply to the bone. The appearance on skeletal scintigraphy is dependent on the time course of the injury. Acute disruption of blood supply creates a photopenic defect. This is commonly seen in femoral neck fractures with capsular disruption in which the femoral head appears photopenic (Fig. 28-16). In the healing phase, neovascularization and osteogenesis occurs at the margin of necrosis, with intense tracer uptake seen on the bone scan.

Trauma

Fractures

Fractures commonly present with pain, deformity, and possible bony displacement in the region of injury. The diagnosis is often established radiographically. When suspected fractures are not confirmed radiographically, bone scintigraphy is one of the imaging modalities used to establish the diagnosis.

The most common occult fractures are fractures of the scaphoid bone, Lisfranc fracture dislocations of the midfoot, and nondisplaced fractures of the femur. Fractures can be detected on a bone scan within 24 hours of injury in 95% of patients under 65 years of age (37). In older and osteoporotic patients, detection of fractures is delayed by 48 to 72 hours and occasionally longer. Bone scintigraphy establishes the diagnosis 7 to 10 days before these fractures can be identified radiographically. This significantly reduces the morbidity associated with delayed diagnosis, particularly for older individuals with occult hip fractures.

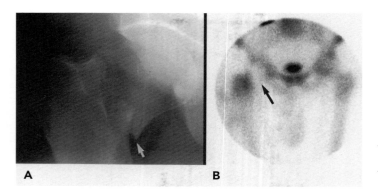

Figure 28-16 Right hip radiograph (**A**) and anterior bone scan image of the pelvis (**B**) in a patient with right hip trauma. The radiograph demonstrates a femoral neck fracture (*white arrow*). The bone scan shows decreased tracer uptake in the femoral head due to disruption of the blood supply (*black arrow*).

Three distinct patterns are visualized on bone scans following a fracture. Initially, diffuse increased uptake of tracer occurs at the fracture site with the fracture line only occasionally visible on delayed images. In the subacute stage, the fracture line is visualized. In the healing phase, increased uptake at the fracture site gradually diminishes over time until it returns to normal (37).

The length of time it takes for the bone scan abnormality to normalize after a fracture depends on the location of the fracture, degree of damage, use of orthopedic fixation devices, and any underlying diseases the patient may have. Compound fractures, open reductions, and orthopedic fixation devices significantly increase the time for the bone scan appearance to normalize.

Fractures that can be missed on plain radiographs include those of the pubic ramus, sacrum, femoral neck, intertrochanteric region, greater trochanter, and the acetabulum (58).

Bone scintigraphy has a 93% sensitivity and 95% specificity for detection of such occult fractures of the hip (33,53). Additional advantages of this imaging modality are early detection of avascular necrosis of the femoral head, availability in smaller hospitals, and the ability to image the whole body to rule out other occult fractures. Recently, magnetic resonance imaging has gained greater acceptance for the detection of femoral neck fractures. This imaging modality allows more rapid delineation of fractures within 24 hours of the injury with significantly better anatomic resolution. Limitations of magnetic resonance imaging include cost, availability, exclusion of patients with pacemakers, aneurysm clips, ocular transplants, and metallic prostheses.

Stress Fractures

When the skeletal system is stressed, via change in activity, active remodeling occurs at an increased rate resulting in stronger osteoid bone. This is a balanced process between resorption of bone and replacement with stronger bone. It has been postulated that an imbalance of these processes leads to stress fractures. Greater resorption causes weakening of trabecular bone, leading to microfractures. Stress fractures are the result of repetitive and prolonged exercise on a bone that is not accustomed to the stress. Stress fractures are commonly found in the tibia and fibula. However, they can occur in any osseous structure and may occur in osteopenic bone around joint implants. Radiographs rarely demonstrate bony changes in the acute phase. Skeletal scintigraphy has now become the diagnostic modality of choice for early detection of this condition.

The scintigraphic appearance of stress fractures varies with the severity of the injury (37). Stress fractures can appear as a linear band of increased uptake along the outer cortex of the bone (Figs. 28-17 and 28-18). As the injury worsens, bone

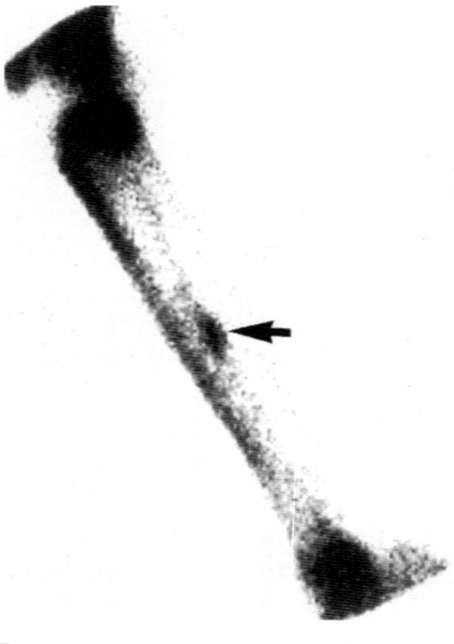

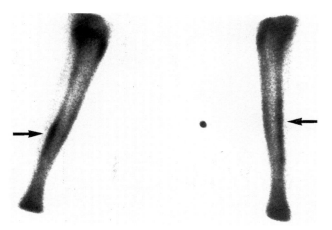

Figure 28-17 Lateral bone scan image of the left shin in an athlete with leg pain. Notice the small fusiform region of increased tracer uptake (*arrow*) involving the posterior cortex of the midtibia representing a stress fracture.

Figure 28-18 Lateral bone scan image of the shins in an athlete with bilateral leg pain. There is elongated, linear abnormal tracer uptake involving the post cortex of both tibias (*arrows*) indicating shin splints.

scans demonstrate a fusiform area with increased uptake extending throughout the entire cortex of the bone. Stress fractures can demonstrate increased vascularity in the blood flow and blood pool phases if they are acute or subacute. After the first few weeks postinjury, bone scans often exhibit increased uptake only on delayed images. This represents ongoing bony repair at the site of stress fracture.

Gallium-67 Citrate Scintigraphy

Gallium-67 citrate scintigraphy is an extremely useful technique for the assessment of infection. Although gallium-67 citrate was initially used to image neoplasms, its value as an infection-imaging agent was first recognized in 1971 (32). Gallium is a group IIIB metal and acts as an iron analog. The reason for uptake of gallium in an area of infection is multifactorial (47). After intravenous administration, gallium binds to serum transferrin, the iron-binding protein of the blood. The gallium–transferrin complex enters the extracellular space of the infection. In an abscess, this space has a high concentration of lactoferrin released by degranulating leukocytes as they attempt to destroy the abscess. Lactoferrin has a higher affinity for gallium than transferrin, and the gallium is transferred to the lactoferrin in the extracellular space of the abscess. A small amount of gallium binds to the lactoferrin in viable circulating leukocytes, and some may bind to siderophores, which are the iron-binding proteins of bacteria. This last mechanism may help to explain how gallium can detect infection in patients with very low white blood cell counts.

Gallium-67 citrate scintigraphy is often a 3- to 4-day procedure. The patient is injected intravenously and scanning begins 24 to 48 hours later. Spot images of a specific body part can be obtained if only a particular region is of clinical concern, such as a localized osteomyelitis. Total-body imaging can be performed in a patient with a fever of unknown origin. Image acquisition usually requires about 1 hour. At this stage, there is often a poor lesion-to-background ratio that improves over time as the background activity is excreted by the kidneys and bowel. Because of this improvement in lesion-to-background ratio, imaging is also routinely performed 48 to 72 hours after injection. At times, images performed several days after injection are needed to best define the abnormality.

Gallium-67 citrate scintigraphy is of value in the evaluation of patients with suspected soft tissue infections. It is of particular value in patients with fever of unknown origin and those with suspected AIDS-related respiratory disease, especially *Pneumocystis carinii* pneumonia. For the purpose of this chapter, we will focus only on gallium's role in the assessment of musculoskeletal infections. As previously mentioned, bone scintigraphy is extremely accurate in diagnosing uncomplicated osteomyelitis but has poor specificity in diagnosing osteomyelitis superimposed on other bone pathology such as fractures, prosthesis insertion, neurotrophic changes, and significant arthritis. Sequential bone/gallium scintigraphy has been successfully used to identify active osteomyelitis in these patients. Gallium is also a bone-scanning agent, and mild increased gallium uptake can be seen in noninfected bone remodeling. Infection is thought to be present when the gallium uptake is extremely intense, more intense than the corresponding bone scan uptake, or spatially incongruent when compared to the bone scan uptake (55). Unfortunately,

these criteria are met in only about 28% of patients (61). Gallium scintigraphy has an accuracy of approximately 75% for the detection of periprostatic infection (39).

Once the diagnosis of osteomyelitis has been made, a gallium scan is useful to access adequate antibiotic therapy and to follow the resolution of the infection. Standard technetium bone scintigraphy should not be used for this purpose because continued bone healing will show tracer uptake for months after the infection has been eradicated.

Indium-111-Labeled Leukocyte Scintigraphy

Indium-111 leukocytes are becoming an increasingly popular imaging technique for the evaluation of patients with infection such as fever of unknown origin, abdominal and pelvic infection, graft infection, and active colitis. In this chapter we will concentrate on this procedure's role in the evaluation of musculoskeletal infections. Indium leukocyte scintigraphy requires the phlebotomy of 50 cm^3 of blood from a patient and then separation of the red blood cells by gravity and/or chemical sedimentation. The "buffy coat" is removed from the red blood cells, and the white blood cell "button" is separated from the plasma by centrifugation. The white blood cell button can be washed with sterile hypotonic water to lyse any remaining red blood cells, and the white cells are then incubated with indium-111 oxine for 30 minutes. Oxine is a lipid-soluble complex that diffuses rapidly through the white cell membrane carrying the indium-111 with it. Once inside the white cell, the indium-111 separates from the oxine, binds intracellularly, and the oxine diffuses out of the cell. When incubation is complete, the labeled white blood cells are resuspended in the patient's plasma and reinjected. The entire labeling process requires 2 to 3 hours to perform. Imaging is usually done 24 hours after injection of the labeled white blood cells; therefore, it is difficult to perform this examination on an emergency basis. As with gallium scintigraphy, total-body imaging or spot images of a specific body part can be obtained. Images at 24 hours demonstrate normally intense activity in the spleen and moderate activity in the liver and bone marrow.

Labeled white cells accumulate in a region of infection because of chemotaxis. There had been concern that antibiotic therapy could effect localization of white blood cells in infection by decreasing the amount of chemoattractants. However, in a study by Datz and Thorne, it was found that antibiotics did not significantly alter the sensitivity of indium white blood cells (89%) when compared to patients who were not (92%) on antibiotics (13). Other factors that potentially could limit chemotaxis, such as hemodialysis, hyperalimentation, hyperglycemia, and steroids, were also found to have no effect on the sensitivity of indium white blood cell scintigraphy (12).

The usual labeling technique creates a mixed white blood cell preparation of tagged leukocytes. Besides polymorphonuclear leukocytes, lymphocytes and monocytes are also labeled. This may explain why the technique has similar sensitivities for acute infection (90%) and chronic infection (86%) (14). This is important in musculoskeletal infections, which tend to be longstanding chronic processes.

Indium-111 leukocyte scintigraphy is very valuable for the diagnosis of osteomyelitis, especially in patients with diabetic

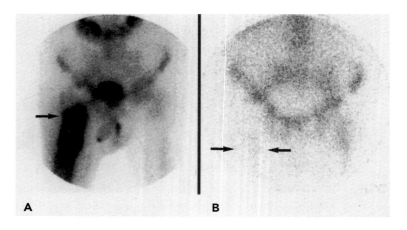

Figure 28-19 Anterior bone scan **(A)** and indium leukocyte scan **(B)** images of the pelvis in a patient with a painful right hip prosthesis 6 months after surgery. The intense uptake on the bone scan (*single arrow*) could be due to infection or postsurgical repair. The lack of abnormal uptake on the leukocyte scan (*double arrows*) rules out infection.

neuropathy, prior trauma, arthritis, or joint prosthesis. These entities might cause changes on radiographs and bone scans that can mimic osteomyelitis. The technique has the most impact in the appendicular skeleton. In the adult, the appendicular skeleton has little normal bone marrow uptake, which could be confused with uptake in infection. Overall, especially when correlated with a bone scan, indium white blood cell scintigraphy has been shown to have a very high sensitivity (88%) and specificity (85%) for the diagnosis of osteomyelitis (60).

In the challenging problem of evaluation of the painful hip prosthesis, radiographs and bone scintigraphy may not differentiate loosening from infection. This is especially true during the first 12 to 18 months after prosthesis insertion. Indium white blood cells have been shown to be extremely valuable in identifying prosthesis infection with an overall accuracy of 82% (36) (Fig. 28-19). However, prosthesis insertion displaces normal bone marrow elements. labeled leukocytes accumulate not only in infection but in normal bone marrow. It has been suggested that the leukocyte scan should be compared to a technetium-99m sulfur colloid bone marrow scan in order to improve its accuracy. This will be discussed in the next section.

Sulfur Colloid Bone Marrow Scintigraphy

As discussed above, indium-111 leukocytes accumulate in both normal bone marrow and sites of infection. If bone marrow distribution is altered, bone marrow uptake can be mistaken for sites of infection. This commonly occurs with a joint prosthesis. When a hip prosthesis is inserted, normal marrow elements may be displaced and compacted at the tip of the prosthesis. There may also be a small amount of marrow left in the trochanters. Patients with sickle cell anemia may have bone pain and symptoms suspicious for osteomyelitis. However, because of altered bone marrow distribution due to expanded erythropoiesis and bone marrow infarctions, indium white blood cell scans can be very difficult to interpret. A bone marrow scan performed with technetium-99m sulfur colloid will demonstrate bone marrow distribution. This agent consists of 0.1- to 0.5-μm-sized colloidal particles. After intravenous injection, the particles are phagocytized in the reticuloendothelial system, specifically the liver, spleen, and bone marrow. By comparing the bone marrow scan with the indium white blood cell scan, the specificity for detection of osteomyelitis is improved. Patients with abnormal uptake on the leukocyte scan, who show similar uptake on the bone marrow scan, are thought not to have bone infection (Fig. 28-20). The abnormal white blood cell uptake therefore is thought to be due to altered bone marrow distribution. If abnormal uptake on the white blood cell scan is not matched by congruent uptake on the bone marrow scan, the finding is suggestive of osteomyelitis (48). Imaging with both indium white blood cell scintigraphy and technetium-99m sulfur colloid bone marrow scintigraphy has significantly improved the specificity

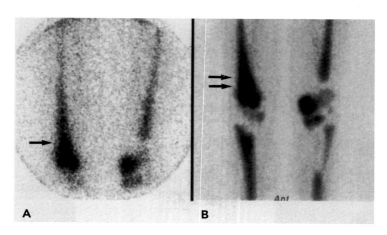

Figure 28-20 Anterior indium leukocyte **(A)** and technetium sulfur colloid bone marrow **(B)** scans of the legs in a sickle cell patient with fever and leg pain suspicious for osteomyelitis. The leukocyte scan shows increased activity in the distal right femur (*arrow*) compared to the left suggesting osteomyelitis. The bone marrow scan, however, shows congruent uptake in the distal femur (*double arrows*) indicating no infection.

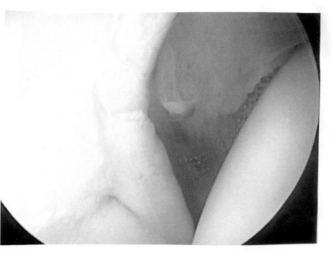

Figure 4-10 Arthroscopic view
tation in the labrum at the anterom
sistent landmark for identifying the
approximately 20% of patients the p
intra-articularly at this level.

rmal inden-
is a con-
lon. In
l lie

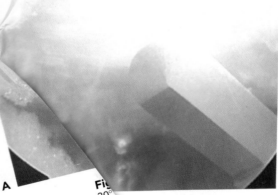

A

Fi
30°

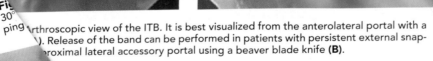

ping Arthroscopic view of the ITB. It is best visualized from the anterolateral portal with a
). Release of the band can be performed in patients with persistent external snap-
roximal lateral accessory portal using a beaver blade knife **(B)**.

B

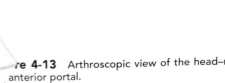

re 4-13 Arthroscopic view of the head–neck junction from
anterior portal.

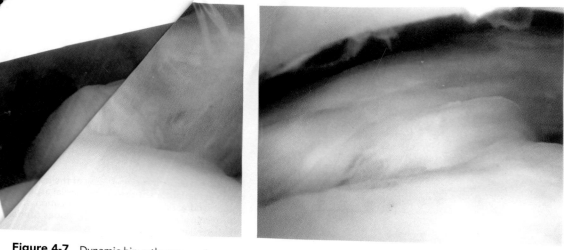

B

Figure 4-7 Dynamic hip arthroscopy demonstrates significant tightening of the ligamentum teres during external rotation **(B)** compared to internal rotation of the hip **(A)**. These findings support the biomechanical role of the ligamentum teres in the stabilization of the hip. (From *Am J Sports Med.* 2003;31, with permission.)

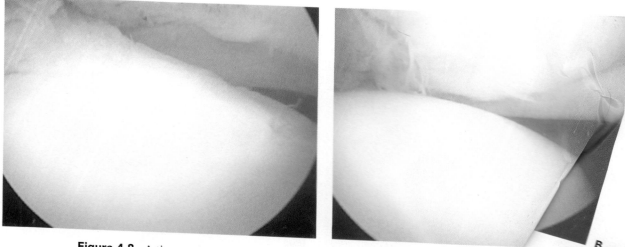

A

B

Figure 4-8 Arthroscopic picture of the fovea capitus where the ligamentum teres origina~~te~~ the medial aspect of the femoral head **(A)** and the transverse acetabular ligament **(B)**.

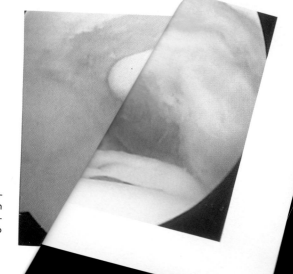

Figure 4-9 Arthroscopic view of the pulvinar or fat pad in the central aspect of the acetabular fossa. The fat pad likely plays a role in joint lubrication and should be treated cautiously during arthroscopic procedures. It is also highly vascular and has a propensity to bleed if it is débrided aggressively.

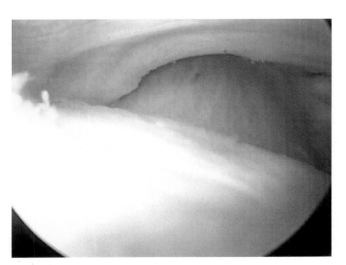

Figure 4-3 Arthroscopic view of the zona orbicularis. These circular fibers are an extension of the iliofemoral ligament and form a circular leash surrounding three quarters of the femoral neck. Its functional role is not well understood.

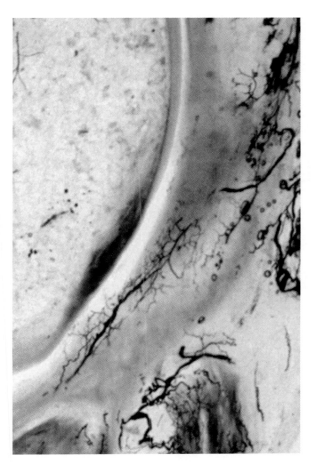

Figure 4-5 The hip labrum is relatively avascular; however, there is increased vascularity seen arising from the capsular attachments. This may have implication for arthroscopic repair of the labrum.

Figure 4-6 Arthroscopic view of the anterior superior labrum demonstrating vascular penetration through the substance of the labrum out to the central articular margin.

Color Plate Section

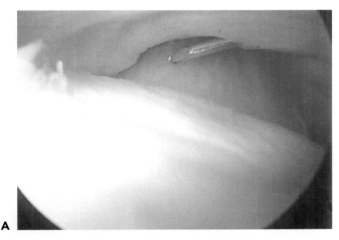

A

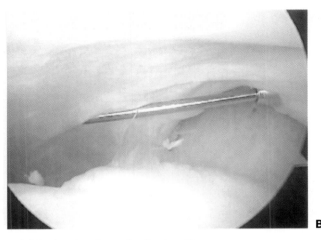

B

Figure 4-14 The distal lateral accessory portal is established under direct visualization. The entry point is at the level of the zona orbicularis and allows for direct access of the anterior femoral head–neck junction.

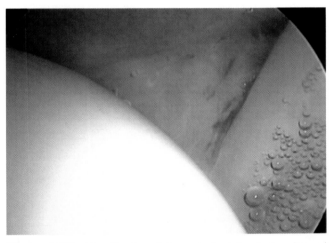

Figure 4-15 Visualization of the anterior triangle is achieved upon entry into the joint through the anterolateral portal.

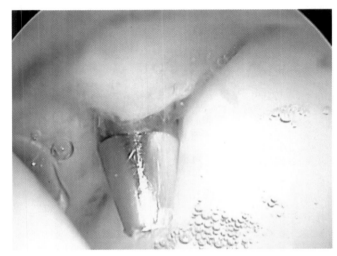

Figure 4-16 The anterior portal can be established under direct visualization from the anterolateral portal. The placement of the portal should be between the lateral and medial limbs of the iliofemoral ligament.

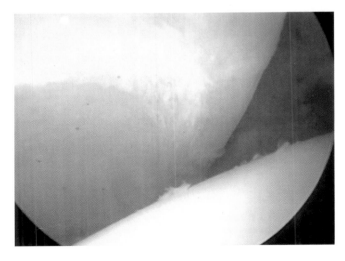

Figure 4-17 Nearly the entire circumference of the labrum can be visualized through the anterolateral portal.

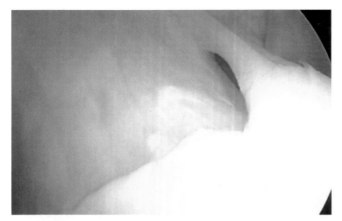

Figure 4-28 View of the anterior femoral neck and associated vincula.

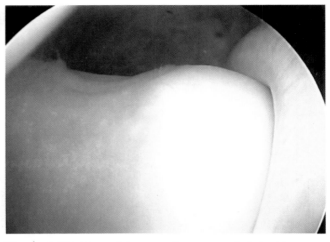

Figure 4-29 View of the normal suction seal of the labrum on the femoral head with the traction released.

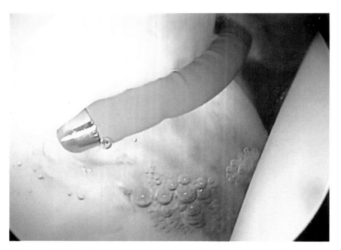

Figure 4-30 Common appearance of an anterosuperior labral tear.

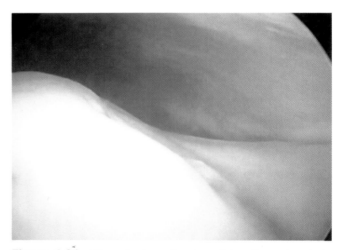

Figure 4-31 View of a large head–neck junction osteophyte resulting in femoroacetabular impingement. This has been previously described by Ganz as the CAM effect (1,22,34).

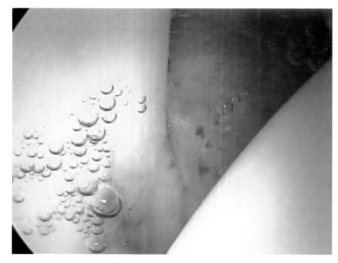

Figure 4-32 Labral bruising associated with excessive capsular laxity and pinching of the labrum between the anteriorly translated femoral head and acetabulum.

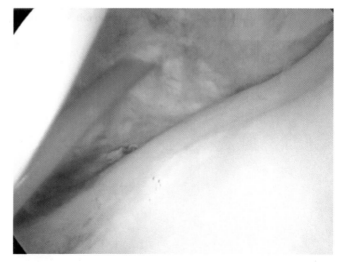

Figure 4-33 The hypoplastic labrum variant may be associated with loss of the normal suction seal and result in increased load across the capsular ligaments.

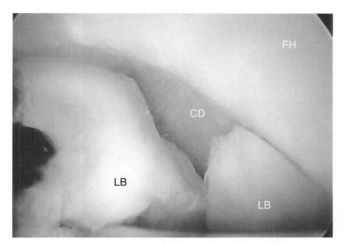

Figure 4-34 Chondral lesion to the femoral head.

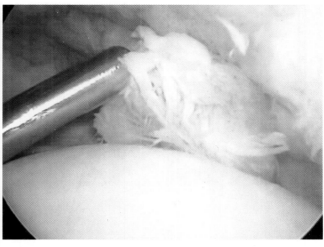

Figure 4-35 Partial tear of the ligamentum teres.

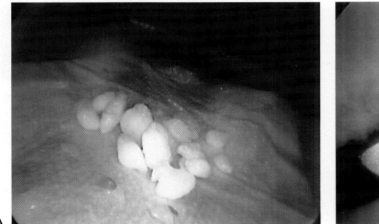

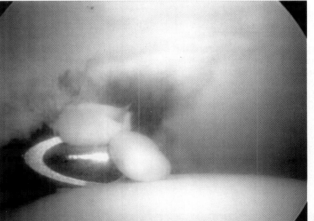

Figure 4-36 **A:** Complete exploration of the joint must be performed to assure removal of all fragments. **B:** Synovial chondromatosis results in numerous loose bodies. (From *Am J Sports Med.* 2003; 31, with permission.)

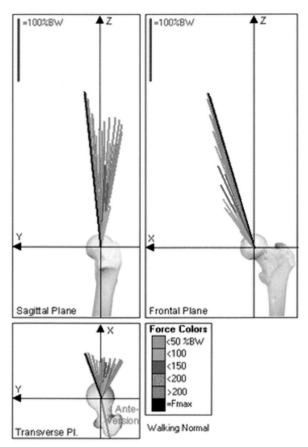

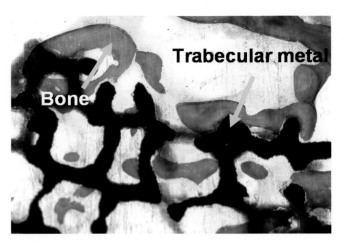

Figure 15-2 Bone ingrowth into tantalum trabecular metal porous coating.

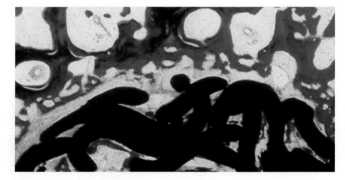

Figure 5-2 Force vectors and points of load transfer on the prosthetic head during level walking for a patient. Positive *x* is directed medially, positive *y* is in the direction of progression (anterior), and positive *z* is superior. (From Bergmann G, ed. *HIP98: Loading of the Hip Joint.* Berlin: Free University of Berlin; 2001, with permission. Compact disc, ISBN 3980784800.)

Figure 15-3 Fibrous tissue formation at the interface of a porous-coated plug that had induced motion of 150 μm in vivo.

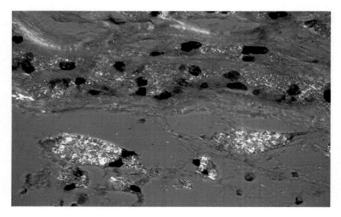

Figure 22-1 Histology of clinical peri-implant interfacial tissue under polarized light. Note macrophages laden with internalized birefringent polyethylene particles. Nuclei appear squished to the right edge of the cell. Birefringence is also observed in other cells in the collagenous tissue. (Micrograph was kindly provided by Prof. Joshua J Jacobs, Rush Medical University, Chicago, IL.)

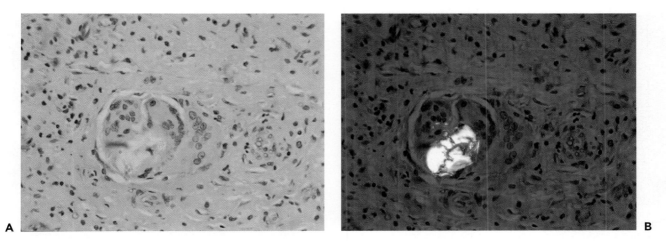

Figure 22-2 Histology of clinical peri-implant interfacial tissue under normal incident **(A)** and polarized light **(B)**. In each figure, a foreign body giant cell has encapsulated a larger fragment of birefringent polyethylene and isolated it from the surrounding tissue. Note the numerous nuclei in the giant cell.

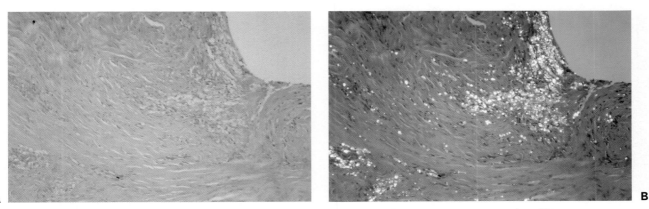

Figure 22-12 Histology of peri-implant granulomatous tissue from a canine uncemented total hip replacement (12 weeks) under normal incident **(A)** and polarized light **(B)**. Birefringent polyethylene debris are dispersed within the tissues.

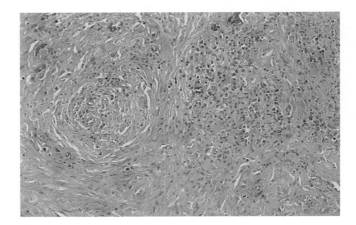

Figure 22-15 Light micrograph of an interfacial membrane from a canine with an uncemented total hip replacement and submicron UHMWPE debris introduced around the implant intraoperatively. Tissues were harvested and analyzed at the end of the 24-week study. Note the significant macrophage infiltrate with intracellular and extracellular wear debris present (magnification, 100×).

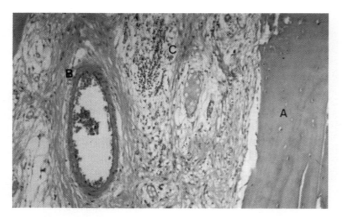

Figure 24-2 Human fresh-frozen cancellous bone allograft. Photomicrograph showing a bone marrow space lined by viable bone trabeculae (A). Note perivascular fibrosis (B) and round cell infiltration (C) (hematoxylin and eosin, 150×).

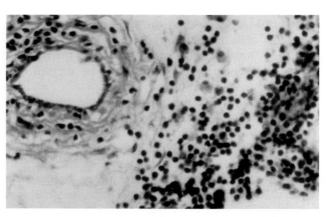

Figure 24-3 Photomicrograph of the specimen in Figure 24-2, obtained at higher magnification. Note an intense perivascular round cell infiltration and histologic features of vasculitis (hematoxylin and eosin, 350×).

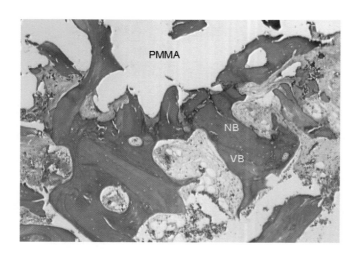

Figure 24-7 Histology image of an autopsy retrieval after impaction grafting demonstrating labeled spaces that had been occupied by cement. Inside is PMMA, then a layer of varying thickness composed of impacted graft.

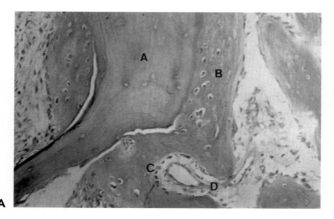

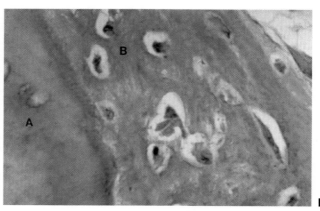

Figure 24-8 Human fresh-frozen cancellous bone allograft. **A:** Low-magnification photomicrograph showing a large complete necrotic cancellous trabeculum (A) lined by newly formed bone (B). Another area shows bone remodeling with active osteoblasts and osteoclasts (C). The marrow is well vascularized (D) (hematoxylin and eosin, 150×). **B:** Higher-magnification photomicrograph of the same area, showing a necrotic trabeculum with dead osteocytes (A) and viable osteocytes on a newly formed trabeculum (B) (hematoxylin and eosin, 400×).

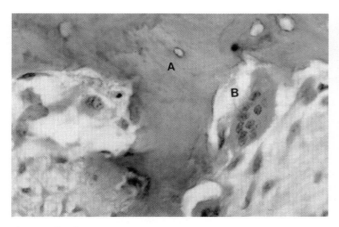

Figure 24-9 Human fresh-frozen cancellous bone allograft. Photomicrograph shows a necrotic bone trabeculum (A) with active osteoclastic resorption (B) (hematoxylin and eosin, 300×).

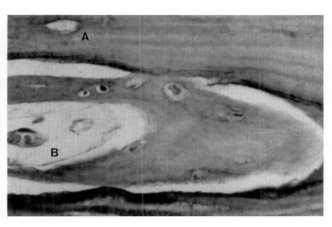

Figure 24-10 Human fresh-frozen cortical bone allograft. Photomicrograph shows a necrotic haversian canal (A) with central capillary revascularization and new bone formation (B) (hematoxylin and eosin, 350×).

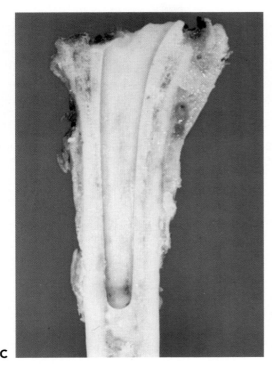

C

Figure 24-11 Fresh-frozen hip allograft composite. **C:** Photograph of the same cut surface showing no evidence of resorption of the allograft about the cement or loosening.

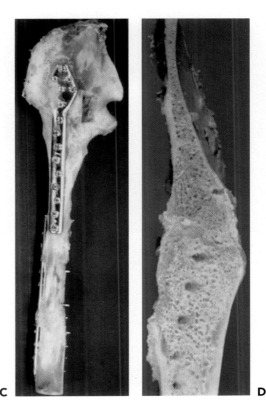

C   D

Figure 24-12 Fresh-frozen intercalary allograft. **C:** Photograph of the same specimen showing both osteotomies. **D:** Photograph of the cut surface of the proximal osteotomy, showing cancellous union.

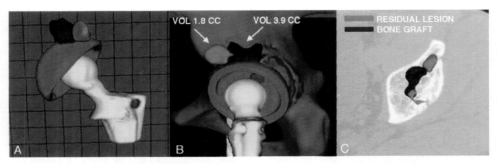

Figure 25-4 An AP **(A)** and lateral **(B)** view of three-dimensional reconstructions of an artifact-suppressed CT scan (VirtualScopics, Inc. Rochester, NY) from the same patient shown in Figure 25-3A,B. Color imaging allows differentiation between the host bone, the allograft and the residual osteolytic lesion. Volumetric measurements are shown (B) for each section. A two-dimensional axial CT scan **(C)** identifies the corresponding region of the ilium superior to the acetabular component. The images suggest that the residual osteolytic lesion remains despite bone-grafting through the screw holes. Further research is required to delineate the clinical significance of such a lesion. Clinical Orthop 2003;417:183–194.

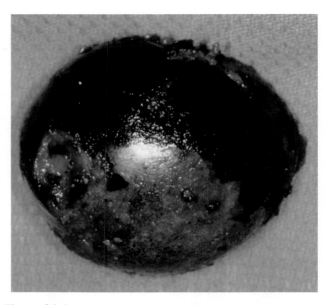

Figure 31-6 Femoral head specimen from patient with ochronosis showing characteristic pigmentation.

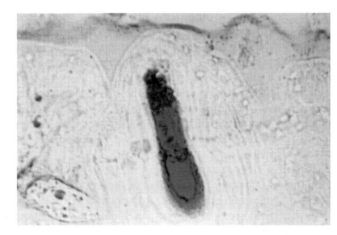

Figure 32-6 An oil red-O stain demonstrating a fat embolus in a subchondral blood vessel. Note proximity to the tide mark. (Courtesy of J. P. Jones, MD.)

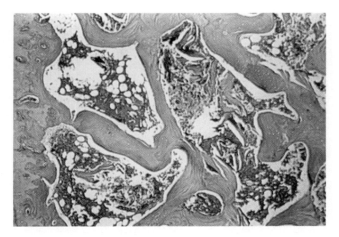

Figure 32-7 Histological section of the subchondral bone exhibiting dead trabeculae with empty osteocyte lacunae and hemorrhagic marrow with necrosis.

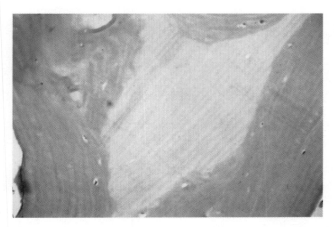

Figure 32-8 Histological section demonstrating lamination of living bone upon a section of dead trabeculae. Note the presence of osteocytes in the lacunae of living bone.

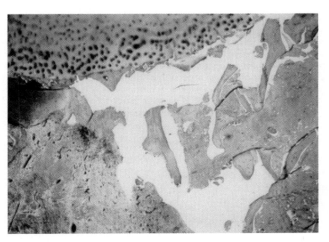

Figure 32-9 Histological section of a subchondral fracture. The articular cartilage is morphologically normal. A small amount of bone appears associated with the cartilage, and the fracture line is through the subchondral bone plate.

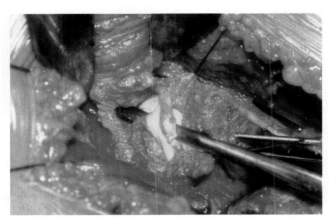

Figure 40-5 Anterolateral labral tear seen at open procedure. (Courtesy of R. Ganz.)

Figure 43-6 A recording of a transcranial Doppler from the middle cerebral artery during total hip arthroplasty. Note the embolic signals depicted in red. (Reprinted from Edmonds CR, Barbut D, Hager D, et al. Intraoperative cerebral arterial embolization during total hip arthroplasty. *Anesthesiology.* 2000;93:315–318, with permission.)

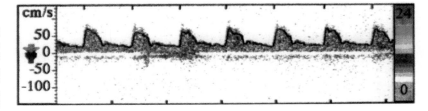

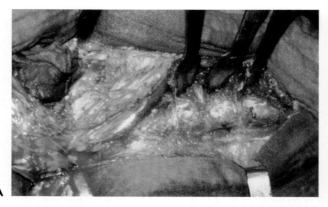

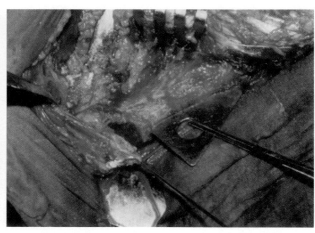

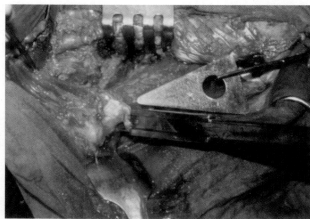

Figure 52-3 A lateral approach to the proximal femur is utilized, with elevation of the vastus lateralis. The hip joint may be approached using the interval between the gluteus medius and tensor fascia lata for palpation of the femoral neck or exposure of the anterior hip capsule **(A)**. The blade track is referenced relative to the femoral shaft using a series of metal wedges of known angulation, and appropriate anterversion of the blade is referenced using a wire placed along the anterior femoral neck, or via direct visualization **(B)**. The blade plate is inserted prior to osteotomy **(C)**, and its correct position is verified radiographically.

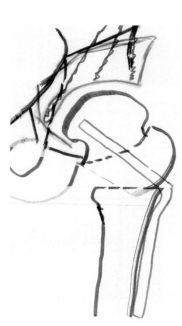

Figure 52-6 Combined periacetabular osteotomy and proximal femoral valgus osteotomy for a Perthes deformity with secondary acetabular dysplasia. A Perthes ostormity of the proximal femur is noted, and secondary acetabular dysplasia is present. This patient was treated with a combined periacetabular osteotomy and a valgus proximal femoral osteotomy, as demonstrated in the preoperative plan **(B)**.

(92%) of the diagnosis of osteomyelitis in these difficult cases when compared to indium white blood cell scanning alone (59%) (62). Accurate comparison of the indium white blood cell and technetium sulfur colloid bone marrow scans is best achieved by computer subtraction. This method improves the accuracy of the technique compared to simple visual comparison (1). This approach, however, obviously requires two scintigraphic procedures, and this may not be practical in a future managed care environment. Indium leukocyte scintigraphy is the best single-imaging procedure currently widely available for the detection of complicated osteomyelitis, especially infected prostheses.

Technetium-99M HMPAO-Labeled Leukocyte Scintigraphy

Leukocytes can be labeled with technetium-99m hexamethylpropyleneamine oxide (HMPAO) using a tagging process similar to indium oxine. Because of its lipophilic properties, technetium-99m HMPAO enters the leukocyte, becomes hydrophilic, and is trapped inside the cell (50). Unlike indium oxine, granulocytes labeling predominates. Labeling the white blood cells with technetium-99m HMPAO instead of indium-111 oxine allows the nuclear radiologist to take advantage of the optimal imaging characteristics of technetium-99m, as well as its lower radiation burden. These factors allow for better quality and higher-resolution images using technetium-99m HMPAO leukocytes when compared to indium-111 leukocytes. The normal distribution of radiotracer on a technetium-99m leukocyte scan is similar to that on an indium leukocyte scan with activity seen in the liver, spleen, and bone marrow. However, there is prominent bowel activity, as well as normal activity seen in the kidneys, bladder, and gallbladder. This bowel activity is not seen until 2 to 4 hours postinjection so imaging must be accomplished within the first 3 to 4 hours (42). This may be another advantage of technetium leukocytes over indium leukocyte scintigraphy, which requires a 24-hour delay before imaging. Technetium leukocyte scintigraphy yields similar overall results for the detection of infection as indium leukocyte scintigraphy with a sensitivity of 87% and a specificity of 81% (60). Specifically for orthopedic infections, technetium leukocyte scintigraphy has a sensitivity, specificity, and accuracy reported as high as 93%, 100%, and 97%,

respectively (10). However, our experience at Wayne State University with technetium leukocyte scintigraphy for the detection of orthopedic infections has not been as optimistic. We have found a similar high sensitivity (86%) but a lower specificity (50%) for this agent and have concerns about the value of this technique compared to indium leukocytes in this patient population.

Radiolabeled Antibody Scintigraphy

A new approach for the detection of sites of infection is the use of radiolabeled antibodies. Techniques have been developed using both radiolabeled nonspecific polyclonal immunoglobulins, as well as radiolabeled monoclonal antibodies. Nonspecific polyclonal immunoglobulins are prepared from pooled human serum gammaglobulin. The agent is labeled with indium-111 in a rapid and simple "shake-and-shoot" procedure unlike the cumbersome technique of labeling leukocytes. There is also no handling of blood products with this technique, unlike leukocyte scintigraphy. Indium-labeled nonspecific antibodies have been shown to be useful in the detection of sites of infection (57). The mechanism of uptake in infection is poorly understood. It seems that tracer accumulation at sites of infection is not due to immunologic properties of the antibody. Uptake is due to protein leakage at the site of inflammation because of capillary permeability. There then appears to be a nonimmunologic physicochemical change in the antibody resulting in polymerization and trapping at the site of infection (56). Imaging can be accomplished 6 to 24 hours postinjection. Images are considered positive if there is abnormal uptake at the site of interest that increases in intensity over time. This technique is still experimental in the United States but has been shown to have an overall sensitivity of 97% and specificity of 85% for the detection of orthopedic infections (45). The authors have previously participated in a multicenter trial evaluating this agent for the detection of periprosthetic infections. Our results demonstrated a significantly higher sensitivity (100%) for polyclonal antibodies compared to technetium leukocytes (50%) (Fig. 28-21). It should be noted that in our experience there is accumulation not only in sites of infection but also at sites of sterile inflammation, giant cell foreign body reactions, and heterotopic ossification. This uptake at sites of sterile inflammation has

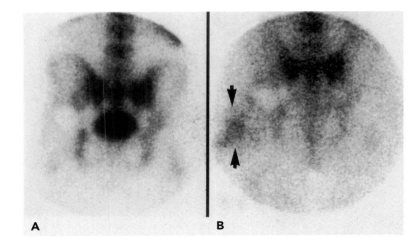

Figure 28-21 Technetium leukocyte **(A)** and indium polyclonal antibody **(B)** scans of the posterior pelvis in a patient with a painful left hip prosthesis. The leukocyte scan does not show abnormal tracer uptake. The polyclonal antibody scan clearly shows abnormal uptake (*arrows*) indicating infection.

been reported by others (45). A similar problem occurs with leukocyte and gallium scintigraphy. More investigation of this agent will be necessary before it can be widely used for the detection of musculoskeletal infections.

Monoclonal antigranulocyte antibodies labeled with technetium-99m have also been developed. These are murine-derived antibodies that react to a nonspecific cross-reacting antigen on the surface of neutrophils (35). In spite of the strong binding of the antibody to the cell membrane, there is no lysis of the cell, and the function of the granulocyte is not altered. The agent can be provided as a ready-to-label, lyophilized kit, allowing an extremely rapid and easy tagging process. Imaging is often performed 6 to 24 hours after injection. Technetium monoclonal antibodies are still experimental in the United States. They have been shown to be very accurate in detecting musculoskeletal infections with a sensitivity of 88% to 95% and specificity of 75% to 85% (4,35). The lower specificity is again thought to be due to the accumulation of the white blood cells–antibody complex at sites of sterile inflammation.

Lung Scintigraphy

Pulmonary embolism is a common medical problem in the postsurgical patient. Fifteen percent of postoperative deaths are related to pulmonary embolism (17). Pulmonary embolism can occur in up to 17% of patients undergoing elective orthopedic surgery, including hip and knee replacements (29). Many times these patients are asymptomatic. The evaluation of suspected pulmonary embolism, history and physical examination, chest radiograph, and arterial blood gases, is often nonconclusive. Ventilation perfusion lung scintigraphy (lung scan) is currently the diagnostic procedure of choice to screen patients for pulmonary embolism (60).

Most pulmonary pathologies cause abnormalities in both lung perfusion and ventilation. Pulmonary embolism, in the absence of pulmonary infarction, classically causes abnormalities only in perfusion, with ventilation remaining normal. Therefore, in order to differentiate pulmonary embolism from other lung pathology, both pulmonary perfusion and ventilation must be assessed.

The ventilation scan is performed either with radioactive gases, such as xenon-133, or with an aerosolized solution of technetium-99m diethylenetriamine pentaacetic acid (DTPA). These agents are inhaled by the patient and are deposited in the lungs proportional to regional ventilation. The perfusion scan is performed by intravenously injecting technetium-99m macroaggregated albumin (MAA), which consists of 10- to 30-μm particles that get trapped in the precapillary beds of the lungs proportional to pulmonary artery blood flow.

Defects seen on both the perfusion scan and the ventilation scan are called "matched defects" and are most likely related to pneumonia, asthma, chronic obstructive pulmonary disease, or other ventilatory pathology. Defects seen only on the perfusion scan without corresponding ventilation abnormalities are called "mismatched defects" and are characteristic of pulmonary embolism. However, results are not reported as positive or negative but in terms of probabilities. "Low probability" (<20% chance of pulmonary embolism), "intermediate probability" (20% to 80% chance of pulmonary embolism), and "high probability" (>80% chance of pulmonary embolism) are the terms most often used and are related to the size and number of mismatched perfusion defects (21) (Fig. 28-22). In a large prospective multicenter trial (PIOPED study) of over 900 patients, it is found that the specificity of a high-probability lung scan was 97% (51). However, as useful and widely performed as the procedure is, the same PIOPED study revealed certain important weaknesses. Only 102 of the 251 patients in this study whose angiograms showed pulmonary embolism had a high-probability study (41% sensitivity) result. Therefore, high-probability scan results miss 59% of patients with pulmonary embolism. A combination of high- and intermediate-probability scan results has a sensitivity of 82% for the detection of pulmonary embolism but a specificity of only 52%. The high-probability scan result also loses specificity in patients with prior episodes of pulmonary embolism (88%) when compared to those without prior pulmonary embolism (98%) (51). In some patients, the defects due to pulmonary embolism may resolve very slowly if at all, especially in the elderly with underlying pulmonary or cardiac disease. Without a prior scan for comparison, lung scintigraphy cannot distinguish the defects due to new acute pulmonary embolism from those unresolved defects due to prior pulmonary embolism.

The lung scan results must not be interpreted by the referring physician without taking into account the patient's clinical

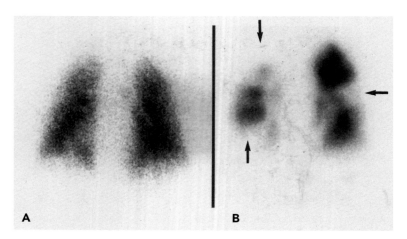

Figure 28-22 Posterior aerosol ventilation (**A**) and macroaggregated albumin (MAA) perfusion (**B**) scans of the lungs. Notice the many defects on the perfusion scan (*arrows*) not seen on the ventilation scan. These multiple mismatched perfusion defects indicate a high probability for pulmonary embolism.

condition. For example, as previously mentioned, without pre-electing the patients, those with a low probability for pulmonary embolism scan result have a 10% to 20% chance of pulmonary embolism. However, in such patients who also have a high clinical suspicion for pulmonary embolism, the posttest probability of pulmonary embolism rises to 40% (49). Similarly, if a patient with a low-probability scan result also has a low clinical suspicion for pulmonary embolism, the posttest probability falls to 4%.

The lung scan results, in conjunction with the clinical suspicion for pulmonary embolism, can be used to decide on the need for pulmonary embolism treatment or further diagnostic testing (52). Patients with a high-probability scan and a high or intermediate clinical suspicion for pulmonary embolism deserve anticoagulation. Patients with a normal perfusion scan or those with a low-probability scan result and a low clinical suspicion for pulmonary embolism need no further testing or treatment. All other patients deserve noninvasive testing for deep venous thrombosis. If deep venous thrombosis is detected, the patient deserves anticoagulation. If deep venous thrombosis is not detected, pulmonary angiography is recommended for a definitive diagnosis of pulmonary embolism unless the lung scan is intermediate and the patient has a low clinical suspicion for pulmonary embolism or the scan is low probability and the clinical suspicion for pulmonary embolism is intermediate.

REFERENCES

1. Achong DM, Oates E. The computer-generated bone marrow subtraction image: a valuable adjunct to combined in-111 WBC/Tc-99m in sulfur colloid scintigraphy for musculoskeletal infection. *Clin Nucl Med.* 1994;19:188–193.
2. Aliabadi P, Tumeh SS, Weissman BN, et al. Cemented total hip prosthesis: radiographic and scintigraphic evaluation. *Radiology.* 1989;173:203–206.
3. Anger HO. Scintillation camera. *Rev Sci Instr.* 1958;29:27–33.
4. Becker W, Bair J, Behr T, et al. Detection of soft-tissue infections and osteomyelitis using a technetium-99m-labeled antigranulocyte monoclonal antibody fragment. *J Nucl Med.* 1994;35:1436–1443.
5. Bilchik T, Heyman S, Siegel A, et al. Osteoid osteoma: the role of radionuclide bone imaging, conventional radiography and computed tomography in its management. *J Nucl Med.* 1992;33:269–271.
6. Blau M, Nagler W, Bender MA. Fluorine-18: a new isotope for bone scanning. *J Nucl Med.* 1962;3:332–334.
7. Bressler EL, Conway JJ, Weiss SC. Neonatal osteomyelitis examined by bone scintigraphy. *Radiology.* 1984;152:685–688.
8. Brown ML. Bone scintigraphy in benign and malignant tumors. *J Nucl Med.* 1993;31:731–738.
9. Charkes ND, Sklaroff DM. Early diagnosis of metastatic bone cancer by photoscanning with strontium-85. *J Nucl Med.* 1964;5:168–179.
10. Copping C, Dagliesh SM, Dudley NJ, et al. The role of ⁹⁹Tcᵐ-HMPAO white cell imaging in suspected orthopaedic infection. *Br J Radiol.* 1992;65:309–312.
11. Corey KR, Kenny P, Greenberg R, et al. The use of calcium 47 in diagnostic studies of patients with bone lesions. *AJR Radium Ther Nucl Med.* 1961;85:955–975.
12. Datz FL. Indium-111-labeled leukocytes for the detection of infection: current status. *Semin Nucl Med.* 1994;2:92–109.
13. Datz FL, Thorne DA. Effect of antibiotic therapy on the sensitivity of indium-111-labeled leukocyte scans. *J Nucl Med.* 1986;27:1849–1853.
14. Datz FL, Thorne DA. Effect of chronicity of infection on the sensitivity of the ¹¹¹In-labeled leukocyte scan. *AJR Am J Roentgenol.* 1986;147:809–812.
15. Davis LP, Porter AT. Nuclear medicine's role in the palliation of painful bone metastases. In: Freeman LM, ed. *Nuclear Medicine Annual 1995.* New York: Raven Press; 1995:169–184.
16. DeNardo GL. The 85-Sr scintiscan in bone disease. *Ann Intern Med.* 1966;65:44–53.
17. Dismuke SE, Wagner EH. Pulmonary embolism as a cause of death. The changing mortality in hospitalized patients. *JAMA.* 1986;255:2039–2042.
18. Eisenberg B, Powe JE, Alavi A. Cold defects in In-111 labeled leukocyte imaging of osteomyelitis in the axial skeleton. *Clin Nucl Med.* 1991;16:103–106.
19. Fogelman I, Carr D. A comparison of bone scanning and radiology in the assessment of patients with symptomatic Paget's disease. *Eur J Nucl Med.* 1980;5:417–421.
20. Fogelman I, Collier BD, Brown ML. Bone scintigraphy. Part 3: Bone scanning in metabolic bone disease. *J Nucl Med.* 1993;34:2247–2252.
21. Gottschalk A, Sostman D, Coleman E, et al. Ventilation-perfusion scintigraphy in the PIOPED study. Part II: Evaluation of the scintigraphic criteria and interpretations. *J Nucl Med.* 1993;34:1119–1126.
22. Handmaker H, Leonards R. The bone scan in inflammatory osseous disease. *Semin Nucl Med.* 1976;6:95–105.
23. Harris WH, Sledge CB. Total hip and total knee replacement. Part 1. *N Engl J Med.* 1990;323:725–731.
24. Harris WH, Sledge CB. Total hip and knee replacement. Part 2. *N Engl J Med.* 1990;323:801–807.
25. Holder LE, Cole LA, Myerson MS. Reflex sympathetic dystrophy in the foot: clinical and scintigraphic criteria. *Radiology.* 1992;184:531–535.
26. Hunter JC, Hattner RS, Murray WR, et al. Loosening of the total knee arthroplasty: detection by radionuclide bone scanning. *AJR Am J Roentgenol.* 1980;135:131–136.
27. Jaszczak RJ, Chang LT, Murphy PH. Single-photon emission computed tomography using multi-slice fan beam collimator. *IEEE Trans Nucl Sci.* 1979;26:610–618.
28. Jones AG, Fracis MD, Davis MA. Bone scanning: radionuclidic reaction mechanisms. *Semin Nucl Med.* 1976;6:3–18.
29. Keenan AM, Palevsky HI, Steinberg ME, et al. An evaluation of preoperative and postoperative ventilation and perfusion lung scintigraphy in the screening for pulmonary embolism after elective orthopedic surgery. *Clin Nucl Med.* 1991;16:13–18.
30. Krishnamurthy GT, Tubis M, Hiss J, et al. Distribution pattern of metastatic bone disease: a need for total body skeletal image. *JAMA.* 1977;237:2504–2506.
31. Lavender JP, Khan RAA, Hughes SPF. Blood flow and tracer uptake in normal and abnormal canine bone: comparisons with Sr-85 microspheres, Kr-81m, and Tc-99m MDP. *J Nucl Med.* 1979;20:413–418.
32. Lavender JP, Loew J, Barker JR, et al. Gallium 67 citrate scanning in neoplastic and inflammatory lesions. *Br J Radiol.* 1971;44:361–366.
33. Lewis SL, Rees JIS, Thomas GV, et al. Pitfalls of bone scintigraphy in suspected hip fractures. *Br J Radiol.* 1991;64:403–408.
34. Libshitz HI. Radiation changes in bone. *Semin Roentgenol.* 1994;1:15–37.
35. Lind P, Langsteger W, Költringer, et al. Immunoscintigraphy of inflammatory processes with a technetium-99m-labeled monoclonal antigranulocyte antibody (Mab BW 250/183). *J Nucl Med.* 1990;31:417–423.
36. Magnuson J, Brown M, Hauser M, et al. In-111 WBC scintigraphy versus other imaging tests in suspected orthopedic prosthesis infection: a comparison. *J Nucl Med.* 1981;28:586.
37. Matin P. Basic principles of nuclear medicine techniques for detection and evaluation of trauma and sports medicine injuries. *Semin Nucl Med.* 1988;2:90–112.
38. McDougall IR, Keeling CA. Complications of fractures and their healing. *Semin Nucl Med.* 1988;2:113–125.
39. Merkel KD, Brown ML, Fitzgerald RH. Sequential technetium-99m HMDP-gallium-67 citrate imaging for the evaluation of infection in the painful prosthesis. *J Nucl Med.* 1986;27:1413–1417.
40. Merkel KD, Fitzgerald RH, Brown ML. Scintigraphic evaluation in musculoskeletal sepsis. *Orthop Clin North Am.* 1984;15:401–416.

41. Miles KA, Harper WM, Finlay DBL, et al. Scintigraphic abnormalities in patients with painful hip replacements treated conservatively. *Br J Radiol.* 1992;65:491–494.

42. Mountford PJ, Kettle AG, O'Doherty M, et al. Comparison of technetium-99m-HM-PAO leukocytes with indium-111-oxine leukocytes for localizing intraabdominal sepsis. *J Nucl Med.* 1990;31: 311–315.

43. Murray IPC. Photopenia in skeletal scintigraphy of suspected bone and joint infection. *Clin Nucl Med.* 1982;7:13–20.

44. O'Donoghue JP, Powe JE, Mattar AG, et al. Three-phase bone scintigraphy. Asymmetric patterns in the upper extremities of asymptomatic normals and reflex sympathetic dystrophy patients. *Clin Nucl Med.* 1993;18:829–836.

45. Oyen WJG, Van Horn JR, Claessens RAMJ, et al. Diagnosis of bone, joint, and joint prosthesis infections with In-111-labeled nonspecific human immunoglobulin G scintigraphy. *Radiology.* 1992;182:195–199.

46. Palestro CJ. Radionuclide imaging after skeletal interventional procedures. *Semin Nucl Med.* 1995;1:3–14.

47. Palestro CJ. The current role of gallium imaging in infection. *Semin Nucl Med.* 1994;2:128–141.

48. Palestro CJ, Roumanas P, Swyer AJ, et al. Diagnosis of musculoskeletal infection using combined In-111 labeled leukocyte and Tc-99m SC marrow imaging. *Clin Nucl Med.* 1992;17: 269–273.

49. Palevsky HI, Alavi A. A noninvasive strategy for the management of patients suspected of pulmonary embolism. *Semin Nucl Med.* 1991;4:325–331.

50. Peters AM. The utility of [^{99m}Tc]HMPAO-leukocytes for imaging infection. *Semin Nucl Med.* 1994;2:110–127.

51. PIOPED Investigators. Value of the ventilation/perfusion scan in acute pulmonary embolism. Results of the prospective investigation of pulmonary embolism diagnosis (PIOPED). *JAMA.* 1990; 263:2753–2759.

52. Ralph DD. The implications of prospective investigation of pulmonary embolism diagnosis. *Radiol Clin North Am.* 1994;32: 679–687.

53. Rizzo PF, Gould ES, Lyden JP, et al. Diagnosis of occult fractures about the hip. Magnetic resonance imaging compared with bone-scanning. *J Bone Joint Surg.* 1993;75:395–400.

54. Rosenthall L, Lepanto L, Rayond F. Radiophosphate uptake in asymptomatic knee arthroplasty. *J Nucl Med.* 1987;28:1546–1549.

55. Rosenthall L, Lisbona R, Hernandez M, et al. ^{99m}Tc-PP and ^{67}Ga imaging following insertion of orthopedic devices. *Radiology.* 1979;133:717–721.

56. Rubin RH, Fischman AJ. The use of radiolabeled nonspecific immunoglobulin in the detection of focal inflammation. *Semin Nucl Med.* 1994;2:169–179.

57. Rubin RH, Fischman AJ, Callahan RJ, et al. In-labeled nonspecific immunoglobulin scanning in the detection of focal infection. *N Engl J Med.* 1989;321:935–940.

58. Ryan PJ, Gibson T, Fogelman I. Bone scintigraphy following intravenous pamidronate for Paget's disease of bone. *J Nucl Med.* 1992; 33:1589–1593.

59. Saha GB. *Fundamentals of Nuclear Pharmacy.* New York: Springer-Verlag; 1992.

60. Schauwecker DS. The scintigraphic diagnosis of osteomyelitis. *AJR Am J Roentgenol.* 1992;158:9–18.

61. Schauwecker DS, Park HM, Mock BH, et al. Evaluation of complicating osteomyelitis with Tc-99m MDP, IN-111 granulocytes, and Ga-67 citrate. *J Nucl Med.* 1984;25:849–853.

62. Seabold JE, Nepola JV, Marsh JL, et al. Postoperative bone marrow alterations: potential pitfalls in the diagnosis of osteomyelitis with In-111-labeled leukocyte scintigraphy. *Radiology.* 1991;180: 741–747.

63. Singh BN, Kesala BA, Mehta SP, et al. Osteomalacia on bone scan simulating skeletal metastases. *Clin Nucl Med.* 1977;6:181–183.

64. Subramanian G, McAfee JG. A new complex of ^{99m}Tc for skeletal imaging. *Radiology.* 1971;99:192–196.

65. Subramanian G, McAfee JG, Blair RJ, et al. Technetium-99m-methylene diphosphonate: a superior agent for skeletal imaging—comparison with other technetium complexes. *J Nucl Med.* 1975; 16:744–755.

66. Tehranzadeh J, Schneider R, Freiberger RH. Radiological evaluation of painful total hip replacement. *Radiology.* 1981;141:355–362.

67. Uren RF, Howman-Giles R. The "cold hip" sign on bone scan. A retrospective review. *Clin Nucl Med.* 1991;16:553–556.

68. Utz JA, Lull RJ, Galvin EG. Asymptomatic total hip prosthesis: natural history determined using Tc-99m MDP bone scans. *Radiology.* 1986;161:509–512.

Magnetic Resonance Imaging

29

Hollis G. Potter   Ian Tsou

Despite a complete physical examination by an experienced clinician and appropriately performed radiographs, the etiology of hip pain may remain unclear. Comprehensive evaluation of the painful hip involves not only detection of osseous pathology, but also assessment of the surrounding soft tissues, including tendons, neurovascular bundles and intracapsular structures, including articular cartilage and labrum. Due to its direct multiplanar capabilities, lack of ionizing radiation, and superior soft tissue contrast, magnetic resonance imaging (MRI) has gained wide acceptance in the assessment of the painful adult hip.

PRINCIPLES OF MRI

Generation of the Signal

While many nuclei are suitable for MRI, including ^{14}N, ^{13}C, and ^{31}P, most clinical units exploit the magnetic properties of ^{1}H due to its copious concentration in soft tissue. These charged hydrogen nuclei have a net spin and induce a local magnetic field; in the absence of an externally applied field, they are randomly oriented. When these individual hydrogen nuclei "magnets" are subjected to a strong external magnet, they orient according to the long axis of the static field (B_0). In order to receive diagnostic information from these nuclei, they need to be raised to a higher energy state. This is done by imparting radiofrequency waves sent into the patient at a specific frequency "tuned" to the hydrogen nuclei, which "excites" tissue magnetization from its lower energy state, M_Z, which is relatively parallel to B_0, to a higher energy state, in the transverse M_{XY} plane. The precessing magnetization causes a change in the magnetic field or flux in the receiver coil, inducing a voltage, which is eventually sent to an analog-to-digital converter. Gradients that are imposed on

the magnetic field create a spatial variation of B_0 amplitude, which allows for individual slice selection as well as spatial encoding of the signal, giving it an anatomic location. The gradients account for the "banging" sound appreciated by the patient in an MRI unit.

Tissue Contrast and Pulse Sequences

When the hydrogen nuclei are "flipped" from the state of longitudinal magnetization (M_Z) to the state of transverse magnetization (M_{XY}), two processes occur simultaneously. Following removal of the radiofrequency pulse, there is an exponential recovery of longitudinal magnetization, known as T1 relaxation time. T1 is also known as the "spin-lattice" recovery, which is conversion of the stored energy in the hydrogen spins to the kinetic energy of other hydrogen nuclei (lattice). Fat protons have a very efficient energy transfer and regain longitudinal magnetization quickly, accounting for the high signal intensity on T1-weighted sequencing. Water has a longer T1 relaxation time due to the lack of larger molecules to take up the additional energy of the excited nuclei, accounting for the lower signal noted.

A simultaneous (and much more rapid) process is T2 decay, which occurs in the transverse plane (M_{XY}). T2 decay reflects the dephasing or loss of "coherence" of the protons and describes the interaction between the excited nuclei (spin-spin). T2 relaxation is a quantifiable measurement that is an exponential decay function and occurs due to rapid dephasing of the unbalanced magnetic dipoles, due to both intrinsic tissue properties within the voxel and extrinsic magnetic field inhomogeneities. Water maintains its phase coherence with less rapid decay of transverse magnetization, resulting in bright signal on a T2-weighted sequence.

One can take advantage of these magnetic parameters to achieve differential soft tissue contrast by altering the repetition rate of successive excitational radiofrequency pulses (repetition time) and the time between the excitational radiofrequency

409

TABLE 29-1
SIMPLIFIED MRI SIGNAL CHARACTERISTICS OF NORMAL TISSUE

	T1	T2	Fat Suppression	Gradient Echo[a]
Cortical bone	Low	Low	Low	Low
Fatty marrow	High	Intermediate	Low	Intermediate
Fluid	Low	High	Very high	High
Cartilage	Intermediate	Intermediate	Higher	Higher
Tendon	Low	Low	Low	Low
Ligament	Low	Low	Low	Low
Labrum	Low	Low	Low	Low
Muscle	Intermediate	Intermediate	Intermediate	Intermediate

[a]For T2*-weighted parameters.

pulse and the center of the obtained echo information (echo time). A T1-weighted sequence typically has a short TR and short TE (on the order of 500 to 600 and 10 to 20 ms, respectively), and a T2-weighted sequence has a long TR and long TE parameters (>2000 and 60 ms, respectively). These parameters form the basis for MR pulse sequences such as spin echo and fast (or turbo) spin echo.

It is important to remember that signal is only obtained from hydrogen nuclei that are "mobil". Thus, cortical bone demonstrates diminished signal intensity on all pulse sequences, and tendons and ligaments, which are primarily composed of type I collagen, allow for little mobility of water due to their highly ordered ultrastructure. Signal can also be affected by paramagnetic substances such as hemosiderin, which act to disturb the magnetic field, creating striking diminished signal intensity on T2-weighted sequences.

Additional pulse sequences may be encountered on routine MRI. Standard hip imaging techniques use fat-suppression to "rescale" the contrast range, allowing for greater conspicuity of fluid in the joint or bone marrow. Although these images are "noisy," they provide important diagnostic information, such as the detection of radiographically occult fractures. Gradient echo techniques have rapid acquisition time and form the basis to noninvasively assess regional vasculature (please refer to the section on MR angiography). Most importantly, the ability of MRI to noninvasively assess articular cartilage has driven much of the recent imaging research. Regardless of the clinically suspected diagnosis, dedicated, previously validated cartilage pulse sequences should be used for imaging of every joint.

Such knowledge of pulse sequences is important as this provides for ready identification of pathology on MR examination of the hip and is the basis for the superior soft tissue contrast of MRI compared to conventional imaging tests. A simplified table of normal MRI signal characteristics is provided in Table 29-1.

Imaging Techniques

Current MRI examination of the hip should include initial assessment of the entire pelvis in order to detect unsuspected pathology, such as sacroiliitis, occult sacral insufficiency fracture, or metastasis. In many institutions, large field-of-view fat-suppression techniques have supplanted

bone scintigraphy for regional assessment of marrow infiltration. Following the initial large field-of-view body coil images, a dedicated surface coil must be placed over the hip in order to provide adequate detail of the cartilaginous surfaces, synovium, and labrum (Fig. 29-1). Ideally, either a dedicated hip or a two-part shoulder coil is recommended in order to achieve high in-plane resolution (in the frequency direction, on the order of 300 to 350 μ), as well as adequate signal to noise. When possible, the hip should be maintained in neutral rotation.

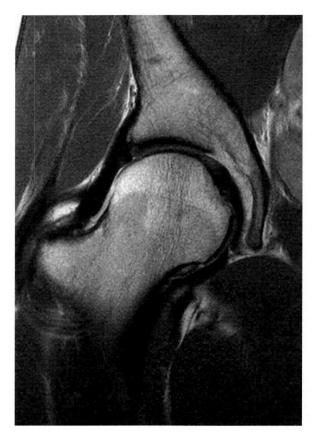

Figure 29-1 Normal surface coil MR image in a 32-year-old woman. Note the ability of the surface coil high-resolution technique to discern the integrity of the articular cartilage, labrum, and surrounding soft tissue structures.

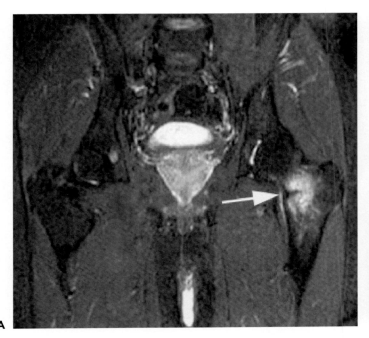

A

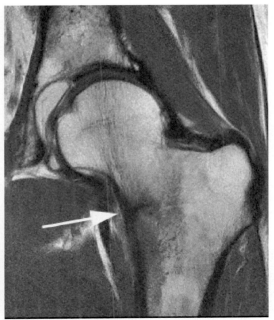

B

Figure 29-2   A: A 56-year-old runner with left hip pain and negative radiographs. Coronal large field-of-view fat-suppressed body coil image discloses the presence of a compressive side femoral neck stress fracture. **B:** Coronal fast spin echo surface coil image discloses the sclerotic fracture line (*white arrow*), as well as endosteal sclerosis and cortical remodeling.

Pulse sequences should be chosen to achieve differential contrast between intracapsular fluid, articular cartilage, and fibrocartilage. While some authors have utilized intra-articular contrast agents for detection of labral tears (34,44), other investigators have found that with adequate spatial resolution, no intra-articular contrast agent is necessary to accurately and reproducibly discern cartilage and labral lesions (37). The decision to convert the normally noninvasive MRI technique to a slightly invasive one (using an intra-articular contrast agent) should be based both on the experience of the MRI radiologist and the confidence of the referring orthopaedic surgeon.

Intravenous contrast injection is typically utilized for MR angiography, particularly arteriography, as well as in cases of suspected osseous infection. Gadolinium is a paramagnetic agent that develops a magnetic moment; with normal dosages and scan times, it primarily acts to shorten T1 relaxation time. Unlike the conventional radiographic contrast agents used for computerized tomography (CT) and angiography, it has a much lower allergic potential and is not nephrotoxic.

DIAGNOSIS BY MRI

Trauma

MRI has largely supplanted bone scintigraphy in detection of radiographically occult hip fractures as it is more sensitive, particularly when evaluating an osteoporotic patient in whom plain films are equivocal (51). The appearance of insufficiency fractures will vary depending on the time interval between

fracture and MRI. Acute fractures are denoted by a bone marrow edema pattern that is accentuated on fat-suppression techniques, with or without cortical displacement and surrounding soft tissue edema. In the subacute and chronic settings, variable amounts of callus are present, thus serving to more accurately assess the age of osseous trauma.

In younger, more active patients, stress fractures may also be disclosed and are manifest as bone marrow edema pattern surrounding the low signal intensity fracture line (Fig. 29-2). Due to its superior soft tissue contrast, MRI shows a wider spectrum of stress reaction to bone, ranging from normal remodeling, accelerated remodeling, fatigue and eventual cortical fracture, reflected as soft tissue periosteal edema, periosteal reaction, cortical fracture, and delayed union. Delayed union is manifest as a cortical fracture line bordered by low signal intensity sclerosis, and typically surrounded by marrow edema. Marrow edema typically resolves within 6 months following a femoral neck stress fracture; persistent edema suggests a new injury or delayed healing (58). Compared to radionuclide bone scan, MRI has been determined to be as sensitive and much more specific in determining the cause of hip pain in endurance athletes, in whom scintigraphy yielded accuracy of 68% for femoral neck stress fractures (32% false positive results), with 100% accuracy using MRI (56). Fredericson et al. have described an MRI grading system which assessed the relative involvement of the periosteum versus the marrow, as well as the presence or absence of a fracture (17). The degree of osseous involvement correlated with clinical symptoms, allowing for appropriate recommendations for rehabilitation and return to activity (17). Additional authors have noted that cortical signal intensity, with or without a fracture line, correlated to a longer time to clinical recovery (81).

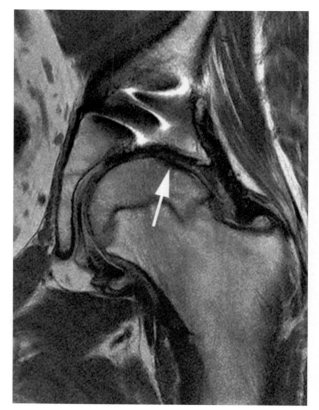

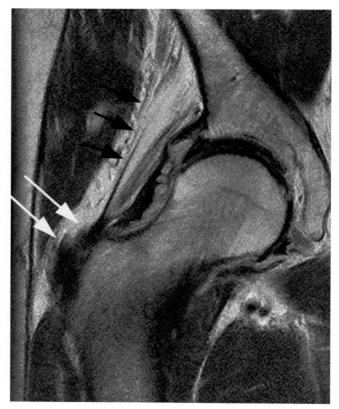

Figure 29-3 Coronal fast spin echo MR image in a 47-year-old patient who had undergone instrumentation for acetabular fracture and persistent left hip pain. Coronal fast spin echo MRI discloses focal osteonecrosis over the lateral, weight bearing aspect of the femoral head (*arrow*). Note the subchondral sclerosis and mild collapse.

Figure 29-4 Abductor tendinosis and atrophy in a 78-year-old woman with complaint of weakness and groin pain. Coronal fast spin echo MR image demonstrates marked tendinosis and partial tear of the gluteus minimus tendon (*white arrows*), as well as considerable fatty infiltration of the muscle (*black arrows*), indicative of atrophy.

With more complex pelvic or acetabular trauma, MRI may be helpful in disclosing injuries to the sciatic nerve, which is at risk for increased iatrogenic injury during fracture reduction and stabilization (47). Despite the presence of standardized instrumentation for acetabular fracture, it is possible to re-image the hip in patients who have persistent symptoms despite apparently anatomic reduction of the fracture on radiographs. Using a modification of commercially available pulse sequences, delayed complications of acetabular or proximal femoral fracture may be disclosed, including osteonecrosis, traumatic chondrolysis, heterotopic ossification or malunion (Fig. 29-3).

In addition to osseous injuries, MRI may also disclose injury to myotendinous structures surrounding the hip joint, which may be difficult to discern from primary joint pain or isolated bursitis. The tendinous attachments of the short external rotators, iliopsoas, gluteus minimus, and gluteus medius muscles are all well demonstrated on surface coil MRI, and insertional tendinosis with or without tear or muscle atrophy may be discerned (Fig. 29-4). Recent attention has been directed toward the gluteus minimus and medius acting as the "rotator cuff of the hip," and increased interest has been directed toward their importance in stabilizing the femoral head within the acetabulum, thus preserving normal hip biomechanics and gait (3,9,26,33). In more symptomatic patients,

primary repair may be necessary to restore normal function (26) (Fig. 29-5).

Articular Cartilage, Labral, and Synovial Evaluation

The ability to noninvasively detect articular cartilage injury has been one of the major advances of MRI in the past decade. While cartilage repair techniques of the hip remain in their infancy, the application of such techniques to standard hip treatment would require a reliable, accurate, and ideally noninvasive means to detect articular cartilage injury and provide an objective assessment of outcome for the repair techniques (8,46). It is important to remember that preservation of joint space on standardized radiographs does not preclude the presence of focal, symptomatic chondral defects of the hip joint (Fig. 29-6). While hip arthroscopy is popular at many institutions, it is an invasive, technically challenging procedure, not without potential morbidity. Previous studies have evaluated conventional contrast arthrography and MR arthrography (12,21,34,44). Mintz et al. studied 92 patients who had high-resolution, noncontrast MRI of the hip followed by arthroscopic surgery, with two independent MR readers (37). Of the 92 patients studied, 84/88 (95%) of labral tears were noted at surgery, and there was 92% interobserver agreement on the

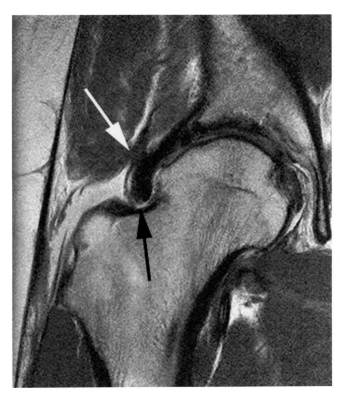

Figure 29-5 Abductor tendon tear in a 53-year-old man. Coronal fast spin echo MR image demonstrates complete detachment of the gluteus minimus tendon (*white arrow*), as well as detachment of the iliofemoral ligament (*black arrow*) and fluid distention of the adjacent greater trochanteric bursa. The gluteus medius tendon was also completely torn. At surgery, a "bald" femoral head was encountered.

MRI studies (37). For articular cartilage defects in the femoral head and acetabulum, there was good (92%) agreement (between MRI and surgery) within one grade using a modified Outerbridge scoring regimen (37,43).

Following trauma, detection of chondral lesions is helpful, particularly in the setting of hip subluxation episodes, where chondral shearing injuries may go undetected on conventional radiographs and CT (42) (Fig. 29-7). Assessment of degenerative patterns of cartilage loss is also useful, particularly in the younger adult patient with acetabular dysplasia in whom arthroplasty is not an immediate option (Fig. 29-8). MRI may help guide timing of more invasive surgical procedures such as an osteotomy or dislocation–debridement in patients with conditions that predispose to early arthrosis, such as femoracetabular impingement syndrome (18,57) (Fig. 29-9).

There are several pitfalls in the MRI detection of labral tears. High in-plane resolution is necessary to discern nondisplaced tears (Fig. 29-10). Similar to findings noted in the knee meniscus and shoulder labrum, there is asymptomatic degeneration of the acetabular labrum in patients of increasing age. Lecouvet et al. studied 200 asymptomatic hips and noted anatomic variations with increasing internal signal intensity, reflecting degeneration, in older patients (35). The use of water-sensitive pulse sequences is therefore helpful in

improving contrast between the high signal intensity of synovial fluid extending to a labral flap tear versus the intermediate signal intensity that is typical of mucoid degeneration of fibrocartilage. As an increased incidence of asymptomatic tears in the labrum is diagnosed with MRI, the utility of high resolution MRI lies in the clinician's ability to combine the information obtained with the MRI with an appropriate physical examination and patient history, in order to direct appropriate management.

Labral tears are made more conspicuous by the detection of paralabral ganglion cysts, which are commonly associated with acetabular dysplasia (Fig. 29-11). Whether traumatic or degenerative in etiology, early detection of labral and cartilage lesions is helpful in guiding management, thus preserving hip arthroscopy as a therapeutic tool.

High resolution noncontrast MRI is also useful in detecting occult synovial disease, as it provides for visualization of the "native" capsule prior to distention by contrast agents. Based on signal characteristics and morphology, most synovial disorders may be noninvasively diagnosed (Fig. 29-12) and their sequela followed (Fig. 29-13).

Osteonecrosis and Transient Osteoporosis

MRI has been demonstrated to be the most sensitive and specific imaging modality for diagnosing osteonecrosis of the femoral head, with sensitivity and specificity range from 94% to 100% and 71% to 100%, respectively (5,16,19,24,39, 45, 66,67,69,72,73). Early and accurate diagnosis of osteonecrosis is critical in management, as treatment modalities such as core decompression and bone grafting have better outcomes if performed in the early stages (14,75). Animal studies of ischemia induced by surgical as well as nontraumatic models in the proximal femora have shown that MRI is able to detect changes within 3 days to 2 weeks after onset of the insult, sooner than any detectable change on plain radiographs (2,7,53). The use of intravenous MRI contrast materials such as gadolinium may help to distinguish between viable repair tissue and necrotic tissue by demonstrating vascularity within the repair tissue but not within the necrotic regions (76). Newer MR techniques such as diffusion imaging have been applied in animal models, and these have shown potential in differentiating reversible ischemia and ischemia leading to osteonecrosis (25). Most importantly, however, the ability to define the necrotic–viable bone interface and confirm the diagnosis of osteonecrosis is a function of spatial resolution, again underscoring the importance of proper imaging techniques with the use of a surface coil.

The typical MRI appearance is a focal, segmental signal abnormality in the subchondral bone of the femoral head. It may have a geographic configuration and may involve any part of the femoral head, although the anterolateral region is characteristically the earliest to be affected (40). The signal intensity within the center of the osteonecrotic lesion varies depending on the stage of the disease. A hypointense signal on both T1- and T2-weighted pulse sequences (equivalent to fibrous tissue) correlates with more advanced stages of osteonecrosis, as opposed to high marrow signal intensity equivalent to fat (hyperintense on T1, intermediate on T2) or blood (hyperintense on T1, hyperintense on T2) (38,54).

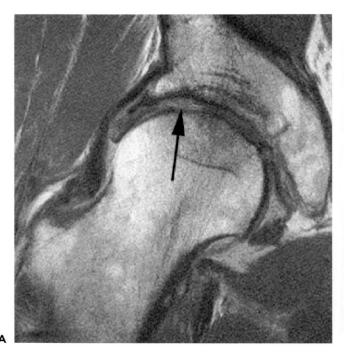

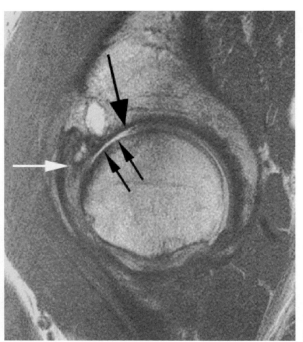

A   B

Figure 29-6 A: A 46-year-old man with preserved joint space on conventional radiographs. Coronal fast spin echo MR image discloses fibrillation and hyperintensity in the cartilage over the immediate weight bearing aspect of the femoral head (*arrow*), as well as abnormal signal in the corresponding lateral aspect of the dome. **B:** Sagittal MR image in the same patient discloses full-thickness cartilage loss over the anterosuperior margin of the femoral head (*small black arrows*), as well as over the anterior aspect of the dome (*large black arrow*). Also note the torn degenerated labrum (*white arrow*), generating soft tissue and intraosseous ganglion cysts.

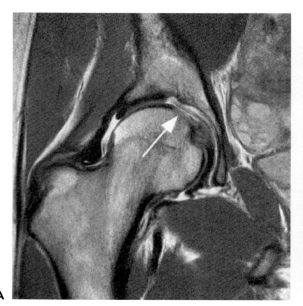

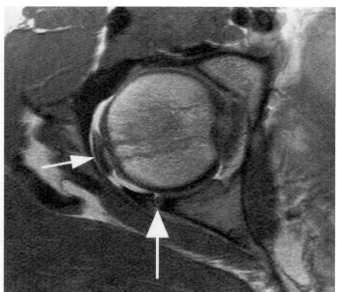

A   B

Figure 29-7 A: Coronal fast spin echo MR image in a 17-year-old lifeguard following a posterior subluxation episode demonstrates a chondral shearing injury (*arrow*) in the immediate suprafoveal aspect of the femoral head. **B:** Axial fast spin echo MR image in the same patient demonstrates a posterior labral tear (*large arrow*) sustained during the posterior subluxation, as well as a free fragment (*small arrow*) of cartilage with a small amount of attached subchondral bone in the lateral joint recess.

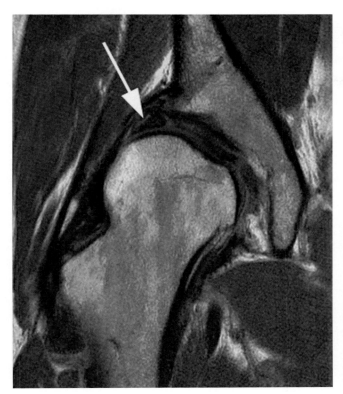

Figure 29-8 A 31-year-old woman with acetabular dysplasia. Coronal fast spin echo MR image demonstrates the presence of acetabular dysplasia with a hyperplastic superior labrum (*arrow*). Note the characteristic subchondral depression and deformity of the shallow fovea with hyperintensity in the adjacent cartilage, but no defect.

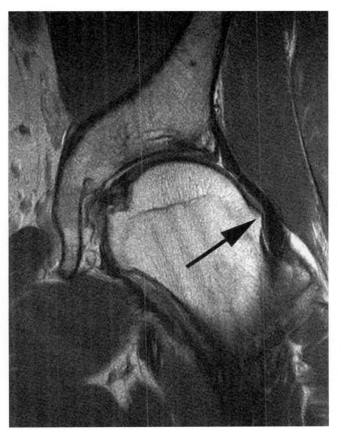

Figure 29-9 Coronal fast spin echo MR image in a patient with impingement syndrome demonstrates characteristic osseous protrusion at the lateral margin of the femoral neck (*arrow*). Moderate cartilage loss was noted on additional images, as well as the presence of an anterior labral tear. The patient successfully underwent arthroscopic ostectomy and debridement.

Generally speaking, a greater volume of low signal intensity subchondral marrow fibrosis on all pulse sequences corresponds to a more unfavorable prognosis, and a greater risk for collapse (Fig. 29-14).

The classic "double line sign," or zone of demarcation at the necrotic–viable bone interface, is present in up to 80% of osteonecrotic femoral heads and is manifest on T2-weighted images as an outer rim of low signal intensity adjacent to an inner band of high signal intensity (38). Histologic analysis of resected femoral heads demonstrates that the peripheral low signal rim consists of fibrous tissue, thickened trabeculae, and cellular debris, whereas the inner, high signal zone consists of necrotic bone and granulation tissue (54). Biopsy of the bone marrow edema pattern has disclosed serous exudate, focal interstitial hemorrhage, and mild fibrosis, rather than extension of the necrotic lesion (31).

Prior studies have attributed diffuse areas of high signal intensity on T2-weighted images (bone marrow edema pattern) as indicative of early changes of osteonecrosis (74,77). This pattern has been more recently demonstrated not to be an early imaging sign of osteonecrosis, but rather progression of disease. Bone marrow edema pattern was rarely detected in stage II, and not at all in stage 0 and stage I disease (27). Other investigators have associated increased edema pattern with impending collapse of the femoral head or development of increased pain (22,23,28,32).

The high sensitivity of MRI in early stages of the disease makes it suitable for detection of asymptomatic cases of osteonecrosis (23,71). In patients who have risk factors predisposing to osteonecrosis, MRI can be used to detect asymptomatic disease (1,6,15,70). MRI is also used to evaluate for osteonecrosis present in the contralateral femoral head of established ipsilateral osteonecrosis, as well as for staging and follow-up of bilateral disease (30,68).

The staging of osteonecrosis is useful in assessing progression of disease and prognostication. Two classifications in use, proposed by the Association Research Circulation Osseous and Steinberg, respectively, both categorize stage 0 as "normal" on all imaging modalities, including MRI, and diagnosed only on histology (63,65). Stage I in both classifications is a preradiographic stage, where abnormal findings are demonstrable on MRI but not on plain radiographs (63,65). More advanced stages include the presence of subchondral flattening, fracture, and joint space narrowing, progressing to advanced degenerative changes. Subchondral fractures may be subtle and are often seen to better advantage in one plane, thus requiring multiplanar assessment, particularly to aid in determining the timing of interventional procedures that are less commonly performed in the presence of fracture (Fig. 29-15).

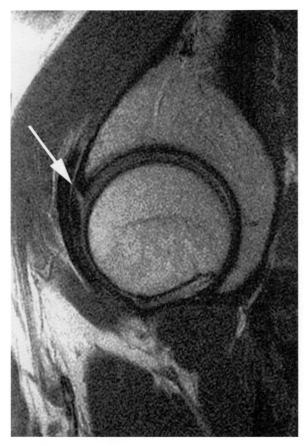

Figure 29-10 Sagittal fast spin echo MR image in a 30-year-old woman discloses a slightly displaced anterior labral tear (*arrow*).

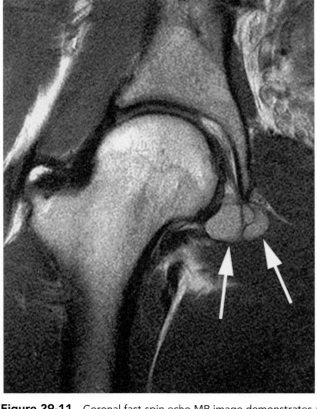

Figure 29-11 Coronal fast spin echo MR image demonstrates a septated ganglion cyst (*arrows*) arising in a 26-year-old patient with an anteroinferior labral tear.

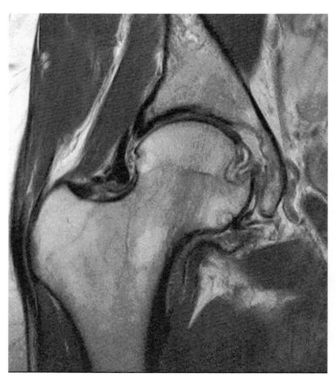

Figure 29-12 Coronal fast spin echo MR image discloses particulate debris in the joint recesses of lower signal intensity, indicative of pigmented villonodular synovitis.

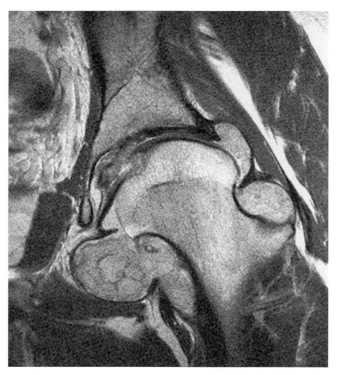

Figure 29-13 A 21-year-old woman with synovial osteochondromatosis. Coronal fast spin echo MR image demonstrates marked distention of the capsule with intermediate signal intensity debris. Note the remodeling of the femoral neck due to the chronic pressure erosion.

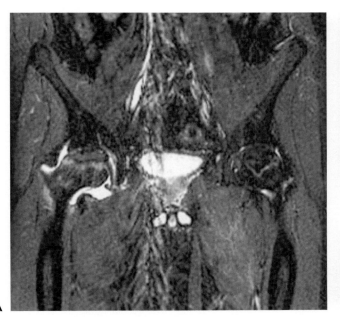
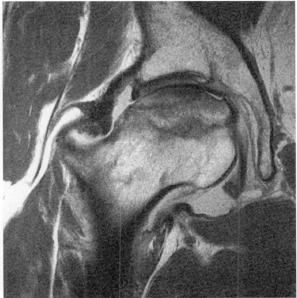

Figure 29-14 **A:** Bilateral osteonecrosis in a 33-year-old man. Coronal large field of view T2-weighted fat-suppressed sequences demonstrates the presence of bilateral osteonecrosis with a large joint effusion on the right side. **B:** Coronal fast spin echo surface coil MR image discloses the presence of marked subchondral sclerosis, manifest as diminished signal intensity on both pulse sequences, with subchondral fracture and collapse.

The prognostic value of MRI is related to its ability to assess extent of involvement of the weight-bearing margin of the femoral head (55). Beltran et al. illustrated the prognostic value of MRI in evaluating early osteonecrosis (stages I and II in the classification by Ficat) prior to core decompression (4).

After core decompression, the majority (86%) of osteonecrotic lesions involving over half of the weight-bearing surface progressed to subchondral collapse, while those involving less than 25% did not, indicating that progression of the osteonecrotic lesion following core decompression was more

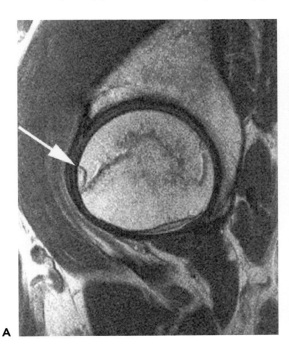
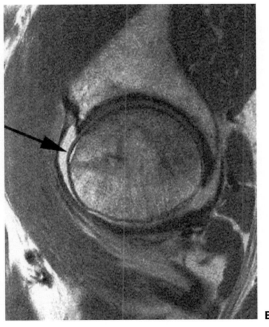

Figure 29-15 **A:** Longitudinal evaluation of a 62-year-old patient with femoral head osteonecrosis. Initial sagittal fast spin echo MR image discloses subtle subchondral fracture and offset of the subchondral plate (*arrow*) at the anterior margin of the necrotic viable bone interface, which precluded core decompression. **B:** Follow-up sagittal MR image obtained 13 months later discloses subchondral fracture at the same site (*arrow*), delaminating subchondral bone and attached cartilage.

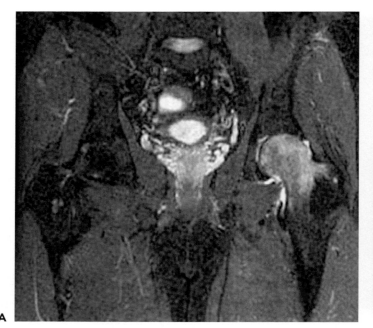

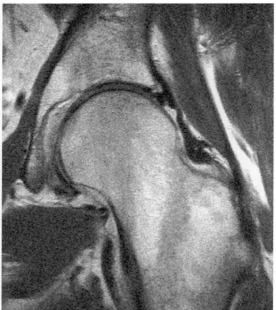

A

B

Figure 29-16 **A:** A 40-year-old man with left hip pain. Coronal large field-of-view, fat-suppressed body coil MR image demonstrates diffuse marrow edema pattern in the proximal left femur. **B:** Subsequent fast spin echo surface coil MR image in the same patient fails to disclose a zone of demarcation that would be indicative of osteonecrosis. The patient was successfully treated for transient osteoporosis.

accurately predicted on the basis of preoperative MRI than conventional radiographs alone (4). Furthermore, conventional radiographs have been shown to overestimate the size of the necrotic segment (62).

For MRI measurement purposes, most techniques are based on the geometry of a sphere or an arc; however, these methods may not be accurate when there is patchy or irregular involvement of the head (10,29,36,62). Manual computer segmentation is superior to extrapolation methods but is time-consuming (20).

Subchondral insufficiency fractures may appear similar to osteonecrosis, as they are a crescentic low signal intensity lines surrounded by high signal on T2-weighted images, but are characteristically more parallel and closely apposed to the articular surface (64,80).

Transient osteoporosis of the hip has been identified as a distinct clinical and radiographic entity. It was initially described in pregnant women (11) but has been shown to be more common in middle-aged men (48). The initial presentation is usually that of acute pain followed by spontaneous resolution with no bony sequela. Radiographic findings include variable osteopenia with preservation of the joint space; radionuclide bone scan depicts diffusely increased, nonspecific radiotracer activity.

MRI demonstrates diffuse bone marrow edema in the proximal femur on fat-suppressed images. On surface coil images, there is no zone of demarcation or collapse (Fig. 29-16). Histological analysis reveals fibrosis, fat necrosis, edema, marrow hyperemia, and reactive bone formation (79). It is important to be able to differentiate transient osteoporosis of the hip from osteonecrosis, as the former is self-limiting with

complete resolution of both clinical symptoms and imaging findings, although the edema pattern on MRI may lag behind clinical recovery.

MR Angiography

MR angiography is a technique that allows for angiographic depiction of vessels with MR parameters. It may be completely noninvasive, utilizing no contrast agent, where contrast is based on the magnetic properties of flow, or more commonly, use gadolinium contrast agents with an intravenous injection. In the setting of instrumentation, gadolinium injection is necessary to provide adequate signal to noise and depiction of the blood vessels. Applications include detection of occult thrombi following fracture (41) or to provide a "roadmap" for free-tissue transfer, such as a vascularized free fibular graft placement for treatment of osteonecrosis. Most recently, MR angiographic techniques have provided insight into the incidence of pelvic thrombosis following total hip arthroplasty and provide superior depiction of pelvic vascular disease compared with conventional Doppler ultrasound or traditional contrast venography obtained by dorsal foot vein cannulation (52) (Fig. 29-17).

MRI of Hip Arthroplasty

Traditionally, MRI was been limited in its ability to assess soft tissues surrounding instrumentation. Potential risks include induction of electrical currents, heating, and displacement of orthopaedic hardware. In addition to potential safety considerations, there is artifact generated by a frequency shift

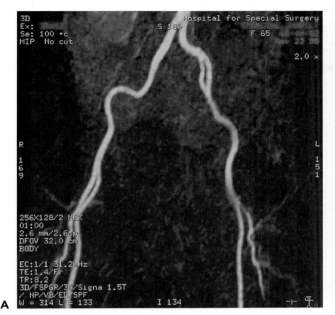

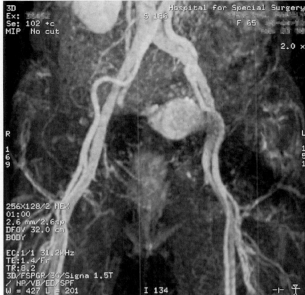

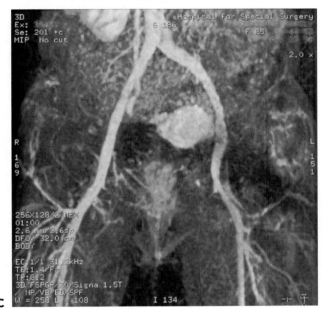

Figure 29-17 A: Contrast enhanced MR angiography in a 65-year-old woman after hip arthroplasty. Initial arteriographic sequence discloses intact arterial flow. **B:** Combined arterial and venographic sequence in the same patient. The focus of enhancement centrally reflects the normally enhancing uterus. **C:** MR venogram obtained following subtraction of the angiographic sequence **(A)** from the combined arteriographic and venographic image **(B)**. (Reprinted from Ryan MG, Westrich GH, Potter HG, et al. Effect of mechanical compression on the incidence of proximal deep venous thrombosis as assessed by magnetic resonance venography. *J Bone Joint Surg.* 2002;84A:1998–2004, with permission.)

induced by the high magnetic susceptibility of the easily magnetized ferromagnetic metallic components and the poorly magnetized diamagnetic soft tissues. The presence of the metal causes a low signal void with rapid signal loss due to prominent T2* decay, surrounding by a mismapping of protons in the frequency direction, accounting for the "flare" of high signal seen adjacent to metal. Fortunately, most orthopaedic instrumentation is nonmagnetic stainless steel and is considered safe for MRI. With some modification, adequate visualization of soft tissues surrounding arthroplasty and instrumentation is possible and is an area of rapidly growing research (49,59,61).

The intensity of the artifact is related to the degree of relative ferromagnetism, with titanium being less ferromagnetic (paramagnetic), thus generating less artifact on MR images, as well as the geometry of the components. The proximal, spherical component of a hip arthroplasty creates greater artifact than that induced by the vertical, linear stem of the femoral component, which is parallel to the long axis of the field.

Such techniques allow for visualization of soft tissues surrounding arthroplasty and have proven clinically useful in the assessment of tendon injury, including iliopsoas and abductor avulsion, localizing heterotopic ossification relative to neurovascular structures, and assessing clinically evident nerve injury (50). In the setting of fulminant infection, MRI may also be helpful in detecting intrapelvic or parapelvic soft tissue abscesses that may serve as a harbinger for recalcitrant infection. Detection of a radiographically occult sacral insufficiency fracture has also proven helpful in unexplained pain following uneventful arthroplasty (Fig. 29-18).

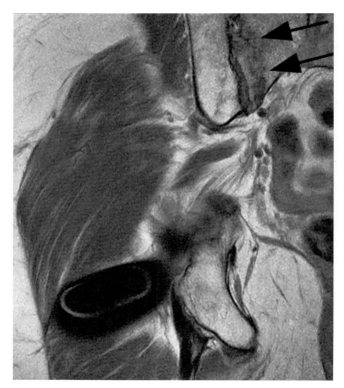

Figure 29-18   A 67-year-old woman after right hip arthroplasty with unexplained pain. Coronal fast spin echo MR image posterior to the arthroplasty discloses a radiographically occult right hemisacral insufficiency fracture (black *arrows*).

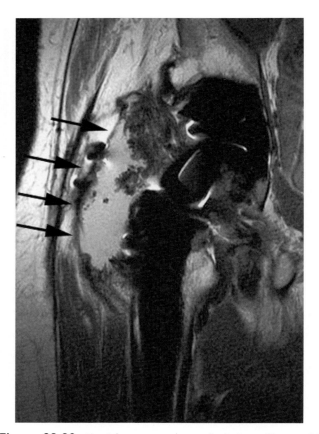

Figure 29-20   Particle wear and metallosis in a 67-year-old woman. Coronal fast spin echo MR image demonstrates the presence of a joint arthroplasty with a large greater trochanteric fluid collection (*arrows*) containing diminished signal intensity debris, indicative of metallic debris from the titanium components of the arthroplasty. The patient successfully underwent revision arthroplasty.

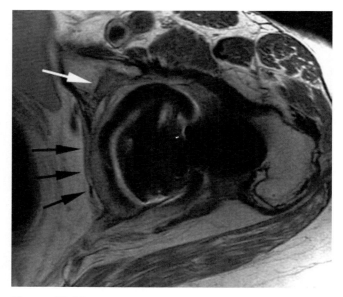

Figure 29-19   Axial fast spin echo MR image in a 71-year-old patient after left total hip arthroplasty demonstrates radiographically occult acetabular osteolysis (*white arrow*). Note the osteolysis affecting the medial wall, creating a mild protrusio deformity (*black arrows*).

Most recently, MRI gained interest in its ability to tomographically and more accurately assess the extent of acetabular osteolysis compared with plain radiographs (49). Osteolysis is typically depicted as areas of intermediate signal intensity within the trabecular bone, and MRI can discern not only the degree of osseous involvement, but also the degree of soft tissue extension, the latter of which is limited on the lower contrast CT techniques (Fig. 29-19). More severe cases of metallosis will impart a striking diminished signal to the dependent portions of the pseudocapsule (Fig. 29-20). Some authors have recommended the use of oblique (45°) radiographic views to impart greater sensitivity to detecting lesion of the posterior wall or column; however, other authors have noted poor interobserver reproducibility in the assessment of osteolysis using plain radiographs (13,60). While modified CT techniques have been shown to be more sensitive in the detection of osteolysis compared to plain radiographs, these techniques generally use higher dosage in order to reduce the beam hardening artifact generated by the arthroplasty (78). The dosage of ionizing radiation becomes an issue in patients requiring serial examinations to quantify the degree of osteolysis, at times to monitor response to pharmaceutical agents aimed at limiting osteoclastic bone resorption. Ultimately, MRI will most likely be most efficacious in detecting early intracapsular synovial disease that precedes the osteoclastic resorption of bone. With further refinement of pulse sequences and surface coils, improved depiction of the soft tissues will be possible and further study would be necessary to further define the clinical application of MRI of arthroplasty.

MRI has proven to be a powerful imaging tool in the assessment of the adult hip. Current techniques mandate high in-plane resolution obtained with a surface coil, standardized cartilage assessment, and multiplanar acquisition. With minor modifications in commercially available software parameters, visualization of the soft tissue envelope surrounding the instrumented hip or arthroplasty is now possible.

REFERENCES

1. Aranow C, Zelicof S, Leslie D, et al. Clinically occult avascular necrosis of the hip in systemic lupus erythematosus. *J Rheumatol.* 1997;24:2318–2322.
2. Babyn PS, Kim HK, Gahunia HK, et al. MRI of the cartilaginous epiphysis of the femoral head in the piglet hip after ischemic damage. *J Magn Reson Imaging.* 1998;8:717–723.
3. Beck M, Sledge JB, Gautier E, et al. The anatomy and function of the gluteus minimus muscle. *J Bone Joint Surg Br.* 2000;82B:358–363.
4. Beltran J, Knight CT, Zuelzer WA, et al. Core decompression for avascular necrosis of the femoral head: correlation between long-term results and preoperative MR imaging. *Radiology.* 1990;175:533–536.
5. Bluemke DA, Zerhouni EA. MRI of avascular necrosis of bone. *Top Magn Reson Imaging.* 1996;8:231–246.
6. Bradbury G, Benjamin J, Thompson J, et al. Avascular necrosis of bone after cardiac transplantation. Prevalence and relationship to administration and dosage of steroids. *J Bone Joint Surg Am.* 1994;76:1385–1358.
7. Brody AS, Strong M, Babikian G, et al. Avascular necrosis: early MR imaging and histologic findings in a canine model. *AJR Am J Roentgenol.* 1991;157:341–345.
8. Brown WE, Potter HG, Marx RG, et al. Magnetic resonance imaging appearance of cartilage repair in the knee. *Clin Orthop Relat Res.* 2004;422:214–223.
9. Bunker TD, Esler CNA, Leach WJ. Rotator cuff tear of the hip. *J Bone Joint Surg Br.* 1997;79B:618–620.
10. Cherian SF, Laorr A, Saleh KJ, et al. Quantifying the extent of femoral head involvement in osteonecrosis. *J Bone Joint Surg Am.* 2003;85A:309–315.
11. Curtiss PH, Kincaid WE. Transitory demineralization of the hip in pregnancy. *J Bone Joint Surg Am.* 1959;41:1327–1333.
12. Czerny C, Hofmann S, Neuhold A, et al. Lesions of the acetabular labrum: accuracy of MR imaging and MR arthrography in detection and staging. *Radiology.* 1996;200(1):225–230.
13. Engh CA Jr, Sychterz CJ, Young AM, et al. Interobserver and intraobserver variability in radiographic assessment of osteolysis. *J Arthroplasty.* 2002;17:752–759.
14. Fairbank AC, Bhatia D, Jinnah RH, et al. Long-term results of core decompression for ischemic necrosis of the femoral head. *J Bone Joint Surg Br.* 1995;77:42–49.
15. Fink B, Degenhardt S, Paselk C, et al. Early detection of avascular necrosis of the femoral head following renal transplantation. *Arch Orthop Trauma Surg.* 1997;116(3):151–156.
16. Fordyce MJ, Solomon L. Early detection of avascular necrosis of the femoral head by MRI. *J Bone Joint Surg Br.* 1993;75:365–367.
17. Fredericson M, Bergman AG, Hoffman KL, et al. Tibial stress reaction in runners. Correlation of clinical symptoms and scintigraphy with a new magnetic resonance imaging grading system. *Am J Sports Med.* 1995;23(4):472–481.
18. Ganz R, Gill TJ, Gautier E, et al. Surgical dislocation of the adult hip. A technique with full access to the femoral head and acetabulum without the risk of avascular necrosis. *J Bone Joint Surg.* 2001;83B:1119–1124.
19. Glickstein MF, Burk DL Jr, Schiebler ML, et al. Avascular necrosis versus other diseases of the hip: sensitivity of MR imaging. *Radiology.* 1988;169:213–215.

20. Hernigou P, Lambotte JC. Volumetric analysis of osteonecrosis of the femur: anatomical correlation using MRI. *J Bone Joint Surg Br.* 2001;83B:672–675.
21. Hodler J, Yu JS, Goodwin D, et al. MR arthrography of the hip: improved imaging of the acetabular labrum with histologic correlation in cadavers. *AJR Am J Roentgenol.* 1995;165:887–891.
22. Huang GS, Chan WP, Chang YC, et al. MR imaging of bone marrow edema and joint effusion in patients with osteonecrosis of the femoral head: relationship to pain. *AJR Am J Roentgenol.* 2003;181:545–549.
23. Iida S, Yoshitada H, Shimizu K, et al. Correlation between bone marrow edema and collapse of the femoral head in steroid-induced osteonecrosis. *AJR Am J Roentgenol.* 2000;174:735–743.
24. Ito H, Matsuno T, Kaneda K. Prognosis of early stage avascular necrosis of the femoral head. *Clin Orthop.* 1999;358:149–157.
25. Jaramillo D, Connolly SA, Vajapeyam S, et al. Normal and ischemic epiphysis of the femur: diffusion MR imaging—study in piglets. *Radiology.* 2003;227:825–832.
26. Kagen II A. Rotator cuff tears of the hip. *Clin Orthop.* 1999;368:135–140.
27. Kim YM, Oh HC, Kim HJ. The pattern of bone marrow edema on MRI in osteonecrosis of the femoral head. *J Bone Joint Surg Br.* 2000;82B:837–841.
28. Koo KH, Ahn IO, Kim R, et al. Bone marrow edema and associated pain in early stage osteonecrosis of the femoral head. Prospective study with serial MR images. *Radiology.* 1999;213:715–722.
29. Koo KH, Kim R. Quantifying the extent of osteonecrosis of the femoral head: a new method using MRI. *J Bone Joint Surg Br.* 1995;77:875–880
30. Kopecky KK, Braunstein EM, Brandt KD, et al. Apparent avascular necrosis of the hip: appearance and spontaneous resolution of MR findings in renal allograft recipients. *Radiology.* 1991;179:523–527.
31. Kubo T, Yamamoto T, Inoue S, et al. Histological findings of bone marrow edema pattern on MRI in osteonecrosis of the femoral head. *J Orthop Sci.* 2000;5:520–523.
32. Kubo T, Yamazoe S, Sugano N, et al. Initial MRI findings of non-traumatic osteonecrosis of the femoral head in renal allograft recipients. *Magn Reson Imaging.* 1997;15:1017–1023.
33. Kumagai M, Shiba N, Higuchi F, et al. Functional evaluation of hip abductor muscles with use of magnetic resonance imaging. *J Orthop Res.* 1997;15:888–893.
34. Leunig M, Werlen S, Ungersbock A, et al. Evaluation of the acetabular labrum by MR arthrography. *J Bone Joint Surg Br.* 1997;79:230–234.
35. Lecouvet FE, Vande Berg BC, Malghem J, et al. MR imaging of the acetabular labrum: variations in 200 asymptomatic hips. *AJR Am J Roentgenol.* 1996;167:1025–1028.
36. Malizos KN, Siafakas MS, Fotiadis DI, et al. An MRI-based semi-automated volumetric quantification of hip osteonecrosis. *Skeletal Radiol.* 2001;30:686–693.
37. Mintz DN, Hooper T, Connell D, et al. Magnetic resonance imaging of the hip: detection of labral and chondral abnormalities using noncontrast imaging. *Arthroscopy.* 2005;21:385–393.
38. Mitchell DG, Kubkel HL, Steinberg ME, et al. Avascular necrosis of the hip: comparison of MR, CT and scintigraphy. *AJR Am J Roentgenol.* 1986;146:1215–1218.
39. Mitchell DG, Rao VM, Dalinka MK, et al. Femoral head avascular necrosis: correlation of MR imaging, radiographic staging, radionuclide imaging, and clinical findings. *Radiology.* 1987;162:709–715.
40. Mont MA, Hungerford DS. Non-traumatic avascular necrosis of the femoral head. *J Bone Joint Surg Am.* 1995;77:459–474.
41. Montgomery KD, Potter HG, Helfet DL. The use of magnetic resonance imaging to evaluate the deep venous system of the pelvis in patients with acetabular fractures. *J Bone Joint Surg.* 1995;77A:1639–1649.
42. Moorman III CT, Warren RF, Hershman EB, et al. Traumatic posterior hip subluxation in American football. *J Bone Joint Surg.* 2003;85A:1190–1196.
43. Outerbridge, RE. The etiology of chondromalacia patellae. *J Bone Joint Surg.* 1961;43B:752–757.
44. Petersilge CA, Haque MA, Petersilge WJ, et al. Acetabular labral tears: evaluation with MR arthrography. *Radiology.* 1996;200:231–235.

45. Poggi JJ, Callaghan JJ, Spritzer CE, et al. Changes on magnetic resonance images after traumatic hip dislocation. *Clin Orthop.* 1995; 319:249–259.

46. Potter HG, Linklater JA, Allen AA, et al. MR imaging of articular cartilage in the knee: a prospective evaluation utilizing fast spin echo imaging. *J Bone Joint Surg.* 1998;80A:1276–1284.

47. Potter HG, Montgomery KD, Heise CW, et al. Magnetic resonance imaging of acetabular fractures: value in detecting femoral head injury, intraarticular fragments and sciatic nerve injury. *AJR Am J Roentgenol.* 1994;163:881–886.

48. Potter H, Moran M, Schneider R, et al. Magnetic resonance imaging in diagnosis of transient osteoporosis of the hip. *Clin Orthop.* 1992;280:323–329.

49. Potter HG, Nestor BJ, Sofka CS, Ho ST, et al. Magnetic resonance imaging of total hip arthroplasty: Evaluation of periprosthetic soft tissue. *J Bone Joint Surg AM.* 2004:86:1947–1954

50. Potter HG, Sofka CM, Peters LE, et al. Evaluation of total hip arthroplasty with magnetic resonance imaging. Presented at: American Academy of Orthopaedic Surgeons 69th Annual Meeting; 13–17 February 2002; Dallas, TX.

51. Rizzo PF, Gould ES, Lyden JP, et al. Diagnosis of occult fractures about the hip. MRI compared with bone scanning. *J Bone Joint Surg.* 1993;75A:395–401.

52. Ryan MG, Westrich GH, Potter HG, et al. Effect of mechanical compression on the incidence of proximal deep venous thrombosis as assessed by magnetic resonance venography. *J Bone Joint Surg.* 2002;84A:1998–2004.

53. Sakai T, Sugano N, Tsuji T, et al. Contrast-enhanced magnetic resonance imaging in a nontraumatic rabbit osteonecrosis model. *J Orthop Res.* 1999;17:784–792.

54. Sakamoto M, Shimizu K, Iida S et al. Osteonecrosis of the femoral head: a prospective study with MRI. *J Bone Joint Surg Br.* 1997;79B:213–219.

55. Shimizu K, Moriya A, Akita T, et al. Prediction of collapse with magnetic resonance imaging of avascular necrosis of the femoral head. *J Bone Joint Surg Am.* 1994;76A:215–223.

56. Shin AY, Morin WD, Gorman JD, et al. The superiority of magnetic resonance imaging in differentiating the cause of hip pain in endurance athletes. *Am J Sports Med.* 1996;24:168–176.

57. Siebenrock KA, Schoeniger R, Ganz R. Anterior femoro-acetabular impingement due to acetabular retroversion. *J Bone Joint Surg.* 2003;85A:278–286.

58. Slocum KA, Gorman JD, Puckett ML, et al. Resolution of abnormal MR signal intensity in patients with stress fractures in the femoral neck. *AJR Am J Roentgenol.* 1997;168:1295–1299.

59. Sofka CM, Potter HG. MR imaging of joint arthroplasty. *Semin Musculoskelet Radiol* 2002;6:79–85.

60. Southwell DG, Bechtold JE, Lew WD, et al. Improving the detection of acetabular osteolysis using oblique radiographs. *J Bone Joint Surg Br.* 1999;81:289–295.

61. Sperling JW, Potter HG, Craig EV, et al. MRI of the painful shoulder arthroplasty. *J Shoulder Elbow Surg.* 2002;11:315–321.

62. Steinberg ME, Bands RE, Pary S, et al. Does lesion size affect the outcome in avascular necrosis? *Clin Orthop.* 1999;367:262–271.

63. Steinberg ME, Hayken GD, Steinberg DR. A quantitative system for staging avascular necrosis. *J Bone Joint Surg Am.* 1995;77B:34–41.

64. Stevens K, Tao C, Lee SU, et al. Subchondral fractures in osteonecrosis of the femoral head: comparison of radiography, CT and MR imaging. *AJR Am J Roentgenol.* 2003;180:363–368.

65. Stulberg BN. Papers from the Fifth International Symposium on bone circulation [editorial]. *Clin Orthop.* 1997;334:2–5.

66. Stulberg BN, Levine M, Bauer TW, et al. Multimodality approach to osteonecrosis of the femoral head. *Clin Orthop.* 1989;240:181–193.

67. Sugano N, Kubo T, Takaoka K, et al. Diagnostic criteria for nontraumatic osteonecrosis of the femoral head: a multicenter study. *J Bone Joint Surg Br.* 1999;81B:590–595.

68. Sugano N, Nishii T, Shibuya T, et al. Contralateral hip in patients with unilateral nontraumatic osteonecrosis of the femoral head. *Clin Orthop.* 1997;334:85–90.

69. Takatori Y, Kokubo T, Ninomiya S, et al. Avascular necrosis of the femoral head. Natural history and magnetic resonance imaging. *J Bone Joint Surg Br.* 1993;75:217–221.

70. Tektonidou MG, Malagari K, Vlachoyiannopoulos PG, et al. Asymptomatic avascular necrosis in patients with primary antiphospholipid syndrome in the absence of corticosteroid use: a prospective study by magnetic resonance imaging. *Arthritis Rheum.* 2003;48:732–736.

71. Tervonen O, Mueller DM, Matteson EL, et al. Clinically occult avascular necrosis of the hip: prevalence in an asymptomatic population at risk. *Radiology.* 1992;182:845–847.

72. Theodorou DJ, Malizos KN, Beris AE, et al. Multimodal imaging quantitation of the lesion size in osteonecrosis of the femoral head. *Clin Orthop.* 2001;386:54–63.

73. Thickman D, Axel L, Kressel HY, et al. Magnetic resonance imaging of avascular necrosis of the femoral head. *Skeletal Radiol.* 1986;15:133–140.

74. Turner DA, Templeton AC, Selzer PM, et al. Femoral capital osteonecrosis: MR finding of diffuse marrow abnormalities without focal lesions. *Radiology.* 1989;171:135–140.

75. Urbaniak JR, Coogan PG, Gunnison EB, et al. Treatment of osteonecrosis of the femoral head with free vascularized fibular grafting. *J Bone Joint Surg.* 1995;77A:681–694.

76. Vande Berg B, Malghem J, Labaisse MA, et al. Avascular necrosis of the hip: comparison of contrast-enhanced and nonenhanced MR imaging with histologic correlation. *Radiology.* 1992;182:445–450.

77. Vande Berg BE, Malghem JJ, Labaisse MA, et al. MR imaging of avascular necrosis and transient marrow edema of the femoral head. *Radiographics.* 1993;13:501–520.

78. White LM, Buckwalter KA. Technical considerations: CT and MR imaging in the postoperative orthopaedic patient. *Semin Musculoskelet Radiol.* 2002;6:5–17.

79. Yamamoto T, Kubo T, Hirasawa Y, et al. A clinicopathologic stuffy of transient osteoporosis of the hip. *Skeletal Radiol.* 1999;28:621–627.

80. Yamamoto T, Schneider R, Bullough PG. Subchondral insufficiency fracture of the femoral head: histolopathologic correlation with MRI. *Skeletal Radiol.* 2001;30:247–254.

81. Yao L, Johnson C, Gentill A, et al. Stress injuries of bone: analysis of MR imaging stating criteria. *Acta Radiol.* 1995;5:34–40.

The Sequelae of Pediatric Hip Disease

30

Stuart L. Weinstein

The majority of childhood hip conditions usually do well for many years regardless of treatment. Yet, many childhood hip disorders lead to degenerative arthritis in adulthood, with resultant clinical disability despite standard up-to-date treatment interventions. This chapter describes the processes of common childhood hip diseases, presents their natural history when known, and reports the results of long-term follow-up of the common treatment modalities in order to identify the processes that may lead to the need for future intervention (285).

DEVELOPMENTAL HIP DYSPLASIA AND DISLOCATION

In the pediatric orthopedic literature, the longstanding terminology of *congenital dysplasia* (or *dislocation*) *of the hip* (CDH) has been replaced by the term *developmental dysplasia* (or *dislocation*) *of the hip* (DDH) (267). The terminology includes congenital and developmental cases, subluxation, dislocation, and dysplasia (156).

The spectrum of DDH variations includes subluxation and dislocation (128,210,211,219). Distinguishing between these two entities is often difficult; hence the term *dysplasia* will be used to encompass these entities and other variations, and the term *dislocation* will be used to refer only to completely unreducible dislocations. For the newborn, the term *dysplasia* refers to any hip with a positive Ortolani sign, which indicates a hip that may be provoked to subluxation, provoked to dislocation, or reduced from either of these positions.

The overwhelming majority of DDH cases are detectable at birth (92,97). However, despite newborn screening programs, some cases are missed, and there is some evidence that a few cases may arise after birth (63,122,123,137,176,202,278,294, 295,304). Another unresolved problem is whether acetabular dysplasia is primary or is secondary to an unrecognized dislocation or subluxation that has spontaneously reduced to "mild" hip instability.

The results of newborn screening programs indicate that 1 in 100 newborn examinations shows evidence of some instability (positive Ortolani or Barlow sign), although the true incidence of dislocation is reported to be between 1 and 1.5 cases per 1000 live births (11,48,81,82,137,201,221,271,278,296). Table 30-1 contains a list of the factors that contribute to DDH.

Completely unreducible dislocations are extremely rare in newborns and are usually associated with other generalized conditions, such as myelodysplasia or arthrogryposis. These teratologic perinatal dislocations account for only 2% of the cases in the newborn (53,54,104,221,258) and are usually manifest by secondary adaptive changes characteristic of the late diagnosed DDH.

If the diagnosis is not made in the nursery, secondary adaptive changes develop and are manifested in the physical findings of limited abduction; asymmetrical gluteal, thigh, or labial folds; apparent femoral shortening; and limb-length inequality (5,17,22,53). In bilateral dislocations, clinical findings include a waddling gait and hyperlordosis of the lumbar spine. The longer the DDH goes undetected, the greater the impairment of femoral head and acetabular development. With increasing age at detection and at reduction, particularly in children over 6 months of age, both intra- and extra-articular obstacles to reduction are increasingly difficult to overcome,

TABLE 30-1

HIGH-RISK FACTORS FOR DEVELOPMENTAL DYSPLASIA OR DISLOCATION OF THE HIP

Breech position
Female gender
Positive family history or ethnic background (e.g., Native American Laplander)
Lower limb uniformity
Torticollis
Metatarsus adductus
Oligohydramnios
Significant persistent hip asymmetry (e.g., abducted hip on one side, adducted hip on the other)
Other significant musculoskeletal abnormalities

and the long-term outcomes for these patients are less predictable (128,287,288,291,292,296).

Natural History

If the diagnosis is not made in the newborn nursery, the hip may follow one of four courses. It may become normal, it may spontaneously relocate but retain dysplastic features, it may go on to subluxation (partial contact between the femoral head and the acetabulum), or it may go on to complete dislocation (11,54,307). The outcome predictability of unstable hips in the nursery is poor, and therefore all newborns with clinical hip instability, as manifested by a positive Ortolani or Barlow sign, should be treated.

In adults, the natural history of untreated complete dislocations varies (60,187,279,282,283). In some cases of complete dislocation, there may be little or no functional disability. The natural history of complete dislocation is dependent on two factors: bilaterality and the presence or absence of a false acetabulum (108,270,282,283,288,292). Wedge and Wasylenko demonstrated only a 24% chance of a good clinical result with a well-developed false acetabulum but a 52%

chance of a good clinical result with a moderately developed or absent false acetabulum (282,283). Completely dislocated hips with well-developed false acetabula are more likely to develop radiographic degenerative joint disease and clinical disability (Fig. 30-1). Factors that lead to the formation or lack of formation of false acetabula remain unknown.

In patients with bilateral complete dislocations, back pain may occur in later adult life (46,60,187,189,282,283,292). This back pain is thought to be secondary to hyperlordosis of the lumbar spine associated with bilateral dislocations (Fig. 30-2).

In unilateral complete dislocations, patients may have limb-length inequality of up to 10 cm, along with flexion–adduction deformities of the hip; secondary valgus deformities of the knee, with attenuation of the medial collateral ligament; and lateral compartment degenerative joint disease (187,270,282,283,288,292). The same factors that are relevant to the development of secondary degenerative disease in the false acetabulum and associated clinical disability in bilateral cases apply to unilateral cases of dislocation.

The natural history of dysplasia and subluxation in untreated patients is extremely important, as the findings can be extrapolated for patients who have these residual problems after treatment (76,178,248,288). Past the neonatal period, the term *dysplasia* has both an anatomic and a radiographic definition. The anatomic definition refers to inadequate development of the femoral head, the acetabulum, or both (53). Thus, all subluxated hips (i.e., those that have some contact between the femoral head and the acetabulum) are by definition anatomically dysplastic. However, in the radiographic definition, the major determining factor is the Shenton line (18,55,282,283) (Fig. 30-3). Radiographic subluxation is heralded by a loss of continuity of the Shenton line: the head is displaced superiorly, laterally, or superolaterally from the medial wall of the acetabulum. In a radiographic dysplasia, the normal Shenton line relationship exists. Unfortunately, these two roentgenographic clinical entities are often not separated in the DDH literature. Many authors have shown that radiographically dysplastic hips are converted to subluxated hips by secondary degenerative changes (55,178,265).

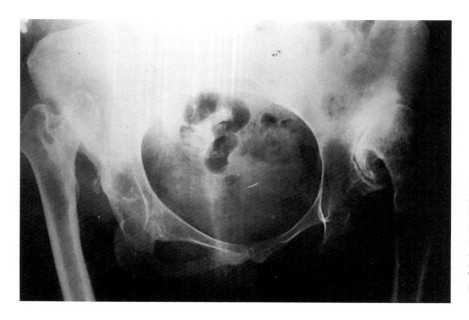

Figure 30-1 Roentgenogram of a 43-year-old woman with complete dislocation of both hips. She is asymptomatic on the right but has disabling symptoms from the left hip. She has no false acetabulum on the right, but she has a well-developed false acetabulum on the left, with secondary degenerative changes. (Reproduced from Weinstein SL. Natural history of congenital hip dislocation [CDH] and hip dysplasia. *Clin Orthop Rel Res.* 1987;225:52.)

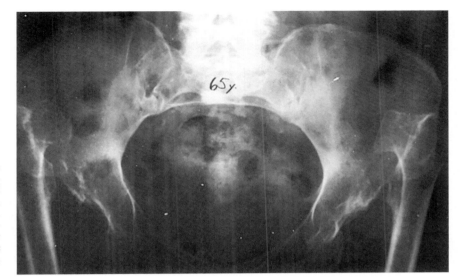

Figure 30-2 This 55-year-old Caucasian woman with bilateral, untreated developmental dislocations of the hips complained of some low back pain but had no hip pain. She had a waddling gait and hyperlordosis. (Reproduced from Weinstein SL. Developmental hip dysplasia and dislocation. In: Morrissy RT, Weinstein SL, eds. *Lovell and Winter's Pediatric Orthopaedics.* 6th ed. Philadelphia: Lippincott Williams & Wilkins; 2005.)

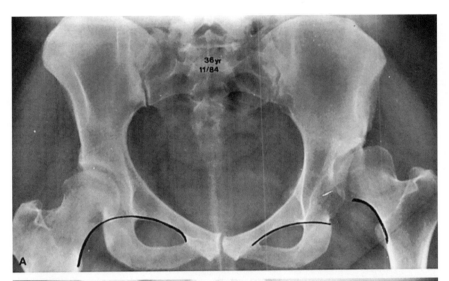

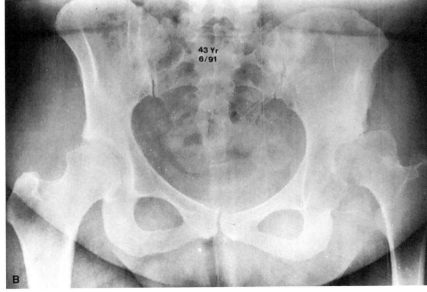

Figure 30-3 Radiographic subluxation and dysplasia. **A:** This 36-year-old woman had bilateral anatomically abnormal (dysplastic) hips. The left hip is radiographically subluxated, with the Shenton line disrupted, and the right hip is radiographically dysplastic, with the Shenton line intact. **B:** Seven years later, there is a marked loss of joint space in the secondary acetabulum of the left hip and very early disruption of the Shenton line on the right. The right hip is asymptomatic, and the left hip is about to undergo total hip arthroplasty. (Reproduced from Weinstein SL. Developmental hip dysplasia and dislocation. In: Morrissy RT, Weinstein SL, eds. *Lovell and Winter's Pediatric Orthopaedics.* 6th ed. Philadelphia: Lippincott Williams & Wilkins; 2005.)

Radiographic subluxation invariably leads to degenerative joint disease and clinical disability (55,178,282,283,288,292) (see Fig. 30-3). The rate of deterioration is directly related to subluxation severity and patient age (55,178).

Although there is considerable evidence that residual radiographic hip dysplasia, particularly in female patients, leads to secondary degenerative joint disease, there are no predictive radiographic parameters (55,100,178,265). Harris (100) reported that symptoms of degenerative joint disease associated with acetabular dysplasia occur early in life and that almost 50% of the patients with acetabular dysplasia in his series had their first reconstructive procedure before the age of 60 years. The reasons for degenerative changes and radiographically dysplastic hips are probably mechanical and related to increased contact stress with time. A certain overpressure (91,182) may correlate with long-term outcome. Aspherical heads (e.g., in secondary aseptic necrosis) tend to experience more symptoms and more severe degrees of overpressure. It appears that radiographic degenerative joint disease correlates with the magnitude of overpressure and the time of exposure.

As physical signs of radiographic hip dysplasia are usually lacking, cases are often diagnosed only incidentally on the basis of roentgenograms taken for other reasons or if the patient presents with symptoms. Stulberg and Harris (265) found that 50% of their patients with radiographic dysplasia and degenerative joint disease had radiographic evidence of dysplasia in the opposite hip. Melvin and associates (187), in their unpublished 30- to 50-year follow-up of DDH, demonstrated that 40% of the patients with DDH had roentgenographic evidence of dysplasia in the opposite hip. Wiberg (298) suggested that there is a direct correlation between the onset of radiographic degenerative joint disease and the amount of dysplasia as measured by the decrease in the center edge (CE) angle.

The primary factor in degenerative joint disease is subluxation, which predictably leads to degenerative joint disease and clinical disability over time (55). The literature on both untreated patients and long-term follow-ups of treated patients suggests that dysplastic patients will eventually develop degenerative joint disease (55,178). Stulberg and Harris (265) demonstrated that there is no roentgenographic picture of degenerative joint disease uniquely associated with pre-existing acetabular dysplasia. In 80% of the patients with dysplasia, the CE angle is usually less than 20°. Investigators also demonstrated that the CE angle, the criterion most commonly used to quantify dysplasia, could be affected by many parameters, including roentgenographic positioning and the changes accompanying the normal development of degenerative joint disease. Secondary degenerative changes in a dysplastic acetabulum may give the hip a normal-appearing CE angle. In their series of 130 patients with primary or idiopathic degenerative joint disease, Stulberg and Harris were able to demonstrate that 48% had evidence of primary acetabular dysplasia and that acetabular dysplasia frequently occurred in women with degenerative joint disease. Further evidence for the association between acetabular dysplasia and degenerative joint disease comes from the population of southern China. An epidemiologic study from Hong Kong demonstrates that where the incidence of childhood hip disease is low, the incidence of adult (nontraumatic) osteoarthritis is also low (116,117).

Wedge and Wasylenko (282,283) reported three peak incidences of pain in subluxation depending on the severity of the subluxation. Patients with the most severe subluxations usually had an onset of symptoms during the second decade of life, those with moderate subluxation experienced the onset during their third and fourth decades, and those with minimal subluxation experienced the onset usually around menopause.

Patients who present soon after symptom onset rarely have the classic signs of degenerative joint disease, such as decreased joint space, cyst formation, double acetabular floor, and inferomedial femoral head osteophytes. The only radiographic feature evident at symptom onset may be increased sclerosis in the weight-bearing area. This increased sclerosis is secondary to osteoblastic stimulation in response to the decreased width of the weight-bearing surface. The increase in the normal per-unit load strains the bone. The mechanism of pain in these instances is purely speculative. In the case of subluxation, the mean age of symptom onset is 36.6 years for women and 54 years for men. Some degenerative radiographic changes become evident approximately 10 years later, at 46.4 years of age for women and 69.6 years of age for men. Patients with subluxated hips usually have symptom onset at a younger age than those with complete dislocations. Progression is rapid after the onset of pain and the start of radiographically evident degenerative disease.

In general, long-term follow-ups of treated patients demonstrate findings that are similar to the natural history presented for subluxation and residual dysplasia (76,178, 248,288). The natural history data for untreated patients with radiographic subluxation seems to correspond to those hips that have developed subluxation after treatment (Figs. 30-3 and 30-4). The long-term problems of residual roentgenographic and anatomic dysplasia after treatment for CDH in the absence of subluxation are more difficult to predict, but good evidence exists for the development of degenerative disease over time (Fig. 30-5).

Avascular necrosis is an iatrogenic complication of the treatment of DDH (178), and the reported incidence after treatment ranges from 0% to 73% (18,61,141,178). Certain patterns of premature physeal arrest, particularly the lateral arrest pattern secondary to physeal plate injury during treatment, may not be evident radiographically for many years (mean, 9 years) after reduction (34,140). There is a strong tendency toward subluxation over time in hips that develop aseptic necrosis.

To summarize, in the treatment of developmental dislocation of the hip, reduction must be obtained and maintained as early as possible to provide the proper stimulus for the resumption of normal hip joint growth and development. Subluxation and total head avascular necrosis must be avoided, as degenerative joint disease is certain to result. Acetabular dysplasia leads to degenerative joint disease with time, although no radiographic parameters are predictive. Normal hip joint anatomy may fail to develop, depending on the age of the patient at reduction and the growth potential of the acetabular cartilage. However, as normal anatomy as can be achieved should be restored (naturally or surgically) by maturity. This should provide the best possible mechanical environment to avoid exceeding the pressure tolerance level of hip joint articular cartilage, thereby avoiding degenerative joint disease.

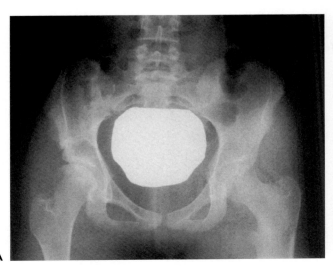
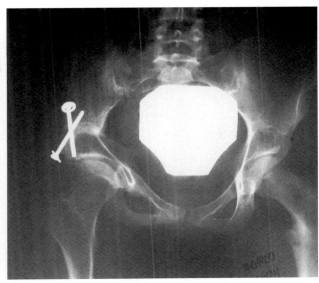

Figure 30-4 A 16-year-old patient with residual dysplasia after treatment for DDH and pain. **A:** Preop AP radiograph. **B:** AP radiograph 2 years postoperative a triple innominate osteotomy. (Reproduced from Weinstein SL. Developmental hip dysplasia and dislocation. In: Morrissy RT, Weinstein SL, eds. *Lovell and Winter's Pediatric Orthopaedics.* 6th ed. Philadelphia: Lippincott Williams & Wilkins; 2005.)

LEGG–CALVÉ–PERTHES DISEASE

Legg–Calvé–Perthes disease, a disorder of the hip in young children, was independently described around the turn of the century by Legg (164), Calvé (36), Perthes (215), and Waldenström (275,277). Despite voluminous literature on the subject, treatment of the condition remains controversial.

Typically, patients present with a history of insidious onset of limp or pain localized to the groin, medial thigh, or knee region. The pain is activity related and usually relieved by rest. On physical examination, patients usually have limited motion, in particular, loss of abduction and medial rotation. They may, in addition, have hip flexion and/or adduction contractors. Thigh, calf, and buttock atrophy may also be evident.

There is considerable epidemiologic, histologic, and radiographic evidence to support the theory that Legg–Calvé–Perthes disease is probably a localized manifestation of a generalized disorder of epiphyseal cartilage manifested in the proximal femur because of its unusual and precarious blood supply (39,43,45,88,98,103,159,223).

From the epidemiologic standpoint, Legg–Calvé–Perthes disease occurs most commonly in children aged 4 to 8 years, but cases have been reported in children as young as 2 years old and in adolescents in their late teens (306). It is more common in boys than girls by a ratio of 4 or 5 to 1 (10). The incidence of bilaterality has been reported as 10% to 12% (306). Several cases of recurrent Legg–Calvé–Perthes disease (180) and bilateral Legg–Calvé–Perthes disease in which one hip remains silent have been reported, so the incidence of bilaterality is probably greater than that recorded in the literature. Although the incidence of a positive family history ranges from 1.6% to 20% (80,88,94,95,212,269,281,305,306), there is no evidence it is an inherited condition.

Transient synovitis has been thought by many investigators to be a precursor of the condition (85). Yet most reports show that only 1% to 3% of patients with transient synovitis ever go on to develop Legg–Calvé–Perthes disease (105,142, 143,197,302,303).

Most current etiologic theories suggest the involvement of vascular embarrassment. Thrombophilia induced by low levels of protein C or S or by resistance to activated protein C has been associated with the development of osteonecrosis and with arterial thrombosis (87). More recent literature has refuted the role of thrombophilia in the cause of Legg–Calvé–Perthes disease, and the cause of the disease remains unknown.

Radiographic Stages

There are four radiographic stages of the disease (138,272). In the *initial stage*, the earliest sign of Legg–Calvé–Perthes disease is failure of the ossific nucleus to grow. This failure results from vascular insult to varying portions of the ossific nucleus and to the deep layers of the epiphyseal cartilage. Widening of the medial joint space becomes evident because of the hypertrophy of the epiphyseal cartilage, which is nourished by synovial fluid. The physeal plate appears irregular, and the metaphyseal region may have areas of increased radiolucency. Another early radiographic sign is the appearance of the subchondral radiolucent zone (the crescent sign) (240,241,273,274). This radiolucency, when present, gives the treating physician an indication of the extent of the necrotic segment.

In the second stage of the repair process, the *fragmentation stage*, the epiphysis appears radiographically to fragment. There are areas of increased radiolucency where there were formerly areas of increased radiodensity within the epiphysis. In the *reossification stage,* there is a return to normal bone density in areas that were previously radiolucent. This stage is sometimes referred to as the "reparative stage." The final radiographic stage is the *healed stage.* Radiographically normal

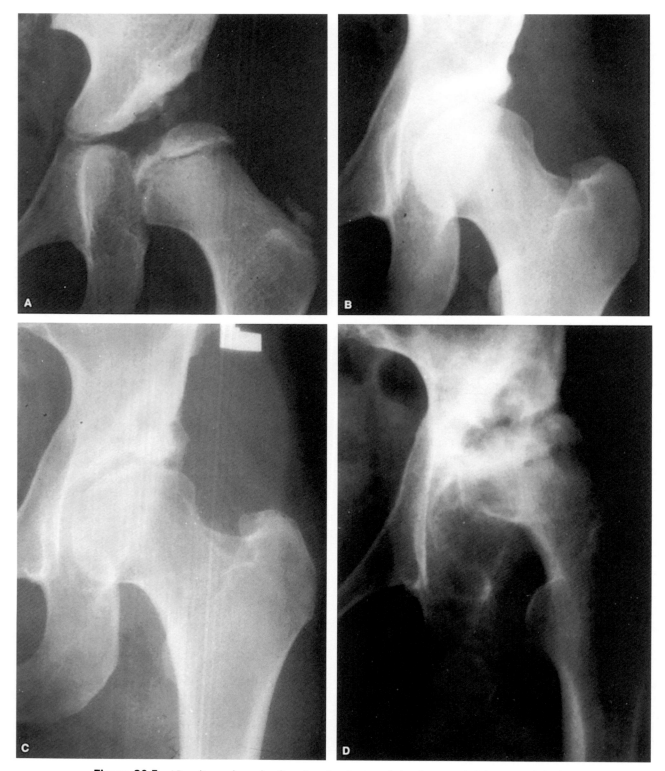

Figure 30-5 AP radiograph made after closed reduction of developmental dislocation of the hip that had been performed when the patient was 2 years, 4 months of age. **A:** At 39 months after reduction, when the patient was 5 years, 7 months of age, the accessory centers of ossification are visible in the acetabular cartilage. **B:** At 15 years after reduction, when the patient was 17 years of age, the Shenton line is intact, and there is mild, acetabular dysplasia. **C:** At 42 years after reduction, when the patient was 44 years of age, degenerative changes are present. **D:** At 51 years after the reduction, when the patient was 53 years of age, the hip was subluxed and has severe degenerative changes (Iowa hip rating, 48 of 100 points). The patient subsequently had a total hip replacement. (Reproduced from Malvitz TA, Weinstein SL. Closed reduction for congenital dysplasia of the hip: functional and radiographic results after an average of 30 years. *J Bone Joint Surg [Am]*. 1994;76:1777.)

bone densities again become radiolucent, and widening of the femoral neck becomes apparent.

Legg–Calvé–Perthes disease cannot be compared with aseptic necrosis after fracture of the neck of the femur or traumatic dislocation of the hip in a young child. In this situation, the vascular insult to the femoral head usually heals rapidly without going through the prolonged stages of fragmentation or repair seen in children with Legg–Calvé–Perthes disease (31,93,223).

Pathogenesis of Deformity

The head deformities that occur in Legg–Calvé–Perthes disease come about in many ways. First, there is growth disturbance as a result of premature closure of the physeal plates (with a resultant deformity such as central physeal arrest), which causes a shortened neck and trochanteric overgrowth (12,29). The repair process itself may cause physical compaction, resulting in structural failure and displacement of tissue elements (86). During the healing process, the femoral head deforms according to the asymmetric repair process and the applied stresses. The molding action of the acetabulum during new bone formation may also be a factor (52,151). With deformity of the femoral head, the acetabulum, particularly the lateral aspect, is deformed secondarily.

The articular cartilage of the femoral head shows changes in shape secondary to the disease process itself. The deepest layer of the articular cartilage, which is nourished by the subchondral blood supply, is often devitalized in Legg–Calvé–Perthes disease (19,20,43,163,168,184). The superficial layers, which are nourished by synovial fluid, continue to proliferate, causing an increase in the thickness of the articular cartilage. With trabecular collapse and fracture and articular cartilage overgrowth, significant head deformities develop that are manifested clinically by the loss of abduction and rotation. Eventually, when the blood supply to the subchondral area is restored, it generally comes from the periphery and moves to the center, restoring enchondral ossification at the periphery first, causing asymmetric growth (184). In addition, there is abnormal ossification in the disorganized matrix of the epiphyseal cartilage. Finally, there is periosteal bone growth and reactivation of the physeal plate along the femoral neck, with abnormally long cartilage columns leading to coxa magna and a widened femoral neck (220,223). The actual deformity that develops is profoundly influenced by the duration of the disease. This in turn is proportional to the extent of epiphyseal involvement, the age at disease onset, the remodeling potential of the patient, the stage of the disease when treatment is initiated, and the type of treatment (289,290,293,297).

Natural History

A fundamental problem in developing treatment plans for patients with Legg–Calvé–Perthes disease is the paucity of natural history data. Catterall (44) compared 46 untreated hips with a matched group of 51 hips treated by a weight-relieving caliper. The 10-year average follow-up in this series is too short to determine the outcome for patients or the natural history of the disease. Most patients with childhood hip disease do well regardless of the radiographic appearance in their early years (43,127,183,195,308).

Catterall also reported on 95 untreated patients gathered from around the British Isles. The average follow-up in this series was only 6 years, and the results were graded according to the grading system of Stundt (266). Unfortunately, very few articles in the literature use this grading system for outcomes, and the follow-up for this group is too short to be defined as natural history.

The only article labeled as natural history in the literature, other than the occasional untreated cases included in various series of treated patients, is not a natural history study but a study of patients treated by different methods from three centers. Stulberg et al. (263) attempted to establish a relationship between residual deformity and degenerative joint disease by identifying clinical and radiographic factors in the active phase of disease that would be predictive of hip deformity in degenerative joint disease.

It is thus evident that long-term natural history data on Legg–Calvé–Perthes disease is not available. Consequently, treatment decision-making is difficult.

Long-Term Follow-up Results

Although much has been learned over the years from retrospective long-term follow-up studies of Legg–Calvé–Perthes disease, these studies suffer from a multitude of faults: small numbers, with many of the original pool of patients not traced; the unavailability of original radiographs; the inclusion of many patients diagnosed between 1910 and 1940, when little was known about the disease, prognostic factors, and radiographic classifications; comparison of patients regardless of the extent of epiphyseal involvement, age at disease onset, age at beginning of treatment, or stage of the disease at treatment initiation; combined treatment modalities; no control groups; different grading systems used to judge clinical and radiographic end results; and, in the majority of series, a lack of any information on inter- and intra-rater reliability (290). Therefore, it is difficult to compare and contrast reported series.

In reviewing long-term follow-up studies, it is apparent, however, that results can improve with time, as femoral head and acetabular remodeling potential continues until the end of growth (43,112).

The 20- to 40-year follow-ups after the first onset of symptoms show that the majority of patients with Legg–Calvé–Perthes disease (70% to 90%) are active and pain-free regardless of treatment. Most patients maintain a good range of motion despite the fact that few have normal-appearing radiographs (Fig. 30-6). Clinical deterioration and symptoms of increasing pain, decreasing range of motion, and loss of function are observed only in those patients with flattened irregular heads at the time of primary healing and in those patients with premature physeal closure as evidenced by neck shortening, head deformity, and trochanteric overgrowth (290).

Beyond 40 years, however, the follow-up studies demonstrate marked reduction in function, with the overwhelming majority of patients developing degenerative joint disease by the sixth or seventh decade of life.

At a 48-year follow-up, McAndrew and Weinstein (183) reported that only 40% maintained an Iowa hip rating of greater than 80 points (Table 30-2). Forty percent of the patients had had an arthroplasty, and an additional 10% were suffering from disabling osteoarthritis symptoms but had not yet had

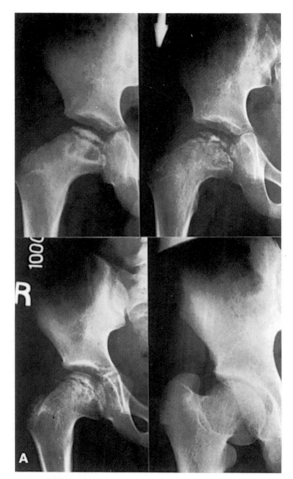

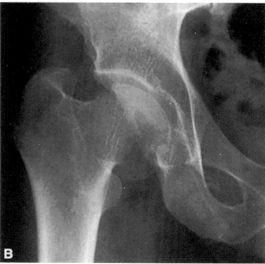

Figure 30-6 **A:** A 6-year-old boy with Catterall group 4 disease. Age 6 years, 2 months—fragmentation stage (*upper left*). Age 6 years, 9 months—early reossification stage (*upper right*). Age 8 years, 9 months—healed (*lower left*). Age 16 years, 2 months—skeletally mature (*lower right*). Patient healed with central physeal arrest pattern. **B:** A 51-year-old patient at 45-year follow-up. He is asymptomatic and has a full range of motion (Iowa hip rating, 95 of 100 points). At maximal fragmentation (*upper right*), the hip is classified as a Catterall group 4, Salter-Thompson type B, and a lateral pillar type C. (Reproduced from Weinstein SL. Legg-Calvé syndrome. In: Morrissy RT, Weinstein SL, eds. *Lovell and Winter's Pediatric Orthopaedics*. 6th ed. Philadelphia: Lippincott Williams & Wilkins; 2005.)

TABLE 30-2
LONGITUDINAL IOWA PERTHES FOLLOW-UP

	IHR >80 Points	Total Hip Replacement
36-year follow-up	93%	8%
48-year follow-up	40%	40%

an arthroplasty. Thus, 50% of the patients had disabling osteoarthritis and pain. The prevalence of osteoarthritis in this group of patients was 10 times that found in the general population in the age range of the patients studied (Figs. 30-7 to 30-9).

Mose (195) followed a group of patients into their seventh decade of life. All those with irregular heads had degenerative joint disease. Of those patients whose heads Mose classified as normal and ball-shaped, none had degenerative joint disease by the middle of the fourth decade, but 67% had severe degenerative arthritis by the middle of the seventh decade. Thus, follow-up studies beyond 40 years demonstrate marked reduction in function, with the overwhelming majority of patients developing degenerative joint disease by the sixth and seventh decades (127,183,195,263,290).

Prognostic Factors

Reviews of the long-term series of patients with Legg–Calvé–Perthes disease have identified two main prognostic factors: patient age at disease onset (more importantly, age at onset of healing) and hip joint deformity.

The most important prognostic factor for outcome is the residual deformity of the femoral head coupled with hip joint incongruity (256). Femoral head deformity and joint congruity are multifactorial problems interrelated with all other prognostic factors. The fundamental disturbance of epiphyseal and physeal cartilage growth is a key factor in deformity. Other factors involved with the development of deformity include the extent of epiphyseal involvement and the varying degrees and patterns of premature physeal closure associated with this condition (218).

Stulberg et al. (263) established a relationship between residual deformity and degenerative joint disease by retrospectively looking at the long-term outcomes of patients from three centers treated by various methods (e.g., bed rest, spica cast, ischial weight-bearing brace, crutches, cork shoe lift on normal side, and combinations of these). By identifying clinical and radiographic factors in the active phase of disease that were predictive of the development of hip deformity, they proposed a radiographic classification of deformity related to long-term outcome (Table 30-3). The more deformity at maturity, the worse the long-term outcome. Patients with aspherical congruency (Stulberg's classes III and IV; see Figs. 30-7 to 30-9) may have a satisfactory outcome for many years, with most patients undergoing significant functional deterioration in the fifth and sixth decades of life (127,183,195,308). It is the Stulberg class V hips that deteriorate earliest, usually with significant symptoms by the end of the fourth decade (127,183,195). While this classification may not have good inter- and intra-rater reliability (199), it still has some intuitive value: the flatter the femoral

TABLE 30-3
STULBERG CLASSIFICATION

Class	Radiographic Features	Congruency
1	Normal hip	Spherical
2	Spherical femoral head, same concentric circle on anteroposterior and frog-leg lateral views but with one more of the following: coxa magna, shorter than normal neck, abnormally steep acetabulum	Spherical
3	Ovoid, mushroom-shaped (but not flat) head, coxa magna, shorter than normal neck, abnormally steep acetabulum	Aspherical
4	Flat femoral head and abnormalities of the head, neck, and acetabulum	Aspherical
5	Flat head, normal neck, and acetabulum	Aspherical incongruency

head and the greater the mismatch in shape between the femoral head and acetabulum, the worse the prognosis for early degenerative joint disease.

Age at disease onset is the second most important factor related to outcome. Eight years seems to be the watershed age in most long-term series, but some authors believe that the prognosis is markedly worse for long-term outcome in patients over 6 years old at disease onset (127,183,290). Age at healing, however, is probably a more important factor. The overall skeletal maturation delay (232) in patients with

Legg–Calvé–Perthes disease and the usual compensation for this delay during the pubertal growth spurt (39) contribute to the more favorable prognosis in the young patient. The more immature the patient at the time of entering the reossification stage, the greater the potential for remodeling. As the shape of the acetabulum is dependent on the geometric pattern within it during growth (14,52,144), and as the acetabulum continues to have significant potential for development up to age 8 or 9 years (35,166,296), if a patient develops a deformity at a very early age, the immature acetabulum will conform to the

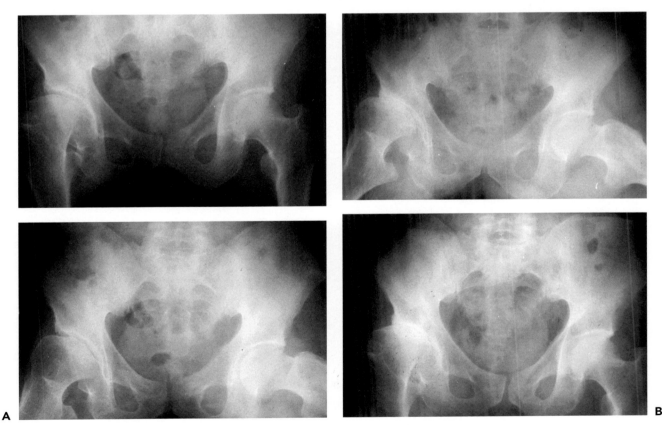

A   **B**

Figure 30-7   Patient with disease onset at 8.5 years of age. **A:** At age 51 years (at the 43-year follow-up), the Iowa hip rating is 90 points. **B:** At 63 years of age, just prior to arthroplasty (55-year follow-up), the Iowa hip rating decreased 21 points to 69. (Reproduced from Weinstein SL. Legg-Perthes disease: results of long-term follow-up. In: *The Hip: Proceedings of the 13th Open Scientific Meeting of the Hip Society.* Baltimore: CV Mosby; 1985:28.)

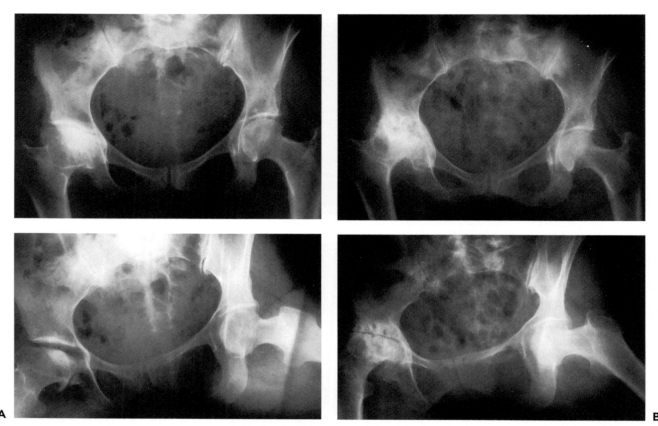

A   B

Figure 30-8   Patient with disease onset at 9.6 years of age. **A:** At 50 years of age (41-year follow-up), the Iowa hip rating is 87 points. **B:** At 62 years of age (53-year follow-up), the Iowa hip rating decreased 12 points to 75. The patient is awaiting arthroplasty. (Reproduced from Weinstein SL. Legg-Perthes disease: results of long-term follow-up. In: *The Hip: Proceedings of the 13th Open Scientific Meeting of the Hip Society*. Baltimore: CV Mosby; 1985:28.)

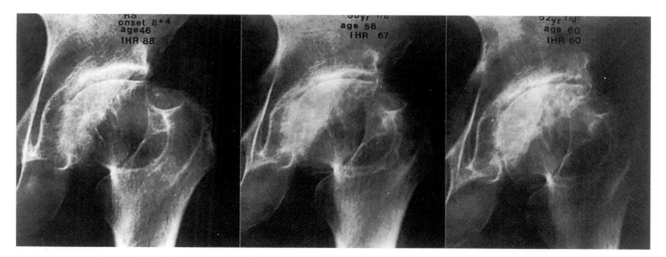

Figure 30-9   This patient had disease onset at 8.3 years of age. At 46 years of age (38-year follow-up), the Iowa hip rating was 88 points (*left*). At 58 years of age (50-year follow-up), there was a loss of 21 points on the Iowa hip rating scale, to 67 (*center*). At 60 years of age, just before arthroplasty, the Iowa hip rating was 60 points (*right*). (Reproduced from Weinstein SL. Legg-Perthes disease: results of long-term follow-up. In: *The Hip: Proceedings of the 13th Open Scientific Meeting of the Hip Society*. Baltimore: CV Mosby; 1985:28.)

altered femoral head shape. This may lead to the development of an aspherical congruency (Stulberg's classes III and IV) that could be compatible with normal function for many years (127,144,183,195,263,308).

Premature physeal arrest secondary to the disease process may have an important impact on outcome (see Fig. 30-6). Interruptions of physeal growth and its resultant effect, which often depend on the age of the patient, may have a significant bearing on the final deformity (50,151).

Treatment

The majority of patients with Legg–Calvé–Perthes disease (60%) do not need treatment (23,43,44,110,111,147,196, 241). Treatment modalities have evolved from the earliest treatments of weight relief until the head was reossified to the present "containment" methods (72,102). The idea underlying containment methods is that, in order to prevent deformities of the diseased epiphysis, the femoral head must be contained within the depths of the acetabulum to equalize the pressure on the head and subject it to the molding action of the acetabulum (33,65,102,145,146,217,229,230,237,238). Containment is an attempt to reduce the forces through the hip joint by actual or relative varisation (26). Considering all methods of containment, it should be realized that the femoral head represents over three fourths of a sphere and the acetabulum less than a hemisphere. Therefore, no method of containment can provide total containment of the femoral head within the acetabulum during all portions of the gait cycle (184,229–231).

All authors would agree that the first treatment modality in Legg–Calvé–Perthes disease is restoration of range of motion, which can be accomplished either by bed rest, with or without traction, or by sequential abduction casts. Once range of motion has been restored, treatment options include nonsurgical and surgical containment.

The treatment of Legg–Calvé–Perthes disease remains controversial, and there is lack of agreement about whether surgical or nonsurgical treatment is more beneficial. The shortage of natural history studies for comparison is another reason it is difficult to resolve this controversy. In addition, the variability of criteria for inclusion of patients in studies, the use of different measures to assess treatment outcomes, the lack of inter- and intra-rater reliability data, and the lack of untreated controls make comparisons difficult.

Brace treatment of Legg–Calvé–Perthes disease, which only 10 to 15 years ago was a common treatment method, is no longer used in North America because of results no better than natural history (73,153,173,227), Although early radiographic anatomic results from the use of an abduction orthosis were reported as comparable to the results of previously used containment, weight-bearing methods, recent reports question the efficacy of this method of management (181,185). As a consequence, many physicians have begun to treat patients with range-of-motion maintenance programs only, including stretching exercises, nighttime abduction splinting, home traction, and combinations of these. Long-term follow-up studies of these nonoperative range-of-motion regimes are needed to determine their efficacy.

The two most widely used methods to maintain containment are femoral osteotomy (9,25,38,51,56,107,169,257) and

innominate osteotomy (37,64,124,213,235,239,257,260). Interest has recently grown in the use of combined femoral and innominate (59,62,205) surgical procedures and in the use of procedures originally thought of as salvage procedures in the primary treatment of Legg–Calvé–Perthes disease (e.g., shelf arthroplasty, Chiari osteotomy, and abduction osteotomy) (16,17,160,300).

To summarize, the etiology of Legg–Calvé–Perthes disease remains unknown, and treatment remains controversial, although most pediatric orthopedic surgeons prefer surgical interventions in children at risk for a poor long-term prognosis. While most surgical procedures are adaptations of procedures initially described for treatment of hip dysplasia, no long-term outcome studies exist to indicate if these procedures will improve the long-term prognosis. Most patients with Legg–Calvé–Perthes disease will develop degenerative joint disease in the fifth and sixth decades of life. Those with greater deformity and incongruency between the femoral head and the acetabulum will develop osteoarthritis at an earlier age.

Long-term series that include patients with uniform treatment matched for age, gender, degree of epiphyseal involvement, and other diagnostic factors and compare them with an untreated control group are required to determine the most effective treatment for Legg–Calvé–Perthes disease.

SLIPPED CAPITAL FEMORAL EPIPHYSIS

Slipped capital femoral epiphysis is a disorder in which there is a displacement of the capital femoral epiphysis from the metaphysis through the physeal plate. The term *slipped capital femoral epiphysis* is actually a misnomer, because the head is held in the acetabulum by the ligamentum teres, and thus it is actually the neck that comes upward and outward while the head remains in the acetabulum. In the majority of cases, there is a varus relationship between the head and neck, but occasionally the slip is into a valgus position, with the head displaced superiorly and posteriorly in relation to the neck (244,251).

Epidemiology

The incidence of slipped capital femoral epiphysis in the general population is about 2 cases per 100,000 (109,130,150, 170,171,200,276). The relative ratio of frequency of slipped capital femoral epiphysis (values normalized to the white population) is 4.5 for Polynesian, 2.2 for black, 1.05 for American Indian, 1.0 for white, 0.5 for Indonesian Malay, and 0.1 for Indo-Mediterranean children. Children who present with unilateral disease are younger than those who present with bilateral disease (171).

The incidence of slipped capital femoral epiphysis in the United States is reported to be higher in blacks, particularly in black female patients, and it is also reported to be higher in the eastern United States (149). The disorder usually occurs in the age range 10 to 16 years in boys (mean, 13.5 years) and 10 to 14 years in girls (mean, 12 years) (109,150,171,222). Seventy percent of affected children have delayed skeletal maturation. Skeletal age may lag behind chronologic age by as much as 20 months (194,255).

Affected patients have a tendency toward obesity (148,149,171,255). Slipped capital femoral epiphysis develops in heavier children at a younger age than lighter children (171). Tall individuals were originally thought to be at higher risk, but this has since been disproved by Sörenson (148,255). The left hip is twice as often affected as the right (109,150,171). Other epidemiologic factors may include seasonal variations and social class (6,150,171).

The incidence of bilaterality is generally accepted to be 25% (range, 20% to 80%) (21,66,130,133,150,160,170,171, 276), but this figure may be low because approximately 50% of bilateral slips are asymptomatic (58,66,130,155,255). This factor becomes important when considering the natural history of the disease. In 82% of the children with sequential bilateral slips, the second slip was diagnosed within 18 months of the first (171).

Pathology

The synovium from patients with slipped capital femoral epiphysis generally exhibits changes characteristic of synovitis (77,121,193). In light microscopy studies, the physis is wide and irregular, sometimes reaching 12 mm in width (the normal width is 2.5 to 6 mm) (126). The resting zone normally constitutes 60% to 70% of the width of the physis, whereas the hypertrophic zone accounts for only 15% to 30% of the width. However, in slipped capital femoral epiphysis, the hypertrophic zone may constitute up to 80% of the physis width. Light microscopy studies document that the actual slip takes place through the zone of hypertrophy, the weakest structural area of the plate, with very occasional extension into the calcifying cartilage (126,188,224). Normal enchondral ossification is disrupted, and there are islands of unorganized cartilage in the proximal metaphysis. The perichondral ring is intact (Fig. 30-10). Electron microscopy of the physis reveals that the cartilage matrix and zone of hypertrophy differ markedly from normal, and histochemical studies of the noncollagenous components of the cartilage matrix reveal an abnormal distribution and accumulation of proteoglycans and glycoproteins in the hypertrophic zone (126,188,224). It remains to be proven, however, whether these changes are primary or secondary.

Etiology

The etiology of slipped capital femoral epiphysis remains unknown. All etiologic agents act either by altering the strength of the zone of hypertrophy or by affecting the shear stress to which the plate is exposed (150). Although trauma may be a contributing factor, and most growth plate fractures occur in an age range similar to that for slipped capital femoral epiphysis (216), it is certainly not the sole etiology, as the pathology of slipped capital femoral epiphysis differs from that seen in physeal fractures.

Several authors have felt that slipped epiphysis is secondary to an inflammatory response or a local or systemic autoimmune response (77,119,193), yet no evidence currently exists that such responses are primary factors. Hormonal and endocrine abnormalities have long been implicated in the etiology of slipped capital femoral epiphysis (2,15,78,101,106, 113–115,139,167,170,190,194,203,204,225,226,233, 245,250,262,299,310). Although there have been no specific endocrine abnormalities detected in patients with slips, there are numerous reports of slipped capital femoral epiphysis

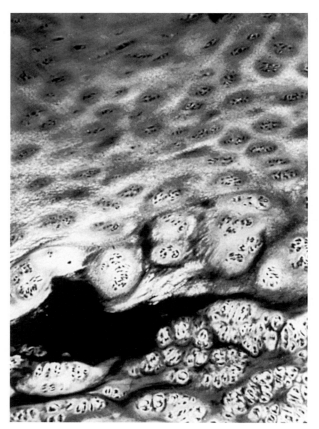

Figure 30-10 Physeal plate from a patient with slipped capital femoral epiphysis. Note slip (cleft) in zone of hypertrophy. Also note the abnormal architecture of the physeal plate. The zone of hypertrophy is increased in width, and the cells are in clusters and clumps.

associated with specific endocrine abnormalities (e.g., primary hypothyroidism, secondary hypothyroidism, and hypogonadism, as well as hypothyroidism in patients who have a growth hormone deficiency and are being treated with growth hormone). Hormonal factors have been reputed to be contributory to slips, as 78% of slips occur during the adolescent growth spurt, and in girls the slip occurs before menarche (255). The male sex prevalence may be accounted for by the fact that boys have a longer and a more rapid growth spurt (113,194). The high correlation with obesity (e.g., in patients with adiposogenital syndrome) has been attributed to an abnormal relationship between growth hormone and sex hormone in which relative predominance is given to the growth effect, leading to a structural weakening of the growth plate (101).

Mechanical factors have also been implicated (194,253,261). Periosteal thinning and femoral anteversion were factors associated with slipped capital femoral epiphysis by Key (152), Chung et al. (47) demonstrated in a cadaver study the importance of the perichondrial fibrocartilaginous complex as a supporting structure, and more recent studies have demonstrated the association of slipped capital femoral epiphysis with proximal femoral retroversion (84).

Thus, while the etiology of slipped capital femoral epiphysis remains unknown, it is probably a multifactorial disorder, with the slip representing the final manifestation of one of several predisposing factors.

Classification

On the basis of the patient's history, physical examination, and roentgenograms, slipped capital femoral epiphysis can be classified into four clinical categories: preslip, acute, acute-on-chronic, and chronic.

In the preslip phase, patients usually complain of weakness in the leg, limping, or exertional pain in the groin, adductor region, or the knee with prolonged standing or walking. On physical examination, the most consistent positive finding is lack of medial rotation. Roentgenographically, there is generalized bone atrophy of the hemipelvis and upper femur only in those patients who limped or limited their activity (disuse osteopenia). There is widening, irregularity, and fuzziness of the physeal plate region (222). A computed axial tomography scan may show evidence of minimal displacement.

An acute slip is an abrupt displacement through the proximal physeal cartilaginous plate in which there was a pre-existing epiphysiolysis (74). Acute slips account for approximately 10% to 15% of the slips in most large reported series (30,171). The clinical criteria for identifying an acute slip include the onset of symptoms within less than 2 weeks. A literature review, however, reveals that 67% of patients with acute slips give a history of mild prodromal symptoms for 1 to 3 months before their acute episode, indicating that they probably had a preslip or mild slip preceding their acute episode (1,30,42, 74,242). The prodromal symptoms—mild weakness, limp, and intermittent groin, medial thigh, or knee pain—were then followed by some history of minor trauma or a direct trauma with immediate increase in pain and inability to use the extremity. The pain is often severe enough to prevent weight bearing. Slips in those patients with a history of mild prodromal symptoms might be better classified as acute-on-chronic slips.

Physical examination demonstrates an external rotation deformity, shortening, and marked limitation of motion secondary to pain caused by marked hip muscle spasm. In general, the greater the amount of slip, the greater the motion restriction.

Patients with chronic slipped capital femoral epiphysis generally have a history of groin or medial thigh pain for months to years and may give a history of exacerbations and remission of the pain or limp. Forty-six percent have knee or lower thigh pain as their initial symptom (41,130). All demonstrate limited motion, particularly medial rotation and shortening, and the majority have thigh and/or calf atrophy. The disease is chronic in 85.5% of cases and acute in 14.5% (171).

A newer and more useful classification of acute slipped capital femoral epiphysis is based on whether the hip is stable or unstable (7,171,172,252). In the stable hip, weight bearing is possible with or without crutches, whereas in the unstable hip, the patient presents with symptoms more like those of a fracture, the pain being so severe that weight bearing is impossible. This classification is probably more important because in a large series of patients with acute symptomatology classified as stable or unstable, all treated with pinning in situ, the incidence of complications (aseptic necrosis) in patients with an unstable slip was significantly greater than in patients with a stable slip. The complications in patients with an unstable slip are most likely secondary to vascular injury caused at the time of the initial displacement (7,171).

Slips can also be classified radiographically by the amount of displacement on the anterior, posterior, or lateral roentgenogram (282). A minimal slip is classified as a slip with a maximal displacement less than one third the diameter of the neck, a moderate slip has a displacement greater than 1 cm but less than half the diameter of the neck, and a severe slip has a displacement greater than half the diameter of the neck. This classification is most important for determining the long-term prognosis, as mild and moderate slips have an excellent long-term prognosis when they are treated by pinning in situ, whereas severe slips tend to deteriorate over time (40,41).

Natural History

Howarth stated that slipped capital femoral epiphysis is probably the most frequent cause of degenerative joint disease of the hip in middle life and is a common source of pain and disability (120), but there are few long-term studies of patients with slipped capital femoral epiphysis, and these include few untreated patients (30,40,41,96,170,206,222,236). The acute episode is followed by a 2- to 3-week period of intolerance to weight bearing. As pain and spasm subside, some motion returns. The hip remains moderately painful in outward rotation, and degenerative changes develop within a few months (222).

In large series of patients with degenerative joint disease, the number of patients with known slipped capital femoral epiphysis is quite small, averaging about 5% (136,198,254). Murray (198), however, reported an association with slipped capital femoral epiphysis in 40% of his 200 patients thought to have primary degenerative joint disease. He described a tilt deformity caused by bone resorption laterally and by new bone formation medially, and he felt this to be compatible with an old slipped capital femoral epiphysis. Stulberg et al. (264) also reported a similar deformity, the pistol grip deformity (also attributed to an old slipped capital femoral epiphysis), in 40% of patients without known prior hip disease undergoing total hip replacement. Resnick (234), however, refuted this theory in a pathologic study of 48 femoral heads of patients with a tilt deformity on roentgenogram; the specimens demonstrated that the deformity was related solely to remodeling changes caused by osteoarthritis.

The severity of deformity correlates with the overall long-term prognosis with respect to degenerative joint disease and function (40,41,131,133,170,206,236). Oram (206) reported on 22 untreated slips, half of which were observed for more than 15 years. Those with moderate slips retained good function for many years, whereas those with severe slips had early degenerative joint disease and poor function. Poor results are occasionally seen even with minimal slips (30,40,41,236).

Carney and Weinstein (40) recently reported on 31 hips in 28 patients with slipped capital femoral epiphysis observed without interventional treatment. The mean duration of patient follow-up from the onset of symptoms was 41 years. The mean patient age was 54 years at review. Complications occurred in four slips: displacement to a severe degree occurred in two hips, and chondrolysis and aseptic necrosis in one hip each. In this natural history group, chondrolysis, defined as early loss of joint space width, was seen in one mild slip, and osteonecrosis, defined as collapse of some portion of the femoral head, was seen in one severe slip. The mean Iowa hip rating for the entire group was 89 points. The mild slips had a mean rating of 92 points, the moderate slips had a mean rating of 87 points, and the severe slips had a mean rating of 75. At the 41-year follow-up, all mild slips had a rating of over 80 points, whereas only 64% of moderate or severe slips had similar ratings. Mild slips had good long-term results, as indicated by their Iowa hip rating and degenerative disease rating. Of the mild slips, 36% had no degenerative changes, but all moderate and severe slips had evidence of degenerative joint disease.

Ordeberg et al. (207,208) studied a series of slipped capital femoral epiphyses never given primary treatment; the cases were investigated 20 to 40 years after diagnosis. Few patients had restrictions in working capacity or social life.

In summary, the natural history of chronic slipped capital femoral epiphysis is favorable provided that displacement is mild and remains so. Jerre (131–133) and Ross et al. (236) reported decreasing good results with greater age at follow-up. Both studies included many patients who did quite well early on but had increasing symptoms and decreasing function with increasing age.

Long-Term Results

Carney et al. (30,41) reported on 155 hips and 124 patients who were reviewed at a mean follow-up of 41 years after the onset of symptoms. The slips were classified by duration of symptoms as acute, chronic, or acute-on-chronic. As determined by the head–shaft angle, 42% of slips were mild, 32% moderate, and 26% severe. Reduction was performed on 39 hips, and realignment in 65 hips. Treatment of chronic slips included symptomatic treatment only in 25%, spica cast in 30%, pinning in situ in 24%, and osteotomy in 20%. The Iowa hip rating and radiographic classification of degenerative joint disease were determined at follow-up, and both worsened with increase in severity of the slip and where reduction or realignment had been done. Osteonecrosis (12%) and chondrolysis (16%) were also more common with increasing severity of the slip. Both reduction and realignment led to poor results. Deterioration over time was most marked with increasing severity of the slip (Table 30-4). The authors reported that the long-term natural history of malunited slips is mild deterioration related to the severity of the slip and complications.

Techniques of realignment are associated with risk of appreciable complications and adversely affect the natural history of the disease. Regardless of the severity of the slip, pin-

ning in situ provided the best long-term function and delay of degenerative arthritis and had a low risk of complications. Although limb-length discrepancy and motion in abduction and internal rotation were affected by the severity of the slip, function was not markedly impaired.

Wilson et al. (301) reviewed the results of 300 hips in 240 patients who had been seen for slipped capital femoral epiphysis at the Hospital for Special Surgery between 1936 and 1960. Of these hips, 187 had been treated by pinning in situ, with good clinical results in 81% and good radiographic results in 77%. The results were poorer (60% good clinical results and 55% good radiographic results) for the 76 hips in which correction of the deformity had been attempted. Hall (96) followed 100 patients from a study of the British Orthopaedic Association as well as an additional 38 hips and reported the results of various types of treatment. The best results were obtained with the use of multiple pins: 16 of 20 patients (80%) had excellent results. The worst results were seen after realignment had been attempted using manipulation or osteotomy. Osteotomy of the femoral neck was followed by a poor result in 36% of the hips and osteonecrosis in 38%.

Patients with slipped capital femoral epiphysis in southern Sweden were followed for more than 30 years (41,77,78, 89,132,174,179). Symptomatic treatment or pinning in situ resulted in high clinical ratings and few radiographic changes, with only 2% of the hips needing a secondary reconstructive procedure. When closed reduction and spica cast were used, the combined rate of osteonecrosis and chondrolysis was 13%, and reconstructive procedures were needed in 35% of the hips. Osteotomy through the femoral neck was followed by a combined rate of osteonecrosis and chondrolysis of 30%, and reconstructive procedures were necessary in 15% of the hips.

In several series, the use of multiple pins in situ resulted in good or excellent results in more than 90% of the hips (41,161,224). The high percentage of good results has been attributed to remodeling of the femoral neck (41,162), but difficulties with removal of pins and a relatively high incidence of unrecognized penetration of the joint space by pins have also been reported (21,41,74,148,204,216). Because of the significant prevalence of early osteoarthritis, reduction by closed or open means is currently not advocated (41,68,106,131,136,150,154).

In the Carney et al. (41) series, 39 slips had been reduced. Their mean Iowa hip rating was 72 points, and the mean radiographic degenerative score was 2.4 out of 3. Osteonecrosis developed in 12 of these hips (31%) and chondrolysis in 11 (28%). For the 116 hips that had not been reduced, the mean Iowa hip rating was 85 points, and the mean radiographic score was 1.7 out of 3. Osteonecrosis developed in 7 hips (6%) and chondrolysis in 14 (12%). Results of this long-term study support the use of pinning in situ as the treatment of choice for slipped capital femoral epiphysis. Twenty-seven hips in which the slip was chronic were so treated, and at the most recent follow-up the mean hip rating was 90 points and the mean radiographic score was 1.5 out of 3. Osteonecrosis developed in one of these hips, and chondrolysis did not develop in any.

In summary, the natural history of the malunited slip is one of mild deterioration related to the severity of the slip and the complications of treatment. Realignment is associated with the risk of substantial complications and adversely affects the natural course of disease. Pinning in situ, regardless of the severity of the slip, provides the best long-term function, has a

TABLE 30-4

IOWA HIP RATING ACCORDING TO THE SEVERITY OF THE SLIPPED CAPITAL FEMORAL EPIPHYSIS

	Average Hip Rating at Follow-Up					
	20–29 Years		30–39 Years		40–49 Years	
Severity	Points	Hips	Points	Hips	Points	Hips
Mild	93	27	93	34	87	30
Moderate	89	15	85	24	80	16
Severe	80	16	80	23	70	9

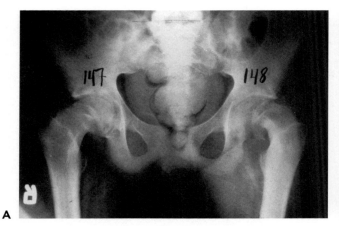

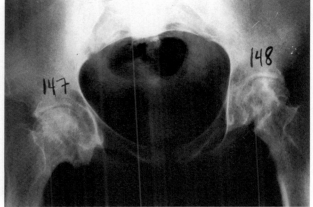

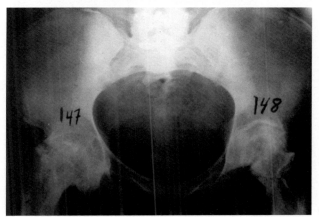

Figure 30-11   Long-term follow-up of pinning in situ.

low risk of complications, and most effectively delays the development of degenerative arthritis. Remodeling of the metaphyseal prominence is noted in many roentgenograms over the course of time.

The factors responsible for the development of aseptic necrosis, the most devastating complication of slipped capital femoral epiphysis, are acute slip, unstable slip, over-reduction of an acute slip, attempt at reduction of the chronic component of an acute-on-chronic slip, placement of pins in the superior lateral quadrant of the femoral head, and osteotomy of the femoral neck (Fig. 30-11) (32,41,49,69,158,170,172,222).

Chondrolysis is manifested clinically as loss of range of motion, pain, limp, and joint contracture (Fig. 30-12). The etiology is unknown. The question of whether it is an autoimmune phenomenon or has some factors interfering with cartilage nutrition is yet to be determined. Risk factors leading to chondrolysis include cast immobilization, unrecognized pin penetration (only if the pin is left in the joint), high slip severity, and long duration of symptoms prior to treatment. The treatment of chondrolysis is difficult, with most patients requiring anti-inflammatory drugs and bed rest with skeletal traction to relieve their contractures. In a worst-case scenario, chondrolysis would require surgical capsulectomy and continuous passive motion (7,41,83,125,186,202,209,280).

Treatment of slipped capital femoral epiphysis is somewhat controversial, but most authors feel that pinning in situ offers the best long-term results, with secondary corrective osteotomies as necessary to relieve mechanical symptoms or

pain once the physis is closed. Slipped capital femoral epiphysis patients generally do well if the slip is of mild or moderate degree, as good congruity between the femoral head and the acetabulum remains. It is only in the severe slips that deterioration and degenerative changes occur over time (Fig. 30-13).

As slips occur at an age when the majority of acetabular development is completed, no adaption to deformity can occur. Mild slips and most moderate slips do well over a long time because there is in general no loss of congruency. Severe slips may cause some incongruity and eventually lead to degenerative disease. Aseptic necrosis and chondrolysis, which may also severely compromise outcome, are associated with a high incidence of degenerative disease.

DEVELOPMENTAL COXA VARA

Coxa vara is a descriptive term used when the angular relationship between the femoral head, the femoral neck, or both, and the femoral shaft is less than normal for the patient's age. This abnormal relationship may be congenital, developmental, or acquired, and it is important to distinguish between these three etiologic groups because each has its own natural history. Congenital coxa vara is present at birth and is assumed to be caused by an embryonic limb bud abnormality; it includes proximal femoral focal deficiency, congenitally short femur, and congenitally bowed femur. Acquired coxa vara includes all entities in which deformity of the proximal femur is secondary

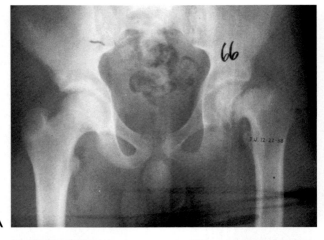

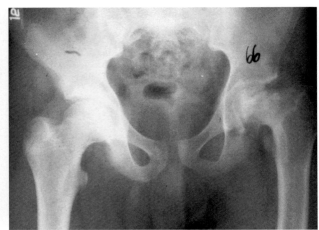

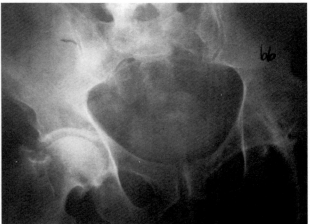

Figure 30-12 Aseptic necrosis after slip.

to an underlying traumatic, metabolic, or other condition, including rickets, fibrous dysplasia, and traumatic closure of the physeal plate.

Developmental coxa vara is an extremely rare condition (1 out of 25,000 live births [134]), and it affects boys and girls equally. It is noted as a defect localized to the cervical region of the proximal femur and is accompanied by a widened and vertically oriented physeal plate (Fig. 30-14). Clinical and radiographic features are not present at birth. About 30% of the cases are bilateral (177,228). A familial tendency has been reported, but the exact mode of inheritance is unknown. The cause of developmental coxa vara is unknown, but many etiologies have been postulated, including embryonic vascular disturbance and regional dysplasia of the proximal femur (28,228,246,309).

Clinically, most patients present to the physician for limb-length inequality or abnormal gait. Parents generally do not seek medical attention until the child is 3 to 7 years of age. The limp or waddling gait (in bilateral cases) is painless and usually progressive. Older children may complain of easy fatigability. Limb shortening is usually evident, and patients are short-statured. Examination of the involved extremity reveals limited abduction and internal rotation, a positive Trendelenburg test, limb shortening, and trochanteric elevation. In bilateral cases, hyperlordosis of the lumbar spine is present, and the patient may have

genu valgum (24,71,165). Limb-length inequalities in developmental coxa vara rarely exceed 2 cm, and the amount of shortening may be asymmetric in bilateral cases.

The diagnosis is made on an anteroposterior radiograph of the femurs and hips by noting the presence of anatomic coxa vara; a widened, vertically oriented physeal plate; a shortened neck; a normal, straight femoral shaft; and a separate triangular ossification center on the inferior part of the femoral neck (see Fig. 30-14). The femoral head is spherical, and the acetabulum generally normal, although mild dysplasia may be apparent in comparison with an opposite normal hip (71,75,214,243,285,309).

Various measurements have been made to quantify the relationship in the proximal femur. These include the head–shaft angle, the neck–shaft angle, and the Hilgenreiner physeal angle (285) (formerly called the Hilgenreiner epiphyseal angle) (see Fig. 30-14). It is best to use the head–shaft angle to follow the progression of deformity, because the neck–shaft angle remains fairly constant even in the face of progressive deformity. The Hilgenreiner physeal angle has been found to be helpful in evaluating and determining the prognostication for patients with developmental coxa vara (285).

The goals of treatment in developmental coxa vara are to promote ossification of the defect and to correct the varus deformity, allowing restoration of the mechanical advantage

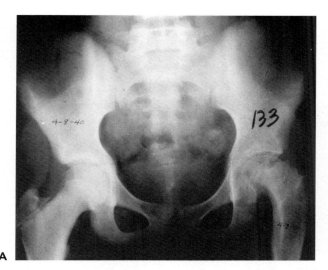

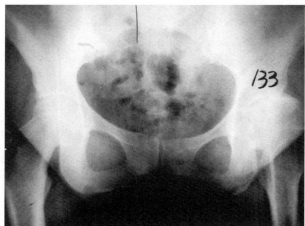

Figure 30-13 Chondrolysis after slip.

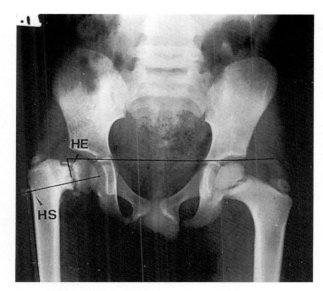

Figure 30-14 Coxa vara development. Note head–shaft angle (HS) and Hilgenreiner epiphyseal angel (HE).

correct the varus deformity, allowing restoration of the mechanical advantage of the hip abductors to improve gait and to equalize limb lengths. In the surgical management, it is important to include internal rotation of the distal segment of the osteotomy to correct the loss of internal rotation seen with developmental coxa vara. One goal of treatment should be to of the hip abductors to improve gait and equalize limb lengths (27). In progressive coxa vara, the natural history suggests that there is increasing deformity, decreasing function, and early degenerative joint disease (Fig. 30-15) (27,118,165, 228,284,285). General indications for surgical treatment include increasing coxa vara and a neck–shaft angle less than 100°. In mild, nonprogressive cases with a neck–shaft angle greater than 100° and a Hilgenreiner physeal angle less than 45°, resolution of the defect may occur as the patient is observed with serial follow-up radiographs (285).

Natural History

The natural history of developmental coxa vara is somewhat varied. Weinstein et al. (285) and Serafin and Szulc (246) demonstrated that the determining factor for progressive varus deformity was the Hilgenreiner physeal angle. Patients demonstrating an angle less than 45° generally healed the femoral neck defect, with arrest of the progression of the varus deformity. Patients with an angle greater than this value were more likely to have varus progression (see Fig. 30-15).

The goals of treatment in developmental coxa vara, as mentioned above, are to promote ossification of the defect and

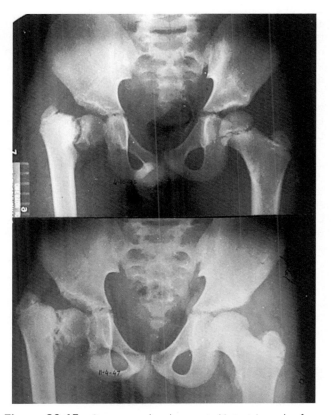

Figure 30-15 Coxa vara development. Note triangular fragment and worsening of condition over a 2-year period (*bottom*).

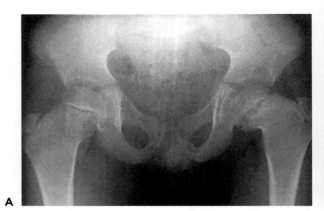
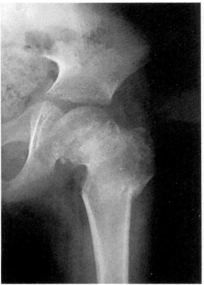

Figure 30-16   **A:** Eight-year-old boy with coxa vara. **B:** Eighteen months after abduction osteotomy.

correct the Hilgenreiner physeal angle to less than 40° at the time of the osteotomy to decrease the potential for recurrence (285).

Indications for surgery include a Hilgenreiner physeal angle greater than 45° to 60°, progressive worsening or decreasing of the neck–shaft angle to below 100°, or the presence of a Trendelenburg gait (285). In patients with a limp and progression in the Hilgenreiner physeal angle to greater than 60°, intertrochanteric or subtrochanteric abduction osteotomy is the treatment of choice (Fig. 30-16) (285). In these patients, the neck–shaft angle should be restored to decrease the shear stress across the vertical defect. With surgery, the defect generally heals, but growth plate arrest may be seen in a significant number of patients, leading to limb-length inequality. Generally, patients older than 5 years at the time of surgery maintain their correction (71,285).

After surgery, the triangular physeal metaphyseal defect generally spontaneously closes in 3 to 6 months. Ninety percent of surgically treated patients will have premature closure of the proximal femoral physeal plate within 2 years after the corrective surgery (243). As trochanteric overgrowth can be a problem, arrest should be considered in younger patients, and distal trochanteric transfer in older patients with a persistent abductor lurch.

Because of the rarity of the condition, few long-term studies are available, and hence outcome data are largely anecdotal. If normal mechanics are corrected by surgery, the main long-term problem is limb-length inequality (57,67,284,285). If the severe progressive varus is left untreated, severe disability may ensue. No other long-term information is available.

SEPTIC ARTHRITIS

Although bone and joint infections in children have been radically altered by the introduction of antibiotics, and the mortality in developed countries has fallen to nearly zero, a successful outcome depends largely on early diagnosis and appropriate management. Unfortunately, infection of the hip continues to be a diagnostic problem and a potentially crippling disease. The longer the delay in diagnosis and treatment, the greater the chances of serious sequelae.

Acute septic arthritis of the hip is a relatively uncommon condition (90,191). Most large centers report only a few cases per year. One third of affected patients are younger than 2 years old, and 49% are younger than 3 years. Septic arthritis is more common in boys by a ratio of 2:1 (129).

Infection spreads to the hip joint by one of three mechanisms (135,192), most commonly by bacteremia that seeds the synovium. The hip joint may also be secondarily infected from osteomyelitis of the intracapsular proximal femoral metaphysis, and a third mechanism is direct penetration into the joint from a puncture or from an adjacent wound. In the infant, the fetal vascular arrangement (the capillaries penetrate the physeal plate into the epiphysis) persists until age 18 months (268). Therefore, in this group there may be spread of infection from the metaphysis directly to the epiphysis and then into the joint. Severe irreparable damage to the physeal plate can occur, with arrest of growth and secondary deformity.

The pathophysiology of primary septic arthritis is complex. Thirty percent of cases have negative cultures yet present clinical signs of septic arthritis indistinguishable from those in patients with positive cultures. The mechanism of cartilage destruction involves release of proteases, peptidases, and collagenases from white blood cells, the synovial cells, and the cartilage itself. In addition, certain organisms release proteolytic enzymes that degrade the cartilage matrix and eventually lead to collagen degradation (8,70,99,259). Unfortunately, the wholesale use of antibiotics by physicians in developed countries often leads to modification of the condition, leading to delayed presentation and frequently a poor outcome. Capsular laxity is followed by subluxation and then dislocation of the joint (Fig. 30-17). Because of the special blood supply to the femoral head, septic necrosis can occur and result in sequestration of the

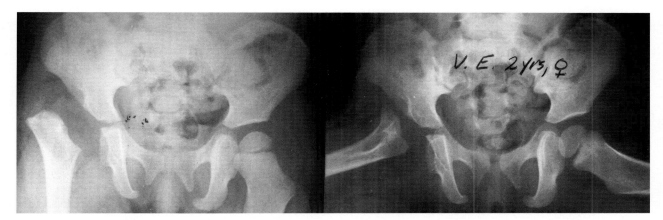

Figure 30-17 Two-year-old child with complete destruction of femoral head and hip dislocation from aseptic necrosis.

ossific growth center. With prompt management, this should be a preventable complication.

In approximately one third of cases of septic arthritis, no bacterial pathogen is identified despite thorough bacteriologic examination. Ninety-four percent of septic arthritis cases involve only a single joint. In children younger than 2 years, *Haemophilus influenzae* (serologic type B) was often the pathogen; however with the advent of vaccination programs it is now rarely seen. In children older than 2 years, *Staphylococcus aureus* is the most common agent (13,79,247). Primary meningococcal arthritis can occur in the absence of meningitis or meningococcemia. In teenagers, *Neisseria gonorrhea* is the most common cause of polyarthritis. With the advent of the *H. influenzae* vaccine, the incidence of this organism causing septic arthritis has been decreasing. In infants and children between 4 weeks and 4 years of age, the most likely organism is *S. aureus* if the patient has been immunized against *H. influenzae*. Without immunization, *H. influenzae* is most likely (4). Group A and group B *Streptococcus* are likely organisms in children younger than 1 year of age.

Diagnosis

Effective treatment depends on the correct diagnosis: localization of the infection, identification of any predisposing cause, and identification of the organism. A high index of suspicion is essential (157,175).

In childhood septic arthritis, the patients generally present as being very ill. They are often lethargic and have a fever. Typically, they complain of pain in the limb and refuse to move the extremity. In the neonatal period, a large majority of the patients may not appear acutely ill, but the infection is indicated by failure to eat or gain weight. Signs include irritability of the hip with diaper changes and restricted motion. The patients generally assume a position of comfort with the hip flexed, externally rotated, and abducted. They may, however, also present with a picture of pseudoparalysis of the extremity. Crease asymmetry (gluteal, thigh, and popliteal) and swelling about the external genitalia or buttock may be apparent. Previous treatment with antibiotics can alter or attenuate symptoms of joint infections and make diagnosis more difficult.

The diagnostic test of choice is joint aspiration. Aspirated fluid should be sent for Gram stain, culture, and leukocyte count. The earlier the infection is diagnosed, the clearer the joint aspirate will be. The white blood count is typically greater than 50,000 cells/mm^3 (3) and is usually in the range of 100,000 (79,249). The one exception is gonococcal arthritis, in which the white blood count is often less than 50,000 cells/mm^3. A white cell count of over 50,000 with greater than 90% polymorphonuclear leukocytes should be considered infectious regardless of the culture results. However, in a large series of culture-proven cases of bacterial septic arthritis, only 44% of the cases had cell counts of over 100,000 cells/mm^3, with 34% of the cases having counts of less than 25,000 cells/mm^3 (79).

Hip joint infections are an orthopedic emergency because of the potential for the development of avascular necrosis as well as the destruction of articular cartilage. The hip joint should be aspirated under fluoroscopic control. Once the diagnosis of septic arthritis has been confirmed, the joint must be surgically drained on an urgent basis.

The general treatment consists of adequate administration of bactericidal antibiotics, drainage, immobilization, and general supportive therapy.

Complications of septic arthritis include complete destruction of the articular cartilage, restricted joint motion, and ankylosis (Fig. 30-18). Damage to the cartilaginous epiphysis and physeal plate may lead to joint deformity, limb-length inequality, and degenerative joint disease. As the proximal femoral physis accounts for approximately 18% of the growth of the limb and 30% of the growth of the femur, septic arthritis in infancy can result in significant limb-length inequality.

The long-term consequences may vary depending on whether there is sufficient cartilage damage to result in total joint destruction. This may lead to the need for early total joint replacement or fusion. The other long-term sequelae are related to partial growth plate arrest patterns that lead to limb-length inequality and proximal femoral growth disturbance problems such as seen in DDH. Coxa vara, coxa breva, coxa magna, and trochanteric overgrowth, for example, can all occur with septic arthritis and depend on the age at which the infection occurs, how developed the acetabulum is, and how much growth remains in the proximal femur and the acetabulum.

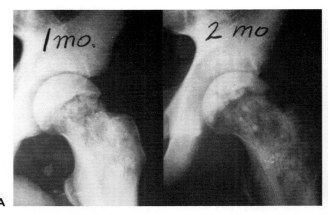
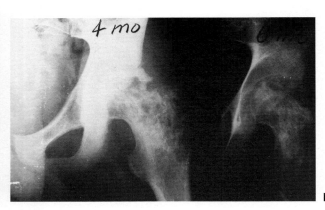

Figure 30-18 Progression of proximal femoral osteomyelitis with secondary septic arthritis progressing to ankylosis over 4 years.

CONCLUSION

The outcomes of pediatric hip conditions discussed in this chapter are multifactorial. The outcomes are related to the pathophysiology of the disease, the age at disease onset, the duration of the condition, and how the duration specifically relates to the stage of femoral head and acetabular development during the disease evolution. An additional factor is residual deformity of the femoral head and neck and whether this can be accommodated for by changes in the shape of the acetabulum. The final factor is the effect of treatment on the condition: whether it alters the natural history and whether complications develop that further alter the natural history.

Age 8 years seems to be the watershed age for prognosis in pediatric hip conditions, as this is the age when the majority of acetabular development is complete. In children younger than 8 years old, deformities in the femoral head as a result of a disease process, such as developmental coxa vara, Legg–Calvé–Perthes disease, or aseptic necrosis secondary to treatment of DDH or septic arthritis, may be accommodated for by secondary changes in acetabular development. After 8 years of age, accommodation of acetabular shape to a deformed femoral head may not be possible. This accommodation factor assumes normal acetabular growth potential, which in a condition such as DDH may not exist.

Slipped capital femoral epiphysis generally occurs during the adolescent growth spurt after the majority of femoral head and acetabular development is complete. The outcomes are related to the relationship between the femoral head and the acetabulum. Mild and moderate degrees of slip are well tolerated, whereas severe slips disrupt this relationship and are subject to the development of early degenerative joint disease.

The short-term outcomes of most pediatric hip conditions are relatively good. However, good long-term outcomes can be assured only with the restoration of normal femoral head and acetabular growth and relationships.

REFERENCES

1. Aadelin RJ, Weiner DS, Hoyt W, et al. Acute slipped capital femoral epiphysis. *J Bone Joint Surg [Am]*. 1974;56:1473–1487.
2. Aceto T, Frasier S, Hayles A, et al. Collaborative study of the effects of human growth hormone deficiency, III: first 18 months of therapy. In: Rati S, ed. *Advances in Human Growth Hormone Research*. Bethesda, MD: National Institutes of Health; 1973:695. DHEW (NIH) 74–612.
3. Ailsby RL, Staheli LT. Pyogenic infections of the sacroiliac joint in children: radioisotope bone scanning as a diagnostic tool. *Clin Orthop*. 1974;100:96.
4. Almquist EE. The changing epidemiology of septic arthritis in children. *Clin Orthop*. 1970;No. 68:96.
5. Ando M, Gotoh E. Significance of inguinal folds for diagnosis of congenital dislocation of the hip in infants aged three to four months. *J Pediatr Orthop*. 1990;10:331–334.
6. Andren L, Borgstrom K. Seasonal variation of epiphysiolysis of the hip and possibility of alimentary causal factor. *Acta Orthop Scand*. 1958;28(1)(entire issue).

7. Aronsson DD, Loder RT. Treatment of the unstable (acute) slipped capital femoral epiphysis. *Clin Orthop.* 1996;No. 322:99–110.
8. Arvidson S, Holme T, Lindholm B. The formation of extracellular proteolytic enzymes by *Staphyloccous aureus. Acta Pathol Microbiol Scand.* 1972;80:835.
9. Axer A, Gershuni DH, Hendel D, et al. Indications for femoral osteotomy in Legg–Calvé–Perthes disease. *Clin Orthop.* 1980;No. 150:78.
10. Barker DJP, Hall AJ. The epidemiology of Perthes' disease. *Clin Orthop.* 1986;No. 209:89–94.
11. Barlow TG. Early diagnosis and treatment of congenital dislocation of the hip. *J Bone Joint Surg [Br].* 1962;44:292–301.
12. Barnes JM. Premature epiphyseal closure in Perthes' disease. *J Bone Joint Surg [Br].* 1980;62:432.
13. Barton LL, Dunkle LM, Habib FH. Septic arthritis in childhood: a 13 year review. *Am J Dis Child.* 1987;141:898.
14. Bellyei A, Mike G. Acetabular development in Legg–Calvé–Perthes disease. *Orthopaedics.* 1988;11:407.
15. Benjamin B, Miller PR. Hypothyroidism as a cause of diseases of the hip. *Am J Dis Child.* 1938;55:1189.
16. Bennett JT, Mazurek RT, Cash JD. Chiari's osteotomy in the treatment of Perthes' disease. *J Bone Joint Surg [Br].* 1991;73:225.
17. Benson MKD, Evans JDC. The pelvic osteotomy of Chiari: an anatomical study of the hazards and misleading radiographic appearance. *J Bone Joint Surg [Br].* 1976;58:163–168.
18. Berkeley ME, Dickson JH, Cain TE, et al. Surgical therapy for congenital dislocation of the hip in patients who are twelve to thirty-six months old. *J Bone Joint Surg [Am].* 1984;66:412–420.
19. Bernbeck R. Kritischenzum Perthes: Problem der Hufte. *Arch Orthop Unfall-Chir.* 1950;44:445.
20. Bernbeck R. Zur Pathogenese der jugendlichen Huftokopfnekrose. *Arch Orthop Unfall-Chir.* 1950;44:164.
21. Billing L, Severin E. Slipping epiphysis of the hip: a roentgenological and clinical study based on a new roentgen technique. *Acta Radiol.* 1959;(suppl):174.
22. Bjerkreim I, Johansen J. Late diagnosed congenital dislocation of the hip. *Acta Orthop Scand.* 1987;58:504–506.
23. Blakemore ME, Harrison MHM. A prospective study of children with untreated Catterall group I Perthes disease. *J Bone Joint Surg [Br].* 1979;61:329.
24. Blockey NJ. Observations on infantile coxa vara. *J Bone Joint Surg [Br].* 1969;51:106.
25. Bohr H, Baadsgaard K, Sager P. The vascular supply to the femoral head following dislocation of the hip joint: an experimental study in new-born rabbits. *Acta Orthop Scand.* 1965;35:264.
26. Bombelli R. Osteoarthritis of the hip. New York: Springer-Verlag; 1983.
27. Borden J, Spencer GE, Herndon CH. Treatment of coxa vara in children by means of a modified osteotomy. *J Bone Joint Surg [Am].* 1966;48:1106.
28. Bos CFA, Sakkers RJB, Bloem JL, et al. Histological, biochemical and MRI studies of the growth plate in congenital coxa vara. *J Pediatr Orthop.* 1989;9:660.
29. Bowen JR, Foster BK, Hartzell CR. Legg–Calvé–Perthes disease. *Clin Orthop.* 1985;No. 185:97–108.
30. Boyer DW, Mickelson MR, Ponseti IV. Slipped capital femoral epiphysis: long-term follow-up and study of one hundred and twenty-one patients. *J Bone Joint Surg [Am].* 1981;63:85–95.
31. Brailsford JF. Avascular necrosis of bone. *J Bone Joint Surg.* 1943;25:249.
32. Brodetti A. The blood supply of the femoral neck and head in relation to the damaging effects of nails and screws. *J Bone Joint Surg [Br].* 1960;42:794–801.
33. Brotherton BJ, McKibbin B. Perthes' disease treated by prolonged recumbency and femoral head containment: a long-term appraisal. *J Bone Joint Surg [Br].* 1977;59:8.
34. Bucholz R, Ogden J. Patterns of ischemic necrosis of the proximal femur in nonoperatively treated congenital hip disease. In: *The Hip: Proceedings of the Sixth Open Scientific Meeting of the Hip Society.* St. Louis: CV Mosby; 1978.
35. Calot F. Ueber neuere Anschauungen in der Pathologie der Hufte auf Grund der Arbeiten der letzen Jahre. *Z Orthop Chir.* 1929;51:134.
36. Calvé J. Sur une forme particuliere de coxalgie greffe, et sur des deformations caracteristiques de l'extremite superieure de femur. *Rev Chir.* 1910;42:54.
37. Canale ST, D'Anca AF, Cotler JM, et al. Innominate osteotomy in Legg–Calvé–Perthes disease. *J Bone Joint Surg [Am].* 1972;54:25.
38. Canario AT, Williams L, Weintraub S, et al. A controlled study of the results of femoral osteotomy in severe Perthes' disease. *J Bone Joint Surg [Br].* 1980;62:348.
39. Cannon SR, Pozo JL, Catterall A. Elevated growth velocity in children with Perthes disease. *J Pediatr Orthop.* 1989;9:285.
40. Carney BT, Weinstein SL. Natural history of untreated chronic slipped capital femoral epiphysis. *Clin Orthop.* 1996;No. 322:43.
41. Carney BT, Weinstein SL, Noble J. Long-term follow-up of slipped capital femoral epiphysis. *J Bone Joint Surg [Am].* 1991; 73:667–674.
42. Casey BH, Hamilton HW, Bobechko WP. Reduction of acutely slipped upper femoral epiphysis. *J Bone Joint Surg [Br].* 1972;54: 607–614.
43. Catterall A. Legg–Calvé–Perthes disease. In: *Legg–Calvé–Perthes Disease.* Edinburgh: Churchill Livingstone; 1982.
44. Catterall A. The natural history of Perthes disease. *J Bone Joint Surg [Br].* 1971;53:37.
45. Catterall A. Thoughts on the etiology of Perthes disease. *Iowa Orthop J.* 1984;4:34.
46. Chapchal GJ. The intertrochanteric osteotomy in the treatment of congenital dysplasia. *Clin Orthop.* 1976;No. 119:54–59.
47. Chung SMK, Batterman SC, Brighton CT. Shear strength of the human femoral capital epiphyseal plate. *J Bone Joint Surg [Am].* 1976;58:94–103.
48. Churgay CA, Caruthers BS. Diagnosis and treatment of congenital dislocation of the hip. *Am Fam Physician.* 1992;45:1217–1228.
49. Claffefy TJ. Avascular necrosis of the femoral head. *J Bone Joint Surg [Br].* 1960;42:802.
50. Clarke NMP, Harrison MHM. Painful sequelae of coxa plana. *J Bone Joint Surg [Am].* 1983;65:13.
51. Coates CJ, Paterson JM, Woods KR, et al. Femoral osteotomy in Perthes disease: results at maturity. *J Bone Joint Surg [Br].* 1990; 72:581.
52. Coleman RC, Slager RF, Smith WS. The effect of environmental influences on acetabular development. *Surg Forum.* 1958;9:775.
53. Coleman SS. *Congenital dysplasia and dislocation of the hip.* St. Louis: CV Mosby; 1978.
54. Coleman SS. Congenital dysplasia of the hip in the Navajo infant. *Clin Orthop.* 1968;No. 56:179.
55. Cooperman DR, Wallensten R, Stulberg SD. Acetabular dysplasia in the adult. *Clin Orthop.* 1983;No. 175:79–85.
56. Cordeiro EN. Femoral osteotomy in Legg–Calvé–Perthes disease. *Clin Orthop.* 1980;No. 150:69.
57. Cordes S, Dickens DRV, Cole WG. Correction of coxa vara in childhood: the use of Pauwels' Y-shaped osteotomy. *J Bone Joint Surg [Br].* 1991;73:3.
58. Cowell H. Significance of the early diagnosis and treatment of slipped capital femoral epiphysis. *Clin Orthop.* 1966;No. 48:89.
59. Craig WA, Kramer WG, Watanabe R. Combined iliac and femoral osteotomies in Legg–Calvé–Perthes syndrome. *J Bone Joint Surg [Am].* 1974;56:1314.
60. Crawford AW, Slovek RW. Fate of the untreated congenitally dislocated hip. *Orthop Trans.* 1978;2:73.
61. Crego CH Jr, Schwartzmann JR. Medial adductor open reduction for congenital dislocation of the hip. *J Bone Joint Surg [Am].* 1948;30:428–442.
62. Crutcher JP, Staheli LT. Combined osteotomy as a salvage procedure for severe Legg–Calvé–Perthes disease. *J Pediatr Orthop.* 1992;12:151.
63. Danielsson LG, Nilsson BE. Attitudes to CDH [guest editorial]. *Acta Orthop Scand.* 1984;55:244–246.
64. Dekker M, VanRens ThJG, Sloff TJJH. Salters pelvic osteotomy in the treatment of Perthes' disease. *J Bone Joint Surg [Br].* 1981;68:282.
65. Denton J. Experience with Legg–Calvé–Perthes disease (LCPD) 1968–1974, at the New York Orthopaedic Hospital. *Clin Orthop.* 1980;No. 150:36.
66. Denton JR. Kulick radiographic grade: a retrospective study of one hundred and twenty-five cases of slipped capital femoral epiphysis. *Clin Orthop.* 1982;No. 162:87.

67. Desai S, Johnson L. Long-term results of valgus osteotomy for congenital coxa vara. *Clin Orthop.* 1993;No. 294:204.

68. DeSmet A, Kuhns L, Fayos J, et al. Effects of radiation therapy in growing long bone. *Am J Roentgenol.* 1976;127:935.

69. Dietz FR. Traction reduction of acute and acute on chronic slipped capital femoral epiphysis. *Clin Orthop.* 1994;No. 302:101.

70. Dingle JT. The role of lysomal enzymes in skeletal tissue. *J Bone Joint Surg [Br].* 1973;55:87.

71. Duncan GA. Congenital and developmental coxa vara. *Surgery.* 1938;3:741.

72. Eyre-Brooke AI. Osteochondritis deformans coxae juvenalis, or Perthes' disease: the results of treatment by traction in recumbency. *Br J Surg.* 1936;24:166.

73. Fackler CD. Nonsurgical treatment of Legg–Calvé–Perthes disease. *Instr Course Lect.* 1989;38:305.

74. Fahey JJ, O'Brien ET. Acute slipped capital femoral epiphysis: review of the literature and report of ten cases. *J Bone Joint Surg [Am].* 1965;47:1105–1127.

75. Fairbank HAT. Infantile or cervical coxa vara. In: *The Robert Jones Birthday Volume: A Collection of Surgical Essays.* London: Oxford University Press; 1928:225.

76. Fairbank JC, Howell P, Nockler I, et al. Relationship of pain to the radiological anatomy of the hip joint in adults treated for congenital dislocation of the hip as infants: a long-term follow-up of patients treated by three methods. *J Pediatr Orthop.* 1986;6:539–547.

77. Ferguson AK, Howorth MB. Slipping of the upper femoral epiphysis: a study of seventy cases. *JAMA.* 1931;97:1867–1872.

78. Fidler M, Brook C. Clipped upper femoral epiphysis following treatment with human growth hormone. *J Bone Joint Surg [Am].* 1974;56:1719–1722.

79. Fink CW, Nelson JD. Septic arthritis and osteomyelitis in children. *Clin Rheum Dis.* 1986;12:423.

80. Fisher RI. An epidemiological study of Legg–Perthes disease. *J Bone Joint Surg [Am].* 1972;54:769.

81. Frankenburg WK. To screen or not to screen: congenital dislocation of the hip [editorial]. *Am J Public Health.* 1981;71:1311–1313.

82. Fredensborg N, Nilsson BE. Overdiagnosis of congenital dislocation of the hip. *Clin Orthop.* 1976;No. 119:89–92.

83. Frymoyer J. Chondrolysis of the hip following Southwick osteotomy for severe slipped capital femoral epiphysis. *Clin Orthop.* 1974;No. 99:120–124.

84. Gelberman RH, Cohen MS, Shaw BA, et al. The association of femoral retroversion with slipped capital femoral epiphysis. *J Bone Joint Surg [Am].* 1986;68:1000–1007.

85. Gershuni DH. Etiology of Legg–Calvé–Perthes syndrome. *Orthop Rev.* 1979;8:49.

86. Glimcher MJ. Legg–Calvé–Perthes syndrome: biological and mechanical considerations in the genesis of clinical abnormalities. *Orthop Rev.* 1979;8:33.

87. Glueck CJ, Glueck DG, Freiberg R, et al. Protein C and S deficiency, thrombophilia, and hypofibrinolysis: pathophysiologic causes of Legg-Perthes disease. *Pediatr Res.* 1994;35:383–388.

88. Goff CW. Legg–Calvé–Perthes syndrome (L.C.P.S.) *Clin Orthop.* 1962;No. 22:93.

89. Goldman AB, Lane JM, Salvati E. Slipped capital femoral epiphysis complicating renal osteodystrophy. *Radiology.* 1978;126:333.

90. Green NE, Edwards K. Bone and joint infections in children. *Orthop Clin North Am.* 1987;18:55.

91. Hadley NA, Brown TD, Weinstein SL. The effect of contact pressure elevations and aseptic necrosis on the long-term outcome of congenital hip dislocation. *J Orthop Res.* 1990;8:504–513.

92. Hadlow V. Neonatal screening for congenital dislocation of the hip: a prospective 21-year survey. *J Bone Joint Surg [Br].* 1988;70:740–743.

93. Haliburton RA, Brockenshire FA, Barber JR. Avascular necrosis of the femoral capital epiphysis after traumatic dislocation of the hip in children. *J Bone Joint Surg [Br].* 1961;43:43–46.

94. Hall D, Harrison MHM. An association between congenital abnormalities and Perthes disease of the hip. *J Bone Joint Surg [Br].* 1978;60:138.

95. Hall DJ. Genetic aspects of Perthes disease: a critical review. *Clin Orthop.* 1986;No. 209:100–114.

96. Hall JE. The results of treatment of slipped femoral epiphysis. *J Bone Joint Surg [Br].* 1957;39:659–673.

97. Hansson G, Nachemson A, Palmen K. Screening of children with congenital dislocation of the hip joint on the maternity wards in Sweden. *J Pediatr Orthop.* 1983;3:271–279.

98. Harper PS, Brotherton BJ, Cochlin D. Genetic risks in Perthes' disease. *Clin Genet.* 1976;10:178.

99. Harris ED, McCroskery PA. The influence of temperature and fibril stability on degradation of cartilage collagen by rheumatoid synovial collagenase. *N Engl J Med.* 1974;290:1.

100. Harris WH. Etiology of osteoarthritis of the hip. *Clin Orthop.* 1986;No. 213:20–33.

101. Harris WR. The endocrine basis for slipping of the upper femoral epiphysis: an experimental study. *J Bone Joint Surg [Br].* 1950;32:5–11.

102. Harrison MHM, Menon MPA. Legg–Calvé–Perthes disease: the value of x-ray measurement in clinical practice with special reference to the broomstick plaster method. *J Bone Joint Surg [Am].* 1966;48:1301.

103. Harrison MHM, Turner MH, Smith DN. Perthes disease treatment with the Birmingham splint. *J Bone Joint Surg [Br].* 1982;64:3.

104. Hass J. Congenital dislocation of the hip. In: *Congenital Dislocation of the Hip.* Springfield, MA: Charles C Thomas, 1951.

105. Haueisen DC, Weiner DS, Weiner SD. The characterization of transient synovitis of the hip in children. *J Pediatr Orthop.* 1986;6:11–17.

106. Heatley FW, Greenwood RH, Boase DL. Slipping of the upper femoral epiphysis in patients with intracranial tumors causing hypopituitarism and chiasmal compression. *J Bone Joint Surg [Br].* 1976;58:169–175.

107. Heikkinen E, Puranen J. Evaluation of femoral osteotomy in the treatment of Legg–Calvé–Perthes disease. *Clin Orthop.* 1980;No. 150:60.

108. Henderson RS. Osteotomy for unreduced congenital dislocation of the hip in adults. *J Bone Joint Surg [Br].* 1970;52:468.

109. Henrikson B. The incidence of slipped capital femoral epiphysis. *Acta Orthop Scand.* 1969;40:365.

110. Herring JA, Kim HT, Browne R. Calvé-Perthes disease, I: classification of radiographs with use of the modified lateral pillar and Stulberg classifications. *J Bone Joint Surg [Am].* 2004;86: 2103–2120.

111. Herring JA, Kim HT, Browne R. Calvé-Perthes disease, II: prospective multicenter study of the effect of treatment on outcome. *J Bone Joint Surg [Am].* 2004;86:2121–2134.

112. Herring JA, Williams JJ, Neustadt JN, et al. Evolution of femoral head deformity during the healing phase of Legg–Calvé–Perthes disease. *J Pediatr Orthop.* 1993;13:41.

113. Hillman JW, Hunter WA, Barrow JA. Experimental epiphyseolysis in rats. *Surg Forum.* 1957;8:566.

114. Hirano T, Stamelos S, Harris V, et al. Association of primary hypothyroidism and slipped capital femoral epiphysis. *J Pediatr.* 1978;93:262.

115. Hirsch P, Hirsch S. Slipped capital femoral epiphysis: occurrence after treatment with chorionic gonadotropin. *JAMA.* 1976;235:751.

116. Hoaglund FT, Healey JH. Osteoarthrosis and congenital dysplasia of the hip in family members of children who have congenital dysplasia of the hip [published erratum appears in *J Bone Joint Surg [Am].* 1991;73:293]. *J Bone Joint Surg [Am].* 1990;72: 1510–1518.

117. Hoagland FT, Yau AC, Wong WL. Osteoarthritis of the hip and other joints in Southern Chinese in Hong Kong. *J Bone Joint Surg [Am].* 1973;55:545.

118. Horwitz T. The treatment of congenital (or developmental) coxa vara. *Surg Gynecol Obstet.* 1948;87:71.

119. Howarth MB. History: slipping of the capital femoral epiphysis. *Clin Orthop.* 1966;No. 48:11.

120. Howarth MB. Slipped capital femoral epiphysis: pathology. *Clin Orthop.* 1966;No. 48:33.

121. Howarth MB. Slipping of the capital femoral epiphysis. *Am J Orthop Surg.* 1965;7:10.

122. Ilfeld FW, Westin GW. Missed or late-diagnosed congenital dislocation of the hip: a clinical entity. *Isr J Med Sci.* 1980;16:260–266.

123. Ilfeld FW, Westin GW, Makin M. Missed or developmental dislocation of the hip. *Clin Orthop.* 1986;No. 203:276–281.

124. Ingman AM, Paterson DC, Sutherland AD. A comparison between innominate osteotomy and hip spica in the treatment of Legg-Perthes disease. *Clin Orthop.* 1982;No. 163:141.

125. Ingram AJ, Clarke MS, Clarke CS Jr, et al. Chondrolysis complicating slipped capital femoral epiphysis. *Clin Orthop.* 1982;No. 165:99–109.

126. Ippolito E, Mickelson MR, Ponseti IV. A histochemical study of slipped capital femoral epiphysis. *J Bone Joint Surg [Am].* 1981; 63:1109–1113.

127. Ippolito I, Tudisco C, Farsetti P. The long-term prognosis of unilateral Perthes disease. *J Bone Joint Surg [Br].* 1987;69:243.

128. Ishii Y, Weinstein SL, Ponseti IV. Correlation between arthrograms and operative findings in congenital dislocation of the hip. *Clin Orthop.* 1980;No. 153:138–145.

129. Jackson MA, Nelson JD. Etiology and medical management of acute suppurative bone and joint infections in pediatric patients. *J Pediatr Orthop.* 1982;2:313.

130. Jacobs B. Diagnosis and natural history of slipped capital femoral epiphysis. *Instr Course Lect.* 1972;21:167–173.

131. Jerre T. Early complication of osteosytheses with a three flanged nail in situ for slipped epiphysis. *Acta Orthop Scand.* 1958;27:126.

132. Jerre T. *Physiolysis of the Hip: Epidemiology, Diagnosis and Long-term Follow-up* [thesis]. Göteborg, Sweden: Göteborg University; 1995.

133. Jerre T. A study in slipped upper femoral epiphysis with special reference to late functional and roentogenological results and the value of closed reduction. *Acta Orthop Scand Suppl.* 1950;6.

134. Johanning K. Coxa vara infantum: clinical appearance and aetiological problem. *Acta Orthop Scand.* 1951;21:273.

135. Johnson AH, Campbell WG, Callahan BC. Infection of rabbit kneejoints after intra-articular injection of *Staphylococcus aureus*. *Am J Pathol.* 1970;60:165.

136. Johnston RC, Larson CB. Results of treatment of hip disorders with cup arthroplasty. *J Bone Joint Surg [Am].* 1969;51:1461.

137. Jones D. An assessment of the value of examination of the hip in the newborn. *J Bone Joint Surg [Br].* 1977;59:318–322.

138. Jonsater A. Coxa plana: a histopathologic and arthrographic study. *Acta Orthop Scand Suppl.* 1953;12:1.

139. Josimovich J, Mintz Z, Finster J. Estrogenic inhibition of growth hormone-induced tibial epiphyseal growth in hypophysectomized rats. *Endocrinology.* 1967;81:1428.

140. Kalamchi A, MacEwen GD. Avascular necrosis following treatment of congenital dislocation of the hip. *J Bone Joint Surg [Am].* 1980;62:876–888.

141. Kalamchi A, Schmidt TL, MacEwen GD. Congenital dislocation of the hip: open reduction by the medial approach. *Clin Orthop.* 1982;No. 169:127–132.

142. Kallio P, Ryoppy S. Hyperpressure in juvenile hip disease. *Acta Orthop Scand.* 1985;56:211–214.

143. Kallio P, Ryoppy S, Kunnamo I. Transient synovitis and Perthes: is there an etiologic connection? *J Bone Joint Surg [Br].* 1986;68:808–811.

144. Kamegaya M, Shinada Y, Moriya H, et al. Acetabular remodelling in Perthes disease after primary healing. *J Pediatr Orthop.* 1992;12:308.

145. Katz JF. Conservative treatment of Legg–Calvé–Perthes disease. *J Bone Joint Surg [Am].* 1967;49:1043.

146. Katz JF. Nonoperative therapy in Legg–Calvé–Perthes disease. *Orthop Rev.* 1979;8:69.

147. Kelly FP, Canale ST, Jones RR. Legg–Calvé–Perthes disease: long-term evaluation of noncontainment treatment. *J Bone Joint Surg.* 1980;62A:400.

148. Kelsey JL. Epidemiology of slipped capital femoral epiphysis: a review of the literature. *Pediatrics.* 1973;51:1042.

149. Kelsey JL, Acheson RM, Keggi KJ. The body builds of patients with slipped capital femoral epiphyses. *Am J Dis Child.* 1972;124:276–281.

150. Kelsey JL, Keggi KJ, Southwick WO. The incidence and distribution of slipped capital femoral epiphysis in Connecticut and southwestern United States. *J Bone Joint Surg [Am].* 1970;52:1203–1216.

151. Keret D, Harrison MHM, Clarke NMP, et al. Coxa plana: the fate of the physis. *J Bone Joint Surg.* 1984;66A:870–877.

152. Key JA. Epiphyseal coxa vara or displacement of the capital epiphysis of femur in adolescence. *J Bone Joint Surg.* 1926;8:53–117.

153. King EW, Fisher RL, Gage JR, et al. Ambulation-abduction treatment in Legg–Calvé–Perthes disease (LCPD). *Clin Orthop.* 1980; No. 150:43.

154. Kirkwood JR, Ozonoff MB, Dteinbach H. Epiphyseal displacement of the metaphyseal fracture in renal osteodystrophy. *Am J Roentgenol.* 1972;115:547.

155. Klein A, Joplin RJ, Reidy JA, et al. Management of the contralateral hip in slipped capital femoral epiphysis. *J Bone Joint Surg [Am].* 1953;35:81–87.

156. Klisic P, Jankovic L, Basara V. Long-term results of combined operative reduction of the hip in older children. *J Pediatr Orthop.* 1988;8:532–533.

157. Kocher MS, Mandiga R, Zurakowski D, et al. Validation of a clinical prediction rule for the differentiation between septic arthritis and transient synovitis of the hip in children. *J Bone Joint Surg [Am].* 2004;86:1629–1635.

158. Krahn TH, Canale ST, Beaty JH, et al. Long term follow-up of patients with avascular necrosis after treatment of slipped capital femoral epiphysis. *J Pediatr Orthop.* 1993;13:154.

159. Kristmundsdottir F, Burwell RG, Harrison MHM. Delayed skeletal maturation in Perthes' disease. *Acta Orthop Scand.* 1987;58:277–282.

160. Kruse RW, Guille JT, Bowen JR. Shelf arthroplasty in patients who have Legg–Calvé–Perthes disease: a study of long-term results. *J Bone Joint Surg [Am].* 1991;73:1338.

161. Lacroix P, Verbrugge J. Slipping of the upper femoral epiphysis: a pathological study. *J Bone Joint Surg [Am].* 1951;33:371–381.

162. Larson CB. Rating scale for hip disabilities. *Clin Orthop.* 1963; No. 31:85.

163. Larsen FH, Reiman I. Calvé-Perthes disease. *Acta Orthop Scand.* 1973;44:426.

164. Legg AT. An obscure affection of the hip joint. *Boston Med Surg J.* 1910;162:202.

165. Le Mesurier AB. Developmental coxa vara. *J Bone Joint Surg [Br].* 1948;30:595.

166. Lindstrom JR, Ponseti IV, Wenger DR. Acetabular development after reduction in congenital dislocation of the hip. *J Bone Joint Surg [Am].* 1979;61:112.

167. Lippe BM, VanHerle AJ, LaFranchi SH, et al. Reversible hypothyroidism in growth hormone deficient children, treated with human growth hormone. *J Clin Endocrinol Metab.* 1975; 40:613.

168. Liu SL, Ho TC. The role of venous hypertension in the pathogenesis of Legg–Perthes disease: a clinical and experimental study. *J Bone Joint Surg [Am].* 1991;73:194.

169. Lloyd-Roberts GC, Catterall A, Salamon PB. A controlled study of the indications for the results of femoral osteotomy in Perthes' disease. *J Bone Joint Surg [Br].* 1976;58:31.

170. Loder RT, Aronson DD, Dobbs MB, et al. Capital femoral epiphysis. *Instr Course Lect.* 2001;50:555–570.

171. Loder RT, Aronson DD, Greenfield ML. The epidemiology of bilateral slipped capital femoral epiphysis. *J Bone Joint Surg [Am].* 1993;75:1141–1147.

172. Loder RT, Richards BS, Shapiro PS, et al. Acute slipped capital epiphysi: the importance of physeal stability. *J Bone Joint Surg [Am].* 1993;75:134–1140.

173. Lovell WW, Hopper WC, Purvis JM. *The Scottish Rite orthosis for Legg–Perthes disease.* Exhibited at American Academy of Orthopaedic Surgeons meeting; Dallas; 1978.

174. Lucas RC. On a form of late rickets associated with albuminuria: rickets of adolescence. *Lancet.* 1883;1:993.

175. Luhmann SJ, Jones A, Schootman M, et al. Differentiation between septic arthritis and transient synovitis of the hip in children with clinical prediction algorithms. *J Bone Joint Surg [Am].* 2004;86:956–962.

176. MacKenzie IG, Wilson JG. Problems encountered in the early diagnosis and management of congenital dislocation of the hip. *J Bone Joint Surg [Br].* 1981;38:38–42.

177. Magnusson R. Coxa vara infantum. *Acta Orthop Scand.* 1954; 23:284.

178. Malvitz TA, Weinstein SL. Closed reduction for congenital dysplasia of the hip: functional and radiographic results after an average of thirty years. *J Bone Joint Surg [Am].* 1994;76:1777–1792.

179. Mankin HJ. Rickets, osteomalacia and renal osteodystrophy. Part I. *J Bone Joint Surg [Am].* 1974;56:101.

180. Martinez AG, Weinstein SL. Recurrent Legg–Calvé–Perthes disease: case report and review of the literature. *J Bone Joint Surg [Am].* 1991;73:1081.

181. Martinez AG, Weinstein SL, Dietz FR. The weight-bearing abduction brace for the treatment of Legg–Perthes disease. *J Bone Joint Surg [Am]*. 1992;74:12.

182. Maxian TA, Brown TD, Weinstein SL. Chronic stress tolerence levels for human articular cartilage: two non-uniform contact models applied to long term followup of CDH. *J Biomech*. 1995;28:159–166.

183. McAndrew MP, Weinstein SL. A long term follow-up of Legg–Calvé–Perthes disease. *J Bone Joint Surg [Am]*. 1984;66:860.

184. McKibbin B. Recent advances in Perthes' disease. In: *Recent Advances in Orthopaedics*. Vol. 2. Edinburgh: Churchill Livingstone; 1975:173–195.

185. Meehan PL, Angel D, Nelson JM. The Scottish Rite abduction orthosis for the treatment of Legg-Perthes disease: a radiographic analysis. *J Bone Joint Surg [Am]*. 1992;74:2.

186. Meier MC, Meyer LC, Ferguson RL. Treatment of slipped capital femoral epiphysis with a spica cast. *J Bone Joint Surg [Am]*. 1992;74:1522–1529.

187. Melvin P, Johnston R, Ponseti IV. Untreated CDH: long term follUp. *Personal communication*, 1970.

188. Mickelson MR, Ponseti IV, Cooper RR, et al. The ultrastructure of the growth plate in slipped capital femoral epiphysis. *J Bone Joint Surg [Am]*. 1977;59:1076–1081.

189. Milgram JW. Morphology of untreated bilateral congenital dislocation of the hips in a seventy-four-year-old man. *Clin Orthop*. 1976;No. 119:112–115.

190. Moorefield WG, Urbaniak JR, Ogden WS, et al. Acquired hypothyroidism and slipped capital femoral epiphysis. *J Bone Joint Surg [Am]*. 1976;58:705–708.

191. Morey BF, Bianco AJ Jr, Rhodes KH. Septic arthritis in children. *Orthop Clin North Am*. 1975;6:923.

192. Morrissy RT, Haynes DW. Acute hematogenous osteomyelitis: a model with trauma as an etiology. *J Pediatr Orthop*. 1989;9:447.

193. Morrissy RT, Kalderon AE, Gerdes M. Synovial immunofluorescence in patients with slipped capital femoral epiphysis. *J Pediatr Orthop*. 1981;1:55.

194. Morsher E. Strength and morphology of growth cartilage under hormonal influence of puberty: animal experiments and clinical study on the etiology of local growth disorders during puberty. *Reconstr Surg Traumatol*. 1968;10:3–104.

195. Mose K. Methods of measuring in Legg-Calvé-Perthes disease with special regard to the prognosis. *Clin Orthop* 1980;No. 150:103.

196. Muirhead-Allwood W, Catterall A. The treatment of Perthes disease: the results of a trial of management. *J Bone Joint Surg [Br]*. 1982;64:282.

197. Mukamel M, Litmanovitch M, Yosipovich Z, et al. Legg–Calvé–Perthes disease following transient synovitis: how often? *Clin Pediatr*. 1985;24:629.

198. Murray RO. The etiology of primary osteoarthritis of the hip. *Br J Radiol*. 1965;38:810–824.

199. Neyt J, Weinstein SL, Spratt K, et al. Stulberg classification system for evaluation of Legg-Calvé-Perthes' disease: intrarater and interrater reliability. *J Bone Joint Surg [Am]*. 1999;81:1209.

200. Ninomiya S Nagasaka Y, Tagawa H. Slipped capital femoal epiphysis: a study of 68 cases in the eastern half of Japan. *Clin Orthop*. 1976;No. 119:172.

201. Noble TC, Pullan CR, Craft AW, et al. Difficulties in diagnosing and managing congenital dislocation of the hip. *Br Med J*. 1978;2(6137):620–623.

202. O'Brien ET, Fahey JJ. Remodeling of the femoral neck after in situ pinning for slipped capital femoral epiphyses. *J Bone Joint Surg [Am]*. 1977;59:62–68.

203. Ogden JA, Southwick WO. Endocrine dysfunction and slipped capital femoral epiphysis. *Yale J Biol Med*. 1977;50:1–16.

204. Oka M, Miki T, Hama H, et al. The mechanical strength of the growth plate under the influence of sex hormones. *Clin Orthop*. 1979;No. 145:264–272.

205. Olney BW, Asher M. Combined innominate and femoral osteotomy for the treatment of severe Legg-Calvé-Perthes disease. *J Pediatr Orthop*. 1985;5:645.

206. Oram V. Epiphysiolysis of the head of the femur: a follow-up examination with special reference to end results and the social prognosis. *Acta Orthop Scand*. 1953;23:100–120.

207. Ordeberg G. *Physiolysis of the Hip* [dissertation]. Lund, Sweden: University Hospital, Department of Orthopaedic Surgery; April 1986.

208. Ordeberg G, Hansson LI, Sandstrom S. Slipped capital femoral epiphysis in southern Sweden: long-term result with no treatment; symptomatic primary treatment. *Clin Orthop*. 1984;No. 191:95–104.

209. Orofino C, Innis JJ, Lowey CW. Slipped capital femoral epiphysis in Negroes: a study of ninety-five cases. *J Bone Joint Surg [Am]*. 1960;42:1079.

210. Ortolani M. Congenital hip dysplasia in the light of early and very early diagnosis. *Clin Orthop*. 1976;No. 119:6–10.

211. Osborne D, Effmann E, Broda K, et al. The development of the upper end of the femur with special reference to its internal architecture. *Radiology*. 1980;137:71–76.

212. O'Sullivan M, O'Rourke, SK, MacAuley, P. Legg–Calvé–Perthes disease in a family: genetic or environmental. *Clin Orthop*. 1985; No. 199:179.

213. Paterson DC, Leitch JM, Foster BK. Results of innominate osteotomy in the treatment of Legg-Calvé-Perthes disease. *Clin Orthop*. 1991;No. 266:96.

214. Pavlov H, Goldman B, Freiberger RH. Infantile coxa vara. *Pediatr Radiol*. 1980;135:631.

215. Perthes G. Uber Arthritis deformans juvenilis. *Dtsch Z Chir*. 1910;10:111.

216. Peterson CA, Peterson HA. Analysis of the incidences of injury to the epiphyseal growth plate. *J Trauma*. 1972;12:275–281.

217. Petrie JG, Bitenc I. The abduction weight bearing treatment in Legg-Perthes disease. *J Bone Joint Surg [Br]*. 1971;53:54.

218. Moller PF. The clinical observations after healing of Calvé-Perthes disease compared with final deformities left by that disease and the bearing of those final deformities on ultimate prognosis. *Acta Radiol*. 1926;5:1.

219. Ponseti IV. Growth and development of the acetabulum in the normal child: anatomical, histological and roentgenographic studies. *J Bone Joint Surg [Am]*. 1978;60:575.

220. Ponseti IV. Legg-Perthes disease. *J Bone Joint Surg [Am]*. 1956; 38:739.

221. Ponseti IV. Morphology of the acetabulum in congenital dislocation of the hip: gross, histological and roentgenographic studies. *J Bone Joint Surg [Am]*. 1978;60:586–599.

222. Ponseti IV, Barta C. Evaluation and treatmnent of slipping of the capital femoral epiphysis. *Surg Gynecol Obstet*. 1948; 86:87.

223. Ponseti IV, Maynard JA, Weinstein SL, et al. Legg-Calvé-Perthes disease: histochemical and ultrastructural observations of the epiphyseal cartilage and the physis. *J Bone Joint Surg [Am]*. 1983;65:797–807.

224. Ponseti IV, McClintock R. The pathology of slipping of the upper femoral epiphysis. *J Bone Joint Surg [Am]*. 1956;38:71–83.

225. Ponseti IV, Sheppard S. Lesions of the skeleton and other mesodermal tissues in rats fed sweetpea seeds. *J Bone Joint Surg [Am]*. 1954;36:1031.

226. Primiano GA, Hughston JC. Slipped capital femoral epiphysis in a true hypogonadal male (Klinefelter's mosaic XY/XXY). *J Bone Joint Surg [Am]*. 1971;53:597–601.

227. Purvis JM, Dimon JH III, Meehan PL, et al. Preliminary experience with the Scottish Rite Hospital abduction orthosis for Legg-Perthes disease. *Clin Orthop*. 1980;No. 150:49.

228. Pylkkanen PV. Coxa vara infantum. *Acta Orthop Scand*. 1960; Suppl 48:1–120.

229. Rab GT. Determination of femoral head containment during gait. *Biomater Med Devices Artif Organs*. 1983;11:31–38.

230. Rab GT, DeNatale JS, Herrmann LR. Three dimensional finite element analysis of Legg-Calvé-Perthes disease. *J Pediatr Orthop*. 1982;2:39–44.

231. Ralis Z, McKibbin B. Changes in shape of the human hip joint during its development and their relation to its stability. *J Bone Joint Surg [Br]*. 1973;55:780.

232. Ralston EL. Legg-Perthes disease and physical development. *J Bone Joint Surg [Am]*. 1955;37:647.

233. Razzano CD, Nelson C, Eversman J. Growth hormone levels in slipped capital femoral epiphysis. *J Bone Joint Surg [Am]*. 1972;54:1224–1226.

234. Resnick D. The tilt deformity of the femoral head in osteoarthritis of the hip, a poor indicator of previous epiphysiolysis. *Clin Radiol.* 1976;27:355.

235. Robinson HJ Jr, Putter H, Sigmond MB, et al. Innominate osteotomy in Perthes disease. *J Pediatr Orthop.* 1988;8:426.

236. Ross PM, Lyne ED, Morawa LG. Slipped capital femoral epiphysis: long-term results after 10–38 years. *Clin Orthop.* 1979;No. 141:176–180.

237. Salter RB. Experimental and clinical aspects of Perthes' disease. *J Bone Joint Surg [Br].* 1966;48:393.

238. Salter RB. Legg-Perthes disease: the scientific basis for the methods of treatment and their indications. *Clin Orthop.* 1980;No. 150:8.

239. Salter RB. The present status of surgical treatment of Legg-Perthes disease. Current concept review. *J Bone Joint Surg [Am].* 1984;66:961–966.

240. Salter RB, Bell M. The pathogenesis of deformity in Legg-Perthes disease: an experimental investigation. *J Bone Joint Surg [Br].* 1968;50B:436.

241. Salter RB, Thompson GH. Legg–Calvé–Perthes disease: the prognostic significance of the subchondral fracture and a two group classification of the femoral head involvement. *J Bone Joint Surg [Am].* 1984;66:479–489.

242. Schein AJ. Acute severe slipped capital femoral epiphysis. *Clin Orthop.* 1967;No. 51:151–166.

243. Schmidt TL, Kalamchi A. The fate of the capital femoral physis and acetabular development in developmental coxa vara. *J Pediatr Orthop.* 1982;2:534.

244. Segal LS, Weitzel PP, Davidson RS. Valgus slipped capital femoral epiphysis: fact or fiction? *Clin Orthop.* 1996;No. 322:91.

245. Selye H, Ventura J. Effect of hypophysectomy and substitution therapy with STH upon experimental bone lathyrism. *Am J Pathol.* 1957;33:219.

246. Serafin J, Szulc W. Coxa vara infantum, hip growth disturbances, etiopathogenesis and long-term. *Clin Orthop.* 1991;No. 272:103.

247. Shaw BA, Kasser JR. Acute septic arthritis in infancy and childhood. *Clin Orthop.* 1990;No. 257:212.

248. Sherlock DA, Gibson PH, Benson MK. Congenital subluxation of the hip: a long-term review. *J Bone Joint Surg [Br].* 1985;67:390–398.

249. Shmerling RH, Delbanco TL, Tosteson AN, et al. Synovial fluid tests: what should be ordered? *JAMA.* 1990;264:1009.

250. Silberberg M, Silberberg R. Steroid hormone and bone. In: Bourne C, ed. *The Biochemistry and Physiology of Bone.* Vol 3. New York: Academic Press; 1971:401.

251. Skinner SR, Berkheimer GA. Valgus slip of the capital femoral epiphysis. *Clin Orthop.* 1978;No. 135:90–92.

252. Smith RB, Ions GK, Gregg PJ. The radiological features of the metaphysis in Perthes disease. *J Pediatr Orthop.* 1982;2:401.

253. Soeur R. Etiology of pathomechanics of slipped upper femoral epiphysis. *J Bone Joint Surg [Br].* 1959;41:618.

254. Solomon L. Patterns of osteoarthritis of the hip. *J Bone Joint Surg [Br].* 1976;58:176–183.

255. Sorensen KH. Slipped upper femoral epiphysis: clinical study on etiology. *Acta Orthop Scand.* 1968;39:499–517.

256. Sponseller PD, Desai SS, Millis MB. Abnormalities of proximal femoral disease. *J Bone Joint Surg [Br].* 1989;71:610.

257. Sponseller PD, Desai SS, Millis MB. Comparison of femoral and innominate osteotomies for the treatment of Legg-Calvé-Perthes disease. *J Bone Joint Surg [Am].* 1988;70:131.

258. Stanisavljevic S. Diagnosis and treatment of congenital hip pathology in the newborn. In: *Diagnosis and Treatment of Congenital Hip Pathology in the Newborn.* Baltimore: Williams & Wilkins; 1964.

259. Steinberg JJ, Sledge CB. Co-cultivation models of joint destruction. In: Dingle JT, Gordon JL, eds. *Cellular Interactions.* Amsterdam: Elsevier/North-Holland Biomedical Press; 1981:263.

260. Stevens P, Williams P, Menelaus M. Innominate osteotomy for Perthes disease. *J Pediatr Orthop.* 1981;1:47.

261. Strange FGS. *The Hip.* London: William Heinemann; 1965.

262. Struntz P. Epiphysiolysis capitus femoris im Alter von 51 Jahren bei Panhypopitutarismus. *Beitr Orthop Traumatol.* 1972;19:231.

263. Stulberg SD, Cooperman DR, Wallensten R. The natural history of Legg-Calvé-Perthes disease. *J Bone Joint Surg [Am].* 1981;63:1095.

264. Stulberg SD, Cordell LD, Harris WH, et al. Unrecognized childhood hip disease: a major cause of idiopathic osteoarthritis of the hip. In: *The Hip: Proceedings of the Third Open Scientific Meeting of the Hip Society.* St. Louis: CV Mosby, 1975.

265. Stulberg SD, Harris WH. Acetabular dysplasia and development of ostoarthritis of the hip. In: *The Hip: Proceedings of the Second Open Meeting of the Hip Society.* St. Louis: CV Mosby; 1974.

266. Sundt H. Malum coxae Calvé-Legg-Perthes. *Acta Chir Scand Suppl.* 1949;148:1.

267. *Surgeons Advisory Statement: CDH Should Be DDH.* Park Ridge, IL: American Academy of Orthopaedic Surgeons; 1991.

268. Trueta J. The normal vascular anatomy of the human femoral head during growth. *J Bone Joint Surg [Br].* 1957;39:358.

269. Vasseur PB, Foley P, Stevenson S, et al. Mode of inheritance of Perthes disease in Manchester terriers. *Clin Orthop.* 1989;No. 244:281.

270. Visser JD. Functional treatment of congenital dislocation of the hip. *Acta Orthop Scand Suppl.* 1984;206:1–109.

271. von Rosen S. Diagnosis and treatment of congenital dislocation of the hip in the newborn. *J Bone Joint Surg [Br].* 1962;44:284–291.

272. Waldenstrom H. The definitive forms of coxa plana. *Acta Radiol.* 1922;1:384.

273. Waldenstrom H. The first stages of coxa plana. *Acta Orthop Scand.* 1934;5:1.

274. Waldenstrom H. The first stages of coxa plana. *J Bone Joint Surg.* 1938;20:559.

275. Waldenstrom H. Der obere Tuberkulose Collumnerd. *Z Orthop Chir.* 1909;24:487.

276. Waldenstrom H. Slipping of the upper femoral epiphysis. *Surg Gynecol Obstet.* 1940;71:198.

277. Waldenstrom H. *Die Tuberkulose des Collum Femoris im Kindersalte ihre Beziehungen zur Huftgelenkentzundung.* Stockholm; 1910.

278. Walker G. Problems in the early recognition of congenital hip dislocation. *Br Med J.* 1971;3:147.

279. Walker JM. Congenital hip disease in Cree-Ojibwa population: a retrospective study. *Can Med Assoc. J* 1977;116:501.

280. Walters R, Simon S. Joint destruction: a sequel of unrecognized pin penetration in patients with slipped capital femoral epiphyses. In: *The Hip: Proceedings of the Eighth Open Scientific Meeting of the Hip Society.* St. Louis: CV Mosby, 1980:145–164.

281. Wansborough RM, Carrie AW, Walker NF, et al. Coxa plana: its genetic aspects and results of treatment with long Taylor walking caliper. *J Bone Joint Surg [Am].* 1959;41.

282. Wedge JH, Wasylenko MJ. The natural history of congenital dislocation of the hip: a critical review. *Clin Orthop.* 1978;No. 137: 154–162.

283. Wedge JH, Wasylenko MJ. The natural history of congenital disease of the hip. *J Bone Joint Surg [Br].* 1979;61:334–338.

284. Weighill FJ. The treatment of developmental coxa vara by abduction subtrochanteric and intertrochanteric femoral osteotomy with special reference to the role of adductor tenotomy. *Clin Orthop.* 1976;No. 116:116.

285. Weinstein JN, Kuo KN, Miller EA. Congenital coxa vara: a retrospective review. *J Pediatr Orthop.* 1984;4:70.

286. Weinstein SL. Bristol-Myers Squibb/Zimmer award for distinguished achievement in orthopaedic research. Long-term follow-up of pediatric orthopaedic conditions: natural history and outcomes of treatment. *J Bone Joint Surg [Am].* 2000;82: 980–990.

287. Weinstein SL. Closed versus open reduction of congenital hip dislocation in patients under 2 years of age. *Orthopedics.* 1990; 13:221–227.

288. Weinstein SL. Congenital hip dislocation: long-range problems, residual signs, and symptoms after successful treatment. *Clin Orthop.* 1992;No. 281:69–74.

289. Weinstein SL. *Legg-Calvé-Perthes Disease.* St. Louis: CV Mosby; 1983.

290. Weinstein SL. Legg-Perthes disease: results of long-term follow-up. In: *The Hip: Proceedings of the Thirteenth Open Scientific Meeting of the Hip Society.* St. Louis: CV Mosby; 1985:28–37.

291. Weinstein SL. The medial approach in congenital dislocation of the hip. *Isr J Med Sci.* 1980;16:272–275.

292. Weinstein SL. Natural history of congenital hip dislocation [CDH] and hip dysplasia. *Clin Orthop.* 1987;No. 225:62–76.

293. Weinstein SL. The pathogenesis of deformity in Legg–Calvé–Perthes disease. In: Uhthoff H, Wiley J, eds. *Behavior of the Growth Plate*. New York: Raven Press; 1988:379–386.

294. Weinstein SL, Mubarak SJ, Wenger DR. Developmental hip dysplasia and dislocation. Part I. *Instr Course Lect*. 2004;53: 523–530.

295. Weinstein SL, Mubarak SJ, Wenger DR. Developmental hip dysplasia and dislocation. Part II. *Instr Course Lect*. 2004;53:531–542.

296. Weinstein SL, Ponseti IV. Congenital dislocation of the hip: open reduction through a medical approach. *J Bone Joint Surg [Am]*. 1979;61:119.

297. Wenger DR. Selective surgical containment for Legg-Perthes disease: recognition and management of complications. *J Pediatr Orthop*. 1981;1:153–160.

298. Wiberg G. Studies on dysplastic acetabula and congenital subluxation of the hip joint. *Acta Chir Scand*. 1939;83[Suppl 58]:1.

299. Wilkens L. Epiphyseal dysgenesis associated with hypothyroidism. *Am J Dis Child*. 1941;61:13.

300. Willett K, Hudson I, Catterall A. Lateral shelf acetabuloplasty: an operation for older children with Perthes disease. *J Pediatr Orthop*. 1992;12:563.

301. Wilson PD, Jacobs B, Schecter L. Slipped upper femoral epiphysis: an end result study. *J Bone Joint Surg[Am]*. 1965;47:1128–1145.

302. Wingstrand H, Bauer G, Brimar J, et al. Transient ischemia of the proximal femoral epiphysis in the child: interpretation of bone scintimetry for diagnosis in hip pain. *Acta Orthop Scand*. 1985;56:197–203.

303. Wingstrand H, Egund N, Carlin NO, et al. Intracapsular pressure in transient synovitis of the hip. *Acta Orthop Scand*. 1985;56: 204–210.

304. Wynne-Davies R. Acetabular dysplasia and familial joint laxity: two etiological factors in congenital dislocations of the hip. *J Med Genet*. 1970;7:315.

305. Wynne-Davies R. Some etiologic factors in Perthes' disease. *Clin Orthop*. 1980;No. 150:12.

306. Wynne-Davies R, Gormley J. The aetiology of Perthes' disease. *J Bone Joint Surg [Br]*. 1978;60:6.

307. Yamamuro T, Doi H. Diagnosis and treatment of congenital dislocation of the hip in newborns. *J Jpn Orthop Assoc*. 1965;39:492.

308. Yrjonen T. Prognosis in Perthes disease after noncontainment treatment: 106 hips followed for 28–47 years. *Acta Orthop Scand*. 1992;63:522.

309. Zadek I. Congenital coxa vara. *Arch Surg*. 1935;30:62.

310. Zubrow A, Lane J, Parks J. Slipped capital femoral epiphysis occurring during treatment for hypothyroidism. *J Bone Joint Surg [Am]*. 1978;60:256–258.

Systemic Diseases Resulting in Hip Pathology

John W. Barrington   *Paul F. Lachiewicz*

The vast majority of hip replacements are performed for routine rheumatologic conditions, such as osteoarthritis or systemic inflammatory arthritis affecting the hip joint. However, there are several other rheumatologic as well as hematologic, metabolic, endocrine, and congenital conditions that result in sufficient hip joint involvement to require surgical intervention. Although total hip arthroplasty has proven to be an effective treatment for the vast majority of conditions that result in loss of the hip joint cartilage, the surgeon treating patients who have systemic illness involving the hip joint must be cognizant of specific features that may affect clinical decision making and treatment recommendations. Such features may affect the patient's ability to tolerate the surgery required, they may alter the technical requirements of the surgery in specific ways, and they may alter the nontypical natural history of the implanted hip arthroplasty in a specific cohort of patients. This chapter reviews several of the most common conditions with which the hip surgeon should be familiar.

SICKLE-CELL HEMOGLOBINOPATHIES

Osteonecrosis of the femoral head is a frequent and important complication of the sickle-cell hemoglobinopathies, which include sickle-cell anemia (hemoglobin S-S genotype), hemoglobin SC disease, hemoglobin S–β-δ-thalassemia disease, and hemoglobin S–β+-thalassemia disease. Concomitant α–thalassemia, which may modify the course of disease, affects about 30% of patients with sickle-cell anemia (47). Although sickle-cell trait occurs frequently in several populations, it is not definitely associated with osteonecrosis of the femoral head.

Prevalence

In a multicenter study of 2590 patients with a sickle-cell hemoglobinopathy, the prevalence of osteonecrosis of one or both femoral heads was 9.8% (253 patients) (33). Through this 3-year study, the prevalence was 13% in the S–β-δ-thalassemia group of patients, 10% in the hemoglobin S-S group, 8.8% in the hemoglobin S-C group, and 5.8% in the S–β+-thalassemia group. Through this 3-year study, the prevalence of osteonecrosis was 8.9%, with the highest incidence among patients with the hemoglobin S-S genotype and α-thalassemia. The median age at diagnosis was 28 years for patients with the hemoglobin S-S genotype and α-thalassemia, 36 years for those with hemoglobin S-S genotype without α-thalassemia, and 40 years for those with hemoglobin S-C genotype. Bilateral involvement of the femoral head is frequent in the sickle-cell hemoglobinopathies, and it developed in 54% of involved patients in this study.

The natural history of osteonecrosis in sickle-cell disease is one of clinical and radiographic progression. A recent study from one center in France found that of 75 hips in adults without collapse (Steinberg stage I and II) at initial presentation, 65 (87%) demonstrated collapse within 5 years of diagnosis, with an average time between diagnosis and collapse of 42 months for stage I hips, and 30 months for stage II hips (28). In a separate report from this same center, with 15-year average follow-up, 80% of hips with the onset of osteonecrosis during childhood were painful and had decreased mobility, limb-length discrepancy, or an abnormal gait (27).

Pathophysiology

The pathophysiology of osteonecrosis in the sickle-cell hemoglobinopathies remains poorly understood. The initial event is probably necrosis of bone marrow and osteocytes, caused by localized sludging of sickled cells in the marrow sinusoids. The subsequent repair process may lead to healing, especially in younger patients, but it may also produce increased intramedullary pressure and ultimately bone resorption, subchondral fracture, and collapse of the femoral head.

Patients with sickle-cell anemia can also have crises, which are often associated with severe polyarthralgia, and occasionally joint effusion and synovitis may occur. Joint effusion and synovitis result from infarction of the synovium. Rarely, patients with sickle-cell anemia present with an inflammatory arthritis of the hip, with protrusio acetabuli, similar to that seen in patients with rheumatoid arthritis.

Other Organ System Involvement

Osteonecrosis of the femoral head in the sickle-cell hemoglobinopathies is frequently associated with other chronic organ system disease. These patients may develop retinopathy, chronic renal disease, cerebrovascular accidents, acute or chronic pulmonary disease (chest syndrome), congestive heart failure, deep vein thrombosis, gallstones, and splenic infarcts. Patients with sickle-cell disease are susceptible to *Salmonella osteomyelitis* because of a defect in the complement pathway. The increased rate of infection that has been reported after total hip arthroplasty is multifactorial and may be related to functional asplenia, an abnormal immune system, and abnormal intraosseous perfusion. Patients also develop chronic skin ulcers in the lower legs and sloughing of the intestinal mucosa, which lead to recurrent episodes of bacteremia and late hematogenously induced prosthetic hip infection.

Life Expectancy

In considering surgical intervention in patients with sickle-cell hemoglobinopathy, it is important to consider the life expectancy and risk factors for early death. In a multicenter study of 3764 patients, the median age at death was 42 years for men and 48 years for women (58). However, 50% of patients with sickle-cell anemia survived past the fifth decade of life. Among patients with hemoglobin S-C disease, the median age at death was 60 years for men and 68 years for women. Patients with renal failure, acute chest syndrome, seizures, and a low level of fetal hemoglobin were associated with an increased risk of early death.

Imaging

In most studies of osteonecrosis of the femoral head in sickle-cell hemoglobinopathies, femoral head osteonecrosis is staged according to the classification of Ficat as described on plain radiographs. In the multicenter study of 2590 patients mentioned previously, osteonecrosis developed in a subgroup of 135 patients, of whom 47% had stage II disease (sclerosis and radiolucent areas), 30% had stage III disease (subchondral lucent line or collapse), and 23% had stage IV disease (late changes) (47). In this study, almost half the patients (47%) in whom osteonecrosis developed had no pain in the hip or limitation of motion at the time of diagnosis. However, one fifth of these patients later developed symptoms. Magnetic resonance imaging (MRI) can detect stage I disease in patients with sickle-cell hemoglobinopathies (Fig. 31-1) and is recommended when a patient presents with pain in the hip, thigh, or knee, and normal radiographs.

Preoperative Preparation

Complications after operative procedures on the hip in patients with sickle-cell anemia are common, and the rate of postoperative complications has been reported to be as high as 50%. Thus, a thorough preoperative medical and hematologic evaluation is required prior to major hip surgery, especially total hip arthroplasty. The operation should be delayed if the patient has any pulmonary problem or leg ulcers.

To decrease the incidence of complications, preoperative transfusion to a hemoglobin level of 10 g/dL, with or without exchange transfusion to decrease the level of hemoglobin S to less than 30%, is generally recommended. In a multicenter, randomized study of transfusion regimens in 692 surgical procedures (72 orthopedic procedures), and in a follow-up study which included 66 additional orthopaedic procedures, it was found that a conservative transfusion regimen (increasing the hemoglobin level to 10 g/dL) was as effective as an aggressive regimen (decreasing the hemoglobin S level to less than 30%) in preventing perioperative complications (71,72). There were only half as many transfusion-related complications in the conservative transfusion group.

For patients undergoing major hip surgery, including total hip arthroplasty, spinal or epidural anesthesia is recommended to decrease blood loss and lower the incidence of thromboembolism. Good oxygenation and hydration throughout the hospitalization is recommended, along with use of a prophylactic antibiotic and some type of thromboembolism prophylaxis. The authors routinely utilize bilateral thigh-high pneumatic compression devices intraoperatively and after total hip arthroplasty in patients with sickle-cell hemoglobinopathies.

Surgical Treatment

Core Decompression

Core decompression has been suggested for the treatment of Ficat stage I (normal radiograph, abnormal MRI scan) and

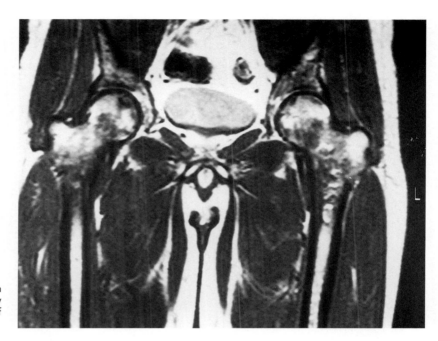

Figure 31-1 An MRI scan of a 32-year-old man with sickle-cell β-thalassemia hemoglobinopathy and left hip pain confirms the diagnosis of osteonecrosis of both hips.

early Ficat stage II idiopathic osteonecrosis of the femoral head. However, few reports of this procedure have included patients with sickle-cell disease, and there is no report of the outcome of core decompression in these patients separately. It has been suggested that the relatively young age of patients with sickle-cell disease and osteonecrosis, along with the greater vascularity of the cancellous bone, may make them reasonable candidates for early intervention with core decompression. One report recommended core decompression for relief of chronic hip pain in a series of 13 hips in ten young patients with a mean age of 15 years (range 9 to 21 years) and a mean follow-up time of 3.7 years. Ten of 11 hips without col-

lapse had improvement in pain, and only three had radiographic progression. Both patients with hips had radiographic progression (65). In another report, core decompression was performed in three patients with early stage II osteonecrosis without collapse, but no patient had relief of pain and all required arthroplasty within 1 year (11). The senior author's personal experience includes four core decompressions in patients with sickle-cell anemia. Two patients with severe pain in the hip and stage I osteonecrosis had complete relief of pain and no progression of osteonecrosis, one at 5 years and the other at 7 years (Figs. 31-2 and 31-3). Two other patients, both with subchondral lucency (early stage III)

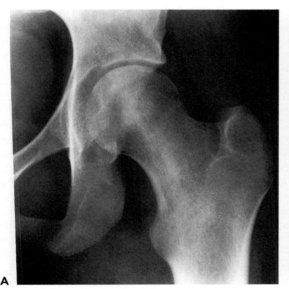
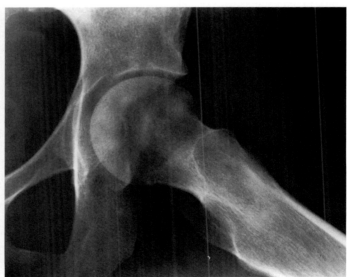

A   B

Figure 31-2 The anteroposterior (AP) **(A)** and lateral **(B)** radiographs of a 22-year-old woman with sickle-cell anemia and left hip pain show stage II osteonecrosis. The diagnosis was confirmed by MRI scan and histologic examination.

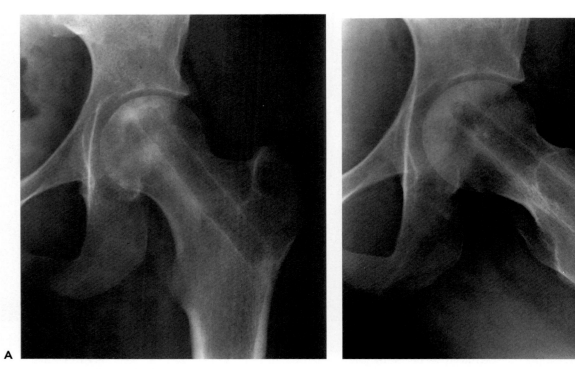

A   **B**

Figure 31-3   The AP **(A)** and lateral **(B)** radiographs 3 years after core decompression. Patient has no pain in the hip and there has been no radiographic progression.

had only some relief of pain, but they have not yet undergone total hip arthroplasty. Longer-term follow-up studies will be required to determine if core decompression truly changes the natural history of the osteonecrosis associated with sickle-cell disease.

Cementation

An alternative new surgical treatment for hips with stage III osteonecrosis has been described in a study from France (27). In 16 hips in ten patients with sickle-cell hemoglobinopathies, the necrotic bone and articular cartilage overlying it were elevated and then injected with low-viscosity acrylic cement to restore the sphericity of the femoral head. At a follow-up time of 3 to 7 years (mean 5 years), two hips had required arthroplasty, one at 1 year and the other at 2 years, but 14 hips were improved. However, some of these patients have pain with walking, or after prolonged activity and limited abduction, with worsening radiographs, indicating that progressive arthritis is present. Further follow-ups from this group and other centers are required before this technique can be recommended.

Prosthetic Hip Resurfacing

Resurfacing of only the osteonecrotic femoral head before acetabular cartilage degeneration has occurred seems an attractive and conservative procedure. Although hemiresurfacing has been successful in short- and medium-term follow-up for osteonecrosis associated with other disorders, it has not been successful in sickle-cell disease. One study reported failure of all four hemiresurfacing procedures in sickle-cell patients (52). One case report described severe protrusio, at only 2 years postoperatively, following hemiresurfacing in a sickle-cell patient (7).

Total Hip Arthroplasty

There is a high prevalence of postoperative complications and a very high rate of failure of all types of hip arthroplasties in patients with sickle-cell hemoglobinopathies. The data in the nine published studies (2,4,9,11,22,24,30,32,50) is summarized in Table 31-1. The prevalence of postoperative complications in these studies ranges from 17% to 100%, with excessive blood loss, sickle-cell crises, wound drainage, and hematoma frequently reported. Hospitalization is prolonged in most studies. One report described difficulty in preparing the femur, which had sclerotic bone and obliteration of the medullary canal and resulted in the intraoperative complication of three perforations and four femoral fractures (11). The rate of infection is very high, 16% to 20% in several studies, probably due to the high incidence of bacteremia. There is a very high rate of failure caused by loosening of all types of hip arthroplasties, ranging from 38% at 5 years to a 50% rate of revision at 10 years. In one series of 13 hips with cemented components, nearly all failed, at a mean follow-up time of 43 months (11). The results with uncemented components were much better, but the follow-up time was only 2 years. In the previously discussed multicenter study of osteonecrosis, 27 patients had a hip arthroplasty, and the probability of survival was only 70% at 4.5 years (47). The senior author has reported 16 primary and revision arthroplasties in these patients, with no early or late infections at a mean follow-up time of 6 years (30). Two young active men had severe polyethylene liner wear with osteolysis requiring reoperation at 7 and 10 years, respectively (Figs. 31-4 and 31-5). Overall, the result was excellent in 9 hips, good in 4, and poor in 2, with 5 hips (33%) requiring reoperation during the follow-up period. One recent study reported the results of 36 bilateral, one-stage bipolar arthroplasties using small

TABLE 31-1
RESULTS OF TOTAL HIP ARTHROPLASTY IN SICKLE-CELL ANEMIA

Author (Year)	Number of Hips (Patients)	Patient Age (Yrs)	Follow-up Time (Yrs)	Early Complications	Infection	Revision or Loosening of Components
Gunderson et al. (1977)	11 (7)	13–26	Not specified	27% (2 fractures of the femur)	0	Not specified
Bishop et al. (1988)	13 primary (11) 4 revision (4)	16–47 (mean 31)	3–13 (mean 7.5)	Not specified	23% [3 of 11 primary (2 early), 1 of 4 revisions]	8% (1 acetabulum at 9 years)
Hanker and Amstutz (1988)[a]	9 primary THR 2 surface replace 2 revision 5 resection 1 arthrodesis	Mean, 32	2–26 (mean 6.5)	100% (including 5 crises and excessive) bleeding	2	50% by 5.4 yrs postoperative
Clarke et al. (1989)	27 (15) 17 primary 10 revision	19–56 (mean, 33)	Minimum 2 yrs. (17 hips)	Femur fracture, 4 crises, 2	0	Femoral 24%, acetabulum 24%[b]
Acurio et al. (1992)	35 (25) 20 THR 11 bipolar 2 Austin-Moore 2 cup	16–45 (mean, 30)	2–18 (mean, 8.6)	49%	20% (10% for THR)	50% revision at 10 yrs
Moran et al. 1993)	22 (14) 15 primary 7 revisions	17–58 (mean, 37); primary; 27–56 (mean, 39) revision	Primary mean, 4.8; revision mean, 5.3	14 in primary cases, 12 in revision cases	8%	31% aseptic failure of primary, 43% failure of revision group
Hickman and Lachiewicz (1997)	15 (10) 8 primary 7 revisions	21–50 (mean 40)	2–12 (mean 6)	75% (including 5 excessive bleeding)	0	20% (2 osteolysis 1 acetabulum at 11 years)
Al-Mousawi et al. (2002)	35 (28)	19–42 (mean 27.5)	5–15 (mean 9.5)	31% (6 crises, 2 excessive bleeding 3 femoral perforations	0 early 1 at 10 yrs	17%
Ilyas and Moreau (2002)	36 (18) all uncemented bipolars	17–39 (mean	2–10 (mean 5.7)	17%	2 (1 deep, 1 superficial)	6%

THR, total hip replacement.
[a]Study included three patients with sickle-cell trait.
[b]Nine of 10 revisions were of loose cemented components.

uncemented femoral components. At a mean follow-up time of 5.7 years, there was no femoral component loosening, but two complications (protrusio; instability) related to the bipolar shell (32). At the present time, cementless components are strongly recommended for all primary and revision total hip arthroplasties in patients with sickle-cell hemoglobinopathies.

GAUCHER'S DISEASE

Gaucher's disease is an autosomal, recessively inherited, systemic lysosomal storage disorder, characterized by the accumulation of glucocerebroside (a complex lipid) in reticuloendothelial cells. Gaucher cell infiltration causes hepatosplenomegaly, pancytopenia, and involvement of bone. There are three forms of the disease, all caused by a genetically induced relative deficiency of glucocerebrosidase. The most common form, type I, spares the central nervous system, is most prevalent among Ashkenazi Jews, and features slow but progressive visceral or bone involvement. The skeletal manifestations of Gaucher's disease are variable and may include osteopenia, fractures, and progressive osteonecrosis of the femoral head (35). MRI demonstrates more extensive involvement of the lower-extremity skeleton than seen on plain radiographs or computed

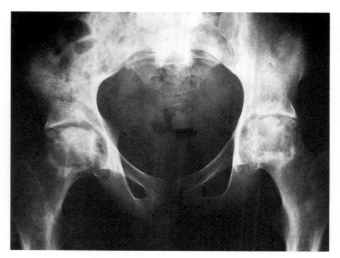

Figure 31-4 Preoperative AP radiograph of the pelvis of a 21-year-old man with sickle-cell disease and endstage osteonecrosis of both femoral heads. Bilateral uncemented total hip arthroplasties were performed for severe pain and disability.

tomography. In one study of 24 patients, MRI showed Gaucher's disease involvement in 15 of 18 femoral heads that were scanned, but only 4 patients had osteonecrosis seen on plain radiographs (62).

In two small series of patients with Gaucher's disease who had total hip arthroplasties, increased intraoperative and postoperative bleeding was often seen (39). There was a high rate

(46%) of aseptic loosening of the cemented components, but no early or late infections in these series. In one study of 15 cemented hips in 8 patients followed for a mean of 7.3 years, 27% of the hips had been revised for loosening (19). One recent multicenter study evaluated 29 total hip arthroplasties in 23 Israeli patients with Gaucher's disease (41). There were 20 primary arthroplasties (mean follow-up time 8.2 years) and 9 revisions (follow-up time not specified). A wide variety of cemented and cementless components were implanted. There was great improvement in pain, quality of life, and function after the primary arthroplasties as determined by a patient questionnaire. The results were not as good after revision. Radiographic loosening was seen in at least 21% of the primary components and 55% of the revision components. There were no hemolytic complications and no early infections. The authors recommended total hip arthroplasty for hip pain and disability associated with Gaucher's disease. There is not enough data to recommend one type of fixation over another.

OCHRONOSIS

Ochronosis, named by Virchow in 1866 from the Greek words ωχρος (yellow, from the color of pigment viewed under the microscope) and νοσος (disease), results from the accumulation of oxidized homogentisic acid in the connective tissues (Fig. 31-6) (54). This accumulation is secondary to alcaptonuria, a rare disorder of tyrosine metabolism resulting in the accumulation and excretion in the urine of large amounts of homogentisic acid. The disease often goes unrecognized until middle life,

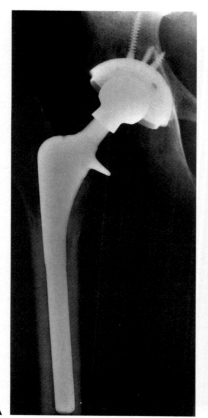
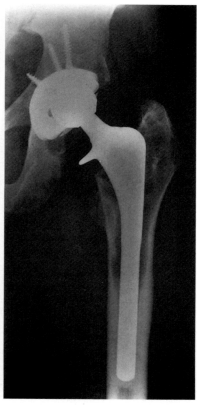

A   B

Figure 31-5 **A:** Ten-year postoperative radiograph of the right hip shows good fixation and no osteolysis. **B:** Ten-year postoperative radiograph of the left hip shows pelvic osteolysis (in ischium) and extensive femoral osteolysis. Patient was asymptomatic, but revision of polyethylene liner and femoral component with bone grafting was performed.

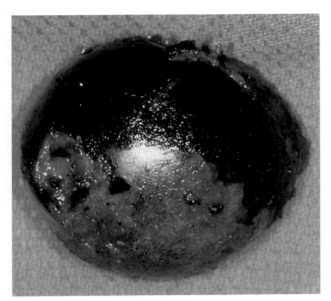

Figure 31-6 Femoral head specimen from patient with ochronosis showing characteristic pigmentation. See Color Plate.

when ochronotic arthritis appears in a majority of the patients, beginning in the fourth decade with back pain and followed in the ensuing 10 years by involvement of the knees and later the shoulders and hips (54). Prior to modern plumbing, darkening of standing urine was often the presenting sign. Discoloration of the sclera and external ears occurs in midlife. Screening tests for homogentisic acid in the urine include reaction with ferric chloride, Benedict's reagent, or saturated silver nitrate and can be confirmed by chromatographic, enzymatic, or spectrophotometric determinations of homogentisic acid (61).

Radiographically, ochronotic arthropathy may be difficult to differentiate from ankylosing spondylitis (34,40). Spinal abnormalities suggestive of ochronosis include dense calcification of the discs with narrowing of the intervertebral space. Radiographically, the involvement of the hip is similar to atrophic osteoarthritis, with generalized cartilage loss and little reactive bone formation (Fig. 31-7) (67). Often there are striking calcifications in adjacent tendons. In a review of the literature, 62 cases of knee involvement and 33 cases of hip involvement were found in the 84 reported cases of ochronotic arthropathy (54). The knees were much more likely to be affected in male patients, but the sex distribution was about equal for the hip. Ochronotic arthropathy can be confirmed with needle biopsy (43). Prior to proceeding with total hip arthroplasty in these patients, cardiac evaluation of any murmurs is recommended. The cervical spine should also be evaluated, as the cervical cord may be at risk for compression from alcaptonuric spondyloarthropathy (38).

HEMOCHROMATOSIS

Hemochromatosis is an iron storage disorder in which excessive intestinal iron absorption results in parenchymal deposition of iron, with eventual organ damage. Signs and symptoms include skin pigmentation, diabetes, liver and cardiac impairment, hypogonadism, and arthropathy. Arthropathy develops in 25% to 50% of the patients, most commonly after the age of 50 (59). The small joints of the hand are usually the first to be involved, but a progressive polyarthritis involving all joints may ensue. In one study of 25 patients with hemochromatosis, 6 were found to have severe hip disease (15). The hip is the most frequently involved large joint; radiographically it appears similar to osteoarthritis. Additionally, there may be chondrocalcinosis and the presence of a subchondral radiolucent wedge (6). The histopathologic evaluation of 19 resected femoral heads with this disorder showed articular cartilage avulsion from the tidemark in 42%, primary or secondary osteonecrosis in 37%, and calcium pyrophosphate deposition in 26% (49). The combined measurements of percent transferrin saturation and

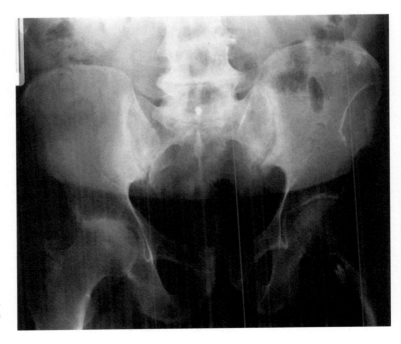

Figure 31-7 The AP pelvis radiographic of a 58-year-old man with ochronosis and hip arthritis. There is also narrowing of multiple intervertebral disc spaces.

serum ferritin levels provide the simplest and most reliable screening tests for the precirrhotic phase of this disease (59). If either test is abnormal, a liver biopsy should be performed. Treatment of hemochromatosis involves removal of excess body iron and support of damaged organs. The life expectancy of untreated patients averages 4.4 years from the time of diagnosis. With treatment, the 5-year survival rate is increased from 33% to 89% (59). Infection with *Yersinia enterocolitica* is a recognized complication of hemochromatosis (15), and prophylaxis with gentamicin or ciprofloxacin should be considered prior to proceeding with hip arthroplasty. In one report of 19 total hip arthroplasties in 15 patients with hemochromatosis, there was no hip pain and improvement in function in 14 patients (49). One patient was nonambulatory due to cemented acetabular component loosening at 10 years. The use of cemented or cementless components should be based on patient age and activity level rather than the pathologic diagnosis.

ACROMEGALY

The clinical syndrome of acromegaly is the result of increased circulating growth hormone in a skeletally mature person. It is usually caused by a pituitary adenoma. The hands, feet, and facial features usually enlarge. In acromegalic arthropathy, which commonly affects the hips, cartilage hypertrophy and hyperplasia initially lead to a distortion of joint geometry and subsequently to a degenerative arthritis similar to primary osteoarthritis. Radiographic widening of the joint space as a result of cartilage hypertrophy is seen early in the course of the disorder. In one report, the patients demonstrated an unusual proboscislike medial osteophyte on the femoral heads, irregular pitting of subchondral bone, osteopenia, and moderate synovial inflammation (33). These pathologic findings suggest that this is a peculiar arthropathy distinct from osteoarthritis. Other than the hips, commonly involved joints are the shoulders, knees, hands, and elbows.

Treatment of acromegaly usually involves treatment of the pituitary tumor by surgical ablation or irradiation. However, this treatment has little effect on the acromegalic arthropathy, which is treated by modalities used in primary osteoarthritis. There is one report of 11 cemented total hip arthroplasties performed in six acromegalic patients with a mean age of 60 years (33). At follow-ups of 1 to 9 years (mean 5.5 years), ten hip arthroplasties had been successful, and one required revision for a broken Mueller femoral component at 5 years. Because of the unusual presence of a large femoral medullary canal and relative osteopenia, a cemented femoral component is recommended.

HEMOPHILIA

Etiology

Clotting disorders result from abnormalities in either the vascular, platelet, or plasma phases of the clotting process. This is complicated by overlap between these three phases. Besides vessel constriction, the vascular phase involves the exposure of tissue elements that promote platelet activation and activate both the extrinsic and intrinsic plasma phases of the clotting process. The majority of musculoskeletal pathology is caused

by X-linked deficiency of factor VIII (classic hemophilia or hemophilia A) or factor IX (Christmas factor or hemophilia B). Repeated hemarthroses lead to synovial hypertrophy, chronic synovitis, cartilage degradation, and eventual arthropathy. The other 11 known plasma coagulation factors may be deficient or absent, but they rarely cause joint hemorrhage without associated trauma (21). Von Willebrand factor, a protein produced by endothelial cells and megakaryocytes, promotes platelet adhesion and serves as a plasma carrier for factor VIII. Factor VIII–related Von Willebrand factor deficiency accounts for less than 1% of hip arthropathy. In a review of 270 hemophiliac patients with orthopedic problems admitted at one center, 236 patients had factor VIII deficiency, 32 patients had factor IX deficiency, and only 2 patients had Von Willebrand's disease (1 of whom required a total hip replacement) (14).

Radiographic Findings

One study reviewed the pelvic radiographs of 34 patients (64 hips) from a population of 175 hemophiliac patients complaining of hip pain (68). Of the hips with an open proximal femoral epiphysis, 80% had a valgus deformity, but none had osteoarthritic changes. Of the skeletally mature hips, 15% had degenerative changes, including protrusio acetabuli in eight hips.

Nonsurgical Management

All joint hemorrhages must be treated with replacement of the deficient clotting factor to a level sufficiently high to stop the hemorrhage. Bed rest is occasionally indicated, but the patient should be encouraged to return to activities as soon as possible. Aspiration has been advocated by some treatment centers but may not be necessary if replacement is instituted quickly. Indications for aspiration include a tense painful joint that does not respond to factor replacement, and pain out of proportion to physical or clinical evaluation, at which point joint sepsis is suspected (especially in the setting of elevated temperature). The two greatest risks to the hip joint in a hemophiliac patient are avascular necrosis and a septic joint, especially in patients who are human immunodeficiency virus (HIV) positive (16).

Surgical Treatment

The chronic synovitis seen in the ankle, knee, and elbow is rarely diagnosed at an early stage in the hip, and therefore hip synovectomy is rarely performed.

Arthroscopic treatment for a wide variety of synovial disorders and loose bodies of the hip has been advocated, but there are no reported results (to our knowledge) of hip arthroscopy for hemophilic synovitis (37).

As a valgus deformity is commonly seen with hemophiliac arthropathy of the hip, a varus osteotomy has been recommended. In one study of 11 varus osteotomies in nine hemophiliac patients with recurrent hemarthrosis and coxa valga, there was clinical improvement in 7 hips (64%), but radiographic progression in 6 hips (55%) at a mean follow-up time of 15 years (74). This procedure could be considered in very young hemophilia patients with coxa valga and no or minimal radiographic arthropathy.

Surgical management of the hemophiliac hip is usually reserved for endstage disease requiring hip arthroplasty. There have been only two published reports with more than 20 patients and more than 5 years of follow-up, of total hip arthroplasty in hemophiliac patients. In one report of 34 hips performed in 27 male patients (at four major hemophilia centers) at a mean follow-up time of 8 years, there was definite or probable loosening of 42% of the cemented femoral components and 65% of the cemented acetabular components (36). There were no revisions and no radiographic loosening of the 7 uncemented hips, but this population had a mean follow-up of only 2.8 years. Complication rates were high for the cemented hips, with 3 hips requiring a resection arthroplasty for infection and a 20% rate of revision for aseptic loosening. Four hips had postoperative bleeding, one hip had anemia, one a deep vein thrombosis, and one developed an inhibitor, but there were no early infections. The other report involved 22 total hip arthroplasties performed at the Oxford Hemophilia Center in 21 patients who had hemophilic arthropathy (53). At a median follow-up of 7.6 years, 5 of the 22 hips had been revised and 3 additional hips had definite radiographic loosening, for a total rate of mechanical failure of 36%. The long-term results of 13 cemented Charnley total hip arthroplasties performed in 11 patients in Malmo have been reported (44). At a mean follow-up time of 10 years (range 6 to 13 years), there had been four revisions: two for loosening and two for late hematogenous infection. Radiographic loosening has been high, seen in six acetabular components and three femoral components.

The possible causes for the high failure rate of the cemented hip arthroplasties include the young age and high activity levels of the patients, the possibility of suboptimal cement technique, the possibility of microhemorrhages at the bone cement interface, and, finally, excessive stress on the hip joint because of involvement of the other lower extremity joints.

Preoperative Preparation

It is generally recommended that total joint arthroplasty in hemophiliac patients should be performed in major centers with experience in managing these patients. By definition, a unit of factor VIII is the activity of factor VIII in 1 mL of fresh-frozen plasma. For a kilogram of body weight, each unit of factor VIII infused will produce a 2% increase in plasma factor VIII level (20). The factor VIII level should be 100% prior to and during surgery, and it should be maintained after surgery at 75% to 100% by continuous infusion for days 1 through 5, at 50% to 74% for days 6 through 10, and at 25% to 49% for days 11 through 15. Patients with inhibitors are resistant to conventional replacement therapy. The severity of the patient's inhibitor status is defined by the number of Bethesda units per milliliter of plasma (12). Inhibitor levels of more than 20 Bethesda units/mL were previously considered a contraindication to surgery. Recent techniques to overwhelm the inhibitor in these severe cases allow surgery to be performed, but the cost is extremely high.

In addition to thorough preoperative medical preparation of the patient, considerable surgical preparation is also required. Depending on the age at which significant bleeding began, the proximal anatomy of the femur can be distorted, and, in the most severe cases, there can be an extremely small femoral medullary canal, valgus and excessive anteversion of the head and neck, and protrusio acetabuli (Fig. 31-8).

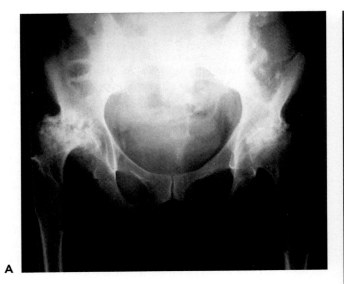
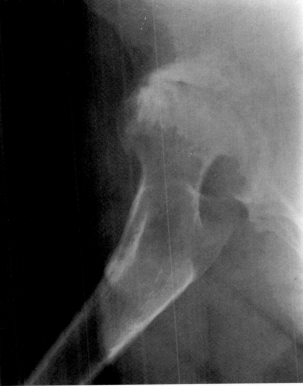

Figure 31-8 The AP pelvis **(A)** and lateral **(B)** radiographs of a 35-year-old man with hemophiliac arthropathy of both hips and valgus deformity of the right femur.

Because the results of cemented hip arthroplasty are poor, prosthetic choice should be directed toward uncemented systems, which require careful preoperative sizing or possibly a custom prosthesis.

Acquired Immunodeficiency Syndrome

Studies from several hemophilia centers suggest that 33% to 92% of persons with hemophilia A and 14% to 52% of persons with hemophilia B have the HIV antibody (63). In the two studies of hip arthroplasty for hemophilic arthropathy, approximately 50% of the patients were known to be seropositive for HIV, contributing to an overall mortality rate at median 7-year follow-up of 20% to 33% (36,53). Patients with CD4 levels of greater than 500, a positive reaction with anergy testing to intradermal skin antigens, platelet count greater than 60,000, absolute leukocyte count greater than 1000, serum albumin greater than 25 g/L, and no history of opportunistic infections or neoplasm have a postoperative complication risk similar to the general population. A surgical rating system has been developed to assist in surgical risk decision making (20,60).

BONE DYSPLASIA

Osteogenesis Imperfecta

Osteogenesis imperfecta is a variably inherited defect in type I collagen cross-linking and secretion which leads to bone fragility, short stature, scoliosis, and ligamentous laxity. Hip pathology in patients with the various types of osteogenesis imperfecta may be related to osteoporosis, fractures, nonunions, or protrusio acetabuli. Because of the increasing life expectancy of these patients, osteoarthritis of the hip and knee may develop in adults who can ambulate. Four cemented total hip arthroplasties have been reported to have a successful clinical (no pain) and radiographic (no loosening) result at a mean follow-up time of 7 years (55). One cemented bipolar arthroplasty had progressive intrapelvic migration, and a resection arthroplasty was required. Total hip arthroplasty in these patients is challenging because of the distorted anatomy, with protrusio acetabuli (seen in approximately 33% of patients [73]) that may require grafting, a small distorted proximal femur, and anterolateral bowing of the femur (seen in 46% to 86% of patients). Cemented, possibly custom-made, components should be considered. There are no reports of cementless components for this disorder. Bipolar components are not recommended.

Diastrophic Dysplasia

This is a rare autosomal recessive skeletal dysplasia characterized by short stature, club feet, scoliosis, and flexion contractures of the hips and knees. Because of the dysplasia and abnormal articular cartilage of the hip joint, arthritis develops in these individuals in early middle age. The disorder is more common in Finland, where the largest series of total hip arthroplasties in diastrophic dysplasia was first reported in 1992 (56), and again in 2003 (26). Forty-one cementless total hip arthroplasties were performed in 24 patients with a

mean age of 37 years. Two patients previously had cemented arthroplasties, and these components had loosened 2 to 3 years after the index procedures. These procedures were technically challenging because of the small medullary canal of the femur, severe anterior bowing in eight femurs (requiring an osteotomy in three), deficient acetabular bone stock (requiring bulk autograft in three), and contractures of the hip flexors and adductors (requiring releases in ten). At a mean follow-up time of 5 years, 11 hips were pain free, 2 had slight pain, and 2 had progressive pain due to loosening of components. However, there was migration of 7 of 15 acetabular components, but most of these were a threaded-ring design. Complications included two femoral nerve palsies and two intraoperative fractures of the femur. In the second report with a mean follow-up of 7.8 years, acetabular loosening was seen in an additional five hips (12%), and there had been no aseptic failures of the femur (26). Careful preoperative planning is necessary for these cases, and nonstandard or custom-made femoral components (31), as well as shortening femoral osteotomy and/or adductor and flexor tenotomies, should be strongly considered because of the size and shape of the femur and long-standing contractures in this dysplasia.

Multiple Epiphyseal Dysplasia and Spondyloepiphyseal Dysplasia

Multiple epiphyseal dysplasia is one of the most common osteochondrodysplasias, usually transmitted as an autosomal dominant trait. It varies widely in severity. The hips are frequently involved most severely, with coxa vara, subluxation, and premature arthritis. Acetabular changes, ranging from severe dysplasia to protrusio acetabuli may be seen (Fig. 31-9). Osteonecrosis of the femoral head may also occur, usually unilaterally, and may result in asymmetric hip disease. Given their similarity, care must be taken to prevent misdiagnosing bilateral Perthes disease rather than late-presenting epiphyseal dysplasia (29). Spondyloepiphyseal dysplasia, existing in both autosomal dominant and X-linked recessive forms, is a group of disorders with dwarfism and involvement of the spine (scoliosis or kyphoscoliosis), knees, feet, and hips. Severe coxa vara, subluxation, and premature arthritis also develop.

In a review of the Mayo Clinic experience with total hip arthroplasty in short-statured people, 14 arthroplasties were in patients with multiple epiphyseal dysplasia and 10 were in patients with spondyloepiphyseal dysplasia (57). There was a high number of complications and there was a high rate of failure. The mean age of the patients was 37 years. The rate of revision was 41% at a mean follow-up time of almost 9 years, but this was thought to result from less-than-optimal prosthesis sizes and cement technique. Miniature Charnley components were most frequently used. Ten uncemented or custom components were used, but the follow-up time was too short to make any strong recommendations concerning the optimum method of fixation.

Periacetabular osteotomy has been recently recommended for a wide variety of hip disorders, including congenital dysplasia, Perthes disease, and epiphyseal dysplasia (70). This osteotomy has been performed in three patients with epiphyseal dysplasia, with good results reported with minimum 2-year follow-up.

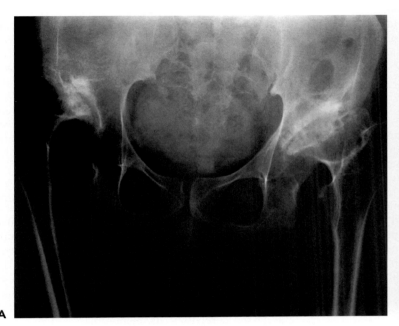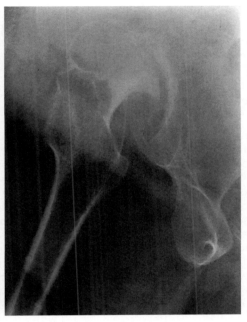

Figure 31-9 The AP pelvis **(A)** and lateral **(B)** radiographs of a 33-year-old man with spondyloepiphyseal dysplasia showing asymmetric hip arthritis. There is a high dislocation of the right hip and severe dysplasia of the left hip.

RENAL FAILURE AND TRANSPLANTATION

Patients with chronic renal failure who are being treated with hemodialysis or chronic ambulatory peritoneal dialysis usually have severe renal osteodystrophy from hyperparathyroidism, osteomalacia, and amyloid deposition. These patients have been reported to have a greater than fourfold risk of hip fracture (3). In reports of total hip arthroplasties placed with modern cement techniques and prostheses, there has been a high rate of deep infection and early loosening of components in patients who continue to receive chronic dialysis. In one retrospective multicenter study of 16 hip arthroplasties in 11 patients who were on chronic dialysis, there was a 45% mortality at a mean follow-up time of only 55 months (42). All but 1 hip had cemented components. Complications were high, including three deep infections (19%), two recurrent dislocations, and one femoral fracture. Ten femoral components were possibly or definitely loose, and 12 acetabular components were possibly or definitely loose.

In another study, from Japan, of a variety of hip arthroplasties in 15 patients on chronic hemodialysis, there was a 35% rate of failure caused by loosening of cemented components (51). Loosening is probably related to osteomalacia and bone resorption at the bone–cement interface. Uncemented components may be a better choice for patients on chronic dialysis.

In another retrospective review of 24 hip arthroplasties performed in 15 patients on chronic renal dialysis, there was a high rate of mechanical loosening (58%) at a mean follow-up time of 8 years (69). There was a high rate of medical complications (66%), and 6 patients (40%) died within an average of

3 years after the index procedure. The results of cementless components were encouraging at short-term (3 to 7 years) follow-up in this report.

Although all reports of total hip arthroplasty in renal dialysis patients emphasize the high perioperative mortality, most recommend the procedure for pain relief and the lack of a better alternative. However, one study reported an in-hospital mortality of 29% (4 of 14 patients) and questioned whether any joint arthroplasty should be performed in these patients (66). A comprehensive registry (United States Renal Data System) has allowed accurate tracking of morbidity and mortality. Of 375,857 patients in the 2000 registry, the mortality after total hip arthroplasty was 0.25% at 30 days and 30% at three years, and this was similar to the overall expected mortality in this population (1).

The early results of cemented total hip arthroplasty for osteonecrosis after renal transplantation were encouraging. However, with longer follow-up, the results in this patient population were less satisfactory because of loosening at the bone–cement interface. In one study of 24 cemented total hip arthroplasties followed for a mean of 86 months, 6 (25%) failed as a result of aseptic loosening (13). There was a high prevalence of dislocation. Iliac crest biopsies of these patients showed high-turnover osteoporosis and hyperosteoidosis, which probably contributed to the high failure rate. However, a 10-year minimum follow-up study of 76 cemented total hip arthroplasties in 50 patients with osteonecrosis following renal transplantation reported a 78% (±11%) survival at 10 years (10). The rate of infection was low (1.3%) despite the use of immunosuppression, but the rate of dislocation was high (16%). The revision-free survival of the cemented implants was longer than the life expectancy of these patients with renal transplants. Uncemented porous-coated total hip arthroplasties may be preferable in this patient population. In one study of 27 cementless hips, all patients had good or excellent hip ratings at a mean of 48 months after surgery (5). In another study, 94% of 53 uncemented total hip arthroplasties were stable at 5 to 8 years (10).

PSORIASIS

Chronic inflammatory arthritis affects less than 10% of patients with psoriasis. Endstage involvement requiring hip surgery in this population is most often due to osteoarthritis with concurrent psoriasis. The most significant question regarding orthopedic procedures in patients with psoriasis is the rate of infection. The use of perioperative antibiotics, previous surgery, diagnosis of rheumatoid arthritis, and the use of corticosteroids are factors that need to be addressed when studying the results of arthroplasty in these patients. There is only one study of hip arthroplasty in patients with psoriasis, reporting 38 patients with 55 Charnley total hip arthroplasties (46). The rate of superficial infection was 9.1% and the rate of deep infection was 5.5%. These arthroplasties were performed in a laminar air enclosure without prophylactic antibiotic therapy. None of these patients had classic psoriatic arthritis, and 11 patients were taking steroids at the time of surgery. Because the organisms were *Staphylococcus aureus*, *Staphylococcus epidermidis*, and *Proteus*, it is unclear what role the lack of preoperative antibiotics may have played in these patients. It is difficult to draw conclusions from studies of total joint arthroplasties in these patients because of the low numbers of patients and extenuating factors (e.g., steroids, lack of preoperative antibiotics, rheumatoid arthritis) (8,46,64). Psoriatic lesions harbor a higher bacterial count than normal skin (18), but routine preoperative skin preparation and perioperative antibiotics appear to be adequate in reducing, if not preventing, infection in these patients (8). Nevertheless, it would seem prudent to obtain a dermatologic consultation for control of the psoriatic lesions in the vicinity of the elective incision prior to proceeding with surgery.

DIABETES MELLITUS

Diabetes mellitus is a common disorder that affects virtually every organ system. Many medical problems of diabetic patients are attributed to involvement of the vascular system. Large vessel involvement causes cerebral, coronary, and peripheral vascular disease. Microvascular involvement causes neuropathy, retinopathy, and renal disease. Preoperative cardiac and peripheral vascular evaluations are recommended for all diabetic patients undergoing total hip arthroplasty. The adverse effects of hyperglycemia on bone strength and fracture healing have been demonstrated in experimental models. Diabetic patients with osteoarthritis of the hip seem to be more osteopenic than nondiabetic osteoarthritic patients. Diabetic patients have an increased susceptibility to infections, which probably results from a defect in the mechanism of phagocytosis.

In one study of 64 Charnley total hip arthroplasties in diabetic patients, four hips (6.5%) developed a deep infection (45). These procedures were performed in a clean-air enclosure, but without prophylactic antibiotics. This rate of infection was significantly higher than in nondiabetic osteoarthritic patients. However, in another study there was no superficial or deep infection in diabetic patients who had 93 total hip arthroplasties performed in a clean-air enclosure with laminar air flow, body-exhaust suits, and a second-generation cephalosporin prophylaxis (48). However, the overall complication rate was high (24.3%) in this patient group, and the most frequent complication (14.2%) was urinary tract infection. There was no increased loosening of cemented prostheses in diabetic patients.

SYSTEMIC LUPUS ERYTHEMATOSUS

Systemic lupus erythematosus (SLE) is a disease in which organs are damaged by pathogenic autoantibodies and immune complexes. Although all ages and both sexes can be affected, the majority of the cases are in women of child-bearing age. The arthritis associated with SLE usually involves the hand and wrist, but any joint is susceptible. Endstage disease in the hip, however, is almost always secondary to avascular necrosis in patients taking corticosteroids. Symptomatic osteonecrosis occurred in 13% of one cohort of 744 patients with SLE (17), and often involved multiple joints. Survival in patients with SLE is approximately 70% over 10 years, with infection and renal failure the leading causes of death (23).

In one report of 43 prosthetic hip replacements in 31 patients with SLE (25), all but 4 patients had osteonecrosis: 1 patient had degenerative disease and 3 others had displaced femoral neck fractures. There were 29 total hip arthroplasties performed, and all but 3 were rated good or excellent at a mean follow-up time of 66 months. Complications included delayed wound healing in 15% and superficial wound infection in 10%. Although no patients who had a total hip arthroplasty required revision, 5 of 14 bipolar arthroplasties required revision. Only five patients (seven hips) with bipolar arthroplasties had a good or excellent result, and there was a high incidence of persistent groin pain in this group of patients. Of these patients, 25% died less than 5 years postoperatively from disease-related complications. Based on their results (published in 1987), these authors recommended cemented total hip arthroplasty for this group of patients.

In a recent report, 26 hip arthroplasties (15 uncemented, 11 other) in 19 patients were followed for a mean of 4.6 years and compared with a matched control group (75). The visual analog pain scores, Harris hip scores, and SF-36 scores were similar in the two groups. In the SLE group, the complications included small calcar cracks in four hips, two early dislocations, one persistent thigh pain, and one asymptomatic cup loosening. No other symptomatic osteolysis or loosening was seen. Longer follow-up may confirm the benefit of cementless fixation, especially on the acetabular side, in this population (74).

CONCLUSIONS

Hip disorders that may require total hip arthroplasty occur frequently in patients with a variety of systemic conditions, including hematologic, metabolic, endocrine, congenital, and rheumatologic disorders. There is often associated multisystem disease, which requires cooperation with specific medical specialists for optimum preoperative preparation of the patient. For patients with specific disorders, such as hemophilia, sickle-cell disease, Gaucher's disease, and chronic renal failure, referral to tertiary care centers that have medical and orthopedic experience with treating these disorders may be prudent. The short- and long-term results of total hip arthroplasties in a patient with any of these conditions are quite different from the results of total hip arthroplasty without these disorders. The surgeon should be aware of underlying pathophysiology and the specific technical problems that may be encountered.

REFERENCES

1. Abbott KC, Bucci JR, Agodoa LY. Total hip arthroplasty in chronic dialysis patients in the United States. *J Nephrol.* 2003;16:34–39.
2. Acurio MT, Friedman RJ. Hip arthroplasty in patients with sickle-cell haemoglobinopathy. *J Bone Joint Surg.* 1992;74B:367–371.
3. Alem AM, Sherrard DJ, Gillen DL, et al. Increased risk of hip fracture among patients with end-stage renal disease. *Kidney Int.* 2000;58: 396–399.
4. Al-Mousawi F, Malki A, Al-Aradi A, et al. Total hip replacement in sickle cell disease. *Int Orthop.* 2002;26:157–161.
5. Alpert B, Waddell JP, Morton J, et al. Cementless total hip arthroplasty in renal transplant patients. *Clin Orthop.* 1992;284:164–169.
6. Axford JS, Bomford A, Revell P, et al. Hip arthropathy in genetic hemochromatosis. Radiographic and histologic features. *Arthritis Rheum.* 1991;34:357–361.
7. Berend KR, Lilly EG. Early acetabular protrusio following hemiresurfacing of the hip for osteonecrosis in sickle cell disease. *J South Orthop Assoc.* 2003;12:32–37.
8. Beyer CA, Hanssen AD, Lewallen DG, et al. Primary total knee arthroplasty in patients with psoriasis. *J Bone Joint Surg.* 1991;73B: 258–259.
9. Bishop AR, Roberson JRS, Eckman JR, et al. Total hip arthroplasty in patients who have sickle-cell hemoglobinopathy. *J Bone Joint Surg.* 1988;70A:853–855.
10. Cheng F, Kilbanoff J, Rohinson H, et al. Total hip arthroplasty with cement after renal transplantation. Long-term results. *J Bone Joint Surg.* 1995;77A:1535–1542.
11. Clarke IJ, Jinnah RH, Brooker AF, et al. Total replacement of the hip for avascular necrosis in sickle cell disease. *J Bone Joint Surg.* 1989;71B:465–470.
12. DeGnore LT, Wilson FC. Surgical management of hemophilic arthropathy. *Instr Course Lect.* 1989;38:383–388.
13. Devlin VJ, Einhorn TA, Gordon SL, et al. Total hip arthroplasty after renal transplantation: long-term follow-up study and assessment of metabolic bone status. *J Arthroplasty.* 1988;3:205–213.
14. Duthie R, Matthew J, Rizza C, et al. *The Management of Musculo-Skeletal Problems in the Haemophilias.* Oxford: Blackwell Scientific; 1972.
15. Faraawi R, Harth M, Kertesz A, et al. Arthritis in hemochromatosis. *J Rheumatol.* 1993;20:448–452.
16. Gilbert MS, Waddell JD. *The Treatment of Hemophilia.* New York: The National Hemophilia Foundation; 1996.
17. Gladman DD, Chaudry-Ahluwalia V, Ibanez D, et al. Outcomes of symptomatic osteonecrosis in 95 patients with systemic lupus erythematosus. *J Rheumatol.* 2001;28:2226–2229.
18. Gladman DD, Keystone EC, Schacter RK. Aberrations in T-cell subpopulations in patients with psoriatic arthritis. *J Invest Dermatol.* 1983;80:286–290.
19. Goldblatt J, Sachs S, Dall D, et al. Total hip arthroplasty in Gaucher's disease. Long-term prognosis. *Clin Orthop.* 1988;228: 94–98.
20. Greene WB, DeGnore LT, White GC. Orthopaedic procedures and prognosis in hemophilic patients who are seropositive for human immunodeficiency virus. *J Bone Joint Surg.* 1990;72A:2–11.
21. Greene WB, McMillan CW. Nonsurgical management of hemophilic arthropathy. *Instr Course Lect.* 1989;38:367–381.
22. Gunderson C, D'Ambrosia RD, Shiji H. Total hip replacement in patients with sickle-cell disease. *J Bone Joint Surg.* 1977;59A:760–762.
23. Hahn BH. Systemic lupus erythematosus. In: Isselbacher KJ, Martin JB, Braunwald E, et al, eds. *Harrison's Principles of Internal Medicine.* Vol 2. New York: McGraw-Hill: 1994:1643–1648.
24. Hanker GJ, Amstutz HC. Osteonecrosis of the hip in the sickle cell disease: treatment and complications. *J Bone Joint Surg.* 1988;70A: 499–506.
25. Hanssen AD, Cabanela ME, Michet CJ. Hip arthroplasty in patients with systemic lupus erythematosus. *J Bone Joint Surg.* 1987;69A:807–814.
26. Helenius I, Remes V, Tallroth K, et al. Total hip arthroplasty in diastrophic dysplasia. *J Bone Joint Surg Am.* 2003;85A:441–447.
27. Hernigou P, Bachir D, Galacteros F. Avascular necrosis of the femoral head in sickle-cell disease: treatment of collapse by the injection of acrylic cement. *J Bone Joint Surg.* 1993;75B:875–880.
28. Hernigou P, Bachir D, Galacteros F. The natural history of symtomatic osteonecrosis in adults with sickle-cell disease. *J Bone Joint Surg Am.* 2003;85A:500–504.
29. Hesse B, Kohler G. Does it always have to be Perthes' disease? What is epiphyseal dysplasia? *Clin Orthop.* 2003;414:219–227.
30. Hickman JM, Lachiewicz PF. Results and complications of total hip arthroplasties in patients with sickle-cell hemoglobinopathies. Role of cementless components. *J Arthroplasty.* 1997;12:420–425.
31. Huo MH, Salvati EA, Lieberman JR, et al. Custom-designed femoral prostheses in total hip arthroplasty done with cement for severe dysplasia of the hip. *J Bone Joint Surg.* 1993;75A:1497–1504.
32. Ilyas I, Moreau P. Simultaneous bilateral total hip arthroplasty in sickle cell disease. *J Arthroplasty.* 2002;17:441–445.
33. Johanson NA, Vigorta VJ, Goldman AB, et al. Acromegalic arthropathy of the hip. *Clin Orthop.* 1983;173:130–139.
34. Kabasakal Y, Kiyici I, Özmen D, et al. Spinal abnormalities similar to ankylosing spondylitis in a 58-year-old woman with ochronosis. *Clin Rheumatol.* 1995;14:355–357.
35. Katz K, Horev G, Grunebaum M, et al. The natural history of osteonecrosis of the femoral head in children and adolescents who have Gaucher disease. *J Bone Joint Surg Am.* 1996;78:14–19.
36. Kelley SS, Lachiewicz PF, Gilbert MS, et al. Hip arthroplasty in hemophilic arthropathy. *J Bone Joint Surg.* 1995;77A:828–834.
37. Krebs VE. The role of hip arthroscopy in the treatment of synovial disorders and loose bodies. *Clin Orthop.* 2003;406:48–59.
38. Kusakabe N, Tsuzuki N, Sonada M. Compression of the cervical cord due to alcaptonuric arthropathy of the atlanto-axial joint. *J Bone Joint Surg.* 1995;77A:274–277.
39. Lachiewicz PF, Lane JM, Wilson PD Jr. Total hip replacement in Gaucher's disease. *J Bone Joint Surg Am.* 1981;63:602–608.
40. Laskar FH, Sargison KD. Ochronotic arthropathy: a review with four case reports. *J Bone Joint Surg.* 1970;52B:653–666.
41. Lebel E, Itzchaki M, Hadas-Halpern I, et al. Outcome of total hip arthroplasty in patients with Gaucher disease. *J Arthroplasty.* 2001;16:7–12.
42. Lieberman J, Fuchs M, Haas S, et al. Hip arthroplasty in patients with chronic renal failure. *J Arthroplasty.* 1995;10:191–195.
43. Linduskovà M, Hrba J, Vykydal M, et al. Needle biopsy of joints: its contribution to the diagnosis of ochronotic arthropathy (alcaptonuria). *Clin Rheumatol.* 1992;11:569–570.
44. Lofqvist T, Nilsson IM, Petersson C. Orthopaedic surgery in hemophilia: 20 years' experience in Sweden. *Clin Orthop.* 1996; 332:232–241.
45. Menon TJ, Thjellesen D, Wroblewski BM. Charnley low-friction arthroplasty in diabetic patients. *J Bone Joint Surg.* 1987;65B: 580–581.
46. Menon TJ, Wroblewski BM. Charnley low-friction arthroplasty in patients with psoriasis. *Clin Orthop.* 1983;176:127–128.
47. Milner PF, Kraus AP, Sebes JI, et al. Sickle cell disease as a cause of osteonecrosis of the femoral head. *N Engl J Med.* 1991;325: 1476–1481.
48. Moeckel B, Huo MH, Salvati EA, et al. Total hip arthroplasty in patients with diabetes mellitus. *J Arthroplasty.* 1993;8:279–284.
49. Montgomery KD, Williams JR, Sculco TP, et al. Clinical and pathologic findings in hemochromatosis hip arthropathy. *Clin Orthop.* 1998;347:179–187.
50. Moran MC, Huo MH, Garvin KL, et al. Total hip arthroplasty in sickle cell hemoglobinopathy. *Clin Orthop.* 1993;294:140–148.

51. Naito M, Ogata K, Shiota I, et al. Total hip arthroplasty in haemodialysis patients. *J Bone Joint Surg.* 1994;76B:428–431.
52. Nelson CL, Walz BH, Gruenwald JM. Resurfacing of only the femoral head for osteonecrosis. Long-term follow-up study. *J Arthroplasty.* 1997;12:736–740.
53. Nelson IW, Sivamurugan S, Latham PD, et al. Total hip arthroplasty for hemophilic arthropathy. *Clin Orthop.* 1992;276:210–213.
54. O'Brien WM, La Du BN, Bunim JJ. Biochemical, pathologic and clinical aspects of alcaptonuria, ochronosis and ochronotic arthropathy. *Am J Med.* 1963;34:813–838.
55. Papagelopoulos PJ, Morrey BF. Hip and knee replacement in osteogenesis imperfecta. *J Bone Joint Surg.* 1993;75A:572–580.
56. Peltonen JI, Hoikka V, Poussa M, et al. Cementless hip arthroplasty in diastrophic dysplasia. *J Arthroplasty.* 1992;7:369–376.
57. Peterson LAF. Little people. In: Morrey B, ed. *Joint Replacement Arthroplasty.* New York: Churchill Livingstone; 1991:749–758.
58. Platt OS, Brambilla DJ, Rosse WF, et al. Life expectancy and risk factors for early death. *N Engl J Med.* 1994;330:1639–1644.
59. Powell LW, Isselbacher KJ. Hemochromatosis. In: Isselbacher KJ, Martin JB, Braunwald E, et al, eds. *Harrison's Principles of Internal Medicine.* Vol 2. New York: McGraw-Hill: 1994:2069–2073.
60. Ragni MV, Crosset LS, Herndon JH. Postoperative infection following orthopaedic surgery in human immunodeficiency virus-infected hemophiliacs with CD4 counts ≤200/mm³. *J Arthroplasty.* 1995;10:716–721.
61. Rosenberg LE. Inherited disorders of amino acid metabolism and storage. In: Isselbacher KJ, Martin JB, Braunwald E, et al, eds. *Harrison's Principles of Internal Medicine.* Vol 2. New York: McGraw-Hill; 1994;2123–2125.
62. Rosenthal DI, Scott JA, Barranger J, et al. Evaluation of Gaucher disease using magnetic resonance imaging. *J Bone Joint Surg.* 1968;68A:802–808.
63. Stehr-Green JK, Evatt BL, Lawrence DN. Acquired immune deficiency syndrome associated with hemophilia in the United States. *Instr Course Lect.* 1989;38:357–365.
64. Stern SH, Insall JN, Windsor RE, et al. Total knee arthroplasty in patients with psoriasis. *Clin Orthop.* 1989;248:108–111.
65. Styles LA, Vichinsky EP. Core decompression in avascular necrosis of the hip in sickle-cell disease. *Am J Hematol.* 1996;52:103–107.
66. Sunday JM, Guille JT, Torg JS. Complications of joint arthroplasty in patients with end-stage renal disease on hemodialysis. *Clin Orthop.* 2002;397:350–355.
67. Tanner KE, Warren NP, Coombs RR. Ochronosis of the hip joint. Case report with biomechanical study. *Scand J Rheumatol.* 1991;20:63–64.
68. Teitelbaum S. Radiologic evaluation of the hemophilic hip. *Mt Sinai J Med.* 1977;44:400–401.
69. Toomey HE, Toomey SD. Hip arthroplasty in chronic dialysis patients. *J Arthroplasty.* 1998;13:647–652.
70. Trumble SJ, Mayo KA, Mast JW. The periacetabular osteotomy. Minimum 2 year followup in more than 100 hips. *Clin Orthop.* 1999;363:54–63.
71. Vichinsky EP, Haberkern CM, Neumayr L, et al. The preoperative transfusion in sickle cell disease study group. A comparison of conservative and aggressive transfusion regimens in the perioperative management of sickle cell disease. *N Engl J Med.* 1995;333:206–213.
72. Vichinsky EP, Neumayr LD, Haberkern C, et al. The perioperative complication rate of orthopedic surgery in sickle cell disease: report of the National Sickle Cell Surgery Study Group. *Am J Hematol.* 1999;62:129–138.
73. Violas P, Fassier F, Hamdy R, et al. Acetabular protrusion in osteogenesis imperfecta. *J Pediatr Orthop.* 2002;22:622–625.
74. Wallny T, Brackmann HH, Hess L, et al. Long-term follow-up after intertrochanteric varus osteotomy for haemophilic arthropathy of the hip. *Haemophilia.* 2002;8:149–152.
75. Zangger P, Gladman DD, Urowitz MB, et al. Outcome of total hip replacement for avascular necrosis in systemic lupus erythematosus. *J Rheumatol.* 2000;27:919–923.

Osteonecrosis: Etiology, Natural History, Pathophysiology, and Diagnosis

32

Roy K. Aaron   Robert R. L. Gray

Osteonecrosis of the femoral head (ONFH) refers to the death of osteocytes and subsequent structural changes leading to femoral head collapse and secondary hip joint osteoarthritis (65). One of the earliest clinical descriptions of ONFH appeared in 1948 and referred to this condition as "coronary artery disease of the hip," a description that is particularly apt in the light of our present understanding of pathogenesis (28). Descriptions of clinical series began appearing in the English literature only in the early 1960s (60,80,81,83,94). The clinical syndrome has undergone several name changes. *Aseptic necrosis* was initially used to distinguish the condition from bone infections. Later, *avascular necrosis* or *ischemic necrosis* presumed a uniform etiology and pathogenesis. The currently accepted term *osteonecrosis* is more neutral in its presumption of causation; it describes the main common feature of this condition, which is bone death (5).

CLINICAL PRESENTATION

Osteonecrosis of the femoral head is now recognized to be a relatively common disorder, although incidence varies with the center reporting. In Japan, a 10-fold increase in the incidence of ONFH was noted from 1965 to 1985, and the number of patients diagnosed with ONFH doubled between 1984 and 1987 (92). ONFH accounts for 5% to 10% of total hip replacements done in the United States (79,124). It occurs in various series in 5% to 25% of patients taking corticosteroids (79). The male-to-female ratio is approximately 4:1, and the mean age of onset is in the fifth decade. ONFH has been reported to be bilateral in 50% or more of cases (18,51,60,81,94). The presentation of symptoms may be asynchronous, but because progression occurs regardless of the temporal appearance of symptoms, a high index of suspicion must be maintained for disease bilaterality. One study reported an incidence of bilaterality, diagnosed by biopsy, of 89% (51). Of the 35 hips studied, 17 were in the preradiographic stage (Ficat stage I); 8 were Ficat stage II, 5 were stage III, and 5 were stage IV. The presence of symptoms in a contralateral hip is not necessary for progression. In a study of asymptomatic contralateral hips in patients with ONFH, 100% of the "silent" hips eventually collapsed (mean time of collapse, 23 months). Further, 83% collapsed in less than 36 months, and 79% underwent total hip replacement in less than 3 years (21).

Pain is the usual presenting symptom; it can be very intense and sudden in onset, as in an infarct, or it can be insidious and chronic. It is most often reported in the groin, but radiating pain to the anterior or anteromedial thigh is common. Less commonly, buttock pain is noted. Pain is

463

present at rest and is worse with hip motion and weight bearing. Patients commonly exhibit an antalgic limp. On physical examination, a corresponding decrease in range of motion, particularly flexion and internal rotation, is observed. In the absence of specific etiologies (e.g., hemoglobinopathies), laboratory studies are normal.

DIAGNOSTIC IMAGING

Radiographs

The roles of diagnostic imaging modalities and staging systems have recently been the subject of an excellent review (104). The typical radiographic appearance of ONFH is one of mottled sclerosis and lucency, usually in the anterosuperior segment of the femoral head (Fig. 32-1A); the progression is to subchondral fracture and eventually to collapse (Fig. 32-1B). In advanced cases, secondary osteoarthritis is observed.

Efforts have been made to develop staging systems based on specific radiographic characteristics. Early staging systems were essentially qualitative (37,81). They provided descriptions of morphologic features but did not grade disease severity within each morphologic category. The most widely used of these systems was devised by Ficat (37). A stage I hip is a symptomatic hip with normal radiographs (preradiographic) but positive diagnostic imaging studies, such as magnetic resonance imaging (MRI) or technetium-99 (^{99}Tc) bone scan. In recent writings, a stage 0 has been added to denote an asymptomatic, preradiographic hip. Stage II hips display the stereotypical alterations in trabecular pattern of mottled sclerosis and lucency without subchondral fracture and without change in femoral head contour. Cyst formation may be observed as well. Stage III hips are hips in which a subchondral fracture (crescent sign) and/or subchondral collapse has occurred, as well as a loss of sphericity and change in contour of the femoral head (Fig. 32-1B). The subchondral fracture can vary from a superficial fracture just below the subchondral plate to deeper incursions into the necrotic bone. A sequestrated segment of dead bone may be observed. Stage IV is synonymous with secondary osteoarthritis. A nonconcentric loss of the articular cartilage space is observed, along with subchondral sclerosis and osteophytes on both sides of the joint.

The Ficat system has been very useful descriptively, but the lack of quantitation of lesion size in stages II and III and of the extent of segmental collapse in stage III does not permit quantitation of disease severity. For example, lesions of the femoral head occupying 10% and 90% of femoral head area are not distinguished from one another, nor are collapsed segments of 1 mm and 9 mm. These distinctions may be important in determining outcome after procedures that conserve the femoral head and therefore in developing guidelines for selecting therapy (108,110–113). As a consequence, the Ficat staging system lacks precision. Intraobserver variability has been reported to be 17.7%, and interobserver differences were noted in 40% of hips (71).

Quantitative radiographic staging systems have been devised to overcome some of these weaknesses. The most useful of these is the University of Pennsylvania system, which stages ONFH in terms of lesion size, extent of subchondral fracture, and depth of collapse in six morphologic stages (107–109) (Table 32-1). This staging system is more precise and reproducible than qualitative systems and is more useful for describing radiographic progression and response to treatment. An international classification system has been devised by the Association for Research in Bone Circulation (ARCO) that takes into account both lesion location and severity of involvement (5). This system is probably too complex for routine clinical use, but it may be useful for reporting results of hip-sparing procedures.

Technetium-99 Scans and Magnetic Resonance Imaging

For many years, ^{99}Tc bone scans were used in the diagnosis of ONFH, especially in the preradiographic stage (Ficat 0 or I, Steinberg 1, ARCO 1 [5]). In the stage of acute infarction, a photopenic defect is seen corresponding to the ischemic segment, followed by an increased uptake of radionuclide corresponding to the repair phase. The method is characterized by high sensitivity, low specificity, and limited spatial resolution (93).

For the most part, bone scans have been supplanted by MRI because of MRI's better precision. The earliest abnormality in OHFH seen with MRI is a low-intensity signal band on both T1-weighted and T2-weighted images (93). In more advanced lesions, the T1 images continue to show a low-

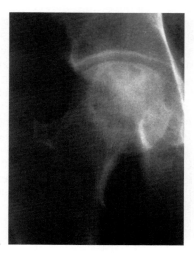

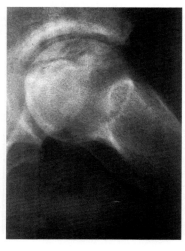

A
B

Figure 32-1 **A:** Ficat stage II lesion exhibiting areas of sclerosis and lucency. No fractures are evident, and the contour of the femoral head is spherical. **B:** Ficat stage III lesion with a subchondral fracture into the substance of the femoral head with a sequestrated segment. No collapse is apparent.

TABLE 32-1

UNIVERSITY OF PENNSYLVANIA SYSTEM FOR STAGING AVASCULAR NECROSIS

Stage	Criteria
0	Normal or nondiagnostic radiograph, bone scan, MRI
I	Normal radiographs; abnormal bone scan and/or MRI
	A. Mild (<15% of femoral head affected)
	B. Moderate (15%–30%)
	C. Severe (>30%)
II	"Cystic" and sclerotic changes in femoral head
	A. Mild (<15% of femoral head affected)
	B. Moderate (15%–30%)
	C. Severe (>30%)
III	Subchondral collapse (crescent sign) without flattening
	A. Mild (<15% of articular surface)
	B. Moderate (15%–30%)
	C. Severe (>30%)
IV	Flattening of femoral head
	A. Mild (<15% of surface and <2 mm depression)
	B. Moderate (15%–30% of surface or 2–4 mm depression)
	C. Severe (>30% of surface or >4 mm depression)
V	Joint narrowing or acetabular changes
	A. Mild ⎰ Average of femoral head involvement,
	B. Moderate ⎱ as determined in stage IV, and
	C. Severe ⎰ estimated acetabular involvement
VI	Advanced degenerative changes

Reproduced from Steinberg ME. Diagnostic imaging and the role of stage and lesion size in determining outcome in osteonecrosis of the femoral head. *Tech Orthopaedics*. 2001;16:6–15.

intensity signal, and the T2 images may exhibit signals of alternating high and low intensity, the so-called double-line sign (Fig. 32-2). It should be noted, however, that a high-intensity signal on T2-weighted images is not necessary for the diagnosis, and one may see a low-intensity signal on both the T1-weighted and T2-weighted images. Comparing MRI to ^{99}Tc bone scans has shown MRI to be more sensitive and specific and to better delineate osteonecrotic lesion location (14,62,84,95,100). The diagnosis of ONFH on coronal MRI sections can be made with about 90% specificity and 95% sensitivity (42,62,95). Abnormalities in the femoral head are only detected by MRI 7 to 10 days after the onset of symptoms, and therefore MRI may not be sensitive in the earliest stage of ONFH (55,95). Excellent correlations between ONFH diagnoses by MRI and by bone biopsy have been reported (63,95,100). Staging methods based on physiological information obtainable from MRI, such as the relative states of hydration and fat content, are under development. It has been suggested that active repair tissue can be differentiated from normal or necrotic bone by variations of the signal on T2-weighted images (63). The MRI appearance of ONFH has also been correlated with the likelihood of segmental collapse (75). Bandlike areas of low signal intensity were strongly correlated with collapse, with a predictive value of a positive test of 31% and of a negative test of 100%. The correlation of bone pathophysiology, MRI images, and clinical behavior should provide interesting and potentially valuable information in the future.

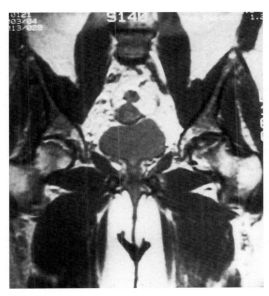

Figure 32-2 T2-weighted magnetic resonance image of bilateral osteonecrosis. Alternating bands of high-intensity and low-intensity signals (the double-line sign) are observed in both femoral heads with differing spatial localization and lesion size.

ETIOLOGY

A number of medical conditions have been associated with ONFH as presumed causes. Because the demographic composition of reporting centers varies widely, it can be difficult to assess the frequency of each cause. In the Democratic Republic of Congo, for example, sickle cell disease is the leading cause of ONFH (6). The frequency of steroid-associated or traumatic ONFH, in another example, would be quite different when reported from a transplant or trauma center as compared with a general hospital population. Distributions of etiologic associations from two separate studies are presented in Table 32-2 (54,60). In another series from Johns Hopkins—a center with a large systemic lupus erythematosus referral population—the incidence of connective tissue diseases is probably closely

TABLE 32-2

ETIOLOGICAL ASSOCIATIONS FROM TWO MEDICAL CENTERS

Etiology	Hospital for Special Surgery (60)		Johns Hopkins Hospital (54)	
	n	%	n	%
Trauma	—	—	15	7
Alcohol	104	39	83	38
Steroids	75	28	99	45
Hyperuricemia	59	22	—	—
Hemoglobinopathy	8	3	6	3
Hyperlipidemia	23	9	—	—
Gaucher's	—	—	4	2
Idiopathic	22	8	11	5

TABLE 32-3

DISEASE ASSOCIATIONS IN 373 PATIENTS WITH ONFH (124)

Etiology	n	%
Rheumatic diseases	134	36
Transplants	14	4
Hemoglobinopathy	12	3
Trauma	11	3
Alcohol	10	3
Malignancy	10	3
Gout	2	—
Asthma	8	2
Other	74	20
Idiopathic	91	24

related to corticosteroid usage (Table 32-3) (124). In a report from Osaka University in Japan, 37% of ONFH cases were thought to be associated with corticosteroids, 23% to be associated with alcohol, and 40% to be idiopathic (92).

Traumatic Osteonecrosis

Osteonecrosis of the femoral head as a consequence of trauma usually involves dislocation of the hip or fracture of the femoral neck. The incidence of ONFH after dislocation is reported to be 10% to 25%, depending on the severity of injury and associated femoral head or acetabular fractures (34,96,116). Prompt relocation may play a role in decreasing the incidence of ONFH. In one series, 52% of hips dislocated for more than 12 hours developed ONFH, compared with 22% of those reduced within 12 hours (22). Displaced intracapsular (femoral neck) fractures have been associated with ONFH in 15% to 50% of cases in several reports (12,41,60,101). Most cases are radiographically evident by 2 to 3 years after fracture. Other attempts have been made to relate fracture type, accuracy of reduction, and time to reduction to the incidence of ONFH, with inconsistent and conflicting results. Displaced fractures or malreductions in either varus or valgus have been associated with higher incidences of ONFH (40% to 85%) than impacted fractures or near-anatomic reductions (12,41). It has been reported that ONFH after femoral neck fractures in the elderly is less symptomatic and has a better prognosis than ONFH associated with other etiologies, with about 50% exhibiting progression (25). ONFH after minor contusive trauma to the hip has also been described (6).

Nontraumatic Osteonecrosis

For patients with nontraumatic ONFH, several etiologic associations have been proposed: dysbarism, corticosteroids, alcohol, and hemoglobinopathies. Other etiologies that are more or less strongly associated include Gaucher's disease, hyperlipidemias, and pregnancy.

Dysbarism

Dysbaric ONFH has two primary causes, one associated with tunnel workers and the other associated with deep sea diving.

Dysbaric ONFH in tunnel workers using compressed air (caisson disease) was quite common in the early part of this century, but it is uncommon now as a consequence of Occupational Safety and Health Administration (OSHA) standards mandating safe working pressures and decompression schedules (68). Standards for safe pressures and decompression have also greatly reduced the incidence of dysbaric ONFH caused by diving. ONFH does not occur below atmospheric pressures of 17 pounds per square inch (psi) and is not believed to be a risk at depths of less than 30 m (67). Naval and commercial divers may have an incidence of 1% to 4%, but not all lesions are symptomatic, and many are not in a juxta-articular location.

Corticosteroids

Steroid-associated ONFH accounts for 10% to 30% of ONFH cases, depending on the center. It has been difficult to separate the effects of corticosteroids from those of underlying associated diseases, particularly in patients with vasculitis or renal failure. A large meta-analysis of 22 series studying steroid-associated ONFH, however, found no correlation between the underlying disease and the osteonecrosis (35). Because ONFH is associated with corticosteroid intake in a number of diverse conditions, including lupus, rheumatoid arthritis, asthma, and organ transplantation, and because patients with Cushing's disease have a higher incidence of ONFH, steroids have long been implicated as an etiologic association in ONFH.

Although it is not certain that the use of steroids presents equal risks in various conditions, clinical attention has been focused on identifying a threshold dose of steroids in determining risk for ONFH. Dose has been expressed as mean daily dose, peak dose, duration of exposure, and cumulative (total) dose. Most studies have suggested an association of ONFH incidence with mean daily or peak dose amounts and have inferred that high doses, even for shorter duration, present more significant risks than cumulative dose or duration of therapy. Table 32-4 presents data on steroid dosages in patients with ONFH from several studies. One study of 161 patients with inflammatory bowel disease treated with corticosteroids reported an incidence of ONFH of 4.3%. The mean daily prednisone dose was 26 mg/d (range, 12 to 34 mg/d), the mean duration of treatment was 42 weeks (range, 20 to 84 weeks), and the mean cumulative prednisone dose was 7000 mg (range, 1800 to 13,500 mg) (117). In a series of 110 patients with steroid-associated ONFH with various diseases, the cumulative prednisone dose was 42 g (32). In a series of patients with steroid-associated ONFH in lupus, the mean daily dose

TABLE 32-4

ONFH AND CORTICOSTEROIDS

Study	Disease	Mean dose (mg/d)	Cumulative dose (g)	Duration (wk)
Cruess (32)	Mixed	—	42	—
Zizic (125)	SLE	>20	45	260
Fischer (39)	Mixed	>25	—	—
Vakil (117)	GI	26	7	42
Felson (35)	Mixed	>20	1.5	—

was greater than 20 mg/d, and the mean cumulative prednisone dose was 45 g, with a mean duration of treatment of 260 weeks (125). In heart transplant patients, no association between the development of ONFH and cumulative prednisone dose was found, but there was an association between ONFH and the peak dose of methylprednisolone (20). The situation may be more complicated in renal transplant patients, but with the use of cyclosporin and reductions in steroid doses, it is probable that ONFH in this population is largely related to the mean daily steroid dose (76). Most patients with ONFH in these and other studies in whom mean daily dose was reported received doses of greater than 20 mg/day, and that dose is generally regarded as presenting a significant risk for ONFH (35,39,117,125). An analysis of 22 studies of steroid-associated ONFH determined there was a 4.6-fold increase in ONFH occurrence for every 10 mg/d increase in oral steroid intake (35). This study reported a strong correlation between mean daily dose and ONFH risk but no correlation between peak dose and ONFH. A threshold cumulative prednisone dose of 2000 mg has been reported to present a risk factor for ONFH, but there are several reports of patients developing ONFH after short-term steroid administration (64).

Alcohol

Osteonecrosis of the femoral head associated with alcohol intake makes up 10% to 40% of ONFH cases in several series (6,60,94,124). Two large studies reported similar percentages: 38% and 39% (Table 32-2). Studies from Japan have determined the relative risks of developing ONFH with varying doses of alcohol (82,92). Individuals consuming more than 400 mL of alcohol per week were at a 9.8-fold greater risk of developing ONFH than those who consumed none, and with consumption over 1000 mL/week the risk rose to 17.9-fold (Table 32-5). In these two studies, the risk of developing ONFH increased with the cumulative dose of alcohol expressed as "drink-years" (weekly alcohol consumption times the number of years of drinking). The relative risks from these two studies, respectively, were <4000 drink-years (3.2 and 2.2), 4000 to 10,000 drink-years (8.3 and 9.7), and >10,000 drink years (31.3 and 12.9).

Hemoglobinopathies

Osteonecrosis of the femoral head has been associated with a number of hemoglobinopathies, most notably sickle cell disease (hemoglobin SS), hemoglobin SC disease, and sickle thalassemia. The incidence of ONFH in sickle cell disease is 4% to 12% (114); in hemoglobin SC disease, the incidence is 20% to 68% (13). In a study of 899 patients with sickle cell disease, 29 were reported to have ONFH, an overall incidence of 3.2%

TABLE 32-5
ONFH AND ALCOHOL (82)

Dose (mL/wk)	Risk
0	1.0
<400	3.3
400–1000	9.8
>1000	17.9

(59). There was a slight predominance in females (male to female, 1:1.6) and in individuals below the age of 25, especially in children between the ages of 6 and 15 years. Twenty-eight of 29 patients (97%) with ONFH had hemoglobin SS. Because 853 of 899 patients had hemoglobin SS, the incidence of ONFH among patients with this electrophoretic pattern was 3.3%. One of 46 patients with hemoglobin SC had ONFH, an incidence of 2.2%. Other studies have suggested that ONFH is more common in hemoglobin SC disease, but this report indicates that the incidence of ONFH is proportionate to the distribution of the electrophoretic pattern of hemoglobin (59). In one study of the natural history of symptomatic osteonecrosis in adults with sickle cell disease, 65 of 75 hips (87%) without collapse of the femoral head at the initial evaluation demonstrated collapse within 5 years after diagnosis (53). The average time between diagnosis and collapse was similar to that for patients with osteonecrosis from other etiologies (see "Natural History" below).

Other Associations

Etiologic associations are less well established for such diverse conditions as hyperlipidemia, pregnancy, pancreatitis, and hyperuricemia. These associations are particularly difficult to establish because idiopathic ONFH constitutes up to 20% of all ONFH in many series. An association has been reported between ONFH and increased circulating pre-β-lipoproteins and hypertriglyceridemia (67). In the Hospital for Special Surgery (New York City) series, hyperlipidemia was found in 28% of patients with steroid-associated ONFH and 69% of those with alcohol-associated ONFH. Patients with hyperlipidemia unassociated with other conditions accounted for 9% of the total ONFH population (60). Several anecdotal reports exist of ONFH associated with pregnancy, but the incidence is unknown and a causal relationship has not been established (29,70). ONFH has also been reported in patients with Gaucher's disease, metastatic or disseminated malignancies, hypersensitivity reactions, and radiation to the femoral head.

NATURAL HISTORY

The natural history of ONFH is usually inferred from patient populations treated with protected weight bearing. Failure criteria vary from study to study, so comparisons among studies must be interpreted broadly. Clinical failure can be expressed as one of several pain scores or by the decision for arthroplasty or other surgical procedures. The assessment of clinical failure is inherently subjective and is a function of the patients' pain tolerance, functional disability, and socioeconomic circumstances and the surgeons' indications for intervention. Radiographic failure can be expressed by one of several scoring systems but has often been reported in imprecise and nonquantitative terms. The reported incidence of radiographic failure is influenced by the relative severity of the scoring system used. With these caveats in mind, comparing results from several studies using different measurements of failure can be enlightening because progression can be demonstrated no matter what measurement is employed.

Early studies reported an overall clinical progression rate of 77% to 98% and a radiographic progression rate of 68% to 75%, with an average of 3 years of follow-up (83,94,97,124).

TABLE 32-6
PROGRESSION OF ONFH—FICAT I

Study	Hips	F/U (mo)	Clinical Failure n (%)	Radiographic Failure n (%)
Steinberg (106)	16	24	—	13 (81)
Stulberg (111)	5	27	4 (80)	4 (80)
Lennox[a]	13	27	8 (62)	13 (100)
Bradway (21)	15	24	13 (87)	15 (100)
Total	49	26	25 (76)	45 (92)

[a]Unpublished data.

TABLE 32-8
PROGRESSION OF ONFH—FICAT III

Study	Hips	F/U (mo)	Clinical Failure n (%)	Radiographic Failure n (%)
Musso (88)	26	18	—	20 (78)
Steinberg (106)	21	24	—	18 (86)
Stulberg (111)	10	27	9 (90)	3 (30)
Hungerford (58)	11	28	11 (100)	10 (91)
Ohzono (89)	36	63	—	36 (100)
Lennox[a]	45	37	39 (87)	42 (93)
Total	149	37	59 (89)	129 (87)

[a]Unpublished data.

From these studies, it was concluded that ONFH is generally progressive and that it progresses usually within 2 to 3 years after the onset of symptoms. More recent studies have reported results by Ficat stage (21,58,88,89,106,111). Progression rates in Ficat I (preradiographic) hips from four studies comprising 49 hips are presented in Table 32-6. An average of 76% of hips progressed clinically and 92% radiographically, with uniformity of results among the studies. Table 32-7 presents progression rates in Ficat II hips compiled from five studies comprising 138 hips. An average of 85% of hips failed clinically and 64% failed radiographically. Ficat III hips exhibited similar failure rates. From six studies, 149 hips exhibited 89% clinical and 87% radiographic failure (Table 32-8). In a review of 21 studies involving 819 hips followed for a mean of 34 months, only 22% had a satisfactory clinical result (86). Of 559 hips in which follow-up radiographs were available, 74% exhibited radiographic progression. Clinical failure and hip loss to arthroplasty occurred in 65% of Ficat I, 69% of Ficat II, and 87% of Ficat III hips. No clinical feature, including corticosteroid intake, affected outcome in terms of hip survival or radiographic progression.

Several studies have examined demographic, clinical, and radiographic features of patients with ONFH, attempting to identify risk factors for more rapid progression. A review of 630 hips with ONFH (of which 84 were conservatively treated) specifically examined risk factors for progression and found that neither corticosteroid administration nor any other etiology correlated with increased risk of hip loss (2). Corticosteroid intake at pharmacologic levels has been referred to as a risk factor for progression; however, although it is a risk factor for the occurrence of osteonecrosis, the literature does not support it as a risk factor for progression (21,88). One study reported that 14 of 18 hips progressed in patients with episodic corticosteroid administration, and 9 of 18 hips progressed in patients requiring continuous steroids (115). The significance was marginal ($p = 0.10$). This study did not report the rate of progression in patients taking corticosteroids compared with other presumptive causes. Progression appears to occur regardless of cause except in the case of elderly patients with ONFH secondary to displaced intracapsular hip fractures, who exhibit about a 50% incidence of clinical and radiographic progression (25).

Studies by our group have examined the time course of clinical and radiographic progression and those clinical and radiographic characteristics that are associated with more rapid progression (4). Clinical progression occurred equally in all three Ficat grades. By the 36-month follow-up, 54% of stage I, 66% of stage II, and 73% of stage III hips required surgery. The mean times to clinical failure were 27 months for stage I, 24 months for stage II, and 21 months for stage III hips. Radiographic progression also occurred equally in all three Ficat grades; by the 36-month follow-up, 94% of stage I, 83% of stage II, and 92% of stage III hips had progressed radiographically. A subsequent study extended these observations. The eventual rate of clinical progression was related to the initial Ficat stage, and radiographic progression was seen in all Ficat stages (3). Overall, 57 hips (71%) progressed clinically, and 91% of hips progressed radiographically (Figs. 32-3 and 32-4). Hips initially presenting as Ficat stage I progressed more rapidly in Ficat stage than did Ficat II and III hips. The radiographic progression of Ficat stage I lesions implies the appearance of a previously preradiographic lesion, whereas the progression of Ficat stage II lesions indicates structural failure (i.e., subchondral fracture). It is possible, therefore, that the radiographic progression of Ficat stage I lesions and the progression of stage II lesions have entirely different prognostic significance. However, the correlation of radiographic and clinical progression and the similar rates of clinical progression in both groups suggest that radiographic progression is significant in Ficat I hips. Within the first 2 years of follow-up, Ficat stage II and III hips exhibited more rapid collapse than Ficat stage I hips, but at the 36-month follow-up, all three groups

TABLE 32-7
PROGRESSION OF ONFH—FICAT II

Study	Hips	F/U (mo)	Clinical Failure n (%)	Radiographic Failure n (%)
Musso (88)	22	18	—	19 (86)
Stulberg (111)	7	27	7 (100)	4 (57)
Hungerford (58)	22	31	21 (95)	19 (86)
Ohzono (89)	70	63	—	33 (47)
Lennox[a]	17	37	11 (65)	14 (82)
Total	138	35	39 (85)	89 (64)

[a]Unpublished data.

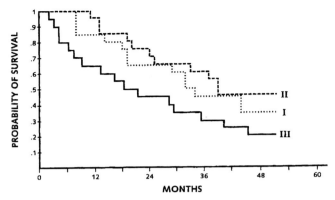

Figure 32-3 Clinical progression. Hips surviving have not undergone total hip replacement. Ficat stage II hips have a significantly better survival probability than Ficat stage III hips ($p = 0.02$). No significant differences were noted in other comparisons. Ficat stage I versus II, $p = 0.52$; Ficat stage I versus III, $p = 0.15$. (Reproduced from Aaron RK, Stulberg B, Lennox D. Clinical and radiographic outcomes in untreated symptomatic osteonecrosis of the femoral head. *Tech Orthop.* 2001;16:1–5.)

exhibited similar rates of progression, with 64% to 72% of hips exhibiting collapse in the three groups. The mean time to collapse was 22 months for Ficat stage I hips, 16 months for Ficat stage II hips, and 20 months for Ficat stage III hips.

Clinical characteristics, including age (considered as a continuous variable), gender, and etiology, did not correlate with either clinical or radiographic progression. However, we did identify certain radiographic risk factors for more rapid progression. Ficat III lesions in patients over the age of 40 did exhibit more rapid clinical and radiographic failure. Segmental collapse of more than 4 mm on initial radiographs was associated with more rapid clinical and radiographic failure than that in hips with an initial collapse of zero to 1 mm. Lesion size over 50% of the femoral head area on the initial anteroposterior (AP) radiograph in Ficat stage III was associated with more rapid clinical failure.

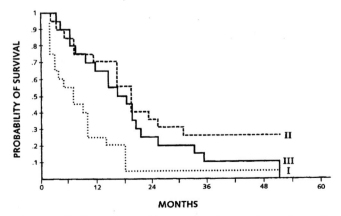

Figure 32-4 Radiographic progression. Substantial radiographic progression is present in all three groups by 18 months follow-up. Ficat stage I hips progress more rapidly than Ficat stage II ($p = 0.004$) and Ficat III ($p = 0.01$) hips. (Reproduced from Aaron RK, Stulberg B, Lennox D. Clinical and radiographic outcomes in untreated symptomatic osteonecrosis of the femoral head. *Tech Orthop.* 2001;16:1–5.)

Other studies have demonstrated that lesion location as well as size may be associated with the outcome of hips treated nonoperatively or with hip-sparing procedures (89,104,105). In particular, the area of subchondral bone involved in the osteonecrotic lesion may be of prognostic significance, an observation that may have a biomechanical explanation (see "Histopathology and Pathomechanics"). Collapse occurred more frequently when the osteonecrotic lesion involved the weight-bearing segment of the femoral head and less often when the lesion was in the medial portion. A subsequent study reported that lesion size as well as location within the femoral head was associated with the propensity of an osteonecrotic lesion to collapse (113). Lesions on the weight-bearing surface of the femoral head involving areas of less than 41% on the AP radiograph or 33% on the lateral radiograph did not collapse. Lesions that progressed to collapse involved more than 61% on either AP or lateral radiographs. However, the predictive accuracy of these measurements is not high.

PATHOPHYSIOLOGY AND PATHOGENESIS

Studies of the pathophysiologic events leading to cell death have focused on the vulnerable microcirculation in the femoral head and the consequences of vascular occlusion. The pathogenesis of ONFH connotes events leading to vascular occlusion, such as intravascular coagulation. It should be recognized that the study of pathogenesis and pathophysiology is hampered by the unavailability of longitudinal studies in humans and the lack of a suitable animal model. Concepts of pathogenesis and pathophysiology are therefore synthesized from a series of unrelated observations of the pathology of human disease or they are extrapolated from animal studies.

Pathophysiology

Examination of the microcirculation of the femoral head has revealed the vulnerability of the blood supply to intravascular occlusion and extravascular compression. Most of the circulation to the weight-bearing area of the femoral head is supplied by the superior retinacular arteries (11). In early ONFH, a diminution in the blood supply from the superior retinacular vessels has been demonstrated (9,10). In later ONFH, extraosseous superior retinacular artery occlusion, neovascularization in the cancellous bone, and decreased vascularity in the area of the subchondral fracture are observed (9,11). Other studies have suggested that interruption of the blood flow in ONFH occurs in intraosseous arteries within the femoral head and that the extent of necrosis is related to the number of arteries involved (90,91). These studies demonstrated that a limited zone of necrosis is accompanied by interruption of the lateral epiphyseal arteries that supply the anterosuperior segment in the femoral head. More extensive zones of necrosis are associated with additional involvement of the superficial and inferior metaphyseal arteries. Impairment of intraosseous circulation has been correlated with histological evidence of osteocyte necrosis (74). This study showed that a 1.6-fold reduction in femoral head blood flow would reduce PO_2 by one third. Interruption of this vulnerable microcirculation,

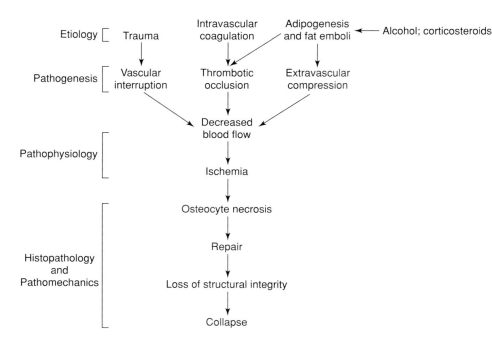

Figure 32-5 A concept of pathogenesis of osteonecrosis that unifies several hypotheses. Many etiologies may contribute to the pathogenic mechanisms of vascular interruption, thrombotic occlusion, or extravascular compression. These mechanisms all may decrease blood flow, leading to ischemia and subsequently to osteocyte necrosis. The presence of necrotic bone induces a repair process in which bone resorption exceeds production, leading to a loss of structural integrity of the subchondral trabeculae and eventually to subchondral collapse.

resulting in ischemia and cell death, could occur in a number of ways, including mechanical interruption from fractures or dislocations, thrombotic occlusion, or extravascular compression.

Pathogenesis

A unifying concept of the pathogenesis of ONFH emphasizes the central role of vascular occlusion and ischemia leading to osteocyte necrosis (Fig. 32-5). Decreased femoral head blood flow can occur through three mechanisms: vascular interruption (fractures or dislocation), extravascular compression (by lipocyte hypertrophy and marrow fat deposition), and thrombotic occlusion (by intravascular thrombi or embolic fat). The mechanical interruption of circulation to the femoral head in hip dislocations or displaced femoral neck fractures is the most obvious and well-understood pathogenic mechanism. The pathogenesis of nontraumatic ONFH is considerably less

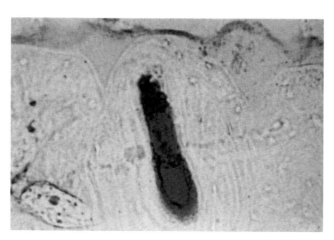

Figure 32-6 An oil red-O stain demonstrating a fat embolus in a subchondral blood vessel. Note proximity to the tide mark. (Courtesy of J. P. Jones, MD.) See Color Plate.

well understood. Some investigators have suggested that embolic fat can occlude the microcirculation and that lipocyte hypertrophy and accumulation of lipids in the subchondral osteocytes contribute to the pathogenesis by extravascular compression (64,66,69,87,120). Intravascular occlusion by fibrin thrombi or embolic fat has been found in a large number of specimens of ONFH, and microcirculatory thrombosis associated specifically with fat emboli has been described (Fig. 32-6) (19,38,66,99,103). Elevated fibrinopeptides and fibrin degradation products indicating the presence of disseminated intravascular coagulation (DIC) have been measured in some cases of ONFH, providing indirect evidence of ongoing thrombosis. DIC, focal intravascular coagulation in the subchondral microcirculation, and ONFH have been observed in human and animal examples of the Shwartzman and Arthus phenomena.

Intravascular Coagulation

Several studies have demonstrated the presence of hypofibrinolysis and thrombophilia in patients with ONFH (46–48). Hypofibrinolysis is usually associated with low levels of stimulated tissue plasminogen activator (tPA), elevated levels of plasminogen activator inhibitor (PAI), and, often, high levels of lipoprotein A. A decrease in the level of antithrombotic protein C or S and resistance to activated protein C (RAP-C) decrease regulation of the prothrombotic factors V and VIII. Both hypofibrinolysis and thrombophilia are accompanied by an increased incidence of thrombotic events. Several reports have linked hypofibrinolysis and thrombophilia to ONFH through the pathogenic mechanism of hypercoagulability and thrombotic occlusion of femoral head circulation (46,47). In one study, 12 of 12 patients (100%) with idiopathic ONFH had coagulation defects. Nine of 12 (75%) had elevated PAI and low tPA, with a corresponding inability to initiate fibrinolysis. Three of 12 patients (25%) had elevated lipoprotein A. Of 18 patients with ONFH associated with specific etiologies, 14 (78%) had elevated lipoprotein A. In a second study, 15 of 18 patients (83%) with idiopathic ONFH had coagulation defects, with the majority (8) having hypofibrinolysis due to elevated lipoprotein A. Of 13 patients with ONFH associated with specific etiologies, 8 (62%) had a variety of coagulation disorders. These observations suggest the hypothesis that patients with these coagulopathies are more susceptible to microcirculatory thrombosis in the femoral head when challenged by epigenetic factors. When heritable thrombophilias are diagnosed in patients with ONFH, it is important that close relatives be tested, because approximately 50% will also have a coagulation disorder that may manifest itself as a thrombotic event, such as thrombophlebitis, pulmonary emboli, ischemic stroke, or myocardial infarction.

Controversy exists concerning the role of both acquired and genetic causes of hypercoagulability in osteonecrosis, and this controversy has recently been summarized, especially with regard to the role of anticardiolipin antibodies (1). The exact role of inherited coagulopathies is still being debated (17,123). Hypercoagulability has not been universally observed in patients with ONFH or Perthes disease and has been seen in other conditions, including bone marrow edema syndrome and osteoarthritis of the hip. Two studies failed to find abnormalities in protein C or S, antithrombin III, or resistance to activated protein C in Perthes disease (72,40). Hypofibrinolysis and elevated levels of Lp(a), on the other hand, have been observed in patients with bone marrow edema syndrome (16). At the present time, this syndrome is recognized as distinct from ONFH in that it is associated with transient osteoporosis and is clinically self-limiting (i.e., does not progress to bone necrosis, subchondral fracture, or collapse). Finally, hypercoagulability and hypofibrinolysis have been observed in patients with osteoarthritis of the hip. Among the more specific findings, elevations in PAI-1 have been observed (30). These studies collectively raise the question of the specificity and sensitivity of the coagulation abnormalities observed in patients with osteonecrosis.

Lipid Accumulation

A number of studies have demonstrated that, particularly after corticosteroid administration, lipids deposit in the marrow extravascular space and within osteocytes and can create an elevation of intraosseous extravascular pressure similar to that seen in ONFH of Gaucher's disease (118). Hypertrophy and proliferation of adipocytes and abnormal lipid metabolism have been found in patients and experimental animals with ONFH secondary to corticosteroid administration (69,119,120). Adipocyte hypertrophy and hyperplasia and intraosseous, extravascular lipid deposition result in intraosseous hypertension and diminished blood flow (118). In addition to this mechanism, adipogenesis may also restrict the number of osteoprogenitor cells by shifting precursors from an osteocytic to an adipocytic pathway. Studies using a cloned mouse bone marrow progenitor cell line have indicated that adipocytes and osteocytes share a common progenitor cell, but in corticosteroid-induced or alcohol-induced adipogenesis, cells shunt from the osteocytic to the adipocytic lineage (121). This is observed in cell-surface lineage markers and reflects the reduced ability of osteocytic cells to effect bone repair.

Intraosseous Hypertension

Using the concept of bone as a Starling resistor, some investigators have focused attention on elevated extravascular intraosseous pressure (IOP) as a pathogenic mechanism in ONFH (37,38,54,56,57). A Starling resistor consists of a rigid-walled chamber through which passes a tube (or tubes) with a flexible wall. Fluid flow through the tube is decreased by elevations of pressure within the chamber. If the chamber represents the intraosseous extravascular space, elevations in pressure in this space can decrease blood flow in the microcirculation passing through it. Elevated bone marrow pressures have been measured within the osteonecrotic femoral head, and this abnormality is associated with decreased venous drainage and stasis (37,38,54,56,57). Pressures have also been shown to be elevated in contralateral asymptomatic and preradiographic hips in patients who subsequently develop biopsy-proven ONFH. Normal resting bone marrow pressures have been measured at about 15 mm Hg, with abnormal recordings being above 30 mm Hg. The infusion of 5 mL of isotonic saline is said to stress the capacity of the vascular system within the bone (54). Infusions into normal femoral heads result in a very transient pressure elevation of about 10 mm Hg, which returns to baseline within a few seconds. In ONFH, this stress test results in sustained elevations in IOP of as much as 30 to 40 mm Hg for more than 5 minutes. Other observers have not found IOP measurements to be reproducible, specific, or sensitive (26,51,77). One study confirmed the observation that IOP above 30 mm Hg is abnormal but suggested that the diagnostic sensitivity of the test in ONFH is low, with 17% of hips with ONFH having IOP below this level (74). Another study, also accepting 30 mm Hg as the upper limit of normal IOP, found 32% of hips with ONFH to fall below this level and concluded that the stress test lacks sufficient precision as a diagnostic tool (77). The experimental increase of IOP, with or without venous occlusion, to 30 to 45 mm Hg increases endosteal, periosteal, and cancellous new bone formation but does not produce osteonecrosis (122). Elevated IOP is seen in osteoarthritis as well as in ONFH and can also be related to elevations in intra-articular pressure and compressive loads (8,33,49,65). Finally, intraosseous hypertension has been found 3 weeks after experimental intraosseous fat embolism (65). These observations have led to the conclusion that elevated IOP, although often observed in ONFH, is not causally related to the pathogenesis of the clinical syndrome (64,65). In this view, elevated IOP is a nonspecific and secondary, but potentially contributory, factor in the pathogenesis of ONFH. The clinical, as opposed to investigational, usefulness of IOP measurement appears to vary widely because of differing perceptions of specificity and sensitivity (26,36,51,54,55,74,77).

HISTOPATHOLOGY AND PATHOMECHANICS

Despite a variety of pathogenic mechanisms, alterations in bone physiology eventually converge to a more or less common and consistent histopathology. Studies suggest that osteocyte necrosis occurs after 2 to 3 hours of anoxia (61). However, 24 to 72 hours are necessary before histologic signs of osteocyte death are apparent (15,67,73). The earliest findings

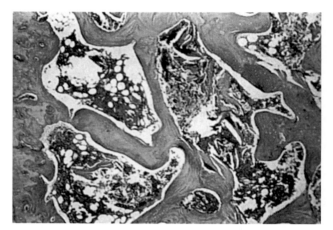

Figure 32-7 Histological section of the subchondral bone exhibiting dead trabeculae with empty osteocyte lacunae and hemorrhagic marrow with necrosis. See Color Plate.

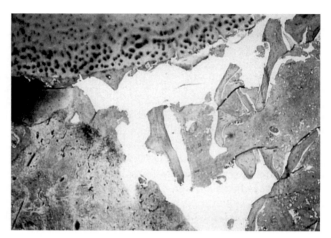

Figure 32-9 Histological section of a subchondral fracture. The articular cartilage is morphologically normal. A small amount of bone appears associated with the cartilage, and the fracture line is through the subchondral bone plate. See Color Plate.

of ONFH on light microscopy are hematopoietic marrow and adipocyte necrosis (67,98). These are followed rapidly by liquefaction necrosis and interstitial edema. The next recognizable event is osteocyte necrosis, reflected by pyknosis of nuclei and subsequently by empty osteocyte lacunae (Fig. 32-7). At this stage, the articular chondrocytes are morphologically and metabolically normal. The necrotic area is surrounded by a zone of reactive hyperemia and fibrous repair (102). Capillary neogenesis and revascularization are believed to occur to a degree in the necrotic zone (43,65). With the entry of blood vessels into the zone of necrosis, a repair process begins consisting of coupled bone resorption and production that produces the radiographic appearance of sclerosis and lucency (27,43–45,73). In the cancellous bone, proliferation of capillaries is observed, and new living bone is laminated onto dead trabeculae, with partial resorption of the dead bone (Fig. 32-8). The repair process appears to be self-limited and to incompletely replace dead with living bone. In the subchondral area, bone formation occurs at a slower rate than does resorption, resulting in the net removal of bone, loss of structural integrity, subchondral fracture, and collapse (Fig. 32-9).

These histopathological changes are reflected in the radiographic appearance of the femoral head (Fig. 32-10). Areas of lucency represent zones of bone resorption; areas of sclerosis are composed of both dead and living bone, with the living reparative bone laminated onto dead trabeculae. Resorption of bone may also cause fractures deep in the femoral head, leading to segmental collapse. It is not the necrosis per se but rather the repair process—particularly bone resorption—that leads to the loss of mechanical integrity of the femoral head, collapse, and joint incongruity. Prior to collapse, the articular cartilage is metabolically and functionally normal, and cartilage degradation does not occur until collapse of the subchondral bone.

Finite element modeling has been used to determine the relative contributions of the subchondral plate and necrotic cancellous bone to subchondral fracture and collapse (24). These studies have demonstrated that a normal subchondral bone plate can provide only modest stress protection to a structurally

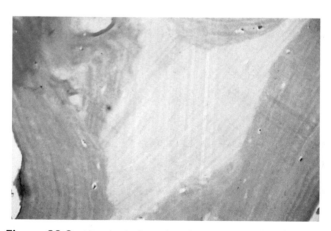

Figure 32-8 Histological section demonstrating lamination of living bone upon a section of dead trabeculae. Note the presence of osteocytes in the lacunae of living bone. See Color Plate.

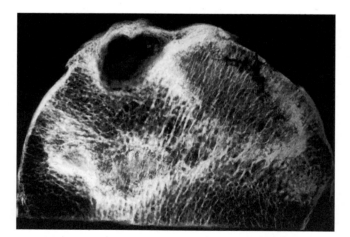

Figure 32-10 Specimen radiograph showing details of sclerotic and lucent zones. The sclerotic zones comprise living bone laminated on dead trabeculae. Subchondral fracture is evident, with 1 mm of collapse.

weakened necrotic segment, whereas structural weakening of the necrotic cancellous bone induces marked stress increases in the overlying subchondral plate. Subchondral collapse is therefore most likely influenced more strongly by the degree of structural weakening of the necrotic cancellous bone as a consequence of trabecular resorption than by the degree of structural loss within the subchondral plate itself. The mechanism underlying the fracture is elevation of shear stresses in the subchondral cancellous bone, which is consistent with a subchondral fracture via shear crack propagation. Studies of the pathomechanics of necrotic subchondral and cancellous bone have recently been summarized, and the effect of lesion size and location upon subchondral collapse has been quantitated (23). The risk of collapse depends on lesion size, particularly the extent of involvement of the subchondral bone, and on the location of the lesion relative to the axis of hip joint loading. The length of subchondral involvement is more predictive of subchondral collapse than is lesion depth or percent volume involvement of the femoral head. According to these data, preferential weighting should be given to the area of subchondral involvement as measured by any one of a number of staging systems. Finite element modeling is applicable not only to assessing collapse risk on a patient-specific basis but also to hip-preserving therapies on an intervention-specific basis. Although beyond the scope of this chapter, the review by Brown (23) discusses the effect of femoral head bone grafting and penetration of core decompression tracks as a function of position and depth of placement.

Opinion is divided as to whether ONFH exhibits the same histopathology regardless of the etiology with which it is associated. Some studies have suggested that ONFH associated with corticosteroid intake, particularly in transplant patients, is characterized by a less complete repair process, with suppressed bone production (73,124). However, in a histomorphometric study of iliac crest biopsies of patients with ONFH from various etiologies, a histologic profile of osteoporosis was observed, including a reduction in trabecular bone volume and osteoid seam width, a decrease in the osteoblastic appositional rate and the bone formation rate, and an increase in total resorptive surface (7). No differences based on presumed etiology were observed among biopsies. These histomorphometric findings could represent metabolic disease that contributes to incomplete bone repair at the osteonecrotic site.

DIAGNOSIS

Core biopsy and histopathologic diagnosis is generally regarded as the standard by which all other diagnostic methods are measured. Although not 100% sensitive because of potential sampling errors and technical and processing artifacts, biopsies are 100% specific (15,110,112). Diagnostic algorithms have been proposed, and two are combined in Figure 32-11 (55,110). The hip to be studied may present with pain or it may be an at-risk hip such as a contralateral hip in a patient with ONFH. AP and frog lateral radiographs should be obtained. If the radiographs are positive for ONFH, the disease should be accurately staged for the purpose of planning treatment. If staging can be done from radiographs alone, no further tests may be needed. Computer tomography is useful for detecting small superficial subchondral fractures with

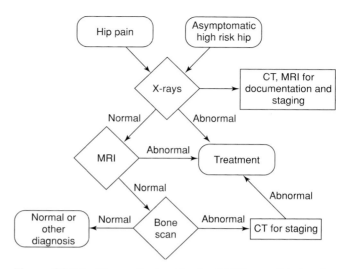

Figure 32-11 Diagnostic algorithm for ONFH consolidating the recommendations of Stulberg et al. (110) and Hungerford and Jones (55).

minimal or no collapse. If the radiographs are negative, an MRI or bone scan should be done. The MRI is generally preferred because it is more accurate, provides a spatial characterization of the lesion, and may be useful in staging. Bone scans allow the detection of ONFH in joints other than the hip during the same study.

The major differential diagnosis of ONFH is transient osteoporosis, or bone marrow edema syndrome. This condition, which occurs in the same age range as ONFH, may also be bilateral. It presents with pain and a corresponding antalgic gait and loss of range of motion. Laboratory studies are normal. Radiographs may show demineralization of the femoral head and neck, and the ^{99}Tc bone scan exhibits increased radionuclide uptake. The MRI provides an important diagnostic distinction. Whereas in ONFH, low signal intensity is observed in both T1-weighted and T2-weighted images, in transient osteoporosis, decreased signal intensity is seen in T1 images and increased signal intensity is seen in T2 images. This pattern is believed to reflect increased water content resulting from bone marrow edema (52). Furthermore, the area of signal alteration in transient osteoporosis is less well defined than in ONFH. The MRI pattern of decreased signal intensity in T1 images and increased signal intensity in T2 images is relatively nonspecific and may be seen in trauma, osteomyelitis, reflex sympathetic dystrophy, and malignancies. The use of T2-weighted images can be useful in differentiating transient osteoporosis from ONFH, especially if a double-line sign is present. The distinguishing characteristics of transient osteoporosis and ONFH have been the subject of a review (50).

CONCLUSIONS

ONFH is a disabling and progressive condition and, if untreated, leads to femoral head collapse requiring total hip replacement. Because hip-preserving therapies are most effective in the earliest stages of ONFH (before subchondral fracture and collapse), the key to successful treatment lies in identifying at-risk populations and quantifying their risk in terms of clinical and pathophysiological characteristics so that a diagnosis can be made before femoral head collapse. In fact, an understanding of the pathogenic and etiological factors in osteonecrosis enables the screening of at-risk individuals. Recognizing the natural history and time to progression facilitates an understanding of the time course and clinical urgency of diagnosis and hip-preserving therapies.

Understanding the pathogenesis of osteonecrosis is likely to have a significant impact on treatment. At the moment, hip-preserving therapies are focused on the structural consequences of osteonecrosis and the prevention of subchondral fracture and collapse. Two studies presented in abstract form have suggested that the administration of bisphosphonates can suppress osteoclastic resorption of subchondral trabeculae and prevent collapse. A better understanding of the pathogenesis of ONFH might focus treatment on earlier stages of the disease in order to reverse mechanisms leading to hypoperfusion and ischemia. Advocates of the role of heritable coagulopathies in osteonecrosis have suggested the use of warfarin or enoxaparin to treat hypercoagulability. Advocates of the mechanism of adipocyte enlargement and intraosseous hypertension have suggested the use of lovastatin for the treatment of local hyperlipidemia and the relief of extravascular compression.

SUMMARY

Osteonecrosis of the femoral head is a relatively common disorder, with estimates suggesting approximately 20,000 new cases per year. Pain is the most common clinical symptom; however, in many hips, a subclinical phase may exist that is asymptomatic but in which imaging studies are positive. Both the subclinical disease and the clinically apparent disease exhibit a high likelihood of clinical and radiographic progression culminating in femoral head collapse, joint incongruity, and pain and requiring surgical intervention (usually total hip arthroplasty). Several predisposing conditions have been identified, but the etiology may be multifactorial, with environmental factors superimposed on genetic or pathologic predispositions. A number of clinical and radiographic staging systems are available. Evidence suggests that quantitation of lesion size and collapse may be important and should be included in any staging system.

REFERENCES

1. Aaron RK, Ciombor DM. Coagulopathies and osteonecrosis. *Curr Opin Orthop.* 2001;12:378–383.
2. Aaron RK, Lennox DW, Stulberg BN. Evaluation of hip-preserving treatment strategies in osteonecrosis of the femoral head. *Trans Orthop Res Soc.* 1994;19:209–236.
3. Aaron RK, Stulberg BN, Lennox DW. Clinical and radiographic outcomes in untreated symptomatic osteonecrosis of the femoral head. *Tech Orthop.* 2001;16:1–5.
4. Aaron RK, Stulberg BN, Lennox DW. The natural history of osteonecrosis of the femoral head and risk factors for progression. In: Urbaniak J, ed. *The Etiology, Diagnosis and Management of Osteonecrosis of the Human Skeleton.* Chicago: American Academy of Orthopaedic Surgeons; 1997:261.
5. ARCO Committee on Terminology and Staging. The ARCO perspective for reaching one uniform staging system of osteonecrosis. In: Schoutens A, Arlet J, Gardeniers JWM, et al., eds. *Bone Circulation and Vascularization in Normal and Pathological Conditions.* New York: Plenum Press; 1993:375–380.
6. Arlet J. Nontraumatic avascular necrosis of the femoral head: past, present, and future. *Clin Orthop.* 1992;277:12–21.
7. Arlot M, Bonjean M, Chavassieux P, et al. Bone histology in adults with aseptic necrosis. *J Bone Joint Surg.* 1983;65A:1319–1327.
8. Arnoldi CC. The relationship between intraosseous and intra-articular pressure. In: Arlet J, Ficat RP, Hungerford DS, eds. *Bone Circulation.* Baltimore: Williams & Wilkins; 1984:213–221.
9. Atsumi T. Bone arteriography of the femoral head of humans in normal and pathological conditions. In: Schoutens A, Arlet J, Gardeniers JWM, et al., eds. *Bone Circulation and Vascularization in Normal and Pathological Conditions.* New York: Plenum Press; 1993:293–299.
10. Atsumi T, Kuroki Y. Role of impairment of blood supply of the femoral head in the pathogenesis of idiopathic osteonecrosis. *Clin Orthop.* 1992;277:22–30.
11. Atsumi T, Yoshikatsu K, Yamano K. A microangiographic study of idiopathic osteonecrosis of the femoral head. *Clin Orthop.* 1989;246:186–194.
12. Barnes R, Brown JT, Garden RS, Nicoll EA, et al. Subcapital fractures of the femur: a prospective review. *J Bone Joint Surg.* 1976;58B:2–24.
13. Barton CJ, Cockshott WP. Bone changes in hemoglobin SC disease. *Am J Radiol.* 1962;88:523–532.
14. Bassett LW, Gold RH, Reicher M, et al. Magnetic resonance imaging in the early diagnosis of ischemic necrosis of the femoral head: preliminary results. *Clin Orthop.* 1987;214:237–248.
15. Bauer TW, Stulberg BN. The histology of osteonecrosis and its distinction from histologic artifacts. In: Schoutens A, Arlet J, Gardeniers JWM, et al. eds. *Bone Circulation and Vascularization in Normal and Pathological Conditions.* New York: Plenum Press; 1993:283–292.
16. Berger CE, Kluger R, Urban M, et al. Elevated levels of lipoprotein(a) in familial bone marrow edema syndrome of the hip. *Clin Orthop.* 2000;377:126–131.
17. Bjorkman A, Svensson PJ, Hillarp A, et al. Factor V Leiden and prothrombin gene mutation: risk factors for osteonecrosis of the femoral head in adults. *Clin Orthop Rel Res.* 2004;425:168–172.
18. Boettcher WC, Bonfiglio M, Hamilton HR, et al. Non-traumatic necrosis of the femoral head, I: relation of altered hemostasis to etiology. *J Bone Joint Surg.* 1970;52A:312–321.
19. Bonfiglio M. Development of bone necrosis lesions. In: Lambertsen CJ, ed. *Underwater Physiology V.* Bethesda, MD: Federation of American Societies for Experimental Biology; 1976:117–132. Proceedings of the Fifth Symposium on Underwater Physiology.
20. Bradbury G, Benjamin J, Thompson J, et al. Avascular necrosis of bone after cardiac transplantation. *J Bone Joint Surg.* 1994;76A:1385–1388.
21. Bradway J, Morrey B. The natural history of the silent hip in bilateral atraumatic osteonecrosis. *J Arthroplasty.* 1993;8:383–387.
22. Brav EA. Traumatic dislocation of the hip. *J Bone Joint Surg.* 1962;44A:1115–1121.
23. Brown TD. Biomechanical aspects of subchondral fracture, core decompression, and bone grafting in femoral head osteonecrosis. *Tech Orthop.* 2001;16:16–23.
24. Brown TD, Baker KJ, Brand RA. Structural consequences of subchondral bone involvement in segmental osteonecrosis of the femoral head. *J Orthop Res.* 1992;10:79–87.
25. Calandruccio RA. Comparison of specimens from nonunion of neck of femur with fresh fractures and avascular necrosis specimens. *J Bone Joint Surg.* 1967;49A:1471–1472.
26. Camp JF, Colwell CW. Core decompression of the femoral head for osteonecrosis. *J Bone Joint Surg.* 1986;68A:1313–1319.
27. Catto M. A histological study of avascular necrosis of the femoral head after transcervical fracture. *J Bone Joint Surg.* 1965;47B:749–753.
28. Chandler FA. Coronary disease of the hip. *J Int Coll Surg.* 1948;2:34–36.
29. Cheng N, Burssens A, Mulier JC. Pregnancy and post-pregnancy avascular necrosis of the femoral head. *Arch Orthop Traumat Surg.* 1982;100:199–210.
30. Cheras PA, Whitaker AN, Blackwell EA, et al. Hypercoagulability and hypofibrinolysis in primary osteoarthritis. *Clin Orthop.* 1997;334:57–67.

31. Chung SMK, Ralston EL. Necrosis of the femoral head associated with sickle-cell anemia and its genetic variants: a review of the literature and study on thirteen cases. *J Bone Joint Surg.* 1969;51A:33–39.

32. Cruess RL. Steroid induced osteonecrosis. *J R Coll Surg Edinb.* 1981;26:69–77.

33. Downey DJ, Simkin PA, Taggart R. The effect of compressive loading on intraosseous pressure in the femoral head in vitro. *J Bone Joint Surg.* 1988;70A:871–877.

34. Epstein HC. Traumatic dislocation of the hip. *Clin Orthop.* 1973;92:116–120.

35. Felson DT, Anderson J. A cross-study evaluation of association between steroid dose and bolus steroids and avascular necrosis of bone. *Lancet.* 1987;1(8538):902–904.

36. Ficat RP. Early diagnosis of osteonecrosis by functional bone investigation. In: Weil UH, ed. *Segmental Idiopathic Necrosis of the Femoral Head.* New York: Springer-Verlag; 1981:17–27. Progress in Orthopaedic Surgery no. 5.

37. Ficat RP. Idiopathic bone necrosis of the femoral head: early diagnosis and treatment. *J Bone Joint Surg.* 1985;67B:3–9.

38. Ficat RP, Arlet J. Functional investigation of bone under normal conditions. In: Hungerford DS, ed. *Ischemia and Necrosis of Bone.* Baltimore: Williams & Wilkins; 1980:29–52.

39. Fisher DE, Bickel WH. Corticosteroid-induced avascular necrosis: a clinical study of seventy-seven patients. *J Bone Joint Surg.* 1971;53A:859–862.

40. Gallistl S, Reitinger T, Linhart W, et al. The role of inherited thrombotic disorders in the etiology of Legg-Calvé-Perthes disease. *J Pediatric Orthop.* 1999;19:12–13.

41. Garden RS. Malreduction and avascular necrosis in subcapital fractures of the femur. *J Bone Joint Surg.* 1971;53B:183–190.

42. Glickstein MF, Burk DL, Schiebler ML, et al. Avascular necrosis versus other diseases of the hip: sensitivity of MR imaging. *Radiology.* 1988;169:213–215.

43. Glimcher MJ, Kenzora JE. The biology of osteonecrosis of the human femoral head and its clinical implications, I: tissue biology. *Clin Orthop.* 1979;138:284–309.

44. Glimcher MJ, Kenzora JE. The biology of osteonecrosis of the human femoral head and its clinical implications, II: the pathological changes in the femoral head as an organ and in the hip joint. *Clin Orthop.* 1979;139:283–312.

45. Glimcher MJ, Kenzora JE. The biology of osteonecrosis of the human femoral head and its clinical implications, III: discussion of the etiology and genesis of the pathological sequelae; comments on treatment. *Clin Orthop.* 1979;140:273– 312.

46. Glueck CJ, Freibert R, Glueck H, et al. Hypofibrinolysis: a common major cause of osteonecrosis. *Am J Hematol.* 1994;45:156–166.

47. Glueck CJ, Freiberg R, Tracy T, et al. Thrombophilia and hypofibrinolysis: pathophysiologies of osteonecrosis. *Clin Orthop.* 1997;334:43–56.

48. Glueck CJ, Glueck HI, Welch M, et al. Familial idiopathic osteonecrosis mediated by familial hypofibrinolysis with high levels of plasminogen activator inhibitor. *Thromb Haemost.* 1994;71:195–198.

49. Goddard NJ, Gosling PT. Intra-articular fluid pressure and pain in osteoarthritis of the hip. *J Bone Joint Surg.* 1988;70B:52–55.

50. Guerra JJ, Steinberg ME. Distinguishing transient osteoporosis from avascular necrosis of the hip. *J Bone Joint Surg.* 1995;77A:616–624.

51. Hauzeur JPH, Pasteels JL, Orloff S. Bilateral non-traumatic aseptic osteonecrosis in the femoral head. *J Bone Joint Surg.* 1987; 69A:1221–1225.

52. Hayes CW, Balkissoon AA. Magnetic resonance imaging of the musculoskeletal system. *Clin Orthop.* 1996;No. 302:297–309.

53. Hernigou P, Bachir D, Galacteros F. The natural history of symptomatic osteonecrosis in adults with sickle-cell disease. *J Bone Joint Surg.* 2003;85;500–504.

54. Hungerford DS. Early diagnosis and treatment of ischemic necrosis of the femoral head. In: Weil UH, ed. *Segmental Idiopathic Necrosis of the Femoral Head.* New York: Springer-Verlag; 1981:29–45.Progress in Orthopaedic Surgery no. 5.

55. Hungerford DS, Jones LC. Diagnosis of osteonecrosis of the femoral head. In: Schoutens A, Arlet J, Gardeniers JWM, et al., eds. *Bone Circulation and Vascularization in Normal and Pathological Conditions.* New York: Plenum Press; 1993:265–275.

56. Hungerford DS, Lennox DW. The importance of increased intraosseous pressure in the development of osteonecrosis of the femoral head: implications for treatment. *Orthop Clin North Am.* 1985;16:635–654.

57. Hungerford DS, Zizic TM. Pathogenesis of ischemic necrosis of the femoral head. *Proc Hip Soc.* 1983;249–262.

58. Hungerford DS, Zizic TM. The treatment of ischemic necrosis of bone in systemic lupus erythematosus. *Medicine.* 1980;59: 143–148.

59. Iwegbu CG, Fleming AF. Avascular necrosis of the femoral head in sickle-cell disease. *J Bone Joint Surg.* 1985;67B:29–32.

60. Jacobs B. Epidemiology of traumatic and nontraumatic osteonecrosis. *Clin Orthop.* 1978;130:51–67.

61. James J, Steijn-Myagkaya GL. Death of osteocytes: electron microscopy after in vitro ischaemia. *J Bone Joint Surg.* 1986;68B: 620–624.

62. Jergesen HE, Heller M, Genant HK. Signal variability in magnetic resonance imaging of femoral head osteonecrosis. *Clin Orthop.* 1990;253:137–149.

63. Jergesen HE, Lange P, Moseley M, et al. Histologic correlation in magnetic resonance imaging of femoral head osteonecrosis. *Clin Orthop.* 1990;253:150–163.

64. Jones JP Jr. Concepts of etiology and early pathogenesis of osteonecrosis. In: Schafer IM, ed. *Instr Course Lect.* 1994;43: 499–512.

65. Jones JP Jr. Etiology and pathogenesis of osteonecrosis. *Semin Arthroplasty.* 1991;2:160–168.

66. Jones JP Jr. Intravascular coagulation and osteonecrosis. *Clin Orthop.* 1992;277:41–53.

67. Jones JP Jr. Osteonecrosis. In: McCarty DJ, ed. *Arthritis and Allied Conditions.* Philadelphia: Lea & Febiger; 1985:1356–1373.

68. Jones JP Jr, Behnke AR Jr. Prevention of dysbaric osteonecrosis in compressed-air workers. *Clin Orthop.* 1978;130:118–128.

69. Kawai K, Tamaki A, Hirohata K. Steroid-induced accumulation of lipid in the osteocytes of the rabbit femoral head: a histochemical and electron microscopic study. *J Bone Joint Surg.* 1985;67A:755–763.

70. Kay NR, Park WM, Bark M. The relationship between pregnancy and femoral head necrosis. *Br J Radiol.* 1972;45:828–831.

71. Kay RM, Lieberman JR, Dorey FJ, et al. Inter- and intraobserver variation in staging patients with proven avascular necrosis of the hip. *Clin Orthop.* 1974;307:124–129.

72. Kealey WDC, Mayne WW, McDonald W, et al. The role of coagulation abnormalities in the development of Perthes' disease. *J Bone Joint Surg.* 2000;82B:744.

73. Kenzora JE, Glimcher MJ. Osteonecrosis. In: Kelley WN, Harris ED, Russy S, et al., eds. *Textbook of Rheumatology.* Philadelphia: WB Saunders; 1981:1755–1782.

74. Kiaer T, Pedersen NW, Kristensen K, et al. Intra-osseous pressure and oxygen tension in avascular necrosis and osteoarthritis of the hip. *J Bone Joint Surg.* 1990;72B:1023–1030.

75. Kokubo T, Takatori Y, Ninomiya S, et al. Magnetic resonance imaging and scintigraphy of avascular necrosis of the femoral head. *Clin Orthop.* 1992;277:54–60.

76. Landmann J, Renner N, Gachter A, et al. Cyclosporin A and osteonecrosis of the femoral head. *J Bone Joint Surg.* 1987;69A: 1226–1228.

77. Learmonth ID, Maloon S, Dall G. Core decompression for early atraumatic osteonecrosis of the femoral head. *J Bone Joint Surg.* 1990;72B:387–390.

78. Lee JS, Koo KH, Ha YC, et al. Role of thrombotic and fibrinolytic disorders in osteonecrosis of the femoral head. *Clin Orthop Rel Res.* 2003;417:270–276.

79. Mankin HJ. Nontraumatic necrosis of bone (osteonecrosis). *N Engl J Med.* 1992;326:1473–1479.

80. Mankin HJ, Brower TB. Bilateral idiopathic aseptic necrosis in adults: Chandler's disease. *Bull Hosp Joint Dis.* 1962;23:42–57.

81. Marcus ND, Enneking WF, Massam RA. The silent hip in idiopathic aseptic necrosis: treatment by bone grafting. *J Bone Joint Surg.* 1973;55A:1351–1366.

82. Matsuo K, Hirohata T, Sugioka Y, et al. Influence of alcohol intake, cigarette smoking, and occupational status on idiopathic osteonecrosis of the femoral head. *Clin Orthop.* 1988;234: 115–123.

83. Merle D'Aubigne RM, Postel M, Mazabraud A, et al. Idiopathic necrosis of the femoral head in adults. *J Bone Joint Surg.* 1965;47B:612–633.
84. Miller IL, Savory CG, Polly DW, et al. Femoral head osteonecrosis. *Clin Orthop.* 1989;274:152–162.
85. Mitchell DG, Steinberg ME, Dalinka MK, et al. Magnetic resonance imaging of the ischemic hip: alterations within the osteonecrotic viable and reactive zones. *Clin Orthop.* 1977;244:60–89.
86. Mont MA, Hungerford DS. Non-traumatic avascular necrosis of the femoral head. *J Bone Joint Surg.* 1995;77A:459–474.
87. Muratsu H, Shimizu T, Kawai K, et al. Alcohol-induced accumulations of lipids in the osteocytes of the rabbit femoral head. *Trans Orthop Res Soc.* 1990;15:49.
88. Musso ES, Mitchell SN, Schink-Ascani M, et al. Results of conservative management of osteonecrosis of the femoral head: a retrospective review. *Clin Orthop.* 1986;207:209–215.
89. Ohzono K, Saito M, Takaoka K, et al. Natural history of nontraumatic avascular necrosis of the femoral head. *J Bone Joint Surg.* 1991;73B:68–72.
90. Ohzono K, Sugano N, Nakamura N, et al. Compared microangiographic images of osteonecrosis of the femoral head and osteoarthritis of the hip. In: Schoutens A, Arlet J, Gardeniers JWM, et al., eds. *Bone Circulation and Vascularization in Normal and Pathologic Conditions.* New York: Plenum Press; 1993:301–312.
91. Ohzono K, Takaoka K, Saito S, et al. Intraosseous arterial architecture in nontraumatic avascular necrosis of the femoral head. *Clin Orthop.* 1992;277:79–88.
92. Ono K, Sugioka Y. Epidemiology and risk factors in avascular necrosis of the femoral head. In: Schoutens A, Arlet J, Gardeniers JWM, et al., eds. *Bone Circulation and Vascularization in Normal and Pathologic Conditions.* New York: Plenum Press; 1993:243–248.
93. Owen RS, Dalinka MK. Imaging modalities for early diagnosis of osteonecrosis of the hip. *Semin Arthroplasty.* 1991;2:169–174.
94. Patterson RJ, Bickel WH, Dahlin DC. Idiopathic necrosis of the head of the femur. *J Bone Joint Surg.* 1964;46A:267–282.
95. Robinson HJ, Hartleben PD, Lund G, et al. Evaluation of magnetic resonance imaging in the diagnosis of osteonecrosis of the femoral head. *J Bone Joint Surg.* 1989;71A:650–663.
96. Roeder LF Jr, DeLee JC. Femoral head fractures associated with posterior hip dislocations. *Clin Orthop.* 1980;147:121–130.
97. Romer U, Wettstein P. Results of treatment of eighty-one Swiss patients with INFH. In: Zinn WM, ed. *Idiopathic Ischemic Necrosis of the Femoral Head in Adults.* Stuttgart: Georg Thieme Publishers; 1971:205–212.
98. Saito S, Inoue A, Ono K. Intramedullary hemorrhage as a possible cause of avascular necrosis of the femoral head. *J Bone Joint Surg.* 1987;69B:346–351.
99. Saito S, Ohzono K, Ono K. Early arteriopathy and postulated pathogenesis of osteonecrosis of the femoral head. *Clin Orthop.* 1992;277:98–110.
100. Seiler JG, Christie MJ, Homara L. Correlation of the findings of magnetic resonance imaging with those of bone biopsy in patients who have stage I or II ischemic necrosis of the femoral head. *J Bone Joint Surg.* 1989;71A:28–32.
101. Sevitt S. Avascular necrosis and revascularization of the femoral head after intracapsular fracture: a combined arteriographic and histologic study. *J Bone Joint Surg.* 1964;46B:270–296.
102. Sissons HA, Nuovo MA, Steiner GC. Pathology of osteonecrosis of the femoral head. *Skeletal Radiol.* 1992;21:229–238.
103. Spencer JD, Brookes M. Avascular necrosis and the blood supply of the femoral head. *Clin Orthop.* 1988;235:127.
104. Steinberg ME. Diagnostic imaging and the role of stage and lesion size in determining outcome in osteonecrosis of the femoral head. *Tech Orthop.* 2001;16:6–15.
105. Steinberg ME, Bands RE, Parry S, et al. Does lesion size affect the outcome in avascular necrosis? *Clin Orthop Rel Res.* 1999;367:262–271.
106. Steinberg ME, Hayken GD, Steinberg DR. The conservative management of avascular necrosis of the femoral head. In: Arlet J, Ficat P, Hungerford D, eds. *Bone Circulation.* Baltimore: Williams & Wilkins; 1984:334–337.
107. Steinberg ME, Hayken GD, Steinberg DR. A new method for evaluation and staging of avascular necrosis of the femoral head. In: Arlet J, Ficat P, Hungerford D, eds. *Bone Circulation.* Baltimore: Williams & Wilkins; 1984:398–403.
108. Steinberg ME, Hayken GD, Steinberg DR. A quantitative system for staging avascular necrosis. *J Bone Joint Surg.* 1995;77B:34–41.
109. Steinberg ME, Steinberg DR. Evaluation and staging of avascular necrosis. *Semin Arthroplasty.* 1991;2:175–181.
110. Stulberg BN, Bauer TW, Belhobek GH, et al. A diagnostic algorithm for osteonecrosis of the femoral head. *Clin Orthop.* 1989;249:176–182.
111. Stulberg BN, Davis AW, Bauer TW, et al. Osteonecrosis of the femoral head. *Clin Orthop.* 1991;268:140–151.
112. Stulberg BN, Levine M, Bauer TW, et al. Multimodality approach to osteonecrosis of the femoral head. *Clin Orthop.* 1989;240:181–193.
113. Sugano N, Takaoka K, Ohsono K, et al. Prognostication of nontraumatic avascular necrosis of the femoral head. *Clin Orthop.* 1994;303:155–164.
114. Tanaka KR, Clifford GO, Axelrod AR. Sickle-cell anemia with aseptic necrosis of the femoral head. *Blood.* 1956;11:98.
115. Tooke SMT, Nugent PJ, Bassett LW, et al. Results of core decompression for femoral head osteonecrosis. *Clin Orthop.* 1988;228:99–104.
116. Upadhyay SS, Moultoj A, Srikrishnamurthy K. An analysis of the late effects of traumatic posterior dislocation of the hip without fractures. *J Bone Joint Surg.* 1983;65B:150–152.
117. Vakil N, Sparberg M. Steroid-related osteonecrosis in inflammatory bowel disease. *Gastroenterology.* 1989;96:62–67.
118. Wang GJ, Cui Q, Balian G. The pathogenesis and prevention of steroid-induced osteonecrosis. *Clin Orthop Rel Res.* 2000;370:295–310.
119. Wang GJ, Lennox DW, Reger SI, et al. Cortisone-induced intrafemoral head pressure change and its response to a drilling decompression method. *Clin Orthop.* 1981;59:274–278.
120. Wang GJ, Sweet D, Reger SI, et al. Fat cell changes as a mechanism of avascular necrosis of the femoral head in cortisone-treated rabbits. *J Bone Joint Surg.* 1977;59A:729–735.
121. Wang Y, Li Y, Mao K, et al. Alcohol-induced adipogenesis in bone and marrow: a possible mechanism for osteonecrosis. *Clin Orthop Rel Res.* 2003;410:213–224.
122. Welch RD, Johnston CE, Waldron MJ, et al. Bone changes associated with intraosseous hypertension in the caprine tibia. *J Bone Joint Surg.* 1993;75A:53–60.
123. Zalavras CG, Vartholomatos G, Dokou E, et al. Genetic background of osteonecrosis: associated with thrombophilic mutations? *Clin Orthop Rel Res.* 2004;422:251–255.
124. Zizic TM, Hungerford DS. Avascular necrosis of bone. In: Kelly WN, Harris ED, Ruddy S, et al., eds. *Textbook of Rheumatology.* Philadelphia: WB Saunders; 1985:1689–1710.
125. Zizic TM, Marcoux C, Hungerford DS, et al. Corticosteroid therapy associated with ischemic necrosis of bone in systemic lupus erythematosus. *Am J Med.* 1985;79:596–603.

Osteonecrosis: Strategies for Treatment

Michael A. Mont   Hari P. Bezwada

Osteonecrosis of the femoral head is a disease affecting young patients (age range usually from 15 to 50 years) that leads to a debilitating arthritis often requiring a total hip replacement for disabling pain. The goals of treatment are often simply to relieve pain, but in the early stages the surgeon can attempt to maintain a congruent hip joint and delay or avoid the need for a total hip replacement. As this disease occurs in a young patient population, it is the authors' philosophy to use procedures aimed at maintaining the femoral head even though further intervention may be necessary. There are many treatment methods that have been utilized for both early and more advanced stages of the disease. Treatment should be based on an evaluation of clinical, radiographic, and intraoperative factors. The authors believe that most of the treatment

determination can be based on the radiographic evaluation, with patient-specific factors and operative details utilized to refine the plan. This chapter elucidates the rationale for utilizing different methods, and each procedure is described in terms of indications, technique, rehabilitation, and expected results.

PATIENT EVALUATION

The following details the important factors necessary to develop a treatment plan for a patient with osteonecrosis of the femoral head utilizing clinical, radiographic, and intraoperative evaluations.

Clinical Evaluation

Patients typically present with groin pain, although 10% to 15% of patients may have nonspecific symptoms such as trochanteric or buttock pain. Groin pain is the clinical hallmark of this disease. It is sometimes reasonable to consider a diagnostic hip injection with a local anesthetic to rule out other pathology such as lumbar disc disease. Often a patient with Occult Osteonecrosis may have nonspecific hip, trochanteric, or buttock symptoms that are coming from the back or another pathological entity.

Patient-Specific Factors

The patient's age, activity level, and general health help to individualize the proposed treatment. The presence of severe systemic illness or a short life expectancy may preclude a major surgical procedure. Similar lesions may not be treated the same way in two patients of different ages and activity levels. For example, a hip with femoral head collapse without acetabular involvement might be best treated with a bone-grafting procedure or resurfacing arthroplasty in a healthy

21-year-old patient. The same radiographic changes in a 72-year-old patient would more likely be treated with a total hip arthroplasty. For large lesions and early collapse lesions, most femoral head–conserving procedures may eventually lead to total hip arthroplasty. The justification for delaying total hip replacement is that an arthroplasty done early will probably not last a patient's lifetime. The expectation is that the head-preserving procedure will delay total hip arthroplasty long enough for technologies to catch up with patient needs. Two other factors come into play, the morbidity associated with the proposed procedure and its impact on the future success of a total hip replacement. In this regard, for example, core decompression might be a better option than vascularized fibular bone grafting for a lesion in which either would be successful, because the core decompression procedure would not make a later hip replacement more difficult. Revision of a bone-grafting procedure may require special surgical equipment or lead to much difficulty during a subsequent total hip arthroplasty (4).

Early diagnosis remains the key to successful treatment. An understanding of the different associated factors for osteonecrosis may help a clinician manage a patient who presents with groin pain and arrive at a proper diagnosis. If a patient presents with risk factors for osteonecrosis and groin pain, it is imperative that evaluation with roentgenograms and magnetic resonance imaging (MRI) performed. Roentgenograms and MRI should be the mainstay in the initial radiographic evaluation of these patients. MRI has an extremely high sensitivity and specificity for this diagnosis, on the order of 99% or greater. Nuclear bone scintigraphy is not as sensitive and may miss the diagnosis in more than 20% of lesions. Scintigraphy was initially thought to be cost-effective. However, one can now obtain a limited cost-effective MRI sequence that can lead to the diagnosis (46). In addition, the authors believe that computed tomography (CT) scans (tomograms) have limited value, and invasive tests, such as intraosseous pressure measurements or core biopsy, are not necessary in making the diagnosis.

See Table 33-1 for a complete list of associated risk factors for osteonecrosis. The most common risk factors are prolonged corticosteroid use (a threshold cumulative dose of 2 g of prednisone) (44) or regular ethanol use (more than 300 g of alcohol a week) (18). Corticosteroids and alcohol account for most of the cases in which a direct causative agent has not been found. Direct causative agents include sickle cell disease or other hemoglobinopathies, myeloproliferative disorders, radiation, dysbarism, and trauma (59).

The role of various clinical factors in terms of treatment outcomes has been debated. Age has not been implicated in various studies as a prognostic factor, but most surgeons will treat a patient younger than 20 years of age differently than a patient who presents with osteonecrosis and is older than 70 years of age. With older patients, it might be more appropriate to try a total hip arthroplasty, for their life expectancy is much less than that of a teenager, they have less activity demands, and the chances of success with a head-sparing procedure, such as bone grafting, would appear to be less. This same type of rationale can be applied to patients with comorbidities. It seems logical that patients with various comorbidities, such as the use of high-dose corticosteroids or alcohol, would be less ideal candidates for head-preserving procedures. However, various studies have not shown a difference in outcomes

TABLE 33-1
LIST OF RISK FACTORS ASSOCIATED WITH OSTEONECROSIS OF THE FEMORAL HEAD

Trauma	Organ transplants
Femoral neck fracture	Renal
Dislocation	Cardiac
Corticosteroids	Liver
Alcohol	Dysbarism
Coagulation disorders	Liver dysfunction
Thrombophilia	Gastrointestinal disorders
Hypofibrinolysis	Myeloproliferative disorders
Systemic lupus erythematosus	Leukemia
and connective tissue	Gaucher disease
disease	Radiation
Hyperlipidemia	Pregnancy
Altered red blood cells	Smoking
Sickle cell anemia	Hyperuricemia
Thalassemia	Chemotherapeutic agents
	Hypersensitivity reactions
	Idiopathic

Reproduced with permission from Chapman MW, ed. *Chapman's Orthopaedic Surgery.* 3rd ed. Philadelphia: Lippincott Williams & Wilkins; 2001.

between various comorbidities, including systemic lupus erythematosus and prolonged corticosteroid use (59,61,66).

One should consider that this disease is often bilateral (range, between 50% and 100%, with bilaterality greater than 80% in large series). When planning treatment, the surgeon may attempt to treat both hips at the same time rather than subject the patient to two separate anesthetic exposures. However, if the intent is to keep a hip from being weight bearing, it might be preferable to separate the procedures by 6 to 12 weeks, depending on the symptomatology and the level of collapse of the hip, so that the patient can maintain the ability to ambulate. If a patient is avoid anything but minimal weight bearing on both hips at the same time, the patient would have to be confined to a wheelchair. In approximately 10% of patients, other joints exhibit osteonecrosis. If a patient has pain in other joints, such as the knee, shoulder, or ankle, the affected joints should be investigated with radiographs and possibly MRI so that a treatment plan for the whole patient can be developed.

There is a debate concerning the treatment of the asymptomatic hip with osteonecrosis. Some reports show less than 50% progression at 5 years' follow-up on asymptomatic hips, (51). While others show a lack of progression in large numbers of patients (51). However, Urbaniak (51) found a greater than 50% rate of progression, a study by Jergesen and Khan (43) found that 14 of 19 asymptomatic hips progressed, 9 within 5 years and 5 beyond 5 years of diagnosis. The authors did not treat asymptomatic hips but acknowledge that a rational argument could be made for empiric treatment of hips that may have a 50% or greater risk of disease progression.

Another factor that is important to consider for the treatment of patients with osteonecrosis of the hip is the duration of symptoms. For example, in a study by Beaule et al. (7), a better prognosis was found for patients who received limited femoral resurfacing and had symptoms for less than 12 months before treatment than for patients with a symptom duration of more than 12 months. Patients with a longer preoperative period of symptoms had a worse acetabular cartilage grading at the time of resurfacing, which was associated with a shorter time to conversion to total hip arthroplasty (7). In a series of core decompressions utilizing multiple percutaneous small-diameter drillings, Mont et al. (66) found that a shorter duration of preoperative symptoms was associated with more successful outcomes. The average preoperative duration of symptoms in the group with successful outcomes was 6 months (80% success, 24 of 30 hips). This can be compared to 11 months in the group of patients with less optimal outcomes (57%, 8 of 15 hips) at a mean follow-up of 2 years (66). In addition, Steinberg et al. (81) studied patients who underwent a total hip arthroplasty for Ficat stage III osteonecrosis and had a mean duration of symptoms of 18 months. Their acetabular cartilage was evaluated both grossly and histologically; 40 of 41 hips had gross acetabular cartilage degeneration, and all hips that had histological samplings were abnormal as well (81). A major tenet for treating this disease is that the earlier the diagnosis and initiation of treatment, the better the results.

In summary, numerous clinical factors including age, etiology and comorbidities can influence the choice of treatment of osteonecrosis of the femoral head. However, radiographic factors and staging should take precedence over these factors. For example, even though a teenager might like to avoid a total hip replacement, this choice may not be appropriate if radiographically detectable arthritic changes are present on both sides of the joint. In the next section we discuss the relevant radiographic factors that should be coupled with these patient-specific factors to create an appropriate treatment plan.

RADIOGRAPHIC EVALUATION

Numerous classification systems have been used to describe the radiographic extent of osteonecrosis of the femoral head. Each system has its limitations, and no single system is presently accepted as the sole guide to treatment. The most commonly used systems are summarized in Table 33-2. In formulating a treatment plan, the authors use four essential roentgenographic findings that have been shown in multiple studies to have prognostic value. First, the lesion should be classified with regard to collapse; is it a precollapse or postcollapse lesion? Precollapse lesions have the best prognosis. Second, the size of the necrotic segment must be assessed, as small lesions have the most favorable results. The next feature of importance is the amount of head depression. Lesions with less than 2 mm of head depression have a more favorable outcome. Finally, acetabular involvement should be characterized, as any sign of osteoarthritis will limit treatment options.

Precollapse versus Postcollapse

Collapse represents mechanical failure of the weakened necrotic bone. Although large areas of collapse can be recognized by a change in the contour of the femoral head, this many not be so obvious in heads without substantial depression. An early indicator is the crescent sign (Fig. 33-1). When collapse is present it is likely that the patient will eventually require a total hip arthroplasty (63,68). On the contrary, hips diagnosed in a precollapse stage have the best chance for head survival for any head-sparing treatment method. (Figs. 33-2 and 33-3).

TABLE 33-2	
RADIOGRAPHIC CLASSIFICATION OF OSTEONECROSIS OF THE FEMORAL HEAD	

Stage	Description
	Ficat and Arlet
I	Normal
II	Sclerotic or cystic lesions, without subchondral fracture
III	Crescent sign (subchondral collapse) and/or step-off in contour or subchondral bone
IV	Osteoarthritis with decreased articular cartilage, osteophytes
	Marcus and Associates; same as Ficat and Arlet except stage III divided into:
III	Crescent sign only
IV	Step-off in contour of subchondral bone
V	Stage IV of Ficat and Arlet
	University of Pennsylvania System of Staging; same as Marcus and Associates except:
V	Divided into early and late arthritis (V and VI)
	Each lesion is divided into A, B, and C depending on the magnetic resonance image size of the lesion (small, moderate, large)
	ARCO
	Three distinct systems published from 1990 to 1992, most recently as follows:
	Same as Steinberg except each lesion also is classified as a, b, or c depending on location (medial, central, or lateral). Quantification of various factors:
A	Amount of head depression
B	Length of crescent arc
C	Size of lesion
	Japanese Investigation Committee on Osteonecrosis; characterized by location of lesion:
A	Medial one-third or less of weight-bearing head
B	Medial two-thirds or less of weight-bearing head
C	Greater than two-thirds of weight-bearing head

Reproduced and modified from Etienne G, Mont MA, Ragland PS. The diagnosis and treatment of nontraumatic osteonecrosis of the femoral head. Instr. *Course Lect.* 2004;53:67–85. Review.

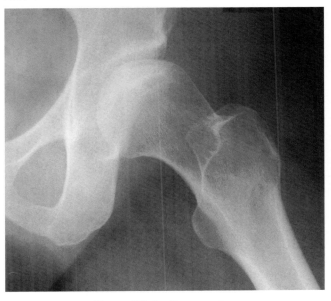

Figure 33-1 Crescent sign.

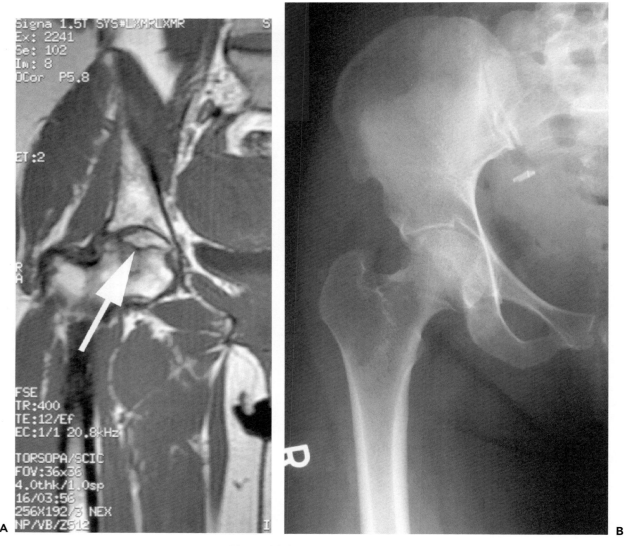

Figure 33-2 Precollapse lesion.

Lesion Size

Multiple studies have shown that the size of the lesion is a major determining factor in both clinical and radiographic outcome (63,72). Small and medium-size lesions have the best prognosis, whereas large lesions fare poorly with all treatment methods. Measurements can be made from MRI scans or from plain radiographs. Steinberg et al. (78) described a method for quantitating the amount of femoral head involvement by MRI. Volumetric measurements are calculated from coronal and axial images. Mild lesions occupy less than 15% of the femoral head, moderate or medium lesions 15% to 30%, and severe lesions more than 30%.

Combined necrotic angle measurements made on standard radiographs can be used in radiographically evident stages of disease (45). To determine this, anteroposterior and lateral views of the hip are obtained. On these radiographs, the arc angles of the surface area with necrosis are measured. The two angles obtained from the anteroposterior and lateral views are then added together. Angles less than 150° are consistent with small lesions, angles between 151° and 250° represent medium-size lesions, and angles greater than 250° correspond to large lesions (Fig. 33-4).

Head Depression

An important feature is the amount of change in head contour. More than 2 mm of head depression confers a worse prognosis. When describing collapse of the femoral head, small lesions are those with less than 2 mm of depression, moderate lesions have 2 to 4 mm of depression, and large lesions have more than 4 mm of depression. Femoral heads with more than 4 mm of head depression are not usually candidates for head-sparing procedures. Berend et al. (8) demonstrated that lesion size and amount of collapse were directly related to poor outcomes following free vascularized fibular grafting for treatment of postcollapse osteonecrosis

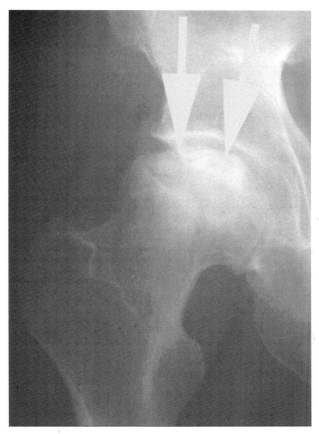

Figure 33-3 Postcollapse lesion.

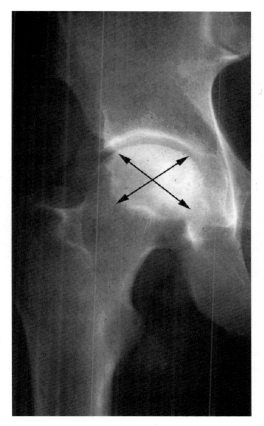

Figure 33-4 Large lesion.

in a study of 224 hips with an overall 64.5% survivorship at a minimum of 5 years (Fig. 33-5).

Acetabular Involvement

Disease with acetabular involvement needs to be recognized. With the early collapse of the femoral head, the joint line may actually appear widened. Therefore, any narrowing of the joint space compared with the opposite side demonstrates acetabular involvement. In patients with arthritis on both sides of the joint, there are few treatment alternatives. Steinberg et al. (82) described two classifications for acetabular involvement: stage V (early or minimal arthritic changes) and stage VI (late or severe arthritic changes). This system, however, may be only moderately useful, as stage V lesions and VI lesions will probably both require reconstructive procedures rather than head-sparing techniques (82). In hips with arthritic changes, treatment directed at only the femoral head will probably not be successful, underscoring the importance of recognizing arthritic changes on plain roentgenograms (or intraoperatively, as described in the next section) (Fig. 33-6).

Intraoperative Assessment

In addition to the clinical and radiographic factors just discussed, intraoperative findings are helpful in directing treatment.

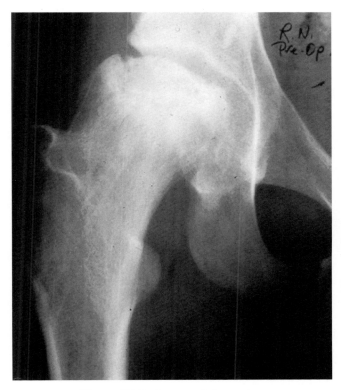

Figure 33-5 Amount of depression.

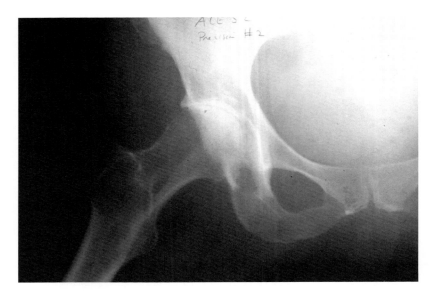

Figure 33-6 Advanced arthritic changes.

Intraoperative findings are a valuable tool for confirming the stage of osteonecrosis previously discovered on imaging studies. For example, one might plan a bone-grafting procedure based on radiographic findings; however, intraoperatively, if it was found that damage to the articular cartilage of the femoral head precluded grafting, this would override the preoperative radiographic staging, and the patient might undergo a resurfacing arthroplasty. Alternatively, one might plan for a resurfacing arthroplasty based on radiographic findings, and if intraoperative assessment demonstrated intact articular cartilage, a femoral head–sparing procedure, such as a bone grafting, could be performed. If it was found intraoperatively that there was gross articular damage on both sides of the joint, a total hip arthroplasty would be indicated.

In summary, preoperative radiographic staging may need to be up-staged or down-staged depending on operative inspection or palpation of the femoral head or acetabulum (Fig. 33-7).

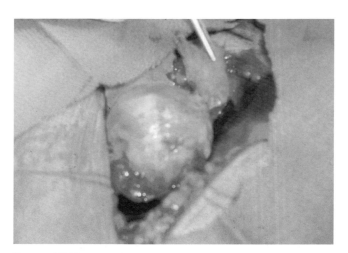

Figure 33-7 Example of cartilage delamination found intraoperatively.

Summary of Preoperative and Operative Evaluation for Treatment Approach

In summary, the four radiographic parameters are of paramount importance in offering treatment to patients with osteonecrosis. These parameters can certainly be modified by specific patient factors as well as intraoperative findings. Small precollapse lesions will be the most successfully treated by methods intended to save the femoral head, whereas patients with end-stage arthritis will not be able to have head-sparing procedures; indeed, they will have few treatment options except for total hip arthroplasty. A treatment algorithm based on these four radiographic parameters is outlined in Table 33-3. This algorithm may be modified based on intraoperative findings and various patient-specific factors. The following section describes all of the various treatment methods outlined in this algorithm table.

OBSERVATION AND MEDICAL MANAGEMENT

For precollapse lesions without symptoms, observation may be appropriate. Jergesen and Khan (43) reported the onset of pain within 5 years in less than one half of symptomatic hips with radiographic evidence of osteonecrosis. Other authors have reported a higher likelihood of progression and poor results from nonoperative management in asymptomatic hips (13,82,83). Thus, the natural history of the asymptomatic lesion is uncertain, and operative intervention remains controversial. If symptoms occur, the likelihood of progression increases dramatically, with the great majority of hips going on to femoral head collapse if left untreated. A recent report demonstrated spontaneous resolution of osteonecrosis in 3 of 13 hips. The authors suggested that spontaneous resolution of osteonecrosis may occur in early, small asymptomatic lesions where there is no evidence of disease in the contralateral hip (87).

For asymptomatic lesions and symptomatic lesions with no radiographic changes, pharmacologic treatment may play a

TABLE 33-3

TREATMENT ALGORITHM BASED ON RADIOGRAPHIC FEATURES

Radiographic Features	Symptoms	Procedure
Normal radiographs Positive MRI	Asymptomatic	Observation, Pharmacologic treatment
Positive MRI Small/medium Precollapse	Symptomatic	Core decompression +/− Bone grafting +/− pharmacologic treatment
Postcollapse <2-mm depression vascularized or nonvascularized	Symptomatic	Bone graft, osteotomy
Postcollapse >2-mm depression (no acetabular involvement)	Symptomatic	Limited femoral resurfacing
Acetabular involvement	Symptomatic	Total hip arthroplasty Consider total hip resurfacing arthroplasty

role. The use of vasodilators, anticoagulants, and lipid-lowering agents has shown promise (20,35,63,90). Recent reports have also suggested potential benefits from systemic alendronate (69). Oral daily alendronate was administered to 11 patients with 14 hips with osteonecrosis. Radiographs, MRIs, and biochemical markers of osteoclastic activity were periodically monitored. There was no evidence of collapse in the alendronate-treated group, while 4 of the 11 hips in the control group went on to collapse at 12 months. There was also a notable decrease in osteoclastic activity in the alendronate-treated group (69).

The choice of various pharmacological medications may be based on the current understanding of the pathophysiology of osteonecrosis in a particular patient. For example, a patient with hypercholesterolemia or hyperlipidemia as an associated risk factor might be best treated with a lipid-lowering agent like lovastatin (22). A patient with known hypertension from renal disease might be considered for treatment with an antihypertensive like verapamil. Patients with inherited coagulation disorders might be considered for anticoagulant treatment. For example, Stanazol, an anabolic steroid, has been utilized for the treatment of osteonecrosis in patients with elevations in lipoprotein A, a thrombophilic factor. Likewise, patients with other coagulation disorders may be treated with various anticoagulants like heparin or sodium warfarin. Certainly these methods require identification of these risk factors in patients with precollapse disease. It is doubtful that any pharmacological treatment would be useful in a patient who already has femoral head collapse (biomechanical compromise).

Protected weight bearing has been advocated by various authors as a treatment method. However, a review of more than 20 studies suggests that this method leads to unsatisfactory results in the greater majority of patients (59). The data pooled from 21 studies indicated successful results in only 22% of hips (182 of 819) at a mean follow-up of 34 months (range, 20 months to 10 years). It also appears that the degree of permitted weight bearing had no impact on the final outcome.

Both basic science and clinical reports have shown that electrical stimulation enhances osteogenesis, and this modal-

ity might be useful as a treatment method for osteonecrosis (5,6,79). However, the US Food and Drug Administration (FDA) has not approved this application. Several different techniques have been reported, including noninvasive pulsed electromagnetic field stimulation, direct-current stimulation of the necrotic area, and noninvasive direct-current stimulation by capacitative coupling. Aaron et al. (1) compared pulsed electromagnetic fields with core decompression in 106 hips and found good or excellent results in 68% of patients treated with electrical stimulation, as compared with 44% in the patients treated with core decompression. Steinberg et al. (80) evaluated electrical stimulation used as an adjunct in 42 patients undergoing core decompression and found no improvement in outcome at 1 year. Yoo et al. (96) reported clinical improvement in 75% of hips (81 of 108) treated with pulsed electromagnetic fields therapy at an average follow-up of 6.9 years. Ultimately, electrical stimulation will require additional study before it becomes a mainstay in the nonoperative treatment of osteonecrosis of the femoral head.

SURGICAL TREATMENT OPTIONS

Core Decompression with or without Bone Grafting

For small and medium-size precollapse lesions, where the contour of the femoral head is maintained, results of core decompression are generally favorable. This is true for lesions that have sclerotic and cystic areas on plain radiographs and those symptomatic lesions with findings only on MRI. It has also been suggested that the results of core decompression are better in predominantly sclerotic disease (91). The rationale for core decompression is that it decreases intraosseous pressure in the femoral head and may immediately relieve the associated pain. Increased intraosseous pressure has been implicated in the pathogenesis of osteonecrosis (30,39).

The results of core decompression have been reported in numerous studies. In a recent review of 54 hips at a minimum follow-up of 10 years, clinical or radiographic failure occurred in only 4 of 13 hips without plain radiographic changes and in none of the 7 hips with sclerotic changes (12). In that study, larger lesions and precollapse lesions with cystic changes did worse. In a study of 128 hips at a mean follow-up of 11 years after core decompression, a successful clinical result was reported in 22 of 25 hips (88%) with normal radiographic appearances (28). Successful results were seen in 36 of the 51 hips (71%) with precollapse disease. Mont et al. (59) reviewed 24 studies of core decompression and found satisfactory clinical results in 741 of 1166 hips (63.5%). In their review of 21 studies of hips managed nonoperatively, only 182 of 819 hips (22.7%) were considered to be successful. For precollapse lesions, there was a 71% success rate in the core decompression group compared with a 34.5% success rate in the nonoperative group.

The most common method of performing a core decompression involves the use of an 8- to 10-mm trephine or cannula inserted under fluoroscopic guidance to penetrate the lesion. Complications can occur if multiple drillings with a large-diameter trephine weaken the femoral head or if the trephine penetrates the femoral head and thus injures the articular cartilage and enters the joint space. In addition, if the entry site is made too low or distal (in the diaphyseal region), a subtrochanteric hip fracture can occur (16,59,62). Recently, a multiple drilling technique has been described as a method similar to core decompression (47,66). Kim et al. (47) compared 35 hips that underwent a multiple drilling technique with 30 hips that underwent a standard core decompression, at a mean follow-up of 60.3 months. The multiple drilling group had a significantly longer time to collapse (mean, 42.3 months vs. 22.6 months; $p = .011$) and a lower rate of collapse (55% vs. 85.7%, $p = 0.03$) than the standard core decompression group (47). Mont et al. (66) utilized multiple percutaneous small-diameter drillings. In their method, a 3.2-mm Steinman pin is inserted percutaneously through the lateral cortex in the metaphyseal region. The pin is then advanced through the femoral neck into the lesion, as previously determined from previous imaging studies, under fluoroscopic guidance. The authors performed two passes into smaller lesions and three passes into larger lesions using a single entry point. Thirty-two of 45 hips (71%) had good or excellent results at a mean 2-year follow-up. Stage I hips (24 of 30 hips, 80%) were more successful than stage II hips (8 of 15 hips, 57%) (66).

Most surgeons place patients on protected weight bearing (approximately 50%) for a period of 6 to 12 weeks postoperatively and then advance them to full weight bearing without impact loading for the first year following surgery.

In summary, satisfactory results can be obtained for small and medium-size precollapse lesions using core decompression. Overall results are not promising in lesions at more advanced stages. The authors believe that core decompression should not be performed in large lesions or when collapse is present except as a possible short-term palliative treatment method (Figs. 33-8 and 33-9 and Table 33-4).

NONVASCULARIZED BONE GRAFTING

In precollapse and early postcollapse disease in which articular cartilage is viable, bone grafting has numerous theoretical

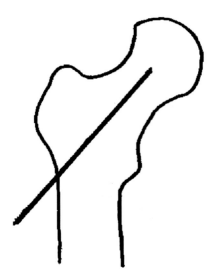

Figure 33-8   Schematic representation of core decompression with a Steinman pin.

advantages. It allows for removal of weak necrotic bone, decompression of the femoral head, and stimulation of repair and remodeling of subchondral bone. Bone grafting also provides for maintenance of articular congruity and prevention of collapse. Cancellous bone and cortical bone can both be utilized.

There are three general methods that have been used for nonvascularized bone grafting of the femoral head: cortical strut grafting through a core track in the femoral head and neck, bone grafting through the articular cartilage (the trapdoor procedure), and bone grafting through the femoral neck or femoral head neck junction (light bulb procedure). These procedures are described in the following subsections.

Cortical Strut Grafting

Cortical grafts can be placed through a core track made in the femoral neck and head. Bone can be harvested from the ilium, tibia, or fibula. Results with this technique have been variable. Buckley et al. (14) reported results for 20 hips in which either structural autografts or allografts were used. These grafts were placed through the track of the core decompression. At an average follow-up of 8 years (range, 2 to 19), there was a 90% success rate for precollapse lesions (Fig. 33-10).

Bone Grafting through Articular Cartilage

Another means for debridement and grafting an osteonecrotic lesion is through the femoral head articular cartilage. A "trapdoor" is made in the articular cartilage, which is lifted to expose the underlying lesion. Necrotic bone is removed, and the cavity is filled with either a cancellous bone graft or a cortical bone graft or a combination of the two (56,60). The articular flap is the held in place with a bioabsorbable screw. In one study, early results using autogenous iliac cortical and cancellous bone grafts combined with demineralized bone matrix showed good or excellent results in 22 of 30 procedures at a mean follow-up of 4.7 years (60). In another study,

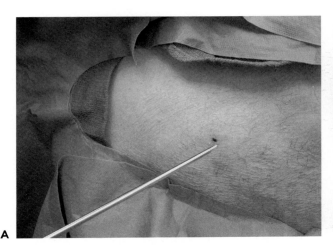
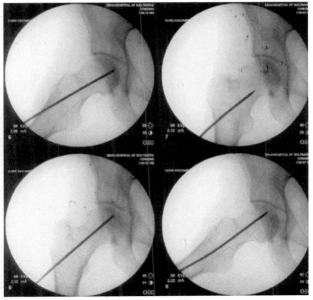

Figure 33-9 **A:** Intraoperative photograph demonstrating the percutaneous multiple small drilling technique. **B:** Intraoperative fluoroscopic views of the multiple small drilling technique.

good results were reported in 8 out of 9 postcollapse hips at a mean follow-up of 3 years (56) (Figs. 33-11 and 33-12).

Bone Grafting through the Femoral Neck

To avoid entering the lesion through the articular cartilage, a window can be made at the base of the head. The necrotic area is removed using burrs and curettes. A bone graft is then placed into the defect. Using this technique, known as the "light bulb" procedure, good results have been reported at long-term follow-up for late precollapse and early postcollapse lesions (71,93). Yamamoto et al. (93) used a combination of iliac crest cortical grafts and cancellous grafts to fill the defects made after removal of the necrotic bone. They reported good or excellent clinical results in 23 of 38 hips at a mean follow-up of 9 years (range, 2 to 15). Using only cancellous

TABLE 33-4
RESULTS OF CORE DECOMPRESSION

Authors	Year	No. of Hips	Success Rate, Stage I, II, III	Overall Success Rate
Aigner et al.	2002	45	96%, 56%, 0%	80%
Simank et al.[a]	2001	94	N	78%
Steinberg et al.[b]	2001	312	72%, 66%, 77%, 64%	
Maniwa et al.[c]	2000	26	N	66%
Chen et al.[d]	2000	25	N	60%
Lavernia et al.	2000	42	100%, 83%, 34%	
Van laere et al.	1998	51	N	39%
Scully et al.	1998	98	100%, 65%, 21%	
Iorio et al.[e]	1998	33	N	70%
Powell et al.	1997	29	N	66%
Mont et al.[f]	1996	1206	N	63.5%

N, not stratified.
[a]Compared outcome to patients who underwent intertrochanteric osteotomy; excluded patients undergoing corticosteroid therapy.
[b]Compared outcome by stage versus size of lesion. Stage I (72%) and small lesions (86%) fared best.
[c]Long-term follow-up (mean, 94 months).
[d]Conversion to THA utilized as endpoint.
[e]Endpoints defined as pain (52% success), collapse (61%), THA (70%).
[f]Compilation of 24 studies.

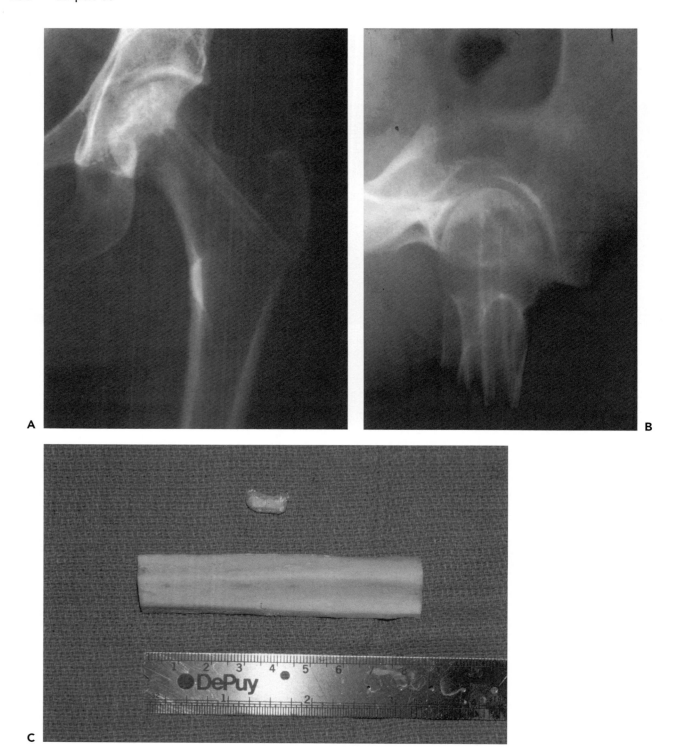

Figure 33-10 **A:** Anteroposterior radiograph following cortical strut grafting for osteonecrosis. **B:** Lateral radiograph following cortical strut grafting for osteonecrosis. **C:** Cortical strut allograft.

bone, Rosenwasser et al. (71) found 13 of 14 hips to be symptom free at a mean follow-up of 12 years (range, 10 to 15).

Mont et al. (61) reported the results of bone grafting through a cortical window at the femoral head neck junction in 21 hips at a mean follow-up of 48 months (range, 36 to 55). The necrotic bone was removed and replaced with bone graft substitute, a combination of demineralized bone matrix, processed allograft bone, and a thermoplastic carrier. Eighteen of 21 hips (86%) were clinically successful at the latest follow-up. Two of these patients had minimal

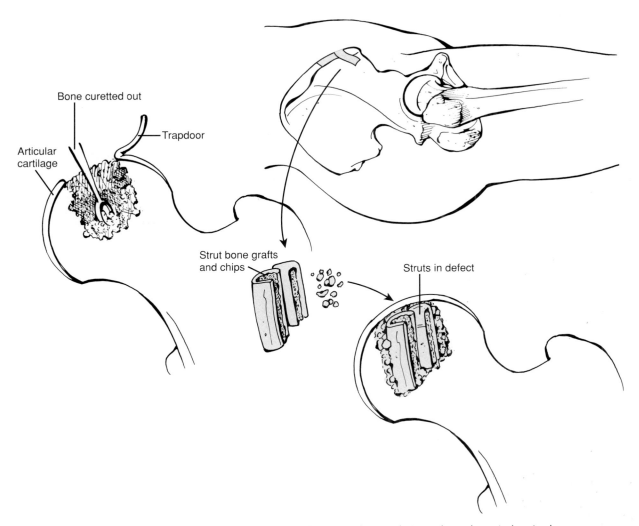

Figure 33-11 Schematic representation of the trapdoor technique through a window in the femoral head cartilage.

roentgenographic progression and less than 2 mm of head collapse.

In general, most surgeons who perform bone grafting procedures upon the femoral head place patients on protected weight bearing, partial weight bearing, or toe-touch weight bearing for a period of 6 weeks postoperatively. Weight bearing is then progressed to partial or 50% weight bearing over the following 6 weeks. Patients usually begin full weight bearing as tolerated by 3 months postoperatively.

In summary, these various bone-grafting techniques can be utilized for precollapse lesions as well as postcollapse lesions but do require that the femoral head articular cartilage be intact. This can be ascertained at the time of surgery during open procedures. In some cases where the femoral head is not visualized directly, it might be prudent to perform an arthroscopic procedure to delineate the status of the femoral head cartilage (9). If the femoral head cartilage is not intact or is found to be delaminated, these bone-grafting procedures might not be efficacious (Fig. 33-7). In this case, other procedures, such as limited femoral head resurfacing or total

hip arthroplasty, would be indicated as more appropriate (Figs. 33-13 to 33-15).

VASCULARIZED BONE GRAFTING

Excellent results for vascularized fibular bone grafting have been reported in early stages of disease. The rationale for vascularized grafting is that it allows for decompression, provides structural support, and enhances the vascular supply. In one report of 88 hips, clinical success was found in 61 hips at a mean of 5.5 years follow-up (76). The best results were seen in small and medium-size precollapse lesions. In another study, 103 hips were followed for at least 5 years (88). Average Harris hip scores improved at all stages. There was a high patient satisfaction rate (81%) among the 75 patients who responded to a questionnaire. The rate of conversion to total hip arthroplasty was 11% (2 of 19) for precollapse lesions, 23% (5 of 22) for postcollapse lesions without depression, and 38% (24 of 62) for more advanced lesions. Berend et al. (8) recently reviewed a

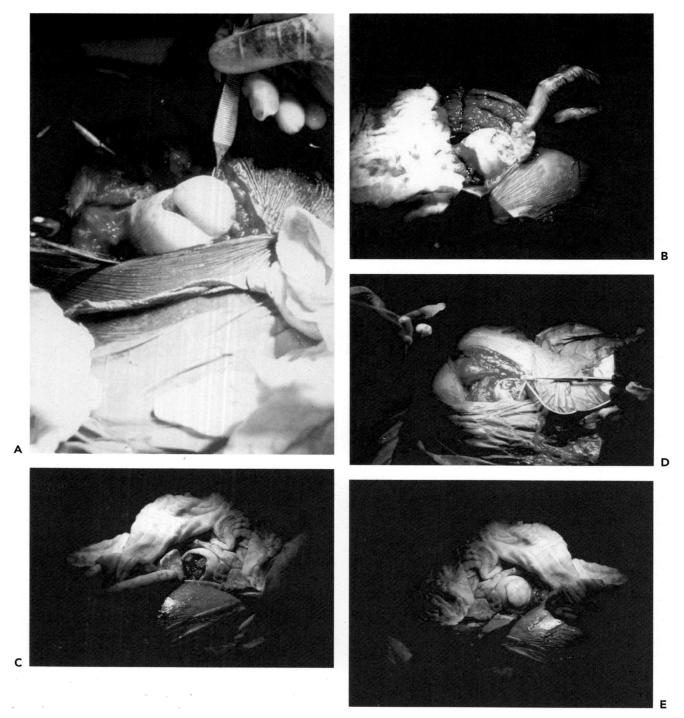

Figure 33-12 **A–E:** Intraoperative photographs demonstrating trapdoor bone grafting through the femoral head cartilage.

consecutive series of 224 postcollapse hips that underwent free vascularized fibular bone grafting at a mean follow-up of 4.3 years (range, 2 to 12 years) and found 63% with good to excellent results. The overall rate of survival was 64.5% at a minimum follow-up of 5 years (8). Yoo et al. (95) reported the results at a minimum follow-up of 10 years (range, 10 to 21 years) for vascularized fibular grafting in 97 hips. Overall satis-

factory clinical results were seen in 78 hips (80.4%), and 63 hips (64.9%) showed radiographic improvement or no change. Only 9 hips were ultimately converted to total hip arthroplasty (95). Plakseychuk et al. (70) directly compared vascularized and nonvascularized fibular grafting in 220 hips. The mean Harris hip score improved by 70% in the vascularized group and by only 36% in the nonvascularized group.

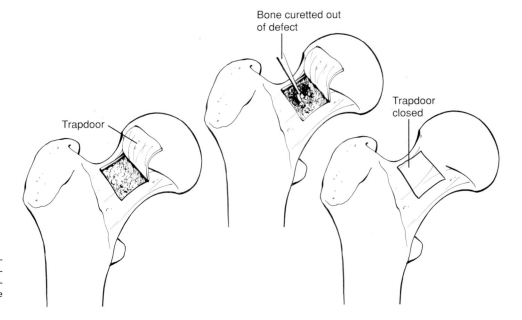

Figure 33-13   Schematic representation of the trapdoor bone-grafting technique through a window in the femoral neck at the head–neck junction.

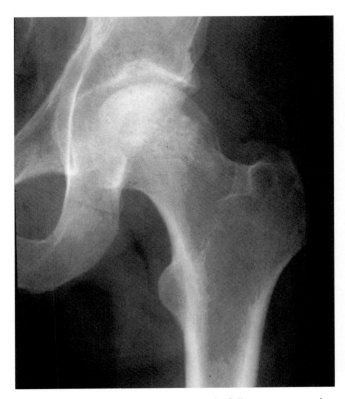

Figure 33-14   Postoperative radiographs following nonvascularized bone grafting through the femoral neck.

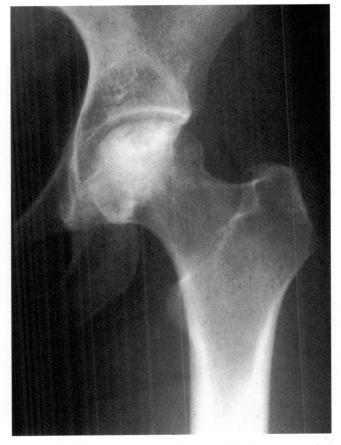

Figure 33-15   Postoperative radiographs following nonvascularized bone grafting through the femoral neck.

TABLE 33-5

RESULTS OF BONE-GRAFTING TECHNIQUES

Author	Year	Procedure Type	Number of Hips	Follow-Up (Yr), Mean (Range)	Clinical Success Rate
Yoo et al.	1992	V	81	5.2 (3–10.8)	91%
Urbaniak et al.	1996	V	64	6 (1–17)	83%
Buckley et al.	1991	C	20	8 (2–19)	90%
Nelson and Clark	1993	C	52	6 (2–12)	77%
Itoman and Yamamoto	1983	W	38	9 (2–15)	61%
Scher and Jakim	1993	T, O	45	5.5 (2.7–10.5)	87%
Rosenwasser et al.	1994	W	15	12 (10–15)	81%
Meyers et al.	1983	T	9	3 (1–9)	89%
Mont et al.	1998	T	24	4.7 (2.5–5)	83%
Mont et al.	2003	W	21	4 (3–4.7)	86%

C, nonvascularized bone grafting through core track; O, with ancillary osteotomy; T, trapdoor, nonvascularized bone graft; V, vascularized fibular graft; W, window in femoral neck, nonvascularized bone graft.

Muscle pedicle bone grafts have been described as a method of treating femoral head osteonecrosis. Meyers (54,55) reported on a muscle pedicle bone graft based on the quadratus femoris that was used to treat femoral neck nonunions and was later adapted to treat osteonecrosis. Yoon et al. (98) reviewed 71 hips that had undergone viable iliac crest bone grafting (9 vessel pedicle and 62 muscle pedicle bone grafts) for osteonecrosis in 52 patients. The overall survivorship was 96%, with good and excellent results in 54 hips (76%), at a mean follow-up of 3.3 years (range, 2 to 5 years).

The rehabilitation following vascularized bone grafting is fairly intensive, with most surgeons placing patients on protected weight bearing for a period of 3 to 6 months postoperatively.

In summary, vascularized grafting procedures require more expertise, and there is also the risk of donor site morbidity. At centers where they are performed often, the results of these procedures appear to be quite satisfactory in hips that do not have significant head depression. The results are worse once head depression is present (Tables 33-5 and 33-6).

TABLE 33-6

SUCCESS RATE AFTER PEDICLE BONE GRAFTS FOR OSTEONECROSIS OF THE FEMORAL HEAD

Authors	Number of Hips	Follow-Up (Yr)	Success Rate (%)
Solonen et al.	13	4.4	61
Urbaniak et al.	103	5.5	70
Ishizuka et al.	31	6.0	77
Sotereanos et al.	88	5.5	69
Soucacos et al.	184	4.7	86
Elsenshenk et al.	80	5.0	87
Judet and Gilbert	68	18.0	52
Hasegawa et al.	31	13.0	65

OSTEOTOMY

There are general two types of osteotomy that can be performed for osteonecrosis of the femoral head; intertrochanteric osteotomies or transtrochanteric rotational osteotomies, which are substantially more complex. All osteotomies are used to move the segment of necrotic bone away from the weight-bearing region. Results with osteotomies are better in small or medium-size lesions (<30% of the femoral head or combined necrotic angle <200°) in the earlier stages of disease. With postcollapse lesions, results are more variable and usually less efficacious.

Mont et al. (62) reviewed 37 corrective varus intertrochanteric osteotomies (with flexion or extension, depending on the location of the lesion) for precollapse lesions and postcollapse lesions without a change in contour of the femoral head. The mean follow-up was 11.5 years. The best results were obtained in small and medium-size lesions in patients who were not receiving high doses of corticosteroids. Scher and Jakim (73) reported long-term results for 55 postcollapse hips treated with valgus intertrochanteric osteotomies and bone grafting. The mean follow-up was 8 years. All patients were younger than 45 years of age, and none required high-dose steroids for an underlying inflammatory disease. Seven hips had gone on to failure as judged by the need of revision or a Harris hip score below 70 points. Drescher et al. (27) reported the results of intertrochanteric flexion osteotomy at a mean follow-up of 10.4 years (range, 3 to 20.3 years). Their 5-year survivorship was 90%. Twenty-seven percent of the hips underwent total hip arthroplasty at an average of 8.7 years following the osteotomy. The survival rates for Ficat stage II hips were higher than for stage III or IV hips, and hips with a necrotic angle greater than 200° fared better than those with a necrotic angle less than 200° degrees (27).

Rotational osteotomies allow for large degrees of translation of the osteonecrotic segment (78,84). Sugioka et al. (84) performed rotational osteotomies in 474 hips and reported a clinical success rate of 78% at a follow-up ranging from 3 to

16 years. Salvage procedures were performed in only 18 hips, of which 10 had extensive lesions and were probably inappropriately indicated for osteotomy. Inao et al. (41) reported the long-term results of a Sugioka-type rotational osteotomy in 14 hips at a mean follow-up of 13.2 years. Three hips were converted to total hip arthroplasty within 5 years of the osteotomy. Of the remaining 11 hips, the clinical and radiographic results were related to the preoperative radiographic stage. Hips with less than 2 mm of initial collapse maintained highly satisfactory results beyond 15 years following the index osteotomy. Hips with more than 2 mm of initial collapse tended to have gradually declining but clinically acceptable results (41). A recent review of rotational osteotomies reported successful results in 18 of 26 hips (78%) at a mean follow-up of 5 years (75). Hasegawa et al. (37) compared the long-term outcomes of pedicle bone grafting versus transtrochanteric rotational osteotomy for the treatment of osteonecrosis and found very similar results for both at 10 years. Other surgeons in the Western Hemisphere have had less successful results. Dean and Cabanela (24) reported only 3 satisfactory results in 18 rotational osteotomies at a mean follow-up of 5 years. Langlais and Fourastier (50) experienced similar results, with 7 failures (39%), 7 fair outcomes, and 7 satisfactory outcomes in 18 rotational osteotomies at a mean follow-up of 5 years. This procedure is clearly more technically demanding than an angular osteotomy. Furthermore, the results are variable, and rotational osteotomy is not routinely performed in the United States (24,42,50).

The rehabilitation following osteotomy is nearly as extensive as that following free vascularized fibular grafting, as patients typically undergo protected weight bearing for a range of 3 to 6 months.

In summary, in well-selected patients, osteotomy may be of value in precollapse or early postcollapse lesions that are small or medium-size. Although osteotomy has a role in these selected patients, the procedure can be difficult to perform and has a high potential for morbidity, including nonunion. Total hip arthroplasty can be performed after osteotomy, but this subsequent procedure may be more difficult than primary arthroplasty (Table 33-7).

TABLE 33-7

SUCCESS RATE AFTER TRANSTROCHANTERIC ROTATIONAL OSTEOTOMY FOR OSTEONECROSIS OF THE FEMORAL HEAD

Authors	Number of Hips	Follow-Up (Yr)	Success Rate (%)
Sugioka et al.	128	2 to 9	77
Eyb and Kotz	39	4.1	59
Tooke et al.	18	3.3	44
Matsuda et al.	52	5.1	69
Sugano et al.	41	6.3	56
Dean and Cabanela	18	5.0	17
Langlais and Fourastier	16	6.5	50
Atumi and Kurokl	18	3.5	94
Noguchi et al.	10	4.3	90
Hasegawa et al.	77	7.0	68

OTHER LESS-OFTEN-UTILIZED ALTERNATIVES TO ARTHROPLASTY

Osteochondral Grafts

Osteochondral allografts have been described in only a few patients (53,55). The procedure requires hip dislocation and the removal of the necrotic bone and overlying cartilage. The defect is packed with an iliac crest cancellous autograft and then capped with an osteochondral allograft. Meyers and Covery (56) reported good or excellent results in 8 of 9 stage III hips at a mean follow-up of 3 years (range, 1 to 9 years).

Arthrodesis

Arthrodesis has generally not been successful in the management of osteonecrosis of the femoral head. One major reason for limited success is the high incidence of bilateral hip involvement. Another reason is that it is difficult to achieve a solid fusion in cases of extensive osteonecrosis, and the method has been reported to carry a 50% risk of pseudoarthrosis (32).

Resection Arthroplasty

Resection arthroplasty of the hip was first described by Girdlestone (34) for the treatment of septic hip arthritis. Milch (57) modified this procedure with an intertrochanteric osteotomy. Although excellent pain relief has been reported, substantial limb shortening does occur, along with some hip weakness. This may be a treatment option for the severely debilitated nonambulatory patient.

LIMITED FEMORAL RESURFACING

Large precollapse lesions and postcollapse lesions with greater than 2 mm of femoral head depression pose a difficult problem. In these more advanced stages, procedures aimed at preservation of the femoral head do not have good results. In the young patient population, total hip arthroplasty may not be a favored option. With femoral head resurfacing arthroplasty, the damaged cartilage on the femoral side is removed, and bone stock is preserved. The viable acetabular articular cartilage is retained without being touched. Resurfacing arthroplasty may be an option for younger patients with postcollapse disease.

Hemiresurfacing is directly related to cup arthroplasty, which was originally invented by Smith-Peterson. The concept of hemiresurfacing is appealing in Ficat and Arlet stage III osteonecrosis because the acetabulum is relatively normal. This technique optimizes durability and achieves maximal surface contact in cases of precision fit. If a subsequent surgery is required, the preservation of the proximal bone stock does not obviate a total hip arthroplasty.

Hungerford et al. (40) reviewed 33 femoral head resurfacings in hips with postcollapse disease. Seven of these hips had early acetabular changes. Preoperatively all hips had an intact joint space of at least 2 mm circumferentially on anteroposterior and lateral radiographs. Twenty-two hips (61%) had good or excellent overall results at a mean follow-up of 10.5 years. The mean interval between limited femoral resurfacing and

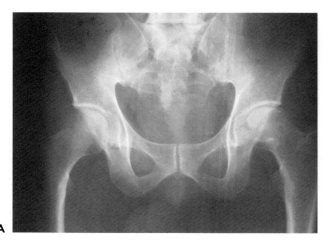
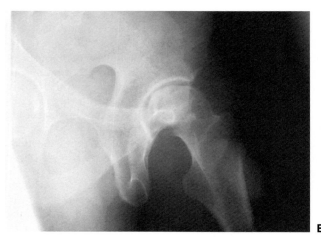

Figure 33-16 A, B: Preoperative anteroposterior and lateral radiographs demonstrating femoral head osteonecrosis without acetabular involvement.

total hip arthroplasty was 60 months. From this review, it was concluded that femoral head resurfacing is a useful interim procedure for more advanced lesions that would otherwise only be treated with total hip arthroplasty.

Amstutz et al. (3) reviewed their experience with 37 hips treated using four different prostheses at a mean follow-up of 7.1 years (range, 1.5 to 18). Twelve hips were revised, 11 for acetabular wear and 1 for femoral loosening. The mean time to revision was 7.4 years, and the probability of survival was 79% at 5 years and 59% at 10 years. Adili and Trousdale (2) reviewed 29 femoral head resurfacings and found a 75% survivorship at 3 years. However, only 62.5% of patients reported satisfaction and good pain relief at last follow-up. Mont et al. (67) compared limited femoral resurfacing and conventional total hip arthroplasty in 60 patients with advanced osteonecrosis and a mean age of 35 years. At a mean follow-up of 7 years, the survivor rates for the femoral resurfacing and

total hip arthroplasty were 90% and 93%, respectively. Patients that underwent limited femoral resurfacing were more active (60% vs. 27%); however, they experienced more groin pain (20% vs. 6%) than patients that underwent total hip arthroplasty (67). Beaule et al. (7) reported the results of 37 limited femoral resurfacings; the overall survivorship was 79% at 5 years and 59% at 10 years. It appeared that the overall survivorship was better when the preoperative symptoms were present for less than 1 year. The average time to conversion to total hip arthroplasty was 7.5 years (7).

Limited femoral resurfacing is a successful method of preserving bone stock while removing damaged cartilage and necrotic bone from the femoral head. It is especially useful in the young patient diagnosed early with postcollapse disease, no joint space narrowing, and no evidence of acetabular articular cartilage damage on radiographs and intraoperative inspection (Table 33-7 and Figs. 33-16 and 33-17).

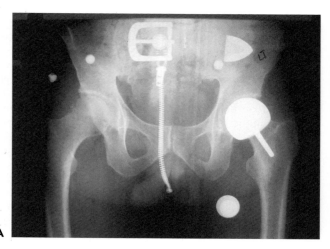
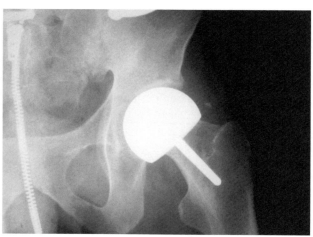

Figure 33-17 A, B: Postoperative anteroposterior and lateral radiographs following limited femoral head resurfacing.

HEMIARTHROPLASTY

Monopolar or unipolar hemiarthroplasty has been plagued by poor results due to stem failure and acetabular destruction. Takaoka et al. (86) reported proximal migration in 12 of 19 Austin-Moore prostheses (63%) at a mean follow-up of 5 years. The authors also noted loosening in 9 of the 18 hips that were inserted without cement. The high failure rate in this series was attributable to inadequate press-fit fixation of a thin cementless stem and to cases in which there was acetabular involvement leading to rapid proximal migration (86). Steinberg (77) reported similar results in a group of patients under the age of 50, in which the revision rate was 47% at a mean follow-up of 7 years. At the time of review, 44% of the unrevised prostheses were rated as fair or poor results. The failure modes were similar to those of Takaoka et al.'s series.

Bipolar hemiarthroplasty became an attractive alternative when the concept of preservation of acetabular cartilage due to increased motion at the prosthetic head and inner bearing insert interface was promulgated. However, several studies have shown little or no motion between the bearings in the prosthesis, suggesting that it behaves much like a unipolar arthroplasty (19,89). Others have shown that a substantial amount of motion occurs at the interbearing interface (10,38,85). Mess and Barmada (52), in a study of Batemen prostheses, showed that in cases in which the prosthesis was placed because of a fracture and the acetabular cartilage was well preserved substantial motion occurred at the outer bearing. In contrast, in cases in which the prosthesis was placed for arthritis, most of the motion occurred at the interbearing interface (52).

Fisher and Capello (31) reported a 20% incidence of groin or buttock pain in 76 patients with bipolar hemiarthroplasties, of whom 64 had osteonecrosis. Lachiewicz and Desman (49) reported 15 good and excellent clinical outcomes in 31 hips (48%) at a mean follow-up of 4.6 years (range, 2 to 11). Cabanela (15) found 10 successful clinical outcomes in 17 patients (59%) that had a Bateman bipolar prosthesis for stage III or IV osteonecrosis at a mean follow-up of 9.2 years. Yamano et al. (94) reported the results of 29 osteonecrotic hips for which an uncemented press-fit bipolar endoprosthesis was placed. At a mean follow-up of 12 years, femoral loosening occurred in 6 hips (21%), 5 hips (17%) developed acetabular protrusion, and osteolysis was seen in 11 hips (38%) (94). A report by Chan and Shih (17) on bipolar hemiarthroplasty versus total hip arthroplasty in patients with bilateral osteonecrosis of the femoral head found no statistical differences in thigh pain, groin pain, osteolysis, dislocation, and revision rates at an average follow-up of 6.4 years (range, 4 to 12). However, osteolysis from polyethylene wear has been reported as a late complication following bipolar hemiarthroplasty (11). In a bipolar hemiarthroplasty, the polyethylene liner is often quite thin, which may contribute to the development of osteolysis. This is one of the major reasons why the authors do not believe that a bipolar hemiarthroplasty is an appropriate approach to the management of this patient population.

In summary, the authors strongly suggest not using this modality for the treatment of osteonecrosis of the femoral head.

TOTAL HIP ARTHROPLASTY

In patients with advanced osteonecrosis with arthritic changes, total hip arthroplasty may be indicated. As stated earlier, total hip replacement may be an appropriate treatment for less extensive lesions in older patients. Although this is the most definitive treatment for the arthritic stage of osteonecrosis, results have not been as good as the results for patients who underwent this treatment for other diseases such as osteoarthritis (6). Earlier studies demonstrated high failure rates (21,26,72). Dorr et al. (25) found a 91% failure rate at 12-year follow-up in 57 hips of patients younger than 45. Patients under the age of 30 had even a worse prognosis. Saito et al. (72) compared the results, at a mean follow-up of 7 years, for 29 hips with osteonecrosis and 63 hips with osteoarthritis. Postoperative hip scores were inferior for the patients with osteonecrosis. Eight of 29 hips (28%) with osteonecrosis required revision, compared with only 4 of the 63 hips (6%) with osteoarthritis. There was also a statistically higher incidence of femoral component loosening detected on radiographs in the osteonecrosis group (72). Schneider et al. (74) reported loosening in 27 of 35 total hip arthroplasties (77%) at a 9-year follow-up.

With improvements in prosthetic designs and newer surgical techniques, better results have recently been reported in patients with osteonecrosis (23,33,92). Fye et al. (33) reported the results of 72 arthroplasties at a mean follow-up of 84 months. Good to excellent results were reported in 94% of all the hips. Using revision as an end point, the likelihood of survival was 96.9%. When radiographic loosening was used as an end point, results were still superior to those previously reported. Xenakis et al. (92) compared results for cementless total hip arthroplasty in 29 patients with osteonecrosis of the femoral head and 29 patients with degenerative joint disease. At a mean follow-up of 7.6 years for the patients with osteonecrosis and 7.1 years for those with osteoarthritis, there were no differences in pain improvement scores. One failure occurred in a patient with osteonecrosis (92). Hartley et al. (36) reported the outcomes of cementless total hip arthroplasty for osteonecrosis in 45 patients. The average age at implantation was 31 years (range, 21 to 40 years). At a mean follow-up of 9.75 years, there were no aseptic failures of the femoral component, and most patients (93%) reported few or no functional limitations. However, 21% of the hips required acetabular revision surgery (36). Kim et al. (43) evaluated cemented versus cementless femoral components in bilateral total hip arthroplasty in patients with osteonecrosis. All patients had a cementless acetabular component. At a mean follow-up of 9.3 years, the average Harris hip scores were very similar for the cemented component group (96 points) and cementless component group (95 points). One cemented stem was revised because of infection, and two cementless stems were revised because of loosening. The prevalence of osteolysis in Gruen zones 1 and 7 was 16% in cemented femurs and 24% in cementless femurs (43). A recent meta-analysis of 44 studies with results for total hip arthroplasty for osteonecrosis in 2037 patients revealed that there were 931 poor outcomes in 2560 hips (36%). Patients with known risk factors such as high-dose steroids, systemic lupus erythematosus, or sickle cell disease had a failure rate of 31%, which was less than the 50% failure rate noted in patients without risk factors (58).

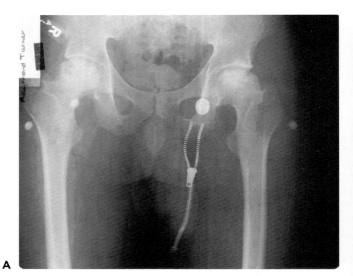

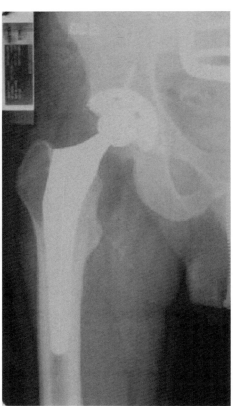

Figure 33-18 **A, B:** Preoperative and postoperative radiographs following THA for osteonecrosis of the femoral head.

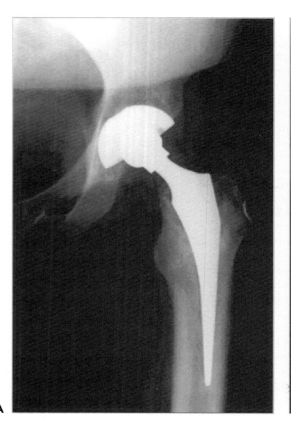

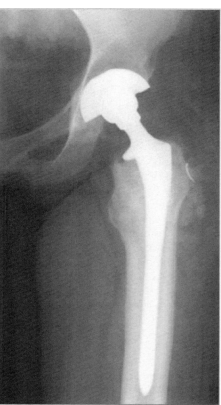

Figure 33-19 **A:** Anteroposterior radiograph demonstrating a failed proximally coated femoral component in a young patient with sickle cell anemia. **B:** Radiograph following revision to an extensively coated femoral component.

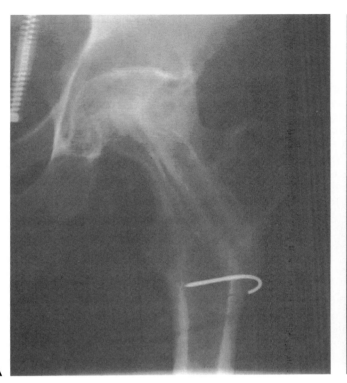
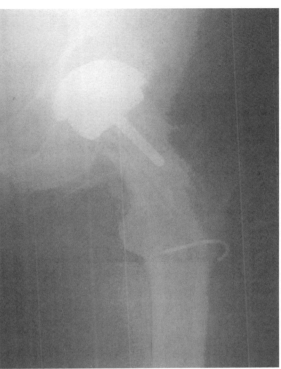

Figure 33-20 **A:** Radiograph of a failed vascularized bone grafting. **B:** Radiograph of the same hip following metal-on-metal resurfacing arthroplasty.

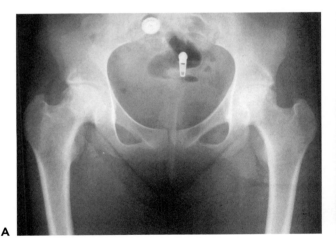
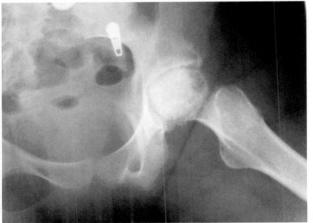
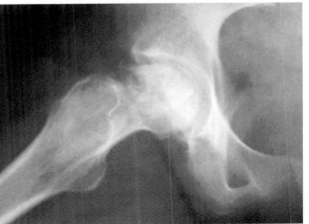

Figure 33-21 **A–C:** Radiographs of a young patient with bilateral hip osteonecrosis.

The authors have utilized a proximally coated, tapered cementless femoral stem (Accolade, Stryker, Allendale, NJ) with a press-fit cementless acetabular component (Trident, Stryker, Allendale, NJ) for advanced osteonecrosis and have seen only one femoral loosening, in a patient with sickle cell disease, with subsequent replacement of the stem by a fully coated cementless stem. From 2000 to 2003, the authors performed 120 cementless total hip arthroplasties for osteonecrosis of the femoral head. The more recent studies lend support to the idea that with improved techniques and implants better results can be anticipated in patients with osteonecrosis requiring total hip arthroplasty. Alternate bearing surfaces and better polyethylene formulations may continue to improve patient outcomes in this population (Figs. 33-18 and 33-19).

METAL-ON-METAL SURFACE ARTHROPLASTY

Surface hip arthroplasty has been an appealing option in this patient population because of the relative conservation of bone stock. However, early experience in the United States with the fully cemented McMinn design was plagued by acetabular component loosening in the short term. Metal-on-metal resurfacing arthroplasty began in 1996 under the aus-pices of an FDA Type II investigational device exemption trial utilizing the Conserve Plus prosthesis (Wright Medical Technology, Arlington, TN). The early results with this device have recently been reported. Amstutz et al. (4) reviewed 400 metal-on-metal hybrid surface arthroplasties performed between November 1996 and November 2000. Of these, 36 were performed for osteonecrosis. The overall component survival rate was at 94.4% at 4 years as assessed by Kaplan-Meier analysis. The results for the group of patients with osteonecrosis did not appear to differ from the overall results. A surface arthroplasty risk index was developed by researchers in order to evaluate patients at risk for early failure. A maximum score was 6 points; the higher the score, the higher the risk of failure. Two points were given for femoral head cysts of >1 cm, 2 points for a patient weight <82 kg, 1 point for previous surgery, and 1 point for high activity as evaluated by the University of California Los Angeles (UCLA) rating system. For patients with a surface arthroplasty risk index of >3, the component survival rate was 89% at four years; for patients with a surface arthroplasty risk index of ≤3, the component survival rate was 97%. The majority of the patients returned to a high level of activity, including participation in sports, as assessed by the UCLA system. Yoo et al. (97) reported 40 hips with osteonecrosis that underwent resurfacing arthroplasty with the Birmingham Hip Resurfacing system. There were no complications, no osteolysis, and no component loosening

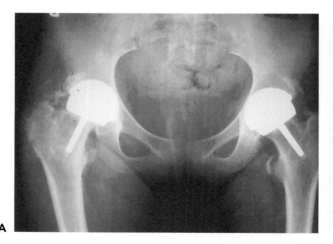

A

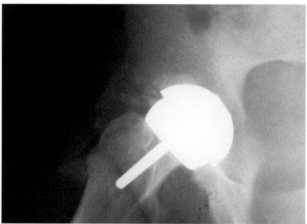

B

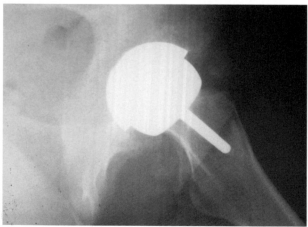

C

Figure 33-22 **A–C:** Postoperative radiographs of the same patient following bilateral metal-on-metal resurfacing arthroplasties.

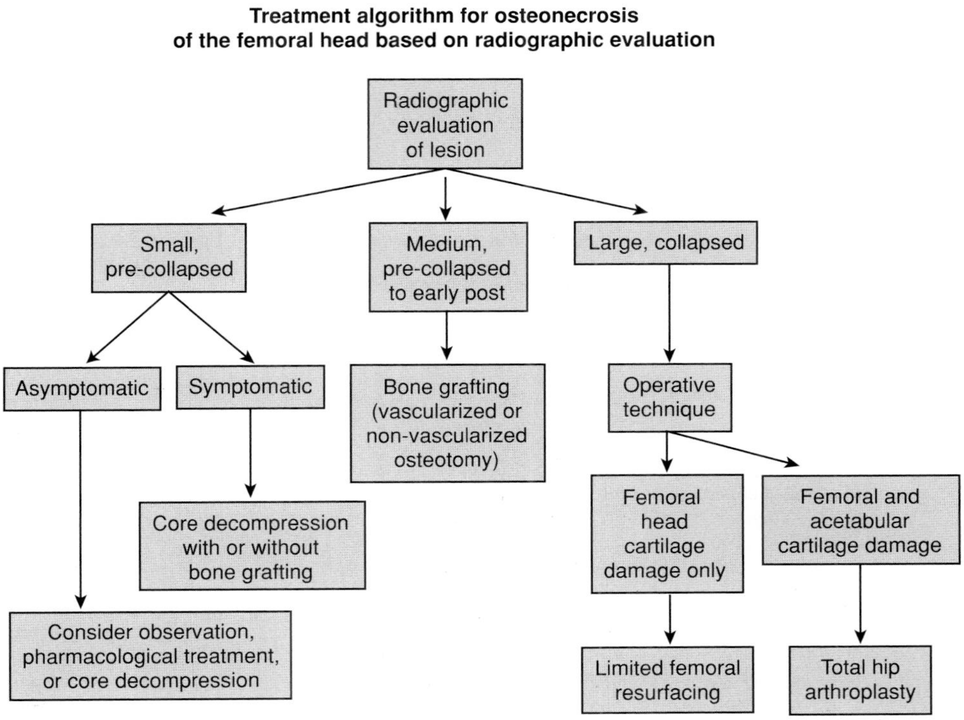

Treatment algorithm for osteonecrosis
of the femoral head based on radiographic evaluation

Figure 33-23 Treatment algorithm for osteonecrosis of the femoral head based on radiographic evaluation.

at a mean follow-up of 4 years. The authors have implanted 27 metal-on-metal total hip resurfacing arthroplasties (Wright Medical Technology, Arlington, TN) for osteonecrosis over the last four years and have had only one failure, from a periprosthetic fracture below the femoral component (Figs. 33-20 to 33-22).

AUTHORS' TREATMENT PHILOSOPHY

Decision making in the treatment of osteonecrosis can be systematic and based on disease stage as manifested by radiographic findings. Treatment options will, in part, be influenced by the surgeon's familiarity with various procedures. As certain treatment modalities have better results for different disease stages, it is important that the treating surgeon shows flexibility and use modalities appropriate for the extent of disease. Patient-related factors, including general health, activity level, and age, may also guide the decision-making process. The possibility that future procedures might be needed should also influence this process. It is not uncommon for a patient with osteonecrosis of the femoral head to require multiple procedures in his or her lifetime.

SUMMARY

In summary, early stage lesions may be treated with core decompression or head-sparing techniques. One may choose to use nonoperative pharmacologic treatment in asymptomatic hips with precollapse lesions. For later stage lesions, before articular cartilage destruction occurs, osteotomies could be considered, as could bone-grafting procedures, both

vascularized and nonvascularized. In situations where there is femoral head cartilage delamination or cartilage loss, but prior to acetabular involvement, femoral head hemiresurfacing could be considered. Once acetabular involvement occurs, the only viable treatment option is total hip arthroplasty. Metal-on-metal resurfacing arthroplasty may be another alternative, but it currently remains investigational (Fig. 33-23).

REFERENCES

1. Aaron RK, Lennox D, Bunce GE, et al. The conservative treatment of osteonecrosis of the femoral head: a comparison of core decompression and pulsing electromagnetic fields. *Clin Orthop.* 1989;249:209–218.
2. Adili A, Trousdale RT. Femoral head resurfacing for the treatment of osteonecrosis in the young patient. *Clin Orthop.* 2003;417:93–101.
3. Amstutz HC. Arthroplasty options for advanced osteonecrosis. *Orthopaedics.* 2000;20:927–928.
4. Amstutz HC, Beaule PE, Dorey FJ, et al. Metal-on-Metal hybrid surface arthroplasty: two to six-year follow-up study. *J Bone Joint Surg [Am].* 2004;86A(1):28–39.
5. Arnoldi CC. Vascular aspects of degenerative joint disorders: a synthesis. *Acta Orthop Scand Suppl.* 1994;261:1–82.
6. Bassett CA, Schink-Ascani M, Lewis SM. Effects of pulsed electromagnetic fields on Steinberg ratings of femoral head osteonecrosis. *Clin Orthop.* 1989;246:172–185.
7. Beaule PE, Schmalzried TP, Campbell P, et al. Duration of symptoms and outcome of hemiresurfacing for hip osteonecrosis. *Clin Orthop.* 2001;385:104–117.
8. Berend KR, Gunneson EE, Urbaniak JR. Free vascularized fibular grafting for the treatment of post-collapse osteonecrosis of the femoral head. *J Bone Joint Surg [Am].* 2003;85:987–993.
9. Berend KR, Vail TP. Hip arthroscopy in the adolescent and pediatric athlete. *Clin Sports Med.* 2001;20:763–778.
10. Bochner RM, Pellicci P, Lyden JP. Bipolar hemiarthroplasty for fracture of the femoral neck: clinical review with special emphasis on prosthetic motion. *J Bone Joint Surg [Am].* 1988;70:1001–1010.

11. Bose WJ, Miller GJ, Petty W. Osteolysis of the acetabulum associated with a bipolar hemiarthroplasty. *J Bone Joint Surg [Am].* 1995;77:1733–1735.
12. Bozic KJ, Zurakowski D, Thornhill TS. Survivorship analysis of hips treated with core decompression for nontraumatic osteonecrosis of the femoral head. *J Bone Joint Surg [Am].* 1999;81:200–209.
13. Bradway JK, Morrey BF. The natural history of the silent hip in bilateral atraumatic osteonecrosis. *J Arthroplasty.* 1993;8:383–387.
14. Buckley PD, Gearen PF, Petty RW. Structural bone grafting for early atraumatic avascular necrosis of the femoral head. *J Bone Joint Surg [Am].* 1991;73:1357–1364.
15. Cabanela ME. Bipolar versus total hip arthroplasty for avascular necrosis of the femoral head: a comparison. *Clin Orthop.* 1990;261:59–62.
16. Camp JF, Colwell CW Jr. Core decompression of the femoral head for osteonecrosis. *J Bone Joint Surg [Am].* 1986;68:1313–1319.
17. Chan YS, Shih CH. Bipolar versus total hip arthroplasty for osteonecrosis in the same patient. *Clin Orthop.* 2000;379:169–177.
18. Chang JD. The relationship between osteonecrosis of the femoral head and alcohol abuse. Paper presented at the Symposium of the Association Research Circulation Osseous; Jeju Island, South Korea; 2003.
19. Chen SC, Badrinath K, Pell LH, et al. The movements of the components of the Hastings bipolar prosthesis: a radiographic study in 65 patients. *J Bone Joint Surg [Br].* 1989;71:186–188.
20. Cheras PA. Role of hyperlipidemia, hypercoagulability, and hypofibrinolysis, in osteonecrosis and osteoarthritis. In: Urbaniak JR, Jones JP Jr, eds. *Osteonecrosis: Etiology, Diagnosis, and Treatment.* Rosemont, IL: American Academy of Orthopaedic Surgeons; 1997:97–104.
21. Cornell CN, Salvati EA, Pellicci PM. Long-term follow-up of total hip replacement in patients with osteonecrosis. *Orthop Clin North [Am].* 1985;16:757–769.
22. Cui Q, Wang CJ, Su CC, et al. The Otto Aufranc award. Lovastatin prevents steroid induced adipogenesis and osteonecrosis. *Clin Orthop.* 1997;344:8–19.
23. D'Antonio JA, Capello WN, Manley MT, et al. Hydroxyapatite coated implants. Total hip arthroplasty in the young patient and patients with avascular necrosis. *Clin Orthop.* 1997;344:124–138.
24. Dean MT, Cabanela ME. Transtrochanteric anterior rotational osteotomy for avascular necrosis of the femoral head: long-term results. *J Bone Joint Surg [Br].* 1993;75:597–601.
25. Dorr LD, Luckett M, Conaty JP. Total hip arthroplasties in patients younger than 45 years: a nine-to-ten year follow-up study. *Clin Orthop.* 1990;260:215–219.
26. Dorr LD, Takei GK, Conaty JP. Total hip arthroplasties in patients less than 45 years old. *J Bone Joint Surg [Am].* 1983;65:474–479.
27. Drescher W, Furst M, Hahne HJ, et al. Survival analysis of hips treated with flexion osteotomy for femoral head necrosis. *J Bone Joint Surg [Br].* 2003;85:969–974.
28. Fairbank AC, Bhatia D, Jinnah RH, et al. Long-term results of core decompression for ischaemic necrosis of the femoral head. *J Bone Joint Surg [Br].* 1995;77:42–49.
29. Fehrle MJ, Callaghan JJ, Clark CR, et al. Uncemented total hip arthroplasty in patients with aseptic necrosis of the femoral head and previous bone grafting. *J Arthroplasty.* 1993;8:1–6.
30. Ficat RP. Idiopathic bone necrosis of the femoral head: early diagnosis and treatment. *J Bone Joint Surg [Br].* 1985;67:3–9.
31. Fisher DA, Capello WN. Bipolar hip prosthesis in intact acetabula. Paper presented at the annual meeting of the Academy of Orthopaedic Surgeons; Atlanta, GA; 1988.
32. Freiherr-von-Salis-Soglio G, Ruff C. Idiopathic femur head necrosis in the adult: results of surgical therapy. *Z Orthop.* 1988;126:492–499.
33. Fye MA, Huo MH, Zatorski LE, et al. Total hip arthroplasty performed without cement in patients with femoral head osteonecrosis who are less than 50 years old. *J Arthroplasty.* 1998;13:876–881.
34. Girdlestone BM. Arthrodesis and other operations for tuberculosis of the hip. *J Bone Joint Surg.* 1925;7:347–374.
35. Glueck CJ, Glueck HI, Welch M, et al. Familial idiopathic osteonecrosis mediated by familial hypofibrinolysis with high levels of plasminogen activator inhibitor. *Thromb Haemost.* 1994;71:195–198.
36. Hartley WT, McAuley JP, Culpepper WJ, et al. Osteonecrosis of the femoral head treated with cementless total hip arthroplasty. *J Bone Joint Surg [Am].* 2000;82:1408–1413.
37. Hasegawa Y, Sakano S, Iwase T, et al. Pedicle bone grafting versus transtrochanteric rotational osteotomy for avascular necrosis of the femoral head. *J Bone Joint Surg [Br].* 2003;85:191–198.
38. Hodgkinson JP, Meadows TH, Davies DR, et al. A radiological assessment of interprosthetic movement in the Charnley-Hastings hemiarthroplasty. *Injury.* 1988;19:18–20.
39. Hungerford DS, Lennox DW. The importance of increased intraosseous pressure in the development of osteonecrosis of the femoral head: implications for treatment. *Orthop Clin North [Am].* 1985;16:635–654.
40. Hungerford MW, Mont MA, Scott S, et al. Surface replacement hemiarthroplasty for the treatment of osteonecrosis of the femoral head. *J Bone Joint Surg [Am].* 1998;80:1656–1664.
41. Inao S, Ando M, Gotoh E, et al. Minimum 10-year results of Sugioka's osteotomy for femoral head osteonecrosis. *Clin Orthop.* 1999;368:141–148.
42. Iwasada S, Hasegawa Y, Iwase T, et al. Transtrochanteric rotational osteotomy for osteonecrosis of the femoral head: 43 patients followed for at least 3 years. *Arch Orthop Trauma Surg.* 1997;116:447–453.
43. Jergesen HE, Khan AS. The natural history of untreated asymptomatic hips in patients who have non-traumatic osteonecrosis. *J Bone Joint Surg [Am].* 1997;79:359–363.
44. Jones JP Jr. Concepts of etiology and early pathogenesis of osteonecrosis. *Instr Course Lect.* 1994;43:499–512.
45. Kerboul M, Thomine J, Postel M, et al. The conservative treatment of idiopathic aseptic necrosis of the femoral head. *J Bone Joint Surg [Br].* 1974;56:291–296.
46. Khanna AJ, Yoon TR, Mont MA, et al. Femoral head osteonecrosis: detection and grading by using a rapid MR imaging protocol. *Radiology.* 2000;217:188–192.
47. Kim SY, Kim DH, Park IH, et al. Multiple drilling compared with standard core decompression for the treatment of osteonecrosis of the femoral head. Paper presented by the Symposium of the Association Research Circulation Osseous; Jeju Island, South Korea; 2003.
48. Kim YH, Oh SH, Kim JS, et al. Contemporary total hip arthroplasty with and without cement in patients with osteonecrosis of the femoral head. *J Bone Joint Surg [Am].* 2003;85:675–681.
49. Lachiewicz PF, Desman SM. The bipolar endoprosthesis in avascular necrosis of the femoral head. *J Arthroplasty.* 1988;3:131–138.
50. Langlais F, Fourastier J. Rotational osteotomies for osteonecrosis of the femoral head. *Clin Orthop.* 1997;343:110–123.
51. Lieberman JR, Berry DJ, Mont MA, et al. Osteonecrosis of the hip: management in the 21st century. *Inst Course Lect.* 2003;52:337–355.
52. Mess D, Barmada R. Clinical and motion studies of the Bateman bipolar prosthesis in osteonecrosis of the hip. *Clin Orthop.* 1990;251:44–47.
53. Meyers MH. Osteonecrosis of the femoral head: pathogenesis and long-term results of treatment. *Clin Orthop.* 1988;231:51–61.
54. Meyers MH. Osteonecrosis of the femoral head treated with the muscle pedicle graft. *Orthop Clin North [Am].* 1985;16:741–745.
55. Meyers MH. The treatment of osteonecrosis of the hip with fresh osteochondral allografts and with the muscle pedicle graft technique. *Clin Orthop.* 1978;130:202–209.
56. Meyers MH, Convery FR. Grafting procedures in osteonecrosis of the hip. *Semin Arthroplasty.* 1991;2:189–197.
57. Milch H. The resection-angulation operation for hip joint disabilities. *J Bone Joint Surg [Am].* 1955;37:699–717.
58. Mont MA, Berry DJ, Lieberman J, et al. Total hip arthroplasty in avascular necrosis of the hip: a meta-analysis study of outcome. Paper presented at the annual meeting of the Harvard Hip Course; Boston, MA; 2003.
59. Mont MA, Carbone JJ, Fairbank AC. Core decompression versus nonoperative management for osteonecrosis of the hip. *Clin Orthop.* 1996;324:169–178.
60. Mont MA, Einhorn TA, Sponseller PD, et al. The trapdoor procedure using autogenous cortical and cancellous bone grafts for

osteonecrosis of the femoral head. *J Bone Joint Surg [Br]*. 1998;80:56–62.

61. Mont MA, Etienne G, Ragland PS. Outcome of nonvascularized bone grafting for osteonecrosis of the femoral head. *Clin Orthop*. 2003;417:84–92.

62. Mont MA, Fairbank AC, Krackow KA, et al. Corrective osteotomy for osteonecrosis of the femoral head. *J Bone Joint Surg [Am]*. 1996;78:1032–1038.

63. Mont MA, Hungerford DS. Non-traumatic avascular necrosis of the femoral head. *J Bone Joint Surg [Am]*. 1995;77:459–474.

64. Mont MA, Jones LC, Sotereanos DG, et al. Understanding and treating osteonecrosis of the femoral head. *Instr Course Lect*. 2000;49:169–185.

65. Mont MA, Pacheco I, Hungerford DS. Radiographic predictors of outcome of core decompression for hips with osteonecrosis stage III. *Clin Orthop*. 1994;354:159–168.

66. Mont MA, Ragland PS, Etienne G. Core decompression of the femoral head for osteonecrosis using percutaneous multiple small diameter drilling. *Clin Orthop Relat Res*. 2004;(429):131–138.

67. Mont MA, Rajadhyaksha AD, Hungerford DS. Outcomes of limited femoral resurfacing arthroplasty compared with total hip arthroplasty for osteonecrosis of the femoral head. *J Arthroplasty*. 2001;16[8 Suppl 1]:134–139.

68. Musso ES, Mitchell SN, Schink-Asani M, et al. Results of conservative management of osteonecrosis of the femoral head: a retrospective review. *Clin Orthop*. 1984;207:209–215.

69. Nishii T, Sugano N, Miki H, et al. Prevention of development of collapse in osteonecrosis of the femoral head by systemic alendronate treatment. Paper presented at the Symposium of the Association Research Circulation Osseous; Jeju Island, South Korea; 2003.

70. Plakseychuk AY, Kim SY, Park BC, et al. Vascularized compared with nonvascularized fibular grafting for the treatment of osteonecrosis of the femoral head. *J Bone Joint Surg [Am]*. 2003;85:589–596.

71. Rosenwasser MP, Garino JP, Kiernan HA, et al. Long term follow-up of thorough debridement and cancellous bone grafting of the femoral head for avascular necrosis: a comparison with osteoarthritis. *Clin Orthop*. 1994;306:17–27.

72. Saito S, Saito M, Nishina T, et al. Long term results of total hip arthroplasty for osteonecrosis of the femoral head: a comparison with osteoarthritis. *Clin Orthop*. 1989;244:198–207.

73. Scher MA, Jakim L. Intertrochanteric osteotomy and autogenous bone grafting of avascular necrosis of the femoral head. *J Bone Joint Surg [Am]*. 1993;75:1119–1133.

74. Schneider E, Ahrendt J, Niethard FU, et al. Save the joint? Replace the joint? Long-term results and considerations in the treatment of femur head necroses in adults. *Z Orthop*. 1989;127:163–168.

75. Shon WY, Lee SH, Hur CY. Sugioka's transtrochanteric rotational osteotomy in the treatment of osteonecrosis of the femoral head. Paper presented at the Symposium of the Association Research Circulation Osseous; Jeju Island, South Korea; 2003.

76. Sotereanos DG, Plakeychuk AY, Rubash HE. Free vascularized fibula grafting for the treatment of osteonecrosis of the femoral head. *Clin Orthop*. 1997;334:243–256.

77. Steinberg ME. Management of avascular necrosis of the femoral head: an overview. *Instr Course Lect*. 1988;37:41–50.

78. Steinberg ME, Bands RE, Parry S, et al. Does lesion size affect the outcome in avascular necrosis? *Clin Orthop*. 1999;367:262–271.

79. Steinberg ME, Brighton CT, Corces A, et al. Osteonecrosis of the femoral head: results of core decompression and grafting with and without electrical stimulation. *Clin Orthop*. 1989;249:199–208.

80. Steinberg ME, Brighton CT, Hayken GD, et al. Electrical stimulation in the treatment of osteonecrosis of the femoral head: a 1-year follow-up. *Orthop Clin North [Am]*. 1985;16:747–756.

81. Steinberg ME, Corces A, Fallon M. Acetabular involvement in osteonecrosis of the femoral head. *J Bone Joint Surg [Am]*. 1999;81:60–65.

82. Steinberg ME, Hayken GD, Steinberg DR. The "conservative" management of avascular necrosis of the femoral head. In: Arlet J, Ficat RP, Hungerford DS, eds. *Bone Circulation*. Baltimore: Williams & Wilkins; 1984:334–337.

83. Stulberg BN, Davis AW, Bauer TW, et al. Osteonecrosis of the femoral head: prospective randomized treatment protocol. *Clin Orthop*. 1991;268:140–151.

84. Sugioka Y, Hotokebuchi T, Tsutsui H. Transtrochanteric anterior rotational osteotomy for idiopathic and steroid induced necrosis of the femoral head: indications and long-term results. *Clin Orthop*. 1992;277:111–120.

85. Suman RK. Prosthetic replacement of the femoral head for fractures of the neck of the femur: a comparative study. *Injury*. 1980;11:309–316.

86. Takaoka K, Nishina T, Ohzono K, et al. Bipolar prosthetic replacement for the treatment of avascular necrosis of the femoral head. *Clin Orthop*. 1992;277:121–127.

87. Thongtrangan I, Laorr A, Saleh KJ, et al. Spontaneous resolution of osteonecrosis of the femoral head. Paper presented at the Symposium of the Association Research Circulation Osseous; Jeju Island, South Korea; 2003.

88. Urbaniak JR, Coogan PG, Gunneson EB, et al. Treatment of osteonecrosis of the femoral head with free vascularized fibular bone grafting: a long-term follow-up study of one-hundred and three hips. *J Bone Joint Surg [Am]*. 1995;77:681–692.

89. Verberne GH. A femoral head prosthesis with a built-in joint: a radiological study of the movements of the two components. *J Bone Joint Surg [Br]*. 1983;65:544–547.

90. Wang GJ, Cui Q. The pathogenesis of steroid induced osteonecrosis and the effect of lipid clearing agents on this mechanism. In: Urbaniak JR, Jones JP Jr, eds. *Osteonecrosis*. Vol. 22. Rosemont, IL: American Orthopaedic Association and American Academy of Orthopaedic Surgeons; 1997:159–166.

91. Warner JJ, Philip JH, Brodsky GL, et al. Studies of osteonecrosis: the role of core decompression in the treatment of nontraumatic osteonecrosis of the femoral head. *Clin Orthop*. 1987;225:104–127.

92. Xenakis TA, Beris AE, Malizos KK, et al. Total hip arthroplasty for avascular necrosis and degenerative osteoarthritis of the hip. *Clin Orthop*. 1997;431:62–68.

93. Yamamoto M, Itoman M, Sagamoto N, et al. Strut bone graft for aseptic necrosis of the femoral head: theory and surgical technique. *Orthop Surg*. 1983;34:902–908.

94. Yamano K, Atsumi T, Kajwara T, et al. Bipolar endoprosthesis for osteonecrosis of the femoral head: a 12-year follow-up of 29 hips. Paper presented at the Symposium of the Association Research Circulation Osseous; Jeju Island, South Korea; 2003.

95. Yoo MC, Cho YJ, Kim KI, et al. Long-term follow-up of free vascularized fibular grafting for osteonecrosis of the femoral head. Paper presented at the Symposium of the Association Research Circulation Osseous; Jeju Island, South Korea; 2003.

96. Yoo MC, Cho YJ, Kim KI, et al. Pulsed electromagnetic fields treatment for the early stages of osteonecrosis of the femoral head. Paper presented at the Symposium of the Association Research Circulation Osseous; Jeju Island, South Korea; 2003.

97. Yoo MC, Cho YJ, Kim KI, et al. Resurfacing arthroplasty in patients with osteonecrosis of the femoral head. Paper presented at the Symposium of the Association Research Circulation Osseous; Jeju Island, South Korea; 2003.

98. Yoon TR, Rowe SM, Moon ES, et al. Viable iliac crest bone grafting for osteonecrosis of the femoral head in young patients under 40 years. Paper presented at the Symposium of the Association Research Circulation Osseous; Jeju Island; South Korea; 2003.

The Neuromuscular Hip

34

Rafael J. Sierra   Miguel E. Cabanela

The hip joint is commonly affected in patients with neuromuscular disorders. As a result of muscle imbalance and the ensuing subluxation or dislocation of the hip joint, painful degenerative arthritis can develop that may ultimately require surgical intervention to improve function and relieve pain.

In general terms, the underlying etiology of the hip dysfunction may be due to either intrinsic or extrinsic factors. Intrinsic muscle imbalance about the hip occurs during childhood and plays a primary role in subsequent hip problems. Extrinsic causes of neuromuscular imbalance occur in stable hips that develop degenerative arthritis in later life. Muscle imbalance in these hips plays a secondary role. The muscle imbalance related to the presence of strong hip flexors and adductors that overpower weaker or absent hip abductors and extensors is the main factor leading to hip instability. However, soft-tissue contractures about the hip and anatomic variations such as coxa valga, increased femoral anteversion, and a more vertical sourcil also play a role in the pathogenesis of this disorder.

Patients who have a neuromuscular disease may need treatment for their hip disease for two general reasons: either the disease process (e.g., cerebral palsy or myelomeningocele) has led to dysplasia of the hip, which in turn has evolved into degenerative arthritis, or the degenerative joint disease has developed independently of the neurologic disease (e.g., Parkinson disease).

Neuromuscular conditions can be divided into two basic categories. The first type of muscle paralysis or paresis is flaccid paralysis or decreased muscle tone, in which the lower motor neurons or peripheral nerves are involved, and the second is spasticity or increased muscle tone, which involves the upper motor neurons or the cortex of the brain. Both flaccid and spastic types are found in intrinsic and in extrinsic disorders. The first type includes conditions such as poliomyelitis, Down syndrome, and myelomeningocele; the second type includes conditions such as cerebral palsy, Parkinson disease, and stroke. Most commonly in the young patient with a neuromuscular hip, successful containment of the hip can be achieved with various treatment modalities such as soft-tissue releases, open reduction, femoral and acetabular osteotomies, or a combination of these procedures. If containment cannot be achieved and hip subluxation or dislocation occurs, hip reduction is not likely to result in pain relief. Cooperman et al. (8) found that half of these hips become painful, most likely because the cartilage of the femoral head has degenerated, and therefore management with a resection arthroplasty, arthrodesis, or total hip arthroplasty (THA) is frequently indicated.

In discussing the neuromuscular hip, certain differences between flaccid and spastic paralysis must be delineated. The spastic muscle has increased tone and often functions in both phases of gait. The flaccid muscle is paralyzed to a greater or lesser degree, but it always functions according to its normal role. Intact sensation is usually present in cerebral palsy, but it may be diminished in adult patients who have suffered a cerebrovascular accident (CVA). Myelomeningocele patients have significant loss of sensation, whereas polio patients have intact sensation. Although diminished sensation itself plays no role in hip instability, its lack is an important consideration in planning surgery as well as determining the prognosis for the joint.

The purpose of this chapter is to review current surgical options in adult patients with neuromuscular hip problems, with a special emphasis on joint replacement, its planning and execution, and possible complications in this group of patients.

PATIENTS WITH INCREASED MUSCLE TONE (SPASTICITY–RIGIDITY)

The major causes of spasticity are cerebral palsy and spinal cord injuries in the child or young adult and cerebrovascular accidents, Parkinson disease, and neuropathic joints in the older adult.

Cerebral Palsy

Hip deformities in cerebral palsy are second in frequency to talipes equinus. The incidence of hip subluxation/dislocation has been reported to be 2.6% to 28% in different series (25,35). Hip dislocation/subluxation is more common with severe or total body involvement. Deformities of the hip joint in patients with cerebral palsy not only produce pain and prevent ambulation but can also interfere with sitting ability and hygiene in the most profoundly affected. As noted, the direct cause of hip instability is muscle imbalance resulting from hip adductors and flexors overpowering the hip abductors and extensors. Femoral anteversion contributes to the problem, as does pelvic obliquity. Hip subluxation/dislocation generally occurs in the child with more severe involvement. Early surgical treatment during childhood consists of muscle releases to obtain balance and early femoral varus rotation or acetabular osteotomies for containment of the femoral head. If early surgical intervention is not performed, the uncovered femoral capital epiphysis becomes deformed from the tremendous pressures generated by the overlying capsule and spastic abductor muscles, leading to painful arthritic changes in adolescents and adults.

In the adult patient, the aim of treatment is to prevent contractures that lead to hip subluxation or dislocation or if end-stage arthritis has occurred to eradicate pain in the affected arthritic joint (Fig. 34-1). Surgical options include resection

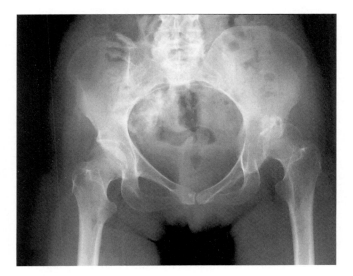

Figure 34-1 Thirty-seven-year-old patient with spastic cerebral palsy. Patient has intractable pain in the left hip.

TABLE 34-1
INTERPOSITIONAL ARTHROPLASTY IN CEREBRAL PALSY

Authors (ref.)	Hips (n)	Patients (n)	Outcome	Heterotopic Ossification
Koffman (22)	16	10	All improved	100%
Baxter and D'Astous (2)	5	4	Good	—
McCarthy et al. (26)	58	34	33 patients with pain relief	98%
Root et al.[a]	15	11	8 patients with pain relief	3 revisions

[a]Unpublished data.

arthroplasty, arthrodesis, interposition arthroplasty, and total hip replacement arthroplasty.

Resection Arthroplasty

Resection arthroplasty needs to be very extensive to relieve pain and deformity reliably and therefore is reserved for patients who are unable to walk and whose functional needs might include improved hygiene and ease of positioning. However, the incidence of recurring pain and heterotopic bone formation and overall poor results have lead several authors to abandon this procedure. McCarthy et al. published the largest series to date in 1988 (26). The authors reported the results of 58 proximal femoral resections in 34 patients, with ages ranging from 15 to 60 years. All of the patients in this study were severely involved. Pain was relieved and sitting improved in 33 of the 34 patients. Ectopic bone was noted in 53 hips. Only 3 hips required revision because of heterotopic bone formation. In 1978, Castle and Schneider (6) also described an extensive proximal femoral resection with interposition arthroplasty with good long-term pain relief, improved sitting, and ease of perineal care in 12 patients (Table 34-1). In this operation, the proximal femur is resected below the lesser trochanter, the capsule is closed over the acetabulum with the detached end of the iliopsoas tendon, and the vastus lateralis is sutured over the stump of the proximal femur. The abductor muscle mass is interposed between the two (Fig. 34-2).

Koffman (22) reported in 1981 the experience at Rancho Los Amigos Hospital. Ten proximal femoral resections where performed in six severely disabled cerebral spastic patients. One of the six patients required a second resection, and one other patient required a THA for continued pain. Almost all patients had heterotopic ossification, and in a few the heterotopic ossifications were symptomatic and interfered with sitting.

Root and Bostrom reported in the first edition of this chapter on 15 proximal femoral resections done at the Hospital for Special Surgery. The first three hips were treated with distal femoral skeletal traction, but because of difficulty in immobilizing these patients and because of significant knee flexion contractures, the authors abandoned skeletal traction in the postoperative period. Three of the 15 hips

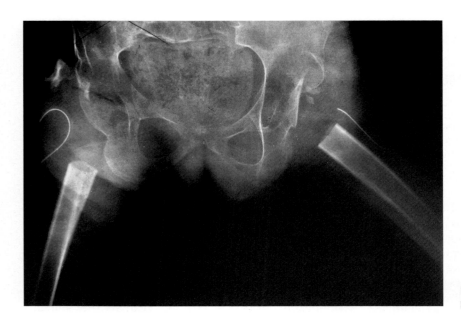

Figure 34-2 Anteroposterior radiograph of a pelvis with bilateral proximal femoral resections.

required revisions because of extensive heterotopic bone formation and pain. To prevent heterotopic ossification, the authors stated that all resections were treated with 600 to 800 rads of radiation to the hip area on postoperative day 1, which has prevented significant heterotopic bone formation in these patients.

Proximal femoral resection is contraindicated in walking patients because the restored limb cannot bear weight. It should not be performed in young, growing children because of upward migration and heterotopic bone formation in this group.

Hip Arthrodesis

Hip arthrodesis is an option that is indicated rarely. In ambulatory patients, it is rarely chosen over THA. Contraindications to hip arthrodesis include a contralateral hip at risk or already involved or the presence of spine deformity. Many of the painful dislocated hips occur in severely involved patients who have bilateral hip dysplasia as well as some grade of spinal deformity, thus ruling out hip arthrodesis as a surgical option (8).

In 2003, investigators at the Santa Casa Medical Hospital in Brasil reported on 14 patients (14 hips) with spastic cerebral palsy and painful unilateral chronic hip dislocations or subluxations that were treated with hip arthrodesis and followed for a mean of 5.3 years (8). Four of these patients were diplegic and ambulators and 7 were bedridden. All were fixed with internal fixation ranging from cancellous screws to rigid fixation using an AO-DCP 4.5-mm plate in 6 hips and the AO cobra plate in 4 hips. Eight hips had postoperative spica casting. The arthrodesis position was a mean of 40° of flexion (20° to 60°), 15° of abduction (0° to 52°), and neutral rotation. Postoperatively, three pseudoarthroses healed with a secondary procedure. The authors reported that all patients were painless at last follow-up. Functional status remained the same or improved a grade in all patients. Five of 7 bedridden patients became sitters, and all preoperative ambulatory patients continued to ambulate in the community.

In 1986, Root et al. (34) reported on eight cerebral palsy patients aged 13 to 34 years who had unilateral hip arthrodeses. All of these patients had painful arthrosis of the hip associated with subluxation or dislocation. Of the original eight patients, six had successful fusions and two required revisions. One of the revisions was ultimately converted to a total hip replacement.

The advantages of a successfully arthrodesed hip are elimination of pain, the ability to sit and stand, and long-term durability. The disadvantages are the high incidence of failure and the need for prolonged postoperative immobilization.

Prosthetic Interposition Arthroplasty

In 1999, Gabos et al. (16) reported the use a prosthetic interposition arthroplasty in 11 nonambulatory patients with severe mental retardation and cerebral palsy. Due to the patients' small proximal femoral diameter and abnormal acetabular contour, 2 custom proximal femoral replacements and 12 humeral replacements (with or without glenoid replacement) were implanted. The level of resection was basocervical ($n = 3$), intertrochanteric ($n = 4$), or subtrochanteric ($n = 7$), dictated by the amount of remaining soft-tissue tension. Patients were immobilized postoperatively in either abduction pillows ($n = 9$) or by bilateral leg casts fixed with broomsticks ($n = 5$) (modified Petrie) for 4 to 6 weeks. Postoperatively 4 hips dislocated. There was 1 clinical failure. This patient had constant pain in a dislocated hip. All other 10 patients had improvement in sitting ability or tolerance at an average of 4 years and 9 months.

Total Hip Arthroplasty

Since the advent of THA, many patients or caretakers choose this option over arthrodesis or proximal femoral resection for the treatment of the painful hip in cerebral palsy. The concerns with THA include the patient's age (patients are usually young), the abnormal muscle strength, the spasticity and contractures that are often present, and poor patient compliance with postoperative regimens. On the other hand, loads across the hip joint may be decreased in this group of patients because they have a low level of activity and often use crutches for ambulation (5).

The indications for performing a total hip replacement in the spastic patient are the following:

■ Hip pain refractory to medication
■ Decreased function in standing, limited sitting, and difficulty with perineal hygiene
■ The potential for standing or walking, transfer ability, or upright sitting in a wheelchair

An absolute contraindication is the presence of ongoing hip infection. Mental retardation is not a contraindication, but patients who are severely retarded and essentially bedridden are not good candidates.

To the authors' knowledge, the first report on THA in patients with cerebral palsy was by Koffman et al. (22). Five THAs were performed on four cerebral palsy patients with total body involvement between 1974 and 1977. Only one patient was ambulatory. The mean age of the patients was 33 years (range, 21 to 57). All patients had pain with walking (the ambulatory patient) or with sitting. Three different designs were used, the Sivash, the LeGrange-Letournel, and the Trapezoidal-28. The average follow-up was 4 years. One patient had a dislocation with subsequent loosening of the acetabular component, and another patient underwent a resection arthroplasty for a painful implant. Arthroplasty was deemed successful in only one patient. The authors reported that the most common complication at that time was heterotopic ossification. Surgery was also challenging, and in fact, the authors recommended that the acetabular component should be more anteverted and the femoral component be slightly retroverted in the nonambulatory patients. Subsequent to this report, Root (33) (1982) and Skoff and Keggi (38) (1986) also reported on THA in selected patients with cerebral palsy. They reported good results.

In 1986, Root (34) also reported on the larger experience at the Hospital for Special Surgery (HSS) with 15 total hips in 15 patients and a follow-up of 2.5 to 12 years. Contractures were released in 11 of 15 hips. All acetabular and femoral components in this series were fixed with cement. Two hips had bone graft augmentation for a deficient acetabulum. A postoperative hip spica cast was used in 13 of 15 patients to prevent dislocations and promote healing of the greater trochanter. Pain relief was complete in 14 of 15 patients. Range of motion was improved in all patients. There were 2 dislocations, and 1 hip subluxated with flexion past 90°. Three patients were reoperated on, 1 acetabular component was revised for recurrent dislocation, 1 femoral component was revised for loosening, and 1 hip was reoperated on for removal of painful trochanteric wires. In 1993, Buly et al. (4), expanded this group to include 18 patients in whom 18 total hips were performed. At an average of 10 years, prosthetic survivorship was 95%.

Weber and Cabanela (43) reported on the Mayo Clinic experience with THA in patients with cerebral palsy. The minimum follow-up was 2 years. There were 10 males and 6 females, and the average age at surgery was 48.5 years (range, 22 to 79). The type of cerebral palsy was hemiplegia in 7 patients, diplegia in 4, quadriplegia in 2, athetoid quadriplegia in 2, and athetoid diplegia in 1. The diagnosis leading to THA was primary degenerative hip disease in 3 patients,

arthritis secondary to hip dysplasia in 8, and failed treatment of a fracture of the femoral neck in 5.

The preoperative pain was severe in 5 patients, moderate in 9, slight in 1, and unknown in 1. Preoperatively, 3 patients were unable to walk, 5 walked indoors only, 6 were community ambulators, and 1 patient could walk an unlimited distance; the walking status of the last patient was unknown. The operation was performed through an anterolateral approach in 8 patients, a transtrochanteric approach in 7, and a posterolateral approach in 1.

Both components were fixed with cement in 12 patients, both were fixed without cement in 2, and a hybrid technique (cup uncemented, femur cemented) was used in another 2 (Fig. 34-3). Soft-tissue releases were performed in 2 patients. One patient was immobilized postoperatively in a spica cast and another in a hip guide brace in order to decrease the potential for instability

After an average of 10 years (range, 2.5 to 21), 15 patients were alive. Pain relief was complete in 11, 2 had slight pain, 1 had moderate diffuse lower-extremity pain, and the last patient had had a revision at 13 years for loosening of both components. Nine patients had improvement in their walking

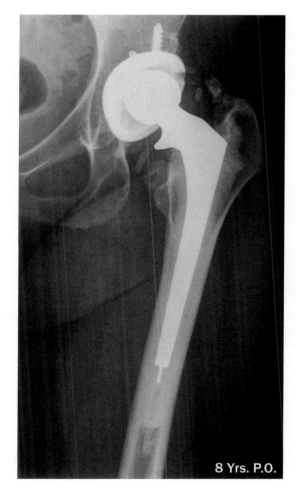

8 Yrs. P.O.

Figure 34-3 Same patient as in Figure 34-1 eight years after hybrid total hip arthroplasty. Patient is doing exceptionally well and has absolutely no symptoms in the hip. Note slight wear on the polyethylene acetabular liner.

status, 5 had no change, and the walking status of 1 patient was unknown. Two of the 5 patients who had no change had had an initial improvement but their walking status later returned to preoperative levels.

Intraoperative complications included trochanteric fracture and one acetabular fracture on press-fit impaction of an uncemented component. One trochanteric avulsion occurred after a transtrochanteric approach, one ulcer on the heel of a patient who wore a cast, one postoperative ileus, and one case of urinary retention. Four patients were reoperated on, 1 for fixation of a trochanteric avulsion, 1 for spasticity (an adductor tenotomy was performed), 1 for removal of painful heterotopic ossification, and 1 for revision of components to resolve loosening (as stated above).

Radiographic follow-up was also satisfactory (11 patients). Ten stems were solidly fixed, and one had some lucency but was not symptomatic. Nine acetabular components were stable, one had a circumferential lucency, and another cup was loose and caused slight pain in a patient who was able to walk independently. The outcome in this group of patients with cerebral palsy managed with THA was satisfactory.

From the literature, one can conclude that THA is a valuable option for the patient with cerebral palsy who has incapacitating pain. Pain relief and function can be improved in the majority of patients. Longevity of the implant can also be expected (>95% at 10 years). Attention should be paid to adductor spasticity that might need an adductor tenotomy at the time of implantation. Placing more anteversion on the socket and placing it a little more horizontal, especially in nonambulatory patients, may afford protection from instability. If instability is a concern intraoperatively, postoperative support with a hip guide orthosis or even a hip spica cast may be needed.

One last topic worth discussing is the treatment of the patient with a preoperative hip subluxation or dislocation. We prefer to use the posterolateral approach because, despite the traditional decreased risk of dislocation with the anterolateral approach, this approach does weaken the abductors (at least temporarily) in patients with already deficient abductors,

whereas the former does not. The acetabular component should be brought down to the true acetabulum rather than placing it in a high hip center, and it should be positioned into slightly more abduction and more anteversion; in addition, at the end of the procedure, the posterior structures (i.e., capsule and external rotators) should be repaired.

Parkinson Disease

The prevalence of Parkinson disease in the general population older than 60 years of age is 1% (15). The incidence rate is 20.5 per 100,000, and concomitant dementia is 3 times more frequent than in a control group (29). Current medical management effectively controls tremors, rigidity, and akinesia; however, impairment of the righting reflexes in the more advanced stages of disease is aggravated by the postural hypotension that is a side effect of levodopa.

Degenerative arthritis of hips in patients with Parkinson disease may occur through natural processes or after hip fractures. There is extensive literature on the treatment of hip fractures in patients with Parkinson disease (Table 34-2 and Table 34-3 [in previous chapter]) (13,24,40,41). In 1983, Eventov et al. (13) reported on 62 Parkinson disease patients with hip fractures, of which 39 were subcapital and 23 were intertrochanteric. Thirty-four patients with subcapital fractures had primary hemiarthroplasty, 11 patients with intracapsular fractures had nail-plate insertion, and 12 refused surgery. Five patients were too medically unstable for surgery. Regardless of fracture type, these patients had high mortality and morbidity rates, with pneumonia being the most frequent complication. Those patients treated with surgery had better functional results and a better quality of life. In 1988, Staeheli et al. (40) reported high rates of complications at 6 months (mostly urinary tract infections and pneumonias) and a high mortality rate (20%) after 50 hemiarthroplasties in 49 Parkinson patients for the treatment of femoral neck fractures (Garden III and IV). Despite this, functional results were good. Eighty percent of the survivors could walk. The authors attributed the good results to the rapid mobilization of the patients

TABLE 34-2
HIP FRACTURES IN PARKINSON DISEASE

Authors (ref.)	Fracture Type	Treatment	Hips (N)	Mortality	Complications
Couglin et al.	Fem neck	Hemiarthroplasty	27	60% at 6 mo[a]	35% dislocation rate[a]
	Intertrochanteric	CRIF	22	27% at 6 mo[a] 47% at 6 mo[b]	
Staeheli et al. (40)	Displaced fem neck	Hemiarthroplasty	50	20% at 6 mo	UTI, 20%, pneumonia, 10%
Eventov et al. (13)	Fem neck	Hemiarthroplasty	34	31% at 3 mo[b]	
	Intertrochanteric	CRIF	11		
Turcotte et al. (41)	Nondisplaced fem neck	In situ pinning	13	14% at 6 mo[b]	
	Displaced fem neck	Hemiarthroplasty	47		5 dislocations[a]
	Intertrochanteric	CRIF	34		
Londos et al. (24)	Nondisplaced fem neck	In situ pinning	8	28% at 2 y[b]	33% healing complications[b]
	Displaced fem neck	CRIF	24		6 nonunions, 3 segmental collapses[a]

CRIF, closed reduction internal fixation; UTI, urinary tract infection; fem, femoral.
[a]Data reflect specific fracture type and treatment.
[b]Data reflect entire study.

TABLE 34-3

HOEHN AND YAHR CLASSFICIATION OF SEVERITY OF PARKINSON DISEASE IN 98 PATIENTS UNDERGOING 107 THAs AT THE MAYO CLINIC BETWEEN 1970 AND 1994

Stage of Parkinson Disease	Characteristics	Primary THA Group[a] (52 patients, 58 hips)	All THAs (98 patients, 107 hips)
I	Unilateral involvement; minimal or no functional impairment	11	14
II	Bilateral or midline; balance not affected	40	52
III	Early loss of equilibrium; mild to moderate disability	6	38
IV	Severe disability, barely able to stand or walk	0	2
V	Confined to bed or wheelchair	0	0
	Unknown	1	1

[a]Subgroup of 52 patients with 58 primary THAs for osteoarthrosis.
Adapted from Weber M, Cabanela ME. Total hip arthroplasty in patients with cerebral palsy. *Orthopedics.* 1999;22:425–427.

postoperatively and to the release of contracted adductor muscles at the time of surgery.

Londos et al. (24) in 1989 recommended internal fixation over primary hip arthroplasty for patients with Parkinson disease and femoral neck fractures. They treated 32 patients with internal fixation. Twenty-four displaced fractures were complicated by six nonunions and three segmental femoral head collapses. In the eight nondisplaced fractures, one case of segmental collapse was diagnosed. Healing complications occurred in 33% of their patients. Three patients with complications required total hip replacement. They compared healing complications to a nonambulatory population of 547 patients with femoral neck fractures. In 151 uncomplicated fractures, healing complications occurred in 8% of them. In 196 patients with displaced fractures, healing complications occurred in 40% of survivors. Although these authors recommended internal fixation over primary arthroplasty in Parkinson disease patients with femoral neck fractures based on the similar outcomes of internal fixation in a general population of displaced fractures, it would seem that perhaps primary arthroplasty should be performed in both population groups for displaced fractures.

Investigators at the Mayo Clinic have also reported the results of total knee, total hip, and total shoulder arthroplasty in this group of patients (10,21,44). Total shoulder replacement in this group of patients relieves pain, but postoperative function is poor and complications are common (21). In total knee arthroplasty, reports from our institution are good, in contrast to other series that demonstrate poor results (10).

Total Hip Arthroplasty

Weber et al. have reported the results of THA in patients with Parkinson disease (44). Between 1970 and 1994, 107 THAs were performed in 98 patients at our institution. Of these, only 58 were done for a diagnosis of osteoarthritis. As for the others, 19 were done for a failed hemiarthroplasty, 10 for aseptic loosening, 7 for femoral neck fracture, 5 for femoral

neck nonunion, 4 for osteonecrosis of the femoral head after fracture, 2 for failed ORIF (open reduction and internal fixation) of fracture, 1 for failed cup arthroplasty, and 1 for failed resection arthroplasty. These THAs accounted for 0.4% of all hip arthroplasties (primary and revision) performed during the same study period at our institution. Parkinson disease was classified according to the severity score described by Hoehn and Yahr (18) (Table 34-3). Thirty-eight patients had a history of falls, and 71 were taking Parkinson medication.

Surgical approaches were anterolateral in 56 hips, transtrochanteric in 36, posterolateral in 12, and direct lateral in 3. Adductor tenotomy (7 hips) and psoas release (1 hip) were performed occasionally.

The complication rate was high (36%) (Table 34-4). Four patients died postoperatively (2 of pneumonia, one of a CVA, and one from pulmonary embolism). At 6 months, two additional patients had died, and at latest follow-up, 51 patients had died. In addition, one other nonfatal pulmonary embolus occurred, one deep wound infection required resection arthroplasty, and six dislocations occurred within 3 months of surgery. All occurred in patients with preoperative diagnoses other than osteoarthritis. Eight patients had nine reoperations, one for deep wound infection (as stated above) and the others for periprosthetic fracture, trochanteric nonunion, trochanteric wire removal, instability, or aseptic loosening of the femoral component, the acetabular component, or both components; the last six reoperations all occurred after a primary arthroplasty. The overall survivorship free of reoperation was 93% at 5 years for the entire group.

For 75 hips followed for a minimum of 2 years (mean, 7.1 years; range, 2 to 21 years), there was significant increase in function and decrease in pain at 1 year postoperatively (Fig. 34-4). Pain relief was satisfactory at latest follow-up, but function continued to deteriorate, as seen by an increased use of gait aids and a decrease in walking distance at last follow-up. Disability related to the underlying Parkinson disease paralleled the decrease in function, as 78% of patients had definite

TABLE 34-4

COMPLICATIONS ASSOCIATED WITH 107 THAs PERFORMED IN 98 PATIENTS AT THE MAYO CLINIC BETWEEN 1970 and 1994

	Primary THA Group (52 patients, 58 hips)	All THAs (98 patients, 107 hips)
Surgical complications		
Dislocation	0	6
Trochanteric nonunion	2	4
Pulmonary embolism	2	2
Deep venous thrombosis	2	3
Deep wound infection	0	1
Hematoma	1	1
Transient peroneal palsy	1	2
Medical complications		
Urinary tract infections	5	8
Pneumonia	0	3
Cerebrovascular accident	0	2
Postoperative confusion	1	4
Ileus	0	1
GI bleed	1	1
Total	15 (26%)	38 (36%)

Note: Six patients (three in the primary group) had two complications each.
Adapted from Weber M, Cabanela ME. Total hip arthroplasty in patients with cerebral palsy. *Orthopedics.* 1999;22:425–427.

neurological progression. At the time of latest follow-up, 57% of patients had progressed to functional stage IV or V.

Of those patients in which radiographs were obtained at a minimum 2-year follow-up (43 patients), heterotopic ossification was rare and never a limiting factor.

Our experience with patients with Parkinson disease has led us to the following conclusions and recommendations:

- Due to patient age, rehab potential, and overall life expectancy, the use of a cemented femoral component is most widely recommended. The use of an uncemented or cemented acetabular component is equally acceptable.
- Preoperative screening for low-grade or asymptomatic infections (urinary tract and chest) should be carried out. Careful monitoring postoperatively, especially for these and other infectious complications, should be strictly done.
- Careful intraoperative testing for instability should be done after components are inserted. Contractures must be dealt with by appropriate capsular resection or release prior to component insertion; we have seldom found it necessary to carry out an adduction tenotomy (usually percutaneous) at the end of the procedure if abduction cannot be obtained. Use of larger diameter heads may also decrease dislocation rates, especially in patients undergoing THA for diagnoses other than osteoarthritis.

Outcome with regard to pain relief is excellent but poor with regard to function because of the inevitable progression of disease.

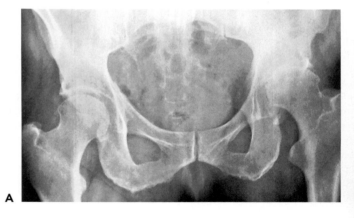

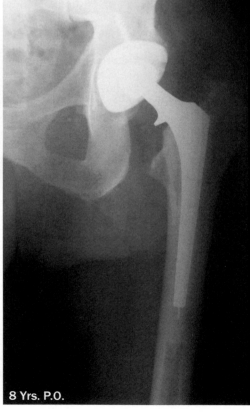

8 Yrs. P.O.

Figure 34-4 **A:** Sixty-nine-year-old patient with moderately advanced Parkinson disease and very symptomatic degenerative disease of the left hip. **B:** Radiograph of the same patient 8 years after hybrid total hip arthroplasty. The patient has had an excellent result as far as the hip is concerned, although there has been considerable worsening of his Parkinson disease.

Upper Motor Neuron Dysfunction (Stroke, Upper Spinal Cord or Brain Injury)

Hip subluxation/dislocation rarely occurs in adult onset spasticity caused by brain or upper spinal cord injury (17). On the other hand, hip joint contractures are frequent, and heterotopic ossification around the hip will decrease range of motion significantly in patients with brain injury (12). Early intensive physical therapy is important for maintenance of hip range of motion. This is especially true in the patient who is comatose for an extended time. Orthoses have proved ineffective in preventing hip contractures. Therefore, the mainstay of treatment includes prone positioning for flexion deformities and gait training and obturator nerve injections for adduction deformity. As many as 50% of patients experience long-term relief with nerve injections (17).

Many patients improve for 3 to 4 months. However, if patients do not continue to improve by 6 months and the adduction contracture results in problems with sitting, hygiene, or ambulatory function, surgery must be considered. Furthermore, patients with severe neurological impairment will probably be wheelchair-bound and will need at least a 90° range of hip flexion for sitting or almost full extension for standing. Usually the hip flexors and adductors are more impaired than the hip extensors and abductors. As a result, simple tenotomies of the involved muscles are helpful in restoring balance in this group of patients. On the other hand, patients with head or spinal injury with ankylosis of the hips due to massive heterotopic ossification will likely need to have this excised to obtain some range of motion to allow sitting or ambulation (12) (Fig. 34-5). Surgical release or lengthening of the tight tendons will improve hip position, but the

relative motion should be maintained postoperatively with a strict regimen of physical therapy. One must also note those patients that walk with an externally rotated affected leg, because adductor tenotomy in these patients is detrimental, as they rely on the adductor musculature for limb progression during the swing phase of gait (17).

Total Hip Arthroplasty

Older stroke patients are more prone to degenerative hip disease and may need treatment with THA. They may require release of contracted adductor or hip flexor muscles at the time of arthroplasty. The adductor tenotomy can be performed percutaneously just before positioning the patient for the hip arthroplasty, and the iliopsoas can be released from its insertion on the lesser trochanter during the exposure of the joint.

Di Caprio et al. (9), reported on the results of THA in patients with a previous stroke. The authors studied 28 hips in 20 patients with a mean age at surgery of 68 years. The diagnosis was osteoarthritis in all hips. The time between the CVA and THA was 22 months. The hip prosthesis was implanted in the affected limb in 15 hips. A modified anterior approach (abductor sparing) was used in all hips. Heterotopic ossification was Brooker class 0 or I in 64% of hips, class II in 14%, class III and IV in 3% each. At an average of 35 months (range, 12 to 80), the average Harris hip score (HHS) was 86 in all hips, and only those patients with Brooker class IV heterotropic ossification demonstrated limitations attributable to decreased range of motion. Seven patients with identifiable risk factors for heterotopic ossification were treated with a single dose of radiation (700 cGy) within 36 hours postoperatively, and none of these developed heterotopic ossification. No dislocations, infections, deep venous thrombosis, or new CVAs occurred in this

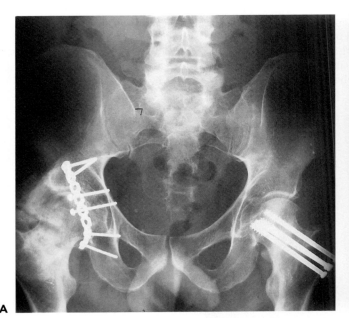

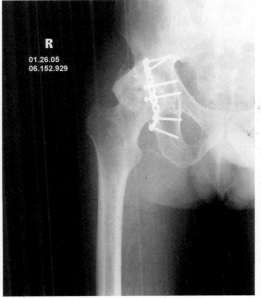

A

B

Figure 34-5   A: Anteroposterior radiograph of the pelvis of a 40-year-old rancher who was involved in a light plane crash in which he sustained a fracture-dislocation of the right hip and fracture of the left femoral neck. He also had a concomitant head injury and was comatose for 2 weeks. Note the significant heterotopic ossification, which virtually eliminated hip joint motion. **B:** Photograph of the same patient at 1 year after excision of heterotopic bone. The patient had recovered 90° of flexion of the hip and had minimal restriction of rotation and abduction. He was very satisfied with his result.

TABLE 34-5
RESULTS OF TOTAL HIP ARTHROPLASTY IN PATIENTS WITH CHARCOT ARTHROPATHY

Authors (ref.)	Cases (N)	Prosthesis Type	Diagnosis	Involvement	Outcome
Ritter and DeRosa (20)	1	McKee/Farrar	Tabes dorsalis	Ataxia	Multiple dislocation
Sprenger and Foley (39)	1	St. George	Tabes dorsalis	No ataxia	Good at 7 years
Baldini et al. (1)	4	Multiple	Tabes dorsalis	Ataxia	Recurrent dislocation and/or loosening
Robb et al. (31)	1	Charnley	Tabes dorsalis	No ataxia	6 dislocations resection arthroplasty
Cabanela, Sierra[a]	2	Charnley, McKee/Farrar	Tabes dorsalis		Multiple dislocations, resection

[a]Unpublished data.

cohort. The authors compared the 22% incidence of severe Brooker class III or IV in this patient cohort with the incidence in their general practice, which was 4% (>3500 THAs), and have instituted postoperative radiation treatment for all patients with a history of CVA who undergo THA.

THA is also recommended for younger patients who, in addition to their head injury, develop painful posttraumatic arthritis or even osteonecrosis of the femoral head. Because the spasticity in these patients is usually quite profound, they should be immobilized for 3 to 4 weeks postoperatively, either in a hip spica cast or in a hip abduction brace, to prevent dislocation or contracture.

Charcot Neuropathic Hip Joint

Neuropathic or Charcot joints present a special problem for the orthopedic surgeon regardless of the specific joint involved. The critical element in treating a patient with a neuropathic hip joint is to establish the diagnosis (1,19,30,31,39) (Table 34-5). The most common etiologies for neuropathic joints include tertiary syphilis, syringomyelia, and diabetes

mellitus, the latter one been the most common. While this has not been clinically proven, there are probably different degrees of neuropathic arthropathy, the worse being that related to tertiary syphilis.

Obtaining an accurate history is essential for making the diagnosis. The physical examination of the patient is also important, especially in relationship to the radiographic findings (Fig. 34-6). Significant radiographic destruction of an essentially asymptomatic or minimally symptomatic joint should alert the clinician, and a diagnosis of neuropathic joint should be entertained.

If the hip remains painless and functional, no treatment is recommended. If pain is present and function is impaired, conservative treatment with protected weight bearing should be extended as long as possible before considering any type of surgical procedure. Treatment with hip arthrodesis results in a rate of nonunion that, historically, has been as high as 100% (19).

THA also has a high failure rate, especially in those patients with significant neurologic findings or ataxia. Although the number of patients treated with THA reported in the literature

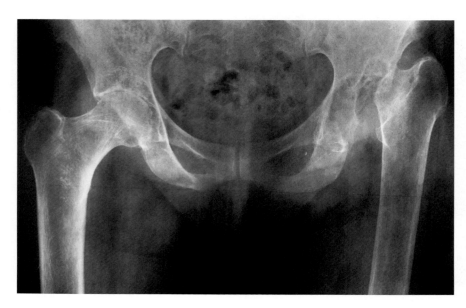

Figure 34-6 Anteroposterior radiograph of a pelvis with a painless left neuropathic hip joint.

is small, probably reflecting the relative low incidence of neuropathic hips, they have mostly done poorly (Table 34-5). The limited evidence strongly indicates that a Charcot hip joint is a contraindication to THA. Of the dozen or so cases reported in the literature, only one patient was stated to have done well with a total hip joint arthroplasty (39). The remainder did poorly even when treated with a broad range of total hip designs. Resorting to resection arthroplasty may be the only viable solution in the treatment of the painful hip in these patients. To the authors' knowledge, there have been no new reports on THA in patients with neuropathic joints since 1988, most likely reflecting the consensus in the joint replacement community regarding THA and neuropathic joints. A review of the Mayo Clinic joint registry yielded the presence of five THAs for which the diagnosis of Charcot arthropathy had been recorded. However, on reviewing the records, only two of the five were truly neuropathic joints and had a history of tabes dorsalis; replacement on both (done in 1979 and 1982) resulted in loosening, multiple dislocations, and eventual removal of the prostheses. No THA has been done at the Mayo Clinic in the last 20 years if a diagnosis of Charcot arthropathy was present.

There may be different grades of neuropathic joints, and the one related to tabes dorsalis is probably the worst one as far as both joint destruction and prognosis after THA.

PATIENTS WITH DECREASED MUSCLE TONE (FLACCID)

The neuromuscular disorders associated with flaccid paralysis include poliomyelitis, myelomeningocele, Charcot-Marie-Tooth, and, in older patients, Down syndrome.

Poliomyelitis

Because poliomyelitis mainly affects the anterior horn cells, sensation is intact and intelligence is not altered. As a result, the patient can cooperate, and the success of muscle balance restoration by release or transfer can be measured. As in the spastic patient, the flexors and adductors overpowering the weaker abductors and extensors cause hip subluxation/dislocation in polio patients. In the young child, coxa valga and excessive femoral anteversion contribute to the development of the hip instability. The flail polio hip rarely dislocates except with marked pelvic obliquity. The hip on the high side is adducted, and the lower hip may have an abduction contracture. In this situation, release of the abductors, as recommended by Eberle (11), may result in reduction just by leveling of the pelvis.

For the most part, the young child with hip subluxation is treated by a combination of procedures to improve muscle balance, with adductor transfers to the ischium or iliopsoas transfers laterally to the greater trochanter (Fig. 34-7) (27,28). If coxa valga and femoral anteversion are associated with the subluxation/dislocation, varus derotation osteotomy is indicated. Acetabular insufficiency can be corrected by pelvic osteotomies such as the Pemberton or shelf-type procedures, the innominate osteotomy of Salter, the sliding osteotomy of Chiari, or the triple osteotomy of Steel. In order to obtain a stable hip, muscle balancing is always necessary and often

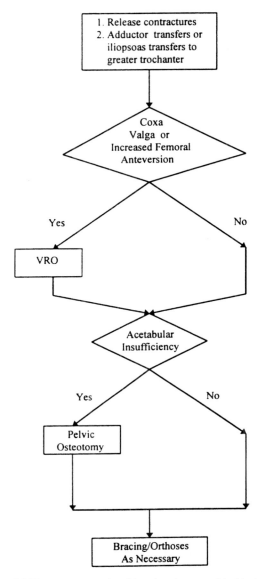

Figure 34-7   Treatment algorithm for the unstable hip in adult patients with poliomyelitis.

must be combined with femoral and pelvic osteotomies. When the contralateral hip has been in abduction, the contracture must be released as well, or the secondary pelvic obliquity could lead to recurrence of the subluxation even after surgical reduction. These operations are generally reserved for children, but in a young adult with similar dysplasia and without arthritic changes a successful, painless reduction can be achieved by the same procedures.

Older polio patients with subluxation of the hips are prone to develop arthritis, whereas the completely dislocated hip is almost never painful. The femoral head deformity seen in spastic subluxation/dislocations does not occur in poliomyelitis. The uncovered femoral head may demonstrate medial flattening as a result of the pressure of the hypertrophied ligamentum teres but not the superolateral flattening associated with the spastic subluxated/dislocated hip.

Total Hip Arthroplasty

In the ambulating adult polio patient, the arthritic painful hip can be very disabling. A Chiari or varus rotational osteotomy may provide pain relief if the arthritis is not advanced. The presence of advanced arthritic changes and decreased range of motion precludes either pelvic or femoral osteotomies. The only other alternatives are hip arthrodesis and THA. In today's world, most patients would strongly prefer a total hip replacement to arthrodesis. As noted earlier, arthrodesis relieves pain and allows sitting and walking. More important for the patient with flaccid paralysis, it does not rely on muscle strength or balance for stability and function. THA provides a functional, painless range of motion and permits sitting and walking. However, if there is a significant loss of muscle power, especially if hip abductors are absent, hip stability is jeopardized. A constrained prosthesis may help to relieve this problem. Arthrodesis should be considered if there is significant muscle weakness.

The authors are aware of only one report (two patients) of hip replacement being performed in the involved extremity of a patient who had residuals from polio and major paralysis. This might be related to the fact that forces across the joints in these patients are substantially decreased, and therefore degenerative disease is relatively rare in these flaccid limbs. Wicart et al. (46) reported on these two patients. One patient had a subluxation of the extremity, while the other had osteonecrosis of the femoral head. They were followed for 1 and 3 years, respectively. The patient with a preoperative subluxation had a postoperative anterior dislocation. Mobility scores improved in the patient who had a preoperative diagnosis of osteonecrosis but remained unchanged in the patient with a preoperative diagnosis of subluxation.

A review from the joint registry at the Mayo Clinic (5) revealed no instance of THA being performed on the involved hip of a patient with residuals of poliomyelitis. However, the senior author has performed five THAs on the contralateral leg of patients afflicted with residuals of polio, and the results for these patients (after follow-up from 2 to 8 years) appeared to be no different from those in the general population of patients who have undergone THA. Although the loads through these hips are not normal, the patients are not very active because of the residual infirmity.

Myelomeningocele

The survival rate for these patients has increased significantly in the last 2 decades because of the emphasis on early closure of the spinal defect and the insertion of a ventricular peritoneal shunt to treat hydrocephalus. Sensory deficits in the lower extremities, as well as frequent pelvic obliquity, complicate the treatment of hip deformities in these children.

The level of the lesion, identified as the lowest active functioning nerve root, determines not only the patient's ability to walk but the risk of developing hip instability. High-level involvement, such as thoracic or high lumbar levels, rarely results in hip instability. Patients with muscle power to L2 walk only with braces and crutches and generally become wheelchair-bound by their adolescent years. Patients with intact L3 and L4 nerve roots have good quadriceps and the potential to be community ambulators, although they may require orthotics. Their prognosis improves if hamstring activity is present as well. The incidence of hip subluxation is greatest in patients with lesions at these levels because hip flexors and adductors remain intact and hip extensors and abductors are absent or weak. According to Sharrard (37), 60% of these children will develop hip subluxation by age 3 if left untreated. Patients with involvement at the L5 level, with strong quadriceps, active hamstrings, and the presence of some abductor or extensor activity, rarely develop hip instability. For the most part, patients with involvement at the S1 level or below never develop hip instability.

There is general agreement in the literature that no attempt should be made to reduce hips if quadriceps function is not present. Contractures should be treated with releases or osteotomies to facilitate the use of braces for standing and sitting. Dislocation in this group, whether unilateral or bilateral, does not become painful in adult life, and sufficient range of motion remains for functioning in a wheelchair. Because dislocation is rare with involvement at L5 and never with involvement at S1, these hips do not present future problems.

Controversy exists as to whether to aggressively treat the dislocated hip of a patient with L3 or L4 level involvement. Some authors recommend no treatment except for the correction of contractures, and others recommend reducing all subluxated or dislocated hips. Open reduction, varus rotational osteotomies, pelvic osteotomy, and any combination of these procedures are often necessary to reduce hips. Some authors recommend iliopsoas transfers to the greater trochanter or an external oblique transfer to the greater trochanter (27,36,47). The goal of these operations is to locate the hip and improve hip abductor strength. In addition, the adductors are often transferred to the ischium to remove a deforming force and reinforce hip extension.

The question whether hip stability is important for ambulation remains unanswered. Root et al. (32) reviewed over 100 myelomeningocele patients. Surgical reduction of the hip above the L2 level uniformly failed. All hips with involvement at the L5 or S1 level were stable. Of 30 hips with involvement at the L3 or L4 level, 60% had persistent instability, including those in which reduction and maintenance of reduction was achieved. Ambulation improved with increased stability of the hips in patients with good quadriceps function.

In 1979, Feiwell et al. (14) reported on 76 patients with myelomeningocele over the age of 5 who failed to achieve hip stability. In the group of patients with midlumbar involvement, stability did not influence ambulation. No hip was painful if there had been no prior surgery, and the presence of subluxation/dislocation instability did not significantly decrease the range of motion. For hip subluxation in these patients, the authors recommended surgical interventions, including adductor tenotomy, medial capsulotomy of the hip, and iliopsoas releases if these structures were contracted. However, the average follow-up was less than 10 years, and no patient was older than 29 years at follow-up.

Total Hip Arthroplasty

In adult patients with myelomeningocele, we are not aware of any study that addresses THA for the treatment of dysplasia or dislocation. Review of the Mayo Clinic joint registry identified three patients all with a low-lumbar-level myelomeningocele who had THA to treat severe pain and instability (45). All the prostheses performed poorly, primarily because of pain and instability, after 5 to 10 years of follow-up. It appears that reasonable muscle power of flexion, abduction, and extension is necessary for a satisfactory outcome. If muscle power is suboptimal, alternatives to THA, such as resection arthroplasty, should be sought. THA should be reserved for patients who have symptomatic arthritis of the hip but preferably without evidence of neuropathic arthropathy and with adequate muscle support around the hip.

Down Syndrome

Hip disease occurs in 8% to 28% of patients with Down syndrome (20). This includes an increased incidence of dislocation, dysplasia, slipped capital epiphysis, Perthes disease, and osteonecrosis of the femoral head. A study of the anatomy of the hip in these patients showed an increase in acetabular depths, a decrease in acetabular anteversion, and an acetabular roof that is more horizontal than usual. This combination of characteristics could create a mechanically stable hip, but the presence of capsular laxity and an increased range of motion, especially in external rotation, appear to make the hip more vulnerable to the development of arthritis. As patients with Down syndrome are living longer, there has been an increased role for THA in the treatment of disabling hip pain in patients with this syndrome who develop end-stage arthritis. If surgical intervention is entertained, one must also remember to obtain cervical spine x-rays in order to rule out gross C1-C2 instability.

The Mayo Clinic joint registry identified seven hips in four patients treated with THA (5). After a duration of 1 to 15 years, the results were excellent for the three hip replacements performed with cement, two uncemented sockets were revised for loosening, and two uncemented constrained sockets were in place (Fig. 34-8). No patient had dislocated. On the basis of this relatively small and anecdotal experience, it would appear that hip replacement in patients with Down syndrome is justifiable if they are reasonably functional and sufficiently symptomatic.

Similar results have also been reported by Kioschos et al. (20). In 1999, these authors reported on nine hip arthroplasties performed on six patients with Down syndrome. The mean age of surgery was 36 years (range, 22 to 47). All patients were mobile and lived at home or in a group residency at the time of the operation. A reamed bipolar prosthesis was used in three hips because of anticipated inability to follow postoperative hip protocol. The remaining six hips were given a standard THA. Two hips were braced, and three were placed in spica casts postoperatively as a precaution. A posterior approach was used, but a trochanteric osteotomy and advancement was necessary in three at the time of arthroplasty. Postoperatively no wound or anesthetic complications occurred. Follow-up averaged 7.75 years. One reamed bipolar dislocated postoperatively on day 5, requiring open reduction, with no subsequent problems with instability. One patient developed acetabular osteolysis, requiring revision. The revision was then complicated by nonunion and superior migration of the trochanter. The authors commented on the poor reliability of hip scores in measuring function in these patients with limited comprehension. However, all patients at last follow-up were fully mobile and had no limitation of function due to their hips.

Charcot-Marie-Tooth Disease

Although patients with Charcot-Marie-Tooth disease rarely develop hip instability, they may develop osteoarthritis in later

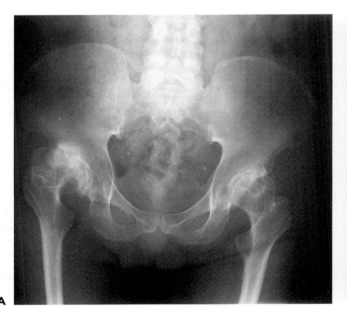
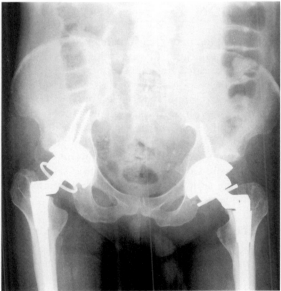

A

B

Figure 34-8   A: Thirty-eight-year-old functional patient with Down syndrome and severe and symptomatic degenerative disease of the hips. The patient has increased ligamentous laxity. **B:** Radiograph of the pelvis of the same patient 1 year after implantation of bilateral uncemented prosthesis. Because of the patient's hyperlaxity, bilateral constrained liners were utilized in this instance to prevent dislocation and poor cognitive function.

years, leading to requiring THA (23,42). The issue of instability after total hip replacement is the same as in the patient with polio. If the muscle weakness is so profound that the arthroplasty is unstable, a constrained device may be necessary.

OTHER PARALYSIS IN THE YOUNG ADULT AND TOTAL HIP ARTHROPLASTY

In 1999, Wicart et al. (46) also reported on 18 cemented arthroplasties performed in 14 patients with neuromuscular hip disorders. This series included not only patients with cerebral palsy (6 hips) but also 1 patient with a paralytic hip after head trauma, 6 patients with spinal medullary disorders (2 Friedrich ataxia, 2 acute anterior poliomyelitis, 1 vascular injury, 1 spinal malformation with sacral agenesis, and 1 cervical spine trauma), and 1 patient with a myotonic muscular dystrophy (Steinert disease). The indication of arthroplasty was a consequence of the paralysis in 14 hips (dislocation in 4, subluxation in 6, 3 complications of surgery for a paralytic hip in childhood, and 1 neurologic hip) and was independent of paralysis in 4 (1 femoral head osteonecrosis and 3 degenerative joint disease). The mean age of patients was 40 years (range, 19 to 64). The mean follow-up was 5.6 years. Eleven patients were ambulatory, and 3 patients were not. A functional initial goal was achieved in all patients. Heterotopic ossification occurred in 3 hips, with no functional consequences. Two nonunions of the trochanter occurred. Four dislocations occurred postoperatively within 4 months, were reduced satisfactorily, and did not recur. Once acetabular loosening occurred at 13 years and was revised. Three femoral components are radiographically loose at last follow-up. The authors concluded that THA in this group gives patients a satisfactory range of motion, relieves pain, and improves function.

CONCLUSION

The treatment of hip pathology in patients with neuromuscular diseases should begin with prevention, especially in those disorders that untreated may cause hip instability. Once instability ensues, these disorders are harder to treat, and complications are more common. In more recent years, THA appears to have found its role in the treatment of these disorders. Patients and families have become more aware of the benefits of THA and prefer this surgical intervention to those that provide less function. Surgeons should be aware of the indications and possible complications in this select group of patients and the appropriate surgical techniques for treating their conditions.

REFERENCES

1. Baldini N, Sudanese A, Toni A. Total prosthetic replacement in tabetic arthropathy of the hip joint. *Ital J Orthop Traumatol.* 1985;11:193–197.
2. Baxter MP, D'Astous JL. Proximal femoral resection-interposition arthroplasty: salvage hip surgery for the severely disabled child with cerebral palsy. *J Pediatr Orthop.* 1986;6:681–685.
3. Bleck EE. The hip in cerebral palsy. *Orthop Clin North Am.* 1980;11:79–104.
4. Buly RL, Huo M, Root L, et al. Total hip arthroplasty in cerebral palsy: long-term follow-up results. *Clin Orthop.* 1993;296:148–153.
5. Cabanela ME, Weber ME. Total hip arthroplasty in patients with neuromuscular disease. *J Bone Joint Surg.* 2000;82:426–432.
6. Castle ME, Schneider C. Proximal femoral resection-interposition arthroplasty. *J Bone Joint Surg [Am].* 1978;60:1051–1054.
7. Cooperman DR, Bartucci E, Dietrick E, et al. Hip dislocation in spastic cerebral palsy: long-term consequences. *J Pediatr Orthop.* 1987;7:268–276.
8. De Morales Barros Fucs PM, Svartman C, Montexuma C, et al. Treatment of the painful chronically dislocated and subluxated hip in cerebral palsy with hip arthrodesis. *J Pediatr Orthop.* 2003;23:529–534.
9. DiCaprio MR, Huo MH, Zatorski LE, et al. Incidence of heterotopic ossification following total hip arthroplasty in patients with prior stroke. *Orthopedics.* 2004;27:41–43.
10. Duffy GP, Trousdale RT. Total knee arthroplasty in patients with Parkinson's disease. *J Arthroplasty.* 1996;11:899–904.
11. Eberle C. Pelvic obliquity and the unstable hip after poliomyelitis. *J Bone Joint Surg [Br].* 1982;64:300–304.
12. Ebinger T, Roesch M, Kiefer H, et al. Influence of etiology in heterotopic bone formation of the hip. *J Trauma.* 2000;48:1058–1062.
13. Eventov I, Moreno M, Geller E, et al. Hip fractures in patients with Parkinson's syndrome. *J Orthop Trauma.* 1983;23:98–101.
14. Feiwell E, Sakai D, Blatt T. The effect of hip reduction on function in patients with myelomeningocele: potential gains and hazards of surgical treatment. *J Bone Joint Surg [Am].* 1978;60:169–173.
15. Frassica FJ, Sim FH. Parkinson's disease. In: Morrey BF, ed. *Reconstructive Surgery of the Joints.* 3rd ed. New York: Churchill Livingstone; 2003:770–773.
16. Gabos PG, Miller F, Galban MA, et al. Prosthetic interposition arthroplasty for the palliative treatment of endstage spastic hip disease in nonambulatory patients with cerebral palsy. *J Pediatr Orthop.* 1999;19:796–804.
17. Gardner MJ, Ong BC, Liporace F, et al. Orthopedic Issues after cerebrovascular accident. *Am J Orthop.* 2002;31:559–569.
18. Hoehn MM, Yahr MD. Parkinsonism: onset, progression and mortality. *Neurology.* 1967;17:427–442.
19. Johnson J. Neuropathic fractures and joint injuries. *J Bone Joint Surg [Am].* 1967;49:1–30.
20. Kioschos M, Shaw ED, Beals RK. Total hip arthroplasty in patients with Down's syndrome. *J Bone Joint Surg [Br].* 1999;81:436–439.
21. Koch LD, Cofied RH, Ahlskog JE. Total shoulder arthroplasty in patients with Parkinson's disease. *J Shoulder Elbow Surg.* 1997;6:24–28.
22. Koffman M. Proximal femoral resection or total hip replacement in severely disabled cerebral-spastic patients. *Orthop Clin North Am.* 1981;12:91–100.
23. Kumar SJ, Marks HG, Bowen JR, et al. Hip dysplasia associated with Charcot-Marie-Tooth disease in the older child and adolescent. *J Pediatr Orthop.* 1985;5:511–514.
24. Londos E, Nilsson LT, Stromqvist B. Internal fixation of femoral neck fractures in Parkinson's disease: 32 patients followed for 2 years. *Acta Orthop Scand.* 1989;60:682–685.
25. Mathews SS, Jones MH, Sperling SC. Hip derangements seen in cerebral palsied children. *Am J Physiol Med.* 1953;32:213–221.
26. McCarthy RE, Simon S, Douglas B, et al. Proximal femoral resection to allow adults who have severe cerebral palsy to sit. *J Bone Joint Surg [Am].* 1988;70:1011–1016.
27. Mustard WT. Iliopsoas transfer for weakness of the hip abductors. *J Bone Joint Surg [Am].* 1952;34A(3):647–650.
28. Carroll NC, Sharord WJ. Longterm follow up of posterior iliopsoas transplantation for paralytic dislocation of the hip. *J Bone Joint Surg [AM].* 1972;54:551–560.
29. Rajput AH. Epidemiology of Parkinson's disease. *Can J Neurol Sci.* 1984;11[suppl 1]:156–159.
30. Ritter M, DeRosa G. Total hip arthroplasty in a Charcot joint: a case report with six year follow-up. *Orthop Rev.* 1977;6:51.
31. Robb JE, Rymaszewski LA, Reeves BF, et al. Total hip replacement in a Charcot joint: brief report. *J Bone Joint Surg [Br].* 1988;70:489.
32. Root L. Total hip replacement in young people with neurologic disease. *Dev Med Child Neurol.* 1982;24:186–188.
33. Root L, Benton LJ, Salvati EA. Reconstructive surgery in the myelomeningocele hip. *Clin Orthop.* 1975;No. 110:261–268.
34. Root L, Goss JR, Mendes J. The treatment of the painful hip in cerebral palsy by total hip replacement or hip arthrodesis. *J Bone Joint Surg [Am].* 1986;68:590–598.

35. Samilson RL, Tsou P, Aamoth G, et al. Dislocation and sub-luxation of the hip in cerebral palsy: pathogenesis, natural history and management. *J Bone Joint Surg [Am]*. 1972;54:863–873.

36. Sharrard WJ. Management of paralytic subluxation and dislocation of the hip in myelomeningocele. *Dev Med Child Neurol*. 1983;25:374–376.

37. Sharrard WJ. Posterior iliopsoas transplantation and the treatment of paralytic dislocation of the hip. *J Bone Joint Surg [Br]*. 1964;46:426–444.

38. Skoff HD, Keggi K. Total hip replacement in neuromuscularly impaired. *Orthop Rev*. 1986;15:154–159.

39. Sprenger TR, Foley CJ. Hip replacement in a Charcot joint: a case report and historical review. *Clin Orthop*. 1982;No. 165:191–194.

40. Staeheli JW, Frassica FJ, Sim FH. Prosthetic replacement of the femoral head for fracture of the femoral neck in patients who have Parkinson disease. *J Bone Joint Surg [Am]*. 1988;70:565–568.

41. Turcotte R, Godin C, Duchesne R, et al. Hip fractures and Parkinson's disease: a clinical review of 94 fractures treated surgically. *Clin Orthop*. 1990;No. 256:132–136.

42. Walker JL, Nelson KR, Heavilon JA, et al. Hip abnormalities in children with Charcot-Marie-Tooth disease. *J Pediatr Orthop*. 1994;14:54–59.

43. Weber M, Cabanela ME. Total hip arthroplasty in patients with low-lumbar-level myelomeningocele. *Orthopedics*. 1998;21:709–712.

44. Weber M, Cabanela ME. Total hip arthroplasty in patients with cerebral palsy. *Orthopedics*. 1999;22:425–427.

45. Weber M, Cabanela ME, Sim FH, et al. Total hip arthroplasty in patients with Parkinson's disease. *Int Orthop*. 2002;26:66–68.

46. Wicart P, Barthas J, Guillaumat M. Replacement arthroplasty of the paralytic hip. *Revue Chir Orthop*. 1999;85:581–590.

47. Yngve DA, Lindseth RE. Effectiveness of muscle transfers in myelomeningocele hips measured by radiographic indices. *J Pediatr Orthop*. 1982;2:121–125.

Metabolic Bone Diseases

35

Eric G. Bonenberger   *Thomas A. Einhorn*

BONE METABOLISM: BASIC PRINCIPLES

Bone differs from the other connective tissues in that it provides both structural and physiologic functions. These characteristics result from bone's unique composition, in which inorganic salts impregnate a well-organized collagen matrix. As a structural component, bone is responsible for protecting the vital organs and providing a rigid framework for the body's shape and locomotion. As an organ, bone serves as the primary site of hematopoiesis and acts as a reservoir for calcium ions, contributing directly to the regulation of extracellular fluid calcium concentrations. To provide these functions, bone is organized into two compartments: a cortical (compact bone) compartment, which provides strength and rigidity, particularly in torsional and bending modes; and a cancellous (trabecular bone) compartment, which serves both to resist compressive loads and to present a high surface-to-volume ratio of bone tissue to extracellular fluids. This latter function enhances bone's metabolic activities and promotes bone remodeling in response to both physiologic as well as mechanical stimuli (59).

The ability of bone to be formed and remodeled and to adapt to its environment is dependent on the cells that regulate

its functions. Osteoclasts, the predominant cell types responsible for bone resorption, are multinucleated giant cells found in cavities on bone surfaces called resorptive pits, or Howship's lacunae. They are characterized by a ruffled border, extensive membrane folding, and abundant mitochondria, rough endoplasmic reticulum, and Golgi complexes. Osteoclasts release protons by a carbonic anhydrase-dependent proton pump, which lowers local pH and thereby facilitates the action of specific acid proteases, which act upon mineral and degrade the extracellular matrix. They respond indirectly to numerous regulatory agents known to induce bone resorption, such as parathyroid hormone (PTH), 1,25-dihydroxyvitamin D_3 (the active metabolite of vitamin D), osteoclast-activating cytokines (e.g., interleukin 1, interleukin 6), and prostaglandin E_2. Because osteoclasts lack receptors for PTH or 1,25-dihydroxyvitamin D_3, their response is believed to be mediated by cells of the osteoblast lineage, which thereby act to influence the localization, induction, stimulation, and inhibition of osteoclastic resorption. Osteoclasts do have receptors for, and respond directly to, calcitonin, colchicine, and α-interferon. Evidence supports the belief that osteoclasts are derived from mononuclear cells originating in bone marrow and other hematopoietic organs (59,138,152).

Osteoblasts are bone-forming cells that synthesize and secrete unmineralized bone matrix (osteoid), participate in bone calcification and resorption, and regulate the flux of calcium and phosphate in and out of bone. Osteoblasts contain intracellular organelles that are typical of cells engaged in protein synthesis; they are also characterized by their abundance of alkaline phosphatase and their ability to synthesize and secrete numerous matrix proteins, including type I collagen, osteocalcin, osteonectin, and specific receptors for proteins such as PTH, 1,25-dihydroxyvitamin D_3, and other bone active hormones. They appear to play a key role in regulating the activity of bone resorption by osteoclasts. Thus, osteoblasts regulate bone remodeling through the control of both bone resorption and formation (59,138).

Once an osteoblast undergoes terminal cell division and is surrounded by a mineralized bone matrix, it becomes an osteocyte. Osteocytes are characterized by a higher nucleus-to-cytoplasm ratio, are arranged concentrically around the central lumen of an osteon and between lamellae, and are uniformly oriented with respect to the longitudinal and radial axes of the lamellae. Osteocytes have extensive cell processes that project through canaliculi, establishing communications with other osteocytes and with osteoblasts that line the surface of bone. Although the function of osteocytes is not clear at this time, several investigators have suggested that osteocytes mediate the transmission of mechanical signals through bone and may also participate in certain bone-resorptive activities (59,138).

The extracellular matrix of bone is an organic substance composed of collagen, noncollagenous proteins, and water. It imparts resilience and flexibility to the tissue. The inorganic component of bone is mineral consisting primarily of calcium and phosphate, mainly in the form of small hydroxyapatite crystals, with the composition $Ca_{10}(PO_4)_6(OH)_2$. It renders bone tissue hard and rigid and accounts for 65% to 70% of its dry weight (13,59,138,152).

Like other cells, a bone cell exhibits a basal level of activity that is modified by systemic hormones and local factors. For example, PTH acts on bone and kidney and indirectly on the gut to increase the rates of calcium flow into the serum and extracellular space and to maintain the body's extracellular calcium concentration at nearly constant levels. The stimulus for PTH release is a drop in the serum ionized calcium concentration. Although the enhancing effect of PTH on bone resorption has been known for some time, this effect is indirect, as receptors for PTH are found only on osteoblasts (59,138). PTH causes cytoskeletal changes in the osteoblast resulting in rounding of the cell, such that it occupies less space on the surface of bone. This configuration allows the osteoclast to gain access to bone surfaces. In addition, it may stimulate osteoblasts to produce factors that activate osteoclasts or increase the recruitment of osteoclast progenitors. Both of these mechanisms will lead to enhanced bone resorption (71,193).

Recent data have helped to advance our knowledge of how osteoblasts regulate bone remodeling and resorption. Lacey et al. have shown that exposure of bone marrow cells and osteoblasts to substances such as PTH, prostaglandin E_2, and 1,25-dyhydroxyvitamin D_3 stimulates osteoclast differentiation and ultimately osteoclast activity through the expression of an osteoclast differentiation factor known as RANK ligand (receptor activator of NF-κB ligand). RANK ligand binds to its receptor, RANK, on the surface of osteoclast precursors. When macrophage colony stimuli factor, a cytokine also produced by bone marrow stromal cells and osteoblasts, binds to its receptor, c-fms, the precursor cell matures into a functioning preosteoclast. This leads to an increase in the number of osteoclasts and hence increased bone resorption. In addition, to further activate bone resorption, RANK ligand can bind RANK on differentiated osteoclasts. Osteoprotegerin, the product of a distinct gene from RANK, inhibits differentiation of osteoclasts by binding RANK as a so-called decoy receptor and preventing its interaction with its ligand (86).

Vitamin D, a steroid hormone that is converted to $25(OH)D_3$ in the liver, then to its active form $1,25(OH)D_3$ in the kidney, plays a role in stimulating biosynthesis of the intestinal and renal calcium-binding proteins and enhances active calcium transport in the gut. How vitamin D is involved in mineralization is not yet known; however, its role in enhancing intestinal calcium and phosphate absorption is

critical to bone and mineral homeostasis. Its activation in the kidney is under the control of PTH, and thus a systemic regulatory control mechanism exists to maintain serum calcium levels (59,112).

Calcitonin, a peptide hormone, is secreted from the parafollicular cells of the thyroid gland in response to an acutely rising plasma calcium concentration. Calcitonin interacts with receptors on the osteoclast, leading to direct inhibition of this cell. The general physiologic role of calcitonin is uncertain, as it seems to play no role in steady-state calcium metabolism (75).

One of the more interesting developments in recent years has been the new knowledge of how bone mass may be regulated through a hypothalamic control mechanism in the central nervous system. According to recent findings, leptin, a small polypeptide hormone secreted primarily by osteoblasts and acting mainly on the hypothalamus, appears to be essential in the control of body weight and, directly or indirectly, gonadal function. Studies have shown that leptin-deficient and leptin-receptor-deficient mice are obese and hypogonadic and demonstrate an increase in bone formation leading to high bone mass. Hence, bone and body mass are physiologically linked through the central nervous system, and pharmacological manipulation of the leptin pathway may prove to be a novel therapeutic approach for the treatment of osteoporosis (64).

OSTEOPOROSIS

Osteoporosis is a pathologic state of bone characterized by decreased bone mass leading to an increased susceptibility to fracture. One major risk factor is a sensitivity of the skeleton to estrogen withdrawal as a result of either natural or surgically induced menopause. Other risk factors include impaired metabolism, long-term calcium deficiency, secondary hyperparathyroidism, and decreased loading of the skeleton. A genetic predisposition (those who are fair skinned, small, or of Northern European ancestry, or have hypermobile joints or scoliosis), or excessive alcohol intake may also lead to the development of osteoporosis. Cigarette smokers show significantly increased incidences of bone loss and hip and vertebral fractures. This may be due in part to the abnormal systemic handling of estrogen metobolites (78) (Table 35-1).

Osteoporosis is so prevalent in the United States that in 2002, approximately 10 million men and women have this condition and an estimated 33 million people have low bone mass (2). Annually, approximately 1.5 million fractures are associated with osteoporosis. This figure includes an estimated 300,000 hip fractures, 700,000 vertebral fractures, 250,000 distal forearm fractures, and 250,000 fractures at other sites (2). Caucasian females older than 50 years of age have a 40% to 50% lifetime risk of sustaining an osteoporotic fracture (3). In 2001 dollars, the cost to the health care system associated with osteoporotic fractures is estimated to be $17 billion. Additionally, each hip fracture currently represents an estimated total medical cost of $40,000 (2001 dollars) (2,120).

On average, peak bone mass is attained between the ages of 16 and 25. The greater this value, the less likely an individual

TABLE 35-1
OSTEOPOROSIS RISK FACTORS

Genetic and Biological	Behavioral and Environmental
Caucasian race	Cigarette smoking
Fair skin and hair	Alcohol excess
Northern European heredity	Inactivity
Scoliosis	Malnutrition
Osteogenesis imperfecta	Caffeine use
Early menopause	Exercise-induced amenorrhea
Slender body build	High-fiber diet
	High-phosphate diet

will reach a critically low level bone loss due to any specific rate of bone loss. Therefore, the less likely the person will be to develop osteoporosis. Bone mass is normally lost at a rate of 0.5% per year in women, and 0.3% per year in men. After menopause (natural or surgical) an accelerated rate of bone loss is noted in women that may reach 2% to 3% and last from 6 to 10 years. This postmenopausal acceleration accounts for the much higher incidence of osteoporosis in women.

Two distinct syndromes of osteoporosis have been described (124). Type I, postmenopausal osteoporosis, affects mainly trabecular bone and occurs most commonly in women within 15 to 20 years after menopause. Type II, senile osteoporosis, affects cortical and trabecular bone equally and occurs in individuals over the age of 70, with a female-to-male ratio of 2:1. It is likely that estrogen plays a role in post-menopausal osteoporosis, whereas aging and long-term calcium deficiency are more integral to senile osteoporosis (Table 35-2).

Clinical Presentation and Diagnosis

Acute fracture often initially brings osteoporosis to the attention of both the patient and the physician. Alternatively, there may be asymptomatic wedge or lumbar compression fractures on a routine lateral chest radiograph. It is important to note that 30% to 50% of bone mineral must be lost before osteopenia is detectable on plain radiographs. The differential diagnosis of radiographic osteopenia includes osteomalacia, endocrine disorders, and disorders of the bone marrow, in addition to osteoporosis (Table 35-3).

Patient Evaluation

Diagnostic accuracy and a staging of the disease for treatment purposes are the goals of patient evaluation. A careful medical

TABLE 35-2
TYPES OF PRIMARY OSTEOPOROSIS

	Type I (Postmenopausal)	Type II (Senile)
Age (years)	51–75	>70
Sex ratio	6:1	2:1

TABLE 35-3
DIFFERENTIAL DIAGNOSIS OF OSTEOPENIA

Primary osteoporosis
  Type I, postmenopausal
  Type II, senile
Osteomalacia
Endocrine disorders
  Cushing's disease
  Diabetes mellitus
  Estrogen deficiency
  Hyperparathyroidism
  Hypogonadism
  Iatrogenic glucocorticoid treatment
  Hyperthyroidism or exogenous thyroid medication
Disuse disorder
  Prolonged immobilization
  Paralysis
Neoplastic disorders
  Leukemia
  Multiple myeloma
Nutritional disorders
  Anorexia nervosa
  High-protein diet
  High-phosphate diet
  Low-calcium diet
Alcoholism
Hematologic disorders
  Sickle-cell anemia
  Thalassemia
Collagen disorders
  Homocystinuria
  Osteogenesis imperfecta

history and physical examination are mandatory, including particular attention to specific risk factors (Table 35-1), systemic causes of osteoporosis (Table 35-4), and known causes of osteomalacia (Table 35-5).

Serum and urine laboratory tests are performed the biochemical basis of the disease process (Table 35-6). Blood tests screen for the presence of hematologic disorders, mineral and electrolyte imbalances, and underlying systemic conditions such as hepatic and renal dysfunction. If the alkaline phosphatase is elevated, fractionation may be necessary, as isoenzymes are secreted by several tissues including bone, kidney, liver, and intestine. In men, measurement of the serum testosterone level should be routine. If nutrient malabsorption is

TABLE 35-4
CAUSES OF SECONDARY OSTEOPOROSIS

Thyroid excess
Parathyroid excess
Hypothalamic hypogonadism
Diabetes mellitus
Steroid exposure (endogenous, iatrogenic)
Multiple myeloma
Leukemia
Prolonged bed rest or inactivity

TABLE 35-5
CAUSES OF OSTEOMALACIA

Vitamin D deficiency
  Dietary
  Malabsorption
    Intestinal disease
    Intestinal surgery
  Insufficient sunlight
Impaired vitamin D synthesis
  Liver disease
  Hepatic microsomal enzyme induction
  Dilantin
  Renal failure
Metabolic acidosis
Fanconi's syndrome
Hypophosphatemia
  Malabsorption
  X-linked hypophosphatemic rickets
  Oncogenic
  Oral phosphate-binding antacid excess
Mineralization inhibition
  Bisphosphonate
  Aluminum
  Fluoride
  Iron
Hypophosphatasia

suspected, the serum carotene level can be measured as an initial screening test. If this is positive, a more complete malabsorption work-up is indicated.

The 24-hour urine collection helps monitor bone resorption. Pyridinoline and deoxypyriodinoline, or the N-telopeptide of type 1 collagen, are peptides predominately found in bone collagen. They are excreted in the urine during bone resorption, and their measurement is a sensitive indicator of bone turnover (149). The 24-hour urine collection is also a means of determining calcium and phosphorus balance. In addition to the metabolites mentioned above, calcium excretion remains an important way to quantify the rate of bone loss. If calcium excretion in the urine is increased, treatment may be indicated to augment total body calcium retention. Thiazide diuretics have been shown effective in maintaining total body calcium levels (103,159). Causes of decreased calcium excretion include a calcium-deficient diet, deficient calcium absorption, or vitamin D deficiency. Phosphorus excretion indicates the effects of PTH on the kidney and is usually elevated when the PTH activity is high.

If hypercalcemia is detected, the patient should be evaluated for primary or secondary hyperparathyroidism. This requires measurement of both serum PTH and 1,25-dihydroxyvitamin D_3 levels. Vitamin D deficiency in patients with hypocalcemia or hypophosphatemia can be evaluated by measuring serum 25-hydroxyvitamin D.

Osteocalcin, also known as γ-carboxyglutamic acid or bone Gla protein (BGP), is another important marker of bone turnover. This protein is synthesized only by osteoblasts and is secreted directly into the circulation. High levels measured in urine or serum suggest a metabolic disorder in which bone is

being formed and degraded. Examples include Paget's disease, renal osteodystrophy, and high-turnover osteoporosis.

Lymphoproliferative malignancies such as multiple myeloma should be considered as this condition is frequently a cause of bone loss and has been shown to mimic osteoporosis radiographically. A serum protein electrophoresis is performed to rule out this (often occult) disease process. If there is an elevated gamma-globulin region, a serum immunoelectrophoresis is ordered. A monoclonal immunoglobin spike would then suggest a diagnosis of multiple myeloma. Urine immunoelectrophoresis may demonstrate the presence of a Bence–Jones protein to confirm a diagnosis of multiple myeloma (Table 35-6).

Radiologic Assessment

Plain radiographs and densitometric scans are both used in the routine evaluation of patients with osteoporosis. Radiographic analysis should include orthogonal images of the thoracolumbosacral spine, because the vertebral bodies are the most common skeletal elements at risk for fracturing.

Bone densitometry is currently the most important tool available for the diagnosis of metabolic bone disease. The most clinically useful methods single and dual energy quantitative computed tomography (QCT), single- and dual-energy x-ray absorptiometry (DXA), and single-photon absorptiometry (SPA). Precision and accuracy of the test, the radiation dose to the patient, and the an atomic sites available for study are the most important parameters in assessing the utility of

TABLE 35-6
LABORATORY TESTS

Routine
Serum
  Complete blood count
  Electrolytes, creatine, blood urea nitrogen
  Calcium, phosphorus, protein, albumin
  Alkaline phosphatase, liver enzymes
  Serum protein electrophoresis
  Thyroid function tests
  Testosterone (men)
24-hour urine
  Calcium
  Pyridinium crosslinks

Special
Serum
  25(OH) vitamin D_3
  1,25(OH)$_2$ vitamin D_3
  Intact parathyroid hormone
  Osteocalcin (bone Gla protein)
Urine
  Immunoelectrophoresis
  Bence–Jones protein

Additional[a]
Gastrointestinal (malabsorption)
Serum carotene
Endocrine
  Plasma cortisol
  Dexamethasone suppression test

[a]Recommended panels for further work-up based on initial history.

TABLE 35-7
TECHNIQUES FOR THE MEASUREMENT OF BONE MASS

Technique	Site	Precision[a] (%)	Accuracy[b] (%)	Examination [Time (min)]	Dose of Radiation (mrem)
Single-energy x-ray absorptiometry	Proximal and distal radius, calcaneus	0.5–2.0	3–5	3–7	1–3
Dual-energy x-ray absorptiometry	Spine, distal radius, hip, total body	0.5–2.0	3–5	3–7	1–3
Quantitative computed tomography	Spine	2–5	5–20	10–15	100–200
Radiographic absorptiometry	Phalanges	1–2	4	2	100

[a]Precision is the coefficient of variation for repeated measurements over a short period of time in young, healthy persons.
[b]Accuracy is the coefficient of variation for measurements in a specimen whose mineral content has been determined by other means.

each of these methods (Table 35-7). These methods, which measure the amount of bone mineral present at a given skeletal site, are accurate and noninvasive and can easily be repeated at 6- to 12-month intervals if necessary.

DXA is the most widely used method for measuring bone mass. An x-ray tube emits and x-ray beam, the attenuation of which is detected by an energy-discriminating photon counter. Bone loss in the radius, calcaneus, hip, spine, or total body can be measured with DXA. Spine and femur scans be performed in about 6 minutes and 3 minutes, respectively, and total body scans take 10 to 20 minutes (93). The radiation dose is very low (1 to 3 mrem). The precision and accuracy are 0.5% to 2% (142) and 3% to 5%, respectively, and high-resolution images are produced (132). In summary, this method can detect small changes in bone mass, with minimal radiation exposure, and with excellent precision, accuracy, and resolution (131).

The informative obtained by a DXA scan shows the bone mineral density (BMD) of the patient and compares it with the normative BMD of other individuals of the same age and sex, as well as with that of younger individuals. These data are reported both as percentages and points on a curve, allowing the physician to determine the degree to which the patient may deviate from the norm.

QCT involves the use a mineral calibration phantom in conjunction with a CT scanner. A lateral CT scan localizes the midplane of two to four lumbar vertebral bodies, and quantitative are readings are then obtained from a region of trabecular bone in the anterior portion of the vertebra. CT determinations of density in the vertebra are then averaged and used to calculate the density of trabecular bone expressed as mineral equivalents of K_2HPO_4 (mg/cm^2) The radiation dose is 100 to 200 mrem, or approximately one tenth of that used in a routine CT study.

In photon absorptiometry, a gamma ray source, a detector, and a system of electronics are used to measure beam attenuation through a section bone. This method is usually applied to the radius with a relatively low radiation dose (10 to 20 mrem). For SPA, precision and accuracy are 1% to 3% and 5%, respectively (58,79).

Bone Biopsy

An extremely useful test in certain metabolic bone disease evaluations is the transiliac bone biopsy. Although invasive, it is associated with minimal pain and inconvenience to the patient, can be performed on an ambulatory basis, and results

in very few complications. It is indicated to establish a diagnosis in patients in whom an occult malignancy is suspected, to distinguish between osteomalacia and osteitis fibrosa cystica in certain hemodialysis patients, or to elucidate the cause of severe osteopenia in patients whose blood and urine test results are insufficiently informative.

By convention, the biopsy is taken from a point 3 cm posterior and 3 cm inferior to the anterior superior iliac spine. The instrument used should produce a cylindrical specimen at least 6 mm in diameter, containing two cortices and an intervening marrow space. Once obtained, the specimen is embedded in methyl methacrylate and cut, processed, and stained using an undecalcified technique. Unstained sections are examined by fluorescence microscopy to determine the dynamic properties of bone. This is made possible by the presence of tetracycline labels. The cellular parameters of bone turnover are assessed by light microscopic examination of hematoxylin and eosin-stained sections. The technique involves preoperative administration of oral tetracycline in two doses that are separated by a specified number of days (e.g., tetracycline 250 mg orally three times a day for 3 days, off for 12 days, repeat for 3 more days, and biopsy between 3 and 7 days later).

Differentiation of mineralized from unmineralized osteoid is achieved using a salt stain such as Von Kossa, in which calcium and phosphorus salts appear dark, whereas unmineralized osteoid appears pale (Fig. 35-1). Through the use of a

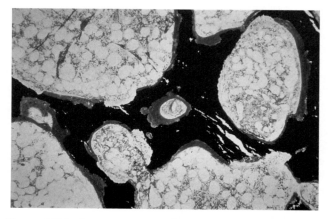

Figure 35-1 Low-power view of osteomalacic bone from a 25-year-old man with metabolic acidosis. Note that mineralized bone appears dark, whereas unmineralized osteoid fails to take up the stain and appears pale (Von Kossa ×25).

computer-assisted calculating system, an optical drawing tube, and an integrated ocular eyepiece, a number of quantitative parameters of bone turnover are measured. This technique, known as histomorphometry, enables the clinician to diagnose the disorder accurately and determine to what extent resorptive or blastic activities are influencing the disease. In patients with renal disease, special stains are used to identify the presence of aluminum in bone as a cause of osteomalacia. This is particularly important because dramatic clinical improvements have been reported after removal of this metal from the bone (92).

Treatment Regimens

Preventive and treatment regimens for osteoporosis continue to evolve, as no single strategy is curative for this condition. This is particularly true for the treatment of primary osteoporosis, for which the etiology is not known. In secondary osteoporosis, however, an underlying cause of the disease can be identified and addressed before agents directed at correcting the skeletal lesion are introduced. Examples of conditions that are usually treatable include endogenous or iatrogenic hyperthyroidism, primary hyperparathyroidism, iatrogenic steroid-induced osteoporosis, and exercise-induced amenorrhea. In other cases, it is not possible to eliminate or reduce the effects of an instigating cause (e.g., steroid-induced osteoporosis), and treatment is extremely difficult. The recommendations offered in this section should be used as guidelines for treating patients with different types of osteoporosis. One must remember, however, that the responses of each patient to treatment may differ, necessitating alterations in management.

Medical treatment for osteoporosis can be broadly divided into anticatabolic and formation-stimulating therapies. Anticatabolic therapies include the use of drugs such as estrogen, calcitonin, and the bisphosphonates. These methods are aimed at producing a direct or indirect reduction in osteoclastic resorbing activity. The formation-stimulating therapies include sodium fluoride and PTH treatment.

The role of dietary calcium supplementation in the prophylactic treatment of osteoporosis appears to be most critical during the childhood and adolescent years, when peak bone mass is being built; today this is the cornerstone of prevention (113). An adequate dietary calcium intake is required at all times, however, to maintain normal skeletal health (Table 35-8). All patients being treated for osteoporosis should take 1.5 g of elemental calcium daily plus one or two multivitamins containing 400 units of vitamin D each. Vitamin D is essential for calcium absorption, but the beneficial role of vitamin D supplementation is unclear in individuals capable of synthesizing adequate vitamin D (ultraviolet light interacting with vitamin D precursors in the skin). Patients who have or are at risk for developing type II osteoporosis should also follow this regimen (38). However, women at risk of developing type 1 osteoporosis are not necessarily afforded protection by calcium supplementation alone (126). Although studies are in progress to determine the best preparation of oral calcium to use to enhance intestinal calcium absorption (e.g., calcium carbonate, calcium citrate, calcium citrate malate, etc.), it is clear that any calcium compound is best absorbed when taken with meals (38). Calcium carbonate absorption is reduced when ingested with meals high in fat or fiber, and this form of calcium requires normal stomach acidity

TABLE 35-8
RECOMMENDED CALCIUM INTAKES

Ages	Amount (mg/day)
Birth to 6 months	210
6 months to 1 year	270
1 to 3 years	500
4 to 8 years	800
9 to 13 years	1,300
14 to 18 years	1,300
19 to 30 years	1,000
31 to 50 years	1,000
51 to 70 years	1,200
71 or older	1,200
Pregnant or lactating	
14 to 18 years	1,300
19 to 50 years	1,000

Source: Dietary Reference Intakes: Applications in Dietary Assessment (2000), page 287. Institute of Medicine, National Academy Press, Washington, D.C.

for adequate absorption. Calcium citrate supplements can be absorbed in the absence of acidity.

Until recently, the most well-accepted treatment for most osteoporotic patients was estrogen replacement therapy. If the patient had no history of breast cancer or heart, thromboembolic, or endometrial disease, and if such therapy was indicated by her gynecologist, then estrogen was considered safe. A recent study may have disproved this notion. The Women's Health Initiative randomized controlled trial demonstrated a higher relative risk for stroke (relative risk [RR] = 1.41), coronary heart disease (RR = 1.29), breast cancer (RR = 1.26), and pulmonary embolism (RR = 2.13) in the group taking estrogen plus progestin. There was an overall protective relative risk in the treatment group for colorectal cancer (RR = 0.63), endometrial cancer (RR = 0.83), and hip fractures (RR = 0.66) (128). Based on these data, the authors only recommend this therapy to patients in whom no other drug treatment can be tolerated.

Alendronate (Fosamax®), a bisphosphonate compound, is the first nonhormonal drug approved for the treatment of this disease. Bisphosphonates are analogues of pyrophosphate that have been shown to have potent inhibitory effects on bone resorption. Alendronate is used in the dose of 10 mg per day or 70 mg once a week, must be taken orally on an empty stomach, and the patient can only drink plain water (no other food or beverage) at the time of dosing. Because of the low bioavailability of this compound from the intestinal tract (approximately 0.7%) no food can be taken at least 30 minutes after dosing. In addition, since some patients experience epigastric pain, the patient may not lie down for at least 30 minutes after dosing so as to avoid gastric reflux and esophagitis. Reports show that alendronate prevents bone loss and is associated with gains in bone mass of up to 10%, and decreases in the risks of hip, distal radial, and vertebral compression fractures of 51%, 44%, and 46%, respectively, within 2 years of intervention (35,90). Another new-generation bisphosphonate, risedronate (Actonel®), decreased the incidence of new vertebral fractures by 41% over 3 years in a randomized controlled trial, with a decreased rate of gastrointestinal side effects such as esophagitis and dyspepsia (67,123). The overall safety profile was similar to placebo.

Raloxifene (Evista®), a second-generation selective estrogen receptor modulator, is a member of a class of drugs that are agonists for bone and the cardiovascular system, but are purported to not affect the breast or the uterus (39). Raloxifene has demonstrated a 2% to 3% increase in bone mineral density over baseline, as compared to a decline with placebo. Also, raloxifene is cardioprotective, reducing overall cholesterol and low-density lipoprotein (LDL) cholesterol levels (6). A randomized clinical trial showed an increase in the bone mineral density of the hip and spine with a reduction in the vertebral fractures in the treated postmenopausal women (5.4% of treated women versus 10.1% in the placebo group) (52).

Calcitonin, a naturally occurring hormonal compound, has been approved by the FDA for several years in an injectable form. The approved dose of injectable salmon calcitonin is 100 units per day. A nasal spray formulation of this compound consists of a dose of 200 units per day. One spray to one nostril per day delivers this dose, and patients should alternate nostrils daily. Calcitonin has been shown to be effective in stabilizing spinal bone mass and decreasing vertebral fractures (25). However, it does not decrease hip fracture risk as it does not affect cortical bone. Additionally, calcitonin has a role in the relief of pain from the microfractures associated with osteoporosis but does not change their rate of healing. Finally, if hypercalcuria accompanies the active osteoporotic state, one to two daily doses of thiazide are given to increase total body calcium retention (103).

Newer pharmacologic approaches aimed at increasing bone mass are now being investigated. These include PTH, parathyroid hormone-related protein (PTHrP), and the targeting of osteoclast integrins to prevent the attachment of those cells to bone. Daily low dosing of PTH and PTHrP increased vertebral bone mass in both animal and human trials, but similar to calcitonin, there were no gains in cortical bone mass (146). However, a recent report of a randomized controlled trial in 1637 postmenopausal women with established osteoporosis has shown increases in vertebral bone mineral density and decreases in the risks of both vertebral and nonvertebral fractures (106). Based on these findings, the FDA has recommended approval of this drug for the treatment of osteoporosis.

The N-terminal fragment of PTH (residues 1 through 34) possess biologic activity and has been named teriparatide. Teriparatide (Forteo; Eli Lilly, Indianapolis, IN) is formed by degradation of the intact PTH in the liver and kidneys. Native PTH is metabolically unstable and, following release from the parathyroid gland, is rapidly degraded, primarily by the liver. Teriparatide is not readily detected in the circulation, and the current assumption is that it is rapidly cleared (91).

Teriparatide is administered via a subcutaneous injection and the absolute bioavailability approaches 95%. The drug has been approved by the U.S. Food and Drug Administration (2000) for the treatment of postmenopausal women with osteoporosis who are at high risk for fracture. This population includes those with a history of osteoporotic fracture, multiple risk factors for fracture, intolerance with osteoporosis therapy,

or failure with therapy. Teriparatide is not recommended for patients at risk for osteosarcomas. This group includes patients with Paget's disease, open epiphyses, and those who have previously undergone skeletal radiation therapy (91). A potential drawback of the routine use of teriparatide is cost. The annual cost of teriparatide is approximately seven times that of bisphosphonates and other antiresorptive treatments (91).

In summary, a careful clinical evaluation of the individual with low bone mass is essential prior to initiating the treatment of osteoporosis. First-line regimens include dietary supplementation (calcium and vitamin D) as well as oral bisphosphonates. Newer drugs, such as teriparatide, should be reserved for higher-risk patients.

HIP FRACTURES AND THE CONTRIBUTION OF OSTEOPOROSIS

Hip fracture is perhaps most serious consequence is related to osteoporosis. One in every six Caucasian women in the United States sustains a hip fracture during her lifetime, and up to 20% of these patients die as a result (34). As mentioned previously, the risk of hip fracture is clearly increased with advancing age and with women. In one report, 87% of patients sustaining a hip fracture were older than 65, and 75% of these patients were women (36). Additionally, it is expected that 33% of women and 15% of men will have sustained at least one hip fracture by age 90 (17).

Risk factors for hip fracture other than skeletal fragility should not be overlooked. In a prospective study of Caucasian women, Cummings et al. (37) reported that a maternal history of hip fracture doubled the risk, and other risk factors including weight loss, relative inactivity, increased caffeine intake, treatment with long-acting benzodiazepines or anticonvulsant drugs, and poor vision were also important. Overall body mass has been found to be a major determinant of the risk of hip fracture in African–American women (62), while thinner Caucasian women are at higher risk for hip fracture (36,53,81). Previous stroke, use of aids in walking, and current (but not prior) alcoholism have also been implicated (55,62).

Femoral neck geometry may be related to the risk of hip fracture (54). Faulkner et al. defined the hip axis length as the length along the femoral neck from the lateral border of the greater trochanter, through the femoral neck, to the inner pelvic prim. A hip axis length one standard deviation longer than average was associated with a twofold increase in the risk for subsequent femoral neck and intertrochanteric fracture, after age adjustment. Moreover, the hip axis length shows no correlation with age or with femoral bone mineral density. Two reports have suggested that taller women have a greater risk of hip fracture (37,99), perhaps because they fall from an increased relative starting point (69,108).

The relationship between low bone mass at several sites, most importantly the femoral neck, and the risk of subsequent hip fracture is well established (1,12,26,32,33,61,72, 74,118,125,,135,154,158). Several investigators have reported a preferentially low bone mineral density of the femoral neck, as measured by dual-photon absorptiometry (1,26), and lower overall bone mass has been associated with greater risk of hip fractures (1,135). Low calcaneal bone density has been reported as an independent risk factor (37,135).

It is important to differentiate between bone mineral content and bone mineral density. Both are quantitative values obtained from densitometric scans. Bone mineral content is measured from as the total mineral in the area of the scan, reported as grams. Bone mineral density, reported as grams per square centimeter, is a measure of the mineral content per given area. This is obtained by dividing the mineral content by the area scanned.

Bohr and Schadt (12) reported that the bone mineral content of the axial skeleton, including the femoral shaft, but not the femoral neck, was significantly reduced in those patients sustaining femoral neck fractures. Several other studies have failed to reproduce these results and have in fact reported that patients with hip fractures are not significantly more osteoporotic than persons of similar age (31,51,85). Other factors, such a tendency to fall and reduced strength of bone, have been implicated as important causes of hip fractures (12).

Several hip fracture patterns have been identified. The femoral neck fracture (intracapsular) occurs through an area that is composed of about 75% cortical bone. However, the intertrochanteric fracture occurs through an area composed of roughly 50% cortical and 50% trabecular bone. Additionally, the stresses in the femur change along a proximal to distal gradient (56). Osteoporosis results in the loss of horizontal trabeculae, which leads directly to an increased susceptibility to fractures of the intertrochanteric portion (46,104).

Several authors have noted that patients with intertrochanteric fractures were older than those with femoral neck fractures (51,57,136,154). Of note, intracapsular fractures occur at approximately the same rate as intertrochanteric fractures (150,154). However, the ratio of intertrochanteric to femoral neck fractures has been reported to increase linearly with age (67). Greenspan et al. (61) found that patients sustaining a trochanteric fracture had relatively low bone mineral density in this region, and they hypothesized that the site-specific bone mineral density may be associated with the type of hip fracture sustained by an elderly patient as a result of a fall. Other investigators have confirmed the finding of preferential bone loss in patients with intertrochanteric fractures (135,154). Seely et al. (135) found a significant association between low appendicular bone mass and intertrochanteric fractures, but not with femoral neck fractures.

In general, the diaphyseal sections of long bones increase in diameter with age, and as a result of cross-sectional expansion, bending strength, torsional strength, and areal and polar moments of inertia are increased (130,140). However, this does not apply to the femoral neck. The femoral neck, which is intracapsular, may undergo endosteal resorption without the benefit of compensatory periosteal apposition. Therefore, it may not be protected by the same cortical expansion mechanism as the remainder of the skeleton. This is probably related to the fact the periosteum is absent from of the proximal femur that is within the hip joint (114,117). The net result is cortical thinning of the femoral neck without an increase in cross-sectional diameter.

Clinically, osteoporosis leads to both a decrease in overall bone mass and an increased susceptibility to fracture. The diagnosis is important for not only prevention of future fractures, but also in determining treatment options. Specifically,

the devices commonly utilized for internal fixation require secure purchase in healthy bone for stable fracture fixation. Barrios et al. (7) reported that healing complications were increased after internal fixation of intertrochanteric fractures in osteoporotic patients. In their prospective study group of 113 patients, 25 of 33 implant failures (76%) occurred in patients with osteoporosis. The greatest risk for failure of fixation was noted in osteoporotic patients with unstable trochanteric fractures. Regarding femoral neck fractures, Sjostedt et al. (139) reported that fixation strength was most dependent on the strength of the bone. They measured the loading-to-failure, postfixation stiffness, and ultimate compression strength of 21 femoral autopsy specimens. A threshold bone mineral content value of 0.4 g/cm^2 was identified, below which failure of osteosynthesis was noted during cyclical loading. These authors recommended a primary arthroplasty in the case of a femoral neck fracture occurring in osteoporotic bone.

In summary, the contribution of osteoporosis to hip fractures is significant for etiologic, diagnostic, therapeutic, and economic implications. Prophylactic treatment regimens for osteoporosis are becoming commonly utilized. Technologic advances in bone densitometry currently aid in the evaluation and diagnosis of osteoporosis. Finally, modification of surgical protocols in patients with osteoporosis should be considered, as internal fixation appears to be associated with a greater risk of implant failure.

OSTEOMALACIA AND RENAL OSTEODYSTROPHY

The prevalence of osteomalacia in the hip fracture population is a matter of some controversy. Hordon and Peacock (71) reported that patients biopsied at the time of femoral neck fracture frequently have histomorphometric abnormalities in cancellous bone. Specifically, they found an overall prevalence of osteomalacia of 12% (9 of 72 patients), diagnosed by double tetracycline labeling of iliac crest biopsies at the time of fracture. Moreover, in this study the prevalences of both osteoporosis and osteomalacia increase with age. These findings are of more than academic importance. Osteomalacia can usually be prevented and treated, once diagnosed; on the other hand, the treatment of established and advanced osteoporosis remains more difficult and controversial.

Osteomalacia is a metabolic disorder characterized by an adequate mineralization of newly formed osteoid. Vitamin D deficiency, vitamin D resistance, intestinal resorption, acquired or hereditary renal disorders, and intoxication with heavy metals, such as aluminum or iron are among the many causes of osteomalacia (Table 35-4). Rickets, the childhood form of osteomalacia, has become rare since the widespread supplementation of dairy products with vitamin D. Identification of the cause of the impairment of mineralization is critical because this will direct treatment and, in many cases, affect the physician's choice of which vitamin D metabolite to use.

The diagnosis of osteomalacia in most patients is confirmed by transiliac bone biopsy. In osteomalacic bone, there is a decreased rate of mineral apposition as determined by tetracycline labeling. In addition, the slower rate of mineralization

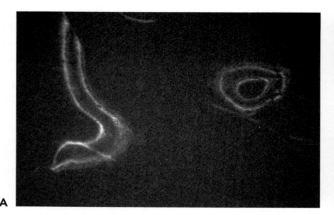 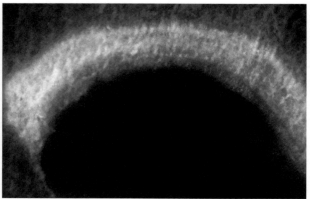

Figure 35-2 High-power unstained fluorescent micrographs of the mineralization fronts from a normal patient **(A)** showing two discrete fluorescent lines, and a patient with osteomalacia **(B)**, whose tetracycline labels appear to be "smudged" (×100). (From Einhorn TA. Osteoporosis and metabolic bone disease. *Adv Orthop Surg.* 1984;8:175–184, with permission.)

results in a "smudged" appearance of these labels, as they do not appear to be separated in time (Fig. 35-2). The major histologic feature of osteomalacia is increase in the width and extent of osteoid seams (Fig. 35-1).

The patient who has osteomalacia often presents with vague complaints such as muscle weakness or diffuse aches and pains. The radiographic presence of pseudofractures or Looser's transformation zones strongly points to a diagnosis of osteomalacia. Looser's zones are radiolucent areas of bone that are the result of multiple microstress fractures that heal by the formation of osteomalacic (unmineralized) bone (Fig. 35-3). Laboratory abnormalities vary in the presence of osteomalacia as a result of different etiologies, but they often include an elevated alkaline phosphatase, low serum calcium, or low inorganic phosphorus level. Analysis of vitamin D metabolites may elucidate the abnormality.

Classically, osteomalacia is caused by a decrease in the vitamin D content in the diet. Those with strict vegetarian diets or diets extremely low in fat are more susceptible. This condition is more common in elderly patients, probably because of the

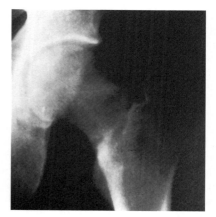

Figure 35-3 Anteroposterior radiograph of the proximal femur of a patient with osteomalacia. Note the presence of a Looser's zone on the inferomedial aspect of the femoral neck. (From Einhorn TA. Osteoporosis and metabolic bone disease. *Adv Orthop Surg.* 1984;8:175–184, with permission.)

"mild malabsorption" of the elderly (121). Treatment is with vitamin D (cholecalciferol).

Anticonvulsant drugs such as phenytoin (Dilantin®) are known to cause osteomalacia by the induction of P-450 mixed-function oxidases in hepatic cells. This causes the conversion of vitamin D to inactive polar metabolites, which reduces the production of 25-hydroxyvitamin D, an essential substrate for the renal conversion to 1,25-hydroxyvitamin D. Treatment involves attempts to eliminate or reduce the dose of phenytoin used by the patient and prescribing 25-hydroxyvitamin D (calcifediol).

Renal stones, hypophosphatemia, and osteomalacia are the major clinical features of distal renal tubular acidosis. This condition, which has a dominant mode of inheritance and variable penetrance, is treated with high doses of vitamin D and sodium bicarbonate.

Patients on hemodialysis for chronic renal failure are also at increased risk for osteomalacia. Osteomalacia in this group of patients may be caused by the intoxication of the skeleton with aluminum. Aluminum containing phosphate-binding antacids are used in hemodialysis to control phosphate accumulation. Of note, phosphate retention will lower serum calcium levels and thus increase PTH production (secondary hyperparathyroidism), leading to osteitis fibrosa cystica. The accumulation of aluminum is believed to interfere directly with skeletal remodeling, including the resorption of bone, synthesis of new matrix, and the deposition of mineral on to the matrix (116). These patients frequently manifest chronic bone pain and susceptibility to pathologic fractures. Aluminum levels can be intermittently controlled with the aluminum-chelating agent deferoxamine, which facilitates mineralization and stimulates osteoid synthesis (92). It is believed that deferoxamine may, in an analogous manner, enhance the union of pathologic fractures secondary to aluminum-associated osteomalacia (116).

In the pediatric population, osteomalacia is referred to as rickets. There are several known hereditary causes of renal rickets in growing children. The most common is X-linked dominant hypophosphatemic rickets, which is usually caused by a renal tubular defect in phosphate reabsorption. Normal growth can be maintained in these patients with early diagnosis and

TABLE 35-9
TREATMENT OF OSTEMALACIA[a]

Disorder	Vitamin D_2 (U)	25(OH)D_3 (μg)	1,25(OH$_2$)D_3 (μg)
Nutritional vitamin D deficiency	50,000 3–5 times/week		
Malabsorption	50,000/day	20–200/day	
Anticonvulsant-induced osteomalacia (Dilantin)	50,000/day	20–200/day	
Renal osteomalacia[b]			1–2/day
Metabolic acidosis[c]			1–2/day
X-linked hypophosphatemia[d]	50,000/day		2–3/day until healing, then 0.5–1.0/day

[a]All patients receive 1.5 g elemental Ca per day.
[b]Renal patients with bone aluminum may require deferoxamine.
[c]To correct acidosis, titrate blood pH with sodium bicarbonate.
[d]Add 1–2 g/day of phosphorus.
From Einhorn TA. Evaluation and treatment methods for metabolic bone diseases. *Contemp Orthop* 1987;14:21–34, with permission.

treatment with phosphate and 1,25-dihydroxyvitamin D. A rare form of osteomalacia that is often associated with a benign tumor of the nasopharyngeal cavity has been reported (21). In this condition, a phosphaturic substance is secreted by the tumor. In general, the treatment strategies for osteomalacia differ depending on the etiology of the condition (Table 35-9).

TOTAL HIP REPLACEMENT AFTER RENAL TRANSPLANTATION

Osteonecrosis has been reported to occur in 5% to 40% of patients who underwent renal transplantation prior to the early 1980s, and the femoral head was the most commonly involved site (10,68,76,88,105). Approximately 50% of cases of osteonecrosis of the femoral head were bilateral. High-dose corticosteroids used for immunosuppression in the perioperative period of the transplant were the cause of most of these cases. With the advent of cyclosporine, corticosteroid use is now much reduced, and few cases of transplant-associated osteonecrosis are seen. Nevertheless, those cases that do occur generally require operative intervention, and an understanding of the condition by the orthopedic surgeon is required.

Patients generally present during the first two years after transplantation with the classic complaints associated with osteonecrosis (thigh or groin pain, stiffness, progressive limitation of movement, and difficulty with ambulation). Surgical procedures that attempt to revitalize the necrotic portion of the femoral head include bone grafting, vascularized free fibula grafts, and core decompression. Other options include intertrochanteric osteotomy, arthrodesis, and total hip arthroplasty (143).

Bradford et al. (14) reported an average time of 20 months (1.7 years) from renal transplantation to the subsequent development of symptoms in a group of 39 patients who developed osteonecrosis of the femoral head after renal transplantation but were not treated with cyclosporine. Radiographic diagnosis of all hips was made an average of 6 months after the patient presented with symptoms.

As noted, there is clear evidence that the development of osteonecrosis after renal transplantation is attributable to corticosteroids (66,76). The addition of cyclosporine A to postoperative treatment protocols has allowed for decreased doses of corticosteroids. Cyclosporine A spares the need for steroids by reducing the number of episodes of rejection, so that fewer steroid boluses are needed. Survival rates, for both patients and grafts, have improved. Landmann et al. (87) reported a substantially reduced incidence of osteonecrosis in patients who received a lower dose of prednisone during the first two months following the transplantation.

Total hip arthroplasty (THA) is considered the treatment of choice for patients with advanced, painful osteonecrosis of the hip after renal transplantation. However, the long-term results of THA in this group of patients have not been promising. Several investigators have reported significantly lower survival of THA in renal transplantation recipients when compared to patients with other diagnosis, including osteoarthritis (29,40,41,119). Deo et al. reported a rate of aseptic loosening in 34 procedures performed on 25 renal transplant patients. The average follow-up was 5 years and the revision rate was 15% at a mean of 8.8 years (40).

Devlin et al. (41) also reported a high rate of complications that long-term follow-up of THA and renal transplant recipients. Of 24 patients, there were 6 (25%) failures to aseptic loosening, 5 dislocations, and 10 hips with heterotopic bone. They found, however, that most patients experienced improved hip function and symptomatic relief of pain as a result of the operation. The high long-term failure rate may be attributed to several factors, including young age and consequently higher levels of activity, a high incidence of bilateral hip involvement (62%), and capsular and soft tissue laxity secondary to corticosteroids, which contributes to dislocation (14). In this series, there was only one deep infection despite immunosuppression. Other investigators have also reported that there was no increase in incidence of infection in these patients (14,40,119).

More recently, Stromboni et al. reported a series 48 of THAs performed on 32 renal transplant recipients with femoral head osteonecrosis. Using the Postel–Merle–d'Aubigne score, 75% of hips scored good, very good, or excellent. Both early and late complications were evaluated. Early complications included 7 wound hematomas, 1 dislocation, and 2 deep infections. A second operation was necessary for seven hips due to aseptic loosening (mean delay 9 years 10 months), for five hips due to septic loosening (mean delay 6 years 8 months). Two hips were revised for instability. In all, 29% of hips required reoperation. These authors concluded that THA enables a good functional outcome in this patient population, but at the high risk of both early and late complications. (147).

Cyclosporine A is currently in a general used for immuno-suppression in patients who have undergone renal transplantation. Therefore, a lower dose of corticosteroids is required postoperatively. The patients studied by Devlin et al. (41) were treated before the widespread use of cyclosporine A, and thus likely received higher doses of prednisone than patients undergoing transplantation today. Specifically, Landmann et al. (87), in a controlled study, reported that during the first 2 months after transplantation, the mean dose of prednisone (per kilogram of body weight per day) was approximately 2.5 times greater in patients receiving conventional immunosuppression as compared with those who received cyclosporine A.

Several authors have reported high dislocation rates after THA in renal transplant recipients; however, the cause of this is unclear (14,41). In their series of 39 patients (60 THAs) Bradford et al. (14) reported 10 dislocations (17%). This is 5 to 8 times the rate of dislocation of THA in nontransplant patients (20,24,30,89,110,160). The authors emphasize the importance of careful repair of the posterior joint capsule after insertion of implants in preventing dislocation.

Cornell et al. (29) reported an overall failure rate of 37%. Other studies have found poor survival rates after THA for a diagnosis of osteonecrosis (23,42,70,144). They attributed their findings to both youth and poor bone quality. The stress limits of the bone–cement interface may be exceeded even in young, normal patients with high activity levels. In addition, ongoing bone necrosis or progressive associated osteoporosis in transplant patients may accelerate mechanical failure. Other investigators have also attributed their poor results after THA to poor bone quality (119). Huffer et al. (73) reported finding reduced bone volume and many of the features of renal osteodystrophy in transplant recipients, including mineralization defects, excessive bone resorption, and reduced bone volume.

Although the results of THA are not as good in renal transplant patients as in patients who have osteoarthritis, the procedure is still considered safe and effective (119). It is generally well tolerated and provides symptomatic relief in the majority of patients.

PAGET'S DISEASE OF BONE

The prevalence of Paget's disease of bone is currently estimated to be approximately 4% in the world's Anglo-Saxon population older than 55 years. Therefore, it is the second most common metabolic bone disease, after osteoporosis. Although the cause is unproven, a viral pathogenesis was proposed in 1974 when viruslike inclusion bodies were found in osteoclasts from affected bone, and research has focused on a slow virus as the causative agent (101). More recent studies have implicated the measles virus of the paramyxovirus family. Additional studies have demonstrated that abnormal virus-infected osteoclasts may generate interleukin 6, a resorptive cytokine from the bone marrow of patients with Paget's disease (9). Brandwood et al. reported on the relationship between gene expression, osteoclastic apoptosis, and Paget's disease. Analysis using human apoptosis cDNA expression arrays revealed that the apoptotic suppressor Bcl-2 showed a marked increase in expression in Pagetic bone. These investigators concluded that in Paget's disease there is an increased expression of genes that are involved in the inhibition of apoptosis, notably Bcl-2. The increase in Bcl-2 may be explained in some patients by mutations in the Bcl-2 gene promoter. Lack of apoptosis leads to an increased relative number of osteoclasts, a hallmark of Paget's disease (16). Population studies recently completed in the United Kingdom, Spain, and New Zealand indicate that the prevalence of Paget's disease may be decreasing (28,44,102). These apparent declines suggest an environmental contribution to the etiology of this disorder. Further laboratory and clinical studies are necessary to unravel the intertwined connections between the potential viral, genetic, and environmental causative factors of this disease.

Extensive osteolysis, large numbers of both osteoclasts and osteoblasts, and the production of a woven-type bone are the histologic hallmarks of pagetic bone. Widened lamellae and disorganized cement lines characterize the newly formed bone, giving it the "mosaic pattern" appearance. Concurrently, the normal fatty or hematopoietic marrow spaces are replaced by loose, highly vascularized fibrous connective tissue. A "burned out" stage ultimately results from decreases in both osteoblastic and osteoclastic activity. Grossly, the affected bones are enlarged, deformed, and densely sclerotic.

Two biochemical markers, serum alkaline phosphatase and urinary pyridinium cross-links, are used to follow the course of the disease and its response to treatment. The high rate of bone turnover in Paget's disease results in an immediate increase in the excretion of type I collagen breakdown products. The compensatory osteoblastic state is marked by an increase in alkaline phosphatase activity.

Most patients are asymptomatic, and Paget's disease is often discovered as an incidental finding on radiographic examinations. Common complaints include bone pain, joint pain, low back pain, and later in the disease, deformities. The technetium-99m methylene-diphosphonate (MDP) bone scan should be done to screen areas of pagetic involvement. Areas that show increased isotopic uptake require radiographic examination to determine the extent and nature of involvement.

In Paget's disease, the radiographic appearance correlates closely with the histologic course. The osteolytic state is seen initially as discrete areas of bone lysis. Subsequently, activation of endosteal erosion leads to expansion of the bone with the compensatory formation of subperiosteal new bone.

Most patients with Paget's disease do not require pharmacologic therapy and can simply be followed clinically. For those patients who have increased pain and poorly controlled indices of bone turnover, three classes of drugs are available: nonsteroidal anti-inflammatory drugs, calcitonin, and the

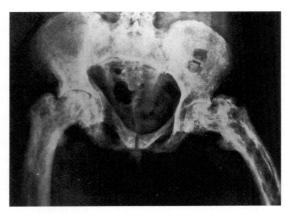

Figure 35-4 Radiographic features of Paget's disease. This patient has bilateral femoral and pelvic involvement. Bilatera coxa vara is present, as well as mild right acetabular protrusion. Early signs of pelvic involvement, particularly the halo of osteoporosis above the acetabulum and a widened iliopectineal line, are present on the left. (From McDonald DJ, Sim FH. Total hip arthroplasty in Paget's disease: a follow-up note. *J Bone Joint Surg.* 1987:69A: 766–772, with permission.)

bisphosphonates. Indomethacin and other related non-steroidal anti-inflammatory agents have been shown to be useful for mild pain symptoms related to Paget's disease.

Patients who have pain and abnormally high alkaline phosphatase activities may be managed with a bisphosphonate. Etidronate disodium was the first bisphosphonate approved by the FDA for the treatment of Paget's disease. It inhibits the ability of osteoclasts to resorb bone. However, high doses and chronic use of etidronate have been shown to inhibit mineralization and may lead to osteomalacia. Most patients are therefore placed on cyclical programs of etidronate therapy in which they are on the drugs for several months at a time and then taken off for long periods of rest. Any patient who sustains a long-bone fracture while using etidronate should be taken off until the fracture heals.

Recently, alendronate has been recommended for the use in the treatment of Paget's disease. It is taken orally at a dosage of 40 mg for 6 months. Adequate calcium intake (1000 to 1500 mg per day, depending on the patient's age) is important during treatment with alendronate. Pamidronate, olpadronate, tiludronate, zoledronate, risedronate, and clodronate are bisphosphonates that have been examined as potentially useful agents for the treatment of Paget's disease (3,19,45,80, 122,148,151,153,161). Route of administration, duration of treatment, cost, and side effects delineate agents within this class more so than efficacy. Intravenous preparations (pamidronate and clodronate) are useful in those who cannot tolerate the gastrointestinal side effects associated with alendronate. Risedronate may become an attractive option because it is an oral agent with efficacy comparable to alendronate, yet fewer gastrointestinal side effects (19,151). Also, the biochemical remission (normalization of serum alkaline phosphatase) was achieved for an average of 33 months after daily doses for only 28 consecutive days (19). To date, prospective, randomized clinical trials that render a particular bisphosphonate as superior to alendronate with respect to side effect profile, efficacy, and cost have not been published.

Calcitonin, a naturally occurring hormone, is the most effective agent for the treatment of Paget's disease. It is given by subcutaneous injection or nasal spray and acts by direct inactivation of osteoclasts. However, almost 60% of patients given calcitonin develop antibodies to it, and the agent may lose its effectiveness over time.

In the polyostotic form of Paget's disease, the pelvis and spine are typically involved. Pelvic lesions are generally well tolerated unless the acetabulum is involved, in which case degenerative joint disease of the hip may develop. Spinal involvement is not as well tolerated. Patients frequently complain of low back pain and present with symptoms of spinal stenosis. Spinal stenosis results when the effected segment becomes progressively deformed, leading to a narrowing of the static canal measurement (65).

Paget's involving the hip is classically seen as coxa vara deformity of the proximal femur (Fig. 35-4). As a result of this altered biomechanical strain environment, there is an increased risk of hip fracture (Fig. 35-5). The treatment of hip fractures and hip degenerative changes in this patient population are discussed below.

A substantial increase in pain in a patient with Paget's disease is strongly suggestive of sarcomatous degeneration, which occurs in less than 1% of patients. Osteogenic sarcoma

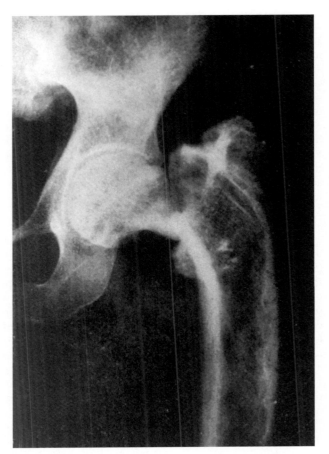

Figure 35-5 Fracture through the neck of the femur in an 80-year-old woman. (From Barry HC. Fracture of the femur in Paget's disease of bone in Australia. *J Bone Joint Surg.* 1967;49A: 1359–1370, with permission.)

is the most common type of sarcoma that occurs in association with this condition. Malignant giant cell tumors, fibrosarcomas, and chondrosarcomas have also been reported (133).

Total Hip Arthroplasty in Patients with Paget's Disease of Bone

Patients with Paget's disease of bone with involvement in the vicinity of joints often develop degenerative joint disease. This process may be related to the biomechanical alteration of the subchondral bone (increased stiffness) as a result of the sclerotic phase of the condition. Operative indications, generally THA, include pain, joint stiffness, and deformity causing severe functional limitation. Symptomatic coxarthrosis has been reported to occur in about 10% of patients with Paget's disease (60). Concentric or medial joint-space narrowing without prominent osteophytes are typical radiographic findings. The pattern of involvement of the hip joint varies depending on whether the pagetoid process involves the femur, the acetabulum, or both.

Intertrochanteric osteotomy has been attempted in the management of patients with paget's disease involving the hip joint (22,111,127). Roper (127) found that osteotomy performed for painful pagetoid arthrosis before the femoral head has collapsed has much the same prognosis as when performed at a similar stage of idiopathic osteoarthrosis. Other authors have also reported similar results.

Total hip arthroplasty is the procedure of choice in the presence of femoral head collapse or significant acetabular involvement. The technical aspects of THA in pagetoid bone must be approached with caution. The difficulties presented to the surgeon include sclerotic bone (which makes reaming difficult), protrusio acetabuli (which makes hip dislocation at surgery difficult), and significant varus deformity. Higher intraoperative blood loss, longer operating time, and an increased rate of heterotopic ossification have been noted in patients with Paget's disease compared to those undergoing THA for diagnoses other than Paget's disease (98). In contrast, other authors have found no increase in blood loss or operating time for THA in patients with Paget's disease (145).

Significant varus deformity of the proximal femur occurs in about one third of affected hips. This likely predisposes to varus placement of the femoral component, leading to an increased incidence of mechanical problems (60). Merkow et al. (98) reported that, of 21 THAs performed on patients with Paget's disease involving the hip, 6 femoral components were inserted in varus angulation. All six of these femora had a preoperative varus deformity. Two patients in this group developed symptomatic mechanical loosening that required loosening that required revision. McDonald and Sim (95) reported that aseptic loosening requiring revision occurred in 8 of 52 hips (15%) at an average of 8.9 years postoperatively. This rate is statistically higher than the authors' over-all experience during the same period of time in patients with diagnoses other than Paget's disease.

A higher incidence of heterotopic ossification after THA in patients with Paget's disease has been reported by several authors (95,98,145), with rates ranging from 28% to 52%. Merkow et al. (98) noted that despite a high prevalence of heterotopic ossification noted on follow-up radiographs (52%), all of these patients had a good or excellent clinical result, including range of motion. These authors recommend perioperative treatment with calcitonin (50 U three times per week for 6 months, beginning 1 to 3 months preoperatively), followed by bisphosphonate treatment for patients with Paget's disease or when a trochanteric osteotomy is planned.

There are many reports of promising early results after THA in patients with Paget's disease involving the hip (95,98,141,145). Good or excellent clinical results have been noted in 74% to 85% of patients treated with cemented THA for degenerative coxarthrosis, and THA appears to be an effective means relieving pain and restoring function in these patients. One studies on the use of porous ingrowth implants has been reported in patients with Paget's disease. Parvizi et al. (115) retrospectively reported on 19 uncemented hip arthroplasties over an average of 7 years. There were no revisions for component loosening and no recognized cases of radiographic loosening. There was radiographic bone ingrowth in all patients and Harris hip scores improved significantly. Intraoperative technical problems (varus deformity, hard sclerotic bone, and increased blood loss) were encountered as was postoperative heterotopic bone formation (6 of 19 hips). These authors concluded that the results of uncemented THA in this patient population were excellent overall with extremely low risk of implant loosening during the first decade after surgery. However, they cautioned that patients and surgeons should be aware of the potential for both increased perioperative blood loss and risk of heterotopic bone formation (115).

Treatment of Fractures in Patients with Paget's Disease of Bone

Femoral fracture is frequently the first presenting feature in Paget's disease. Fractures in pagetoid bone may heal with abundant callus and at least as rapidly as in normal bone (8). However, refracture is occasionally seen, and therefore callus is not considered a reliable sign of union. Union is most reliably assessed by a lack of mobility at the fracture site, lack of pain on weight bearing, and radiographic evidence of trabeculae crossing the fracture line. In the sclerotic phase of Paget's disease, both delayed unions and nonunions are encountered more frequently (97). The reported incidence of nonunion of femur fractures has ranged from 14% to 40% (8,15,43), with subtrochanteric and femoral neck fractures being particularly problematic.

The femur is the bone most commonly fractured in patients with Paget's disease, fractures of the proximal femur often occur as a result of trivial trauma, comparable to that which causes fractures of the femoral neck in elderly women (8,63). Grundy reported on 63 femur fractures in 48 patients with Paget's disease. In 22 patients, there was a history of increasing pain in the limb for weeks to months prior to fracture. There was a mild injury, such as a fall caused by tripping, in 35 fractures, a moderate injury in 11 fractures, and in 17 fractures, the patient denied any trauma and reported that the leg simply gave away. There were no cases of severe trauma in this series.

Multiple stress fractures at the femoral neck, resulting from very minor trauma, may cause deformity and eventually a vertical type fracture of the femoral neck (109). This predisposes the patient to developing a coxa vara deformity. The results of internal fixation for femoral neck fractures have been disappointing, with most failures attributed to soft bone (15,43). In Bradley and Nade's series, 7 of 9 patients with femoral neck fractures managed by internal fixation collapsed into varus and went on to implant failure, nonunion, and revision surgery. Thus, hemiarthroplasty has been advocated by some (43). However, others have reported unsatisfactory results after hemiarthroplasty because of the acetabular involvement in most patients with Paget's disease (8,15,109). Bradley and Nade reported that patients with femoral neck fractures managed by hemiarthroplasty subsequently showed protrusio acetabuli, which was manifest early and was rapidly progressive and disabling so that the patient became nonambulatory. As a result, THA, with a longstem femoral component, is recommended.

Barry (8) hypothesized that there was a predilection for fractures to occur in the subtrochanteric region of the femur. In his series of 70 femur fractures in 59 patients with Paget's disease, 26 occurred just below the lesser trochanteric. Other investigators have noted similar findings (15,43,63). Disappointing results have been reported in patients treated nonoperatively (43,63), as controlling the position of the fracture is difficult. Dove (43) reported that 89% treated conservatively developed a varus deformity. In Grundy's series (63), fractures with greater initial displacement were more likely to heal in varus after conservative treatment. Patients with subtrochanteric fractures are at a biomechanical disadvantage, as this is the point of maximal stress and bowing of the femur. Hence, the insertion of an intramedullary nail is technically demanding.

It is now widely accepted that fractures of the femur should be treated operatively. Options include intramedullary nailing and plate fixation. Interlocked intramedullary nails control both rotation and angulation (15,63). However, some investigators have noted technical problems with the insertion of a nail at the point of maximal bowing of the femur, and they recommended the use of a two-piece pin and plate configuration (43). Grundy advocates the use of an intramedullary nail to control angulation, noting that nail-plate is difficult because of the hardness of the bone. Bradley and Nade (15) also recommended the use of an intramedullary nail, with osteotomy to allow distal placement when necessary. They reported a high rate of implant failures using plate fixation, as the pagetoid process appears to "grow past" the end of the implant. Finally, Barlow and Thomas (5) reported the results of three patients with subtrochanteric fractures treated closed intramedullary nailing. One patient required a diaphyseal osteotomy to correct severe deformity and enable implant insertion. All fractures, including the osteotomy, united, at average of 10 weeks. There were no difficulties with proximal locking screw insertion in the presence of varus neck angulation.

Patients undergoing fractures should be taken off etidronate and placed on calcitonin until fracture healing is complete. This helps prevent the development of a nonunion, which might otherwise occur because chronic etidronate may inhibit the mineralization of newly formed fracture callus matrix. The use of newer-generation bisphosphonates during the period of fracture management in patients has not yet been assessed. Reports of the use of calcitonin in the healing of fractures in pagetic bone suggest that this hormone may promote healing by controlling resorptive activities (100).

BONE DENSITOMETRY IN THE EVALUATION OF PERIPROSTHETIC REMODELING OF BONE AFTER TOTAL HIP REPLACEMENT

Bone remodeling is an expected sequela after insertion of a femoral prosthesis, and it results in a characteristic redistribution of bone adjacent to the prosthesis. In some cases, bone loss is substantial and progressive and is characterized by extensive resorption proximally, with a gradient from proximal to distal (49,50,94). Stress shielding has been thought to be responsible for most of the changes in bone density after THA, with patterns of stress and remaining bone reduced by the implant. More recently, osteolysis associated with wear debris has been implicated in the etiology of periprosthetic bone loss.

Resorption of bone from the proximal femur is an important factor contributing to failure of both cemented and noncemented THA. Prosthetic loosening, subsidence, and fracture of the femur or the prosthesis are associated with bone loss (18,27,144). Bone mineral density, however, cannot be adequately assessed by standard radiographs. Changes in density must be greater than 30% to be observed with certainty on plain radiographs, and precision and accuracy are poor (4,157). In order to quantitatively assess progressive changes in periprosthetic bone quality as a way to determine when an unfavorable situation is developing in a prosthetic joint, a better method for evaluating bone is needed. The ability to make such accurate assessments may aid surgeons in knowing when to intervene to preserve bone stock for a revision procedure. Also, it may aid prosthesis manufacturers in their efforts to redesign and improve their implants.

DXA, the most recent development in bone densitometry, provides a noninvasive means for the quantitative assessment of bone mineral content and density of the proximal femur in vivo. Conventionally, DXA has been used for the diagnosis and monitoring metabolic bone disease, in which the primary regions of interest are the femoral neck and the lumbar spine. The use of special orthopaedic software supplied by the manufacturer identifies sites in the proximal femur with clinical relevance after THA (Fig. 35-6). This enables the determination of loss (or gain) of periprosthetic bone. Furthermore, DXA requires only a small volume of bone, and thus it is appropriate for the evaluation of an osteoporotic femoral shaft, around either a cemented or noncemented prosthesis. DXA software also allows for the measurement of bone mineral density adjacent to metal implants, and hence for the identification and analysis of regional percentage variations in bone mineral density over the length of the proximal femur (Fig. 35-7). The entire femoral component, as well as surrounding bone and soft tissue, may be included in an anteroposterior scan. Local soft tissue can be subtracted from the scan based on a standardized soft tissue "baseline." Similarly, areas of the scan in which the x-ray beams are attenuated by the implant may be subtracted from the scan results.

Furthermore, DXA provides both the accuracy and precision necessary to detect and quantify changes that occur after

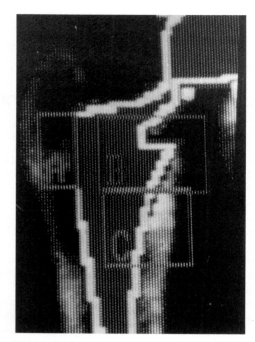

Figure 35-6 Computer-generated image of a femoral stem after scanning by DXA. The regions of interest are shown for determination of bone mineral content and density. (From Bobyn JD, Mortimer ES, Glassman AH, et al. Producing and avoiding stress shielding: laboratory and clinical observations of noncemented total hip arthroplasty. *Clin Orthop.* 1992;274:79–96, with permission.)

THA. Error attributable to nonuniform soft tissue distribution and observer bias is virtually eliminated. Kiratli et al. (83) showed that the DXA technique was accurate for determination of bone mineral content and density, with error below 1%. The precision error in vivo in this study was 2% to 4.5%, attributed mainly to variable patient position and nonhomogeneous distribution of soft tissue. In the clinical setting, patient positioning is probably the greatest variable.

It is well accepted that the initial bone stock in the femur has an important has an important influence on the extent of resorptive bone remodeling. Accordingly, some authors advocate routine preoperative analysis of bone density, with DXA, to predict the extent of bone remodeling after THA, especially for patients with poor bone stock or those at risk for osteoporosis (49). However, at the present time, the use DXA to determine which patients should be recommended for cemented versus noncemented arthroplasties has not been fully demonstrated.

After the implantation of extensively porous-coated implants, there is a concern about the adverse affects of remodeling. Several investigators have used DXA to quantitate the absorptive remodeling changes characteristic of periprosthetic bone after a cementless THA (49,82,83,96). Engh et al. (49) reported that compared to the femora obtained at autopsies of five elderly patients who had had an AML (anatomic medullary locking) prosthesis in situ for 17 to 84 months, the bone mineral content of the contralateral normal femur was 7% to 52% higher, as determined by anteroposterior DXA analysis. In addition, the periprosthetic mineral loss was greatest at the most proximal level, with a predictable gradient in

the loss of bone from proximal to distal. Kilgus et al. (82) utilized DXA to confirm earlier reports that stiffer femoral implants with more extensive porous coating produce greater stress remodeling and result in the increased occurrence of marked bone resorption (11,47,48). McGovern et al. (96) reported a strong linear correlation between area densities as determined by DXA analysis of femora with porous-coated prostheses in situ for at least 6 years and volumetric cortical densities of sectioned specimens measured by videodensitometry. This finding helps confirm the role of DXA for quantification of gross remodeling after noncemented THA.

Bone remodeling changes are most pronounced in the first 2 postoperative years, after which time bone remodeling continues, but at much slower rate. Kiratli et al., using DXA, retrospectively reported bone losses of 13% to 24% in the first 2 years after THA (84). The density of both cortical and cancellous bone adjacent to the proximal portion of extensively porous-coated implants is decreased. In partially porous-coated implants, increases in cortical bone density and thickness were observed at the junction of the proximal porous coating and the distal smooth portion (50).

Periprosthetic bone remodeling has been further studied in femora implanted with both cemented and uncemented components. Venesmaa et al. used DXA at intervals for 5 years following cemented THA in 15 patients. A reduction in BMD of 5% to 18% occurred all Gruen zones during the first 3 months following implantation. The bone loss continued in for up to six months in almost all Gruen zones. However, from 1 to 5 years, only minor changes in BMD were noted. At the end of 5 years, the mean greatest bone loss (26%) was seen in the femoral calcar region. The reduction in mean BMD was 5% in

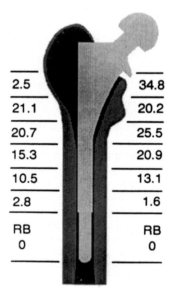

Figure 35-7 A comparison of the differences (percent decreases) in the regional bone mineral densities of the proximal femur after implantation of extensively porous-coated femoral stems with those of hips and the contralateral femur that did not undergo surgery. (From Kilgus DJ, Shimaoka EE, Tipton JS, et al. Dual-energy x-ray absorptiometry measurement of bone mineral content around porous-coated cementless femoral implants: methods and preliminary results. *J Bone Joint Surg.* 1993;75B:279–287, with permission.)

men, 16% in women. These investigators also observed that lower preoperative BMD correlated with higher postoperative bone loss. Like Kiratli et al., these authors concluded that after a phase of acute bone loss, further bone loss was minimal (155).

In a similar report published by Venesmaa et al., uncemented femora were evaluated for 3 years following implantation. Bone loss was documented in the initial 3 months following surgery. At the end of the first year, the most pronounced decrease in bone mineral density was noted in the femoral calcar (Gruen zone 7). During the second postoperative year, a slight restoration of periprosthetic bone loss was observed. During the third year, no significant changes in BMD were recorded. These authors surmised that early bone loss noted during the first 3 postoperative months was caused by limited weight bearing on the operative limb and stress shielding. The subsequent restoration of BMD may be a sign of successful osteointegration between bone and implant (156).

In conclusion, DXA provides a precise and accurate means for the evaluation of periprosthetic bone remodeling after THA. In comparison with other means of measuring and quantifying bone mineral content, such as dual photon absorptiometry, DXA provides superior resolution of images as well as better precision, with shorter scanning time and a relatively low radiation dose. Furthermore, DXA may be performed with relatively low volumes of bone, as in osteoporotic femora. DXA software also allows for the "subtraction" of surrounding soft tissue and metal implants. The literature has supported its utilization to evaluate the magnitude and rate of bone response after THA, particularly for noncemented femoral prostheses.

OSTEOLYSIS AND THE ROLE OF BISPHOSPHONATES

Bone stock following both cemented and uncemented total hip arthroplasties often undergoes resorptive remodeling in the years following implantation. This is concerning to both surgeon and patient as the end result, aseptic loosening, develops in as many as 20% of hips (134). Currently, it is accepted that wear debris generated from the artificial bearing surface initiates a macrophage-mediated inflammatory response, leading to osteoclast activation and bone resorption at the implant–bone interface (134).

Discovering a pharmacological agent capable of interrupting the cascade that leads to osteolysis, aseptic loosening, and ultimately to implant failure and revision is the goal of clinical and basic science researchers. Recent work has focused on harnessing the antiresorptive properties of bisphosphonates. This class of drugs has been successfully used to treat osteoporosis and Paget's disease. Shanbhag et al. (137), performed a trial in which 24 adult canines were randomized into three groups after undergoing a right uncemented THA. Group I was the control group. Groups II and III received a particle cocktail of ultrahigh molecular weight polyethylene (90%), titanium alloy (5%), and cobalt chrome alloy (5%). The mixture was introduced intraoperatively into the proximal femoral gap. The group III canines received 5 mg of alendronate each from postoperative day 7 until sacrifice (24 weeks). Radiographs obtained preoperatively, postoperatively, and at the time of sacrifice were evaluated for periprosthetic osteolysis. Interfacial

tissues were examined histologically and assayed for prostaglandin E_2 and interleukin 1. Periprosthetic radiolucencies with endosteal scalloping were evident in 1 of 8 of the control canines (group 1) and 6 of 7 from the debris-only canines (group II). In contrast, these radiographic abnormalities were present in only one of the 8 debris plus alendronate canines (group III). Tissue analysis indicated that macrophage population and both prostaglandin E_2 and interleukin 1 levels were elevated significantly in both experimental groups. This work suggests that continuous oral alendronate administration effectively inhibited osteolysis for the 24 week duration of the study (137). A similar study, conducted using rats and the synthetic bisphosphonate TRK-530, yielded similar results. This agent is unique in that in addition to the traditional bisphosphonatelike mechanism of action, it also has been shown to decrease the level of tumor necrosis factor alpha in the bone marrow of rats. Therefore, this TRK-530 may also inhibit the cytokine mediated inflammatory response associated with polyethylene induced osteolysis (77).

Few clinical studies have been conducted to evaluate the safety and efficacy of bisphosphonates used to prevent osteolysis in humans following THA. In a prospective randomized trial, Nehme et al. compared the outcomes of daily alendronate and calcium (20 patients) administration versus placebo (18 patients) after cemented THA. The study group was followed for two years postoperatively after the unilateral THA. Using x-ray biphotonic absorptiometry (DPX) and conventional radiographs taken at postoperative intervals, these authors reported that DPX demonstrated a significant reduction in BMD in both groups. In each group, bone loss was similar during the early postoperative period, reaching maximum loss at 3 months. After this time, a difference in periprosthetic bone remodeling was noted. In the placebo group, bone loss reached a plateau at 6 months, then BMD started to recover progressively, reaching 12.7% bone loss at 2 years. However, in the drug treatment group, there was no plateau. BMD increased continuously form the 3 months and reached 6.9% bone loss at 2 years follow-up. These investigators concluded that alendronate and calcium may preserve bone stock. Short comings included a small number of patients and a lack of long-term follow-up (107).

One recent clinical trial found that oral alendronate has little or no effect on the preservation of bone stock following THA. Rubash et al. conducted a multicenter, randomized, double-blind, placebo-controlled study of daily oral alendronate for the prevention and treatment of periprosthetic osteolysis in patients with THA and established osteolysis. One hundred twenty-three patients with THA and femoral osteolysis, as detected on plane radiographs, were enrolled at 16 centers in the United States. The study groups were given either placebo, alendronate 10 mg orally, or alendronate 35 mg orally. Duration of treatment was either 6 or 18 months. Plane radiographs were taken at baseline and months 6 and 18, which were digitized and quantitative measurements were made of the lesion area, and depth and length of the interface between the lesion and the prosthesis. The primary endpoint was the change from baseline in primary (largest) lesion area. Changes from baseline in total lesion area and total lesion–prosthesis interface length, and primary lesion depth were secondary end points. Other end points included hip pain, as measured on a visual analog scale, and radiologist's assessment of osteolysis progression. Data analysis revealed that treatment with alendronate did not appear to have an effect on quantitative osteolytic measurements. Alendronate 35 mg may have an effect on pain at 6 months. This was not seen at 18 months, nor with any of the other treatment regimens. These authors surmised that the lack of a treatment effect may be due to the lack of sensitivity of the methodology in detecting changes in osteolytic lesions or the heterogeneity in the rate of progression of osteolysis in the study patients. Techniques such as quantitative CT may be of value in future studies (129).

In summary, initial animal and human data indicates that bisphosphonates may play a useful role in preserving bone stock and avoiding revision surgery. Further studies are necessary to establish guidelines for dosage and duration of these agents following THA.

REFERENCES

1. Aloia JF, McGowan D, Erens E, et al. Hip fracture patients have generalized osteopenia with a preferential deficit in the femur. *Osteoporos Int.* 1992;2:88–93.
2. *America's Bone Health: The State of Osteoporosis and Low Bone Mass in Our Nation.* Washington, DC: National Osteoporosis Foundation; February 2002;1–55.
3. Ang G, Feiglin D, Moses AM. Symptomatic and scintigraphic improvement after intravenous pamidronate treatment of Paget's disease of bone in patients with normal serum alkaline phosphatase levels. *Endocr Pract.* 2003;9:280–283.
4. Ardran GM. Bone destruction not demonstrable by radiography. *Br J Radiol.* 1951;23:107.
5. Barlow IW, Thomas NP. Reconstruction nailing for subtrochanteric fractures in the pagetic femur. *Injury.* 1994;25:426–428.
6. Barrett-Connor E, Grady D, Sashegyi A, et al. Raloxifene and cardiovascular events in osteoporotic postmenopausal women. Four-year results from the MORE (Multiple Outcomes of Raloxifene Evaluation) randomized trial. *JAMA.* 2002;287:847–857.
7. Barrios C, Lars-Ake B, Walheim G. Healing complications after internal fixation of trochanteric hip fractures: the prognostic value of osteoporosis. *J Orthop Trauma.* 1993;7:438–442.
8. Barry HC. Fractures of the femur in Paget's disease of bone in Australia. *J Bone Joint Surg.* 1967;49A:1359–1370.
9. Bender IB. Paget's disease. *J Endocrinology.* 2003;29:720–723.
10. Bewick M, Stewart PH, Rudge C, et al. Avascular necrosis of bone in patients undergoing renal allotransplantation. *Clin Nephrol.* 1976;5:66–72.
11. Bobyn JD, Mortimer ES, Glassman AH, et al. Producing and avoiding stress shielding: laboratory and clinical observations of non-cemented total hip arthroplasty. *Clin Orthop.* 1992;274:79–96.
12. Bohr H, Schadt O. Bone mineral content of femoral bone and the lumbar spine measured in women with fracture of the femoral neck by dual photon absorptiometry. *Clin Orthop.* 1983;179:240–245.
13. Boskey AL. Noncollagenous matrix proteins and their role in mineralization. *Bone Miner.* 1989;6:111–123.
14. Bradford DS, Janes PC, Simmons RS, et al. Total hip arthroplasty in renal transplant recipients. *Clin Orthop.* 1983;181:107–113.
15. Bradley CM, Nade S. Outcome after fractures of the femur in Paget's disease. *Aust N Z J Surg.* 1992;62:39–44.
16. Brandwood CP, Hoyland JA, Hillarby MC, et al. Apoptotic gene expression in Paget's disease: a possible role for Bcl-2. *J Pathol.* 2003;201:504–512.
17. Brody JA. Prospects for an aging population. *Nature.* 1985;315:463–466.
18. Brown IW, Ring PA. Osteolytic changes in the upper femoral shaft following porous-coated hip replacement. *J Bone Joint Surg.* 1985;67B:218–221.
19. Brown JP, Hosking DJ, Ste-Marie L, et al. Risedronate, a highly effective, short-term oral treatment for Paget's disease: a dose-response study. *Calcif Tissue Int.* 1999;64:93–99.
20. Cabanela ME, Campbell DC, Henderson ED. Total hip arthroplasty: the hip. *Mayo Clin Proc.* 1979;54:559.
21. Cai Q, Hodgson SF, Kao PC, et al. Brief report: inhibition of renal phosphate transport by a tumor product in a patient with oncogenic osteomalacia. *N Engl J Med.* 1994;330:1645–1649.
22. Chambers GM, Pearson JR. Femoral osteotomy in Paget's disease affecting the hip joint. *Br J Clin Pract.* 1970;24:107.
23. Chandler HP, Reineck FT, Wixson RL, et al. Total hip replacement in patients younger than thirty years old. *J Bone Joint Surg.* 1981;63A:1426–1434.
24. Charnley J, Cupic Z. The nine and ten year results of the low friction arthroplasty of the hip. *Clin Orthop.* 1973;95:9.
25. Chestnut CH, Silverman S, Andriano K, et al. A randomized trial of nasal spray salmon calcitonin in postmenopausal women with established osteoporosis: the prevent recurrence of osteoporotic fractures study. PROOF Study Group. *Am J Med.* 2000;109:267–276.
26. Chevalley T, Rizzoli V, Nydegger D, et al. Preferential low bone mineral density of the femoral neck in patients with a recent fracture of the proximal femur. *Osteoporos Int.* 1991;1:147–154.
27. Cooke PH, Newman JH. Fractures of the femur in relation to cemented hip prostheses. *J Bone Joint Surg.* 1988;70B:386–389.
28. Cooper C, Schafheutle K, Dennison E, et al. The epidemiology of Paget's disease in Britain: is the prevalence decreasing? *J Bone Min Res.* 1999;14:192–197.
29. Cornell CN, Salvati EA, Pellicci PM. Long-term follow-up of total hip replacement in patients with osteonecrosis. *Orthop Clin North Am.* 1985;16:757–769.
30. Coventry MB, Beckenbaugh RD, Nolan DR, et al. 2012 total hip arthroplasties: a study of postoperative course and early complications. *J Bone Joint Surg.* 1974;56A:273
31. Cummings SR. Are patients with hip fractures more osteoporotic? *Am J Med.* 1985;78:487–494.
32. Cummings SR, Black DM, Nevitt MC, et al. Appendicular bone density and age predict hip fracture in women. *JAMA.* 1990;263:665–668.
33. Cummings SR, Black DM, Nevitt MC, et al. Bone density at various sites for prediction of hip fractures. *Lancet.* 1993;341:72–75.
34. Cummings SR, Black DM, Rubin SM. Lifetime risks of hip. Colles', or vertebral fracture and coronary heart disease among white postmenopausal women. *Arch Intern Med.* 1989;149:2445–2448.
35. Cummings SR, Black DM, Thompson DE, et al. Effect of alendronate on risk of fracture in women with low bone mineral density but without vertebral fractures: results from the Fracture Intervention Trial (FIT). *JAMA.* 1998;280:2077–2082.
36. Cummings SR, Kelsey JL, Nevitt MC, et al. Epidemiology of osteoporosis and osteoporotic fractures. *Epidemiol Rev.* 1985;7:178–208.
37. Cummings SR, Nevitt MC, Browner WS, et al. Risk factors for hip fracture in white women. *N Engl J Med.* 1995;332:767–773.
38. Dawson-Hughes B, Dallal GE, Krall EA, et al. A controlled trial of the effect of calcium supplementation on bone density in postmenopausal women. *N Engl J Med.* 1990;323:878–883.
39. Delmas PD, Bjarnason NH, Mitlak BH, et al. Effects of raloxifene on bone mineral density, serum cholesterol concentration, and uterine endometrium in postmenopausal women. *N Engl J Med.* 1997;337:1641–1647
40. Deo S, Gibbons MH, Emerton M, et al. AHRW Total hip replacement in renal transplant patients. *J Bone Joint Surg.* 1995;77B:299–302.
41. Devlin VJ, Einhorn TA, Gordon SL, et al. Total hip arthroplasty after renal transplantation: long-term follow-up study and assessment of metabolic bone status. *J Arthroplasty.* 1988;3:205–213.
42. Dorr LD, Taki GK, Conaty JP. Total hip arthroplasties in patients less than forty-five years old. *J Bone Joint Surg.* 1983;65A:474.
43. Dove J. Complete fractures of the femur in Paget's disease of bone. *J Bone Joint Surg.* 1980;62B:12–17.

44. Doyle T, Gunn J, Anderson G, et al. Paget's disease in New Zealand: evidence for declining prevalence. *Bone.* 2002;31:616–619.

45. Eekhoff ME, Zwinderman AH, Haverkort DM, et al. Determinants of induction and duration of remission of Paget's disease of bone after bisphosphonate (olpadronate) therapy. *Bone.* 2003;33:831–838.

46. Einhorn TA. Bone strength: the bottom line. *Calcif Tissue Int.* 1992;51:333–339.

47. Engh CA, Bobyn JD. The influence of stem size and extent of porous coating on femoral bone resorption after primary cementless hip arthroplasty. *Clin Orthop.* 1988;231:7–28.

48. Engh CA, Bobyn JD, Glassman AH. Porous-coated hip replacement: the factors governing bone ingrowth, stress shielding, and clinical results. *J Bone Joint Surg.* 1987;69B:45–55.

49. Engh CA, McGovern TE, Bobyn JD, et al. A quantitative evaluation of periprosthetic bone-remodeling after cementless total hip arthroplasty. *J Bone Joint Surg.* 1992;74A:1009–1020.

50. Engh CA, McGovern TF, Schmidt LM. Roentgenographic densitometry of bone adjacent to a femoral prosthesis. *Clin Orthop.* 1993;292:177–190.

51. Eriksson SAV, Widhe TL. Bone mass in women with hip fractures. *Acta Orthop Scand.* 1988;59:19–23.

52. Ettinger B, Black DM, Mitlak BH, et al. Reduction of vertebral fracture risk in postmenopausal women with osteoporosis treated with raloxifene. Results from a 3-year randomized clinical trial: Multiple Outcomes of Raloxifene Evaluation (MORE) investigators. *JAMA.* 1999;282:637–645.

53. Farmer ME, Harris T, Madans JH, et al. Anthropometric indicators and hip fracture: the NHANES I epidemiologic follow-up study. *J Am Geriatr Soc.* 1989;37:9–16.

54. Faulkner KG, Cummings SR, Black D, et al. Simple measurement of femoral geometry predicts hip fracture: the study of osteoporotic fractures. *J Bone Miner Res.* 1993;8:1211–1217.

55. Felson DT, Kiel DP, Anderson JJ, et al. Alcohol consumption and hip fractures: the Framingham Study. *Am J Epidemiol.* 1988;128:1102–1110.

56. Fielding JW, Cochran GV, Zickel RE. Biomechanical characteristics and surgical management of subtrochanteric fractures. *Orthop Clin North Am.* 1974;5:629–650.

57. Gallagher JC, Melton LJ, Riggs BL, et al. Epidemiology of fractures of the proximal femur in Rochester, Minnesota. *Clin Orthop.* 1980;150:163–171.

58. Genant HK, Block JE, Steiger P, et al. Advances in bone densitometry. In: Genant HK, Kanis JA, eds. *Osteoporosis Including New Diagnostic Techniques.* Washington, DC: The American Society for Bone and Mineral Research; 1989;1–15.

59. Gill SS, Einhorn TA. Bone metabolism and metabolic bone disease. In: Beaty JH, ed. *Orthopaedic Knowledge Update 6 Home Study Syllabus.* Rosemont, IL: American Academy of Orthopaedic Surgeons; 1998;149–165.

60. Graham J, Harris WH. Paget's disease involving the hip joint. *J Bone Joint Surg.* 1971;53B:650–659.

61. Greenspan SL, Myers ER, Maitland LA, et al. Trochanteric bone mineral density is associated with type of hip fracture in the elderly. *J Bone Miner Res.* 1994;9:1889–1894.

62. Grisso JA, Kelsey JL, Strom BL, et al. Risk factors for hip fracture in black women. *N Engl J Med.* 1994;330:1555–1559.

63. Grundy M. Fractures of the femur in Paget's disease of bone: their etiology and treatment. *J Bone Joint Surg.* 1970;52B:252–263.

64. Haberland M, Schilling AF, Rueger JM, et al. Brain and bone: central regulation of bone mass. A new paradigm in skeletal biology. Current Concepts Review. *J Bone Joint Surg.* 2001;83A:1871–1876.

65. Hadjipavlou A, Lander P. Paget disease of the spine. *J Bone Joint Surg.* 1991;73A:1376–1381.

66. Harris RR, Niemann KMW, Diethelm AG. Skeletal complications after renal transplantation. *South Med J.* 1974;67:1016–1019.

67. Harris ST, Watts NB, Genant HK, et al. Effects of risedronate treatment on vertebral and nonvertebral fractures in women with postmenopausal osteoporosis: a randomized controlled trial. Vertebral Efficacy with Risedronate Therapy (VERT) study group. *JAMA.* 1999;282:1344–1352.

68. Hawking KM, van den Bosch BF, Wilmink JM. Avascular necrosis of bone after renal transplantation [letter]. *N Engl J Med.* 1976;294:397.

69. Hayes WC, Myers ER, Morris JN, et al. Impact near the hip dominates fracture risk in elderly nursing home residents who fall. *Calcif Tissue Int.* 1993;52:192–198.

70. Hedley AK, Kim W Prosthetic replacement in osteonecrosis of the hip. *Instr Course Lect.* 1983;32:265–271.

71. Hordon LD, Peacock M. Osteomalacia and osteoporosis in femoral neck fracture. *Bone Miner.* 1990;11:247–259.

72. Horsman A, Nordin C, Simpson M, et al. Cortical and trabecular bone status in elderly women with femoral neck fracture. *Clin Orthop.* 1982;166:143–151.

73. Huffer WE, Kuzela D, Popovtzer MM, et al. Metabolic bone disease in chronic renal failure. II: Renal transplant patients. *Am J Pathol.* 1975;78:385–397.

74. Hui SL, Slemenda CW, Johnston CC. Baseline measurement of bone mass predicts fracture in white women. *Ann Intern Med.* 1989;111:355–361.

75. Hurley DL, Tiegs RD, Wahner HW, et al. Axial and appendicular bone mineral density in patients with long-term deficiency or excess of calcitonin. *N Engl J Med.* 1987;317:537–541.

76. Ibels LS, Alfrey AC, Huffler WE, et al. Aseptic necrosis of bone following renal transplantation: experience in 194 transplant recipients and review of the literature. *Medicine.* 1978;57:25–15.

77. Iwase M, Kim KJ, Kobayashi Y, et al. A novel bisphosphonate inhibits inflammatory bone resorption in a rat osteolysis model with continuous infusion of polyethylene particles. *J Orthop Res.* 2002;20:499–505.

78. Jenson J, Christiansen C, Rodbro P. Cigarette smoking, serum estrogens, and bone loss during hormone replacement therapy early after menopause. *N Engl J Med.* 1985;313:973–975.

79. Johnston CC Jr, Slemenda CW, Melton LJ. Clinical use of bone densitometry. *N Engl J Med.* 1991;342:1105–1109.

80. Joshua F, Epstein M, Major G. Bisphosphonate resistance in Paget's disease of bone. *Arthritis Rheum.* 2003;48:2321–2323.

81. Kelsey JL, Hoffman S. Risk factors for hip fracture. *N Engl J Med.* 1987;316:404–406.

82. Kilgus DJ, Shimaoka EE, Tipton JS, Eberle RW. Dual-energy x-ray absorptiometry measurement of bone mineral content around porous-coated cementless femoral implants: methods and preliminary results. *J Bone Joint Surg.* 1993;76B:279–287.

83. Kiratli BJ, Heiner JP, McBeath AA, et al. Determination of bone mineral density by dual x-ray absorptiometry in patient with uncemented total hip arthroplasty. *J Orthop Res.* 1992;10:836–844.

84. Kiratli BJ, Heiner JP, McKinley N, et al. Bone mineral density of the proximal femur after uncemented total hip arthroplasty. *Trans Orthop Res Soc.* 1992;17:238.

85. Krolner B, Nielsen P. Bone mineral content of the lumbar spine in osteoporotic women: cross-sectional and longitudinal studies. *Clin Sci.* 1982;62:329–336.

86. Lacey DL, Timms E, Tan HL, et al. Osteoprotegerin ligand is a cytokine that regulates osteoclast differentiation and activation. *Cell.* 1998;93:165–176.

87. Landmann J, Renner N, Gachter A, et al. Cyclosporin A and osteonecrosis of the femoral head. *J Bone Joint Surg.* 1987;69A:1226–1228.

88. Levine E, Erken EH, Price HL, et al. Osteonecrosis following renal transplantation. *AJR Am J Roentgenol.* 1977;128:985.

89. Lewinnek GE, Lewis JL, Tarr R, et al. Dislocations after total hip replacement arthroplasties. *J Bone Joint Surg.* 1978;60A:217.

90. Liberman UA, Weiss SR, Broll J, et al. Effect of oral alendronate on bone mineral density and the incidence of fractures in postmenopausal osteoporosis. *N Engl J Med.* 1995;333:1437–1443.

91. Madore GR, Sherman PJ, Lane JM. Parathyroid hormone. *JAAOS.* 2004;12:67–71.

92. Malluche HH, Smith AJ, Abreo K, et al. The use of deferoxamine in the management of aluminum accumulation in bone in patients with renal failure. *N Engl J Med.* 1984;311:140–144.

93. Mazess R, Collick B, Trempe J, et al. Performance evaluation of a dual-energy x-ray bone densitometer. *Calcif Tissue Int.* 1989;44:228–232.

94. McCarthy CK, Steinberg GG, Agren M, et al. Quantifying bone loss from the proximal femur after total hip arthroplasty. *J Bone Joint Surg.* 1991;73B:774–778.

95. McDonald DJ, Sim FH. Total hip arthroplasty in Paget's disease: a follow-up note. *J Bone Joint Surg.* 1987;69A:766–772.

96. McGovern TF, Engh CA, Zettl-Schaffer K, et al. Cortical bone density of the proximal femur following cementless total hip arthroplasty. *Clin Orthop.* 1994;306:145–154.
97. Merkow RL, Lane JM. Paget's disease of bone. *Orthop Clin North Am.* 1990;21:171–189.
98. Merkow RL, Pellicci PM, Hely DP, et al. Total hip replacement for Paget's disease of the hip. *J Bone Joint Surg.* 1984;66A:752–758.
99. Meyer HE, Tverdal A, Falch JA. Risk factors for hip fracture in middle-aged Norwegian women and men. *Am J Epidemiol.* 1993;137:1203–1211.
100. Meyers MH, Singer FR. Osteotomy for tibia vara in Paget's disease under cover of calcitonin. *J Bone Joint Surg.* 1978;60A:810–814.
101. Mills BG, Singer FR. Nuclear inclusions in Paget's disease of bone. *Science.* 1976;194:201–202.
102. Morales-Piga AA, Bachiller-Corral FJ, Abraira V, et al. Is the clinical expressiveness of Paget's disease of bone decreasing? *Bone.* 2002;30:399–403.
103. Morton DJ, Barrett-Connor EL, Edelstein SL. Thiazides and bone mineral density in elderly men and women. *Am J Epidemiol.* 1994;139:1107–1115.
104. Mosekilde L, Viidik. Correlation between the compressive strength of iliac and vertebral trabecular bone in normal individuals. *Bone.* 1985;6:291–295.
105. Murray WR. Hip problems associated with organ transplants. *Clin Orthop.* 1973;95:217.
106. Neer RM, Arnaud CD, Zanchetta JR, et al. Effect of parathyroid hormone (1-34) on fractures and bone mineral density in postmenopausal women with osteoporosis. *N Engl J Med.* 2001;344:1434–1441.
107. Nehme A, Maalouf G, Tricoire JL, et al. Effect of alendronate on periprosthetic bone loss after cemented primary total hip arthroplasty: a prospective randomized study. *Rev Chir Orthop Reparatrice Appar Mot.* 2003;89:593–599.
108. Nevitt MC, Cummings SR. Type of fall and risk of hip and wrist fractures: the study of osteoporotic fractures. *J Am Geriatr Soc.* 1993;41:1226–1234.
109. Nicholas JA, Killoran P. Fracture of the femur in patients with Paget's disease: results of treatment in twenty-three patients. *J Bone Joint Surg.* 1965;47A:450–161.
110. Nicholson OR. Total hip replacement-an evaluation of the results and techniques, 1967–1972. *Clin Orthop.* 1973;95:217.
111. Nicoll EA., Holden NT. Displacement osteotomy in the treatment of osteoarthritis of the hip. *J Bone Joint Surg.* 1961;43B:50.
112. Norman AW, Roth J, Orci L. The vitamin D endocrine system: steroid metabolism, hormone receptors and biological response. *Endocr Rev.* 1982;3:331–366.
113. Ott SM. Bone density in adolescents. *N Engl J Med.* 1991;325:1646–1647.
114. Pankovich AM. Primary internal fixation of femoral neck fractures. *Arch Surg.* 1975;110:20–26.
115. Parvizi J, Schall DM, Lewallen DG, et al. Outcome of uncemented hip arthroplasty components in patients with Paget's disease. *Clin Orthop.* 2002;403:127–134.
116. Phelps KR, Einhorn TA, Vigorita VJ, et al. Fracture healing with deferoxamine therapy in a patient with aluminum associated osteomalacia. *Trans Am Soc Artif Intern Organs.* 1986;32:198–200.
117. Phemister DB. The pathology of ununited fractures of the neck of the femur with special reference to the head. *J Bone Joint Surg.* 1939;21:681–693.
118. Pogrund H, Makin M, Robin C, et al. Osteoporosis in patients with fractures femoral neck in Jerusalem. *Clin Orthop.* 1977;124:165–172.
119. Radford PJ, Doran A, Greatorex RA, et al. Total hip replacement in the renal transplant recipient. *J Bone Joint Surg.* 1989;71B:456–459.
120. Ray NF, Chan JK, Thamer M, et al. Medical expenditures for the treatment of osteoporotic fractures in the United States in 1995: report from the National Osteoporosis Foundation. *J Bone Miner Res.* 1997;12:16–23.
121. Recker RR. Calcium absorption and achlorhydria. *N Engl J Med.* 1985;313:70–73.
122. Rendina D, Postiglione L, Vuotto P, et al. Clodronate treatment reduces serum levels of interleukin-6 soluble receptor in Paget's disease of bone. *Clin Exp Rheum.* 2002;20:359–364.
123. Reginster J, Minne HW, Sorenson H, et al. Randomized trial of the effects of risedronate on vertebral fractures in women with established postmenopausal osteoporosis: Vertebral Efficacy with Risedronate Therapy (VERT) study group. *Osteoporos Int.* 2000;11:83–91.
124. Riggs BL, Melton LJ III. Evidence for two distinct syndromes of involutional osteoporosis. *Am J Med.* 1983;75:899–901.
125. Riggs BL, Wahner HW, Seeman E, et al. Changes in bone mineral density of the proximal femur and spine with aging: differences between the postmenopausal and senile osteoporosis syndromes. *J Clin Invest.* 1982;70:716–723.
126. Riis B, Thomsen K, Christiansen C. Does calcium supplementation prevent postmenopausal bone loss? A double-blind, controlled clinical study. *N Engl J Med.* 1987;316:173–177.
127. Roper BA. Paget's disease at the hip with osteoarthrosis: results of intertrochanteric osteotomy. *J Bone Joint Surg.* 1971;53B:660–662.
128. Rossouw JE, Anderson GL, Prentice RL, et al. Risks and benefits of estrogen plus progestin in healthy postmenopausal women. Principal results from the Women's Health Initiative randomized controlled trial. *JAMA.* 2002;288:321–333.
129. Rubash H, Dorr L, Jacobs J, et al. Does alendronte inhibit the progession of periprosthetic osteolysis? Presented at: Orthopaedic Research Society Annual Meeting; 2004; San Francisco.
130. Ruff CB, Hayes WC. Subperiosteal expansion and cortical remodeling of the human femur and tibia with aging. *Science.* 1982;217:945–948.
131. Sartoris DJ, Resnick D. Current and innovative methods for noninvasive bone densitometry. *Radiol Clin North Am.* 1990;28:257–278.
132. Sartoris DJ, Resnick D. Dual-energy radiographic absorptiometry for bone densitometry: current status and perspective. *Am J Roentgenol.* 1989;152:241–246.
133. Schajowicz F, Aranjo ES, Berenstein M. Sarcoma complicating Paget's disease of bone. *J Bone Joint Surg.* 1983;65B:299–307.
134. Schwarz EM, Benz EB, Lu AP, et al. Quantitative small-animal surrogate to evaluate drug efficacy in preventing wear debris-induced osteolysis. *J Orthop Res.* 2000;18:849–855.
135. Seely DG, Browner WS, Nevitt MC, et al. Which fractures are associated with low appendicular bone mass in elderly women? *Ann Intern Med.* 1991;115:837–842.
136. Sernbo I, Johnell O. Changes in bone mass and fracture type in patients with hip fractures. *Clin Orthop.* 1989;238:139–147.
137. Shanbhag AS, Hasselman CT, Rubash HE. The John Charnley Award. Inhibition of wear debris mediated osteolysis in a canine total hip arthroplasty model. *Clin Orthop.* 1997;344:33–43.
138. Silver JJ, Majeska RJ, Einhorn TA. An update on bone cell biology. *Curr Opin Orthop.* 1994;5:50–59.
139. Sjostedt A, Zetterberg C, Hansson T, et al. Bone mineral content and fixation strength of femoral neck fractures: a cadaver study. *Acta Orthop Scand.* 1994;65:161–165.
140. Smith CB, Smith DA. Relations between age, mineral density and mechanical properties of human femoral compacta. *Acta Orthop Scand.* 1976;47:496–502.
141. Sochart DH, Porter ML. Charnley low-friction arthroplasty for Paget's disease of the hip. *J Arthroplasty.* 2000;15:210–219.
142. Sorenson JA, Hanson JA, Mazess RB. Precision and accuracy of dual energy x-ray absorptiometry. *J Bone Miner Res.* 1988;3:S126.
143. Springfield DS, Ennelking WJ. Surgery for aseptic necrosis of the femoral head. *Clin Orthop.* 1978;130:175.
144. Stauffer RN. Ten year follow-up of total hip replacement. *J Bone Joint Surg.* 1982;64A:983.
145. Stauffer RN, Sim FH. Total hip arthroplasty in Paget's disease of the hip. *J Bone Joint Surg.* 1976;58A:476–178.
146. Stewart AF. PTHrP(1-36) as a skeletal anabolic agent for the treatment of osteoporosis. *Bone.* 1996;19:303–306.
147. Stromboni M, Menguy F, Hardy P, et al. Total hip arthroplasty and femoral head osteonecrosis in renal transplant recipients. *Rev Chir Orthop Reparatrice Appar Mot.* 2002;88:467–474.
148. Theriault RL. Zoledronic acid (Zometa) use in bone disease. *Expert Rev Anticancer Ther.* 2003;3:157–166.

149. Uebelhart D, Gineyts E, Chapuy MC, et al. Urinary excretion of pyridinium crosslinks: a new marker of bone resorption in metabolic bone disease. *Bone Miner.* 1990;8:87–96.

150. Uitewaal PJ, Lips P, Netelenbos JC. An analysis of bone structure in patients with hip fracture. *Bone Miner.* 1987;3:63–73.

151. Umland EM, Boyce EG. Risedronate: a new oral bisphosphonate. *Clin Ther.* 2001;23:1409–1421.

152. Vaes G. Cellular biology and biochemical mechanism of bone resorption: a review of recent developments on the formation, activation, and mode of action of osteoclasts. *Clin Orthop.* 1988;231:239–271.

153. Vasireddy S, Talwalker A, Miller H, et al. Patterns of pain in Paget's disease of bone and their outcomes on treatment with pamidronate. *Clin Rheum.* 2003;22:376–380.

154. Vega E, Mautalen C, Gomez H, et al. Bone mineral density in patients with cervical and trochanteric fractures of the proximal femur. *Osteoporosis Int.* 1991;1:81–86.

155. Venesmaa PK, Kroger HP, Jurvelin JS, et al. Periprosthetic bone loss after cemented total hip arthroplasty: a prospective 5-year dual energy radiographic absorptiometry study of 15 patients. *Acta Orthop Scand.* 2003;74:31–36.

156. Venesmaa PK, Kroger HP, Miettinen HJ, et al. Monitoring of periprosthetic BMD after uncemented total hip arthroplasty with dual-energy X-ray absorptiometry: a 3-year follow-up study. *J Bone Min Res.* 2001;16:1056–1061.

157. Vose GP. Factors affecting the precision of radiographic densitometry of the lumbar spine and femoral neck. In: Whedon GD, Neuman WE Jenkins DW, eds. *Progress in Development of Methods in Bone Densitometry.* Washington, DC: NASA; 1966;47–63.

158. Vose GP, Lockwood RM. Femoral neck fracturing-its relationship to radiographic bone density. *J Gerontol.* 1965;20:300–305.

159. Wasnich RD, Benfante RJ, Yano K, et al. Thiazide effect on the mineral content of bone. *N Engl J Med.* 1983;309:344–347.

160. Woo RYG. Morrey BE. Dislocations and recurrent subluxations following total hip arthroplasty. *Orthop Trans.* 1981;5:436.

161. Zhang ZL, Meng XW, Xing XP, et al. Prospective study of pamidronate disodium in treatment of Paget's disease of bone. *Zhon Yi Xue Za Zhi.* 2003;83:1653–1656.

Primary Tumors and Tumorlike Conditions of the Hip

36

Erik N. Zeegen　　*Philip Z. Wirganowicz*　　*Francis P. Cyran*　　*Jeffrey J. Eckardt*

The hip is a common location for primary bone tumors and tumorlike conditions. Lesions around the hip joint may produce symptoms such as groin pain, buttock pain, or even referred pain to the knee and prompt patients to seek medical attention. However, some lesions may be clinically silent and only discovered incidentally or after a patient sustains a pathologic fracture. It is important for the hip surgeon to have a familiarity with the presenting features, differential diagnosis, and treatment options for benign bone tumors, tumorlike conditions of bone, and various malignant bone tumors.

The diagnostic workup of bone tumors requires a systematic approach comprising a thorough history and physical exam, comprehensive imaging studies, and, in select situations, biopsy of the lesion in question. Biopsies should only be performed by the surgeon who will be performing the definitive surgical treatment of the lesion. Mankin et al. showed that improper biopsies of sarcomas by nonorthopedic oncologists can result in significant complications and potentially adversely affect the oncologic and functional outcome for the patient (42). It is critical early on in the diagnostic process to determine if the tumor in question is benign or malignant, as this will determine the type of treatment necessary. In general, most benign bone tumors may be treated with a curettage and bone grafting, and malignant bone tumors should be treated with a wide resection. The goals of treatment of malignant bone tumors are first and foremost to achieve a wide resection in order to minimize the risk of local recurrence—which, if it occurs, often portends a fatal outcome—and secondarily to preserve the function of the affected extremity.

In the 1960s and 1970s, amputation was the principle surgical technique used in treating malignant bone tumors. However, over the last 30 years, there have been substantial advances made in the treatment of bone and soft-tissue sarcomas. Specifically, there have been such vast improvements in chemotherapeutic regimens, radiation treatments, imaging modalities, reconstructive materials, and surgical techniques that limb-sparing surgery is now the mainstay of surgical treatment for malignant bone tumors and has been shown to be as safe as amputation in terms of oncologic outcome (14,59,67).

Patients who are told there may be a tumor around their hip, whether it is benign or malignant, often become filled with anxiety about the potential loss of limb and/or life. It is important for the hip surgeon to be familiar with the more common benign and malignant bone tumors that occur around this joint so that a prompt diagnosis may be made and an appropriate and effective treatment method planned and executed.

DIAGNOSIS

An accurate diagnosis of bone tumors involves a thorough history and physical, various imaging modalities, and, in certain situations, biopsy of the lesion in question.

History

The most common presenting complaints in patients with bone tumors include pain and a noticeable mass. Often there is a history of trauma to the area, and often patients believe the trauma caused the mass. While this may be true in select cases, more often than not the trauma merely brought the mass to the patient's attention and was already there well before the traumatic event. Sometimes, the lesion is noted as an incidental finding on plain radiographs or on physical exam. It is important to obtain a detailed history in regards to the nature of the pain. Pain that occurs at rest and pain that awakens the patient at night certainly are more worrisome for a malignant process than pain that is only activity related. There are also certain pain patterns that should be looked for. For instance, pain at night that is relieved by aspirin or nonsteroidal anti-inflammatory medications is quite typical for an osteoid osteoma. Aside from the diagnostic entity, the pain characteristics may shed light on the integrity of the bone. For example, in patients with known radiolucent lesions around the hip, groin pain with weight-bearing activities should raise concern for an impending pathologic fracture.

If the patient has a mass, it is important to ascertain as much about the mass as possible. How long the mass has been noticeable, has it increased in size, and if so, over what period of time? Is it soft or hard? Does it hurt? A rapidly growing, firm, painful, large mass is more suggestive of an aggressive, perhaps malignant, process than a slow-growing, soft, nonpainful, smaller mass. A mass that goes up and down in size throughout the course of a day may represent a hemangioma.

Constitutional symptoms should also be sought by the physician. Fatigue, decreased appetite, and weight loss raise concerns that a malignant process may be present. While fevers and chills suggest an infection, patients with Ewing sarcoma also often present with fevers, in addition to an elevated WBC count and sedimentation rate.

The patient's past medical history should also be reviewed, and any past carcinoma, sarcoma, or benign bone or soft-tissue history with potential malignant degeneration risks should be noted. For instance, a patient who has been having groin pain with weight bearing and has a history of lung cancer is likely to have a metastatic lung carcinoma lesion around the hip. If the patient is suspected of having a metastatic carcinoma lesion, it is crucial to know the tissue of origin, as certain tumors, such as renal cell and to a lesser degree thyroid carcinoma, tend to be hypervascular and should be embolized prior to any surgical intervention. Patients who have a prior history of a soft-tissue sarcoma, who received radiation to the area, and who now have pain are of concern. If there was significant periosteal stripping at the time of surgery to achieve wide margins, pain after a couple of years may be indicative of an impending pathologic fracture. If it has been 10 to 20 years since the radiation and the patient has new pain and a mass, a radiation-induced sarcoma should be ruled out. Patients who have a known history of multiple enchondromatosis or hereditary multiple osteochondromatosis and who have a new onset of pain at rest or at night should be worked up for a possible chondrosarcoma. Similarly, patients who have a history of neurofibromatosis and have an enlarging, painful soft-tissue mass should be evaluated further to rule out the possibility of a malignant peripheral nerve sheath tumor.

Physical Exam

Although the physical exam may not always be revealing, it certainly is critical in the diagnostic workup. A thorough exam can often pick up subtle findings that may be missed with a short, cursory exam focused just on the hip. The examiner should assess the patient's vital signs, noting particularly whether or not there is a fever. The examiner should also record the blood pressure, heart rate, respiratory rate, and patient's weight as a baseline, especially if the patient will be having surgery. The examiner should inspect the patient's skin, noting any café au lait spots, including the pattern of any spot. Spots with jagged, irregular borders that have a "Coast of Maine" appearance are seen in patients with McCune-Albright syndrome, whereas a smoother border with a "Coast of California" appearance is found in patients with neurofibromatosis. A complete exam should be performed, including the eyes, ears, nose, and throat; neck; lungs; heart; and abdomen. Metastatic disease may manifest with symptoms in any one of these locations, and therefore a thorough exam is crucial. A rectal exam should also be performed, and any palpable masses in the rectum, ischiorectal fossa, or prostate in male patients should be noted.

A complete musculoskeletal exam should also be carried out. Malignant primary bone tumors and metastatic carcinomas may spread to bones, and therefore the axial and appendicular skeletal system should be examined, and any masses, areas of tenderness, or limits in range of motion should be noted. A thorough neurological exam should be performed to uncover any focal deficits in the cranial or peripheral nerve distributions. Upper motor neuron lesions should also be looked for, as these may indicate an area of central nervous tumor involvement.

The hip should be examined last. The examiner should observe the patient's gait, noting the gait pattern and looking for signs of abductor weakness and/or antalgia. The examiner should assess leg lengths with the patient in the standing position, noting whether the pelvis is level. With the patient in the supine position, the examiner should inspect the hip, noting any masses or areas of fullness or adenopathy in the inguinal region. The examiner should assess the overlying skin, noting any prior incisions, areas of prior irradiation, or ulcerations. The examiner should then assess the hip motion, noting the flexion, external and internal rotation, abduction, adduction, and extension, as well as any flexion contractures. Pain at the extremes of motion may reflect an intra-articular process. Because deep tumors around the hip joint can extend along the pelvis and thigh, the examiner should palpate the iliac crest and buttock, noting any areas of tenderness or fullness. Furthermore, because they are adjacent joints to the hip, the knee and sacroiliac joints should also be examined.

Imaging

There are several imaging modalities used today to characterize a tumor around the hip joint. These include plain radiographs, computed tomography (CT) scans, magnetic resonance imaging (MRI) scans, technetium-99 bone scans, ultrasound, angiography, and even positron emission tomography (PET) scans. Plain radiographs remain the most informative, cost-effective, and readily obtainable studies. The plain x-ray is particularly useful for assessing bony abnormalities but sometimes may show soft-tissue masses, especially ones that have undergone some degree of mineralization.

A careful examination of the x-ray can reveal a significant amount of information about the lesion in question, and the clinician should be able to formulate a fairly accurate and concise differential diagnosis. Each tumor has specific characteristics that can be delineated on a plain x-ray. For instance, the location of the tumor within the bone is quite revealing. Certain tumors occur within the epiphysis, metaphysis, or diaphysis. For example, chondroblastomas are epiphyseal, osteosarcomas metaphyseal, and Ewing sarcoma diaphyseal. Furthermore, some tumors are cortically based (osteoid osteomas), surface based (osteochondromas), centrally located within the intramedullary space (enchondromas), or eccentrically located in the intramedullary space (giant cell tumors). Radiographic evaluation and characterization of bone tumors has been described extensively by Enneking et al. (18) using four parameters that are helpful in coming up with a differential diagnosis.

1. *Where is the lesion located within the bone?* (That is, is it epiphyseal, metaphyseal, diaphyseal, surface based, cortically based, intramedullary, etc.)
2. *What is the lesion doing to the bone?* (Large destructive lesions with irregular borders, cortical disruption, and associated soft-tissue masses are generally malignant, whereas small lesions confined to the bone are generally benign.)
3. *How is the host bone responding to the lesion?* (In fast-growing, aggressive malignant tumors, the bone cannot keep pace with the tumor to react to it, and therefore the lesion has a permeative or moth-eaten border appearance. In contrast, in slow-growing, benign tumors, the host bone has a chance to react to the tumor and form a well-defined sclerotic rim around the lesion.)
4. *What is the periosteal reaction to the lesion?* (The periosteal reaction can be used as an indicator of the tumor's aggressiveness. Tumors that break through the cortex may do so with the periosteum intact. In slow-growing lesions, the periosteum sleeve remains intact and is able to keep pace with the tumor and form new periosteal bone on top of the expanding tumor. This creates the appearance of a Codman's triangle, a lamellated periosteal reaction. This is most commonly seen in osteosarcomas. An "onion skin" pattern is often seen in diaphyseal regions, such as with Ewing sarcoma. In fast-growing tumors that expand rapidly beyond the periosteal sleeve's capacity to keep up, a "sunburst" pattern may be seen.)

Other features on plain radiographs that are helpful in diagnosing the tumor are the internal characteristics of the lesion. For instance, cartilage tumors have a mineralization pattern with well-defined punctuate densities that form arcs and rings. Bone-forming tumors, on the other hand, have osteoid mineralization that is more amorphous or "cloudlike." Bone cysts, intraosseous lipomas, and giant cell tumors tend to have no significant mineralization within the lesion. Finally, fibrous dysplasia has a typical "ground glass" appearance.

If the etiology of the tumor remains unclear on the plain radiographs, cross-sectional imaging such as MRI and/or CT scanning may be helpful. MRI scans are helpful in characterizing the osseous extent of the tumor, identifying any associated soft-tissue masses, and characterizing the internal characteristics of the lesion. For instance, the presence of fluid-fluid levels is highly suggestive of an aneurysmal bone cyst component. Bright signal on T1 sequences is suggestive of a fatty lesion. Bright signal on T2 sequences suggests water content and is often be associated with cartilage lesions. Furthermore, MRI scans can help assess the relationship of the tumor to key neurovascular structures to help with preoperative planning.

CT scans are best used to evaluate the overall bony architecture and also cortical integrity to assess for impending pathologic fractures. Furthermore, in cartilage lesions, CT scans are ideal for evaluating the endosteal surface to look for endosteal scalloping, which can be associated with chondrosarcomas. Finally, CT scans are helpful in determining the relationship of mineralized soft-tissue lesions to the underlying bone. For instance, CT scans are quite useful in delineating osteochondromas, parosteal osteosarcomas, and myositis ossificans. For instance, on the CT scan, osteochondromas will demonstrate a confluency of the intramedullary contents of the underlying bone into the exostosis. Parosteal osteosarcomas will tend to have a "pasted on" appearance, most often behind the knee. Finally, areas of myositis ossificans will have a clear separation of soft tissue between itself and the underlying bone, and the pattern of mineralization of the lesion will demonstrate an area of radiolucency surrounded by peripheral mineralization. CT scans are also essential for monitoring the chest, abdomen, and pelvis for metastatic disease. The lung is the most common site of metastatic disease for most sarcomas. The retroperitoneal space is a common site of metastatic disease for some liposarcomas.

Additional imaging modalities include ultrasound, angiography, and radionuclide scanning. Ultrasound is often used to quickly determine if a mass is solid or fluid filled and occasionally is used as image guidance for needle biopsy. Angiography is most helpful in assessing the anatomic relationship of major vascular structures to large tumors, particularly for preoperative planning. Furthermore, in highly vascular lesions such as renal cell carcinoma metastases, angiography can be used to assess the vascularity and then embolize the lesion so that blood loss may be minimized during excision. Finally, radionuclide scanning (e.g., technetium-99 whole-body bone scanning) is useful for surveying the entire skeletal system for potential sites of other lesions that may not be clinically apparent. PET is another type of scanning that has been used lately to survey the body for potential sites of soft-tissue nodal sites of disease. There are some centers now using this modality in patients with soft-tissue sarcomas, such as synovial, epithelioid, and clear cell sarcomas, for staging purposes as well as for surveillance following treatment (31). PET scanning cannot accurately distinguish benign versus malignant tumors (19,31), but some studies have shown that it can demonstrate tumor responsiveness to treatment therapy (71). It has also been used in some studies to follow the clinical responsiveness of osteosarcomas and has been combined with MRI to differentiate posttherapy tumor changes from residual tumor and to even look for potential sites of recurrence (6,7).

Biopsy

Biopsies are indicated in cases of suspected malignant tumors, certain aggressive benign tumors, and lesions that cannot be determined using imaging studies alone. There are certain lesions that have classic radiographic appearances—such as those of nonossifying fibromas and osteochondromas—that may make biopsy unnecessary unless the patient is having significant pain associated with the lesion or the diagnosis is questioned. Biopsies may be performed in an open or closed fashion. Closed biopsies include fine needle aspirates (FNA) and core needle biopsies. Open biopsies may be excisional or incisional.

Before considering biopsy techniques, it is important to understand the biology of tumors and the classification of margins in relationship to this biology. Sarcomas grow centrifugally (away from the center), with the most immature portion of the tumor at its periphery; the center is the most mature portion and is often necrotic. At the interface between the expanding tumor and normal surrounding tissue is a reactive zone with some satellite tumor cells, neovascular tissue, and inflammatory tissue. There may or may not be a well-defined capsule surrounding the reactive zone and tumor. Based on this tumor biology, a classification of resections has been developed. An *intralesional* resection cuts through tumor and leaves gross or microscopic tumor behind. A *marginal* resection removes the tumor, but cuts through the reactive tissue and likely leaves behind microscopic tumor satellite lesions in the reactive zone. A *wide* resection removes the entire tumor and reactive zone with a normal cuff of tissue all the way around both and has little chance of leaving behind microscopic disease. A *radical* resection removes the entire muscle compartment that contains the tumor. A hip disarticulation and a hemipelvectomy are examples of radical resections for malignant tumors around the hip.

There are several biopsy techniques. The least invasive biopsy is a needle biopsy. This can be done under direct vision for large, obvious soft-tissue lesions or with the aid of CT guidance for bone lesions with an associated soft-tissue mass extension. If a bone lesion has a surrounding cortex completely intact, needle biopsy is not feasible. The advantage of a needle biopsy is that it can be done under local anesthetic and does not require an open surgical procedure, thereby avoiding many of the complications associated with open biopsy, such as tumor spread, wound healing problems, and bleeding. The diagnostic accuracy of needle biopsy has been shown to be 70% to 80% (15,28,68,72,74). Despite these logistical advantages, this technique has a lower rate of accuracy than open biopsy, mainly because of the small sample size obtained. Possible outcomes of a needle biopsy are lack of diagnosis, indeterminate diagnosis, and even potential error in the diagnosis of the lesion or of the histological grade. The surgeon must have a reasonable idea of what the diagnosis will be prior to the biopsy. If the biopsy results are nondiagnostic or the pathology seems discordant with the presumed diagnosis, an open biopsy should be performed. The management of patients who, after core needle biopsy, have a diagnosis of a bone or soft-tissue tumor is best carried out by an experienced musculoskeletal oncologist working in close collaboration with an experienced musculoskeletal pathologist. Placement of the needle track should be carefully planned and discussed by the surgeon and the radiologist prior to the biopsy because this track needs to be excised at the time of the definitive excision.

Excisional biopsies are reserved for lesions that are known to be low-grade benign lesions that have a low propensity for local recurrence or metastasis. Excisional biopsies are acceptable for lipomas, osteochondromas (provided the perichondrial sleeve and cartilage cap are excised as well), unicameral bone cysts, and nonossifying fibromas. If the nature of the tumor is unclear, the biopsy should be incisional, and several key principles should be kept in mind. First, the biopsy track will be considered contaminated with tumor once the biopsy has been performed. Therefore, the biopsy track and overlying skin incision must be excised with the tumor itself at the time of definitive resection. With that in mind, the placement of the biopsy incision and the approach to the tumor are critical. The incision should be kept as small as possible and be longitudinal along the lines of extensile exposure. Transverse incisions should be avoided, as these may require such wide biopsy track excision as to make limb-sparing surgery impossible. The biopsy track should be the shortest distance to the tumor but should not violate more than one compartment to get to it. Furthermore, normal neurovascular intervals used in hip surgery should be avoided to prevent contamination of neurovascular structures. Rather than developing planes between muscles, a single muscle should be incised to get directly to the tumor for sampling. Meticulous hemostasis is emphasized to minimize the risk of hematoma and thus tumor spread and contamination. Use of thrombin-soaked Gelfoam or methylmethacrylate plugs for bone windows should be used to minimize postoperative bleeding. Drains may be used but should be brought out of the skin in line with the incision close to the end of the incision. If sutured into place, the sutures should be kept close to the drain, and large "throws" of the needle should be avoided. When sampling the tumor, the periphery of the tumor, which is the most viable and thus the most representative portion, should be biopsied. The tissue should be sent for frozen section to ensure that there is adequate tissue for diagnosis. The tissue should also be sent for culture (aerobic, anaerobic, fungal, and mycobacterial).

If the lesion is within the bone and the cortex is completely intact, a cortical window must be made to sample the lesion. The window should be oblong in shape, and sharp corner edges must be avoided to minimize stress risers in the bone and thereby lessen the risk of pathologic fracture (10). Following the biopsy, the limb should be protected from full weight bearing, as the bone has been structurally compromised by the tumor and the cortical window. Use a large angled curette to remove tumor from within the bone cavity. It is often helpful to obtain an intraoperative radiograph with the curette in the lesion to confirm and document that the curette is in the correct location.

Staging

The stage of a tumor is based on the tumor's histological grade, the local involvement of the tumor, and whether or not the tumor has spread to other anatomic sites such as the lungs. Although a staging system is predominantly based on the local characteristics of the tumor, its main purpose is to predict the development of metastases. Staging does not, however, predict the risk of local recurrence. Risk factors for tumor local recurrence include inadequate surgical margins, less than 90% tumor necrosis in high-grade tumors after preoperative chemotherapy, and patients who already have a local recurrence at the time of presentation. There are several staging classifications, but the most commonly used and widely accepted for musculoskeletal tumors is the Enneking system, which is used by the Musculoskeletal Tumor Society. This system provides standardized descriptions of tumors so that surgeons may communicate with one another or with medical oncologists or radiation oncologists in an efficient and standardized manner. It also provides prognostic information that can help guide necessary treatment. Furthermore, a standardized staging system allows for critical analysis and comparison of tumors in large cohorts of patients and thus permits evaluation of the effects of chemotherapy, radiation, and/or surgical treatment.

The histologic grade of a tumor indicates the "aggressiveness" of the tumor and the risk of metastatic disease. The grade is assessed by the pathologist based on the histologic features of the tumor (nuclear atypia, pleomorphism, mitotic activity) and how well differentiated the tumor is relative to the tissue of origin. The grading scale is from 1 to 3. Low-grade tumors (grade 1) have less than a 15% risk of metastatic spread whereas high-grade tumors (grades 2 and 3) have greater than a 15% risk of metastatic spread.

The local extent of the tumor is categorized according to whether the tumor is confined to the compartment of origin or extends beyond it into another compartment. For bone sarcomas, the tumor is designated intracompartmental (an A lesion) if it is still within the confines of the bone, and it is designated extracompartmental (a B lesion) if it extends beyond the confines of the cortex and out into the soft tissues. Large tumor size has also been correlated with metastatic potential but is not currently used as a criterion for staging bone sarcomas.

Low-grade lesions are thus referred to as stage I lesions, and high-grade lesions are referred to as stage II lesions. Each stage can be subdivided into A or B, depending on the anatomic extent of the tumor, as described above. All tumors with metastatic lesions are considered stage III tumors irrespective of the tumor grade. A high-grade osteosarcoma of the proximal femur with a large soft-tissue mass coming out of the bone would be classified as a stage IIB lesion.

Benign bone tumors are classified in a similar fashion, using Arabic rather than Roman numerals for the stage. In terms of histologic grading, all benign tumors are considered to be grade 0. Stage 1 tumors are *latent* tumors with no propensity for enlargement or spread outside their site of origin, such as an enchondroma or osteochondroma after skeletal maturity. Some stage 1 tumors may heal spontaneously, such as an involuting, nonossifying fibroma or a simple bone cyst. Stage 2 tumors are *active* lesions that continue to grow, expand, and even deform the bone but remain within the confines of the bone. Examples include aneurysmal bone cysts and osteoblastomas. Stage 3 tumors are *aggressive* lesions that grow and extend beyond the confines of the bone and have a high chance of local recurrence if not adequately treated. A classic example of a stage 3 benign tumor is a giant cell tumor that has eroded through the cortex and has an associated soft-tissue mass.

TREATMENT

Not all bone tumors require surgery. Lesions that have a classically benign appearance and are asymptomatic and not at risk

for pathologic fracture may be observed closely with serial imaging studies. A nonossifying fibroma of the distal tibia is an example of such a tumor that usually is found incidentally, causes no symptoms, and often involutes in early adulthood. If observation is chosen, serial imaging studies should be obtained on a frequent and regular basis so that secondary malignant degeneration or an increase in the size and/or cortical involvement of the lesion can be picked up sooner rather than later. Most benign tumors are treated with an intralesional curettage and packing of the cavity with either bone graft (autogenous or allogenic) or methylmethacrylate. Malignant tumors generally require wide resection, which can be achieved with either amputation or limb salvage surgery.

Surgical Considerations for Benign Bone Tumors

Most stage 1 and 2 benign tumors can be adequately treated with intralesional curettage and filling of the defect with either bone graft (autogenous or allogenic) or methylmethacrylate Osteochondromas may be removed with a marginal excision so long as the cartilage cap and perichondrial sleeve are removed. Stage 3 lesions may be treated with intralesional curettage, but local adjuvant therapy such as phenol cauterization or liquid nitrogen cryotherapy should be used as well to extend the margin of tumor excision beyond the curettage. Phenol is usually applied to the borders of the curettage cavity and will extend the zone of necrosis on the order of millimeters. Liquid nitrogen, on the other hand, extends the zone of necrosis on the order of a centimeter beyond the curettage cavity. Not only can the cryotherapy result in injury to adjacent neurovascular structures and articular cartilage, but the freezing can also increase the risk for pathologic fracture. No matter which local adjuvant is used, the defect should be packed with polymethylmethacrylate, as this provides an immediately stable construct. Furthermore, the heat of polymerization also extends the zone of necrosis beyond the curettage. Finally, local recurrences (indicated by a radiolucent line) are easier to visualize on plain radiographs around a cement packing than an area of bone graft. Because of the high stresses placed on the proximal femur, lesions that have been curetted and packed with bone graft or bone cement should be prophylactically stabilized with either a hip screw and side plate or intramedullary device to prevent pathologic fracture. In cases of extensive bone loss or local recurrence, en bloc resection should be performed, and the joint reconstructed with either an endoprosthesis or osteoarticular allograft.

Surgical Considerations for Malignant Bone Tumors

In the early 1970s, malignant bone tumors were treated with amputation alone. The 5-year disease-free survival was only 15% to 20% for patients with osteosarcomas and 5% to 10% for those with Ewing sarcoma. Today, with neoadjuvant chemotherapy, radiation, sophisticated imaging modalities, and improved surgical resection and reconstructive techniques, most patients are able to undergo limb preservation surgery and maintain a functional extremity and expect a 60% to 70% 5-year survival (3,16,17,20,23,38,47,50,54–56,73).

Multiple studies have shown no difference in patient survival between limb salvage and amputation (16,21,32,66,70).

Around the hip joint, resections of the proximal femur can be reconstructed with a metallic endoprosthesis, an osteoarticular allograft, or a combination thereof known as an alloprosthetic composite (APC). Each technique has its own unique set of advantages and disadvantages.

Osteoarticular allografts were used frequently in the 1970s. They have the unique advantage of achieving a "biologic" reconstruction, sparing the uninvolved portion of the joint and restoring bone stock. Disadvantages include inability to bear weight (it can take a year, sometimes longer, for the allograft–host junction to heal), fracture, nonunion, infection (including the theoretical use of infectious disease transmission), joint instability, and arthritic degeneration. In one of the largest series of allografts, there was a 19% fracture rate, 17% nonunion rate, 11% infection rate, and 6% rate of joint instability (41). Most of these complications occurred during the first 3 years after implantation. It is in this early period—during which the allograft is at high risk for failure—that many patients with malignant tumors are still undergoing chemotherapy and radiation. Some patients may not even survive beyond this time. Patients for whom osteoarticular allografts are used should therefore be carefully selected to minimize the risk of these complications. If the osteoarticular allograft does last beyond this critical early period, it may develop arthritic changes that subsequently require a resurfacing arthroplasty. In the series published by Mankin, 16% of the osteoarticular allografts went on to require a resurfacing joint arthroplasty (41).

Allografts may be combined with metallic endoprostheses to create what is known as an alloprosthetic composite (APC). This composite reconstruction has certain advantages over allografts alone and metal endoprostheses alone. In contrast to osteoarticular allografts, the metal and polyethylene do not collapse or have arthritis develop and rarely fracture. The allograft portion of the composite restores bone stock and retains soft-tissue attachments for the insertion of muscle tendons, which is more difficult to achieve using an endoprosthesis alone. Although this type of reconstruction often results in a good or excellent functional outcome, the surgical procedure is more complex and technically challenging than those for either an osteoarticular allograft or an endoprosthesis alone.

The use of endoprostheses also has evolved during the last 25 years. The current model includes modular segments, forged stems, a kinematic rotating hinge for constructs around the knee, a circumferential porous coating around the prosthesis at the bone–prosthesis junction, and loopholes for critical soft-tissue attachments (a rotator cuff, hip abductors, or an extensor mechanism). The advantages of the current modular metallic endoprosthesis include availability, intraoperative flexibility to fill the surgical defect, and immediate structural stability to allow for immediate weight bearing. This form of reconstruction has also been shown to result in excellent hip function with long-term durability (29,30,39,53,59,60). However, this type of reconstruction has its own unique complications, including loosening, fatigue fracture, dislocation, dissociation of the modular components, and infection.

The initial endoprostheses were custom made on a case-by-case need. During the time that the endoprosthesis was being manufactured, the patient was given chemotherapy prior to surgery, and it was discovered that patient survival was dramatically improved. Because of this, neoadjuvant chemotherapy is now given to patients with high-grade spindle cell sarcomas such as osteosarcoma and some high-grade chondrosarcomas. Chemotherapy is also an integral part of the treatment of small, round cell tumors such as Ewing sarcoma, non-Hodgkin lymphoma, PNET, and rhabdomyosarcoma. Chemotherapy is aimed at reducing the tumor size locally as well as attacking microscopic metastatic disease. Radiation may also help reduce the tumor size in the local area so that limb-sparing surgery may be achieved.

The significant advances in adjuvant treatments such as chemotherapy and irradiation made over the last 20 to 30 years have resulted in increased numbers of patients who are long-term disease-free survivors, have kept their extremity, and have come to expect a high level of function in the extremity. Despite these higher expectations, the orthopedic oncologist must keep in mind that the primary goal is to achieve local control in order to save the patient's life. Consequently, the risk of local recurrence should not be greater with limb salvage surgery than with amputation, nor should long-term survival be compromised to maintain function of the extremity. Local recurrence is usually associated with a fatal outcome, and therefore limb-sparing surgery should not be considered if wide margins cannot be achieved.

Even though limb-sparing surgery has become the rule rather than the exception, there are several contraindications (some relative and some absolute) that must be closely adhered to. Neurovascular involvement is perhaps the most significant. If a major nerve, such as the sciatic nerve, is involved with the tumor and must be resected to achieve a wide margin, salvage of an extremity with an insensate foot with no motor function is not reasonable. There are some lesser nerves (e.g., the peroneal nerve), however, that can be resected with the tumor to achieve wide margins and still maintain a functional limb with the assistance of braces or tendon transfers. Involved major vessels may be resected with the tumor and then reconstructed with a vein graft or synthetic graft. Pathologic fracture may preclude limb salvage surgery, as the fracture hematoma spreads tumor cells along tissue planes, making wide resection difficult. This has previously been considered an absolute contraindication to limb-sparing surgery. However, there have been several studies showing that in select cases in which the tumor responds favorably to chemotherapy and the entire fracture hematoma can be widely excised, limb-sparing surgery had no increased risk for local recurrence or fatal outcome than amputation (2,64,65). Inadequate soft-tissue coverage may sometimes preclude limb salvage. If the tumor resection results in a large soft-tissue defect, muscle flaps and skin grafts may be necessary to cover the defect. However, in the setting of prior irradiation, the flap and/or skin graft may not heal well and may make limb salvage difficult. An improper biopsy incision may also preclude limb-sparing surgery. Because the biopsy track must be excised at the time of definitive surgery, if the biopsy has been performed through an improper orientation (e.g., transverse), it will be difficult to excise the tumor and biopsy track and still have a viable soft-tissue envelope for subsequent reconstruction. Furthermore, if the biopsy track violated more than one muscle compartment, limb salvage will be extremely difficult to achieve in that gaining wide margins would be nearly impossible without performing an amputation.

Technical Aspects of Surgery for Benign Lesions

In select situations (e.g., synovial osteochondromatosis), the patient should be placed in the supine position to utilize the anterior Smith-Peterson approach. However, the majority of lesions of the hip can be approached with the patient in the lateral position. In this position, the tissue planes are more easily defined, as gravity allows the muscle tissue to fall away from the planes of dissection. For this approach, the incision should be centered over the vastus ridge and then extend proximally, heading anteriorly toward the anterior superior iliac spine. The avascular plane between the abductors and the sartorius is utilized to gain access to the anterior hip capsule. The capsule is then opened, and the anterior aspect of the femoral neck may be identified. A cortical window may be made with a high-speed burr. It must be big enough to accommodate a large angled curette to remove the lesion. The window should be ovoid and have rounded edges to minimize stress risers. The lesion must be adequately curetted out to normal appearing bone. Local adjuvants such as phenol or liquid nitrogen should be used as indicated (such as for giant cell tumors) to extend the zone of necrosis beyond the curettage. The lesion will need to be packed with allograft or polymethylmethacrylate, depending on the age of the patient and tumor type. However, the packing should be done after any fixation is introduced into the hip. Because of the high stresses placed on the hip, a hip screw and side plate should be routinely placed for prophylactic internal fixation when the lesion involves the femoral neck and/or intertrochanteric region. The iliotibial band is split, and the vastus lateralis is elevated off the posterior intermuscular septum and then "L'd" at the vastus ridge. When elevating the vastus musculature off the posterior septum, the perforating artery branches should be identified and ligated to minimize blood loss. Transection of these vessels can result in significant bleeding, as the cut vessels retract deep into the posterior compartment and are difficult to find for coagulating or tying off to achieve hemostasis. If methylmethacrylate is used for packing, intraoperative x-rays should be obtained to verify that no cement extrusion into the joint has occurred.

Technical Aspects of Surgery for Malignant Lesions

As with benign lesions, most malignant tumors around the hip may be approached with the patient in the lateral decubitus position. Unlike conventional total hip arthroplasty surgery, however, the approach for a proximal femoral resection is dependent on the location, size, and extent of the tumor. Furthermore, the tumor may significantly distort the normal anatomy and displace key structures away from their normal location. For instance, tumors of the proximal femur with large posterior soft-tissue components may displace the sciatic nerve anteriorly and laterally so that the nerve is much more vulnerable to injury during the superficial dissection. Each approach, therefore, is slightly different and must be well planned preoperatively. The key to a successful limb salvage surgery for tumors around the hip is having a key understanding of the location and extent of the tumor, and having a thorough knowledge of the surrounding anatomy, and, perhaps most importantly, being creative in how to navigate through the soft-tissue planes, all the while keeping in mind what will be needed for the subsequent soft-tissue reconstruction after the tumor has been resected.

There are several key structures around the hip that must be kept in mind when planning and executing a limb salvage procedure. The greater trochanter and abductor muscles are the "centerpiece" of the dissection, as most exposures are either posterior or anterior to these structures. If possible, the greater trochanter and attached abductor muscles should be preserved for possible later reattachment to the implant with either cerclage wires or with a cable grip system. The acetabular labrum should also be preserved, as it helps with stability of the bipolar component. Key neurovascular structures include the sciatic nerve and femoral artery, vein, and nerve. The sciatic nerve must be identified in the retrogluteal region and mobilized away from the tumor and protected during the resection. The superficial femoral artery and vein should be identified anteriorly just medial and deep to the sartorius. The superficial vessels should be protected, but the profunda vessels can be ligated as needed just distal to their takeoff from the common femoral vessels. If the superficial vessels need to be taken with the tumor, the artery may be reconstructed by a vascular surgeon with either with a vein graft or synthetic graft.

The typical exposure begins with a long lateral incision distal to the greater trochanter, which then is extended anteriorly from the greater trochanter up toward the anterior superior iliac spine. Anterior and posterior skin flaps are created to improve visualization. Electrocautery should be used to optimize hemostasis and minimize the risk of tumor spread. Proximal to the greater trochanter, the exposure is anterior to the abductor musculature. The superficial dissection is carried down between the sartorius and tensor fascia lata. If the superficial vessels need to be mobilized, the dissection must proceed medial and deep to the sartorius. The deep dissection is carried down between the rectus femoris and the gluteus medius. The iliopsoas is detached from the lesser trochanter. At the greater trochanter, depending on the extent of the tumor within the proximal femur, the abductors may taken off the greater trochanter, keeping the abductors in continuity with the vastus lateralis as one soft-tissue sleeve, or a trochanteric osteotomy may be performed just distal to the trochanteric ridge, thereby keeping the abductors attached to the greater trochanter. Distal to the greater trochanter, the dissection is posteriorly based. The short external rotators, quadratus femoris, and gluteus maximus tendon are detached from the posterior femur, thereby opening up the retrogluteal space. The sciatic nerve can then be exposed and mobilized so it can be protected. After the anterior and posterior dissections have been completed, the hip capsule should be exposed circumferentially and can then be opened up so that the femoral head may be dislocated. The acetabular labrum should be preserved if a bipolar hemiarthroplasty is going to be used.

At this point, the level of the femoral osteotomy is determined. Based on preoperative imaging, the distance from a fixed anatomic landmark, such as the greater or lesser trochanter, to a point 3 to 4 cm below the distal-most extent of the tumor as seen on preoperative MRI studies is determined. Prior to making the osteotomy, the distance from the patient's femoral head to the osteotomy should be measured so that this distance may be reestablished with the endoprosthesis. The osteotomy is made with a either an oscillating saw or a Gigli saw. The specimen is passed off to the back table. The intramedullary contents of the distal osteotomy segment are curetted and sent for frozen section to confirm that there is no tumor present. Once this margin is confirmed to be negative, the intramedullary canal is prepared for the endoprosthetic stem with reamers. The stem should be 2 mm less than the last reamer used in order to allow for a 2-mm cement mantle. The patient's femoral head is measured with a caliper to determine the bipolar shell outer diameter. The acetabulum may then be trialed to determine the optimal bipolar shell outer diameter. A trial reduction is performed with the modular pieces put together. The hip should have a supple range of motion and be stable anteriorly and posteriorly. Leg lengths should be equal, and there should not be undue tension on the sciatic nerve. The real components are then assembled and cemented into place using modern third-generation cementing technique.

The wound is closed over large suction drains to prevent the accumulation of a hematoma or seroma. The drains should be sutured into place at the skin so that they are not accidentally removed by the patient or medical personnel, and they should be left in place until the output is less than 30 cc per day. The patient should be kept at bed rest in balanced suspension for 10 to 14 days before mobilization is initiated. Once the patient is allowed to mobilize, an abduction brace should be worn for 8 weeks to protect the abductor mechanism. A pseudocapsule eventually forms around the prosthesis, attaching to the circumferential porous coating. The abductor musculature scars down onto this pseudocapsule, thereby allowing for functional abduction of the hip. Once this process has completed, most patients achieve excellent abduction strength and can walk without an abductor limp. Total hip precautions must be followed indefinitely to minimize the risk of dislocation.

For lesions of the proximal femur that extend into the hip joint or for lesions of the pelvis, an internal hemipelvectomy may be performed. This entails removal of the entire innominate bone as well as the head and neck of the femur. The femoral nerve and vessels and sciatic nerve must be preserved in order to maintain a functional lower extremity. Following this resection, there is a significant defect that may be left alone or reconstructed with either an endoprosthesis or allograft prosthetic composite. In our experience, patients in whom no reconstruction has been performed do remarkably well. The femur will migrate proximally into the pelvis and eventually form a fibrous pseudarthrosis, leaving the patient with a significant leg-length discrepancy. With a properly fitted shoe lift, the patient may ambulate. Most patients require the use of a cane or other ambulatory assist device, but some walk quite well without any such assistance.

BENIGN TUMORS

Osteoid Osteoma

This lesion is one of the benign bone-forming lesions. It is a small, round lesion that has a central osteoblastic mass, known as the "nidus," surrounded by a radiolucent zone, which is then surrounded by an outer sclerotic rim. This pattern gives

this lesion a "bull's-eye" appearance on radiographs. Although it is histologically identical to an osteoblastoma, an osteoid osteoma is by definition less than 1.5 cm, thereby distinguishing it from an osteoblastoma. The classic presentation includes pain at night that is relieved with nonsteroidal anti-inflammatory medications (NSAIDs). It typically occurs in patients between the ages of 10 and 25. The lesion is usually cortically based and most commonly occurs around the proximal femur, often in the medial calcar region. While the lesion is often not able to be visualized on plain films, the cortical-thickening response to the lesion can often be seen (Fig. 36-1). Tc-99m bone scans and/or CT scans are often necessary to identify the lesion. The lesion is usually best seen on CT scans, which are almost always required for making the diagnosis and planning surgical treatment (if this treatment option is chosen). On CT scanning, the lesion appears as a central lucent nidus with a surrounding sclerotic rim of bone (Fig. 36-2).

Initial treatment includes nonsteroidal anti-inflammatory medications. It is believed that the tumor produces prostaglandins that tend to increase at night and thereby elicit the night pain. The NSAID of choice should have a long enough half-life (i.e., 8–12 hours) to relieve the night pain and let the patient sleep through the night. However, it is not uncommon for patients to present with a history of taking NSAIDS for up to 1 to 2 years without relief. On occasion, the lesion may "burn out" or spontaneously resolve.

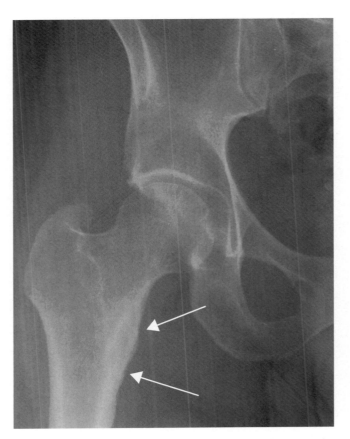

Figure 36-1 Radiograph of an osteoid osteoma lesion in the right proximal femur (*arrows*). The lesion is characterized by a cortical thickening with a sclerotic border and lytic central nidus, giving a bull's-eye appearance.

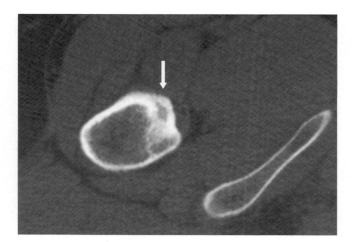

Figure 36-2 CT scan of the lesion shown in Figure 36-1. The lesion is cortically based, and the surrounding sclerosis and the central nidus are well visualized (*arrow*).

However, most patients cannot tolerate the pain and taking NSAIDS for a long period of time, and surgical intervention is then recommended. In order to successfully excise this small lesion, it is imperative that the surgeon know its exact location prior to and during surgery. This requires utilizing identifiable landmarks such as the greater or lesser trochanters to reference from in order to localize the lesion intraoperatively. The distance from these landmarks to the lesion can be measured on the preoperative CT scan, and this can then be used intraoperatively to localize the lesion. Often, the overlying cortex is thickened, which helps identify the area. The lesion should be opened up with a high-speed burr, and then the nidus may be excised with the use of large angled curettes. Grossly, the nidus has a reddish appearance and may be soft or hard, depending on how mature the lesion is. If the lesion involves a high-stress area in the proximal femur, following excision the hip should be prophylactically stabilized with internal fixation. A dynamic hip screw is the recommended implant, as it is easy to use and offers excellent stability. If the lesion is located in the medial calcar, it is best approached from the anterior aspect of the hip. The patient is positioned laterally. The incision starts distal to the vastus ridge in line with the femur and extends proximally to the greater trochanter and then gently curves anteriorly toward the anterior superior iliac spine. The iliotibial band and fascia lata are incised. The tensor fascia lata muscle is split in line with its fibers and is elevated off the underlying gluteus medius, and the tensor fascia lata is then retracted anteriorly. The gluteus medius is retracted posteriorly, and the avascular plane between these two muscles is developed down to the anterior hip capsule, which is opened in order to expose the anterior and medial cortex. The lesion can then be excised by making a cortical window. The vastus lateralis is then elevated off the lateral aspect of the femur in a subperiosteal fashion from posterior to anterior so that the side plate of the dynamic hip screw may be applied directly to the femur.

Over the past several years, several institutions have treated this lesion successfully with CT-guided percutaneous radiofrequency ablation. As initially described by Rosenthal et al., the lesion is localized under CT guidance, and then a radiofrequency probe is percutaneously inserted into the lesion under CT guidance and heated to 90°C for 6 minutes. This is typically performed under general or spinal anesthesia and is done in an outpatient setting. In their most recent report on 263 patients, Rosenthal et al. reported a 91% success rate at a minimum of 2 years follow-up when the procedure was performed as the initial treatment. For recurrent lesions, the procedure had the significantly lower success rate of 60% (57). This method has been compared to operative treatment, and there was no difference in the rates of recurrence between these two treatment methods (58). As this less invasive treatment method has become popular for treating osteoid osteomas, its use has also been extended to the treatment of other benign bone tumors and tumorlike conditions as well as some difficult-to-access malignant tumors.

Osteoblastoma

This is another bone-forming benign tumor. It is similar to an osteoid osteoma, except it is generally larger in size, typically between 2 and 6 cm in diameter. Unlike osteoid osteomas, the classic history of night pain relieved by anti-inflammatories is not present with osteoblastomas. The pain is often deep and aching, and if located around the hip joint, it will often cause a limp. If the tumor has compromised the cortical integrity of the proximal femur, activity-related pain may be present. On occasion, these lesions may weaken the surrounding cortex and result in pathologic fracture.

Radiographically, the lesion has a mixed lytic and blastic appearance, with a central ossified region surrounded by a lucent halo, which in turn is surrounded by a sclerotic rim. The reactive outer sclerotic rim is not as distinct as with osteoid osteomas. The lesion may expand the bone and is often associated with internal mineralizations. Secondary aneurysmal bone cysts occur among osteoblastomas 15% of the time and may cause more bone expansion than an osteoblastoma by itself. CT scans are often necessary to determine the extent of the lesion and to assess the amount of cortical involvement (if any). On MRI, there is often a significant amount of surrounding edema, which makes it sometimes difficult to distinguish this benign condition from a malignant one. These lesions most commonly occur in the metaphysis but on occasion may extend into the epiphysis. They are rarely diaphyseal. They may also occur in the spine, mostly in the posterior elements.

Treatment of these lesions around the hip requires extensive intralesional curettage through a cortical window using a high-speed burr to remove the entire lesion and get out into normal surrounding bone. Therefore, local adjuvants such as phenol, hydrogen peroxide, or liquid nitrogen should be used to extend the zone of tumor necrosis beyond the curettage. The resulting defect may then be packed with bone graft. Lesions in the proximal femur are in an area of high stress and should be prophylactically stabilized with internal fixation following curettage and bone grafting. Following intralesional curettage, the local recurrence rate is about 10% to 20%. If a recurrence occurs, the diagnosis of a sclerosing osteosarcoma should be considered, as it is sometimes difficult to distinguish (histologically and radiographically) an aggressive osteoblastoma from a low-grade osteosarcoma.

Osteochondroma

This is the most common benign tumor of bone, comprising approximately one-third of all benign bone tumors and one-tenth of all bone tumors. This lesion is a cartilage-capped bone projection on the external surface of the bone. It develops from an aberrant focus of growth cartilage. By definition, the intramedullary contents of the underlying bone are contiguous with the bony projection of the lesion (Fig. 36-3). The cartilage cap, made up of hyaline cartilage, is the source of growth, which occurs via enchondral ossification. Because it follows a pattern of enchondral ossification, the lesion continues to enlarge until the end of skeletal growth, at which point it tends to involute or become ossified. The thickness of the cap varies with the age of the patient. Skeletally immature patients have a very thick and active cap, whereas skeletally mature patients have a thin cap that in some cases is completely ossified. The cap is best visualized on MRI scans.

The most common age at presentation is in the second decade of life. Because many lesions remain asymptomatic, the exact incidence and age of presentation may not be accurately determined. The most common presenting symptom is a painful bony lump adjacent to a large joint. Pain is often a result of inflammation of an overlying bursa or tendon. If prominent enough, the lump can be quite tender if even just bumped against a hard object. Because osteochondromas often occur in adolescents, another common presenting complaint is the uncosmetic appearance of the prominence. Other issues related to osteochondromas are joint deformity (particularly around the elbow, wrist, and ankle), limited range of motion, and neurovascular impingement. Around the hip, osteochondromas may result in an inability to fully extend the hip or may present with sciatica-type symptoms.

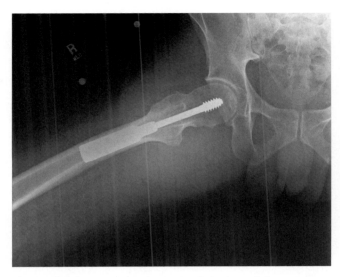

Figure 36-4   Lateral radiograph of the hip of the patient in Figure 36-3 following excision of the osteochondroma and prophylactic fixation with a dynamic hip screw.

Osteochondromas typically occur at the ends of bones in the metaphyseal region and grow away from the adjacent joint. They may be pedunculated or sessile based and may occur as a single lesion or multiple lesions. Hereditary multiple osteochondromas is an autosomal dominant condition with varying degrees of penetrance. Malignant degeneration is approximately 1% in single osteochondromas. In patients with multiple lesions, however, the risk of malignant degeneration varies from 10% to 30%. When malignant degeneration occurs, the lesion is most often a secondary low-grade chondrosarcoma, although on rare occasions a high-grade dedifferentiated chondrosarcoma may develop. Signs of malignant degeneration include a change in symptoms (e.g., pain in a lesion that had been previously asymptomatic), change in the size of the lesion after skeletal maturity, and an enlarging cartilage cap or a cap that measures more than 2 cm in thickness at the time of presentation in a skeletally mature patient.

Most osteochondromas may be treated nonoperatively. If the lesion is an incidental finding and is painless and has a cartilage cap less than 2 cm, it may be observed with serial exams and radiographs. If the lesion is symptomatic or has features concerning for malignancy, it should be excised. For lesions excised around the proximal femur, prophylactic internal fixation should be performed to prevent pathologic fracture after the mass has been excised and the cortex left disrupted (Fig. 36-4). On occasion, a previously asymptomatic pedunculated osteochondroma may fracture through the stalk and become painful. In this situation, the lesion may be excised and the stalk burred down to a smooth surface on the bone.

Enchondroma

This is a benign intramedullary cartilage lesion that is often an incidental finding discovered on a radiograph taken when the patient complains of hip pain. The hand is the most common location, and less than 10% of all enchondromas occur around

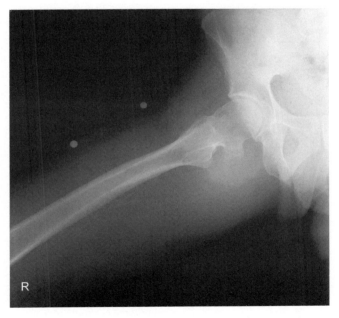

Figure 36-3   Lateral radiograph of right hip demonstrating an osteochondroma arising from the posterior femoral neck. The lesion was causing mechanical symptoms in the patient's hip joint.

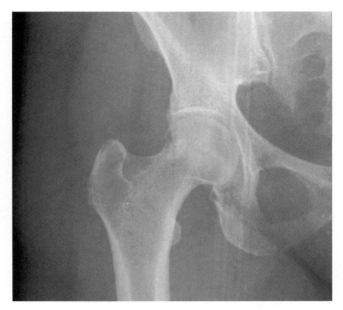

Figure 36-5   Radiograph of the hip showing an enchondroma of the femoral neck. The lesion has stippled calcifications. There is no endosteal scalloping, cortical thinning, or bony expansion, which supports the diagnosis of a benign chondroid lesion.

the hip joint. Enchondromas may occur as a single lesion or as multiple lesions in Ollier's disease (multiple enchondromas) or Maffucci's disease (multiple enchondromas with soft-tissue hemangiomas). The risk of malignant transformation for a single enchondroma is less than 1%. However, in the setting of multiple enchondromas, the risk of malignant transformation can be as high as 25% in Ollier's disease and even up to or greater than 50% in Maffucci's disease.

Plain radiographs and computed tomography (CT) are usually the two best imaging modalities to determine the chondroid nature of the lesion. Typically, the enchondroma is seen on plain films as an intramedullary lesion with a zone of radiolucency filled with chondroid matrix that is classically described as "popcorn calcifications" (Fig. 36-5). It usually does not expand the bone, nor does it cause endosteal scalloping or cortical thinning (features more consistent with chondrosarcomas). In short tubular bones (such as the phalanges), there may be some bony expansion and cortical thinning, and often the patient presents with a pathologic fracture through the lesion. MRI may help in delineating the extent of the tumor. Furthermore, the lesion is typically dark on T1 sequences and bright on T2 sequences due to the water content of the cartilage of the tumor. Almost all enchondromas display increased tracer uptake on bone scans.

Enchondromas are typically not painful. Painful lesions without evidence of fracture should be highly suspect for malignant transformation. Chondroid lesions that show bony expansion and/or endosteal scalloping should also be suspected for malignant degeneration. The CT scan is the imaging study of choice for assessing the relationship of the tumor and the surrounding bone, looking for signs of malignant transformation such as cortical thinning and endosteal scalloping, and assessing the cortical integrity and risk of pathologic fracture (Fig. 36-6).

If the lesion is felt to be a classic enchondroma, neither biopsy nor surgery is indicated. The lesion should be followed with serial radiographs to make sure the lesion is not changing. At the time of initial presentation, a CT scan should be obtained as a baseline study. If there are any changes noted over time on the radiographs, or if the patient becomes symptomatic, a repeat CT scan may be obtained for comparative analysis. If the lesion is going to be openly biopsied, it is quite difficult on frozen section for even the most experienced pathologist to differentiate a highly cellular benign enchondroma from a low-grade chondrosarcoma. Furthermore, there is often tumor heterogeneity, and there may be sampling error at the time of biopsy, which could lead to a false-negative biopsy. Nonetheless, the surgeon should have a good idea of the nature of the lesion preoperatively so that the appropriate surgical treatment may be planned in advance. For instance, if there is a question of malignancy preoperatively, the surgeon should treat the lesion with aggressive curettage, extend the margins with a high-speed burr, and add a local adjuvant such as phenol or hydrogen peroxide or else perform a wide resection.

Giant Cell Tumor of Bone

This tumor is considered to be one of the more aggressive benign lesions of bone. Although of unknown etiology, it is named after the multinucleated giant cell seen in this lesion, while the basic cell type of this tumor is the spindle-shaped stromal cell. The giant cells, like osteoclasts, are a result of fusion of proliferating mononuclear cells. In fact, older literature referred to this tumor as an osteoclastoma because of this histologic appearance. Many other lesions, both benign and malignant, have a giant cell component, leading to potential

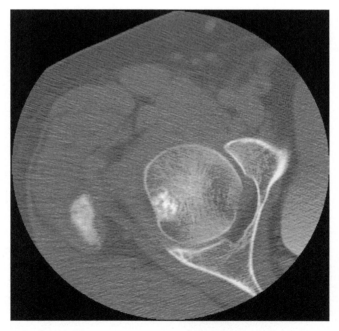

Figure 36-6   CT scan of the enchondroma in Figure 36-5, showing the stippled calcifications and a well-defined border. There are no features of endosteal scalloping, cortical thinning, or bony expansion.

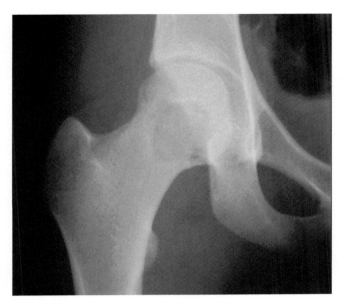

Figure 36-7 Radiograph of a patient with a lytic lesion of the femoral head and neck. The lesion has ill-defined margins and has no internal matrix. This lesion was initially felt to be a benign bone cyst, but the final pathology proved it to be a giant cell tumor.

diagnostic confusion. Eighty percent of giant cell tumors occur in persons over the age 20 years, and the peak incidence occurs in the third decade of life. Most giant cell tumors are eccentrically located epiphyseal lesions that abut the subchondral cartilage. Radiographically, they are lytic tumors with a poorly demarcated margin adjacent to normal bone (Fig. 36-7).

Approximately 10% of giant cell tumors occur about the region of the hip. Common symptoms include pain or limited range of motion. A palpable soft-tissue mass is infrequent, although soft-tissue extension of the tumor still contained by periosteum is a common feature.

Treatment consists of an aggressive curettage followed by adjuvant therapy with either cryosurgery or phenol cauterization, filling of the defect (either with methylmethacrylate or bone graft), and prophylactic internal fixation for lesions around the proximal femur (Fig. 36-8). Lesions about the acetabulum and pelvis may be treated in a similar fashion, although on occasion resection or irradiation may be indicated (61). Prior to the use of adjuvant therapy, the rate of local recurrence of giant cell tumors of bone was approximately 50% (9,11,24). Phenol is a benzylic alcohol that is a surface-acting agent causing chemical cauterization. It kills tumor cells that are contained within the bone interstices and remain after curettage. Marcove et al. introduced the use of liquid nitrogen in the treatment of giant cell tumors (44). They carefully poured liquid nitrogen into the cavity created by the curettage, which extended the area of necrosis up to 2 cm beyond the border of the cavity. This very effectively caused tumor necrosis; however, necrosis of the adjacent normal bone may lead to either pathologic fracture or delayed healing of bone graft if used to fill the defect (40). The zone of necrosis can be reduced to a few millimeters by the use of a liquid nitrogen spray. Because both phenol and surface-applied liquid nitrogen have a limited zone of necrosis, it must be emphasized that the use of adjuvants is not a substitute for

adequate and complete curettage. The curettage must extend to the level of normal-appearing bone, and then the adjuvants should be used. The combination of aggressive curettage and use of adjuvant therapy has reduced the rate of local recurrence for giant cell tumors to less than 5% in primary tumors treated by orthopedic oncologists (1,8,22). The remaining bone defect usually needs to be filled with either bone graft or methylmethacrylate. Bone graft has the advantage of being a biologic reconstruction; however, the limb needs to be protected from full weight bearing until there is complete incorporation of the graft. In contrast, the use of bone cement allows for early weight bearing, and the heat produced by cement polymerization has the added benefit of additional tumor kill by thermal necrosis (36). Bone cement has the theoretical disadvantage of having less long-term durability and reducing the amount of shock absorption if placed in a subchondral location. Irradiation has been used in the treatment of giant cell tumors, but its use is now reserved for lesions that are considered to be unresectable.

A CT scan of the affected area should be obtained soon after treatment as a baseline for evaluating for recurrent tumor. The median time for recurrence is 16 to 18 months,

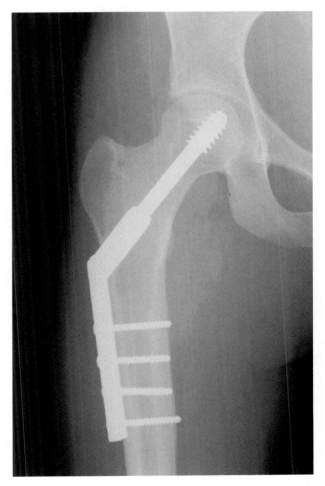

Figure 36-8 Radiograph of same patient in Figure 36-7 with a local recurrence of a giant cell tumor 1 year after curettage, prophylactic internal fixation, and allograft packing of what was initially thought to be a benign bone cyst.

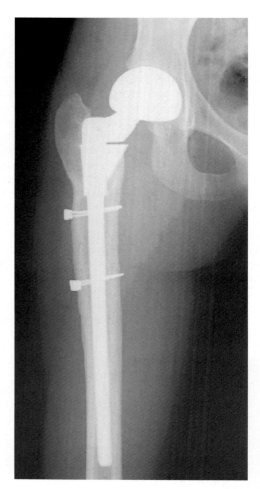

Figure 36-9 Radiograph of same patient in Figures 36-7 and 36-8 following resection of femoral head and neck and reconstruction with a modular, uncemented bipolar hemiarthroplasty.

although recurrence may occur many decades after primary treatment. Local recurrence may be associated with malignant degeneration, especially if irradiation was used previously. Giant cell tumors of bone are capable of metastasis, primarily to the lung, or of implantation into soft tissues at the time of surgery. Care must be taken at the time of the primary surgery to prevent tumor from spilling into the soft tissues. Chest radiographs or lung CT scans should be obtained at regular intervals to assess for metastatic disease.

Chondroblastoma

Chondroblastomas are rare tumors that have radiographic and histologic similarities to giant cell tumors of bone. The basic stromal cell of a chondroblastoma appears similar to a giant cell tumor; however, a chondroid matrix is produced by these cells, which distinguishes this tumor as a distinct entity. The lesion is most common in the second decade of life. Chondroblastomas are epiphyseal lesions, and they may occur in areas of secondary ossification such as the greater trochanter of the hip (Fig. 36-10). They are lytic lesions that may extend to the subarticular surface. They may be sharply delineated from the surrounding normal bone by a thin rim

of reactive sclerosis. Thin, septated trabeculations may be seen. The lesions most commonly present with pain caused by impending or frank pathologic fracture. There may be referred pain in the area of the knee when the chondroblastoma affects the hip region.

For those lesions that occur about the hip, chondroblastomas have a predilection for the triradiate cartilage. Nearly 25% of all chondroblastomas occur about the region of the hip, and approximately 50% of these occur in the region of the triradiate cartilage.

Treatment consists of thorough curettage, bone grafting, and internal stabilization, as indicated. In cases where the lesion has destroyed much of the articular surface, excision and joint reconstruction may be necessary (Fig. 36-11). This lesion is less aggressive than a giant cell tumor, and recurrence is rare with proper treatment. There have been cases of soft-tissue implantation that occurred at the time of original surgery, so care must be taken to prevent tumor spillage. In addition, there have been cases reported of metastasis to the lungs. As a result, regular clinical follow-up is necessary to determine any local or distant recurrence.

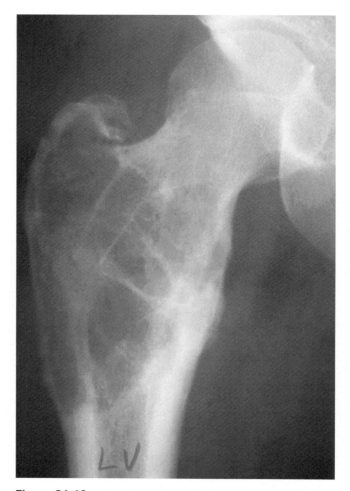

Figure 36-10 AP radiograph of right hip demonstrating a large chondroblastoma involving the greater trochanter and peritrochanteric region. It is a lytic lesion containing thin septations and is usually epiphyseal in location but may be located in areas of secondary ossification, as in this case.

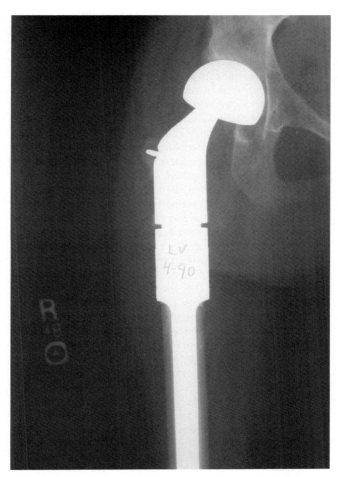

Figure 36-11 Radiograph of the patient in Figure 36-10, whose femur required resection and reconstruction with a proximal femur endoprosthesis.

Eosinophilic Granuloma

This lesion is characterized by the presence of Langerhans histiocytic cells and not eosinophils, as the name suggests. Histiocytosis X (Langerhans cell histiocytosis) is the generalized name for this lesion, which consists of three clinical syndromes of varying severity (37). Eosinophilic granuloma may be unifocal or polyostotic, and it is the most benign of these lesions. Hand–Schüller–Christian disease and Letterer–Siwe disease are more severe variants of histiocytosis X (the latter being usually fatal at an early age as a result of acute, widespread dissemination of the histiocytic cells). Pain is the usual presenting complaint, and there is occasionally a palpable mass. Most lesions are radiographically lytic and well demarcated without a sclerotic border. They tend to be diaphyseal lesions, but they are also common in the ilium. This location may lead to focal collapse of the hip about the acetabulum, leading to a leg-length discrepancy and early degenerative changes. Clinically, the lesion may be mistaken for a chronic bone abscess or osteomyelitis as a result of the presence of a necrotic center at the time of surgery, and histologically it may appear as an abscess because of the presence of eosinophilic clusters. These lesions are most commonly noted in the first and second decades of life, although no treatment may have

been instituted until adulthood. There is a decreased incidence with each successive decade of life.

Treatment is instituted according to severity and necessity (5,25). The lesions may heal spontaneously or, in some cases, following the injection of methylprednisolone acetate. In areas of impending pathologic fracture, curettage, bone grafting, and internal fixation may be needed. Irradiation in low doses has been found to be curative; however, because of the risk of treatment-associated sarcoma in later life, irradiation is usually reserved for lesions that are inaccessible to injection or are difficult to approach surgically. If there has been collapse of the acetabulum leading to a lack of congruency of the hip joint, then total hip arthroplasty may be necessary.

Synovial Osteochondromatosis

Synovial (osteo)chondromatosis is a rare condition of cartilaginous metaplasia of the subsynovial connective tissue. Multiple cartilaginous loose bodies are formed within the joint when the pedunculated metaplastic foci become detached. Although the knee is the most common location, other large joints, including the hip, may be affected. Patients may present with joint swelling and pain, mechanical symptoms such as locking and giving way, or a sensation of loose bodies within the joint. It is most common in middle age (40 to 60 years) (46). Radiographically, multiple small intra-articular opacities with some calcification are seen. There may be a joint effusion or a soft-tissue mass in association with this condition.

Treatment is directed toward complete removal of the affected synovium with a total synovectomy. In cases of limited areas of synovial involvement, this can be performed arthroscopically; however, in most cases, including those involving the hip, this excision should be performed by an open synovectomy. If degenerative changes are seen within the joint, then a total hip arthroplasty can be performed. In rare cases, synovial chondromatosis can cause other problems, including hip joint subluxation (27) and secondary degeneration to a chondrosarcoma (26,51).

Pigmented Villonodular Synovitis

Pigmented villonodular synovitis (PVNS) is a rare condition of unclear etiology. In this condition, the joint synovium is thickened and hypertrophied in a neoplastic type of proliferation. There is an abundance of hemosiderin deposition in the tissue, which produces the pigmentation. The disease is mostly monoarticular, and the hip is the second most common location after the knee. The disease presents with a limp, which may be associated with pain. Overall range of motion is usually spared, although there may be pain at the extremes of motion. A routine work-up of these patients fails to reveal any evidence of trauma, infection, or inflammatory arthritis as the source of the symptoms. Joint fluid is typically hemosiderin stained (brownish), with cell count and glucose, protein, and immunoglobulin levels within normal range. Radiographically, the joint with PVNS shows some degree of joint-space narrowing, although it is not as severely affected as in degenerative arthritis. More specifically, PVNS is characterized by cyst formation on both sides of the joint articulation with subchondral sclerosis. The cystic changes bordered by sclerosis are out of proportion to the degree of joint-space narrowing compared to osteoarthritis. The disease presents at a younger age (third and fourth decades) than osteoarthritis. Two forms of PVNS exist, nodular and diffuse (33,69). The diffuse form, which affects the entire joint synovium, is found in approximately 90% of affected individuals. The nodular form is limited to a portion of the synovium.

Histologically, there is a hyperplasia of the synovial cells, which creates a villus type of appearance. The cells frequently contain hemosiderin staining. Histiocytes and giant cells are seen frequently, and mitotic figures are common. Inflammatory cells are scarce.

Treatment consists of a complete synovectomy in the diffuse form, although this is difficult to perform around the hip and leads to frequent recurrence (12). In addition, because the disease presents with signs of joint degeneration, total hip arthroplasty is frequently recommended as treatment (63). The nodular form is much more easily treated by excision of the affected tissue. Excision of the nodule is usually curative. Some authors have recommended intra-articular brachytherapy using radioactive isotopes (49). We have limited experience with this form of treatment, and in general we do not recommend its use for lesions about the hip.

MALIGNANT TUMORS

Osteosarcoma

Osteosarcomas are the most common primary sarcoma of bone. Only multiple myeloma occurs with greater frequency as a primary malignancy in bone. Osteosarcomas are spindle cell neoplasms that produce osteoid. As a result, although a tumor

may have a predominance of other elements, such as chondroid or fibromatoid tissue, the presence of osteoid identifies the lesions as an osteosarcoma. Because of the histologic variability, osteosarcomas are differentiated into chondroid, fibromatoid, and osteoid subtypes, according to the predominant cellular subtype. Peak incidence is in the late teens and early adulthood. Osteosarcomas usually present with pain or a palpable mass of variable duration. Radiographically, osteosarcomas are lytic, metaphyseal lesions that may be permeative. There may be areas of osteoblastic activity (Fig. 36-12). These lesions break through the overlying cortex and extend into the soft tissues. As they do so, there is periosteal elevation, which causes the classic Codman triangle. In cases of rapid tumor growth, the soft-tissue extension may show areas of bone spicules that are perpendicular to the shaft. Most osteosarcomas present as stage IIB lesions (i.e., high-grade, extracompartmental tumors). However, it is estimated that approximately 10% to 20% of patients with conventional high-grade osteosarcoma will have radiographic evidence of metastatic disease at diagnosis (MSTS stage III). Prior to the advent of modern chemotherapeutic regimens, there was a 15% to 20% 5-year survival rate for osteosarcomas treated with amputation. Currently, long-term survival is over 50% for all patients presenting with an osteosarcoma at treating institutions specializing in orthopedic oncology. In those patients who are without known metastatic disease (stage III) at the time of presentation, the long-term survival rate is over 75%. The most common location for osteosarcomas is about the knee, with the proximal femur and pelvis the second most common location.

Classically, osteosarcomas are considered to originate from central medullary lesions; however, some osteosarcomas may arise from the bone surface, such periosteal and parosteal osteosarcomas. These osteosarcoma variants tend to be less

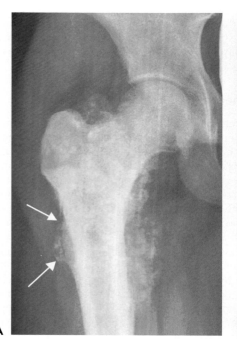
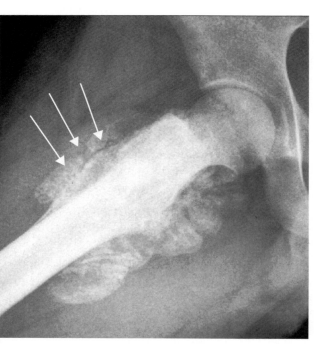

A   B

Figure 36-12   AP (**A**) and lateral (**B**) radiographs of a patient with an osteosarcoma of the right proximal femur. Note the mixed radiodense and radiolucent regions of the lesion in the metaphysis as well as the Codman's triangle (*white arrows*) and large posteromedial soft tissue mass.

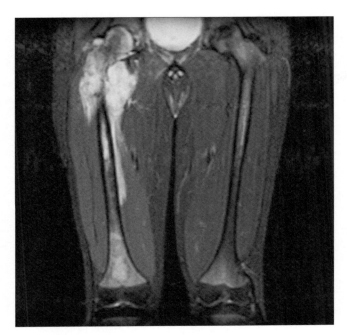

Figure 36-13 MRI of the osteosarcoma shown in Figure 36-12. Note the large soft-tissue mass around the proximal femur as well as the skip lesion in the distal femur. The patient required a total femur resection for complete wide resection.

aggressive. On the other hand, telangiectatic osteosarcomas are a particular variant that have an even worse prognosis than conventional osteosarcomas. These are more difficult to diagnose because of their different radiographic appearance and their microscopic and gross histologic similarities to an aneurysmal bone cyst.

Osteosarcomas may occur as primary tumors or as a secondary malignant transformation from other pre-existing lesions. Common predisposing conditions include Paget disease and sites of previous irradiation. The incidence of treatment-associated osteosarcomas (radiation induced) is as high as 20% in some studies, and patients are at increased risk throughout the remainder of their lives. The mean time interval between receiving radiation and the development of secondary osteosarcoma is approximately 15 years. Because radiation is used for a variety of conditions—both benign and malignant—long-term morbidity from its use must be considered whenever radiotherapy is contemplated. It is recommended that radiation be used in those lesions that are considered to be radiosensitive, such as Ewing sarcoma, or those lesions that are considered to be surgically unresectable. In patients with known Paget disease, the onset of increased pain or swelling should be highly suspect for malignant degeneration. The risk of malignant transformation in those patients with Paget disease is 1%. The osteosarcomas that occur as secondary lesions tend to be more aggressive and have a worse prognosis than routine primary osteosarcomas.

After a biopsy has confirmed the diagnosis, neoadjuvant chemotherapy is instituted. Preoperative studies, including plain radiographs, CT scans of the extremity and lungs, MRIs, and scanograms, are obtained. The CT and MRI scans are used to determine the intramedullary extent of the tumor, the soft-tissue extension, and the presence of skip lesions (Fig. 36-13). These imaging studies are used to determine appropriateness of performing a limb salvage procedure. These imaging studies should be performed at the time of diagnosis to serve as a baseline and may be repeated during preoperative chemotherapy to assess the tumor's responsiveness. Immediately prior to surgery, an

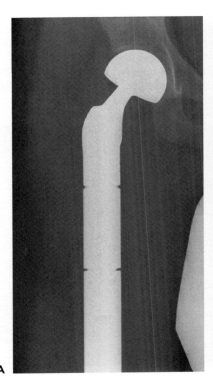

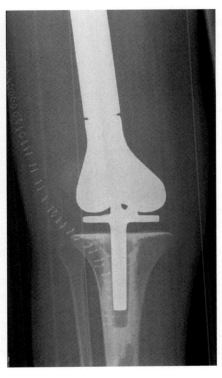

Figure 36-14 AP radiographs of the hip **(A)** and knee **(B)** of the patient in Figures 36-12 and 36-13 showing a total femoral endoprosthesis.

A   B

MRI should be done to determine the extent of the tumor and thus be able to plan the approach and resection level so as achieve a wide margin. Following the resection, the large segmental defect may be reconstructed with various options. The most common techniques involve modular endoprostheses, osteoarticular allografts, and allograft–prosthetic composites. No study has demonstrated one technique to be superior to the others. However, there has been a trend to avoid use of allografts because of the high complication rates associated with their use. In a recent study by Zeegen et al., there was noted to be a fourfold increase in the number of endoprosthetic reconstructions and a 50% decrease in the use of allograft reconstructions for limb preservation surgery at Massachusetts General Hospital (75). Several studies have shown endoprosthetic metallic prostheses to have good durability. With the current modular design, several studies have shown good durability and low complication rates. Henshaw and Malawer reported an overall 10-year implant survival rate of 88% for all anatomic locations (proximal humerus, proximal femur, distal femur, and proximal tibia) (29). Per location, the 10-year implant survival rate was 100% for proximal femur, 98% for proximal humerus, 90% for distal femur, and 78% for proximal tibia (29). In several other studies, the endoprosthetic reconstructions around the shoulder and hip have had greater survival rates than the distal femoral and proximal tibial reconstructions (30,39,41,53,59,60).

Chondrosarcoma

Chondrosarcomas are identified by the presence of proliferating cartilaginous cells. These tumors may also produce other stromal elements, and areas may be myxomatous or calcified, or they may have fibrosarcomatous cells. In contrast to osteosarcomas, chondrosarcomas tend to be less aggressive and to have a slower clinical course. Metastases are less frequent and generally occur later in the disease process, although these lesions have a high propensity for local recurrence. Chondrosarcomas may develop as primary, de novo lesions; however, it is far more common for these lesions to arise as secondary chondrosarcomas from pre-existing lesions (62). Enchondromas, especially multiple enchondromas, are the most common pre-existing lesion leading to secondary chondrosarcomas. Chondrosarcomas may arise from osteochondromas, but this occurs less commonly. Chondrosarcomas develop primarily in adults and the elderly. The proximal femur, ilium, and periacetabular region constitute a frequent location for chondrosarcomas. These lesions usually present with pain, and the onset of pain in a known pre-existing lesion is strongly suggestive of malignant degeneration.

Radiographically, chondrosarcomas frequently have the appearance typical of medullary destruction, combined with areas of mottled calcifications (Figs. 36-15 and 36-16). Endosteal scalloping may be seen with chondrosarcomas; however, this finding alone is less suggestive of malignancy. Malignant degeneration of an osteochondroma should be considered when the cartilaginous cap exceeds 2 cm in thickness or if there is a change in the thickness of the cap that occurs after skeletal maturity. Secondary degeneration from an enchondroma is usually preceded by growth of the lesion, a

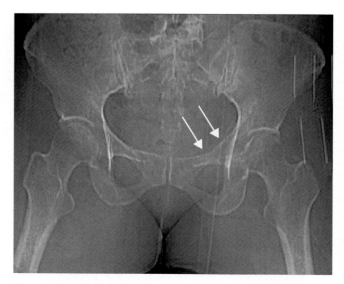

Figure 36-15 Radiograph of the pelvis revealing a subtle area of stippled calcifications with an expansile soft-tissue mass along the medial border of the superior pubic ramus.

change in the calcification pattern, periosteal reaction, or endosteal scalloping.

The mainstay of treatment in high-grade chondrosarcomas involves wide surgical resection of the lesion. With the exception of high-grade lesions, chondrosarcomas generally do not respond to adjuvant therapies such as chemotherapy and radiation. Local spread of tumor cells or an intralesional excision of a chondrosarcoma has a high likelihood of local recurrence; therefore, particular care must be taken not to enter the tumor at the time of the resection. In addition, in those cases where the diagnosis is uncertain and an intralesional procedure is being performed (e.g., curettage of a presumed enchondroma), the wound should be packed off to minimize tumor spillage in case the ultimate pathology indicates malignancy.

The treatment of low-grade chondrosarcomas remains controversial. Some authors have advocated intralesional excision

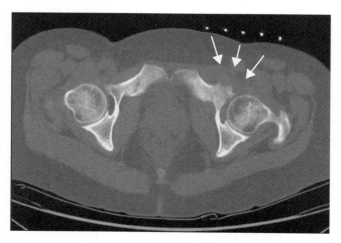

Figure 36-16 CT scan of the lesion in Figure 36-15. An open biopsy revealed this to be a high-grade chondrosarcoma.

with local adjuvant therapy in an effort to preserve the joint by avoiding wide resection. For instance, Marco et al. demonstrated a low local recurrence rate in 58 patients with low-grade intramedullary chondrosarcomas of a long bone treated with intralesional excision (43). Others in the Musculoskeletal Tumor Society, however, believe that even low-grade chondrosarcomas have a nonnegligible metastatic potential and should be treated with wide resection. For instance, Lee et al. retrospectively reviewed 227 patients with chondrosarcomas treated at Massachusetts General Hospital (35). Of the 86 patients who had a low-grade chondrosarcoma, 3 went on to develop pulmonary metastases, and 2 of these patients died. The authors of this study concluded that failure to perform a wide resection is associated with a higher likelihood of local recurrence, which in turn is associated with a high rate of metastasis and death.

Ewing Sarcoma

Although the exact etiology of Ewing tumors is unclear, it is suspected that the primary cell type may be either neuroectodermal (13) or undifferentiated mesenchymal in origin. Characteristic histology shows a small, round-cell tumor that has little intervening stroma. The cells appear uniform, with little pleomorphism or anaplasia and few mitotic figures. The proximal femur and ilium are the most common locations for Ewing sarcomas. The peak age incidence is in the second decade. Pain is the most common presenting sign, and occasionally a mass is palpable. These tumors may also have systemic symptoms, including fevers, chills, elevated white blood cell count and erythrocyte sedimentation rate, and anemia. The radiographs show a lytic process that is permeative, with poor margination and possible cortical expansion (Fig. 36-18). There may be prominent periosteal reaction caused by spread of tumor beyond the cortex. This typically appears as lamellations ("onion skinning").

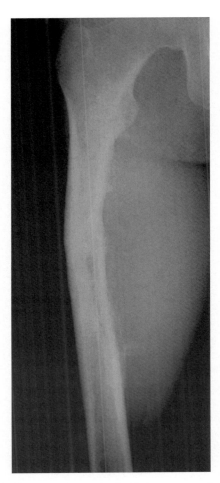

Figure 36-18   AP radiograph of a Ewing sarcoma involving the proximal femur. Note the diaphyseal location, periosteal reaction with lamellations ("onion skinning"), and pathological fracture.

Because of the systemic symptoms, the radiographic appearance, and the gross pathologic appearance of the tumor (which mimics pus), Ewing sarcoma may be mistaken for osteomyelitis. A large soft-tissue mass is common (Fig. 36-19).

Previously, these tumors were among the most lethal of osseous tumors. Fortunately, with newer chemotherapeutic agents in conjunction with radiation, there has been a dramatic improvement in long-term survival rates. These tumors are extremely sensitive to chemotherapy and radiation, and it is common for the entire soft-tissue extension to melt away and for the bone involvement to appear normal after medical treatment. As a result, an MRI should be obtained prior to treatment to assess medullary extent of tumor and possible neurovascular involvement. Medullary extent determines the proper level of resection, and neurovascular involvement with tumor prior to treatment may preclude limb salvage surgery. The role of surgical resection has been questioned because of the excellent response to medical therapy in most Ewing sarcomas, but it is generally believed that wide resection after medical therapy is indicated (4,50,52,73). For many Ewing sarcomas of the proximal femur and hip, wide resection followed by reconstruction using a limb salvage technique is successful. For those lesions within the pelvis, an internal hemipelvectomy or formal hemipelvectomy may be indicated.

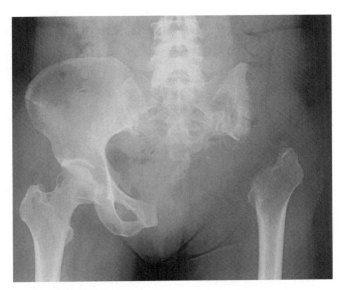

Figure 36-17   Postoperative radiograph of the patient in Figures 36-15 and 36-16 after an internal hemipelvectomy. After a period of non-weight-bearing, the proximal femur forms a pseudarthrosis with the soft tissues of the pelvis. The patient is now able to ambulate with a cane in the contralateral hand and a large shoe lift to compensate for the leg-length discrepancy.

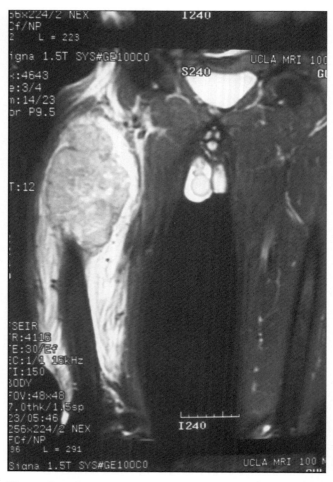

Figure 36-19 MRI of the patient in Figure 36-18 showing the large soft-tissue mass and extensive periosteal reaction.

Malignant Fibrous Histiocytoma

This neoplasm is composed of malignant cells that may show variable areas of fibrous or histiocytic cells. Because of the fibrous component, these tumors may appear remarkably similar to fibrosarcomas. The cells are arranged in a whirling storiform pattern, in contrast to the classic herringbone pattern of fibrosarcomas. The presence of histiocytes distinguishes this lesion. The cytoplasm of these cells has a foamy appearance, their nuclei may be indented or folded, and the nucleoli are large. Many malignant tumors have either fibrous or histiocytic components, and the presence of either chondroid or osteoid elements excludes the diagnosis of malignant fibrous histiocytoma. This tumor is more commonly seen as a soft-tissue malignancy; however, when it occurs in bone, the histologic appearance is similar to that of a soft-tissue tumor.

Malignant fibrous histiocytomas occur over a wide age spectrum; however, most are seen in patients over the age of 20 years. The proximal femur and pelvis represent a common location for these tumors. Symptoms of pain or swelling are common, and the duration of symptoms is usually several months. Radiographically, these tumors are poorly margined, and they may show cortical perforation, soft-tissue

extension, and periosteal reaction. The tumors have an overall malignant appearance on radiographs, although they have no distinguishing characteristic features. Treatment consists of neoadjuvant chemotherapy followed by wide excision, with reconstruction as indicated. These tumors are relatively radioresistant. Overall prognosis for many malignant fibrous histiocytomas remains somewhat guarded, with long-term survival approximately 50%.

Myeloma

Myeloma is the most common primary malignant tumor of bone. However, the orthopedic surgeon is infrequently called upon to manage these tumors. This tumor is composed of plasma cells. When the tumor occurs in only one site, it is called a plasmacytoma. When there is polyostotic involvement, then this lesion is called multiple myeloma. These tumors are usually seen in patients above the age of 50 years, and it is very rare to see a patient with myeloma below the age of 40 years. Symptoms are usually related to increasing pain of several months' duration (48). Fatigue, malaise, and weight loss are common. The initial presentation may be a pathologic fracture. Occasionally, other presenting symptoms occur, including neurologic compromise or polyneuropathy, renal compromise, bleeding diatheses, and fever. A soft-tissue mass

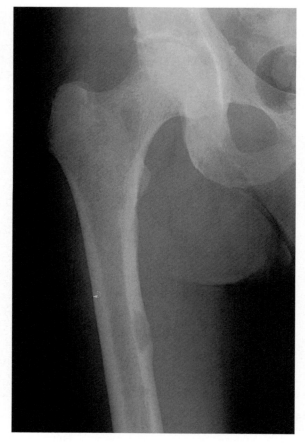

Figure 36-20 Radiograph of the proximal femur showing a punched-out lytic lesion in the medial cortex of the diaphysis in a patient with diffuse multiple myeloma.

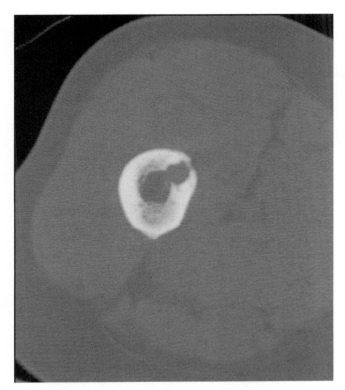

Figure 36-21 CT scan of the patient in Figure 36-20. This shows significant cortical destruction, with anteromedial cortical disruption. Because of pain with weight bearing and the location in the proximal femur, this was felt to represent an impending pathological fracture.

may be palpable. Blood tests may show anemia, a significantly elevated erythrocyte sedimentation rate, and hypercalcemia. When tested, Bence-Jones proteins in the urine may be found in approximately 50% of patients. Immunoelectrophoresis of serum and urinary proteins provide critical information for the diagnosis. The pelvis is the third most common location after the spine and ribs, and the proximal femur is the location fifth in frequency for myelomas. Radiographically, myelomas present with a lytic lesion of bone. There is little surrounding sclerosis, and the lesions are well demarcated, giving them the appearance of a punched-out lesion (Figs. 36-20 and 36-21). The cortex may be slightly expanded. Histologically, myelomas consist of uniformly packed cells with little intervening stroma. The cells have the appearance of a plasma cell with abundant, granular basophilic cytoplasm and an eccentrically placed nucleus. This gives these cells the appearance of a fried egg.

The overall prognosis for patients with myeloma is bleak, and many patients with myeloma die within 2 years of diagnosis. A plasmacytoma is considered to be the precursor for disseminated disease. Radiation is the treatment of choice for solitary lesions or patients at risk for pathologic fracture in non-weight-bearing extremities. Chemotherapy is reserved for multiple lesions. Orthopedic intervention is needed in cases of pathologic fracture, impending pathologic fracture in weight-bearing bones (Fig. 36-22), and neurologic compromise (to achieve spinal decompression). Surgical resection has not been shown to be of benefit for long-term survival.

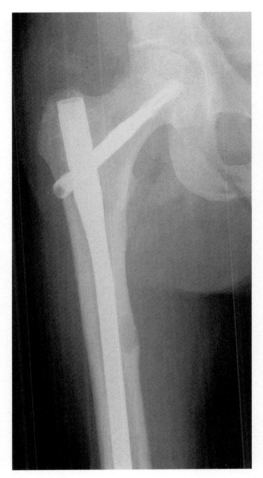

Figure 36-22 Postoperative radiograph of the patient in Figures 36-20 and 36-21 following prophylactic intramedullary nailing. The patient was treated with radiation therapy to the right femur approximately 3 weeks after the surgery.

TUMORLIKE CONDITIONS OF BONE

Aneurysmal Bone Cyst

This condition is probably related to a reactive nonneoplastic process and is best not considered a primary bone tumor. The exact etiology, however, is unknown. It has been suggested that aneurysmal bone cysts occur as a result of a vascular disturbance within bone (44). In addition, the lesion frequently regresses after incomplete excision. Aneurysmal bone cysts may occur as primary lesions, or they may be associated with other conditions, such as giant cell tumors, fibrous dysplasia, chondromyxoid fibromas, and chondroblastomas. Radiographically, they appear as lytic lesions with expansion of the overlying cortex. The cortex appears as an egg shell over the lesion (Fig. 36-23). Pathologic fractures are common. On MRI and/or CT scans, fluid-fluid levels are commonly seen (Fig 36-24). Because the lesions are blood filled, when the patient rests for a prolonged period, such as during a CT scan, the blood begins to separate into its components, which are then distinguishable. The radiographic appearance may mimic that of other lesions, such as giant cell tumors; however, nearly 80% of patients with

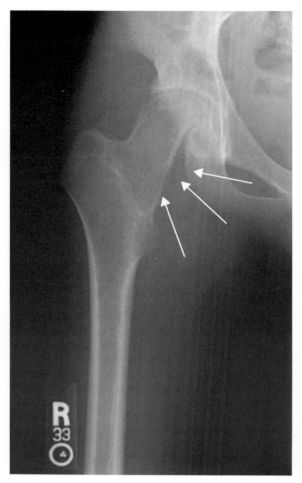

Figure 36-23 AP radiograph showing an expansile radiolucent lesion of the femoral head and neck. The thinned cortex remains barely intact (*arrows*). This proved to be an aneurysmal bone cyst.

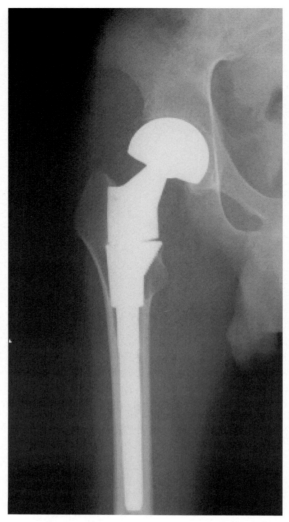

Figure 36-25 AP radiograph of the patient in Figures 36-20 and 36-21 following excision and bipolar hemiarthroplasty. Preoperatively, the patient underwent angiogram and embolization of the lesion to minimize the risk of excessive bleeding.

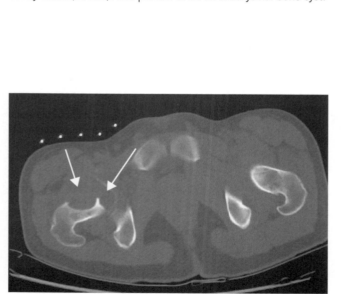

Figure 36-24 CT scan of the patient in Figure 36-23 showing an expansile lesion of the femoral head and neck with a thinned overlying cortex. Fluid-fluid levels are frequently seen in aneurysmal bone cysts and can be seen here (*arrows*).

aneurysmal bone cysts are under the age of 20. In contrast, over 80% of patients with giant cell tumors are over the age of 20. Also, a diagnosis of recurrent aneurysmal bone cyst should be questioned: it is more likely a giant cell tumor with an aneurysmal bone cyst component. Treatment consists of curettage, bone grafting, and internal fixation when structural integrity is compromised (34). Some authors have advocated the use of adjuvant therapies such as cryosurgery (40,45) and polymethylmethacrylate cement (40). When treated appropriately, the risk of recurrence is low.

Fibrous Dysplasia

Fibrous dysplasia arises from an abnormality in bone development. The exact etiology, however, is unknown. As the name suggests, the principal histologic feature of this lesion is abnormal fibrous tissue within bone. The disease develops in childhood but usually does not become symptomatic until the second decade of life. The upper femur is the most common location for fibrous dysplasia, occurring in about one third of cases. Many cases are asymptomatic and are discovered incidentally on radiographs. When symptomatic, fibrous dysplasia presents with pain or pathologic fracture in the affected extremity or joint. There may also be bone or joint deformity, leg-length discrepancy, or limited and asymmetric range of joint motion. Rarely, a patient will present with Albright syndrome, the triad of polyostotic fibrous dysplasia, café-au-lait spots, and precocious puberty.

The radiographic appearance of fibrous dysplasia shows a well-demarcated zone of slightly expanded cortex and a mildly sclerotic rim. The central portion of the lesion typically has a homogeneous rarefaction, classically described as a ground glass appearance (Fig. 36-26). If the condition has existed for long, there may be bony deformity from repeated minor pathologic fractures. In the proximal femur, this produces the well-described "shepherd's crook." Histologically, there is a proliferation of fibroblasts with an abundance of collagen matrix. There are also islands of osteoid and reactive bone formation. The trabeculae are randomly arranged, giving the appearance of scattered alphabet characters or "Chinese letters." Osteoblasts are not present at the periphery

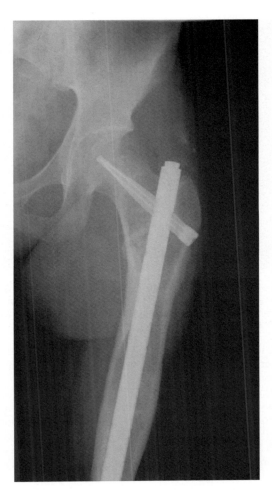

Figure 36-27 Postoperative radiograph of the patient in Figure 36-26 following open biopsy, curettage and allograft packing, and prophylactic fixation with a third-generation intramedullary nail.

of the trabeculae, which distinguishes fibrous dysplasia from a rare condition called "osteofibrous dysplasia."

Treatment is usually conservative, unless an impending pathologic fracture necessitates stabilization. In this case, curettage and bone grafting are usually performed. Treatment may be supplemented with prophylactic internal fixation when needed (Fig. 36-27) (34). Total hip arthroplasty is indicated if degenerative joint symptoms are present. The fibrous dysplasia is curetted, and bone grafting is performed as needed. Irradiation has been used as a form of treatment, but the benefit is questionable, and there is increased incidence of sarcomatous degeneration secondary to the radiotherapy. Therefore, irradiation is not recommended for the treatment of any fibrous dysplasia lesion.

Paget Disease

The cause of Paget disease is unknown, although a viral etiology is suspected. Paget disease most commonly affects middle-aged to older individuals. Any bone may be affected, but the proximal femur, hip, and pelvis are common locations. Active and latent forms of the disease process have been described. In the active form, bone metabolism is increased in both resorption and reparation. Early in the disease, bone resorption predominates.

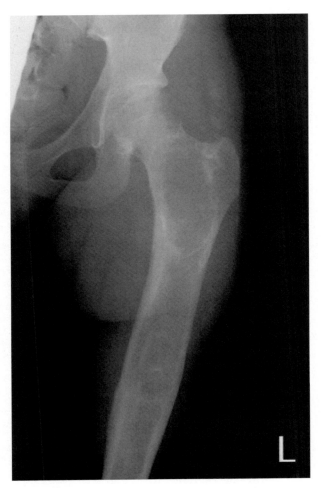

Figure 36-26 Radiograph showing a radiolucent lesion of the left proximal femur with slight bony expansion and a ground glass appearance to the matrix within the lesion.

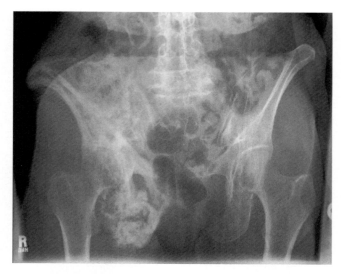

Figure 36-28 Radiograph of a patient with extensive Paget disease involving the right hemipelvis. The patient developed new onset of pain, and radiographs demonstrated a large mass of the ischium and inferior pubic ramus, which proved to be a secondary osteosarcoma.

In the latent form of Paget disease, the bone becomes more sclerotic and relatively less active. With progression of the disease, the bone may develop deformity, hence the older term "osteitis deformans." Histologically, broad trabeculae are present, frequently with immature lamellar bone. An increased fibrovascular stroma is present, and prominent osteoclast activity may be seen. Paget disease is usually treated with medical management, except in cases of secondary degenerative arthritis as a result of deformity. The surgical treatment is then joint arthroplasty. In rare cases of Paget disease, malignant transformation to an osteosarcoma can occur (Fig. 36-28). Radiographically, this transformation may be difficult to diagnose because of the underlying abnormal bone appearance. Bone scans may be difficult to interpret in the case of malignancy because the various stages of the Paget-disease process exhibit different activity levels. Malignancy should be suspected in patients who have a

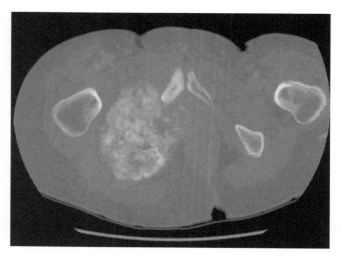

Figure 36-29 CT scan of the patient in Figure 36-28 with Paget disease showing the large mass that proved to be a secondary osteosarcoma.

change in the level of pain in an extremity affected by Paget disease or if there are radiographic changes, including cortical expansion or disruption and pathologic fracture.

REFERENCES

1. Aboulafia AJ, Rosenbaum DH, Sicard-Rosenbaum L, et al. Treatment of large subchondral tumors of the knee with cryosurgery and composite reconstruction. *Clin Orthop Relat Res.* 1994:189–199.
2. Abudu A, Sferopoulos NK, Tillman RM, et al. The surgical treatment and outcome of pathological fractures in localised osteosarcoma. *J Bone Joint Surg [Br].* 1996;78:694–698.
3. Bacci G, Ferrari S, Longhi A, et al. Neoadjuvant chemotherapy for high grade osteosarcoma of the extremities: long-term results for patients treated according to the Rizzoli IOR/OS-3b protocol. *J Chemother.* 2001;13:93–99.
4. Bacci G, Toni A, Avella M, et al. Long-term results in 144 localized Ewing's sarcoma patients treated with combined therapy. *Cancer.* 1989;63:1477–1486.
5. Bollini G, Jouve JL, Gentet JC, et al. Bone lesions in histiocytosis X. *J Pediatr Orthop.* 1991;11:469–477.
6. Bredella MA, Caputo GR, Steinbach LS. Value of FDG positron emission tomography in conjunction with MR imaging for evaluating therapy response in patients with musculoskeletal sarcomas. *AJR Am J Roentgenol.* 2002;179:1145–1150.
7. Brenner W, Bohuslavizki KH, Eary JF. PET imaging of osteosarcoma. *J Nucl Med.* 2003;44:930–942.
8. Capanna R, Fabbri N, Bettelli G. Curettage of giant cell tumor of bone: the effect of surgical technique and adjuvants on local recurrence rate. *Chir Organi Mov.* 1990;75:206.
9. Capanna R, Sudanese A, Baldini N, et al. Phenol as an adjuvant in the control of local recurrence of benign neoplasms of bone treated by curettage. *Ital J Orthop Traumatol.* 1985;11:381–388.
10. Clark CR, Morgan C, Sonstegard DA, et al. The effect of biopsy-hole shape and size on bone strength. *J Bone Joint Surg [Am].* 1977;59:213–217.
11. Dahlin DC, Cupps RE, Johnson EW Jr. Giant-cell tumor: a study of 195 cases. *Cancer.* 1970;25:1061–1070.
12. Descamps F, Yasik E, Hardy D, et al. Pigmented villonodular synovitis of the hip: a case report and review of the literature. *Clin Rheumatol.* 1991;10:184–190.
13. Devaney K, Abbondanzo SL, Shekitka KM, et al. MIC2 detection in tumors of bone and adjacent soft tissues. *Clin Orthop Relat Res.* 1995:176–187.
14. DiCaprio MR, Friedlaender GE. Malignant bone tumors: limb sparing versus amputation. *J Am Acad Orthop Surg.* 2003;11:25–37.
15. Dupuy DE, Rosenberg AE, Punyaratabandhu T, et al. Accuracy of CT-guided needle biopsy of musculoskeletal neoplasms. *AJR Am J Roentgenol.* 1998;171:759–762.
16. Eckardt JJ, Eilber FR, Dorey FJ, et al. The UCLA experience in limb salvage surgery for malignant tumors. *Orthopedics.* 1985;8:612–621.
17. Eilber F, Giuliano A, Eckardt J, et al. Adjuvant chemotherapy for osteosarcoma: a randomized prospective trial. *J Clin Oncol.* 1987;5:21–26.
18. Enneking WF, Spanier SS, Goodman MA. Current concepts review: the surgical staging of musculoskeletal sarcoma. *J Bone Joint Surg [Am].* 1980;62:1027–1030.
19. Feldman F, van Heertum R, Manos C. 18FDG PET scanning of benign and malignant musculoskeletal lesions. *Skeletal Radiol.* 2003;32:201–208.
20. Ferguson WS, Goorin AM. Current treatment of osteosarcoma. *Cancer Invest.* 2001;19:292–315.
21. Gebhardt MC, Goorin A, Traina J, et al. Long-term results of limb-salvage and amputation in extremity osteosarcoma. In: Yamamuro T, ed. *New Developments for Limb Salvage in Musculoskeletal Tumors.* New York: Springer; 1989:99–109.
22. Gitelis S, Mallin BA, Piasecki P, et al. Intralesional excision compared with en bloc resection for giant-cell tumors of bone. *J Bone Joint Surg [Am].* 1993;75:1648–1655.
23. Glasser DB, Lane JM, Huvos AG, et al. Survival, prognosis, and therapeutic response in osteogenic sarcoma: the Memorial Hospital experience. *Cancer.* 1992;69:698–708.

24. Goldenberg RR, Campbell CJ, Bonfiglio M. Giant-cell tumor of bone: an analysis of two hundred and eighteen cases. *J Bone Joint Surg [Am]*. 1970;52:619–664.

25. Greis PE, Hankin FM. Eosinophilic granuloma: the management of solitary lesions of bone. *Clin Orthop Relat Res*. 1990:204–211.

26. Hamilton A, Davis RI, Nixon JR. Synovial chondrosarcoma complicating synovial chondromatosis: report of a case and review of the literature. *J Bone Joint Surg [Am]*. 1987;69:1084–1088.

27. Hardacker J, Mindell ER. Synovial chondromatosis with secondary subluxation of the hip: a case report. *J Bone Joint Surg [Am]*. 1991;73:1405–1407.

28. Hau A, Kim I, Kattapuram S, et al. Accuracy of CT-guided biopsies in 359 patients with musculoskeletal lesions. *Skeletal Radiol*. 2002;31:349–353.

29. Henshaw RM, Malawer MM. Review of endoprosthetic reconstruction in limb-sparing surgery. In: Malawer MM, Sugarbaker PH, ed. *Musculoskeletal Cancer Surgery: Treatment of Sarcomas and Allied Disorders*. Dordrecht: Kluwer Academic Publishers; 2001:383–403.

30. Horowitz SM, Glasser DB, Lane JM, et al. Prosthetic and extremity survivorship after limb salvage for sarcoma: how long do the reconstructions last? *Clin Orthop*. 1993;No. 293:280–286.

31. Ioannidis JP, Lau J. 18F-FDG PET for the diagnosis and grading of soft-tissue sarcoma: a meta-analysis. *J Nucl Med*. 2003;44:717–724.

32. Ivins J, Taylor W, Golenzer H. A multi-institutional cooperative study of osteosarcoma. In: Yamamuro T, ed. *New Developments for Limb Salvage Surgery in Musculoskeletal Tumors*. New York: Springer; 1989:61–69.

33. Jaffe HL, Lichtenstein L, Sutro CJ. Pigmented villonodular synovitis, bursitis and tenosynovitis: a discussion of the synovial and bursal equivalents fo the tenosynovial lesion commonly noted as xanthoma, xanthogranuloma, giant cell tumor or myeloplaxoma of the tendon sheath, with some consideration of the tendon sheath lesion itself. *Arch Pathol*. 1941;31:731.

34. Jaffe KA, Dunham WK. Treatment of benign lesions of the femoral head and neck. *Clin Orthop Relat Res*. 1990:134–137.

35. Lee FY, Mankin HJ, Fondren G, et al. Chondrosarcoma of bone: an assessment of outcome. *J Bone Joint Surg [Am]*. 1999;81:326–338.

36. Leeson MC, Lippitt SB. Thermal aspects of the use of polymethylmethacrylate in large metaphyseal defects in bone: a clinical review and laboratory study. *Clin Orthop Relat Res*. 1993:239–245.

37. Lichtenstein L. Histiocytosis X: integration of eosinophilic granuloma of bone, Letterer-Siwe disease, and Schuller-Christian disease as related manifestations of a single nosologic entity. *AMA Arch Pathol*. 1953;56:84–102.

38. Link MP, Goorin AM, Horowitz M, et al. Adjuvant chemotherapy of high-grade osteosarcoma of the extremity: updated results of the Multi-Institutional Osteosarcoma Study. *Clin Orthop*. 1991; No. 270:8–14.

39. Malawer MM, Chou LB. Prosthetic survival and clinical results with use of large-segment replacements in the treatment of high-grade bone sarcomas. *J Bone Joint Surg [Am]*. 1995;77:1154–1165.

40. Malawer MM, Dunham W. Cryosurgery and acrylic cementation as surgical adjuncts in the treatment of aggressive (benign) bone tumors: analysis of 25 patients below the age of 21. *Clin Orthop Relat Res*. 1991:42–57.

41. Mankin HJ, Gebhardt MC, Jennings LC, et al. Long-term results of allograft replacement in the management of bone tumors. *Clin Orthop*. 1996:86–97.

42. Mankin HJ, Mankin CJ, Simon MA. The hazards of the biopsy, revisited. Members of the Musculoskeletal Tumor Society. *J Bone Joint Surg [Am]*. 1996;78:656–663.

43. Marco RA, Gitelis S, Brebach GT, et al. Cartilage tumors: evaluation and treatment. *J Am Acad Orthop Surg*. 2000;8:292–304.

44. Marcove RC, Lyden JP, Huvos AG, et al. Giant-cell tumors treated by cryosurgery: a report of twenty-five cases. *J Bone Joint Surg [Am]*. 1973;55:1633–1644.

45. Marcove RC, Sheth DS, Takemoto S, et al. The treatment of aneurysmal bone cyst. *Clin Orthop Relat Res*. 1995:157–163.

46. Maurice H, Crone M, Watt I. Synovial chondromatosis. *J Bone Joint Surg [Br]*. 1988;70:807–811.

47. Meyers PA, Heller G, Healey J, et al. Chemotherapy for nonmetastatic osteogenic sarcoma: the Memorial Sloan-Kettering experience. *J Clin Oncol*. 1992;10:5–15.

48. Mundy GR, Yoneda T. Facilitation and suppression of bone metastasis. *Clin Orthop Relat Res*. 1995:34–44.

49. Murnaghan JJ, Salonen DC. Pigmented villonodular synovitis. *Curr Opin Orthop*. 1995;6(6):8–12.

50. Nesbit ME Jr, Gehan EA, Burgert EO Jr, et al. Multimodal therapy for the management of primary, nonmetastatic Ewing's sarcoma of bone: a long-term follow-up of the First Intergroup study. *J Clin Oncol*. 1990;8:1664–1674.

51. Perry BE, McQueen DA, Lin JJ. Synovial chondromatosis with malignant degeneration to chondrosarcoma: report of a case. *J Bone Joint Surg [Am]*. 1988;70:1259–1261.

52. Pritchard DJ. Indications for surgical treatment of localized Ewing's sarcoma of bone. *Clin Orthop Relat Res*. 1980:39–43.

53. Roberts P, Chan D, Grimer RJ, et al. Prosthetic replacement of the distal femur for primary bone tumours. *J Bone Joint Surg [Br]*. 1991;73:762–769.

54. Rosen G, Caparros B, Huvos AG, et al. Preoperative chemotherapy for osteogenic sarcoma: selection of postoperative adjuvant chemotherapy based on the response of the primary tumor to preoperative chemotherapy. *Cancer*. 1982;49:1221–1230.

55. Rosen G, Marcove RC, Caparros B, et al. Primary osteogenic sarcoma: the rationale for preoperative chemotherapy and delayed surgery. *Cancer*. 1979;43:2163–2177.

56. Rosen G, Marcove RC, Huvos AG, et al. Primary osteogenic sarcoma: eight-year experience with adjuvant chemotherapy. *J Cancer Res Clin Oncol*. 1983;106(suppl):55–67.

57. Rosenthal DI, Hornicek FJ, Torriani M, et al. Osteoid osteoma: percutaneous treatment with radiofrequency energy. *Radiology*. 2003;229:171–175.

58. Rosenthal DI, Hornicek FJ, Wolfe MW, et al. Percutaneous radiofrequency coagulation of osteoid osteoma compared with operative treatment. *J Bone Joint Surg [Am]*. 1998;80:815–821.

59. Rougraff BT, Simon MA, Kneisl JS, et al. Limb salvage compared with amputation for osteosarcoma of the distal end of the femur: a long-term oncological, functional, and quality-of-life study. *J Bone Joint Surg [Am]*. 1994;76:649–656.

60. Safran MR, Kody MH, Namba RS, et al. 151 endoprosthetic reconstructions for patients with primary tumors involving bone. *Contemp Orthop*. 1994;29:15–25.

61. Sanjay BK, Frassica FJ, Frassica DA, et al. Treatment of giant-cell tumor of the pelvis. *J Bone Joint Surg [Am]*. 1993;75:1466–1475.

62. Schmale GA, Conrad EU 3rd, Raskind WH. The natural history of hereditary multiple exostoses. *J Bone Joint Surg [Am]*. 1994;76: 986–992.

63. Schwartz HS, Unni KK, Pritchard DJ. Pigmented villonodular synovitis: a retrospective review of affected large joints. *Clin Orthop Relat Res*. 1989:243–255.

64. Scully SP, Ghert MA, Zurakowski D, et al. Pathologic fracture in osteosarcoma: prognostic importance and treatment implications. *J Bone Joint Surg [Am]*. 2002;84A:49–57.

65. Scully SP, Temple HT, O'Keefe RJ, et al. The surgical treatment of patients with osteosarcoma who sustain a pathologic fracture. *Clin Orthop*. 1996:227–232.

66. Simon MA. Limb-salvage for osteosarcoma. In: Yamamuro T, ed. *New Developments for Limb Salvage in Musculoskeletal Tumors*. New York: Springer; 1989:71–72.

67. Simon MA, Aschliman MA, Thomas N, et al. Limb-salvage treatment versus amputation for osteosarcoma of the distal end of the femur. *J Bone Joint Surg [Am]*. 1986;68:1331–1337.

68. Skrzynski MC, Biermann JS, Montag A, et al. Diagnostic accuracy and charge-savings of outpatient core needle biopsy compared with open biopsy of musculoskeletal tumors. *J Bone Joint Surg [Am]*. 1996;78:644–649.

69. Smith JH, Pugh DG. Roentgenographic aspects of articular pigmented villonodular synovitis. *Am J Roentgenol Radium Ther Nucl Med*. 1962;87:1146–1156.

70. Tomita K, Aotake Y, Sugihara M, et al. Overall results and functional evaluation of limb salvage for osteosarcoma. In: Yamamuro T, ed. *New Developments for Limb Salvage in Musculoskeletal Tumors*. New York: Springer; 1989:53–57.

71. Vernon CB, Eary JF, Rubin BP, et al. FDG PET imaging guided re-evaluation of histopathologic response in a patient with high-grade sarcoma. *Skeletal Radiol*. 2003;32:139–142.

72. Welker JA, Henshaw RM, Jelinek J, et al. The percutaneous needle biopsy is safe and recommended in the diagnosis of musculoskeletal masses. *Cancer.* 2000;89:2677–2686.

73. Wilkins RM, Pritchard DJ, Burgert EO Jr, et al. Ewing's sarcoma of bone: experience with 140 patients. *Cancer.* 1986;58:2551–2555.

74. Yao L, Nelson SD, Seeger LL, et al. Primary musculoskeletal neoplasms: effectiveness of core-needle biopsy. *Radiology.* 1999;212:682–686.

75. Zeegen EN, Aponte-Tinao LA, Hornicek FJ, et al. Survivorship analysis of 141 modular metallic endoprostheses at early followup. *Clin Orthop Relat Res.* 2004:239–250.

Metastatic Disease about the Hip

37

Joseph H. Schwab   *Patrick J. Boland*

INTRODUCTION AND SCOPE OF THE PROBLEM

Carcinoma metastatic to bone is the most common malignant tumor of bone. It is estimated that the incidence of metastatic bone disease is 40 times the incidence of primary bone sarcomas (33). The true incidence of metastatic bone disease is unknown, but Jaffe reported an incidence of nearly 90% at autopsy in patients who succumbed to osteophilic carcinomas (38). Tumors that tend to be osteophilic are lung, breast, prostate, renal, and thyroid carcinoma. Seventy percent of all cancer deaths in this country are due to lung, breast, and prostate cancer (40). It is estimated that 350,000 people in the United States die each year with bone metastasis, and many more live with bone metastasis (53). Roughly 1 million people develop cancer each year in the United States. Nearly 50% of people with visceral cancer will develop bone metastasis at some time during the course of their disease (70). The axial

and proximal appendicular skeleton are the most common sites of skeletal metastasis. Galasko reported the incidence of pelvic metastasis as 66%, and nearly half of his patients had femoral metastasis (24). Haberman et al. reported 306 cases of pathologic fractures or impending fractures, of which 66% occurred in the hip area (27).

Once carcinoma has spread to bone, it is considered incurable except in the rarest of cases. However, survival time after the development of bone metastasis is quite variable. Average survival times have been reported as low as 3 months for lung carcinoma up to 19 months for breast and thyroid carcinoma (19). Patients with skeletal metastasis alone fare better than patients with skeletal and visceral metastasis (54). Marco et al. reported 12 months as the average survival with skeletal metastasis alone versus 3 months with both skeletal and pulmonary metastasis (46). The extent of skeletal metastasis is also an important consideration. Patients with multiple bony metastases have a worse prognosis than patients with a solitary bony metastasis (42,54).

The nonsurgical management of skeletal metastasis is improving as systemic therapies continue to evolve. Exciting new areas of drug development focusing on growth factor inhibitors are beginning to show favorable clinical results (37,39,75). However, the early success of these treatments is based on their ability to slow the progression of systemic disease. The hope is that these patients will liver longer with their disease. As patients live longer, they are more likely to accumulate complications associated with metastatic bone disease. One of the most feared complications of cancer is pain, the most common manifestation of bone metastasis (11). The goal of surgical management in this patient population is to mitigate pain and provide a stable limb upon which the patient can

559

immediately weight bear. A prerequisite to treating these patients is an understanding of the biomechanical implications of destructive bony lesions. Further, familiarity with the pathogenesis and complications of skeletal metastasis are important in order to provide optimum care for these patients.

PATHOGENESIS

The mechanisms that lead to skeletal metastasis are the focus of intense molecular biologic research. However, the basis for skeletal metastasis was postulated over 100 years ago by Paget. He promulgated the "seed and soil" theory of metastasis according to which cancer cells interact with the local tissue environment to facilitate tumor growth (57). In order to metastasize, the tumor cell must be able to clear many different hurdles. First, it must break free from its connective tissue milieu. In order to spread distally, it must then find passage in a blood or lymphatic vessel. Once the tumor cell finds an acceptable end organ, it must then breakthrough the endothelial lining of the vessel and basement membrane before entering into the substance of the organ.

All of these steps require an extremely complex interplay between the tumor cell and its environment. Tumor cells produce a variety of growth factors that impact their local environment, including PTHrP, IL-1, IL-6, prostaglandin E2, and TNF (37). These factors help the tumor cell find an acceptable place to grow. It has been shown that tumors that express PTHrP are more likely to metastasize to bone tumors of the same histology that do not express PTHrP (63). The expression of growth factors seems to play an important part in cancer honing in on bone. This helps to explain why hematogenous skeletal metastasis is so common despite only 5% to 10% of cardiac output going to bone (14). Once the tumor cells have nested in bone, they produce cytokines such as IL-6 and PTHrP, both of which are known to stimulate osteoclasts (37). Breast cancer cells have been shown to produce several cytokines that increase RANKL expression on osteoblasts and stimulate osteoclasts (15,43). However, there are important mechanical considerations regarding the vascular spread of tumor cells to the pelvis and proximal femur. Ewing stressed the importance of circulatory anatomy in the development of metastatic disease (17). Batson described the valveless, extracaval, paravertebral venous plexus that extends from the pelvis to the base of the skull. The fact that it is valveless and outside the thoracic and abdominal cavity makes it sensitive to the Valsalva maneuver. During a Valsalva maneuver, the blood in this system can stagnate and flow in a retrograde direction. This allows more time for cells in the blood to interact with the local tissues near the plexus. The breast and prostate utilize Batson's plexus for drainage (3).

CLINICAL FEATURES

Pain is the most common presenting complaint of a patient with metastatic disease. However, it is important to note that up to 50% of patients with bone metastasis will not have any symptoms referable to their metastasis (22). Typically, the pain is described as a dull ache that is worse at night. The pain is often not relieved by rest, which helps in making the diagnosis.

As the tumor progresses, the pain becomes pronounced with weight bearing. Pain is described as "biologic" or "mechanical" in nature. Biologic pain stems from the presence of the tumor cells in bone and the factors they secrete. Tumor cells are known to secrete cytokines, neuropeptides, and inflammatory mediators that stimulate pain receptors in and around bone. The presence of the tumor within bone can increase the intraosseous pressure, which again stimulates pain receptors. Mechanical pain, also referred to as "functional pain," is associated with structural weakening of bone. As the tumor progresses, the remaining normal bone is forced to bear more of the load. This leads to greater strain and stretching of intraosseous and periosteal mechanoreceptors, leading to pain. Gross and microscopic fractures can also be sources of significant pain.

A careful history and physical examination is essential for pinpointing the origin of the pain. Tumor involving the femoral head, acetabulum, or pubic rami typically is felt in the groin. Patients frequently report hip pain when referring to symptoms in the sacroiliac area. Rest pain in the groin increased by weight bearing or attempted active flexion suggests proximal femoral or pubic rami pathology, and tenderness over the pubic rami helps differentiate pubic from intertrochanteric or neck disease. Upper lumbar spine pathology may also cause groin or anterior thigh pain. Pain with passive stretch of attached muscles may indicate an avulsion fracture. Careful palpation may indicate a pubic ramus fracture. Obvious deformity usually accompanied by severe pain is diagnostic of a fracture. However, an impending fracture can be very difficult to diagnose. Rest pain made worse with activity is the most important nonradiographic finding indicative of impending fracture.

Not all hip pain in a patient with cancer is directly caused by the tumor. A careful history may uncover other treatable conditions. Many of these patients will be immunocompromised, and this will predispose them to conditions such as joint sepsis and herpes zoster infections. Several chemotherapy regimens include intravenous corticosteroids, which places these patients at increased risk for avascular necrosis of the hip. Of course, osteoarthritis and osteoporotic fractures are also common in this patient population.

HYPERCALCEMIA

Hypercalcemia of malignancy is the most common paraneoplastic syndrome in cancer (52). It is more common in squamous cell lung carcinoma, breast cancer, multiple myeloma, and renal cell carcinoma. Hypercalcemia has been reported in up to 49% of patients with breast cancer (26,62). Hypercalcemia is caused by two distinct mechanisms. The first mechanism involves tumor secretion of PTHrP in an endocrine fashion. The PTHrP causes the equivalent of secondary hyperparathyroidism. The second mechanism involves tumors cells stimulating osteoclasts in a paracrine fashion, and it is the most common mechanism by which hypercalcemia of malignancy occurs. Renal insufficiency can also contribute to hypercalcemia of malignancy, often aggravated by dehydration. Patients often become lethargic, fatigued, and anorexic. They complain of nausea and exhibit disorientation. If left untreated, these patients will become comatose and eventually die of cardiac arrhythmia (64).

The first line of treatment should be rehydration using normal saline. Removing hypercalcemia-producing agents, such as thiazide diuretics, is imperative. Once the patient has been rehydrated, he or she can be given loop diuretics for the hypercalciuric properties (73). Intravenously administered bisphosphonates have been FDA approved for this condition, and they are now the treatment of choice for hypercalcemia, along with rehydration.

BONE MARROW REPLACEMENT

Anemia, leukocytopenia, and thrombocytopenia are often found in the patient with metastatic cancer. One of the causes of these entities is complete marrow replacement, leading to myelophthisis. The marrow is either replaced by tumor or destroyed by chemotherapy or radiation therapy. Prostate cancer is notorious for replacing the marrow with sclerotic bone. This can make it very difficult to ream. One should consider a high-speed drill in this setting. Broaches should be used with great caution to avoid fracture.

DIAGNOSTIC EVALUATIONS

The evaluation of patients with metastatic disease begins with a thorough history and physical examination and proceeds in a systematic way with appropriate imaging studies and laboratory tests.

Plain Radiography

Clinical decisions are based in large part on the appearance of the plain x-rays, and plain radiography is the most cost-effective means of evaluating a painful metastatic bone lesion. However, it should be remembered that 30% to 50% of the bone must be destroyed before it will be appreciated on plain x-rays. Bone metastasis is either lytic, blastic, or mixed. The appearance of these lesions is a direct result of what the tumor is doing to the balance between osteoblasts and osteoclasts. Lung tumors tend to favor the osteoclasts, and they appear as lytic lesions. Prostate cancer tends to be blastic, and breast cancer often has a mixed appearance. The main purpose of obtaining plain films is to evaluate the structural integrity of the bone. This is best done by evaluating the cortical bone. Radiographs of the pelvis should include Judet views in order to evaluate the integrity of the anterior and posterior columns. When surgery is planned, the entire length of the femur should be viewed to help determine the most appropriate stem to use. The tip of the stem should bypass the most distal lesion by at least two cortical diameters.

Bone Scintigraphy

Bone scintigraphy involves attaching a radionucleotide such as technetium-99m to an osteophilic substrate such as methylene diphosphate. The diphosphate will localize to areas of increased osteoblastic activity as it is incorporated into hydroxyapatite during mineralization. Technetium bone scans should be used as the primary screening modality for occult bony metastasis (28). The sensitivity of bone scans has been shown to range from 64% to 100% (9,10,13,21,25,32). Multiple myeloma is notorious for negative bone scans owing to its failure to evoke an osteoblastic response. In very aggressive lesions, such as some lung carcinomas, the progression of tumor is so swift that little or no osteoblastic response is elicited, resulting in a false-negative scan.

Computed Tomography

Computed Tomography is an excellent tool for evaluating the structural integrity of the pelvis and hip. It provides the most information about the condition of the cortical bone in the femur. It also provides very useful information about the dome of the acetabulum and the anterior and posterior columns (46). We obtain CT scans in many of our patients who have functional pain emanating from the pelvis or proximal femur.

Magnetic Resonance Imaging

Although MRI provides excellent detail and contrast between normal and abnormal tissue, it is less helpful than plain radiographs or CT in evaluating metastatic disease about the hip. The MRI often exaggerates the degree of bony involvement and may not be as good for evaluating the structural integrity of the bone. While it is important to know the extent of marrow involvement, which is clearly shown with MRI, this imaging modality is less helpful in surgical planning. MRI is useful if one suspects an occult fracture in the hip that does not show up on CT scan (66).

Positron Emission Tomography

The use of PET scans to evaluate cancer patients is becoming more common. One of two radiopharmaceuticals is utilized to evaluate bone metastasis: ^{18}F-Fluoride or [^{18}F] fluorodeoxyglucose. Fluoride is a nonspecific bone tracer, and it accumulates in areas of increased osteoblastic activity. Unlike the previous imaging modalities, [^{18}F] fluoro-deoxyglucose scanning takes advantage of differences in metabolic activity to distinguish tumor cells from normal cells. Tumor cells tend to be more metabolically active than normal cells, and they require more glucose. In a study of 110 patients with bony metastasis, PET scans had a sensitivity very similar to that of bone scintigraphy; however, the accuracy of PET scans was nearly 98%, compared with 61% for bone scans (7).

Arteriography

Arteriography coupled with embolization should be considered in cases of thyroid carcinoma and renal cell carcinoma (Fig. 37-1). These tumors tend to be quite vascular, and there is real danger of exsanguination even in experienced hands.

Evaluation of the Unknown Primary

Patients over the age of 40 with a poorly marginated bony lesion are more likely to have a metastatic carcinoma than a primary sarcoma. However, the source of the metastasis is not always known. Three percent to 4% of patients who present with metastatic carcinoma have an unknown primary

1-year survival of 40% after hip arthroplasty for metastatic disease in a series of 299 patients. Patients with breast and prostate cancer survived the longest, with the median survival in prostate over 1 year. Aggressive management with durable reconstruction is therefore indicated (69).

Bone Biomechanics

The collagen and mineral composition of bone as well as its structural properties determine the overall strength of bone. The mineral content determines the tensile yield strength as well as the compressive strength (65). After the yield point has been reached, collagen has the greatest impact on the tensile properties of bone (6). The shape and distribution of trabecular and cortical bone determine the structural properties of bone. It is important to think about the integrity of the "normal" bone before considering what the metastasis is doing to the overall biomechanics of the bone. Many cancer patients are in a catabolic state, and their nutrition is not be optimized. This will have an impact on the bone's ability to remodel and heal normally. Radiation and chemotherapy have an adverse effect on the bone's ability to repair and remodel itself (60). If a patient has osteopenia or osteoporosis, the structural properties of bone will be compromised. Hipp et al. evaluated the impact of lytic and blastic metastasis on the mechanical properties of bone. Both types of metastasis weakened the bone, but lytic lesions weakened the bone to a greater degree. Lytic lesions disrupted the mineral, organic, and structural components of the bone, leading to losses in strength and stiffness. Blastic lesions disrupted the trabecular framework of the bone, which was detrimental to the bone's overall stiffness and fatigue properties, while sparing bone strength (35). Small lytic lesions in the cortex cause an accumulation of stress in the bone surrounding the hole, which is known as a "stress riser." If a cortical lytic lesion measures 20% of the overall bone diameter, the bending strength of bone is reduced by 40% (48). If a lytic lesion is greater in size than the overall bone diameter, it is known as an "open section defect." Such a defect is associated with a 90% reduction in bending strength. Lytic lesions tend to be most detrimental to the bone's ability to withstand torsion. Torsional forces are applied when a person pivots or rises from a chair during transfers (48).

Impending Fractures

Prophylactic fixation of an impending fracture is preferable to fixing a pathologic fracture. It allows the procedure to be performed in a semi-elective setting without the sequelae of fracture, including pain, immobility, and hemorrhagic anemia. Zickel reported that prophylactic fixation of subtrochanteric fractures led to shorter hospital stays, earlier ambulation, and longer survival when compared with the group fixed after the fracture had occurred (78).

While most would agree with prophylactic fixation, there is little agreement on the proper criteria for an impending fracture. Snell and Beals considered a lytic femoral cortical lesion of 2.5 cm sufficient (72). Parrish and Murray felt that a lesion measuring at least 50% of the bone diameter and accompanied by increasing pain was an indication for surgery (58). Fidler reported that destruction of at least 50% of the cortex was an indication (18). In their study of subtrochanteric fractures,

Zickel and Mourandian concluded that the size of the lesion was not a useful predictor (78). Harrington proposed the following criteria for predicting fractures: (a) a lytic lesion greater than 2.5 cm in the proximal femur, (b) a lytic lesion involving more than 50% of the cortical bone circumferentially, and (c) avulsion of the lesser trochanter associated with a lytic lesion (30). However, Keene reported that lesions in the proximal femur were often difficult to measure, and in those lesions that could be measured, there was no correlation between size and fracture risk in the proximal femur (41).

Mirels proposed a weighted scoring system to help predict fracture (Table 37-1). He performed a retrospective review of 78 patients with breast cancer who were treated with irradiation but without prophylactic fixation. The scoring system is based on 4 categories. Each category has a possible score of 3, making a score of 12 the highest possible and 4 the lowest. The first criterion is the location of the metastasis. Three locations are possible, including the upper limb, lower limb, and peritrochanteric. Pain is the second criterion, and it is rated as mild, moderate, or functional (with weight bearing). The quality of the lesion is considered next. The lesion is described as blastic, mixed lytic and blastic, or purely lytic. The size of the lesion is the final criterion. A score of 1 is given if the lesion is less than one third the diameter of the bone on plain x-ray, a score of 2 is given for a lesion between one third and two thirds the diameter of the bone, and lesions greater than two thirds the diameter of the bone are given a score of 3. Two groups were formed in his study based on whether a fracture occurred or not. The nonfracture group had scores ranging from 4 to 9. The fracture group had scores ranging from 8 to 12. Mirel proposed that a score of 9 was associated with a significant risk of fracture (57%). Subset analysis of this study showed that functional pain was the most predictive of fracture. The author also noted that patients with functional pain had lesions greater than two thirds the diameter of the bone. The site of disease did not seem to be helpful in predicting fracture, and no patients with purely blastic lesions fractured (50). It is therefore apparent that in none of these systems are

TABLE 37-1

A WEIGHTED SCORING SYSTEM TO QUANTIFY THE RISK OF SUSTAINING A FRACTURE

Variable	Score 1	2	3
Site	Upper limb	Lower limb	Peritrochanteric
Pain	Mild	Moderate	Functional
Lesion	Blastic	Mixed	Lytic
Size	<1/3	1/3–2/3	>2/3

Score	Patients (N)	Fracture rate (%)
0–6	22	0
7	19	5
8	12	33
9	7	57
10–12	18	100

Adapted from Mirels H. Metastatic disease in long bones: a proposed scoring system for diagnosing impending pathologic fractures. *Clin Orthop.* 1989;249:256.

the recommendations entirely satisfactory, and they should be used merely as guidelines.

Hipp performed a biomechanical analysis of lytic lesions in the proximal femur using cadavers (34). He created the lesions and imaged them with plain films and CT scan. The cadaver hips were then stressed to failure. He then asked surgeons to evaluate the scans and describe the extent of the lytic lesions before predicting the loss in weight-bearing capacity of the bones. Only modest agreement existed between the surgeons in describing the extent of bone lysis. There was no relation between their estimated reduction in weight-bearing capacity and that measured in the laboratory (34). Hipp emphasized that the fracture risk was a function of the anticipated load applied to the bone and the capacity of the bone to bear weight. It thus becomes clear that load reduction by protected weight bearing is critical in helping to prevent fracture.

At Memorial Sloan Kettering, we use the following as a general guideline for prophylactic fixation in the proximal femur: (a) functional pain after radiotherapy; or (b) endosteal cortical destruction of greater than 50%; or (c) a cortical defect larger than the diameter of the bone or larger than 2.5 cm. Again, these are only guidelines, and the treatment of these patients must be individualized.

SURGICAL MANAGEMENT

Pathologic fractures about the hip are almost always treated surgically. The exceptions to this principle occur when the patient has less than 1 month to live and when the patient's general condition would prevent the patient from tolerating a surgical procedure. These patients should be treated with pain management and best supportive care.

The entire femur should be evaluated radiographically in order to determine the appropriate length of the prosthesis to be inserted. In addition, both humeri should be filmed, as strong upper limbs will be necessary for crutch ambulation. Embolization should be considered for renal and thyroid carcinoma.

In the case of solitary metastasis, the lesion should be biopsied to confirm the diagnosis. Wide resection of the proximal femur should follow. A long-stem proximal femoral replacement should be utilized for reconstruction.

Most lesions will be multicentric, and every effort should be made to remove as much tumor as possible. This helps to reduce tumor bulk and will thus improve the effectiveness of radiation therapy. Removing gross tumor will also help to reduce pain. Surgical adjuvants such as liquid nitrogen should

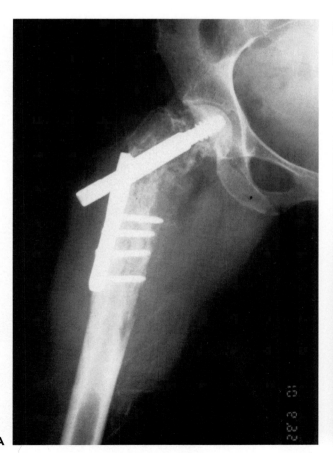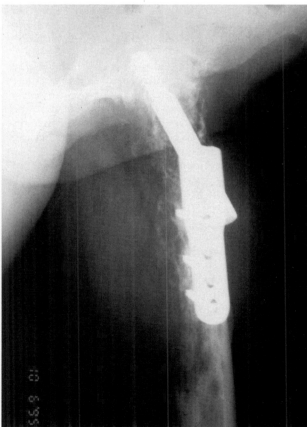

A   B

Figure 37-2 Anteroposterior **(A)** and lateral **(B)** radiographs of the proximal femur demonstrating loss of fixation and tumor progression in a patient with metastatic breast cancer. One year earlier the patient suffered a pathologic intertrochanteric fracture, which was stabilized with a sliding screw and side plate.

be considered. This is particularly true when the tumor has proven to be resistant to chemotherapy and radiotherapy. Residual tumor left behind can progress and lead to fixation failure, especially when a plate and screws are utilized for fixation (Fig. 37-2). Methylmethacrylate should be used liberally to help provide compressive strength and to secure intramedullary fixation. Methylmethacrylate is strongest in compression. It is ideally suited to help buttress the medial cortical bone of the proximal femur, which is most susceptible to compressive loads.

In a report of 24 transcervical fractures treated with a variety of fixation methods, none went on to union (23). Therefore, it is our recommendation that most transcervical fractures be treated with replacement rather than fixation. At Memorial Sloan Kettering we favor cemented, long-stem bipolar hemiarthroplasty for disease on the femoral side of the hip. We subscribe to the philosophy of "one bone, one operation" in this patient population. As mentioned previously, these patients are not considered curable. The patients are as healthy as they are likely going to be at the time you are seeing them. They may not be in a position to tolerate revision surgery at a later date.

Habermann found gross or microscopic disease of the acetabulum in 19 of 23 patients treated for femoral head and neck disease. He recommended total hip arthroplasty for all patients being treated for femoral head and neck disease. We recommend careful preoperative plain film and CT evaluation coupled with intraoperative inspection and finger palpation of the subchondral acetabular bone. If an acetabular deficiency is noted, then total hip arthroplasty should be considered (27).

Prior to reaming the femoral shaft and inserting methylmethacrylate into it, the medullar cavity should be vented with a 1/4-inch dill bit. Venting the femur helps to prevent fat and monomer embolization. The vent hole should be placed at least two medullary diameters above the final resting place of the prosthesis tip to prevent a stress riser from occurring (61). The anesthesiologist should be made aware that reaming and cement insertion are imminent and should optimize the patient's oxygenation and intravascular fluid volume (59).

Intertrochanteric Fractures

We favor joint replacement arthroplasty for intertrochanteric hip fractures (44). However, there are advocates for open curettage, replacement of defects with methylmethacrylate, and stabilization with plate and screws. If this last method is used, it is important to replace medial cortical defects with methylmethacrylate to prevent fixation failure. The hip screw should be inserted prior to cement polymerization. Again, we favor cemented long-stem bipolar hemiarthroplasty after curettage of gross tumor. Excision of the head and neck eliminates these areas as potential sources of tumor invasion and failure. The long cemented stem also achieves three-point fixation and prophylactically stabilizes the entire femur, making failure unlikely. To achieve optimal hip function, every attempt is made to preserve the muscular attachments to the proximal femur. This is accomplished by preserving the outer shell of bone in the proximal femur. A trochanteric claw and cables may be necessary.

Subtrochanteric Fractures

Subtrochanteric fractures pose a particularly difficult problem with regard to fracture reduction (Fig. 37-3). We recommend open curettage followed by direct reduction using bony landmarks as a guide to appropriate realignment. The femur should be reamed and methylmethacrylate inserted into the bony defects left after curettage. Satisfactory results have been reported using intramedullary fixation rods (27,78). However, for the reasons previously outlined, we recommend long-stem hemiarthroplasty in most of these cases (Fig. 37-4).

If the bone destruction is particularly severe, then proximal femoral replacement should be performed (Fig. 37-5).

Acetabular Fractures

Metastasis to the pelvis is common, for reasons described earlier. When painful lesions are found in the ilium and pubic rami, they can usually be managed with radiation and protected weight bearing. Pathologic fractures in the weight-bearing portions of the pelvis and acetabulum can be very difficult to manage. Frequently there is extensive bony destruction, making reconstruction difficult. Further, these lesions have often been irradiated, making healing less likely. If no tumor can be identified on CT scan, then postirradiation fracture ought to be considered in the differential diagnosis (12).

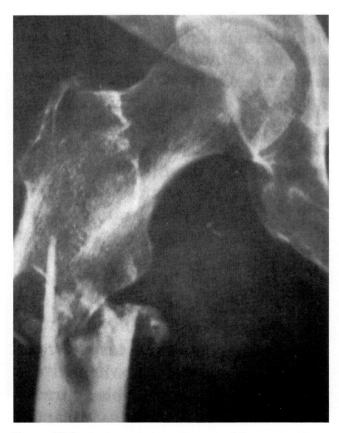

Figure 37-3 Anteroposterior radiograph of the proximal femur showing a pathologic subtrochanteric fracture.

volved with tumor. In class 1 lesions, a cemented total hip arthroplasty is the preferred method of treatment. The subchondral bone should be accessed through a cortical window created to allow the advancement of a curette to facilitate tumor removal. Methylmethacrylate can be inserted into the bony defect left after tumor curettage. The acetabular component can be placed in its usual position, resting on the intact cortices of the acetabulum. Fixation can be reinforced with long acetabular screws.

Class 2 lesions can be managed using some of the principles applied to protrusio acetabuli. In these lesions, the acetabular rim is intact. A flanged acetabular cup should be utilized to transfer loads to the intact acetabular rim and away from the medial wall. A barrier such as wire mesh should be inserted into the medial defect to prevent extravasation of cement into the pelvis.

Class 3 lesions involve the medial wall, superior dome, and lateral cortices, and they pose a particularly difficult problem for the reconstructive surgeon. Again, the key to stabilization is to transfer loads from the areas involved with tumor to the

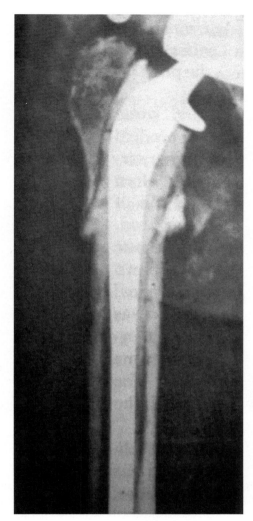

Figure 37-4 Postoperative radiograph following resection of the femoral head and neck and stabilization of the fracture with a long stem, bipolar prosthesis, and methylmethacrylate.

These patients usually complain of groin pain made worse with ambulation. Passive range of motion of the hip may not elicit pain if no tumor is present on the femoral side of the hip. If untreated, these tumors will progress to fracture, with significant migration of the femoral head a possible sequela.

Initially, these patients can be treated with protected weight bearing and radiation therapy. Cheng et al. reported success with conservative treatment alone (8). Surgical treatment is indicated if pain persists after at least 4 weeks of conservative management, a coexisting femoral lesion requires surgery, or a displaced fracture or fracture–dislocation occurs.

Harrington placed metastatic lesions of the acetabulum into three classes based on whether the lateral, superior, and/or medial cortices of the acetabulum are intact (29). In class 1 lesions, the trabecular bone about the acetabulum is involved with tumor, but all three cortices remain intact. In class 2 lesions, there is destruction of the medial wall of the acetabulum. Class 3 lesions involve all three cortices of the acetabulum.

Principles of surgical fixation are based on transferring loads from the areas involved with tumor into areas unin-

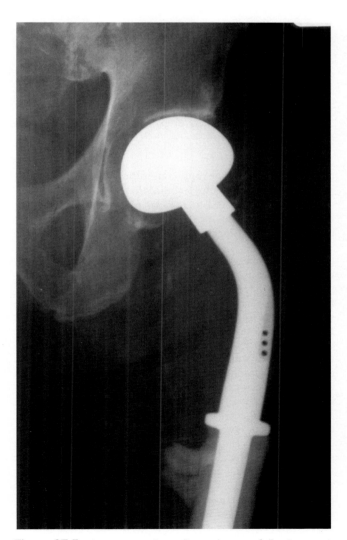

Figure 37-5 Anteroposterior radiograph status following proximal femoral replacement.

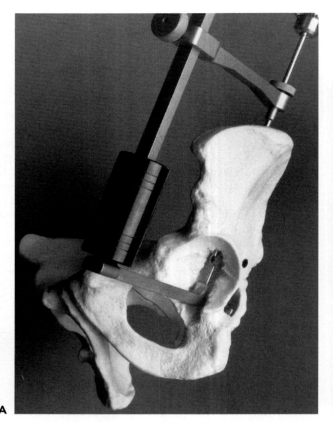
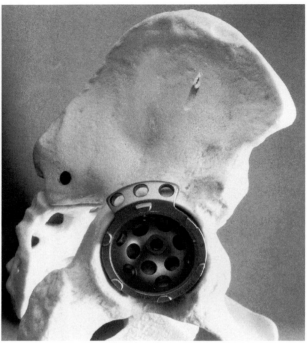

A   B

Figure 37-6 **A:** Targeting device used for inserting a pin from the iliac crest to the deficient posterior acetabulum. **B:** Healey flanged protrusio cup (Biomet, Warsaw, IN).

areas not involved. We apply a modification of the method proposed by Harrington to stabilize these lesions.

The patient is placed in a lateral position with his or her waste over the break in the table. Flexion of the table will allow better access of the iliac crest. The leg should be prepped free, and the skin well above iliac crest should be included in the prep. A posterolateral incision with an extended posterior arm to allow better acetabular visualization is used. Careful exposure of the bone surrounding the acetabulum will often reveal large defects. All gross tumor is removed. Significant bleeding should be anticipated prior to this portion of the procedure. Rapid removal of gross tumor followed by packing of the defects is done to minimize blood loss. The argon beam coagulator is also useful in controlling surface bony bleeding. Further, the temporary insertion of methylmethacrylate can serve as an effective hemostatic maneuver. Harrington recommends inserting pins or screws in a retrograde fashion into the overlying healthy bone. This effectively transfers the forces generated at the hip articulation to the overlying healthy bone. If there are defects in the superior dome only, then we also insert our pins or screws in a retrograde fashion. However, for more extensive lesions, we utilize an antegrade insertion technique starting at the iliac crest. Anterior and posterior incisions are made over the iliac crest. Large threaded Steinmann pins are inserted in an antegrade fashion into the lateral wall of the hemipelvis. The pins are inserted so that they traverse the deficient areas, thereby stabilizing them. The anterior and posterior columns are reconstructed in this manner. A guide can be used to help insert the

pins into appropriate position (Fig. 37-6). While the pins are being inserted, care must be taken to protect the sciatic nerve in the sciatic notch. Methylmethacrylate is then packed around the pins. Insufficiencies of the medial acetabular wall are reconstructed with a cemented, flanged acetabular cup (46) (Fig. 37-7). A femoral component is placed using techniques outlined previously. Radiation therapy is started 2 to 3 weeks after surgery if the wound is healing well.

Harrington reported a retrospective review of 59 patients with metastatic disease to the acetabulum. The mean survival was 29 months. After 6 months, 37 of the remaining 51 patients reported minimal to no pain. Fifty-four patients were ambulating with or without a gait aid in the immediate postoperative period. Five patients developed component loosening as a result of tumor progression (29).

Marco et al. reported the experience at Memorial Sloan Kettering with the use of a modified Harrington technique (46). After 3 months, 41 of 55 patients survived, and 83% demonstrated significant pain reduction. Ambulation was restored in 9 of 18 patients who were bedridden prior to surgery. Fourteen of 17 patients maintained their ability to ambulate in the community. Twenty-one patients had more than 1 year follow-up. Fourteen (67%) of those patients continued to experience pain relief, and 12 (57%) remained ambulatory in the community or household. This study demonstrated that, despite a relatively short life expectancy following surgery, the positive effect on overall function and pain relief validated surgical intervention in this patient population.

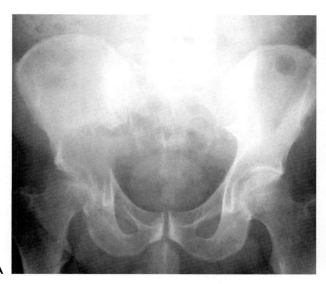 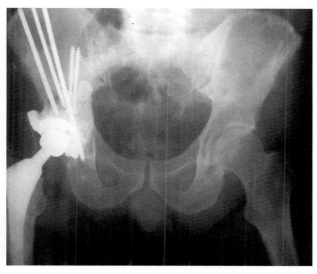

Figure 37-7 A: Metastatic carcinoma with marked destruction of the acetabulum. **B:** Reconstruction with pins, screws, methylmethacrylate, and a total hip arthroplasty using a flanged acetabular cup.

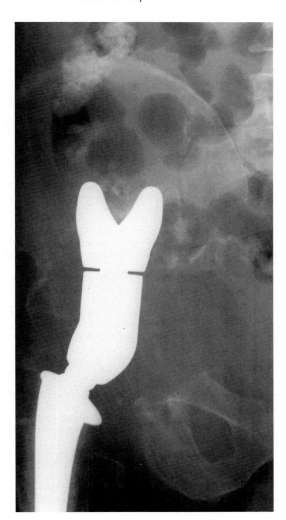

Figure 37-8 A saddle prosthesis (Waldermar-Link, Hamburg, Germany) used to reconstruct the hip following curettage of extensive metastatic disease.

At times, the extent of bony destruction is such that the only reconstructive options are a saddle prosthesis (Waldemar Link, Hamburg, Germany) (Fig. 37-8) and resection arthroplasty. These techniques may be helpful in select patients with intermediate-term life expectancy.

Finally, nerve blocks and anterolateral cordotomy should be considered in patients with intractable pain who are not surgical candidates (1).

REFERENCES

1. Arbit E, ed. *Management of Cancer Related Pain*. Mt. Kisco, NY: Futura; 1993.
2. Arcangeli G, Giovinazzo G, Saracino B, et al. Radiation therapy in the management of symptomatic bone metastases: the effect of total dose and histology on pain relief and response duration. *Int J Radiat Oncol Biol Phys*. 1998;42:1119.
3. Batson O. The role of the vertebral veins in the spread of metastasis. *Ann Intern Med*. 1942;16:38–45.
4. Blitzer P. Reanalysis of the RTOG study of the palliation of symptomatic osseous metastasis. *Cancer*. 1985;55:1468.
5. Bonarigo BC, Rubin P. Nonunion of pathologic fractures after radiation therapy. *Radiology*. 1967;88:889–898.
6. Burstein AH, Zika JM, Heiple KG, et al. Contribution of collagen and mineral to the elastic-plastic properties of bone. *J Bone Joint Surg*. 1975;57:956.
7. Bury T, Barreto A, Daenen F, et al. Fluorine-18 deoxyglucose positron emission tomography for the detection of bone metastases in patients with non-small cell lung cancer. *Eur J Nucl Med*. 1998;25:1244–1247.
8. Cheng DS, Seitz CB, Eyre HJ. Nonoperative management of femoral, humeral and acetabular metastasis in patients with breast cancer. *Cancer*. 1980;45:1533–1537.
9. Citrin DL, Bessent RG, Greig WR. A comparison of the sensitivity and accuracy of the 99TCm-phosphate bone scan and skeletal radiograph in the diagnosis of bone metastases. *Clin Radiol*. 1977;28:107–117.
10. Citrin DL, Tormey DC, Carbone PP. Implications of the 99mTc diphosphonate bone scan on treatment of primary breast cancer. *Cancer Treat Rep*. 1977;61:1249–1252, .
11. Cleeland CS. The impact of pain on the patient with cancer. *Cancer*. 1984;54[11 Suppl]:2635–2641.
12. Cooper KL, Beabout JW, Swee RG. Insufficiency fractures of the sacrum. *Radiology*. 1985;156:15–20.

13. Crippa F, Seregni E, Agresti R, et al. Bone scintigraphy in breast cancer: a ten-year follow-up study. *J Nucl Biol Med.* 1993;37(2): 57–61.
14. Cumming JD, Nutt ME. Bone-marrow blood flow and cardiac output in the rabbit. *J Physiol (Paris).* 1962;162:30–34.
15. de la Mata J, Uy HL, Guise TA, et al. Interleukin-6 enhances hypercalcemia and bone resorption mediated by parathyroid hormone-related protein in vivo. *J Clin Invest.* 1995;95:2846–2852.
16. Didolkar MS, Fanous N, Elias EG, et al. Metastatic carcinomas from occult primary tumors: a study of 254 patients. *Ann Surg.* 1977;186:625–630.
17. Ewing J, ed. *Neoplastic Diseases.* Philadelphia: Saunders; 1928.
18. Fidler M. Incidence of fracture through metastasis in bones. *Acta orthop Scand.* 1981;52:623–627.
19. Finkelstein JA, Zaveri G, Wai E, et al. A population-based study of surgery for spinal metastases: survival rates and complications. *J Bone Joint Surg [Br].* 2003;85:1045–1050.
20. Gainor B, Buchart P. Fracture healing in metastatic bone disease. *Clin orthop.* 1983;178:297.
21. Galasko CS. The detection of skeletal metastases from mammary cancer by gamma camera scintigraphy. *Br J Surg.* 1969;56: 757–764.
22. Galasko CS. Diagnosis of skeletal metastases and assessment of response to treatment. *Clin Orthop Relat Res.* 1995;312:64–75.
23. Galasko CS. Pathologic fractures secondary to metastatic cancer. *J R Coll Surg Edinb.* 1974;19:351–362.
24. Galasko CS. Skeletal metastases and mammary cancer. *Ann R Coll Surg Engl.* 1972;50:3–28.
25. Galasko CS. The value of scintigraphy in malignant disease. *Cancer Treat Rev.* 1975;2:225–272.
26. Galasko CS, Burn JI. Hypercalcaemia in patients with advanced mammary cancer. *Br Med J.* 1971;3(774):573–577.
27. Habermann ET, Sachs R, Stern RE, et al. The pathology and treatment of metastatic disease of the femur. *Clin Orthop Relat Res.* 1982;169:70–82.
28. Hamaoka T, Madewell JE, Podoloff DA, et al. Bone imaging in metastatic breast cancer. *J Clin Oncol.* 2004;22:2942–2953.
29. Harrington K. The management of acetabular insufficiency secondary to metastatic malignant disease. *J Bone Joint Surg [Am].* 1981;63A:653–664.
30. Harrington K, ed. *Metastatic Bone Disease.* St. Louis: Mosby; 1988.
31. Harrington K. Orthopaedic Management of extremity and pelvic lesions. *Clin Orthop.* 1995;312:136–147.
32. Haubold-Reuter BG, Duewell S, Schilcher BR, et al. The value of bone scintigraphy, bone marrow scintigraphy and fast spin-echo magnetic resonance imaging in staging of patients with malignant solid tumours: a prospective study. *Eur J Nucl Med.* 1993;20: 1063–1069.
33. Higinbotham NL, Marcove RC. The management of pathological fractures. *J Trauma.* 1965;5:792–798.
34. Hipp J. Predicting pathologic fracture risk in the management of metastatic bone defects. *Clin Orthop.* 1995;312:120–135.
35. Hipp J, Rosenberg A, Hayes W. Mechanical properties of trabecular bone within and adjacent to osseous metastasis. *J Bone Miner Res.* 1992;7:1165.
36. Hortobagyi GN, Theriault RL, Lipton A, et al. Long-term prevention of skeletal complications of metastatic breast cancer with pamidronate. Protocol 19 Aredia Breast Cancer Study Group. *J Clin Oncol.* 1998;16: 2038–2044.
37. Hynes NE, Lane HA. ERBB receptors and cancer: the complexity of targeted inhibitors. *Nat Rev Cancer.* 2005;5:341–354.
38. Jaffe H, ed. *Tumors and Tumorous Conditions of Bones and Joints.* Philadelphia, Lea & Febiger, 1958.
39. Janne PA, Engelman JA, Johnson BE. Epidermal growth factor receptor mutations in non-small-cell lung cancer: implications for treatment and tumor biology. *J Clin Oncol.* 2005;23:3227–3234.
40. Jemal A, Murray T, Ward E, et al. Cancer statistics, 2005. *CA Cancer J Clin.* 2005;55:10–30.
41. Keene JS, Sclinger BS, McBeath AA, et al. Metastatic breast cancer in the femur: a search for the lesion at risk for fracture. *Clin Orthop.* 1986;203:282–288.
42. Koizumi M, Yoshimoto M, Kasumi F, et al. Comparison between solitary and multiple skeletal metastasis lesions of breast cancer patients. *Ann Oncol.* 2003;14:1234–1240.
43. Kurihara N, Bertolini D, Suda T, et al. IL-6 stimulates osteoclast-like multinucleated cell formation in long term human marrow cultures by inducing IL-1 release. *J Immunol.* 1990;144: 4226–4230.
44. Lane JM, Sculco TP, Zolan S. Treatment of pathologic fractures of the hip by endoprosthetic replacement. *J Bone Joint Surg.* 1980;62A: 954–959.
45. Lipton A, Small E, Saad F, et al. The new bisphosphonate, Zometa (zoledronic acid), decreases skeletal complications in both osteolytic and osteoblastic lesions: a comparison to pamidronate. *Cancer Invest.* 2002;20[Suppl 2]:45–54.
46. Marco RA, Sheth DS, Boland PJ, et al. Functional and oncological outcome of acetabular reconstruction for the treatment of metastatic disease. *J Bone Joint Surg [Am].* 2000;82:642–651.
47. Matsubrayshi TK, Koga H, Nishiyama Y, et al. The reparative process of metastatic bone lesions after radiotherapy. *Jpn J Clin Oncol.* 1981;11:253–264.
48. McBroom RC, Cheal E, Hayes W. Strength reductions from metastatic cortical defects in long bones. *J Orthop Res.* 1988;6:369.
49. McMillan JH, Levine E, Stephens RH. Computed tomography in the evaluation of metastatic adenocarcinoma from an unknown primary site: a retrospective study. *Radiology.* 1982;143:143–146.
50. Mirels H. Metastatic disease in long bones. *Clin Orthop.* 1989;No. 249:256–264.
51. Moertel CG. Adenocarcinoma of unknown origin. *Ann Intern Med.* 1979;91:646–647.
52. Mundy GR. Hypercalcemia of malignancy revisited. *J Clin Invest.* 1988;82:1–6.
53. Mundy GR. Metastasis to bone: causes, consequences and therapeutic opportunities. *Nat Rev Cancer.* 2002;2:584–93.
54. Nathan SS, Healey JH, Mellano D, et al. Survival in patients operated on for pathologic fracture: implications for end-of-life orthopedic care. *J Clin Oncol.* 2005;23:6072–6082.
55. Nissenblatt MJ. The CUP syndrome (carcinoma unknown primary). *Cancer Treat Rev.* 1981;8:211–224.
56. Nystrom JS, Weiner JM, Wolf RM, et al. Identifying the primary site in metastatic cancer of unknown origin: inadequacy of roentgenographic procedures. *JAMA.* 1979;241:381–383.
57. Paget S. The distribution of secondary growths in cancer of the breast. *Lancet.* 1889;1:571–573.
58. Parrish FM, Murray JA. Surgical treatment of secondary neoplastic fractures: a retrospective study of ninety-six patients. *J Bone Joint Surg [Am].* 1970;52A:665–686.
59. Patterson BH, Healey JH, Cornell CN, et al. Cardiac arrest during hip arthroplasty with cement. *J Bone Joint Surg [Am].* 1991;73A:271–277.
60. Pelker RF, Friedlander G, Panjabi M, et al. Chemotherapy-induced alterations in the biomechanics of rat bone. *J Orthop Res.* 1985;3:91.
61. Pellicci PS, Sakati EA, Wilson PD. Revision arthroplasty of the hip. In: *Surgery of the Musculoskeletal System.* New York: Churchill Livingstone; 1990:3083–3115.
62. Plunkett TA, Smith P, Rubens RD. Risk of complications from bone metastases in breast cancer. implications for management. *Eur J Cancer.* 2000;36:476–482.
63. Powell GJ, Southby J, Danks JA, et al. Localization of parathyroid hormone-related protein in breast cancer metastases: increased incidence in bone compared with other sites. *Cancer Res.* 1991;51:3059–3061.
64. Ralston SH, Gallacher SJ, Patel U, et al. Cancer-associated hypercalcemia: morbidity and mortality: clinical experience in 126 treated patients. *Ann Intern Med.* 1990;112:499–504.
65. Reilly DB, Burstein A, Frankel V, et al. The elastic modulus for bone. *J Biomech.* 1974;7:271.
66. Rizzo PF, Gould E, Lyden JP, et al. Diagnosis of occult fractures about the hip: magnetic resonance imaging compared with bone-scanning. *J Bone Joint Surg.* 1993;75:1879.
67. Rougraff BT. Evaluation of the patient with carcinoma of unknown origin metastatic to bone. *Clin Orthop Relat Res.* 2003; 415(suppl):S105–109.
68. Rougraff BT, Kneisl JS, Simon MA. Skeletal metastases of unknown origin: a prospective study of a diagnostic strategy. *J Bone Joint Surg [Am].* 1993;75:1276–1281.
69. Schneiderbauer MM, von Knoch M, Schleck C, et al. Patient survival after hip arthroplasty for metastatic disease of the hip. *J Bone Joint Surg [Am].* 2004;86A:1684–1689.

70. Silverberg E. Cancer statistics, 1986. *CA Cancer J Clin.* 1986;36:9–25.
71. Simon MA, Bartucci EJ. The search for the primary tumor in patients with skeletal metastases of unknown origin. *Cancer.* 1986;58:1088–1095.
72. Snell WB, Beals RK. Femoral metastasis and fractures from breast cancer. *Surg Gynecol Obstet.* 1964;119:22–24.
73. Stewart AF. Clinical practice: hypercalcemia associated with cancer. *N Engl J Med.* 2005;352:373–379.
74. Theriault RL, Lipton A, Hortobagyi GN, et al. Pamidronate reduces skeletal morbidity in women with advanced breast cancer and lytic bone lesions: a randomized, placebo-controlled trial. Protocol 18 Aredia Breast Cancer Study Group. *J Clin Oncol.* 1999;17:846–854.
75. Tibes R, Trent J, Kurzrock R. Tyrosine kinase inhibitors and the dawn of molecular cancer therapeutics. *Annu Rev Pharmacol Toxicol.* 2005;45:357–384.
76. Tong DG, L, Hendrickson F. The palliation of symptomatic osseous metastases: final results of the study by the Radiation Therapy Oncology Group. *Cancer.* 1982;50:893.
77. Vargha ZG, A, Boland J. Single-dose radiation therapy in the palliation of metastatic disease. *Radiology.* 1969;93:1181.
78. Zickel RM, WH. Intramedullary fixation of pathologic fractures and lesions of the subtrochanteric region of the femur. *J Bone Joint Surg.* 1976;58A:1061–1066.

Arthritis and Allied Conditions

38

Calvin R. Brown, Jr.

PRINCIPLES OF INFLAMMATION

The human immune system consists of a number of cell types and organs that, because they act as a defense against infection by pathogenic microorganisms, are essential for our survival. Although an individual's immune system can respond to an almost unlimited number of foreign antigens, it does not normally respond to the individual's own tissues. This property, known as "self-tolerance," is a fundamental feature of normal immune function (12). When self-tolerance fails, the resulting autoimmune reaction can be the basis for many arthritic disorders that may affect the hip.

INFLAMMATORY CELLS

The cells of the immune system originate from pluripotent stem cells and through differentiation give rise to the lymphoid and myeloid lineage (45). Specificity within the immune system is provided by lymphocytes, which express a large number of different molecules on their surfaces. These molecules interact with specific antigens, allowing lymphocytes to distinguish between self and nonself. This specific immune response can be further subdivided into cellular and humoral systems. Humoral immune responses depend on antibody molecules secreted by lymphocytes of the B-cell lineage. Cellular immune responses are independent of immunoglobulins and are primarily directed by T lymphocytes.

The myeloid lineage consists of monocytes (macrophages) and neutrophils, which provide nonspecific inflammatory mediators and phagocytic function. In addition, monocytes and certain other cells are specialized to present foreign antigens to T cells and thus contribute to specific immune responses (31).

Although the immune system protects the individual against invasion by agents that are perceived as foreign, in many diseases the immune system can be injurious to the organism. In some cases, this immunopathology is an unavoidable byproduct of the immune system's attack of an infectious organism or other antigen, such as in septic arthritis and gout, respectively. Immune injury can also result from inappropriate targeting by the immune system of self components, which results from failure of normal regulation (12). Several potential mechanisms could result in autoimmunity, although most of these possibilities have yet to be demonstrated in human disease (13).

INFLAMMATORY MEDIATORS

Once the immune response has been initiated, cells of the immune response need to communicate in order to coordinate the subsequent inflammatory response. This communication is accomplished through two sets of molecules—a series of cell surface adhesion molecules that regulate communication between cells that are in direct contact and a series of soluble proteins, the cytokines, that allow communication between cells that are in proximity but do not directly contact each other (47). There are at least 20 molecules in each series already identified, and the number continues to increase, indicating the multitude and complexity of these interactions (4).

Stimuli leading to inflammation cause the release of arachidonic acid from membrane phospholipids and the oxidation of arachidonic acid to prostaglandins, leukotrienes, and thromboxanes, which are collectively known as "eicosanoids."

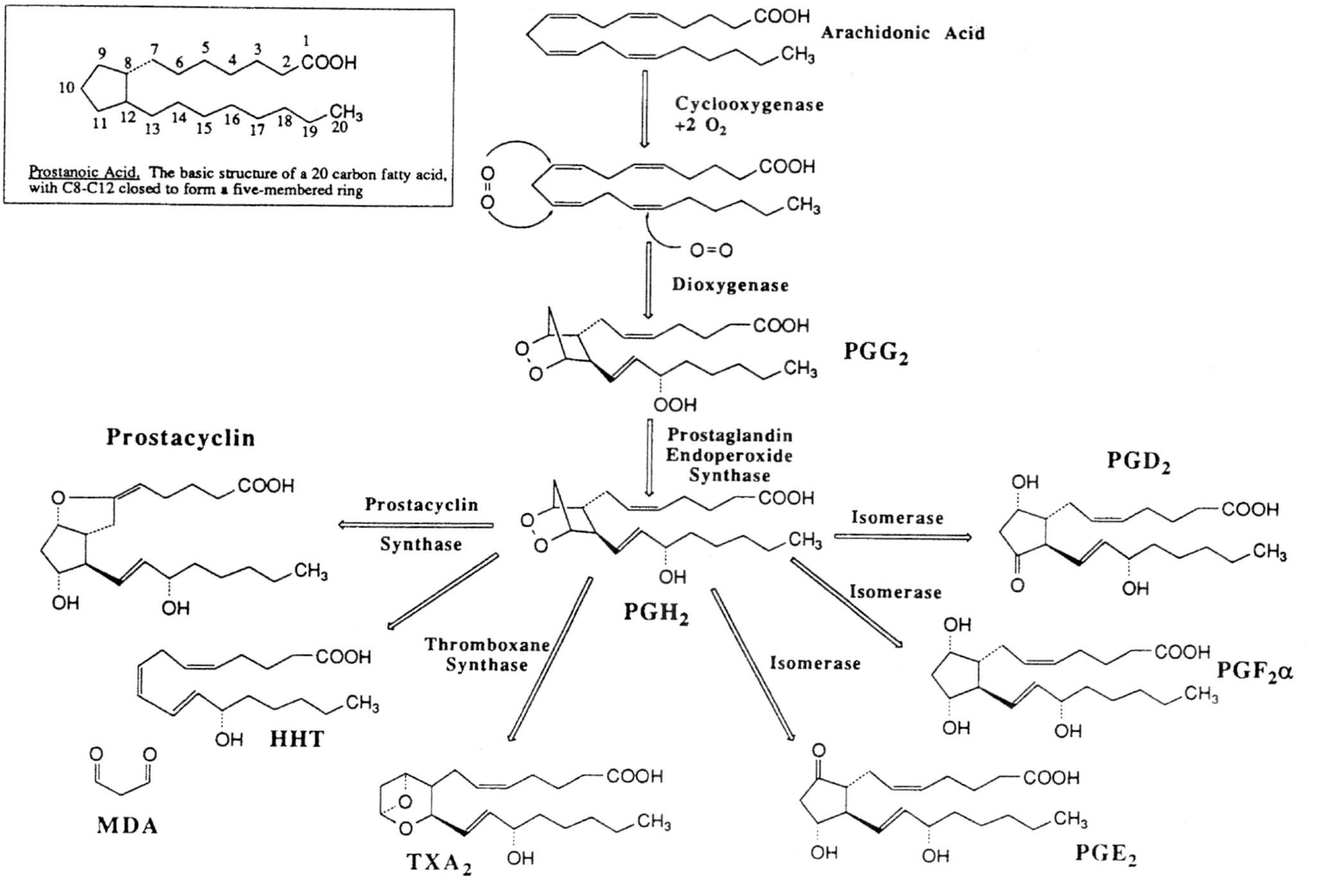

Figure 38-1 The cyclooxygenase pathway of arachidonic acid metabolism.

Arachidonic acid is converted to prostaglandin E_2 (PGE$_2$) (Fig. 38-1). Recent evidence indicates that there are at least two distinct cyclooxygenase enzymes. The previously known cyclooxygenase 1 is constitutively produced and is necessary for normal function of several organs, for example, stomach and kidney. The newly discovered cyclooxygenase 2 is inducible by inflammatory cytokines, and it is found primarily in inflammatory cells (22). Most (if not all) current nonsteroidal anti-inflammatory drugs (NSAIDs) block both cyclooxygenases and can therefore lead to gastrointestinal complications. Currently, a new class of NSAIDs is being sought that will inhibit only the inducible cyclooxygenase, thus avoiding the side effects of the current NSAIDs. Different types of cells may produce predominantly one type of prostaglandin. Prostaglandin E_2 appears to be the major cyclooxygenase product derived from human rheumatoid synovial cells.

Arachidonic acid can also be metabolized via the lipoxygenase pathway (Fig. 38-2). The lipoxygenases have a limited tissue distribution, predominantly in platelets and myeloid cells (29). Although specific inhibitors of lipoxygenase are not currently available, they are being studied for possible clinical use. A variety of cytokines are able to influence the ability of cells to produce eicosanoids, and they probably act as the communication between specific immunity and the inflammatory response.

There are a wide variety of other mediators, including histamine, serotonin, and components of the complement and coagulation systems. Inflammation is also accompanied by the cellular release of enzymes known as proteinases that can degrade connective tissue and extracellular matrix. More detailed understanding of immune system function has resulted in elucidation of multiple cytokines, small molecular weight proteins that mediate communication between cells. This system is normally self-regulated; however, pathophysiologic consequences, resulting in inflammatory arthritis, may arise from unregulated action or inappropriate production of a particular cytokine. Understanding of this system and the chemical nature of these molecules has lead to development of a therapeutic class of particularly effective treatments, known as "biologic response modulators," that inhibit cytokines through various strategies (14).

CLINICAL CONDITIONS OF THE HIP

Approach to the Patient

With few exceptions, any joint disorder may initially present in the hip. Arthritis of the hip can therefore present a diagnostic challenge to even the most experienced clinician, and in

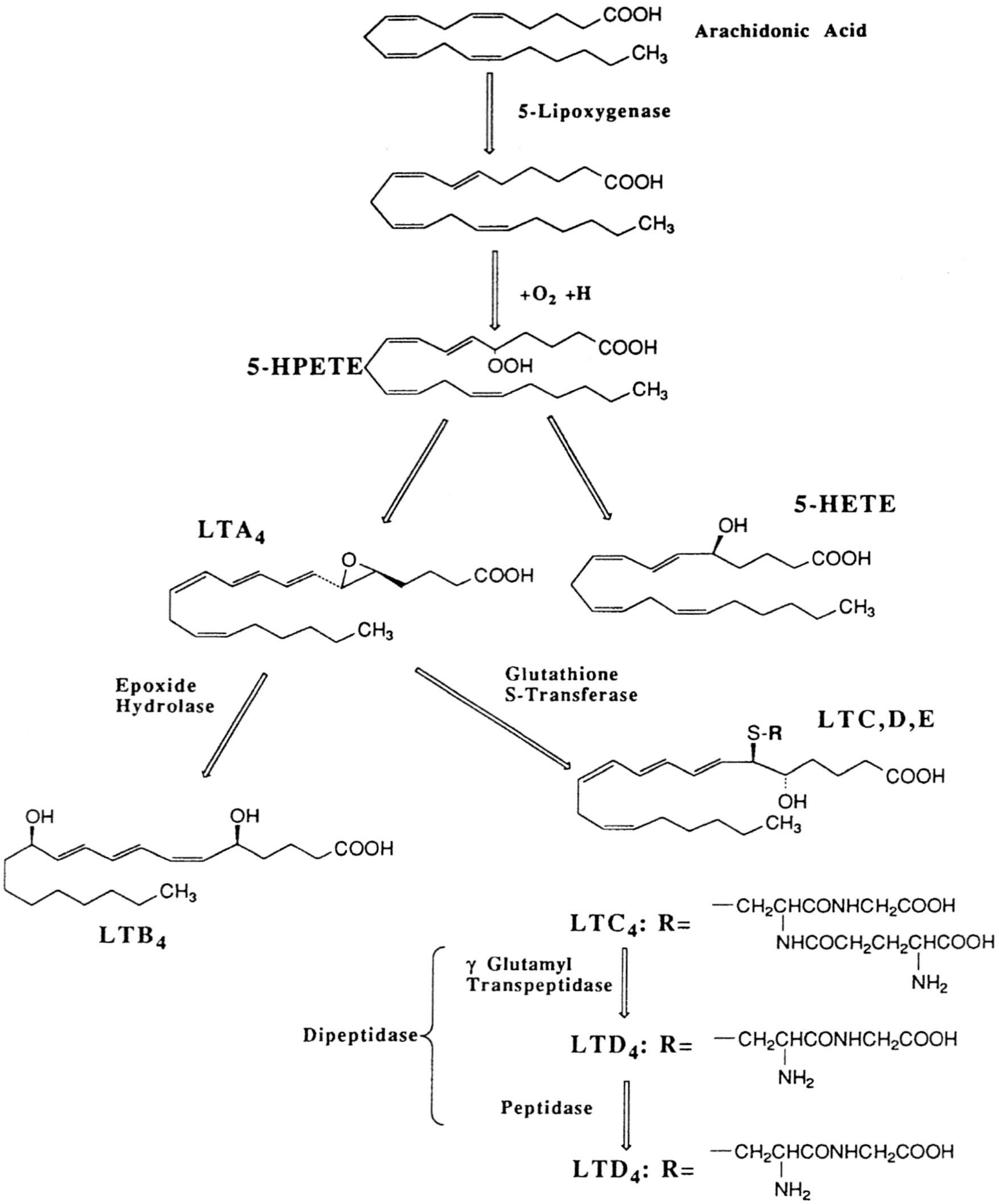

Figure 38-2   The 5-lipoxygenase pathway of arachidonic acid metabolism.

some cases it can remain incompletely understood even after a thorough evaluation. Fortunately, it is almost always possible to identify those patients who require vigorous evaluation and treatment to prevent rapid disease progression.

Confronted with a patient with pain in the hip, the physician must be sure to localize the hip joint as the anatomic site of the abnormality. Bone pain, tendonitis or bursitis, neuropathic or referred pain, and soft-tissue infections can simulate

arthritis and must be differentiated. The most important issue in evaluating hip complaints is whether the hip joint is the sole site of involvement (monoarthritis) or is occurring in the setting of multiple joint involvement (polyarthritis), and distinct differential diagnoses can be deduced based on this characterization (2). Another important fact to obtain with the history is the acuity of onset. Extremely rapid onset of pain (over seconds or minutes) suggests a fracture, loose body, or trauma.

Acute onset over several hours to 1 week is typical of most forms of inflammatory arthritis, particularly bacterial infection and crystal-induced synovitis, whereas a more protracted onset suggests structural disease. Finally, determining whether the underlying process is mechanical or inflammatory is very useful. This question is most reliably answered by a synovial fluid white blood cell count, and, whenever possible, attempts to obtain fluid should be made. But because the hip is not readily accessible to aspiration, historical patterns are again useful. Waxing and waning of disease activity unrelated to patterns of use, morning stiffness, and gelling suggest inflammation. Pain that occurs only after use, improves with rest, and involves weight bearing suggests mechanical disease (39).

Combining the historical factors above with the number of involved joints allows the generation of a more concise differential diagnosis. For example, acute inflammatory monoarthritis of the hip deserves special attention because immediate benefit may result from identification and treatment of the underlying disease. In most cases, a working diagnosis of infection, crystal-induced arthritis, or onset of a potentially chronic inflammatory arthritis will be made.

Whereas constitutional symptoms and a remote source of infection suggest septic arthritis, a history of recurrent self-limited attacks suggests crystal-induced arthritis. Chronic monoarticular inflammation raises special concern for chronic infections or tumors. Noninflammatory monoarticular arthritis of the hip implies structural disease, most commonly osteoarthritis. Exceptions to this include young patients, in whom dysplasia, slipped epiphysis, or spontaneous osteonecrosis should be suspected. Sudden onset of symptoms should arouse suspicion of the possibility of fracture related to osteopenia, adjacent destructive process such as tumor, or avascular necrosis (34). An algorithmic approach to the patient with symptoms in one or several joints is summarized in Figure 38-3. The approach to a patient with symptoms in many (more than five) joints (referred to as polyarthralgia) is summarized algorithmically in Figure 38-4.

Arthritis of the hip in the setting of other joint involvement implies polyarthritis. Careful inquiry may be necessary to elicit evidence of antecedent or coincident involvement of additional joints. A history of inflammatory symptoms in multiple joints for more than a month suggests a chronic

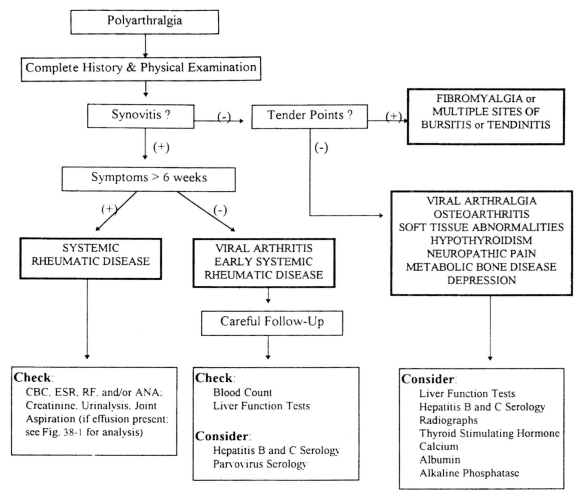

Figure 38-3 An initial approach to the patient with polyarticular joint symptoms. CBC, complete blood cell count; ESR, erythrocyte sedimentation rate; RF, rheumatoid factor; ANA, antinuclear antibodies.

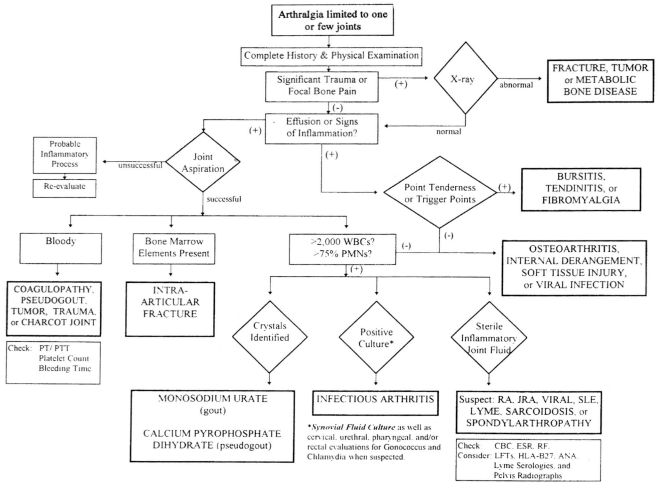

Figure 38-4 An initial approach to the patient with symptoms in one or a few joints. The majority of diagnoses will be determined by the history and physical examination. WBCs, white blood cells; PMNs, polymorphonuclear neutrophils; PT, prothrombin time; PTT, partial thromboplastin time; RA, rheumatoid arthritis; JRA, juvenile rheumatoid arthritis; SLE, systemic lupus erythematosus; CBC, complete blood cell count; ESR, erythrocyte sedimentation rate; RF, rheumatoid factor; LFTs, liver function tests; ANA, antinuclear antibodies.

inflammatory arthritis. Multiple arthralgias of short duration may accompany the onset of many illnesses. Truly migratory disease suggests gonococcal infection or rheumatic fever. The patient should be specifically questioned about recurrent pain or morning stiffness in the low back. Sacroiliitis with radiographic changes suggests ankylosing spondylitis or Reiter disease (see later). Spondylitis is usually clinically apparent before the development of associated structural disease of the hip. Polyarticular peripheral arthritis usually represents rheumatoid arthritis. Psoriatic arthritis, the arthritis associated with psoriasis, is distinguished by a characteristic skin rash and the fact that there is usually involvement of just a few joints. Last, like noninflammatory monoarthritis, noninflammatory polyarthritis implies osteoarthritis (39).

Osteoarthritis

Osteoarthritis (OA) is the most common cause of musculoskeletal pain and disability. It has been estimated that 2% to 3% of the adult population suffer regular pain from OA. In

addition to the hip, the main joints involved by OA are the hand, foot, and knee (17). About one third of adults in the United States between 25 and 74 years of age have radiographic evidence of OA involving at least one of these sites, the prevalence rising directly with age (Table 38-1). The prevalence of

TABLE 38-1

PREVALENCE OF RADIOGRAPHIC OSTEOARTHRITIS IN THE HIP

Age	Sex	Prevalence
<55	Men	1%
	Women	1%
55–65	Men	3%
	Women	2%
>65	Men	6%
	Women	4%

hip OA has a linear association with age, and it has roughly equal incidence in both sexes (or possibly a modest male preponderance). Although OA is worldwide in distribution, hip OA is said to be relatively uncommon in some African and Asian populations.

The risk factors for OA can be divided into those that appear to reflect a generalized predisposition to the disorder and those that reflect abnormal biomechanical loading at the hip. Generalized susceptibility is reflected by the age association, positive family history, diabetes, and hypertension. Local biomechanical factors include associations with abnormalities in joint shape (resulting from congenital or acquired abnormalities in joint shape, such as congenital dislocations of the hip), Legg-Calvé-Perthes disease, and slipped capital epiphysis. Surprisingly, obesity has not proven to be associated with hip OA, as it has with knee OA. Osteoporosis and smoking appear to have a negative association, slightly decreasing the risk (44).

Osteoarthritis is a disorder of the entire joint, involving the cartilage, bone synovium, and capsule. Opinion varies as to which of these tissue components is most important in the pathogenesis of the condition, but there is general agreement that the articular cartilage is the most obvious target tissue. Focal areas of damage to the integrity of the articular cartilage with fibrillation and loss of volume are one of the main hallmarks of OA. Mechanical factors clearly play a major role in dictating the site and severity of these lesions.

Early human OA is difficult to study, but much has been learned from animal models. There is gradual loss of cartilage matrix components. Initially, this loss appears to be caused mainly by loss of proteoglycans, although some changes in the integrity of the collagen network may be necessary (23). Destruction of the matrix is probably mediated by several proteinases. Much recent attention has focused on the metalloproteinases and their natural tissue inhibitor, known as "TIMP." Enzyme activity seems to be controlled by a balance in secretion between the enzyme and TIMP. The balance of these factors is controlled by the chondrocyte, and imbalance may be the final common pathway involved in cartilage destruction.

Cartilage repair can occur. In experimental animals, superficial lesions show little response, but lesions that extend to the subchondral bone are repaired with a viable matrix of fibrocartilage (51). In humans, osteotomy may be followed by the formation of a new joint surface of a fibrocartilage type.

There is an increase in the vascularity and activity of subchondral bone, with areas of relative sclerosis and porosis (cysts). These factors may be associated with raised interosseous pressure, which may be a factor in the pain experienced by patients with OA. Osteoarthritis is nearly always accompanied by changes at the joint margin, which include outgrowths of cartilage as well as osteophyte formation. Osteophytes can occur as an independent, age-related change, without evolution to OA. Extensive thickening of the capsule is common, and patchy synovitis may be seen in any stage of the disease. Periarticular disorders such as trochanteric bursitis may accompany OA, presumably as a result of the abnormal mechanics of the damaged hip joint.

The main symptoms of OA are joint pain and stiffness. The pain is generally related to activity and tends to be worse at the end of the day. Pain is usually felt in the anterior groin

TABLE 38-2

AMERICAN COLLEGE OF RHEUMATOLOGY CLASSIFICATION CRITERIA FOR OSTEOARTHRITIS OF THE HIP

Clinical criteria
1. Hip pain +
2a. Internal rotation <15 +
2b. ESR <44 mm/h
or
3a. Internal rotation >15 +
3b. Morning stiffness <60 min +
3c. Age >50 y +
3d. Pain on internal rotation

Clinical and radiographic criteria
1. Hip pain + at least 2 of the following:
2a. ESR <20 mm/h
2b. Radiographic osteophytes
2c. Radiographic joint space narrowing

ESR, erythrocyte sedimentation rate.

area but can radiate around posteriorly. Postactivity pain or sharp pains related to a particular movement may occur. Stiffness in the morning is usual but generally lasts less than 30 minutes, which helps distinguish OA from other arthropathies.

The American College of Rheumatology has developed descriptive criteria that distinguish OA of the hip from other rheumatic disorders of this joint (Table 38-2).

The plain radiograph is still the standard by which the presence of OA is determined (Fig. 38-5). It is, however, a very insensitive indicator of joint pathology (48). Some hip OA can be detected only on oblique or lateral views, the standard anteroposterior view appearing normal. Magnetic resonance imaging is useful for assessing soft-tissue and bony changes but is, as yet, disappointing as a means of detecting subtle

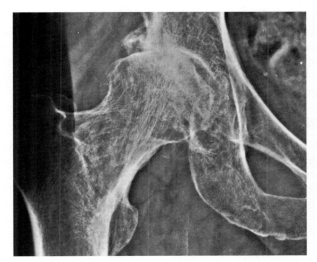

Figure 38-5 This hip radiograph shows typical changes of osteoarthritis, including bone sclerosis, subarticular cysts, narrow joint space, osteophytes, and sclerosis of the femoral shaft and neck.

changes in the articular cartilage. Scintigraphy is a sensitive but nonspecific way of detecting the activity of OA. Activity on a simple bone scan reflects some aspect of abnormal joint physiology. Scintigraphic abnormalities seem to precede changes on the radiograph.

In the management of OA of the hip, reassurance and education are important for many patients. Knowing that the disease is not rheumatoid arthritis and that it is unlikely to cause severe disability is helpful. Understanding that it is better to go on using the joint rather than protect it too much is important.

Physical therapy should be available to all patients. They should be taught and encouraged to do gentle exercises each day to maintain muscle strength and full range of motion. Of all published trials of nonmedicinal and noninvasive therapies for hip osteoarthritis, those involving aerobic activity have consistently shown the most benefit. Topical irritants (capsaicin), laser therapy, acupuncture, transcutaneous nerve stimulation, and pulsed electromagnetic fields have all been studied, with either inconsistent or inadequate data to evaluate their role in OA of the hip (40). On the other hand, it is a widely held clinical opinion that hydrotherapy seems particularly helpful in hip disease.

Reduction of stress on joints can relieve pain and may affect outcome favorably. Obese patients should be helped to lose weight. Use of a cane in the contralateral hand can reduce loading on the hip by 30% to 60%. Shoe adjustments to correct leg-length inequality or angulation deformities can be valuable.

Drugs are probably overused. Several studies have shown simple analgesics are helpful and perhaps equal to NSAIDs (7). NSAIDs do relieve pain and stiffness to a significant degree in some patients, at least in the short term. As yet, no drug has been proved to have chondroprotective value in human OA. Studies of glucosamine and chondroitin sulfate, either alone or in combination, have shown they provide some relief of symptoms, but again they have not been proven to regenerate articular cartilage (25).

Very little is known about the long-term outcome of patients with OA. Many patients probably stabilize, and what literature there is suggests that symptomatic improvement is common. The determinants of a poor outcome are unknown, although joint instability and obesity are possibly indicators of a poor prognosis. It is reasonable to provide most patients who do not have these features with a relatively optimistic prognosis.

Rheumatoid Arthritis

Rheumatoid arthritis (RA) is a chronic inflammatory disease that causes progressive disability. It is recognized worldwide, with an incidence that varies in different populations, ranging from 0.2 to 0.4 per 1000 per year. It occurs in women more than men, but recent studies have suggested that the incidence in women may be decreasing. The decrease has been attributed to the use of oral contraceptives and postmenopausal estrogens; the exact mechanism by which this occurs is unknown (27).

The pathology of RA is characterized by the infiltration of the synovium with mononuclear phagocytes, lymphocytes, plasma cells, and polymorphonuclear leukocytes. As the disease progresses, the synovium becomes massively edematous and hypertrophic, and innumerable villous projections of synovial tissue protrude into the joint space. If RA persists and progresses, the patient will accumulate manifestations related to structural damage in addition to those related to ongoing synovitis. It is critical to distinguish between these two because their clinical management differs. Synovitis is a potentially reversible condition and is dealt with pharmacologically and by other nonsurgical means. The clinician follows its manifestations and orchestrates intervention based on fluctuations in symptoms and findings related to the presence and severity of synovitis. Structural damage to the articular surface of the hip characterized by cartilage loss and erosion of periarticular bone is an irreversible process, and its development is the end result of the inflammatory process.

RA is not always the same disease—there may be a benign form limited to synovitis alone and an aggressive form with structural damage occurring within the first 2 years of disease onset (24). The problem is to identify patients with the aggressive form at an early stage, before joint damage has occurred. Accurate predictors of outcome are being sought.

In 1987, the criteria for the classification of RA, which had served as a standard for 30 years, were revised (Table 38-3) (5). The presence of unequivocal evidence of chronic synovial inflammation is required. By definition, RA cannot be diagnosed until the condition has been present for at least several weeks. Other conditions causing synovitis must be excluded. It should be noted that there is no laboratory test or histologic or radiographic finding that alone conclusively indicates a definitive diagnosis of RA, but each may be a part of the overall characteristic picture.

TABLE 38-3

1987 AMERICAN COLLEGE OF RHEUMATOLOGY CRITERIA FOR THE CLASSIFICATION OF RHEUMATOID ARTHRITIS

1. Morning stiffness in and around the joints, lasting at least 1 hour before maximal improvement.
2. At least three joint areas simultaneously have had soft-tissue swelling or fluid (not bony overgrowth) observed by a physician. The 14 possible areas are right or left PIP, MCP, wrist, elbow, knee, ankle, and MTP joints.
3. At least one area swollen (as defined above) in a wrist, MCP, or PIP joint
4. Simultaneous involvement of the same joint areas (as defined in 2) on both sides of the body (bilateral involvement of PIPs, MCPs, or MTPs) is acceptable without absolute symmetry.
5. Subcutaneous nodules, over bony prominences, or extensor surfaces, or in juxta-articular regions, observed by a physician.
6. Demonstration of abnormal amounts of serum rheumatoid factor.
7. Radiographic changes typical of rheumatoid arthritis which must include erosions or unequivocal bony decalcification localized in or most marked adjacent to the involved joints.

PIP, proximal interphalangeal (joint); MCP, metacarpophalangeal (joint); MTP, metatarsophalangeal (joint).
For the diagnosis of RA, four of the seven criteria are required. Criteria 1 through 4 must have been present for at least 6 weeks.

Although commonly involved in RA, the early manifestations of hip disease are often not apparent, even to a skilled examiner. The joint location, deep within the pelvis, obscures evidence of palpable distension or synovial thickening. In addition, early involvement is often asymptomatic, although subtle reduction of range of motion may be observed. The initial dysfunction is usually difficulty in putting on sock and shoe on the affected side. When symptoms do develop, they characteristically occur in the groin or thigh, but they may also be felt in the low back or knee. If cartilage destruction does occur, its symptoms may accelerate more rapidly than in other joints (3).

Rheumatoid factor is found in the serum of about 85% of patients with RA and in about 5% of healthy normal individuals. The detection of the factor is of clinical value, because its presence tends to correlate with severe and unremitting disease. However, serial titers are of no value in following the disease process. Rheumatoid factor can occur in several other inflammatory disorders associated with synovitis, so it cannot be relied upon alone for diagnosis. A new autoantibody, anti-cyclic citrullinated protein (anti-CCP) seems to have greater specificity and appear earlier in the course of RA and therefore may be useful in the differential diagnosis of early polyarthritis (33). The erythrocyte sedimentation rate (ESR) is a measure of the rate at which red blood cells settle, and it is related to several factors in the serum. It is rare for a patient with active RA to have a normal ESR, and the rate usually varies according to the degree of inflammation (37). The C-reactive protein (CRP) is one of the acute-phase reactants, and it may also be used to monitor the level of inflammation.

Plain radiographs continue to be the mainstay of the diagnosis and differentiation of RA of the hip and are very important for the selection of appropriate therapy as well. Uniform joint-space loss, periarticular osteopenia, and marginal erosion are the classic signs (Fig. 38-6). Late in the course of RA, typical degenerative findings may be superimposed on these classic RA characteristics. Although bone scans sensitively reflect the presence of abnormalities in the joint, with rare exception they do not, in and of themselves, lead to a specific diagnosis. They can be useful in detecting and documenting a pattern of multiple joint involvement that is suggestive of RA

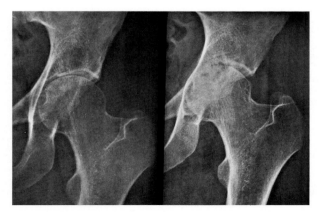

Figure 38-6 Radiographs of the hip joint in rheumatoid arthritis. Early disease shows some central loss of joint space and early protrusio acetabuli (*left*). At a later stage, loss of joint space is much more marked, and erosions are present (*right*).

(37). Magnetic resonance imaging can demonstrate synovitis in the hip, but this finding must be combined with the finding of synovitis elsewhere to make a diagnosis. In fact, isolated synovitis of the hip alone should lead to the suspicion of other diagnoses (15).

The treatment of RA has improved dramatically in recent years, as a result of increased knowledge of immune system function and the biologic response–modifying agents that have been developed based on this knowledge. General measures of education, adequate rest, and physical and occupational therapy are an important base of therapy for all patients. Use of orthotics, such as resting wrist splints, dynamic wrist splints, and cane crutches, as well as other physical aids, is individualized.

Medications are very important in the management of patients with RA. Four major classes are used: corticosteroids, NSAIDs, various disease-modifying antirheumatics that are thought to modify fundamental pathologic processes responsible for chronic inflammation, and the aforementioned biologic response modifiers. The range of clinical improvement seen with drug therapy is extremely broad and includes both patients who experience marked reductions in synovitis and patients who are totally resistant to therapy. The reasons for such variable response remain unknown. Regardless of the duration of therapy, in the majority of patients there is a slowly progressive return of joint inflammation if medications are discontinued, so treatment should be ongoing.

Although aspirin was the standard of therapy for many years, numerous NSAIDs have been developed that have efficacy similar to aspirin but a lower risk of gastrointestinal side effects. These agents are generally prescribed as baseline therapy in every newly diagnosed patient with RA unless contraindicated. In appropriate dosage, these agents can decrease pain and swelling, but they are not capable of preventing cartilage destruction or bone erosion and are therefore used primarily to reduce synovitis and relieve symptoms (8). They may be adequate therapy alone in treating patients with the more mild or benign cases, where symptoms of synovitis exist without evidence of bone or cartilage damage.

The use of corticosteroids is controversial, and the exact mechanism of action has not been identified. Low daily doses (10 mg or less of prednisone or its equivalent) are sometimes used as an alternative to NSAIDs or when the latter are contraindicated. It should be remembered that although they do provide symptom relief, corticosteroids, like NSAIDs, do not prevent cartilage or bone damage (28). The potential for toxicity related side effect such as skin thinning, weight gain, and steroid-induced osteopenia exists. For these reasons, steroids, if required, should be used at the minimal dose needed for efficacy and usually in combination with disease-modifying agents to prevent joint erosion and deformity.

Patients who do not respond adequately to symptomatic therapy or who have any evidence of bone or cartilage damage become candidates for disease-modifying antirheumatic drugs (DMARDs). There is a trend toward earlier use of these agents in an attempt to control the inflammatory process as soon as possible in hopes that this will reduce joint destruction. Table 38-4 lists many of the DMARD agents currently in use (20). Although direct comparisons of DMARDs usually fail to demonstrate significant differences, clinical experience suggests methotrexate may be the most effective treatment, at

TABLE 38-4
SLOW-ACTING ANTIRHEUMATIC DRUGS CLASSIFIED BY TOXICITY

Milder	Moderate	Very toxic
Auranofin	Azathioprine	Cyclosporine
Hydroxychloroquine	Methotrexate	
Sulfasalazine		

least for the control of symptoms (20). Alternative approaches to therapy are being sought, including combination therapies and more aggressive approaches (6).

With the advent of the biologic response modulators, there is now an effective therapy for the many patients who fail to show a complete or even adequate response to DMARDs. At the current time, inhibition of the cytokine tumor necrosis factor-α (TNF-α) appears to be the most effective strategy, and there are a number of different medications that accomplish this. Etanercept is a recombinant TNF receptor that binds up circulating TNF. Infliximab and adalimumab are monoclonal antibodies that bind TNF directly. Each of these must be given parenterally, either by subcutaneous injection or intravenous infusion. Anakinra inhibits another cytokine, interleukin-1, by binding to and therefore antagonizing its receptor on the cell. It has shown somewhat less efficacy on average than the TNF inhibitors. Table 38-5 summarizes these agents and their administration. All share the propensity to increase risk of minor infections such as viral upper respiratory illness, and in the presence of a serious bacterial infection they must be immediately discontinued due to increased risk of sepsis as well. Patients should also be screened for potential latent or active tuberculosis due to risk of activation of this infection. No data exist, but an increased risk of early or late postoperative infections has not been noted or observed.

It must be remembered that RA is a systemic disease, and it has the potential to cause many complications beyond the commonly affected joints. Discussion of many of these goes beyond the scope of this chapter, but the complication of atlantoaxial subluxation is of particular relevance to patients who may undergo general anesthesia. Disruption of the odontoid transverse ligament by synovial inflammation can lead to instability of the cervical atlantoaxial joint, making the spinal cord vulnerable during intubation and extubation. Lateral cervical spine films in extension and flexion can screen for this instability (30).

Juvenile Rheumatoid Arthritis

Juvenile rheumatoid arthritis (JRA) may develop at any age during childhood. Diagnosis of definite JRA requires at least 6 consecutive weeks of objective synovitis. Alternative nomenclature to JRA includes the term "juvenile chronic polyarthritis," used by some European investigators, and the simpler "juvenile arthritis." Juvenile rheumatoid arthritis can be subclassified into three onset subtypes: pauciarticular, polyarticular, and systemic. Whether these subtypes are distinct diseases resulting from different causes or varying responses to common factors is unknown. No laboratory test is diagnostic for JRA, although the presence of rheumatoid factors or antinuclear antibodies may assist in classifying subtypes (10).

About 10% of children with JRA have a systemic onset, with spiking fever, diffuse lymphadenopathy, and transient arthritis that is maximal with fever spikes. Chronic polyarthritis develops in most. Polyarticular onset, involving five or more joints, occurs in 40% of children with JRA. Rheumatoid factors are detected in only 10% to 15%, but antinuclear antibodies are found in 40% to 60% (52). Systemic and polyarticular JRAs are associated with growth disturbances from the effects of inflammation on epiphyseal growth, resulting in overgrowth or undergrowth of long bones (53). Pauciarticular onset, involving four or fewer joints, occurs in up to 50% of children with JRA. Many of these present with only one swollen joint, frequently the knee.

Juvenile rheumatoid arthritis frequently has a better prognosis than the adult form. Many children undergo a permanent remission of their arthritis, and others who have persistent synovitis do not seem to develop bone erosion or cartilage damage as frequently as is observed with adults. Destructive disabling arthritis occurs in as many as 50% of those with consistent positive rheumatoid factor but in perhaps only 10% to 15% of rheumatoid factor–negative patients (10,52).

TABLE 38-5
BIOLOGICAL RESPONSE MODIFIERS

	Etanercept	Infliximab	Adalimumab	Anakinra
Class	sTNFR construct	TNF-α mAb	TNF-α mAb	IL-1Ra
Recombinant construct	Human	Chimeric	Human	Human
Half-life	4.3 days	8–10 days	10–20 days	4–6 hours
Primary binding target	TNF-α	TNF-α	TNF-α	Type I IL-1R
Administration	25 mg sc 2x/wk	3–10 mg/kg q4–8 wk iv + MTX	40 mg sc eow[a]	100 mg/d sc

[a]Some patients not taking concurrent methotrexate may derive additional benefit from increasing the dosing frequency to 40 mg every week.

Many children with objective arthritis complain little of joint pain, particularly if they are less than 10 years old. Rather, they limit any motion that would result in pain. Although aspirin remains the single most effective, and least expensive, medication for JRA, public acceptance in the United States has been severely compromised by its association with Reye syndrome. Many children with JRA are now treated with other NSAIDs. Ibuprofen, tolmetin, naproxen, and fenoprofen have been approved for use in patients under 14 years of age. For children over 14, any of the NSAIDs can be used (18). If JRA is incompletely responsive to aspirin or other NSAIDs after several months, gold therapy may be added. Methotrexate should be considered for the treatment of severe, longstanding, or rapidly progressive JRA (52), and the biologic agents have been shown to be comparably effective in children and adults.

Seronegative Spondyloarthropathies

The seronegative spondyloarthropathies are a series of interrelated rheumatic disorders that affect the spine and peripheral joint of the lower extremity, including the hip in particular. Most, but not all, of these disorders show an increased prevalence among individuals who have inherited the human lymphocyte antigen (HLA)-B27 gene. Ankylosing spondylitis, Reiter syndrome, and psoriatic arthritis are the most commonly recognized diagnostic entities in this category. All are characterized by chronic synovitis in involved joints (27). The pathology of this synovitis is virtually identical to rheumatoid arthritis, so synovial biopsy will not differentiate these conditions from RA, and clinical diagnosis is necessary.

Ankylosing spondylitis is characterized by involvement of the sacroiliac joints and peripheral joints. Therefore, back pain and stiffness are prominent features, particularly at onset. Inflammatory involvement of entheses, where ligaments attach to bone, causes multiple tender skeletal sites. Eventual calcification of the anterior spinous ligament leads to spinal rigidity. The first symptoms sometimes result from involvement of the hips and shoulders. Accurate assessment of hip range of motion is important because the hips are involved at some stage of the disease in one third of patients. Hip involvement is usually bilateral and potentially more crippling than involvement of any other joint. Some degree of flexion contracture at the hip is common at later stages of the disease, giving rise to the characteristic rigid gait with some flexion at the knees to maintain erect posture. The characteristic radiologic appearance of the spine is useful to confirm the diagnosis. HLA-B27 typing can be used as an aid to the diagnosis, but an overwhelming majority of patients can be diagnosed clinically on the basis of history, examination, and radiographic studies (49).

Reiter syndrome is the development of an asymmetric arthritis involving a small number of joints, frequently accompanied by eye, mucous membrane, and skin inflammation, following infection in the genitourinary or gastrointestinal tract. Arthritis usually appears within 1 to 3 weeks of the inciting urethritis or diarrhea, and it involves a few joints in an asymmetric pattern; knees, ankles, feet, and wrists are most commonly involved, and hip involvement is relatively rare. Inflammation of entheses, particularly the Achilles tendon, is common. Eventually, up to 70% of patients show radiographic involvement of the sacroiliac joints. Soft-tissue swelling is prominent around joints, but bone density is surprisingly well preserved even in chronic joint disease. HLA-B27 is present in 80% of patients (32). Despite the fact that this syndrome is triggered by infection, the joint inflammation is sterile, and Reiter syndrome is not a septic process. Recently, Reiter syndrome has been recognized in association with human immunodeficiency virus (HIV) infection (9).

An increased prevalence of inflammatory arthritis has been recognized in association with psoriasis, leading to the concept of psoriatic arthritis (36). Inflammation of the peripheral joints and spine occurs in varying patterns, but sacroiliitis is not as prevalent as in the other spondyloarthropathies. The diagnosis is made when there is evidence of psoriasis of the skin or nails in conjunction with chronic inflammatory polyarthritis. Nail involvement, including pitting, hyperkeratosis, or lysis of the nail bed, is an early and strongly suggestive clue (21). The psoriatic synovium is identical to rheumatoid synovium, and synovial fluid findings are similar among all chronic polyarthropathies, including rheumatoid arthritis and the spondyloarthropathies.

Given that the synovial reaction in the spondyloarthropathies is similar to that in rheumatoid arthritis, it would seem that the treatments should be similar. Most patients with spondyloarthropathies respond to NSAIDs, but indomethacin seems to have a better response in patients with spondyloarthropathies than in those with RA. Virtually all of the DMARDs have been tried in patients with spondyloarthropathies with some success, but they are more successful in patients with RA (43). On the other hand, the biologic response modifiers, when used, have proven remarkably effective (41).

Although the data are few, patients with both conditions seem to benefit from joint replacement identically.

Other Inflammatory Arthropathies

The crystal-induced arthritides—gout and pseudogout—present usually as a single, acute, swollen, and exquisitely tender joint, the so-called *hot* joint. Although isolated case reports of both conditions describe presentation in the hip, in clinical practice they are quite rare. Both are associated with fever and elevated white blood cell count, and thus they simulate a septic joint. The only reliable means of differentiating between the crystal-induced arthritides and sepsis is synovial fluid analysis, showing the presence of crystals or a positive culture, respectively (50). Pseudogout, or calcium pyrophosphate deposition disease, may be associated with calcification of the articular cartilage visible on plain radiographs. Because hip aspiration is difficult, it is fortunate that acute arthritis of the hip is quite rare. All of the connective tissue disorders can be accompanied by inflammatory arthritis, and the potential for hip involvement exists. Fortunately, arthritis of any site, including the hip, is rarely a presenting manifestation, and therefore the obvious systemic manifestations of these conditions make the diagnosis obvious.

Lyme disease is a complex multisystem illness caused by the tick-borne spirochete *Borrelia burgdorferi*. Although the illness has been reported in 47 states, most cases have occurred along the northeastern coast from Massachusetts to Maryland, in the Midwest in Wisconsin and Minnesota, and on the West

Coast in California and Oregon. Lyme disease is widely disseminated throughout Europe. Three to 30 days after the tick bite, a characteristic red, annular skin rash called "erythema migrans" occurs, usually at the site of the tick bite. Within days, the organism spreads through the bloodstream to cause a similar skin rash at other sites, migratory joint pain, and eventually meningitis and cardiac infection. Fortunately, the various manifestations can usually be treated successfully with oral antibiotics. For early Lyme disease, doxycycline, 100 mg twice daily for 10 to 30 days, is sufficient. Intravenous ceftriaxone, 2 g/day, is commonly used for late or established infections (47).

PRINCIPLES OF MEDICAL MANAGEMENT

The therapeutic goals in treatment of arthritis of the hip focus on reducing pain and improving function. Nonsteroidal anti-inflammatory drugs have been the mainstay of medical management, but their use has been associated with risks (8). Consequently, interest in other medicinal and nonmedicinal therapies has emerged.

Nonmedicinal Management

Many nonmedicinal, nonsurgical treatments have been used to treat patients with various arthritides of the hip. Because osteoarthritis is far and away the most prevalent condition, most trials have focused on this diagnosis. However, the number of published controlled trials is surprisingly small. In fact, no experimental studies of superficial heat and cold, orthotic devices, vibration, or weight loss exist. Single, well-designed studies suggest that topically applied capsaicin and low-energy laser treatment reduce pain associated with knee osteoarthritis, but no data specifically address the role of these therapies in hip arthritis (40). Of all nonmedical therapies for which data has addressed efficacy in osteoarthritis of the hip, exercise had the strongest evidence of beneficial effect. Exercise programs varied from simple exercises done at home to a sophisticated supervised program that included education, strengthening, and aerobics (35).

Nonsteroidal Anti-Inflammatory Drugs

Increasing awareness of the risk of NSAIDs has led to a reappraisal of their use in noninflammatory conditions such as osteoarthritis (19). In a randomized, double-blind comparison of acetaminophen versus analgesic and anti-inflammatory doses of ibuprofen, comparable benefit was found among all three groups (7). Subsequent studies have shown comparable benefit from mild, nonnarcotic analgesics. Based on this evidence, analgesics are now recognized as appropriate therapy for noninflammatory arthritis of the hip.

NSAIDs nevertheless remain drugs of preference for many patients and physicians and are used every day by millions of patients. In contrast to the studies showing comparable results for analgesics and NSAIDs are studies showing that patients frequently prefer NSAIDs to acetaminophen based on perceived increased efficacy (38). The prototypic NSAID has been acetylsalicylic acid. Subsequently, several preparations from several chemical categories were available

for use. The specific choice of drug for a specific arthritic disorder is primarily a function of physician-prescribing behavior. Traditionally, salicylates have been the first drugs used for both inflammatory and degenerative arthropathies. However, aspirin does not seem to be tolerated as well as other NSAIDs, and patient compliance with the complex aspirin dosing regimen may be problematic. Thus, for ease of administration, other NSAIDs, especially once-daily or twice-daily drugs, are frequently utilized.

NSAIDs work in part by reducing the production of proinflammatory prostaglandins of the E series (1). However, nonspecific NSAIDs also inhibit the formation of prostacyclin and thromboxane, and the resulting effects of this inhibition contribute to the overall clinical effects of these compounds. So-called Cox-2 inhibitors were developed to minimize the risk of gastrointestinal bleeding because they do not inhibit thrombaxone and prostacyclin, but questions as to their potential risk in exacerbation cardiovascular thrombosis has been raised, so their recommendations for use are currently undergoing significant restriction. All NSAIDs are almost completely absorbed after oral administration, metabolized in the liver, and excreted in the urine, factors which must be taken into consideration when prescribing NSAIDs for patients with physiologic dysfunction of these organ systems. The most clinically important side effects result from drug effects on gastrointestinal tissues, including esophagitis, gastritis, peptic ulcer, perforation, and gastrointestinal hemorrhage. All of these effects are likely to be the result of a systemic depletion of prostaglandins, which are known to be critical for maintenance of normal gastrointestinal physiology. The therapeutic approach to the arthritis patient with risk for NSAID-associated gastrointestinal toxicity is controversial. Misoprostol, a prostaglandin analog, has been shown to inhibit the development of significant gastric ulcers in NSAID-treated patients. On the basis of these data, misoprostol may be used in conjunction with NSAIDs in patients at risk for gastrointestinal complications, including the elderly and those with a prior history of ulcer disease. Although the histamine (H_2) receptor antagonists (cimetidine, ranitidine) may improve the symptoms of dyspepsia in NSAID-treated patients, they have not been shown to reduce the frequency of gastric erosions. Proton pump inhibitors reduce esophageal reflux and gastrointestinal bleeding in the NSAID-treated patient (16). In patients with risk factors for gastrointestinal hemorrhage and without risk factors for cardiovascular disease, a Cox-2–specific inhibitor could be used.

All NSAIDs have the ability to induce reversible impairment of renal function, and this may occur more frequently in patients who have heart failure, diabetes, hypertension, or atherosclerosis or in patients with hypovolemia or hypoalbuminemia. Indomethacin may be the NSAID most commonly associated with this adverse reaction. Although sulindac has been profiled as a renal-sparing drug in some studies, this has not been confirmed (11).

Corticosteroids

Therapeutic administration of corticosteroids produces rapid, potent, and reliable suppression of inflammation. This suppression, however, is evanescent and therefore not suitable for long-term treatment. However, this short-term efficacy and versatility have made corticosteroids a key element in the treatment of rheumatic conditions characterized by inflammation. Because of the multiple preparations and dosing regimens, along with the great variety of clinical applications, significant medical art is required to correctly prescribe corticosteroids. In general, increasing doses and dosing frequency corresponds to enhanced inflammatory suppression, more rapid onset of therapeutic benefit, and increased side effects. Available corticosteroid preparations all affect bone metabolism by decreasing calcium absorption from the gastrointestinal tract. In the face of rheumatic diseases that in themselves hasten calcium loss from bones, accelerated osteoporosis and fractures can occur (28). Exogenous administration of corticosteroids can shut down native adrenal corticosteroid production, which can lead to Addisonian crisis and shock in situations such as hypovolemia, sepsis, and surgery. The inhibitory effect of corticosteroids on immune responses also results in an increased risk of infection by opportunistic microorganisms such as *Mycobacterium tuberculosis*, *Pneumocystis carinii*, and fungi. Easy bruisability, impaired wound healing, glaucoma, cataract formation, hypertension, and diabetes all result from long-term use (42). These side effects are related to dose, and they occur equally with oral and parenteral routes of administration.

For rapid control of self-limited processes such as gout, the choice of corticosteroid and the tapering schedule are not as vital as with long-term use, defined as greater than 2 weeks. In prolonged suppression of rheumatic disease, the desired dose is the minimum necessary to suppress disease activity. Tapering should be gradual to avoid a disease flare, with serial reductions of prednisone by 2.5 to 5.0 mg/day every few weeks to months.

Oral or parenteral therapy with corticosteroids is not indicated in OA of the hip. Intra-articular injections, using fluoroscopic guidance, may be beneficial when used judiciously in the management of acute joint flares, but they should be infrequent and no more often than 4 times per year.

Other Pharmacologic Agents

The treatment of rheumatoid arthritis and other systemic rheumatic diseases has changed over the last 20 years with the introduction of the slow-acting antirheumatic drugs (SAARDs) (20). In addition, appreciation of the need to treat rheumatoid arthritis early before cartilage damage occurs has led to a much more aggressive approach, including early use of these agents. If these agents are to be used at an early stage, it is especially important to recognize their potentially more serious adverse effects. The decision as to which drug or combination of drugs to use in an individual—a decision influenced by a number of factors—goes beyond the scope of this chapter. Perhaps, then, the most appropriate recommendation is that at the first recognition of a chronic inflammatory condition specialty consultation or referral should be entertained.

REFERENCES

1. Abramson S, Weissman G. The mechanisims of action of nonsteroidal antiinflammatory drugs. *Clin Exp Rheumatol.* 1989;7(suppl):163–170.
2. American College of Rheumatology Ad Hoc Committee on Clinical Guidelines. Guidelines for the initial evaluation of the adult patient with acute musculoskeletal conditions. *Arthritis Rheum.* 1996;39:1–8.
3. Anderson RJ. Rheumatoid arthritis. In: Schumacher HR, ed. *Primer on the Rheumatic Diseases.* Atlanta: Arthritis Foundation; 1993:90–95.
4. Arai KI, Lee F, Miyajima A, et al. Cytokines: coordinators of immune and inflammatory response. *Ann Rev Immunol.* 1990;59:783–836.
5. Arnett FC, Edworthy SM, Bloch DA, et al. The American Rheumatisim Association 1987 revised criterion for the classification of rheumatoid arthritis. *Arthritis Rheum.* 1988;31:315–324.
6. Boers M, Ramsden M. Long acting drug combinations in rheumatoid arthritis: a formal overview. *J Rheumatol.* 1991;18:316–324.
7. Bradley JD, Brandt KD, Katz BP, et al. Comparison of an anti-inflammatory dose of ibuprofen, an analgesic dose of ibuprofen, and acetominophen in the treatment of patients with osteoarthritis of the knee. *N Engl J Med.* 1991;325:87–91.
8. Brooks PM, Day RO. Drug therapy: nonsteroidal anti-inflammatory drugs—differences and similarities. *N Engl J Med.* 1991;324:1716–1725.
9. Calabrese LH, Kelley DM, Meyers A, et al. Rheumatic symptoms and human immunodeficiency virus infection. *Arthritis Rheum.* 1991;34:257–263.
10. Cassidy JT, Petty RE. *Textbook of Pediatric Rheumatology.* New York: Churchill Livingstone; 1990.
11. Clive DM, Stoff JS. Renal syndromes associated with nonsteroidal antiinflammatory drugs. *N Engl J Med.* 1984;310:563–572.
12. Cohen PL, Eisenberg RA. Lpr and gld: single gene models of systemic autoimmunity and lymphoproliferative disease. *Annu Rev Immunol.* 1991;9:243–270.
13. Cooper MD. Current concepts. B lymphocytes: normal development and function. *N Engl J Med.* 1987;238:1452–1456.
14. Cush JJ, Kavanaugh AF. Biologic intervention in rheumatoid arthritis. *Rheum Dis Clin North Am.* 1995;23:797–816.
15. Dalinka MK, Kricun ME, Zlatkin MB, et al. Modern diagnostic imaging in joint disease. *Am J Roentgenol.* 1988;152:229–240.
16. Ekstrom, P, Carling, L, Wetterhus, S, et al. Prevention of peptic ulcer and dyspeptic symptoms with omeprazole in patients receiving continuous non-steroidal anti-inflammatory drug therapy: a Nordic multicentre study. *Scand J Gastroenterol.* 1996;31:753–758.
17. Felson DT. Osteoarthritis. *Rheum Dis Clin North Am.* 1990;16:499–512.
18. Fink CW. Medical treatment of juvenile arthritis. *Clin Orthop.* 1990;No. 259:60–69.
19. Fries JF, Williams CA, Bloch DA. The relative toxicity of nonsteroidal antiinflammatory drugs. *Arthritis Rheum.* 1991;34:1353–1360.
20. Furst DE. Rational use of disease modifying antirheumatic drugs. *Drugs.* 1990;39:19–37.
21. Gladman DD, Shuckett R, Russel ML, et al. Psoriatic arthritis: an analysis of 220 patients. *Q J Med.* 1987;62:127–141.
22. Goetzl EJ, Goldstein IM. Arachadonic acid metabolites. In: McCarty DJ, Koopman WJ, eds. *Arthritis and Allied Conditions.* Philadelphia: Lea & Febiger; 1993:479–494.
23. Hardingham T, Bayliss M. Proteoglycans of articular cartilage: changes in aging and disease. *Semin Arthritis Rheum.* 1990;20[Suppl 1]:12–33.
24. Harris ED Jr. Rheumatoid arthritis: pathophysiology and implications for therapy. *N Engl J Med.* 1009;322:1277–1289.
25. Hochberg MC, McAlindon T, Felson DT. Systemic and topical treatments. In: Felson DT, conference chair. Osteoarthritis: new insights, II: treatment approaches. *Ann Intern Med.* 2000;133:726–729.
26. Hochberg MC, Spector TD. Epidemiology of rheumatoid arthritis: update. *Epidemiol Rev.* 1990;12:247–252.
27. Kahn MA, van der Linden SM. A wider spectrum of spondyloarthropathies. *Semin Arthritis Rheum.* 1990;20:107–113.
28. Kimberly RP. Glucocortocoid therapy for rheumatic diseases. *Curr Opin Rheumatol.* 1992;4:325–331.
29. Konig W, Schonfeld W, Raulth M, et al. The neutrophil and leukotrienes: role in health and disease. *Eicosanoids.* 1990;3:1–22.
30. Kramer J, Jolesz F, Kleefield J. Rheumatoid arthritis of the cervical spine. *Rheum Dis Clin North Am.* 1991;17:757–772.

31. Kuby J. *Immunology*. New York: WH Freeman; 1992.

32. Lahesmanna-Rantala R, Tovianen A. Clinical spectrum of reactive arthritis. In: Tovianen A, Tovianen P, ed. *Reactive Arthritis*. Boca Raton, FL: CRC Press; 1988:1–13.

33. Lee, DM, Schur, PH. Clinical utility of the anti-CCP assay in patients with rheumatic diseases. *Ann Rheum Dis*. 2003;62:870–874.

34. Liang MH, Sturrock RD. Evaluation of musculoskeletal symptoms. In: Klippel JH, Dieppe PA, eds. *Rheumatology*. London: Mosby-Yearbook Europe; 1994:50–65.

35. Minor MA, Hewett JE, Webel RR, et al. Efficacy of physical conditioning exercise in patients with rheumatoid arthritis and osteoarthritis. *Arthritis Rheum*. 1989;32:1396–1405.

36. Moll JMH, Wright V. Familial occurrence of psoriatic arthritis. *Ann Rheum Dis*. 1973;32:181–201.

37. Pincus T. A pragmatic approach to cost-effective use of laboratory tests and imaging procedures in patients with musculoskeletal symptoms. *Prim Care*. 1993;20:795–814.

38. Pincus, T, Koch, G, Lei, H, et al. Patient Preference for Placebo, Acetaminophen (Paracetamol) or Celecoxib Efficacy Studies (PACES): two randomised, double blind, placebo controlled, crossover clinical trials in patients with knee or hip osteoarthritis. *Ann Rheum Dis*. 2004;63:931–939.

39. Polley HF, Hunder GG. *Rheumatological Interviewing and Physicial Examination of the Joints*. Philadelphia: WB Saunders; 1978.

40. Puett DW, Griffin MR. Published trials of nonmedicinal and noninvasive therapies for hip and knee osteoarthritis. *Ann Intern Med*. 1994;121:133–140.

41. Rudwaleit M, Listing J, Brandt J, et al. Prediction of a major clinical response (BASDAI 50) to TNF-α blockers in ankylosing spondylitis. *Ann Rheum Dis*. 2004;63:665–670.

42. Schaghecke R, Kornely E, Santen RT, et al. The effect of long-term glucocorticoid therapy on pituitary-adrenal responses to exogenous corticotropin-releasing hormone. *N Engl J Med*. 1992;326:226–230.

43. Schumacher HR. *Primer on the Rheumatic Diseases*. Atlanta: Arthritis Foundation; 1993.

44. Schumacher JR. Secondary osteoarthritis. In: Moskowitz RW, Howell DS, Goldberg VM, et al., eds. *Osteoarthritis: Diagnosis and Management*. Philadelphia: WB Saunders; 1992:367–398.

45. Schwartz BD. *Immunology*. Kalamazoo, MI: The Upjohn Company; 1991.

46. Springer TA. Adhesion receptors of the immune system. *Nature*. 1990;346:425–434.

47. Steere AC. Lyme disease. *N Engl J Med*. 1989;321:586–596.

48. Summers MN, Haley WE, Reveille JD, et al. Radiographic assessment and psychologic variables as predictors of pain and functional impairment in osteoarthritis of the knee or hip. *Arthritis Rheum*. 1988;31:204–209.

49. Taurog JD. Genetics and immunology of the spondyloarthropathies. *Curr Opin Rheumatol*. 1989;1:144–150.

50. Terkeltaub RA. What stops a gouty attack? *J Rheumatol*. 1992;19:8–10.

51. Vignon E, Arlot M, Hartmann D, et al. Hypertrophic repair of articular cartilage in experimental osteoarthritis. *Ann Rheum Dis*. 1983;142:82–88.

52. Wallace CA, Levinson JE. Juvenile rheumatoid arthritis: outcome and treatment for the 1990s. *Rheum Dis Clin North Am*. 1991;17:891–906.

53. White PH. Growth abnormalities in children with juvenile rheumatoid arthritis. *Clin Orthop*. 1990;259:46–50.

Septic Arthritis

Michael R. O'Rourke   *Marnold T. Berman*
Louis Quartararo

39

Sepsis in the native adult hip is an uncommon problem that has an increased incidence in the elderly and immunocompromised population. Early diagnosis is important to minimize the injury to the articular cartilage and prevent secondary arthritis. The hip accounts for 13% of all septic joints, second only to the knee joint (66). Adult mortality from infectious coxitis is reported at 13% (9,27). Pyogenic arthritis and sepsis in an arthritic joint can pose difficult management problems since the risk of infection of a total joint replacement is higher.

Sepsis following joint arthroplasty is the most common infection of the adult hip. This chapter focuses only on sepsis of the native hip without previous arthroplasty.

ETIOLOGY

Mechanism of Infection

Septic arthritis of the hip is more common in the pediatric population, in part because of the unique vascular architecture of the proximal femur. Unlike in adults, joint sepsis in the skeletally immature patient is commonly the result of hematogenous osteomyelitis of the metaphysis that has spread to the joint through local communication. Metaphyseal closed-loop end arterioles have slower flow and predispose this area to the deposition of bacteria (Fig. 39-1). The adult hip is more resistant to this hematogenous mode of infection after closure of the physis and anastomosis between metaphyseal and epiphyseal blood vessels (see Fig. 39-1D).

Hematogenous spread, although less common in adults, is still the most common route of infection of the hip. Common sources of infection include bacteremia resulting from a urinary tract infection, pneumonia, diverticulitis, endocarditis, and skin infections (8). The route of hematogenous spread of bacteria to the adult hip is generally through the synovium. Bacteria in blood lodge directly in the abundant arterial and capillary arcades of synovial membrane.

In addition to an arterial bacteremia as a source for hematogenous spread, retrograde venous flow may also lead to bacterial seeding of the hip. Normal venous return from the hip flows into the veins of Batson plexus around the bladder, rectum, prostate, and uterus (Fig. 39-2) (83). Batson plexus is a valveless venous system that may allow retrograde flow with Valsalva maneuvers. This retrograde flow predisposes the hip to bacterial seeding from these pelvic sources.

Direct inoculation of the hip joint can occur as a result of trauma, diagnostic procedures, and therapeutic procedures. Arthrography, hip aspiration, and steroid injection are common culprits. Femoral vessel puncture, as when blood is drawn or during angiography, can result in inadvertent puncture of the hip capsule and subsequent infection (31,68,76). Gunshot wounds to the hip also are responsible for directly seeding the hip. In particular, transabdominal gunshot wounds violating both the hip joint and the gastrointestinal (GI) tract can have devastating effects if not treated properly by diverting colostomy and immediate arthrotomy (14).

Previous nonarthroplasty surgical procedures are a source of infection, such as open reduction internal fixation for acetabular fractures and proximal femur fractures. These injuries may be complicated by conditions that cause pain in the hip and mask an underlying infection (e.g., posttraumatic arthritis), nonunion, malunion, or osteonecrosis of the femoral head. Infection as a cause of failure or as a concomitant problem should be kept high on the differential when evaluating and treating these patients.

Extension from nearby or distant foci may result in hip sepsis (22). Retroperitoneal and intra-abdominal abscesses may spread along the iliopsoas tendon to the hip joint (51). The iliopsoas muscle crosses the anterior hip capsule as it courses

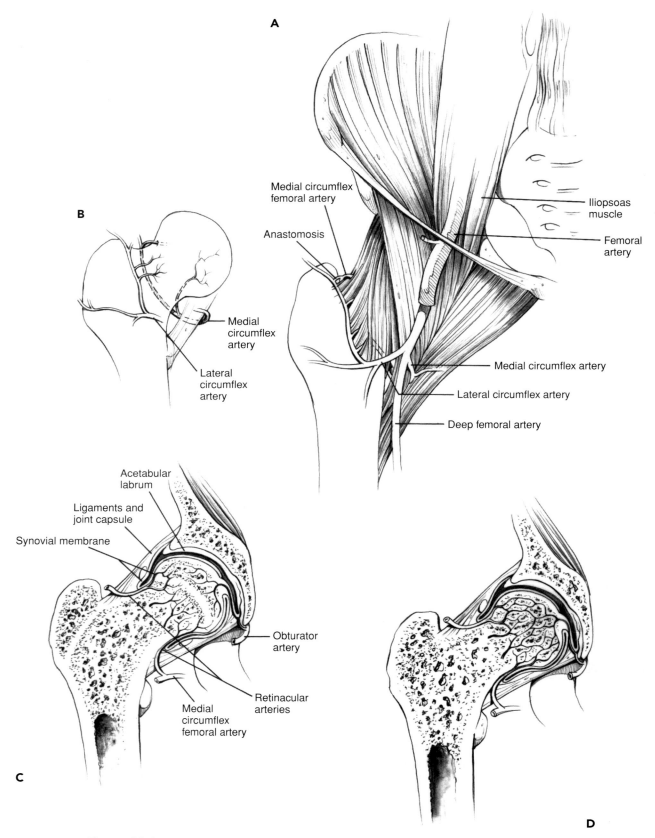

Figure 39-1 Blood supply to the adult and pediatric femoral head. **A,B:** Arterial anatomy. **C:** Coronal section, pediatric hip. Note physeal block to arterial anastomosis. **D:** Coronal section, adult hip with anastomosis. (Adapted from Netter F. *Atlas of Human Anatomy*. 1989.)

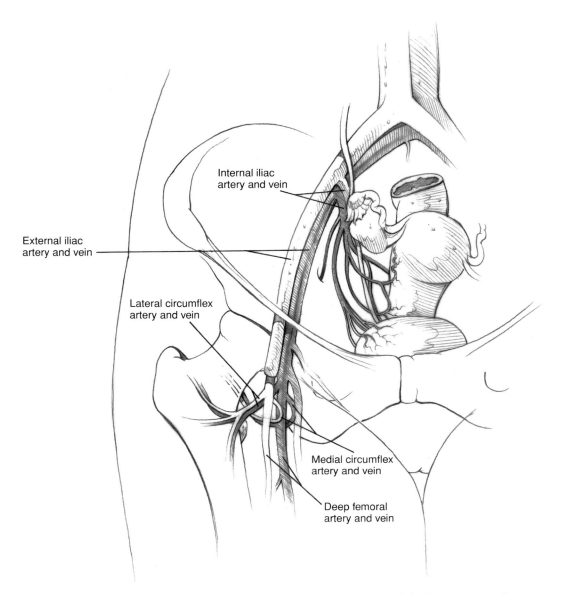

Figure 39-2 Batson plexus draining pelvic vicera and venous drainage of the hip. Retrograde flow from venous blood in the common iliac vein may seed the hip. (Adapted from Netter F. *Atlas of Human Anatomy.* 1989.)

to its insertion on the lesser trochanter. The capsule is thinnest anteriorly, between the iliofemoral and pubofemoral ligaments, and it is prone to the spread of bacteria through this point. Furthermore, the iliopsoas bursa communicates directly with the hip joint in 15% of the population, and infection of this bursa from surrounding abscesses or infections results in hip sepsis (Fig. 39-3) (4,76,79). Other bursae found to communicate with the hip joint include the greater trochanteric bursa and the ischiotrochanteric bursa (75). Infection around these bursae can result in hip infections.

Other nearby sources of infection extending to the hip include skin decubiti (8,53), pelvic fractures associated with rectal tears (55), genitourinary injuries (18), ureter injuries following stent insertion (90), Crohn disease with GI–hip capsule fistulae (29,72), and ruptured diverticulitis (59).

Microbiology

Staphylococcus aureus is the most prevalent cause of septic arthritis of the hip, responsible for 40% to 75% of cases (8,60). Next most common are the *Streptococcus* species (32,49,61,73,76). Gonococcus, although the most common cause of septic arthritis in all joints, rarely affects the hip joint (2,50,69,78). Gram-negative bacilli are an increasingly common pathogen, accounting for 12% of hip sepsis cases in one series (66). These organisms include *Pseudomonas* species, *Escherichia coli*, *Salmonella* species, *Klebsiella* species, *Enterobacter* species, and *Proteus* species (3,11,67,70,76). When present, these organisms are associated with a poor prognosis. Other common pathogens include *Haemophilus influenzae* (76), *Campylobacter* species (41,88), *Listeria* species (81), and

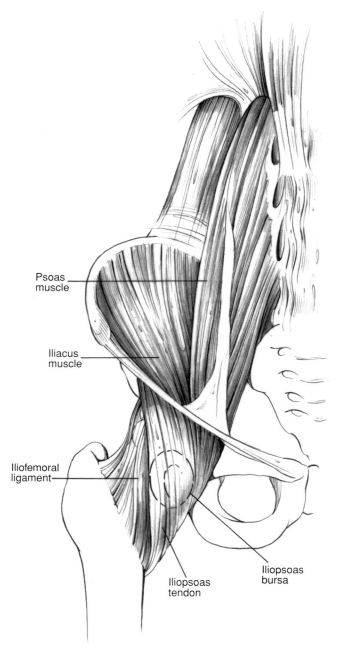

Psoas
muscle

Iliacus
muscle

Iliofemoral
ligament

Iliopsoas
tendon

Iliopsoas
bursa

Figure 39-3 Anatomy of the iliacus muscle, psoas muscle, iliopsoas tendon, and iliopsoas bursa in relationship to the hip joint. (Adapted from Netter F. *Atlas of Human Anatomy.* 1989.)

Branhamella species (20). Anaerobic bacteria, such as *Bacteroides fragilis* (58) and *Bacteroides melaninogenicus* (82), among others, are being isolated with increasing frequency because of better culture techniques and the increasing incidence of immunosuppression in the population. These account for less than 5% of all septic joints (76).

Mycobacterium tuberculosis is rare in modern societies, yet it is also increasing with the recent resurgence of pulmonary tuberculosis in immunocompromised patients. Atypical mycobacterial infections are extremely rare (76). Other opportunistic infections, including those caused by *Coxiella burnetii* (19), *Nocardia asteroids* (64), *Mycoplasma* (56,87), and *Kingella kingae* (21,45,92), have been recently reported.

Fungal infections of the hip are most commonly caused by *Candida* species (74,89), but *Cryptococcus* (12) and *Coccidioides* (76) are also found. These infections are usually contracted via extension from nearby foci of infection rather than by hematogenous spread, which is the way most of the bacterial infections are acquired.

Infection with spirochetes such as *Treponema pallidum* (syphilis) or *Borrelia burgdorferi* (Lyme disease) may also occur in the hip. *Treponema pallidum* usually results in destruction of the hip joint indirectly by the neuropathic arthropathy associated with tertiary syphilis (76).

Parasitic infections have recently been reported in the foreign literature. These include schistosomiasis (28) and echinococciasis (39).

Viruses can result in a transient synovitis with symptoms similar to those of joint sepsis. The infection is self-limiting in most cases and requires no treatment (25,52).

PATHOPHYSIOLOGY

The synovial membrane is a highly vascular, highly permeable connective tissue lining of the joint. The absence of a capillary-limiting membrane accounts for its high permeability. An ultrafiltrate of plasma through these capillaries results in the production of normal synovial fluid. Synovial fluid provides nutrients and removes waste from the articular cartilage. Disruption of the normal production and flow of this fluid can be disastrous, resulting in destruction of the cartilage and joint. The chondrocytes play a role in the defense against infection. Articular chondrocytes have been shown to produce defensin proteins when challenged with Gram-negative organisms (86).

Bacterial organisms traveling in the bloodstream may lodge in the synovium and then enter the joint. A damaged synovium increases the susceptibility of the joint to a hematogenous infection. Once in the joint, bacteria proliferate rapidly, resulting in inflammatory cellular infiltration, immune complex formation, and an inflammatory fibrinous exudate. The fibrin adheres to the articular cartilage, disrupts nutrient exchange, and can also isolate pockets of infection. The inflammatory reaction results in the production of proteolytic enzymes. The interruption of normal exchange of the nutrients and waste, coupled with the inflammatory formation of proteolytic enzymes, destroys the articular cartilage. Exposed subchondral bone is susceptible to osteomyelitis, particularly in cases with osteonecrosis or delayed diagnosis. The joint capsule is similarly attacked by enzymes and weakened, resulting in soft-tissue abscess formation. Rarely, the hip will subluxate or dislocated as a result of sepsis (60). Adhesions may form within the joint, resulting in fibrous, then bony, ankylosis of the hip (76).

Nonpyogenic organisms (e.g., mycobacteria and fungi) incite a different sequence of events resulting in joint destruction. A granulomatous reaction occurs in the synovium in response to the joint infection. The synovium thickens and produces fibrin "rice bodies" and an effusion. Proteolytic digestion does not occur. Cartilage is destroyed slowly by chronic granulation tissue, first at the periphery of the joint, then later throughout the joint as the granulation tissue dissects between the articular cartilage and bone. Caseous necrosis of bone occurs, and soft-tissue abscesses and sinus tracts may form (76).

PREDISPOSING FACTORS

Many conditions, both local and systemic, may predispose the joint to infection. Normally, the joint is able to effectively fight bacterial invasion. The joint's defenses are weakened by local disease, chronic systemic illness of the host, or both.

Local articular disorders resulting in a predilection for infection include osteoarthritis (23), avascular necrosis (33,63), hemophilia, previous trauma, seronegative arthritides (7), sickle cell disease, neuropathic arthropathy, and crystal-induced arthritis (76). These conditions may result in alteration of the normal joint environment, interrupting the exchange of nutrients and waste, or may produce a substance irritating to the joint. Synovial permeability may thus increase, allowing bacterial invasion. Hemophilia and trauma may result in a hemarthrosis, which may easily be seeded through damaged blood vessels.

Chronic systemic disease and immunosuppression clinically result in an increased incidence of hip infections. The chronic diseases include diabetes mellitus (3,32,34), alcoholism (34,58), cirrhosis (32,34,88), end-stage renal disease (74), malignancy, systemic lupus erythematosus (34,70), rheumatoid arthritis (23), malnutrition, and human immunodeficiency virus (HIV) (78). The immunocompromised state may result from treatment with steroids, chemotherapeutic drugs, and radiation therapy (64,76). Diabetics and alcoholics have a sluggish white blood cell response. Alcoholics and cirrhotics have altered complement protein production. End-stage renal disease patients may have less than optimal immune system function as the result of uremia and pancytopenia. Patients with rheumatoid arthritis and systemic lupus erythematosus may have decreased complement and antibody function. Malignancy results in overall weakening of the immune mechanism. Elderly, malnourished patients have a decreased number of T cells and an increased antibody response. Thus, many of the chronic illnesses are associated with immunosuppression, either as the result of a disease or as the result of a treatment. The primary sources of hematogenous seeding of the hip joint under immunosuppressed conditions are the genitourinary tract, lung, and skin (8).

DIAGNOSIS

Early diagnosis and treatment of hip sepsis is important, as the final outcome is determined by the extent of infection and the amount of joint destruction present. The diagnosis may be clinically obvious by history and physical, but in up to 50% of cases the presentation is atypical and the diagnosis uncertain (27). Further tests are then required.

History

The history is the first clue to the diagnosis. Most patients present with pain in the groin and inner thigh, occasionally radiating to the knee. The pain is present at rest and with activity. Fever is present with most pyogenic infections (except those caused by gonococcus). A single joint involvement is typical but not the rule. Symptoms suggesting a concurrent source of infection are often present, usually in the lung, urinary tract, or skin (8). Prodromal symptoms of malaise, weight loss, anorexia, and chills may be present, indicating the presence of bacteremia. A thorough history should be obtained, including a review of systems and a potential history of IV drug use, alcoholism, or diseases associated with immunosuppression. Prior surgical procedures or percutaneous procedures of the involved hip should raise the possibility of an iatrogenic infection.

Pain occurs acutely in most cases and is the result of joint capsule distension and secondary muscle spasm. When the pain if subacute or insidious in onset, the diagnosis may be delayed, leading to increased morbidity and mortality (8,14). This may occur in the following scenarios:

- The organism is Gram-negative.
- The patient is elderly, debilitated, or immunosuppressed and thus unable to mount an adequate inflammatory response to infection (8).
- The infection is caused by nonpyogenic organisms, such as mycobacteria or fungi. These organisms usually infect immunosuppressed or chronically ill patients and are associated with nonarticular joint pain, malaise, and other constitutional symptoms.
- The infection is acquired by extension from a nearby focus, and the hip capsule is eroded from the outside in. Thus no increase in joint pressure occurs, and pain is minimized.

Delay in diagnosis may also occur with hip sepsis superimposed on a hip with pre-existing disease. Patients with avascular necrosis, rheumatoid arthritis, and osteoarthritis often complain of "flare-ups," or occasional exacerbations of symptoms. Care must be taken to rule out hip sepsis in these patients when there is an increase in pain and concomitant systemic symptoms (23).

Physical Examination

Severe pain with attempts at any hip motion and typical positioning of the hip in about 45° of flexion, slight abduction, and external rotation are the classic signs of an acutely infected hip joint. This position is one of minimal intra-articular pressure and thus minimal pain. Usually the patient is unable to walk at all or has a severe antalgic pattern (shortened time in stance phase). Tenderness, erythema, and warmth over the hip are not often present; however, if present, they suggest a soft-tissue abscess extension. Some organisms, such as *Neisseria gonorrhea*, are associated with a rash.

A general physical evaluation should be conducted to detect potential local and systemic septic etiologies, including an assessment of the skin, mucosal membranes, rectum, lungs, heart, and abdomen. Involvement of an experienced physician able to detect abnormalities such as a cardiac murmur should be sought.

Chronic infections of the hip have a wider range of presentations on physical exam. Pain motion and contractures will be present but may be less dramatic than with a typical acute infection. Pronounced muscle atrophy is often present in the affected limb, indicating the chronicity of the process. The ambulatory patient will have an antalgic gait. Cutaneous manifestations may be more evident, such as palpable swelling, tenderness, and erythema. Cutaneus fistulae may develop and confirm the diagnosis of a chronic infection.

Radiologic Examination

In the evaluation of a suspected septic hip, the radiographic evaluation is generally limited to plain radiographs (AP pelvis and lateral of the proximal femur) and a fluoroscopic-guided or ultrasound-guided hip aspiration. The diagnosis of acute joint sepsis is based on the history and physical, with confirmation by a joint fluid evaluation. The purpose of the plain radiographs is to determine the joint space remaining and the potential for associated osteomyelitis. Ordering other examinations, such as a magnetic resonance imaging (MRI) scan, may delay the time to the definitive treatment. In cases where the diagnosis is difficult, unclear, or chronic, other imaging modalities may be helpful for detecting a joint effusion, soft-tissue thickening, a periarticular abscess, or osteomyelitis. These imaging modalities include ultrasound, MRI, computed tomography (CT), and types of nuclear medicine scanning (bone scanning, sulfur colloid scanning, and indium-labeled white blood cell scanning).

On a plain radiograph, early signs of infection (within 1 to 2 weeks) include soft-tissue swelling and widening of the teardrop interval. Radiographs may remain entirely normal for up to 2 weeks. The teardrop interval is measured from the lateral margin of the teardrop to the most medial aspect of the femoral head. In the absence of degenerative joint disease, a widening of 1 mm or more when compared with the opposite hip may be consistent with hip joint fluid (80). Pneumoarthropathy, or air in the joint, has been reported as an early radiographic manifestation of Gram-negative septic arthritis of the hip joint (11,57,66,83). Late x-ray findings include erosion and absorption of surrounding bone. Destruction of the femoral head and acetabulum are seen in far advanced, untreated cases. Dislocation and subluxation of the hip are also observed in severe cases (60).

Articular tuberculosis and fungal infections display more subtle x-ray findings. Nonpyogenic infections lack the early destruction of articular cartilage seen in pyogenic infections. Early x-ray findings may show only soft-tissue swelling. The articular cartilage is well preserved until very late in the disease course. Late disease may show bony destruction and abscess formation (76). Careful examination of the chest radiograph may aid in the diagnosis of tubercular or fungal joint sepsis. The majority of patients with fungal infections have pulmonary involvement, and 50% to 75% of patients with tubercular joint infections have pulmonary manifestations (76).

Ultrasound is a very useful modality in early detection of joint fluid. Minor fluid collections as small as 1 or 2 mL can be accurately detected (95). The quality of the fluid is also revealing; hyperechoic fluid and a thickened, hypertrophic capsule are diagnostic of septic arthritis (24,71,95). An echo-free effusion virtually rules out septic arthritis (95). Ultrasound should be used more often as a diagnostic tool, as it is much more sensitive and much cheaper than studies such as CT, MRI, and nuclear scans (43). Some authors consider it the method of choice for detecting joint effusions (24,71,95).

CT is a valuable modality in the evaluation of patients with acute septic arthritis of large joints. The quality of this imaging modality has increased significantly. A CT scan can be obtained quickly at relatively low cost. CT scans have been shown to identify periarticular soft-tissue swelling as early as 36 hours after onset of symptoms. They are also superior to plain radiographs for defining early articular bone erosion and for distinguishing adjacent osseous foci of infection in the abdomen and pelvis. CT scanning also may be used to guide needle aspiration of the hip joint (65).

An MRI scan, with its superior ability to clearly define soft-tissue pathology, may be helpful in defining early cartilage erosion and adjacent soft-tissue and bony involvement in infection. In the presence of an acute hip infection, the time required to obtain the study is not justified if the diagnosis is clear. On the other hand, MRI can helpful in the evaluation of a painful hip when the clinical picture is not felt to be consistent with an acutely infected hip or in a situation of chronic sepsis to determine the extent of involvement of the bone and adjacent soft tissues.

Nuclear scans using technetium, gallium, and indium, for example, are very sensitive in defining disease processes in the hip but are not specific. In one retrospective series of patients with a "cold" bone scan (decreased uptake in the involved joint), 22% of these patients had a septic joint at the time of surgery. It is believed that the pressure caused by a large hip effusion may impair profusion of the structures within the capsule (54,85,91). Therefore, nuclear scans, whether positive or negative, are not diagnostic of hip sepsis, and aspiration should be performed if clinically indicated.

Laboratory Examination

Systemic laboratory tests generally include peripheral white blood cell count, along with differential, erythrocyte sedimentation rate (ESR) and C-reactive protein (CRP). The ESR and CRP are nonspecific indicators of inflammation. They have a relatively high sensitivity and a moderate specificity. Mild anemia is often present in patients with septic hips, who must be carefully differentiated from patients with hip pain and severe anemia, which is suggestive of malignancy (5). The white blood cell count may or may not be elevated and is thus of questionable significance. However, the differential often shows an increased percentage of polymorphonuclear leukocytes. Blood cultures are positive in 50% of nongonococcal hip infections and in 20% of gonococcal hip infections. Cultures from the various possible sites of primary infection (genitourinary tract, sputum, skin, and throat) are recommended and may aid in the identification of the organism.

Joint Aspiration

Joint aspiration is the single most important test in the establishment of the diagnosis of hip septic arthritis (83). Once the diagnosis is established and the organism isolated, proper antibiotic treatment can be selected. Joint fluid is obtained by needle aspiration under strict sterile technique. An 18-gauge or larger spinal needle is inserted into the hip joint using one of three standard approaches (Fig. 39-4). All

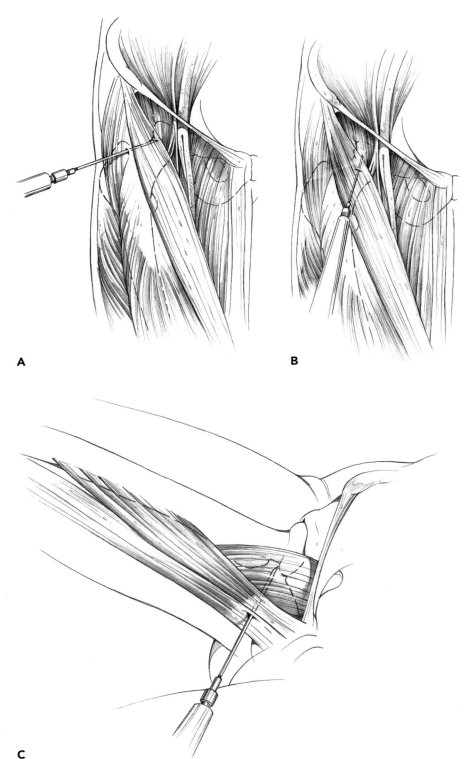

A

B

C

Figure 39-4 A: The lateral approach involves insertion of the spinal needle just inferior and anterior to the greater trochanter, at a 45° angle to the thigh, aimed superiorly. The needle is advanced medially and proximally for 5 to 10 cm into the joint. **B:** The anterior approach involves insertion of the needle at 2.5 cm distal and 2.5 cm lateral to the point at which the femoral artery crosses the inguinal ligament. The femoral pulse is easily palpable at this point in most people. The needle is advanced medially and proximally for 5 to 7.5 cm into the joint. **C:** The medial approach is performed with the leg flexed and abducted. The needle is placed inferior to the abductor longus tendon and directed toward the anterior tip of the greater trochanter. (Adapted from Crenshaw AH, ed. *Campbell's Operative Orthopaedic*. 8th ed. St Louis: Mosby Yearbook, Inc; 1992.)

insertions are best performed under fluoroscopic guidance and with the introduction of contrast into the joint to confirm needle placement. The hip should be aspirated dry. If no fluid is obtained, then nonbacteriostatic saline should be introduced into the hip and withdrawn (76). The presence of a draining sinus track makes aspiration of the joint impossi-

ble. Sinus drainage should not be sent for culture. True results are obtained only by joint biopsy in these cases (76). Collected fluid should be sent for Gram stain and culture (aerobic, anaerobic, acid fast, and fungal), cell count and differential, and chemical analysis—particularly glucose, protein, and lactic acid. The fluid should also be assessed grossly for volume, color, clarity, viscosity, and capacity to form a mucin clot.

The normal hip has a volume of 1 to 2 mL of fluid. This fluid is clear, straw-colored, and viscous, and it forms a firm mucin clot. Total white blood cell count is from 0 to 200, with less than 10% neutrophils. Protein is less than 2.5 g/dL, and glucose equals the serum glucose. Synovial fluid from a septic hip with pyogenic organisms is usually turbid or grossly purulent and malodorous, with decreased viscosity and a poor mucin clot. White blood cell count is elevated to 100 to 250,000, with 90% neutrophils. Protein ranges from 2.5 to 8 g/dL, and glucose is approximately 90 mg/dL lower than serum glucose. Lactic acid is elevated as compared with plasma. Gram stains are positive. Nonpyogenic organisms have a slightly different profile (1). Organism stains are often equivocal, and cultures must be carefully reviewed, with follow-up at 4 to 6 weeks if initially negative. If the clinical picture suggests joint sepsis, and cultures are negative, synovial biopsy is indicated (76).

There are many clinical entities that produce effusions, and differentiation of these entities can be made clinically upon analysis of synovial fluid. Group 1 (noninflammatory effusions) includes avascular necrosis, degenerative joint disease, and traumatic arthritis. These lack the constitutional symptoms seen in septic arthritis. Group 2 and group 3 (including systemic lupus erythematosus, seronegative arthritides, and scleroderma) have classic syndromes and characteristic features associated with them (1,76).

TREATMENT

Acute joint sepsis should be considered an emergency since irreparable cartilage damage ensues within 48 hours. In the preantibiotic era, the goal of treatment was survival of the patient, as nearly two thirds of the patients died. Those who survived had severely compromised extremity function. Today, mortality is much lower (13%), and the treatment goals are elimination of infection and preservation of joint function (1,27,76). This is accomplished by antibiotic therapy, joint drainage, physical therapy and rehabilitation, and reconstructive surgery.

Joint drainage is a mainstay of treatment for a septic joint. Evacuation of the joint is necessary to remove the inflammatory fluid and relieve the pressure. The inflammatory fluid contains many toxins and proteolytic enzymes that destroy the articular cartilage. Increased intra-articular pressure compromises circulation to the femoral head and surrounding structures. This results in osteonecrosis and pressure necrosis of soft tissues and decreased penetration of the joint by circulating antibiotics. The joint can be drained by repeated arthrocentesis, arthroscopy, or arthrotomy.

Adjuvant treatments to protect the remaining cartilage are being evaluated. Use of an adenosine A2A agonist may decrease the articular damage associated with the immune response to a joint infection (17). Systemic administration of steroids may have cartilage protective effects when treating septic joints in conjunction with appropriate antibiotic treatment (40,77). Hyperbaric oxygen has been used postoperatively in anaerobic infections with success (58).

Acute Infection

Arthrocentesis

Repeated arthrocentesis has been used successfully by a few authors (33,66); however, it is very difficult and generally not recommended by most as the best drainage mechanism. A sensitive organism (such as gonococcus), an early diagnosis, and a relatively healthy host are usually necessary factors for this technique to work.

Hip Arthroscopy

Hip arthroscopy has been used successfully to treat septic arthritis of the hip. Arthroscopic lavage and debridement, coupled with postoperative suction and drainage or closed-tube drainage, has been shown to be as effective a treatment as open arthrotomy, with a much lower morbidity and an earlier return of joint mobility (10,13,16,46,93). In the hands of an experienced arthroscopist, this technique may soon be the treatment of choice.

Kim et al. reported results for 10 patients aged 3 to 36 years with acute hip infections treated by arthroscopy in the supine position. All patient sustained resolution of the infection and had an excellent clinical result (average Harris hip score of 97) at 59 months postoperatively (46).

Open Debridement

Open surgical drainage is the present gold standard of hip drainage. An arthrotomy allows complete release of intra-articular fluid, exposure to irrigate, and access for tissue biopsy. It also allows for femoral head resection in advanced cases.

The arthrotomy can be performed via one of several approaches. The choice of approach is based largely on the surgeon's preference, with factors such as future surgical reconstruction and skin integrity taken into account (76,83). The posterolateral, anterolateral (Watson-Jones), and direct anterior are all commonly used approaches for open irrigation. The posterior approach requires protection of the medial circumflex artery to minimize the chance of causing femoral head necrosis. For surgeons who are comfortable performing joint arthroplasty through the posterolateral approach, using the same surgical plane for irrigation and debridement has advantages if the patient needs further reconstructive procedures. The advantages of the anterior approach are the internervous plane and the safety of the proximal femoral blood supply.

The capsule is left open following irrigation and debridement. Removing a window of the capsule ensures decompression of the joint cavity during the postoperative period. The wound may be packed open, closed loosely over suction, or closed over a closed-tube irrigation–suction system. Open packing of a wound allows drainage, but there is an increased risk of superinfection and cartilage desiccation. Delayed primary closure can be performed at a later date based on wound inspection. Any soft-tissue abscesses or fistulous tracks should be débrided at the time of surgery.

Postoperatively, gentle active and passive range of motion is then instituted. Depending on the degree of hip pain and destruction, the patient may be placed in balanced suspension or in light Bucks traction until acute pain is gone and the patient has control of the leg (i.e., can raise it off of the bed against gravity).

Antibiotics

Antibiotic treatment should be started immediately after fluid is obtained. Antibiotic selection is based on the Gram stain results and the clinical setting. If the Gram stain shows Gram-positive organisms in pairs, a penicillinase-resistant penicillin (nafcillin) or a second-generation cephalosporin (cephazolin) is initiated. Vancomycin is generally reserved for documented resistant strains of *Staphylococcus aureus*. *Staphylococcus epidermitis* is rarely a pathogen without previous implants; however, one should be aware that up to 90% of these species are resistant to penicillinase-resistant penicillin. If the Gram stain is consistent with *Streptococcus* species, penicillin G is instituted. In the setting of a negative Gram stain, an extended spectrum cephalosporin (such as ceftriaxone) should be instituted. Delay in antibiotic treatment until results of cultures and sensitivities are available is unwise. When cultures and sensitivities are available, the antibiotics may be tailored to the specific organism.

The optimal duration of antibiotic treatment is not known. Antibiotics should be administered parentally for at least 4 weeks. The antibiotics penetrate the inflamed synovium readily from the bloodstream (30). Intra-articular injection or infusion of antibiotics is unnecessary and may lead to a chemical synovitis or toxicity to the chondrocytes. The use of polymethylmethacrylate beads impregnated with antibiotics (gentamicin, tobramycin, and/or vancomycin) and inserted into the dead space after resection has proven to be effective in producing high concentrations of antibiotics locally (36,76).

A longer duration of antibiotic treatment is required under certain circumstances. *Staphylococcus aureus*, Gram-negative bacilli, and anaerobic organisms may require an additional 2 weeks of antibiotic treatment. Six weeks of antibiotic treatment is also required if bony involvement (i.e., osteomyelitis) is suspected. If fungi are the causative organisms, 6 to 12 weeks is required. *Mycobacterium* requires 6 to 24 months of antibiotic treatment. In any circumstance, antibiotics may be switched from the parental to the oral route once clinical signs of sepsis have abated and serial CRP levels have decreased toward normal. Occasionally, a repeat joint aspiration may be necessary to determine the effectiveness of the original surgical drainage and antibiotic regimen.

Acutely Infected Arthritic Hip and Pyogenic Arthritis

Decisions regarding the management of the patient with a septic joint in the face of absent cartilage can be more difficult. Decisions regarding the reconstruction must be considered when planning the treatment of the infection. The optimal result for the patient with a septic arthritic hip would include resolution of the infection and reconstruction with a total joint arthroplasty in a timely manner. The timing between treatment of the sepsis and placement of a joint arthroplasty is debatable. Alternatively, achieving ankylosis in a young patient or a patient with a significant risk of sepsis with joint arthroplasty may be preferable to a resection arthroplasty.

Debridement and Fusion

Arthrodesis is recommended by some in young, active patients (76). However, fusion is very difficult to achieve, and arthrodesis is not a necessary or an adequate means of obtaining a good result in hip infection (26).

Resection Arthroplasty

In some patients, such as the elderly or immunocompromised, patients with severe joint destruction, and patients requiring motion of the hip, resection arthroplasty, or Girdlestone, may be performed (Fig. 39-5). A Girdlestone may be a definitive operation or it may be one step in a two-stage total hip replacement procedure or muscle flap procedure. Long-term results of Girdlestone arthroplasty show that it is an excellent procedure for patients with low ambulatory demands (patients who are elderly, bedridden, or paraplegic) and that it is a good procedure for relief of pain in all groups (84). Ambulatory groups showed excellent pain relief, control of infection, and restoration of the ability to squat and sit cross-legged. Ambulatory status, however, was not fully restored (48,84).

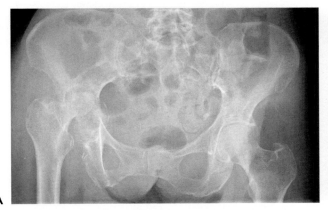
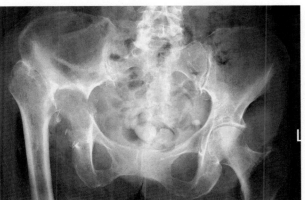

Figure 39-5 **A:** Radiographs illustrating a 75-year-old woman with severe medical cormorbidities who developed right hip sepsis following complications from a right femoral artery catheterization. Previous right groin abscess irrigation and debridement by a vascular surgeon resulted in a complete femoral nerve palsy. **B:** The right hip infection was treated with a resection arthroplasty that resulted in resolution of the infection and pain. She is able to walk with a cane for short distances and uses a walker when walking one to two blocks.

Despite resection of the hip, infection can recur, especially when infection is caused by *E. coli*, *Pseudomonas*, *Proteus*, or *Streptococcus* group D (83). When infection persists, radical debridement is required. If this is still unsuccessful, the options available include hip disarticulation, vastus lateralis muscle flap, or acceptance of a chronically draining hip. Hip disarticulation is associated with problems of wound healing, and it does not leave the patient with a functional joint (or extremity, for that matter). The vastus lateralis muscle flap is utilized to fill the dead space in the hip after debridement and is successful in promoting healing (48,76). A draining hip is aesthetically unpleasing, requires constant wound care, and is a source of protein loss in the already ill (and usually malnourished) patient (76).

Two-Stage Arthroplasty

The functional outcome is better with joint arthroplasty than with resection arthroplasty (6). For patients with an unacceptable functional result with a Girdlestone, total hip replacement can be performed once infection is eradicated (Fig. 39-6) (6,15,35,38,42,44). Many of the series that have reported the results of joint replacement following a history of native hip sepsis show a variable interval between the treatment and resolution of the infection and the joint arthroplasty. Cherney

and Amstutz reported results for 33 patients with previous joint infections treated with hip arthroplasty (15). Ten of these patients were native joint infections and were associated with a higher failure rate at 2- to 7-year follow-up (4 of 10 failed). With one exception, the time between debridement and joint arthroplasty in these patients was 12 to 72 months. Kim et al. reported results for 170 hips with previous childhood sepsis (age range, 1 to 11 years) converted to total replacements at an average age of 42 years (47). Two hips in one patient who had conversion to an arthroplasty at 7 years developed recurrent infections. All other patients (>10 years between joint sepsis and arthroplasty) had successful procedures without recurrence of infection.

Immediate resection with antibiotic spacer placement followed by a staged joint arthroplasty is the treatment of choice for an infected joint, with success rates of approximately 80%. Presumably, a similar treatment philosophy could be applied to the treatment of septic arthritis. Septic arthritis of the knee treated with resection, antibiotic spacer placement, and staged total knee replacement (average, 3 months from debridement/spacer) has been reported, with no recurrent infection at 4- to 5-year follow-up (62). Hernigou et al. reported results for 10 septic hips in patients with sickle cell disease treated with a resection, local antibiotics, and staged

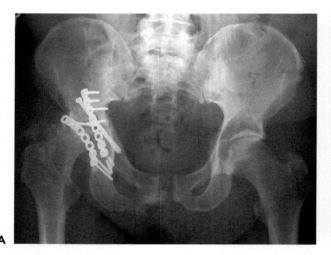

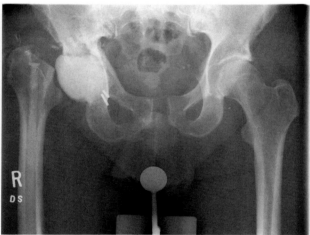

A   B   C

Figure 39-6   Radiographs of a 67-year-old male who had an open reduction and fixation of a displaced acetabualar fracture 2 years prior. **A:** Evaluation for presumed posttraumatic arthritis revealed purulence with *Staphylococcus epidermidis*. **B:** Resection and placement of an antibiotic spacer was performed. **C:** Conversion to a total hip was performed after a 6-week course of antibiotics and 4 weeks off antibiotics, without recurrence.

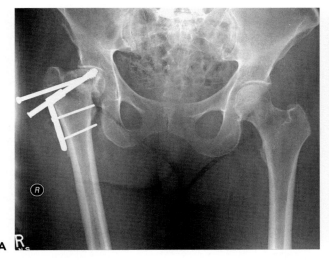
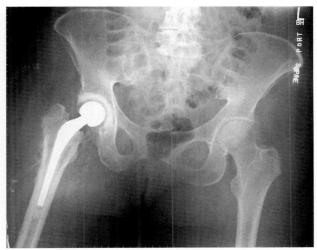
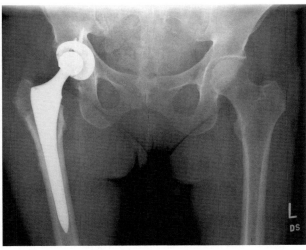

Figure 39-7 Radiographs of a 68-year-old woman who had a failed internal fixation of a femoral neck fracture complicated with avascular necrosis. **A:** Evaluation for infection was positive for *Staphylococcus epidermidis*. **B:** Placement of a PROSTALAC (DePuy, Warsaw, IN). **C:** Conversion to a total hip following 6 weeks of antibiotics and an infection-free period of 4 weeks off antibiotics.

total hip at 2 to 12 years. Two of 10 hips developed an infection of the arthroplasty, and the remaining patients had near-normal hip function (35).

Temporary prosthesis placement (e.g., PROSTALAC) for the interval period between resection and conversion to total hip is an alternative and may allow for maintenance of soft-tissue tension and improved stability (Fig. 39-7) (94). Hsieh et al. found that 9 of 63 patients (14%) treated with resection and bead placement dislocated, compared with 1 of 56 patients (1.8%) treated with an articulated spacer prior to reimplantation (37).

CONCLUSION

Septic arthritis in the adult hip is an increasing problem with a significant mortality rate (13%). It must be diagnosed and treated early. If clinical, laboratory, or radiographic evidence even remotely suggests hip sepsis, the joint must be aspirated. Hip aspiration and identification of the microorganism are of paramount importance, and culture samples must be carefully taken and prepared. Antibiotics should be started immediately after Gram stain results are back, and they should be tailored to the specific organism when cultures grow out. Open

arthrotomy or arthroscopic debridement is performed on an emergent basis to protect the cartilage. In situations in which sepsis is present and the joint has been destroyed, the options include fusion, Girdlestone resection, or staged resection followed by joint arthroplasty.

REFERENCES

1. Andreoli TE, Carpenter CJ, Plum F, et al., eds. *Cecil's Essentials of Medicine.* Philadelphia: WB Saunders; 1990.
2. Ang-Fonte GZ, Rozboril MB, Thompson GR. Changes in non-gonococcal septic arthritis: drug abuse and methicillin-resistant *Staphylococcus aureus. Arthritis Rheum.* 1985;28:210–213.
3. Apple JS, Halvorsen RA, Chapman TM, et al. *Klebsiella pneumoniae* arthritis of the hip in a diabetic patient. *South Med J.* 1984;77:229–231.
4. Ash N, Salai M, Aphter S, et al. Primary psoas abscess due to methicillin-resistant *Staphylococcus aureus* concurrent with septic arthritis of the hip joint. *South Med J.* 1995;88:863–865.
5. Aston JW Jr. Pediatric update no. 16. The orthopaedic presentation of neuroblastoma. *Orthop Rev.* 1990;19:929–932.
6. Balderston RA, Hiller WD, Iannotti JP, et al. Treatment of the septic hip with total hip arthroplasty. *Clin Orthop Relat Res.* 1987;221:231–237.
7. Barker CS, Symmons DP, Scott DL, et al. Joint sepsis as a complication of sero-negative arthritis. *Clin Rheumatol.* 1985;4:51–54.

8. Bettin D, Dethloff M, Karbowski A. [Joint destruction and infection in advanced age]. *Z Orthop Ihre Grenzgeb.* 1994;132:472–475.
9. Bettin D, Schul B, Schwering L. Diagnosis and treatment of joint infections in elderly patients. *Acta Orthop Belg.* 1998;64:131–135.
10. Blitzer CM. Arthroscopic management of septic arthritis of the hip. *Arthroscopy.* 1993;9:414–416.
11. Bliznak J, Ramsey J. Emphysematous septic arthritis due to *Escherichia coli. J Bone Joint Surg [Am].* 1976;58:138–139.
12. Bosch X, Ramon R, Font J, et al. Bilateral cryptococcosis of the hip: a case report. *J Bone Joint Surg [Am].* 1994;76:1234–1238.
13. Bould M, Edwards D, Villar RN. Arthroscopic diagnosis and treatment of septic arthritis of the hip joint. *Arthroscopy.* 1993;9:707–708.
14. Brien EW, Brien WW, Long WT, et al. Concomitant injuries of the hip joint and abdomen resulting from gunshot wounds. *Orthopedics.* 1992;15:1317–1319; discussion 1319–1320.
15. Cherney DL, Amstutz HC. Total hip replacement in the previously septic hip. *J Bone Joint Surg [Am].* 1983;65:1256–1265.
16. Chung WK, Slater GL, Bates EH. Treatment of septic arthritis of the hip by arthroscopic lavage. *J Pediatr Orthop.* 1993;13:444–446.
17. Cohen SB, Gill SS, Baer GS, et al. Reducing joint destruction due to septic arthrosis using an adenosine2A receptor agonist. *J Orthop Res.* 2004;22:427–435.
18. Cooke CP 3rd, Levinsohn EM, Baker BE. Septic hip in pelvic fractures with urologic injury: a case report, review of the literature and discussion of the pathophysiology. *Clin Orthop.* 1980;147: 253–257.
19. Cottalorda J, Jouve JL, Bollini G, et al. Osteoarticular infection due to *Coxiella burnetii* in children. *J Pediatr Orthop B.* 1995;4:219–221.
20. Craig DB, Wehrle PA. *Branhamella catarrhalis* septic arthritis. *J Rheumatol.* 1983;10:985–986.
21. Davis JM, Peel MM. Osteomyelitis and septic arthritis caused by *Kingella kingae. J Clin Pathol.* 1982;35:219–222.
22. De Boeck H, Noppen L, Desprechins B. Pyomyositis of the adductor muscles mimicking an infection of the hip: diagnosis by magnetic resonance imaging: a case report. *J Bone Joint Surg [Am].* 1994;76:747–750.
23. Donell S, Williamson DM, Scott DL. Septic arthritis complicating hip osteoarthritis. *Ann Rheum Dis.* 1991;50:722–723.
24. Dorr U, Zieger M, Hauke H. Ultrasonography of the painful hip: prospective studies in 204 patients. *Pediatr Radiol.* 1988;19:36–40.
25. Dzioba RB, Barrington TW. Transient monoarticular synovitis of the hip joint in adults. *Clin Orthop.* 1977;126:190–192.
26. Evrard J, Hourtoulle P, Roure JL, et al. [Hip arthrodeses for septic arthritis: critical study]. *Rev Chir Orthop Reparatrice Appar Mot.* 1985;71:87–93.
27. Evrard J, Soudrie B. [Primary arthritis of the hip in adults]. *Int Orthop.* 1993;17:367–374.
28. Fachartz OA, Kumar V, al Hilou M. Synovial schistosomiasis of the hip. *J Bone Joint Surg [Br].* 1993;75:602–603.
29. Femminineo AF, LaBan MM. Paraparesis in a patient with Crohn disease resulting from septic arthritis of the hip and psoas abscess. *Arch Phys Med Rehabil.* 1988;69[3 Pt 1]:223–225.
30. Frimodt-Moller N, Riegels-Nielsen P. Antibiotic penetration into the infected knee: a rabbit experiment. *Acta Orthop Scand.* 1987;58:256–259.
31. Fromm SE, Toohey JS. Septic arthritis of the hip in an adult following repeated femoral venipuncture. *Orthopedics.* 1996;19: 1047–1048.
32. Gomez-Rodriguez N, Ferreiro JL, Willisch A, et al. [Osteoarticular infections caused by *Streptococcus agalactiae*: report of 4 cases]. *Enferm Infecc Microbiol Clin.* 1995;13:99–103.
33. Habermann ET, Friedenthal RB. Septic arthritis associated with avascular necrosis of the femoral head. *Clin Orthop.* 1978:134: 325–331.
34. Hamza M, Elleuch M, Meddeb S, et al. [Arthritis and osteomyelitis caused by *Salmonella typhimurium* in a case of disseminated lupus erythematosus]. *Rev Rhum Mal Osteoartic.* 1990;57:670.
35. Hernigou P, Odent T, Manicom O, et al. [Total hip arthroplasty for the treatment of septic hip arthritis in adults with sickle-cell disease]. *Rev Chir Orthop Reparatrice Appar Mot.* 2004;90:557–560.
36. Hovelius L, Josefsson G. An alternative method for exchange operation of infected arthroplasty. *Acta Orthop Scand.* 1979;50:93–96.
37. Hsieh P-H, Shih C-H, Chang Y-H, et al. Two-stage revision hip arthroplasty for infection: comparison between the interim use of antibiotic-loaded cement beads and a spacer prosthesis. *J Bone Joint Surg [Am].* 2004;86:1989–1997.
38. Hughes PW, Salvati EA, Wilson PD Jr, et al. Treatment of subacute sepsis of the hip by antibiotics and joint replacement: criteria for diagnosis with evaluation of twenty-six cases. *Clin Orthop Relat Res.* 1979;No. 141:143–157.
39. Izbekov AT, Godzhaev AG, Maliukov GT. [Echinococcosis of the spine and hip joint]. *Khirurgiia (Mosk).* October 1987:53–57.
40. Jafari HS, Saez-Llorens X, Paris M, et al. Dexamethasone attenuation of cytokine-mediated articular cartilage degradation in experimental lapine Haemophilus arthritis. *J Infect Dis.* 1993;168:1186–1193.
41. Joly P, Boissonnas A, Fournier R, et al. [Septic arthritis caused by *Campylobacter fetus*]. *Rev Rhum Mal Osteoartic.* 1986;53:223–226.
42. Jupiter JB, Karchmer AW, Lowell JD, et al. Total hip arthroplasty in the treatment of adult hips with current or quiescent sepsis. *J Bone Joint Surg [Am].* 1981;63:194–200.
43. Kang B, Zhu TB, Du JY, et al. Ultrasound diagnosis of effusion of the hip. *J Tongji Med Univ.* 1993;13:156–160.
44. Katz LM, Lewis RJ, Borenstein DG. Successful joint arthroplasty following *Proteus morganii (Morganella morganii)* septic arthritis: a four-year study. *Arthritis Rheum.* 1987;30:583–585.
45. Kiang KM, et al. Outbreak of osteomyelitis/septic arthritis caused by *Kingella kingae* among child care center attendees. *Pediatrics.* 2005;16:e206–213.
46. Kim SJ, Choi NH, Ko SH, et al. Arthroscopic treatment of septic arthritis of the hip. *Clin Orthop Relat Res.* 2003;407:211–214.
47. Kim YH, Oh SH, Kim JS. Total hip arthroplasty in adult patients who had childhood infection of the hip. *J Bone Joint Surg [Am].* 2003;85A:198–204.
48. Klein N, Moore T, Capen D, et al. Sepsis of the hip in paraplegic patients. *J Bone Joint Surg [Am].* 1988;70:839–843.
49. Lam K, Bayer AS. Serious infections due to group G streptococci: report of 15 cases with in vitro–in vivo correlations. *Am J Med.* 1983;75:561–570.
50. Lee AH, Chin AE, Ramanujam T, et al. Gonococcal septic arthritis of the hip. *J Rheumatol.* 1991;18:1932–1933.
51. Levitin B, Rubin LA, Rubenstein JD. Occult retroperitoneal abscess presenting as septic arthritis of the hip. *J Rheumatol.* 1982; 9:904–908.
52. Lohmander LS, Wingstrand H, Heinegard D. Transient synovitis of the hip in the child: increased levels of proteoglycan fragments in joint fluid. *J Orthop Res.* 1988;6:420–424.
53. Lortat-Jacob A, Lortat-Jacob S, Jouanin T, et al. [Arthritis of the hip in paraplegic patients: apropos of 8 cases]. *Rev Chir Orthop Reparatrice Appar Mot.* 1984;70:383–388.
54. Mack JM, Sziklas JJ, Rosenberg RJ, et al. Recovery of femoral head perfusion after drainage of septic joint. *Clin Nucl Med.* 1987;12: 850–851.
55. Magen AB, Moser RP Jr, Woomert CA, et al. Septic arthritis of the hip: a complication of a rectal tear associated with pelvic fractures. *AJR Am J Roentgenol.* 1991;157:817–818.
56. McDonald MI, Moore JO, Harrelson JM, et al. Septic arthritis due to *Mycoplasma hominis. Arthritis Rheum.* 1983;26:1044–1047.
57. Meredith HC, Rittenberg GM. Pneumoarthropathy: an unusual radiographic sign of Gram-negative septic arthritis. *Radiology.* 1978;128:642.
58. Merle-Melet M, Mainard D, Regent D, et al. An unusual case of hip septic arthritis due to *Bacteroides fragilis* in an alcoholic patient. *Infection.* 1994;22:353–355.
59. Messieh M, Turner R, Bunch F, et al. Hip sepsis from retroperitoneal rupture of diverticular disease. *Orthop Rev.* 1993;22:597–599.
60. Milgram JW, Rana NA. Resection arthroplasty for septic arthritis of the hip in ambulatory and nonambulatory adult patients. *Clin Orthop.* 1991;272:181–191.
61. Nakata MM, Silvers JH, George WL. Group G streptococcal arthritis. *Arch Intern Med.* 1983;143:1328–1330.
62. Nazarian DG, de Jesus D, McGuigan F, et al. A two-stage approach to primary knee arthroplasty in the infected arthritic knee. *J Arthroplasty.* 2003;18[7 Suppl 1]:16–21.
63. Nuovo MA, Sissons HA, Zuckerman JD. Case report 662. Bilateral avascular necrosis of femur, with supervening suppurative arthritis of right hip. *Skeletal Radiol.* 1991;20:217–221.

64. Ostrum RF. *Nocardia* septic arthritis of the hip with associated avascular necrosis: a case report. *Clin Orthop.* 1993;288:282–286.

65. Rafii M, Firooznia H, Golimbu C. Computed tomography of septic joints. *J Comput Tomogr.* 1985;9:51–60.

66. Rampon S, Lopitaux R, Meloux J, et al. [Non-tuberculous infectious coxitis in adults]. *Rev Rhum Mal Osteoartic.* 1981;48(1):77–81.

67. Reboli AC, Bryan CS, Farrar WE. Bacteremia and infection of a hip prosthesis caused by *Bacillus alvei. J Clin Microbiol.* 1989;27:1395–1396.

68. Resnik CS, Sawyer RW, Tisnado J. Septic arthritis of the hip: a rare complication of angiography. *Can Assoc Radiol J.* 1987;38:299–301.

69. Rubinow A. Septic arthritis of the hip caused by *Neisseria gonococcae. Clin Orthop.* 1983;181:115–117.

70. Shiota K, Miki F, Kanayama Y, et al. Suppurative coxitis due to *Salmonella typhimurium* in systemic lupus erythematosus. *Ann Rheum Dis.* 1981;40:312–314.

71. Shiv VK, Jain AK, Taneja K, et al. Sonography of hip joint in infective arthritis. *Can Assoc Radiol J.* 1990;41:76–78.

72. Shreeve DR, Ormerod LP, Dunbar EM. Crohn's disease with fistulae involving joints. *J R Soc Med.* 1982;75:946–948.

73. Small CB, Slater LN, Lowy FD, et al. Group B streptococcal arthritis in adults. *Am J Med.* 1984;76:367–375.

74. Specht EE. *Candida* pyarthrosis of the hip and renal homotransplant: report of a case treated by femoral head and neck resection and 5-fluorocytosine. *Clin Orthop.* 1977;No. 126:176–177.

75. Steinbach LS, Schneider R, Goldman AB, et al. Bursae and abscess cavities communicating with the hip: diagnosis using arthrography and CT. *Radiology.* 1985;156:303–307.

76. Steinberg ME, ed. *The Hip and Its Disorders.* Philadelphia: WB Saunders; 1991.

77. Stricker SJ, Lozman PR, Makowski AL, et al. Chondroprotective effect of betamethasone in lapine pyogenic arthritis. *J Pediatr Orthop.* 1996;16:231–236.

78. Strongin IS, Kale SA, Raymond MK, et al. An unusual presentation of gonococcal arthritis in an HIV positive patient. *Ann Rheum Dis.* 1991;50:572–573.

79. Strugo R, Tovar R, Zimlichman R. [Psoas abscess mimicking septic arthritis of the hip]. *Harefuah.* 1995;128:216–219, 263.

80. Sweeney JP, Helms CA, Minagi H, et al. The widened teardrop distance: a plain film indicator of hip joint effusion in adults. *AJR Am J Roentgenol.* 1987;149:117–119.

81. Thangkhiew I, Ghosh MK, Kar NK, et al. Septic arthritis due to *Listeria monocytogenes. J Infect.* 1990;21:324–325.

82. Tibrewal SB, Kenwright J. Septic arthritis of the hip due to bacteroides-melanogenicus. *J R Soc Med.* 1990;83:117–118.

83. Tronzo RG, ed. *Surgery of the Hip Joint.* New York: Springer-Verlag; 1987.

84. Tuli SM, Mukherjee SK. Excision arthroplasty for tuberculous and pyogenic arthritis of the hip. *J Bone Joint Surg [Br].* 1981;63B:29–32.

85. Uren RF, Howman-Giles R. The "cold hip" sign on bone scan: a retrospective review. *Clin Nucl Med.* 1991;16:553–556.

86. Varoga D, Pufe T, Harder J, et al. Production of endogenous antibiotics in articular cartilage. *Arthritis Rheum.* 2004;50:3526–3534.

87. Verinder DG. Septic arthritis due to mycoplasma hominis: a case report and review of the literature. *J Bone Joint Surg [Br].* 1978;60B:224.

88. Watine J, Martorell J, Bruna T, et al. In vivo pefloxacin-resistant *Campylobacter fetus* responsible for gastro-intestinal infection and bacteremia associated with arthritis of the hip. *Yonsei Med J.* 1995;36:202–205.

89. Wegmann T, Monegat J, Haegi V, et al. [Candida coxitis (author's trans.)]. *Dtsch Med Wochenschr.* 1979;104:635–637.

90. Williams PH, Odurny A. Case report: septic arthritis of the hip following ureteric stent insertion. *Br J Radiol.* 1995;68:534–536.

91. Williamson BR, Sistrom CL. Femoral and acetabular photopenia associated with septic hip arthritis. *Clin Nucl Med.* 1991;16:52.

92. Yagupsky P. *Kingella kingae*: from medical rarity to an emerging paediatric pathogen. *Lancet Infect Dis.* 2004;4:358–367.

93. Yamamoto Y, Ide T, Hachisuka N, et al. Arthroscopic surgery for septic arthritis of the hip joint in 4 adults. *Arthroscopy.* 2001;17:290–297.

94. Younger AS, Duncan CP, Masri BA, et al. The outcome of two-stage arthroplasty using a custom-made interval spacer to treat the infected hip. *J Arthroplasty.* 1997;12:615–623.

95. Zieger MM, Dorr U, Schulz RD. Ultrasonography of hip joint effusions. *Skeletal Radiol.* 1987;16:607–611.

Soft-Tissue Disorders about the Hip

40

Michael J. Archibeck

Although orthopedic surgeons have become quite familiar with the nonoperative and surgical treatment of hip joint disorders, soft-tissue ailments about the hip account for a large portion of patients presenting with hip complaints. An understanding of the diagnosis and treatment of these soft-tissue disorders will serve the physician well when treating such patients. This chapter reviews trochanteric bursitis, iliopsoas syndrome, tendonitis, the snapping hip, labral pathology, and nerve entrapment syndromes about the hip.

TROCHANTERIC BURSITIS

While many bursae exist about the hip, the trochanteric bursa is known to commonly become inflamed and painful. The trochanteric bursa is located deep to the fascia lata and covers a variable surface area of the gluteus medius, lateral greater trochanter, and vastus lateralis complex. Although the bursal tissue can become inflamed and painful, surrounding tissues have also been shown to contribute to the pain syndrome. Such tissues include the gluteus medius and minimus tendinous insertions into the greater trochanter (34). Bird et al. found tears or tendonitis of the gluteus medius to be present on magnetic resonance imaging (MRI) in over 63% of patients with clinically diagnosed trochanteric bursitis (5).

Trochanteric bursitis is associated with other disease processes such as lumbar spine disease, intra-articular hip pathology, rheumatoid arthritis, leg-length discrepancies, and ipsilateral lower extremity atrophy (53,65). Trochanteric bursitis is also common after total hip replacement. In such cases, it is felt to be secondary to irritation of local tissues from scarring, sutures, or hardware.

Other bursae about the hip can be a source of pain as well. Ischial bursitis has been described and presents with sitting intolerance or a mass in the buttock (1,37). The iliopsoas bursa can be symptomatic as well, as discussed later.

Often referred to in the literature as *greater trochanteric pain syndrome* (GTPS) (59), trochanteric bursitis most commonly affects middle-aged and elderly patients. It can result from antecedent trauma but is frequently insidious in its onset. It is more common in females than males (5). Patients generally describe lateral-sided hip pain in the region of the greater trochanter. The pain can radiate down the lateral thigh toward the knee (59). Pain is often described to be present with prolonged sitting and is often present at rest as well as with activity. Sleeping on the side is typically painful.

Physical examination findings in GTPS can include an antalgic gait. Palpation of the trochanter during gait can demonstrate crepitation or snapping. A Trendelenburg sign has been described as indicative of gluteus medius tendon involvement (5). Supine exam often demonstrates normal range of motion. Pain is often present with external rotation of the hip, especially in positions that tighten the iliotibial band (extension and adduction). Tenderness directly over the trochanter is the most common physical examination finding in GTPS. Pain with resisted abduction can indicate involvement of the abductor tendons as well.

While the diagnosis is generally made based on history and physical examination, occasionally adjunctive tests are available from referring physicians or are ordered to determine the etiology of hip pain of unknown origin. Plain radiography is generally normal, although calcifications and lateral trochanteric irregularities can be present. MRI findings can include a distended bursa, edema adjacent to the trochanter, and/or abductor tendinosis (5,34,38) (Fig. 40-1). Bird et al. found that in 24 female patients with clinically diagnosed GTPS, MRI demonstrated gluteus medius tears or tendonitis in over 63% (5). Technicium-99 bone scan scintography can also show mild localized uptake in the region of the lateral greater trochanter (Fig. 40-2) (2). Sonography has been successfully used to evaluate gluteus medius and minimus tendinopathy as well (9). Although not the imaging technique of choice, computed tomography (CT) scan can demonstrate a distended trochanteric bursa (71).

Other disease processes that can result in lateral-sided hip pain include radicular pain (L2, L3 nerve roots) (69), lesions of the greater trochanter, intra-articular hip pathology, and infection. Septic trochanteric bursitis can occur and has been described as a complication of injection (28,75).

The mainstay of treatment for trochanteric bursitis is nonoperative. Exercises include stretching of the iliotibial band and strengthening of the abductor musculature. Nonsteroidal anti-inflammatories can be useful. Physical therapists are generally very helpful in guiding the patient's exercise program. Many patients have found modalities such as localized ultrasound helpful as well.

The use of localized injection has been very successful in the treatment of GTPS (14,60). The injection generally includes a local anesthetic and a corticosteroid. This is generally injected adjacent to the lateral aspect of the greater trochanter at the point of maximal tenderness. Injections can be repeated at 3- to 4-month intervals if successful. Injections can also be diagnostic—if the local anesthetic, which typically lasts for 2 to 6 hours, is effective at relieving the patient's pain, the diagnosis of GTPS is likely. Ege Rasmussen identified an excellent response in two thirds of 36 cases of GTPS and some improvement in the remaining patients (14). Shbeeb found relief in 77%, 69%, and 61% of 75 patients at 1, 6, and 26 weeks postinjection, respectively (60). A case of necrotizing fasciitis has been described as a complication of trochanteric bursa injection (28).

On an exceedingly rare occasion, GTPS may be refractory to conservative measures. In such cases, one should be mindful of

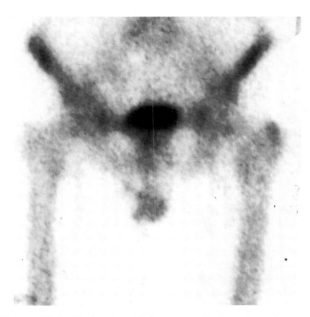

Figure 40-2 Technetium-99 bone scan findings in patient with trochanteric bursitis of the left hip.

a potentially incorrect diagnosis and re-evaluate other potential causes of pain. Several surgical procedures have been described for persistent trochanteric bursitis. Most techniques include excision of the inflamed trochanteric bursa, removal of any trochanteric prominences (including hardware), and some form of iliotibial band release or lengthening. The literature on these procedures is limited to a few noncontrolled, nonrandomized series with a limited number of patients. Zoltan et al. reported on excision of an elliptical portion of the iliotibial band over the trochanter and resection of the bursa with success in four of five patients (76). Slawski and Howard reported on a simple longitudinal release of the iliotibial band over the trochanter and excision of the bursa with improvement in five of five patients (62). Govaert et al. reported on a trochanteric reduction osteotomy in 12 hips, with improvement in all (20). Kagan coined the term "rotator cuff tears of the hip" to refer to chronic attenuation or partial tears of the gluteus medius and found that seven patients managed with surgical reattachment of gluteus medius were all satisfied (32). Endoscopic débridement has been reported as a treatment option for trochanteric bursitis and calcific tendonitis of the gluteus medius, with good results reported in a few small series of patients (6,19,35). Patients should be warned prior to any surgical intervention for bursitis that complete pain relief is unpredictable even with hardware removal.

ILIOPSOAS SYNDROME

Inflammation of the iliopsoas bursa and/or tendon, often referred to as "iliopsoas syndrome," is an often unrecognized source of groin pain or anterior hip snapping (33). It has been associated with rheumatoid arthritis or osteoarthritis of the hip, synovitis of the hip, and even the aftermath of total hip replacement (22,68).

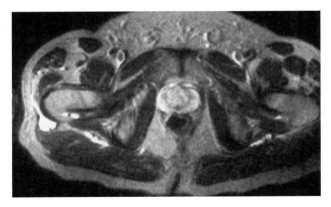

Figure 40-1 MRI findings in patient with trochanteric bursitis of the right hip. Note fluid in the greater trochanteric bursa on T2-weighted image. (Courtesy of C. Tillotson.)

The diagnosis of iliopsoas syndrome is generally made by history and physical examination. History generally includes groin pain and/or snapping with hip extension and rotation. It can be accompanied by a groin mass, which on occasion can cause compression syndromes of the inguinal compartment (68). Physical exam findings can include pain with active straight leg raise or pain on resisted hip flexion in a sitting position. Snapping and/or pain can be elicited as the hip is extended and inwardly rotated from a flexed, adducted, externally rotated position. The groin should be examined for tenderness and/or a mass.

Imaging techniques that have been described for evaluation of iliopsoas syndrome include real-time ultrasound, MRI, CT, and bursography (25,33,40,68,74). Findings generally include an enlarged iliopsoas bursa. The iliopsoas bursa has been found to communicate with the hip joint in many cases and can be associated with hip effusion (74). Wunderbaldinger concluded that although ultrasound is the most cost-effective diagnostic test, MRI is the most accurate (74).

While nonoperative treatment is the treatment of choice, conservative management strategies have not been well documented. As is the case for most soft-tissue ailments, general treatment approaches include rest, nonsteroidal anti-inflammatories, stretching, and strengthening. Johnston et al. reported on an exercise regimen of hip rotation exercises and stretching, with improvement in seven of nine patients (32). Injections can be useful as well.

Iliopsoas tendonitis following total hip replacement is a well-described complication (10,26,70). Its etiology can include impingement on an overhanging cementless acetabular component or an overhanging femoral component collar. Groin pain on resisted hip flexion is suggestive. The diagnosis can be confirmed by local injection of the iliopsoas bursa or tendon sheath. Nonoperative modalities, as described earlier, are the appropriate initial treatment. If unsuccessful, surgical release of the iliopsoas tendon has been reported to be successful in a few published cases (10,26).

OTHER SOURCES OF TENDONITIS

While iliopsoas tendonitis or syndrome has been well described, other, less common sources of tendonitis can be symptomatic as well. Adductor tendonitis and rectus abdominis tendopathy has been reported in soccer and hockey players (45,72). Treatment again includes nonoperative and, less commonly, operative treatment options (45). Calcific tendonitis of the medial and lateral heads of the rectus femoris and the anterior inferior iliac spine (ASIS) can be symptomatic (52,57). Other reported tendinopathies include involvement of the obturator internus or the gluteus maximus (29,56).

Another, poorly described source of pain is that of hip abductor muscular pain. This pain, referred to as "abductor pain syndrome," is located in the lateral hip region proximal to the trochanter. This syndrome involves overuse injury of the gluteus medius and minimus and can include trochanteric bursitis (4). Treatment includes nonoperative modalities such as physical therapy, nonsteroidal anti-inflammatories, and occasionally injection of trigger points or bursitis (4).

THE SNAPPING HIP

One relatively common complaint about the hip is snapping. It can be painful or painless. The etiology of the snapping hip, also referred to as "coxa sultans," has been divided into extra-articular sources and intra-articular sources. Intra-articular sources are discussed in the next section.

Generally, extra-articular sources of snapping include snapping of the iliotibial band over the prominent trochanter and snapping of the iliopsoas over the iliopectineal eminence at the anterior pelvic brim. Other, less common sources of extrinsic hip snapping include snapping of the biceps femoris at its origin.

Snapping of the iliotibial band over the trochanter is the most common etiology of the snapping hip (Fig. 40-3). The fascia that incorporates the tensor fascia lata and gluteus maximus form a confluence over the trochanter. This cord of the iliotibial band can snap over the prominence of the trochanter as the hip flexes and extends or rotates. It can often be reproduced by the patient by adducting the hip and going from an externally rotated position to internal rotation.

The diagnosis can be confirmed with imaging techniques if the etiology remains unknown. Real-time sonography can be used to identify the temporal relationship between jerky tendon motion and snapping. The etiology may include snapping of the iliopsoas tendon over the pelvic rim or iliotibial band snapping over the trochanter (8,50).

Treatment may not be necessary if asymptomatic. It painful or disruptive, nonoperative management includes a program of iliotibial band stretching, nonsteroidal anti-inflammatories, and injections. On the rare occasion that these are inadequate, surgical treatment has been described. As in treatment for trochanteric bursitis, this generally includes resection of the trochanter bursa and release of the iliotibial band. Kim et al. reported on three patients treated with Z-plasty of the iliotibial band, with only one patient able to return to full activities; they concluded that this technique yielded less than optimal results (36). However, Brignall and Stainsby reported on the same technique used in eight patients, all of whom had successful results (7).

While reported less frequently than iliotibial band snapping, snapping of the iliopsoas tendon over the iliopectineal eminence of the pelvic brim has been studied extensively (Fig. 40-4). Patients typically complain of snapping in the groin noted with extension of the hip. Supine physical examination can often reproduce the snap when the hip is moved from flexion to extension in an abducted, externally rotated position (67).

Imaging techniques used to identify snapping of the iliopsoas tendon have included bursography with live fluoroscopy as well as ultrasonography (31). Using these imaging techniques, the etiology of the snapping has been delineated as catching of the iliopsoas over the iliopectineal eminence or a portion of the lesser trochanter (58). Treatment again generally includes nonoperative modalities such as stretching, nonsteroidal anti-inflammatories, and occasionally injections into the iliopsoas tendon sheath. If these are inadequate, surgical treatments have been reported. Dobbs et al. reported on nine adolescent patients who underwent fractional lengthening of the iliopsoas tendon at the musculotendinous junction via a

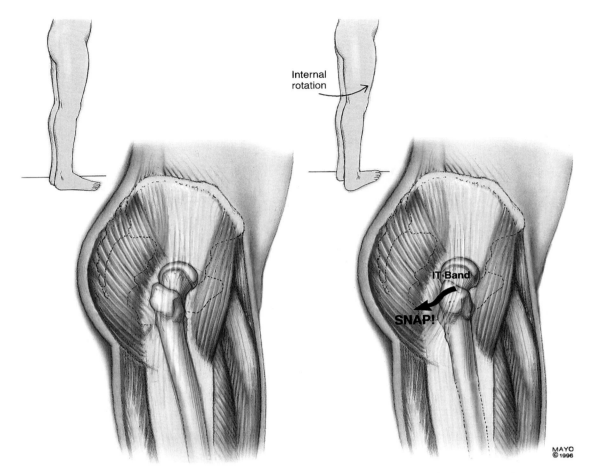

Figure 40-3 Snapping iliotibial band. The iliotibial band subluxates over the greater trochanter, causing a snapping sensation over the lateral hip.

modified ilioinguinal approach, with only one having persistent snapping (11). Gruen et al. studied 11 patients who failed nonoperative modalities and were treated with fractional lengthening of the iliopsoas tendon, with resolution of the symptoms in all patients (24). Taylor et al. performed release of the iliopsoas tendon via a medial approach in 14 patients, with resolution in 10, improvement in 5, and no change in 1 (67). Jacobson and Allen reported on 20 hips that underwent lengthening of the iliopsoas tendon via a step cut of the tendinous portion, with improvement in all but one patient (31). Schaberg et al. reported on lengthening of the iliopsoas tendon and partial release with minimal resection of the lesser trochanteric bony ridge, with good results (58).

LABRAL PATHOLOGY

Soft-tissue disorders within the capsule of the hip joint can involve the synovium (pigmented villonodular synovitis, synovial chondromatosis) or, more commonly, the labrum. Labral injuries can result in intrinsic snapping of the hip. Pigmented villonodular synovitis and synovial chondromatoses are reviewed in Chapter 36, on primary tumors of the hip. Pathologic tears of the labrum are an increasingly recognized

phenomenon. The etiology of labral tears can be posttraumatic, secondary to acetabular dysplasia, or idiopathic. Labral tears can be a source of intrinsic hip snapping, as mentioned previously.

Posttraumatic labral tears can be related to hip dislocation, subluxation, or acetabular fractures (42). Others have postulated that sudden twisting or pivoting motions put athletes at risk for labral tears (48). Labral tears can be identified at the time of surgical fixation of acetabular fractures, can cause persistent joint space widening following closed reduction of a hip dislocation, or can simply present as hip pain or snapping following hip injury. If suspected, the diagnosis can generally be confirmed with MRI scan or magnetic resonance (MR) arthrography (13). If an osteochondral loose body is suspected following hip dislocation, CT scan may be more appropriate.

Labral tears associated with acetabular dysplasia have been well documented (12,27). It has been hypothesized that acetabular dysplasia leads to higher localized forces on the superior and anterior articular cartilage and labrum, resulting in an elevated risk of secondary osteoarthritis and labral hypertrophy and tears (12,41). These labral tears are felt to be a precursor to osteoarthritis, as the ability of the labrum to more evenly distribute forces and fulfill its "joint-sealing" function has been compromised (27,41,48,49). In their series of 75 periacetabular osteotomies, Ganz et al. found labral

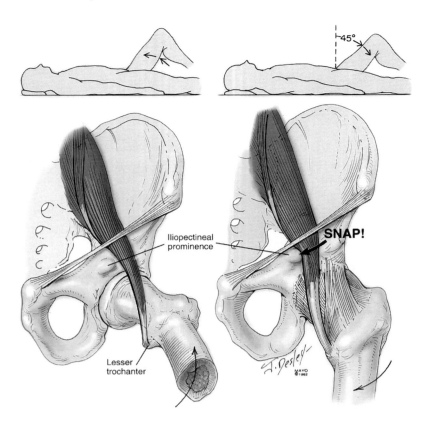

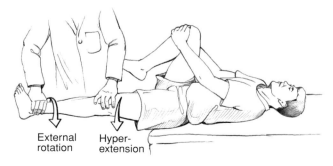

Figure 40-4 Snapping iliopsoas tendon. The iliopsoas tendon snaps over the iliopectineal prominence of the pelvis as the hip is extended, causing a snapping sensation in the groin.

lesions to be present in 21% of cases (Fig. 40-5) (61). Physical examination in a patient with a labral lesion can include a positive aprehension test (Fig. 40-6). Another exam finding of labral pathology is the impingement sign, this test is performed with the patient supine. The hip is internally rotated as it is passively flexed to about 90° and adducted (41). Diagnosis of such lesions include plain radiographic evaluation and diagnosis of acetabular dysplasia (described in detail in Chapter 27). MR arthrography can assist in the diagnosis of labral pathology. Treatment of these lesions can include joint-preserving options such as periacetabular and/or proximal femoral osteotomies if the secondary osteoarthritis is limited and labral tear resection (61).

Idiopathic labral tears, not associated with trauma or acetabular dysplasia, have been reported as well. Presenting symptoms include groin pain or hip snapping that is sudden in onset and relatively short in duration. Physical examination is characterized by a labral test described by Fitzgerald (17). With the patient supine, the hip is taken from a fully flexed, abducted, externally rotated position to an extended, adducted, internally rotated position. This will generally elicit pain in patients with an anterior labral tear. The reciprocal maneuver, going from a flexed, adducted, internally rotated position to an extended, abducted, externally rotated position, can elicit pain with a posterior labral tear (17). Plain radiography in this scenario is generally unrevealing. MRI scan alone can miss many labral tears (13). The use of MR arthrography with injection of saline solution or diluted gadolinium improves the sensitivity (51,64). An intra-articular injection of local anesthetic with or without a corticosteroid allows confirmation of an intra-articular source of pain.

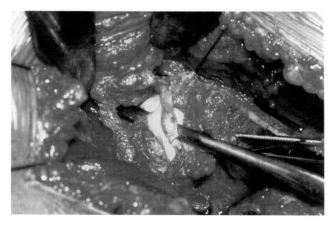

Figure 40-5 Anterolateral labral tear seen at open procedure. (Courtesy of R. Ganz.) See Color Plate.

Figure 40-6 Hip apprehension test for labral pathology.

Fitzgerald reported on 56 hips in 55 patients treated for acetabular labral tears (17). Most patients were between 20 and 50 years old. Mechanical pain associated with a hip click following minor trauma was characteristic in this group of patients. The pain was generally noticed as discrete episodes of pain associated with pivoting or twisting of the hip. Sixty-one percent described a click in association with the pain. Arthrography was performed in 50 of the patients and demonstrated a tear in 44. MRI was helpful in eliminating other potential sources of pain but did not often show the labral tear. Fitzgerald's treatment protocol included injection of the hip with local anesthetic and corticosteroid followed by 4 weeks of protected weight bearing, with success in 13% of patients. The remaining 87% underwent surgical treatment. An open labral resection was performed in 92% of the cases. Arthroscopy was performed in the remaining 8%. Fitzgerald found an anterior tear in 92% of the 42 hips and a posterior tear in 8%. Adjacent chondromalacia of the femoral head was present in a third of the hips. In 45 hips, a partial excision of the labrum was performed. Eighty-eight percent were improved (64).

Arthroscopy of the hip has more recently been used to both confirm the diagnosis and treat tears of the acetabular labrum (13,27,44,46). McCarthy et al. reported on 13 hips in 10 elite athletes treated with arthroscopy for labral tears, with all 13 having anterior tears and 2 having additional posterior tears. Twelve of the 13 arthroscopies were successful, with recurrence of symptoms in one patient (47).

NERVE ENTRAPMENT SYNDROMES ABOUT THE HIP

Piriformis syndrome is a rare, controversial disorder characterized by compression of the sciatic nerve as it exits the greater sciatic foramen and passes beneath the piriformis muscle. The controversy stems from an unclear cause, similarities to more recognizable causes of sciatica, lack of consistent objective findings, and its relative rarity (55). Piriformis syndrome is a diagnosis of exclusion, and any investigation should seek to exclude more common causes of radicular symptoms.

Symptoms can include buttock pain that may extend down the leg in a radicular fashion and intolerance to sitting. Physical examination should seek out other potential causes of sciatica, such as lumbar spine pathology. Exam findings have included tenderness at the sciatic notch and pain with flexion, adduction, and internal rotation of the hip (3). Electrodiagnostic studies can be of assistance and generally, although not always, demonstrate extrapelvic compression of the sciatic nerve (3,16).

Treatment of piriformis syndrome can include nonsteroidal anti-inflammatories, physical therapy, and occasionally injections. Such treatment has been reported to be successful in approximately 80% of patients (16). If ineffective, surgical release of the piriformis with or without neurolysis has been reported as successful (3,16,18,55).

Other nerve entrapment syndromes about the hip have been described as well. Entrapment syndrome of the superior gluteal nerve by the superior fibers of the piriformis has been described and can present as claudication-type buttock pain with abductor weakness and Trendelenburg gait (54). Obturator neuropathy was diagnosed in 22 patients with EMG

at the Mayo Clinic (Rochester, MN) and is generally treated conservatively (63). Grant et al. reported on two cases of obturator neuropathy as a result of intrapelvic extrusion of cement during total hip replacement (21). Cluneal nerve entrapment has been described as a compression of the medial superior cluneal nerve at its osseofibrous orifice at the posterior iliac crest, resulting in low back and buttock pain (43). Nerve blocks can be helpful and surgery is occasionally indicated (43,66).

Meralgia paresthetica is a well-described mononeuropathy of the lateral femoral cutaneous nerve (LFCN) caused by entrapment or neuroma formation as the nerve exits the pelvis in the region of the anterior superior iliac spine (30). The anatomy of the LFCN in this region is highly variable (23). Symptoms of meralgia paresthetica include numbness, pain, and dysesthesias of the anterolateral thigh. The disease process can be spontaneous, the result of repetitive trauma, or iatrogenic, following procedures such as pelvic osteotomies, bone graft harvest, or compression by hip-positioning devices (39). Examination findings include a distribution of pain or numbness in the distribution of the LFCN (anterolateral thigh) and can include a Tinel sign medial to the anterior superior iliac spine. The differential diagnosis includes radiculopathy (15). Treatment includes removal of the source of external compression or aggravating factors (e.g., belt), local anesthetic or corticosteroid injections, rest, and anti-inflammatories. Surgical treatment options include sectioning of the nerve or neurolysis with transposition. The superiority of any one surgical treatment remains controversial (73).

REFERENCES

1. Akisue T, Yamamoto T, Marui T, et al. Ischiogluteal bursitis: multimodality imaging findings. *Clin Orthop.* 2003;406:214–217.
2. Allwright SJ, Cooper RA, Nash P. Trochanteric bursitis: bone scan appearance. *Clin Nucl Med.* 1988;13:561–564.
3. Benson ER, Schutzer SF. Posttraumatic piriformis syndrome: diagnosis and results of operative treatment. *J Bone Joint Surg [Am].* 1999;81:941–949.
4. Bewyer DC, Bewyer KJ. Rationale for treatment of hip abductor pain syndrome. *Iowa Orthop J.* 2003;23:57–60.
5. Bird PA, Oakley SP, Shnier R, et al. Prospective evaluation of magnetic resonance imaging and physical examination findings in patients with greater trochanteric pain syndrome. *Arthritis Rheum.* 2001;44:2138–2145.
6. Bradley DM, Dillingham MF. Bursoscopy of the trochanteric bursa. *Arthroscopy.* 1998;14:884–887.
7. Brignall CG, Stainsby GD. The snapping hip: treatment by Z-plasty. *J Bone Joint Surg [Br].* 1991;73(2):253–254.
8. Choi YS, Lee SM, Song BY, et al. Dynamic sonography of external snapping hip syndrome. *J Ultrasound Med.* 2002;21:753–758.
9. Connell DA, Bass C, Sykes CA, et al. Sonographic evaluation of gluteus medius and minimus tendinopathy. *Eur Radiol.* 2003;13:1339–1347.
10. Della Valle CJ, Rafii M, Jaffe WL. Iliopsoas tendinitis after total hip arthroplasty. *J Arthroplasty.* 2001;16:923–926.
11. Dobbs MB, Gordon JE, Luhmann SJ, et al. Surgical correction of the snapping iliopsoas tendon in adolescents. *J Bone Joint Surg [Am].* 2002;84A:420–424.
12. Dorrell JH, Catterall A. The torn acetabular labrum. *J Bone Joint Surg [Br].* 1986;68:400–403.
13. Edwards DJ, Lomas D, Villar RN. Diagnosis of the painful hip by magnetic resonance imaging and arthroscopy. *J Bone Joint Surg [Br].* 1995;77:374–376.
14. Ege Rasmussen KJ, Fano N. Trochanteric bursitis: treatment by corticosteroid injection. *Scand J Rheumatol.* 1985;14:417–420.
15. Erbay H. Meralgia paresthetica in differential diagnosis of low-back pain. *Clin J Pain.* 2002;18:132–135.

16. Fishman LM, Dombi GW, Michaelsen C, et al. Piriformis syndrome: diagnosis, treatment, and outcome: a 10-year study. *Arch Phys Med Rehabil.* 2002;83:295–301.

17. Fitzgerald RH, Jr. Acetabular labrum tears: diagnosis and treatment. *Clin Orthop.* 1995;311:60–68.

18. Foster MR. Piriformis syndrome. *Orthopedics.* 2002;25:821–825.

19. Fox J. The role of arthroscopic bursectomy in the treatment of trochanteric bursitis. *Arthroscopy.* 2002;18:E34.

20. Govaert LH, van der Vis HM, Marti RK, et al. Trochanteric reduction osteotomy as a treatment for refractory trochanteric bursitis. *J Bone Joint Surg [Br].* 2003;85:199–203.

21. Grant P, Roise O, Ovre S. Obturator neuropathy due to intrapelvic extrusion of cement during total hip replacement: report of 2 patients. *Acta Orthop Scand.* 2001;72:537–540.

22. Grindulis KA. Rheumatoid iliopsoas bursitis. *J Rheumatol.* 1986;13:988.

23. Grossman MG, Ducey SA, Nadler SS, et al. Meralgia paresthetica: diagnosis and treatment. *J Am Acad Orthop Surg.* 2001;9:336–344.

24. Gruen GS, Scioscia TN, Lowenstein JE. The surgical treatment of internal snapping hip. *Am J Sports Med.* 2002;30:607–613.

25. Harper MC, Schaberg JE, Allen WC. Primary iliopsoas bursography in the diagnosis of disorders of the hip. *Clin Orthop.* 1987;221:238–241.

26. Heaton K, Dorr LD. Surgical release of iliopsoas tendon for groin pain after total hip arthroplasty. *J Arthroplasty.* 2002;17:779–781.

27. Hickman JM, Peters CL. Hip pain in the young adult: diagnosis and treatment of disorders of the acetabular labrum and acetabular dysplasia. *Am J Orthop.* 2001;30:459–467.

28. Hofmeister E, Engelhardt S. Necrotizing fasciitis as complication of injection into greater trochanteric bursa. *Am J Orthop.* 2001;30:426–427.

29. Hottat N, Fumiere E, Delcour C. Calcific tendinitis of the gluteus maximus tendon: CT findings. *Eur Radiol.* 1999;9:1104–1106.

30. Ivins GK. Meralgia paresthetica, the elusive diagnosis: clinical experience with 14 adult patients. *Ann Surg.* 2000;232:281–286.

31. Jacobson T, Allen WC. Surgical correction of the snapping iliopsoas tendon. *Am J Sports Med.* 1990;18:470–474.

32. Johnston CA, Lindsay DM, Wiley JP. Treatment of iliopsoas syndrome with a hip rotation strengthening program: a retrospective case series. *J Orthop Sports Phys Ther.* 1999;29:218–224.

33. Johnston CA, Wiley JP, Lindsay DM, et al. Iliopsoas bursitis and tendinitis: a review. *Sports Med.* 1998;25:271–283.

34. Kagan A 2nd. Rotator cuff tears of the hip. *Clin Orthop.* 1999;368:135–140.

35. Kandemir U, Bharam S, Philippon MJ, et al. Endoscopic treatment of calcific tendinitis of gluteus medius and minimus. *Arthroscopy.* 2003;19:E4.

36. Kim DH, Baechler MF, Berkowitz MJ, et al. Coxa saltans externa treated with Z-plasty of the iliotibial tract in a military population. *Mil Med.* 2002;167:172–173.

37. Kim SM, Shin MJ, Kim KS, et al. Imaging features of ischial bursitis with an emphasis on ultrasonography. *Skeletal Radiol.* 2002;31:631–636.

38. Kingzett-Taylor A, Tirman PF, Feller J, et al. Tendinosis and tears of gluteus medius and minimus muscles as a cause of hip pain: MR imaging findings. *AJR Am J Roentgenol.* 1999;173:1123–1126.

39. Kitson J, Ashworth MJ. Meralgia paraesthetica: a complication of a patient-positioning device in total hip replacement. *J Bone Joint Surg [Br].* 2002;84:589–590.

40. Kozlov DB, Sonin AH. Iliopsoas bursitis: diagnosis by MRI. *J Comput Assist Tomogr.* 1998;22:625–628.

41. Leunig M, Siebenrock KA, Ganz R. Rationale of periacetabular osteotomy and background work. *Instr Course Lect.* 2001;50:229–238.

42. Leunig M, Sledge JB, Gill TJ, et al. Traumatic labral avulsion from the stable rim: a constant pathology in displaced transverse acetabular fractures. *Arch Orthop Trauma Surg.* 2003;123:392–395.

43. Maigne JY, Doursounian L. Entrapment neuropathy of the medial superior cluneal nerve: nineteen cases surgically treated, with a minimum of 2 years' follow-up. *Spine.* 1997;22:1156–1159.

44. Mason JB. Acetabular labral tears in the athlete. *Clin Sports Med.* 2001;20:779–790.

45. Martens MA, Hansen L, Mulier JC. Adductor tendinitis and musculus rectus abdominis tendopathy. *Am J Sports Med.* 1987;15:353–356.

46. McCarthy JC. Hip arthroscopy: applications and technique. *J Am Acad Orthop Surg.* 1995;3:115–122.

47. McCarthy J, Barsoum W, Puri L, et al. The role of hip arthroscopy in the elite athlete. *Clin Orthop.* 2003;No. 406:71–74.

48. McCarthy J, Noble P, Aluisio FV, et al. Anatomy, pathologic features, and treatment of acetabular labral tears. *Clin Orthop.* 2003;No. 406:38–47.

49. McCarthy JC, Noble PC, Schuck MR, et al. The watershed labral lesion: its relationship to early arthritis of the hip. *J Arthroplasty.* 2001;16[8 Suppl 1]:81–87.

50. Pelsser V, Cardinal E, Hobden R, et al. Extraarticular snapping hip: sonographic findings. *AJR Am J Roentgenol.* 2001;176:67–73.

51. Petersilge CA, Haque MA, Petersilge WJ, et al. Acetabular labral tears: evaluation with MR arthrography. *Radiology.* 1996;200:231–235.

52. Pope TL Jr, Keats TE. Case report 733. Calcific tendinitis of the origin of the medial and lateral heads of the rectus femoris muscle and the anterior iliac spine (AIIS). *Skeletal Radiol.* 1992;21:271–272.

53. Raman D, Haslock I. Trochanteric bursitis: a frequent cause of "hip" pain in rheumatoid arthritis. *Ann Rheum Dis.* 1982;41:602–603.

54. Rask MR. Superior gluteal nerve entrapment syndrome. *Muscle Nerve.* 1980;3:304–307.

55. Rodrigue T, Hardy RW. Diagnosis and treatment of piriformis syndrome. *Neurosurg Clin North Am.* 2001;12:311–319.

56. Rohde RS, Ziran BH. Obturator internus tendinitis as a source of chronic hip pain. *Orthopedics.* 2003;26:425–426.

57. Sarkar JS, Haddad FS, Crean SV, et al. Acute calcific tendinitis of the rectus femoris. *J Bone Joint Surg [Br].* 1996;78:814–816.

58. Schaberg JE, Harper MC, Allen WC. The snapping hip syndrome. *Am J Sports Med.* 1984;12:361–365.

59. Shbeeb MI, Matteson EL. Trochanteric bursitis (greater trochanter pain syndrome). *Mayo Clin Proc.* 1996;71:565–569.

60. Shbeeb MI, O'Duffy JD, Michet CJ Jr, et al. Evaluation of glucocorticosteroid injection for the treatment of trochanteric bursitis. *J Rheumatol.* 1996;23:2104–2106.

61. Siebenrock KA, Leunig M, Ganz R. Periacetabular osteotomy: the Bernese experience. *Instr Course Lect.* 2001;50:239–245.

62. Slawski DP, Howard RF. Surgical management of refractory trochanteric bursitis. *Am J Sports Med.* 1997;25:86–89.

63. Sorenson EJ, Chen JJ, Daube JR. Obturator neuropathy: causes and outcome. *Muscle Nerve.* 2002;25:605–607.

64. Steinbach LS, Palmer WE, Schweitzer ME. Special focus session. MR arthrography. *Radiographics.* 2002;22:1223–1246.

65. Swezey RL. Pseudo-radiculopathy in subacute trochanteric bursitis of the subgluteus maximus bursa. *Arch Phys Med Rehabil.* 1976;57:387–390.

66. Talu GK, Ozyalcin S, Talu U. Superior cluneal nerve entrapment. *Reg Anesth Pain Med.* 2000;25:648–650.

67. Taylor GR, Clarke NM. Surgical release of the "snapping iliopsoas tendon." *J Bone Joint Surg [Br].* 1995;77:881–883.

68. Toohey AK, LaSalle TL, Martinez S, et al. Iliopsoas bursitis: clinical features, radiographic findings, and disease associations. *Semin Arthritis Rheum.* 1990;20:41–47.

69. Traycoff RB. "Pseudotrochanteric bursitis": the differential diagnosis of lateral hip pain. *J Rheumatol.* 1991;18:1810–1812.

70. Trousdale RT, Cabanela ME, Berry DJ. Anterior iliopsoas impingement after total hip arthroplasty. *J Arthroplasty.* 1995;10:546–549.

71. Varma DG, Parihar A, Richli WR. CT appearance of the distended trochanteric bursa. *J Comput Assist Tomogr.* 1993;17:141–143.

72. Weinstein RN, Kraushaar BS, Fulkerson JP. Adductor tendinosis in a professional hockey player. *Orthopedics.* 1998;21:809–810.

73. Williams PH, Trzil KP. Management of meralgia paresthetica. *J Neurosurg.* 1991;74:76–80.

74. Wunderbaldinger P, Bremer C, Schellenberger E, et al. Imaging features of iliopsoas bursitis. *Eur Radiol.* 2002;12:409–415.

75. Yamamoto T, Iwasaki Y, Kurosaka M. Tuberculosis of the greater trochanteric bursa occurring 51 years after tuberculous nephritis. *Clin Rheumatol.* 2002;21:397–400.

76. Zoltan DJ, Clancy WG Jr, Keene JS. A new operative approach to snapping hip and refractory trochanteric bursitis in athletes. *Am J Sports Med.* 1986;14:201–204.

Nonoperative Management of Osteoarthritis of the Hip

David S. Hungerford   *Marc W. Hungerford*

According to the National Health Interview Survey, 185,000 total hip arthroplasties were carried out in 2002. The same survey estimated that 43 million Americans suffer from physician-diagnosed arthritis. While obviously not all of these have involvement of the hip, it is clear that for every patient who has the level of symptoms to justify a total hip replacement, there are dozens who have symptomatic osteoarthritis (OA) of the hip but whose symptoms and/or disability have not yet risen to that level. These patients frequently present themselves to physicians seeking some relief. It is the purpose of this chapter to review the nonoperative modalities that have some scientific evidence of efficacy and that deserve to be a part of the armamentarium in treating this disease.

GOAL OF NONOPERATIVE MANAGEMENT

First, it is important for patients to understand something about their disease. Many patients present to the physician because of symptoms for which they do not have a diagnosis. Their primary concern is that their symptoms may be a sign of something serious, even life-threatening. Most importantly, they are looking for reassurance that there is a specific cause for their symptoms and some idea of what the future holds. Many have multiple possible sources for symptoms that could be referable to the area of the hip, particularly arthritis of the lumbar spine. In fact, many patients who self-refer to an orthopedist for what they consider to be "hip disease" do not have anything wrong with the hip. Fully 10% of our new patients have no physical or radiographic evidence of hip disease. The two most common diagnoses among this group of patients are lumbar spine disease and greater trochanteric bursitis. For these patients, establishing the diagnosis and making the proper referral is the first step in nonoperative management.

For many other patients, the earliest symptoms lead to a concern about their source more than a concern for the reduction of symptoms. No patient wants to hear his or her doctor say, "You should have come sooner," or learn that some preventive measures could have delayed progression but now more aggressive intervention is necessary. It is important to ask patients what it is that they hope to get out of the contact or, if appropriate, the proposed treatment. In some instances, nothing is necessary other than reassurance and establishing the diagnosis.

Most patients who present for initial evaluation want symptomatic improvement. Most can also get improvement through one or more of the measures outlined in this chapter. Even for patients with more severe and disabling symptoms, a response to nonoperative management can be very satisfying to both patient and physician. There are obviously patients whose disease is so advanced and who have symptoms so severe that immediate surgical intervention, without passing through a period of nonoperative management, is fully justified.

Nonetheless, many patients, even with significant disease, can respond to nonoperative management. There are also patients with severe disease and disability whose medical condition is so precarious that operative intervention poses an unacceptable risk. For them, nonoperative management is all that is available, and some improvement is almost always possible.

The primary goal of treatment for osteoarthritis is to reduce symptoms. Most patients also want to improve function. The typical response to joint pain is to eliminate or reduce the activities that produce it. The first thing to be discontinued is usually sport, then exercise. Gradually, walking distance is shortened and stair climbing curtailed. With the reduction in activity comes an increase in weight. It is not uncommon for patients to have put on 20 to 30 lbs by the time they present to the surgeon looking for answers, in some cases much more. The additional weight and deconditioning are frequently accompanied by further disability.

PHYSICAL MODALITIES

OA of the hip leads to limitation of activity, loss of strength around the affected joint, stiffness, loss of motion, and generalized deconditioning. One of the goals of nonoperative management is to halt this downward trend and in many cases to reverse it. The risk/benefit ratio is so attractive, especially for elderly patients, coupling general health benefits with the absence of side effects, that it argues for giving these modalities a prominent role in any program to treat OA. This section includes a brief review of these modalities, including strengthening exercises, ROM, aerobic conditioning, and weight control/reduction.

Weight Reduction

Many patients with symptomatic OA of the hip are overweight. Most have put on significant weight since their hip became symptomatic. It has been documented that weight reduction and strength increase can reduce the symptoms of arthritis. It is still controversial whether obesity is a cause of OA, but the obese have a significantly higher incidence of self-reported symptomatic arthritis. Mehrotra et al., writing in the *American Journal of Preventive Medicine*, reported that roughly 26% of patients with a body mass index (BMI) less than 25 self-reported arthritis, compared with roughly 44% of those with a BMI greater than 30 (52).

Reducing weight and improving exercise tolerance can reduce symptoms. Messier et al. reported on a controlled study of 316 community-based subjects with OA of the knee whom he divided into four arms (53): healthy life style (control), exercise alone, diet alone, and exercise plus diet. Improvement was measured by the Western Ontario and McMaster University Osteoarthritis Index (WOMAC), a timed 6-minute distance walk, and stair climbing. Diet alone produced no improvement, exercise improved only the timed 6-minute distance walk, whereas diet plus exercise resulted in improvement in all three parameters.

Exercise

Lin, Davey, and Cochrane reported the effectiveness of a 12-month community-based water exercise program on measures of self-reported health and physical function in people over 60 years old with knee–hip OA (41). Sixty-six subjects in the exercise group were compared with 40 age-matched nonexercisers who were offered monthly educational material about OA and quarterly follow-up telephone calls. Seventy percent of the exercise group completed the 12-month program, and 77% of the exercise group and 89% of the control group completed both pre- and postprogram outcome measures. The exercise group had statistically significant improvement in WOMAC scores, hip and knee range of motion, physical function, perception of pain, and ability to ascend and descend stairs, compared with the nonexercising group.

Foley et al., in a similar study, compared a gym-based exercise program to a water-based program and found improvements in both programs, with no significant differences (28). Compliance with both programs was similar, and both achieved significant gains compared with controls.

In a huge service to the medical community, which is trying to sort out the evidence for and against various possible programs, the MOVE group of distinguished physicians, including rheumatologists, physiatrists, generalists, orthopedic surgeons, and an epidemiologist, evaluated the medical literature on the subject and concluded a four-round Delphi panel evaluation of the data, ending with 10 evidence-based propositions (65). These recommendations appear in Table 41-1. The quality of the evidence appears in the second column, with 1 representing the highest quality and 4 the lowest. The strength of the recommendation appears in column 3, with A the strongest and D the weakest.

Heat, Diathermy, Ultrasound

Although there is some literature concerning these modalities in treating gonarthrosis, there is no literature concerning their use in hip OA. Since many of the articular structures of the knee are superficial, and ligaments, capsules, muscles, and tendons are subcutaneous in the knee and deep in the hip, this may account for the difference. The evidence for use in the knee is not strong, but it is absent for hip OA, and their use should not be considered.

Assistive Devices

Brand and Crowninshield, in a sophisticated three-dimensional biomechanical study of the forces across the hip, estimated a 40% reduction in force with the use of a cane in the opposite hand (9). However, while up to 50% of patients with significant symptoms for rheumatoid arthritis and OA possess an assistive device, one third did not use the device (79). Negative perception, lower level of symptoms, and unsatisfactory results contributed to nonuse. It behooves the physician to encourage the patient to use appropriate assistive devices and give instructions on proper use.

Acupuncture

Acupuncture is extensively used for controlling pain in a wide variety of conditions, but there is extremely little literature regarding its use in the management of OA of the hip. There are thee studies that are worth mentioning. The first, published in *Acupuncture Medicine*, showed beneficial effects in

TABLE 41-1
PROPOSITIONS, CATEGORY OF EVIDENCE, AND STRENGTH OF RECOMMENDATION

Proposition	Category of Evidence (1–4)	Strength of Recommendation (A–D)
Both strengthening and aerobic exercise can reduce pain and improve function and health status in patients with knee and hip OA.	Knee 1B Hip 4	A C (extrapolated from knee OA)
There are few contraindications to the prescription of strengthening or aerobic exercise in patients with hip or knee OA.	4	C (extrapolated from adverse event data)
Prescription of both general (aerobic fitness training) and local (strengthening) exercises is an essential, core aspect of management for every patient with hip or knee OA.	4	D
Exercise therapy for OA of the hip or knee should be individualized and patient-centered, taking into account factors such as age, comorbidity, and overall mobility.	4	D
To be effective, exercise programs should include …	4	D
advice and education to promote a positive lifestyle change with an increase in physical activity.	1B	A
Group exercise and home exercise are equally effective …	1A	A
and patient preference should be considered.	4	D
Adherence is the principal predictor of long-term outcome from exercise in patients with knee or hip OA.	4	D
Strategies to improve and maintain adherence should be adopted, e.g., long-term monitoring/review and inclusion of spouse/family in exercise.	1B	A
The effectiveness of exercise is independent of the presence or severity of radiographic findings.	4	Not recommended
Improvements in muscle strength and proprioception gained from exercise programs may reduce the progression of knee and hip OA.	4	D

what was intended to be a "controlled" study (31). However, the control group received advice and exercises while the study group received 25 minutes of acupuncture therapy once a week for 6 weeks. This did not control for the placebo effect of the active intervention. The second study compared placement of the needles according to the traditional Chinese acupuncture theory to random placement of the needles in the same general area (27). Improvements in standardized outcome measures were achieved equally in both groups, but again there was no control for the placebo effect of an active intervention. Finally, one study compared acupuncture and hydrotherapy (both conjoined with patient education) with patient education alone (71). Both the active interventions produced symptomatic and function improvement compared with education alone. The only conclusion is that some intervention is better than no intervention at all. The role of acupuncture in the treatment of OA of the hip will have to await more extensive and better conducted trials before one can conclude that acupuncture deserves a place in the armamentarium.

Interferential Stimulation

This form of electrical stimulation is reported to be useful for numerous painful conditions, including low back pain, fibromyalgia, and trochanteric bursitis. However, there are no reports of its use in treating OA of the hip, and its use should not be considered.

Transcutaneous electrical nerve stimulation (TENS) has been reported as beneficial for a number of clinical painful conditions, including OA of the knee. There is, though, only one reported study of a novel stimulation of the subcutaneous nerves over the radial, median, and saphenous nerves in patients with clinically diagnosed OA of the hip (19). Acceptable pain relief was obtained in 60% of the patients. Yet the same results were obtained in control patients in whom needles were placed but whose nerves were not stimulated. The authors concluded that placement of the needles appears to have evoked a sizable placebo response. It is studies like this that must call into question any physical, or indeed any treatment, modality evaluated using studies that lack adequate and appropriate controls.

PHARMACOLOGIC MODALITIES

Analgesics

The mainstay for analgesic management of symptoms has been acetaminophen (ACET). This has long been considered the first line of treatment by primary care physicians and rheumatologists. It still has an important role to play, particularly for intermittent symptom flares. Patients are likely to self-medicate with this over-the-counter (OTC) drug. Patients can be reassured that taking up to 2 or even 3 g of acetaminophen per day for short periods of time is quite safe, as long as they do not have liver or kidney disease (4). Even long-term dosage at this level is unlikely to produce serious side effects. Aspirin and OTC NSAIDs, in addition to acetaminophen, are commonly used by patients with arthritis for intermittent or short-term self-medication. Fries and Bruce reviewed 5692 patients with rheumatoid arthritis and 3124 patients with OA from 12 databank centers, with 36,262 patient-years of observation, who were taking either aspirin, acetaminophen, or OTC ibuprofen (IBU) (29).

They concluded that "OTC use of ASA, IBU, or APAP (acetaminophen) carries little risk of serious GI toxicity for most persons." Individuals at higher risk for GI complications had a higher incidence of GI complications than the baseline.

NSAIDs

Mechanism of Action

The family of nonsteroidal anti-inflammatory drugs (NSAIDs) inhibits the arachidonic cascade of inflammation by blocking the cyclo-oxygenase (COX) enzymatic conversion of arachidonic acid to prostaglandin. The problem is that prostaglandins are involved in many normal tissue processes, including tissue homeostasis (e.g., mucosal defense and repair). COX-1, which produces the normal tissue prostaglandins, is inhibited by the standard NSAIDs. COX-2 is an inducible enzyme that appears in areas of injury and inflammation. The class of COX-2 inhibitors was developed in an effort to avoid the side effects of the nonspecific COX inhibitors, specifically gastric and renal complications.

NSAIDs in general and the COX-2 inhibitors specifically have been mass marketed to the public, resulting in a multi-billion-dollar industry. Physicians are under pressure to prescribe "the latest," and patients are resistant to the physician recommendation to take regular doses of OTC NSAIDs or acetaminophen, which they have often already tried, in a hit or miss pattern, and found to be ineffective. Already in the 1990s, NSAIDs had become the "de facto" treatment of choice. A survey of the practice patterns of general practitioners revealed that only 10% would prescribe a pure nonopioid analgesic for uncomplicated OA (47). The rest chose sub anti-inflammatory or full anti-inflammatory doses of NSAIDs.

Most clinical studies show NSAIDs to be more effective than placebo or simple analgesics (acetaminophen), but some studies show little difference. Bradley et al. randomized 182 knees into three groups—OTC level NSAID, therapeutic level NSAID, and acetaminophen—and found no difference (8). Even in those studies that do show a statistically significant difference, the improvements in pain and function scores are only in the 10% to 20% range.

Efficacy Differences between NSAIDs

There have been so many clinical studies done involving NSAIDs that it is possible to find support for almost any one NSAID versus another. However, there is no compelling evidence that any one NSAID is better than another (3,12,22, 32,44,84). COX-2 inhibitors lead to fewer withdrawals due to intolerance and complications than COX-1 inhibitors but have not been found to be more effective therapeutically that the nonspecific COX inhibitors (25).

Toxicity of NSAIDs

Because of the ubiquity of prostaglandins in normal tissues, it should not be surprising that inhibition of prostaglandin production might cause unwanted side effects. Long-term NSAID consumption may cause fluid retention, worsen congestive

heart failure, cause a decline in renal function (or exacerbate renal failure), worsen liver failure, or cause or exacerbate hypertension. However, the dominant side effects occur in the gastrointestinal tract. GI complications of NSAIDs have been referred to as the "second most deadly rheumatic disease" (29). Upper GI complications include dyspepsia, ulceration, hemorrhage, perforation, and death. Increased risk factors include advanced age, longevity of treatment, increased dose, prior history of peptic ulcer disease, concomitant use of corticosteroids or anticoagulants, and poor general health. Because the effects of NSAIDs are additive, only one NSAID should be taken at a time. It is sobering to consider a 1998 publication that estimated 107,000 hospitalizations and 16,500 deaths annually in the United States alone from complications of NSAID therapy (70).

Withdrawal of Two COX- 2 Inhibitors

The dominant story in conservative management of OA of the hip or knee is the decimation of the NSAID market by the withdrawal of Vioxx by Merck in September 2004. This voluntary withdrawal of rofecoxib (Vioxx) was based on the interim analysis of 3-year data from a prospective, randomized, placebo-controlled clinical trial, the APPROVe (Adenomatous Polyp Prevention on Vioxx) trial. This study involved patients with recurrent colorectal polyps who were placed on 25 mg of Vioxx for 3 years. The interim review at 18 months showed no increased incidence of cardiovascular events compared with placebo, but patients who had completed 36 months of the study did show an increase (7.2/1000 vs. 5.3/1000). In 2000, the VIGOR study showed an increase in myocardial infarction (MI) compared with Naprosyn (0.1% vs. 0.4%) but not a difference in myocardial deaths (4). Four percent of the study subjects had a history of MI, angina, cerebrovascular accident, transient ischemic attack, angioplasty, or coronary bypass and met the criteria of the U.S. Food and Drug Administration (FDA) for the use of aspirin for secondary cardiovascular prophylaxis. None were taking low-dose aspirin therapy. They comprised 38% of the MI group. When they were removed from the analysis, there was no difference in the MI rate. Furthermore, a study comparing the effectiveness of rofecoxib and three NSAIDs other than Naproxen did not show any increased incidence of cardiovascular events (21). The exact mechanism of this action is unknown. Bextra was also withdrawn voluntarily in April 2005.

The publicity that followed has put this entire class of drug under suspicion in the mind of the public. In 2003, the last full year of sales, Vioxx sales topped $2.5 billion; Bextra sales, in 2004, topped $1.3 billion; and the whole class of COX-2 inhibitors exceeded $8 billion. One might imagine that, with its two competitors off the market, sales of Celebrex, the only COX-2 inhibitor left, would go through the roof. On the contrary, sales of Celebrex dropped 50%, indicating the depth of the public mistrust of these drugs. In our experience, many patients are reluctant to accept a prescription for any of the NSAIDs, including the nonspecific COX inhibitors and even OTC NSAIDs.

The withdrawal, which was voluntary, has produced a massive public awareness campaign by trial lawyers searching for patients who can claim harm by virtue of taking the drugs in question. Subsequent to the withdrawal, there have been some criticisms questioning the conclusions and also questioning whether the benefits outweigh the risks, particularly since the COX-1 inhibitors, which remain on the market, have a significantly increased risk of upper GI bleed compared with the COX-2 inhibitors. The FDA advisory panel, meeting in February 2005, actually recommended that that both Vioxx and Bextra be brought back to the market with a "black box" warning about the increased cardiovascular risks. As of this writing, neither manufacturer has chosen to pursue that route, nor has the FDA acted on that advice.

The controversy has sparked a lot of debate, both in the medical literature and in the press. The president of the Arthritis Foundation, writing on the foundation's website, said, "This might be the time to even begin to think about surgery."

Rational Use of NSAIDs

OA is a chronic disease. There is no convincing evidence of disease modification from chronic use of NSAIDs (10). Symptoms of OA are evanescent. Many patients will get satisfactory relief of symptoms with OTC NSAIDs or ACET. They should be encouraged to get such relief. Complications of NSAIDs are proportional to dose, length of time that they are taken, and age of the patient. Patients should be started on the lowest possible dose, and the medication should be discontinued as soon as possible. Periodic attempts should be made to reduce or even eliminate the dosage. NSAIDs should be used with great caution in the elderly, if at all. Two important studies underscore the rationale of not using NSAIDS on a chronic basis for the control of OA symptoms. Dieppe et al. carried out a 2-year study comparing diclofenac versus placebo (23). Only 57% of the participants completed the study. There were a higher number of dropouts due to lack of efficacy in the placebo group and a higher number of dropouts in the study group due to intolerance. An equal number in both groups withdrew because of lack of compliance (15%). At the end of the study, 52% in the diclofenac group reported improvement, compared with 45% in the placebo group. Williams et al. did another long-term study comparing Naprosyn and acetaminophen. Only 35% of the participants completed the study! As in the prior study, withdrawal in the ACET group was higher due to lack of efficacy and in the Naprosyn group due to side effects. Few differences in efficacy were found between the groups (85).

Hyaluronans

Intra-articular hyaluronans injections are a well-recognized treatment modality for gonarthrosis. However, there is very little literature on the use of hyaluronans for OA of the hip. There are only three open-label pilot studies involving small numbers of patients (18,54,77). However, all three showed positive results using objective measurement criteria, and all indicated that larger prospective randomized studies were justified to determine the place of the treatment in the nonoperative armamentarium.

Intra-Articular Steroids

Although long-acting intra-articular steroid injections are frequently used for OA of the knee, and although there are many controlled reports of positive therapeutic response, this treatment has not been routinely used for OA of the hip. The difference may well be that the hip injection does not lend itself to office practice and must be guided by ultrasound or fluoroscopy. In fact, the authors could only find one controlled study of corticosteroid injection for the hip. Kullenberg et al., reporting in 2004 in the *Journal of Rheumatology*, described their experience with 80 patients divided into two equal groups (39). One group received 80 mg triamcinolone acetonide intra-articularly under fluoroscopic guidance and the other group received 1% mepivacaine. The treatment group experienced significant pain relief, functional improvement, and increased range of motion. Rest pain was greatly relieved. The control group remained unchanged from the baseline. Positive results were maintained out to the study's 12 weeks of follow-up. This article suggests that intra-articular injection of the hip with corticosteroids deserves to be more widely employed than it currently is.

However, there is one disconcerting publication concerning this topic. In 2005, Kaspar and de V de Beer reported four deep infections after total hip replacement in 40 patients who had received an intra-articular corticosteroid injection in the preoperative period, compared with no infections in 40 case-matched controls who had not had an intra-articular injection (38).

Chondroprotective Agents

Over the past decade, treatment modalities claiming "chondroprotective" capabilities have appeared. Such proposed agents are also called disease-modifying osteoarthritis drugs (DMOADs). Although no agreed-upon definition exists, Ghosh and Brooks proposed that a chondroprotective agent should (a) enhance chondrocyte macromolecule synthesis; (b) enhance synthesis of hyaluronans; (c) inhibit degradative enzymes; (d) mobilize deposits of thrombin, fibrin, lipids, and cholesterol in vessels surrounding the joint; (e) reduce joint pain; and (f) reduce joint synovitis (30). With these guidelines in mind, we will examine the evidence for several agents.

Some of these fall into a relatively new class of agents call "nutraceuticals," which are nutritional supplements that have pharmacologic properties. Many of our most important pharmaceuticals have their origin in plants, such as digoxin, penicillin, and Coumadin. However, many physicians are deeply skeptical about the use of natural remedies. This skepticism is based on concerns about patient self-diagnosis and self-treatment as well as the lack of scientific testing of claims. Because these substances are relatively unregulated, there is no requirement for rigorous scientific testing prior to marketing. This lack of regulation also poses problems regarding purity and quality control. Even so, patients are being bombarded with and responding to claims about the results of using herbs, nutraceuticals, and nutritional supplements. Glucosamine and chondroitin sulfate sales in the United States are estimated at $600 million. Sales of all nutraceuticals and vitamin supplements in the United States exceeded $12 billion in 1999.

Many physicians took offense at the title of the book by Theodosakis et al. published in 1997, *The Arthritis Cure*, because they know no "cure" exists (73). The Arthritis Foundation initially took the position that there was little or no scientific evidence for the efficacy of glucosamine and chondroitin sulfate, and the offense felt by physicians translated into a discounting of the very reasonable recommendations in the book. In 1998 Gerald Weissmann, a past president of the Arthritis Foundation, appeared on national television (the program *Dateline NBC*) and compared glucosamine and chondroitin sulfate to "snake oil in my father's generation"; he also accused physicians who recommended them of "abdicating responsibility," even to the point of malpractice. Patients, on the other hand, pushed up sales of the book until it reached the bestseller list. Weissmann's tirade and subsequent physician skepticism totally ignored the dozens of recent articles that had been published in peer-reviewed journals reporting on the positive effects of glucosamine and chondroitin sulfate in tissue culture, animal models of arthritis, veterinary clinical trials, and human comparative or placebo-controlled trials. The vast majority of clinical trials for these two molecules have involved the knee alone, with a few less well controlled studies that included both hip and knee osteoarthritis patients. However, considering the basic science of articular cartilage, articular cartilage degeneration, and the clinical natural history of OA, it does not involve a leap of faith to draw the inference that what has a positive effect on OA of the knee, on the metabolism of chondrocytes in culture, and on animal models of articular degeneration might be a reasonable therapeutic agent for OA of the hip. Following is a brief summary of the basic science for these two molecules and a brief review of the clinical experience, although most of this experience concerns OA of the knee.

Glucosamine

The book mentioned above and numerous media articles have drawn attention to the use of oral glucosamine sulfate as treatment for OA. What is more surprising than the spate of new interest in this compound is the lack of recognition of its usefulness, given the wealth of laboratory and clinical support already published. In 1994, McCarty decried the complete lack of interest in glucosamine as a treatment for arthritis in light of the fact that (a) culture studies dating back to the 1950s have shown it to enhance the secretion of mucopolysaccharides in cartilage-derived fibroblasts, (b) animal studies demonstrated a beneficial effect in both prevention and treatment of arthritis, and (c) human trials demonstrated not only efficacy of the compound but also a complete lack of serious side effects (50). When these findings are contrasted with the questionable effects of NSAIDs on cartilage, together with the high rate of complications of these compounds, a strong argument emerges for consideration of glucosamine as a first-line agent in the treatment of arthritis (51).

Rationale for Glucosamine

Glucosamine is a simple amino sugar that serves as a substrate for the synthesis of both glycosaminoglycans and hyaluronic acid. Glucosamine is synthesized directly by the chondrocyte but, when supplemented, can be used directly to synthesize larger macromolecules. Most preparations are derived from chitin in crustacean shells. In vitro and animal models show a variety of effects that can be broadly classified as substrate, transcriptional, "antireactive," and "antiarthritic" effects.

As far back as 1956, Roden noted an increased production of glycosaminoglycans and collagen when glucosamine sulfate was added to cartilage-derived fibroblast cell cultures (66). Other studies confirmed this effect (82,83). Karzel later demonstrated that glucosamine sulfate was efficiently incorporated into mucopolysaccharides (37). These studies demonstrated a specific effect for glucosamine sulfate; N-acetyl glucosamine was far less active and glucuronic acid was without effect (40).

Jimenez et al. demonstrated that glucosamine not only can act as a simple substrate but can also affect gene transcription within the chondrocyte (36). Chondrocyte cultures, incubated with 50 μmgm glucosamine showed a twofold increase in perlecan and aggrecan mRNA levels and a moderate increase in stromelysine mRNA. The same authors showed a dose-dependent down-regulation of metalloproteinase I and II mRNA in the same model (metalloproteinase I and II are important enzymes in the degradation of cartilage).

Glucosamine may be even more effective in up-regulating cartilage metabolism in arthritic or stressed cartilage. Lippiello et al. found an increase in GAG synthesis in arthritic cartilage explants under various types of stress when exposed to glucosamine, compared with young or nonstressed explants (43). Looking at a biologic marker for Type II cartilage degradation, Christgau et al. determined that patients with higher rates of cartilage turnover (higher levels of CTX-II in the urine) benefited the most from glucosamine supplementation (16). Glucosamine also increases the synovial production of hyaluronic acid, a substance that has itself been shown to have anti-inflammatory effects, induce anabolic activity in chondrocytes, decrease joint pain, and increase mobility in in vivo and clinical studies (49).

Animal studies have demonstrated that glucosamine has an "antireactive effect": it prevents an inflammatory response to certain irritants known to cause inflammation in rats but has no inhibitory effects on inflammation caused by inflammatory mediators such as bradykinin, serotonin, and histamine (69). Specifically, and importantly, glucosamine did not show any inhibition of the cyclo-oxygenase system, thus lending some credibility to the claim of gastrointestinal tolerability. In fact, glucosamine may stimulate the production of protective mucopolysaccharides in the gastric mucosa and therefore may even be useful in ulcer therapy (55).

Hua et al. used high-dose (300 mg/kg) oral glucosamine sulfate to suppress adjuvant arthritis in Wistar rats (35). Treated animals demonstrated suppression of synovial hyperplasia, cartilage destruction, and inflammatory cell infiltration. They concluded that high-dose glucosamine sulfate might be a novel anti-inflammatory agent for the treatment of rheumatoid arthritis.

Therapeutic efficacy for glucosamine has been demonstrated in animal models for inflammatory arthritis, mechanical arthritis, immunoreactive arthritis, and generalized inflammation (69). Although its efficacy in these models was lower than that of indomethacin, its toxicity was significantly lower. Therefore, the overall therapeutic margin was much more favorable. Based on these basic science effects, glucosamine may have a place in the therapy of inflammatory arthritis in addition to OA.

Human Studies

Contrary to perception in the United States, glucosamine sulfate has been heavily studied in human arthritis sufferers in the past 25 years. Studies were performed in many countries, including Italy (20), Germany (5,26,58), Spain (45), Portugal (72), China (62), and the Philippines (61). Subjects suffered from arthritis of the hand, spine, shoulders, hips, and knees. The results were consistent: all studies showed a beneficial effect of the study drug. Improvement in pain occurred slowly over a period of several weeks. Subjects continued to improve while taking the study drug, as compared with patients taking placebo, who did not improve. Subjects also maintained improvement for weeks to months after the drug was discontinued. Response to treatment was high, ranging from 56% to over 90% (61,72). Equally important, no study encountered significant side effects with glucosamine. All studies reported diminution of pain, some improvement of mobility, and no significant side effects (5,26,58). Since the early 1980s, numerous controlled studies, including 13 double-blind studies (20,24,33,45,57,59–62,64,78), have been carried out. At least 5 double-blind, single-joint, placebo-controlled studies using a validated outcome tool have been performed (57,59,60,63,64).

Criticism of the older literature on glucosamine has centered on the small numbers of patients studied, the short time periods of those studies, and the relative lack of studies independent of corporate sponsorship (14). Methodological concerns, specifically the failure of most studies to specifically control for NSAID use, were also raised. Recent meta-analyses should help dispel some of the concern over the quality of the clinical evidence. Towheed et al., writing for the Cochrane Database, evaluated 16 regulated clinical trials (RCTs), 12 comparing glucosamine with placebo and 4 comparing it with an NSAID (74). The authors concluded that glucosamine was both safe and effective. McAlindon et al. reviewed 6 studies of glucosamine involving 911 patients (48). Combined results showed a moderate treatment effect for glucosamine.

Glucosamine may be an effective symptomatic treatment for OA of the knee, but does it have a chondroprotective effect? Perhaps the most convincing evidence comes from a pair of very similar long-term studies. Reginster et al. randomized 212 patients to either glucosamine sulfate (1500 mg/day) or placebo and followed them for 3 years (63). Standardized weight-bearing knee radiographs were obtained, and the minimum medial tibiofemoral joint space was measured using digital image analysis. The patients on placebo showed progressive joint space narrowing of approximately 0.1 mm/year, whereas those on glucosamine did not. WOMAC scores worsened slightly in the placebo group and improve in the glucosamine group. Reginster et al. allowed the use of several different NSAIDs as rescue medications, and some commentators were concerned that increased knee extension due to symptomatic relief in the glucosamine group could skew the results. To address some of these perceived deficiencies, Pavelka et al. performed a very similar study with nearly identical results (60). In this study, 202 patients were randomized to glucosamine sulfate or placebo. Only Tylenol was used for rescue analgesia. Minimal tibiofemoral compartment width at a standard degree of knee flexion and WOMAC and Lequesne scores were used as endpoints. Progressive joint space narrowing was noted in the placebo group, whereas joint preservation occurred in the glucosamine group. Lequesne and WOMAC scores also showed statistically significant improvement in the treatment group.

Unfortunately, comparable studies have not been done for OA of the hip. A group of physicians from the EULARS group carried out a thee-round Delphi panel discussion of treatment for OA of the hip and concluded that "symptomatic, slow acting disease modifying drugs SYSDMO (glucosamine sulfate, chondroitin sulfate, diacerhein, avocado soybean unsaponifiable, and hyaluronic acid) have a symptomatic effect and low toxicity, but effect sizes are small , suitable patients are not well defined, and clinically relevant structure modification and pharmacoeconomic aspects are not well established" (86).

Chondroitin

Chondroitin sulfate (galactosaminoglycuronoglycan sulfate) is a mucopolysaccharide that, together with keratan sulfate and a protein core, forms aggrecan. Aggrecan, in turn, associates with hyaluronan to form a hydroscopic macromolecule largely responsible for the physical elasticity of cartilage. During aging, the ratio of keratan sulfate to chondroitin sulfate in aggrecan increases, reflecting a relative loss of chondroitin. Also, chondroitin sulfate from diseased cartilage is shorter in length than normal (29).

As a nutraceutical, chondroitin exhibits anti-inflammatory properties similar to those of other glycosaminoglycans and gag (group-specific antigen) precursors (2). In humans, it is well tolerated, has few side effects, and has reasonable bioavailability (67). Further, as with other gag precursors, stimulatory effects on cartilage have been reported (37). Chondroitin sulfate has also been shown to neutralize catabolic processes, such as IL-1 production and metalloprotease activation, in human OA chondrocyte tissue culture (46).

Several randomized, controlled trials demonstrating a beneficial effect of chondroitin sulfate have been published (7,13,68,75,76,80,83). Morreale et al., in a rigorous study comparing chondroitin and diclofenac showed a more rapid response to diclofenac but a more profound and long-lasting response to chondroitin (56). The chondroitin group maintained their symptomatic improvement 3 weeks after discontinuation of the drug, whereas symptoms in patients treated with diclofenac returned immediately after cessation of therapy.

There is even some credible evidence that chondroitin alters the course of disease in humans. Studying 120 patients with knee OA, Uebelhart et al. found the group given chondroitin sulfate had better functional outcomes and less joint space narrowing on standard radiographs at 1 year than did the control group (75). Verbruggen et al. have also reported on two studies in which patients with erosive arthritis of the hand who were given chondroitin suffered less progression and fewer new lesions than did the controls (80,81).

Glucosamine–Chondroitin Synergy

Looking back to the definition of a "chondroprotective agent" supplied by Ghosh and Brooks, it is clear that neither glucosamine alone nor chondroitin alone satisfy all the criteria. However, since glucosamine acts mostly as a stimulant to GAGS production and chondroitin mostly as an inhibitor of degradative enzymes affecting articular cartilage, it is reasonable to suppose they could have a synergistic effect. Lippiello et al. published a dramatic study in a rabbit instability model of knee OA (44). The authors compared glucosamine alone, chondroitin alone, their combination, and the carrier. Although glucosamine and chondroitin each was noted to have a chondroprotective effect, their combination almost completely prevented the onset of OA.

Because of the significant promise glucosamine and chondroitin seem to hold for the treatment of OA, the NIH funded a 24-week, five-arm trial comparing glucosamine, chondroitin, their combination, and an NSAID versus placebo. The study has been concluded, but the results are pending at the time of this writing.

Several other amino sugars or glycosaminoglycans are commercially available for the treatment of OA. These include glycosaminoglycan-peptide association complex (Rumalon), glycosaminoglycan polysulfuric acid (GAGPS or Arteparon), and sodium pentosan polysulfate (Cartrofen). While these compounds enjoy some laboratory and clinical support, they have not gained the popularity of, nor been as well studied as, glucosamine, chondroitin, and hyaluronic acid.

The recent report by Clegg and co workers of the extensive NTH funded trial of glucosamine and chondroitin alone and in combination compared to placebo and celebrex has spread confusion and doubt about the efficacy of these compounds. The Abstract that was published on the meeting web site prior to the presentation of the study to the American College of Rheumatology meetings in San Diego in Nov. 2006 concluded that "Combination of G (Glucosamine) and CS (Chondroitin Sulfate) is effective in treating moderate to severe knee pain due to OA". However in his podium presentation, Dr. Clegg concluded that both compounds were ineffective alone or in combination. This report and those conclusions received extensive coverage in the lay press. However, when the work was published in the New England Journal of Medicine (NEJM) in February 2006, the conclusions were more in line with the original abstract. (18) It appeared in the study that the combination of Glucosamine and chondroitin was effective in patients with more severe WOMAC scores, but not in patients with WOMAC scores in the mild range (100–300).

It is hard to ignore the whole body of evidence, much of which has been presented above, clinical, cell culture, in vivo data and the effect on experimental arthritis and conclude that there is no place for these compounds in the therapeutic armamentarium. The Clegg article was accompanied in the NEJM with an editorial by Marc Hochberg, Chief of Rheumatology at the University of Maryland (34). He concluded that "Three months of treatment is a sufficient period for the evaluation of efficacy: if there is no clinically significant decrease in symptoms by this time, the supplements should be discontinued." This has been, and continues to be our practice since first beginning to use these agents 10 years ago.

Dangers of "Nutraceuticals"
Most of the studies cited in the previous paragraphs were performed in countries where glucosamine and chondroitin are considered pharmaceuticals and are regulated accordingly. In the United States, these substances are considered "nutritional supplements" and are therefore not regulated by the FDA. The nutritional supplement industry is regulated by the Dietary Supplement Health Education Act, which simply requires the percentage of active ingredient to match the label claim. There is no requirement for safety, efficacy, or bioavailability of the product. Recent investigations have even cast doubt on the accuracy of the label claim percentage (1). Furthermore, several studies have shown that high-molecular-weight chondroitin sulfate is poorly absorbed and much less permeable into the chondrocyte (1,15). Until the FDA takes a more serious position on these agents, it will be incumbent upon the physician to investigate the purity and efficacy of individual formulations before recommending them to patients.

Other agents primarily directed at inhibiting enzymatic or inflammatory cartilage destruction are being investigated. These include Orgotein (bovine superoxide dismutase) interleukin-1 receptor antagonist, S-adenosyl methionine, and Cartrofen (sodium pentosan polysulfate). Although some encouraging data have been presented, these compounds should be considered investigational at this time.

REPORT OF THE EULAR STANDING COMMITTEE FOR INTERNATIONAL CLINICAL STUDIES INCLUDING THERAPEUTICS (ESCISIT)

A guideline development committee consisting of 23 experts in the field of OA (18 rheumatologists, 4 orthopedic surgeons, and 1 epidemiologist) was commissioned by ESCISIT to agree on 10 key propositions for the management of OA of the hip. Their report was published in 2004 and is worth reading in its entirety (86). The propositions were developed by the group as a whole through three Delphi panel-type rounds and then evaluated using the published peer literature and subjecting it quality grading. Eight of the 10 propositions concern the nonoperative management of hip OA. They are listed according to category (general, nonpharmacological, and pharmacologic/invasive) and are reported below:

1. Optimal management of hip OA requires a combination of nonpharmacological and pharmacological treatment modalities.
2. Treatment of hip OA should be tailored according to:
   (a) Hip risk factors (obesity, adverse mechanical factors, physical activity, dysplasia)
   (b) General risk factors (age, sex, comorbidity, comedications)
   (c) Level of pain intensity, disability, handicap
   (d) Location and degree of structural damage
   (e) Wishes and expectations of the patient.
3. Nonpharmacological treatment of hip OA should include regular education, exercise, appliances (thick insoles), and weight reduction if obese or overweight.
4. Because of efficacy and safety, paracetamol (acetaminophen) (up to 4 g/day) is the oral analgesic of first choice for mild–moderate pain and, if successful, is the preferred long-term oral analgesic.
5. NSAIDs, at the lowest effective dose, should be added or substituted in patients who respond inadequately to paracetamol. In patients with increased gastrointestinal risk, nonselective NSAIDs plus a gastroprotective agent, or a selective COX-2 inhibitor (coxib) should be used.
6. Opioid analgesics, with or without paracetamol, are useful alternatives in patients in whom NSAIDs, including COX-2 inhibitors, are contraindicated, ineffective, and/or poorly tolerated.
7. SYSADOA (DMOADS) (glucosamine sulphate, chondroitin sulphate, diacerhein, avocado soybean unsaponifiable, and

hyaluronic acid) have symptomatic effect and low toxicity, but effect sizes are small, suitable patients are not well defined, and clinically relevant structure modification and pharmacoeconomic aspects are not well established.

8. Intra-articular steroid injections (guided by ultrasound or x-ray) may be considered in patients with a flare that is unresponsive to analgesics and NSAIDs.

The committee ended by determining areas of future needed research, many of which would be useful in further evaluating some of the committee's recommendations.

SUMMARY

Many patients with OA of the hip can be significantly benefited by applying the nonoperative modalities that are the subject of this chapter. Generalists, internists, and rheumatologists are generally aware of at least some of these methods and do apply them, although in a somewhat haphazard way. In our experience, many of the patients who self-refer for evaluation of hip pain and who have hip OA have never tried these modalities or even had any of them recommended. Moreover, many patients who are physician referred have not been through any sustained or effective attempt at a conservative regime but have been referred "for surgery." Surgery should be a last resort, in most instances employed only when reasonable nonoperative methods have failed. Orthopedic surgeons owe it to their patients and to themselves to employ these methods where they have not yet been tried. Even if they eventually fail, their use offers physicians an opportunity to get to know their patients and at the same time lets the patients know that their physicians are really interested in their well-being and do not just see them as just another "case."

REFERENCES

1. Adebowale A, Cox DS, Zhongming L, et al. Analysis of glucosamine and chondroitin sulfate content in marketed products and the Caco-2 permeability of chondroitin sulfate raw materials. *JAMA.* 2000;3:37–44.
2. Baici A, Bradamante P. Interaction between human leukocyte elastase and chondroitin sulfate. *Chem Biol Interact.* 1984;51:1–11.
3. Bellamy N, Buchanan WW, Chalmers A, et al. A multicenter study of tenoxicam and diclofenac in patients with osteoarthritis of the knee. *J Rheumatol.* 1993;20:999–1004.
4. Benson GD, Koff RS, Tolman KG. The therapeutic use of acetaminophen in patients with liver disease. *Am J Ther.* 2005;12: 133–141.
5. Bohne W. Glokosamine in der conservativen Arthosebehandlung. *Med Welt.* 1969;30:1668–1671.
6. Bombardier C, Laine L, Reicin, A. Comparison of upper gastrointestinal toxicity of rofecoxib and naproxen in patients with rheumatoid arthritis. VIGOR Study Group. *N Engl J Med.* 2000;343:1520–1528; 2 pp. following 1528.
7. Bourgeois P, Chales G, Dehais J, et al. Efficacy and tolerability of chondroitin sulfate 1200 mg/day vs. chondroitin sulfate 3 × 400 mg/day vs. placebo. *Osteoarthritis Cartilage.* 1998;6[Suppl A]:25–30.
8. Bradley JD, Brandt KD, Katz BP, et al. Comparison of an antiinflammatory dose of ibuprofen, an analgesic dose of ibuprofen, and acetaminophen in the treatment of patients with osteoarthritis of the knee [see comments]. *N Engl J Med.* 1991;325:87–91.
9. Brand RA, Crowninshield RD. The effect of cane use on hip contact force. *Clin Orthop Relat Res.* 1980;147:181–184.
10. Brandt KD. The mechanism of action of nonsteroidal antiinflammatory drugs. *J Rheumatol Suppl.* 1991;27:120–121.
11. Brandt KD, Palmoski M. Organization of ground substance proteoglycans in normal and osteoarthritic knee cartilage. *Arthritis Rheum.* 1976;19:209–215.
12. Breshnihan B, Hughes G, Essigman WK. Diflunisal in the treatment of osoteoarthrosis: a double blind study comparing diflunisal with ibuprofen. *Curr Med Res Opin.* 1978;5:556.
13. Bucsi L, Poor G. Efficacy and tolerability of oral chondroitin sulfate as a symptomatic slow-acting drug for osteoarthritis (SYSADOA) in the treatment of knee osteoarthritis. *Osteoarthritis Cartilage.* 1998;6[suppl A]:31–36.
14. Callaghan JJ, Buckwalter JA, Schenck RC Jr. Argument against use of food additives for osteoarthritis of the hip. *Clin Orthop Relat Res.* 2000;No. 381:88–90.
15. Cho SY, Sim JS, Jeong CS, et al. Effects of low molecular weight chondroitin sulfate on type II collagen-induced arthritis in DBA/1J mice. *Biol Pharm Bull.* 2004;27:47–51.
16. Christgau S, Henrotin Y, Tanko LB, et al. Osteoarthritic patients with high cartilage turnover show increased responsiveness to the cartilage protecting effects of glucosamine sulphate. *Clin Exp Rheumatol.* 2004;22:36–42.
17. Clegg DO, Reda DJ, Harris CL, Klein MA, et al. Glucosamine, chondroitin sulfate, and the two in combination for painful knee osteoarthritis. *N Engl J Med.* 2006 Feb. 23;354(8):795–808.
18. Conrozier T, Bertin P, Mathieu P, et al. Intra-articular injections of hylan G-F 20 in patients with symptomatic hip osteoarthritis: an open-label, multicentre, pilot study. *Clin Exp Rheumatol.* 2003;21: 605–610.
19. Cottingham B, Phillips PD, Davies GK, et al. The effect of subcutaneous nerve stimulation (SCNS) on pain associated with osteoarthritis of the hip. *Pain.* 1985;22:243–248.
20. Crolle G, D'Este E. Glucosamine sulphate for the management of arthrosis: a controlled clinical investigation. *Curr Med Res Opin.* 1980;7:104–109.
21. Daniels B, Seidenberg B. Cardiovascular safety profile of rofecoxib in controlled clinical trials. *Arthritis Rheum.* 1999;42(suppl): S143–143.
22. De Blecourt JJ. A comparative study of ibuprofen ("Brufen") and indomethacin in uncomplicated arthritis. *Curr Med Res Opin.* 1975;3:477.
23. Dieppe P, Cushnaghan J, Jasani MK, et al. A two-year, placebo-controlled trail of non-steroidal anti-inflammatory therapy in osteoarthritis of the knee joint [see comments]. *Br J Rheumatol.* 1993;32:595–600.
24. Drovanti A, Bignamini AA, Rovati AL. Therapeutic activity of oral glucosamine sulfate in osteoarthrosis: a placebo-controlled double-blind investigation. *Clin Ther.* 1980;3:260–72.
25. Edwards JE, McQuay HJ, Moore RA. Efficacy and safety of valdecoxib for treatment of osteoarthritis and rheumatoid arthritis: systematic review of randomised controlled trials. *Pain.* 2004;111:286–296.
26. Eichler J, Nöh E. Behandlung der Arthrosis deformans durch Beeinflussung des Knorpelstoffwechsels. *Orthop Praxis.* 1970;6: 225–229.
27. Fink MG, Kunsebeck HW, Wippermann B. Effect of needle acupuncture on pain perception and functional impairment of patients with coxarthrosis [in German] J Z Rheumatol. 2000;59:191–199.
28. Foley A, Halbert J, Hewitt T, et al. Does hydrotherapy improve strength and physical function in patients with osteoarthritis: a randomized controlled trial comparing a gym based and a hydrotherapy based strengthening programme. *Ann Rheum Dis.* 2003;62:1162–1167.
29. Fries JF, Bruce B. Rates of serious gastrointestinal events from low dose use of acetylsalicylic acid, acetaminophen, and ibuprofen in patients with osteoarthritis and rheumatoid arthritis. *J Rheumatol.* 2003;30:2226–2233.
30. Ghosh P, Brooks P. Chondroprotection: exploring the concept [editorial]. *J Rheumatol.* 1991;18:161–166.
31. Haslam R. A comparison of acupuncture with advice and exercises on the symptomatic treatment of osteoarthritis of the hip: a randomised controlled trial. *Acupunct Med.* 2001;19:19–26.
32. Hedner T. Comparative evaluations of NSAIDs and other analgesics in osteoarthrosis. In: *Pharmacological Treatment of Osteoarthritis.* 2nd ed. Uppsala, Sweden: Almqvist and Wiksell; 1989:173–198.
33. Hehne HJ, Blasius K, Ernst HU. Therapy of gonarthrosis using chondroprotective substances: prospective comparative study of

glucosamine sulphate and glycosaminoglycan polysulphate [in German]. *Fortschr Med.* 1984;102:676–682.

34. Hochberg MC. Nutritional supplements for knee osteoarthritis–still no resolution. *N Engl J Med.* 2006 Feb 23;354(8):858–60

35. Hua J, Suguro S, Hirano S, et al. Preventive actions of a high dose of glucosamine on adjuvant arthritis in rats. *Inflamm Res.* 2005;54:127–132.

36. Jimenez S, Dodge G. The effects of glucosamine sulfate on human chondrocyte gene expression. *Osteoarthritis Cartilage.* 1997;5:72.

37. Karzel K, Domenjoz R. Effects of hexosamine derivatives and uronic acid derivatives on glycosaminoglycane metabolism of fibroblast cultures. *Pharmacology.* 1971;5:337–345.

38. Kaspar S, de V de Beer J. Infection in hip arthroplasty after previous injection of steroid. *J Bone Joint Surg [Br].* 2005;87:454–457.

39. Kullenberg B, Runesson R, Tuvhag R, et al. Intraarticular corticosteroid injection: pain relief in osteoarthritis of the hip? *J Rheumatol.* 2004;31:2265–2268.

40. Kutzim H. Über ^{14}C-markiertes Glukosamin. Report of the Nuclear Medicine Laboratory. Bonn: University Clinic of Bonn; 1970.

41. Lin SY, Davey RC, Cochrane T. Community rehabilitation for older adults with osteoarthritis of the lower limb: a controlled clinical trial. *Clin Rehabil.* 2004;18:92–101.

42. Lippiello L. Glucosamine and chondroitin sulfate: biological response modifiers of chondrocytes under simulated conditions of joint stress. *Osteoarthritis Cartilage.* 2003;11:335–342.

43. Lippiello L, Woodward J, Karpman R, et al. In vivo chondroprotection and metabolic synergy of glucosamine and chondroitin sulfate. *Clin Orthop.* 2000;No. 381:229–240.

44. Lister BJ, Poland M, DeLapp RE. Efficacy of nabumetone versus diclofenac, naproxen, ibuprofen, and piroxicam in osteoarthritis and rheumatoid arthritis. *Am J Med.* 1993;95(2A):2S–9S.

45. Lopes Vaz A. Double-blind clinical evaluation of the relative efficacy of ibuprofen and glucosamine sulphate in the management of osteoarthrosis of the knee in out-patients. *Curr Med Res Opin.* 1982;8:145–149.

46. Mathieu P. A new mechanism of action of chondroitin sulfates ACS4-ACS6 in osteoarthritic cartilage [in French]. *Presse Med.* 2002;31:1383–1385.

47. Mazzuca SA, Brandt KD, Anderson SL, et al. The therapeutic approaches of community based primary care practitioners to osteoarthritis of the hip in an elderly patient. *J Rheumatol.* 1991;18:1593–1600.

48. McAlindon TE, LaValley MP, Gulin JP, et al. Glucosamine and chondroitin for treatment of osteoarthritis: a systematic quality assessment and meta-analysis. *JAMA.* 2000;283:1469–1475.

49. McCarty MF. Enhanced synovial production of hyaluronic acid may explain rapid clinical response to high-dose glucosamine in osteoarthritis. *Med Hypotheses.* 1998;50:507–510.

50. McCarty MF. The neglect of glucosamine as a treatment for osteoarthritis: a personal perspective. *Med Hypotheses.* 1994;42:323–327.

51. McKenzie LS, Horsburgh BA, Ghosh P, et al. Osteoarthrosis: uncertain rationale for anti-inflammatory drug therapy [letter]. *Lancet.* 1976;1(7965):908–909.

52. Mehrotra C, Naimi TS, Serdula M, et al. Arthritis, body mass index, and professional advice to lose weight: implications for clinical medicine and public health. *Am J Prev Med.* 2004;27:16–21.

53. Messier SP, Loeser RF, Miller GD, et al. Exercise and dietary weight loss in overweight and obese older adults with knee osteoarthritis. The Arthritis, Diet, and Activity Promotion Trial. *Arthritis Rheum.* 2004;50:1501–1510.

54. Migliore A, Tormenta S, Martin LS, et al. Open pilot study of ultrasound-guided intra-articular injection of hylan G-F 20 (Synvisc) in the treatment of symptomatic hip osteoarthritis. *Clin Rheumatol.* 2005;24:285–289.

55. Moriga M, Aono M, Murakami M, et al. The activity of N-acetylglucosamine kinase in rat gastric mucosa. *Gastroenterol Jpn.* 1980;15:7–13.

56. Morreale P, Manopulo R, Galati M, et al. Comparison of the anti-inflammatory efficacy of chondroitin sulfate and diclofenac sodium in patients with knee osteoarthritis. *J Rheumatol.* 1996;23:1385–1391.

57. Muller-Fassbender H, Bach GL, Haase W, et al. Glucosamine sulfate compared to ibuprofen in osteoarthritis of the knee. *Osteoarthritis Cartilage.* 1994;2:61–69.

58. Mund-Hoym WD. The treatment of hip and knee joint arthroses [in German]. *ZFA (Stuttgart).* 1980;56:2153–2159.

59. Noack W, Fischer M, Forster KK, et al. Glucosamine sulfate in osteoarthritis of the knee. *Osteoarthritis Cartilage.* 1994;2:51–59.

60. Pavelka K, Gatterova J, Olejarova M, et al. Glucosamine sulfate use and delay of progression of knee osteoarthritis: a 3-year, randomized, placebo-controlled, double-blind study. *Arch Intern Med.* 2002;162:2113–2123.

61. Pujalte JM, Llavore EP, Ylescupidez FR. Double-blind clinical evaluation of oral glucosamine sulphate in the basic treatment of osteoarthrosis. *Curr Med Res Opin.* 1980;7:110–114.

62. Qiu GX, Gao SN, Giacovelli G, et al. Efficacy and safety of glucosamine sulfate versus ibuprofen in patients with knee osteoarthritis. *Arzneimittelforschung.* 1998;48:469–474.

63. Reginster JY, Deroisy R, Rovati LC, et al. Long-term effects of glucosamine sulphate on osteoarthritis progression: a randomised, placebo-controlled clinical trial. *Lancet.* 2001;357(9252):251–256.

64. Reichelt A, Forster KK, Fischer M, et al. Efficacy and safety of intramuscular glucosamine sulfate in osteoarthritis of the knee: a randomised, placebo-controlled, double- blind study. *Arzneimittelforschung.* 1994;44:75–80.

65. Roddy E, Zhang W, Doherty M, et al. Evidence-based recommendations for the role of exercise in the management of osteoarthritis of the hip or knee: the MOVE consensus. *Rheumatology (Oxford).* 2005;44:67–73.

66. Roden L. Effect of hexosamines on the synthesis of chondroitin sulphuric acid in vitro. *Ark Kemi.* 1956;10:345–352.

67. Ronca F, Palmieri L, Panicucci P, et al. Anti-inflammatory activity of chondroitin sulfate. *Osteoarthritis Cartilage.* 1998;6[Suppl A]:14–21.

68. Rovetta G. Galactosaminoglycuronoglycan sulfate (matrix) in therapy of tibiofibular osteoarthritis of the knee. *Drugs Exp Clin Res.* 1991;17:53–57.

69. Setnikar I, Cereda R, Pacini MA, et al. Antireactive properties of glucosamine sulfate. *Arzneimittelforschung.* 1991;41:157–161.

70. Singh G. Recent considerations in nonsteroidal anti-inflammatory drug gastropathy. *Am J Med.* 1998;105(1B):31S–38S.

71. Stener-Victorin E, Kruse-Smidje C, Jung K. Comparison between electro-acupuncture and hydrotherapy, both in combination with patient education and patient education alone, on the symptomatic treatment of osteoarthritis of the hip. *Clin J Pain.* 2004;20:179–185.

72. Tapadinhas MJ, Rivera IC, Bignamini AA. Oral glucosamine sulphate in the management of arthrosis: report on a multi-centre open investigation in Portugal. *Pharmatherapeutica.* 1982;3:157–168.

73. Theodosakis JA, Adderly B, Fox B. *The Arthritis Cure.* New York: St. Martin's Press; 1997.

74. Towheed TE, Anastassiades TP, Shea B, et al. Glucosamine therapy for treating osteoarthritis. *Cochrane Database Syst Rev.* 2001;No. 1:CD002946.

75. Uebelhart D, Thonar EJ, Delmas PD, et al. Effects of oral chondroitin sulfate on the progression of knee osteoarthritis: a pilot study. *Osteoarthritis Cartilage.* 1998;6[Suppl A]:39–46.

76. Uebelhart D, Thonar EJ, Zhang J, et al. Protective effect of exogenous chondroitin 4,6-sulfate in the acute degradation of articular cartilage in the rabbit. *Osteoarthritis Cartilage.* 1998;6[Suppl A]:6–13.

77. Vad VB, Sakalkale D, Sculco TP, et al. Role of hylan G-F 20 in treatment of osteoarthritis of the hip joint. *Arch Phys Med Rehabil.* 2003;84:1224–1226.

78. Vajaradul Y. Double-blind clinical evaluation of intra-articular glucosamine in outpatients with gonarthrosis. *Clin Ther.* 1981;3:336–343.

79. Van der Esch M, Heijmans M, Dekker J. Factors contributing to possession and use of walking aids among persons with rheumatoid arthritis and osteoarthritis *Arthritis Rheum.* 2003;49:838–842.

80. Verbruggen G, Goemaere S, Veys EM. Chondroitin sulfate: S/DMOAD (structure/disease modifying anti-osteoarthritis drug) in the treatment of finger joint OA. *Osteoarthritis Cartilage.* 1998;6[Suppl A]:37–38.

81. Verbruggen G, Goemaere S, Veys EM. Systems to assess the progression of finger joint osteoarthritis and the effects of disease modifying osteoarthritis drugs. *Clin Rheumatol.* 2002;21:231–243.

82. Vidal y Plana RR, Bizzarri D, Rovati AL. Articular cartilage pharmacology, I: in vitro studies on glucosamine and non steroidal antiinflammatory drugs. *Pharmacol Res Commun.* 1978;10(6):557–69.

83. Vidal y Plana RR, Karzel K. Glucosamine: its importance for the metabolism of articular cartilage, II: studies on articular cartilage [in German]. *Fortschr Med.* 1980;98:801–806.

84. Ward DE, Veys EM, Bowdler JM, et al. Comparison of aceclofenac with diclofenac in the treatment of osteoarthritis. *Clin Rheumatol.* 1995;14:656–662.

85. Williams HJ, Ward JR, Egger MJ. Comparison of naproxen and acetaminophen in a two-year study of treatment of osteoarthritis of the knee. *Arthritis Rheum.* 1993;36:1196–1206.

86. Zhang W, Doherty M, Arden N, et al. EULAR evidence based recommendations for the management of hip osteoarthritis: report of a task force of the EULAR Standing Committee for International Clinical Studies Including Therapeutics (ESCISIT). *Ann Rheum Dis.* 2005;64:669–681.

Preoperative Medical Evaluation

42

Anthony B. Fiorillo   Francis X. Solano, Jr.

This chapter acquaints the reader with an approach to the patient undergoing hip replacement, describes strategies for preoperative assessment, and discusses the management of common medical conditions in the perioperative period.

The preoperative assessment of patients undergoing hip replacement follows the basic principles of preoperative assessment of patents undergoing anesthesia and noncardiac surgery. Inherent in this population are comorbid conditions that may increase their surgical risk. The goal of preoperative assessment is to identify the patient's known and occult med-

ical conditions, optimize medical care, and intervene with therapy to improve the surgical outcome. An added benefit is the chance for the assessing physician to express to the patient the risks and benefits of surgery given his or her comorbid conditions.

Often patients are willing to accept a higher surgical risk to obtain an improved quality of life and in particular to decrease chronic pain and increase mobility and functional capacity.

The most important elements of the preoperative assessment are the history and physical examination. A history can predict fitness in 96% of surgical patients (64). Limitations of functional capacity make assessing cardiovascular risk assessment by history difficult in orthopedic patients. It is important to determine the duration of functional. Functional status has been shown to be reliable for perioperative and long-term prediction of cardiac events (39,49). If the patient has not had a recent exercise test, functional capacity can be estimated from the ability to perform the activities of daily living. Functional capacity can be expressed in metabolic equivalent (MET) levels; the oxygen consumption (VO_2) of a 70-kg, 40-year-old man in a resting state is 3.5 mL per kg per minute, or 1 MET. Functional capacity has been classified as excellent (greater than 10 METs), good (7 to 10 METs), moderate (4 to 7 METs), poor (less than 4 METs), or unknown. Perioperative cardiac and long-term risks are increased in patients unable to meet a 4-MET demand during most normal daily activities (52). In one series of 600 consecutive patients undergoing major noncardiac procedures, perioperative myocardial ischemia and cardiovascular events were more common in patients reporting poor exercise tolerance (inability to walk four blocks or climb two flights of stairs) even after adjustment for baseline characteristics known to be associated with increased risk (49). The likelihood of a serious complication occurring was inversely related to the number of blocks that could be walked ($p = 0.006$) or the flights of stairs that could be

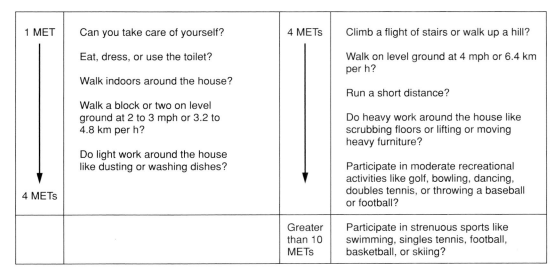

1 MET	Can you take care of yourself?	4 METs	Climb a flight of stairs or walk up a hill?
	Eat, dress, or use the toilet?		Walk on level ground at 4 mph or 6.4 km per h?
	Walk indoors around the house?		Run a short distance?
	Walk a block or two on level ground at 2 to 3 mph or 3.2 to 4.8 km per h?		Do heavy work around the house like scrubbing floors or lifting or moving heavy furniture?
4 METs	Do light work around the house like dusting or washing dishes?		Participate in moderate recreational activities like golf, bowling, dancing, doubles tennis, or throwing a baseball or football?
		Greater than 10 METs	Participate in strenuous sports like swimming, singles tennis, football, basketball, or skiing?

MET indicates metabolic equivalent.
*Adapted from the Duke Activity Status Index (7) and AHA Excercise Standards (27).

Figure 42-1 Examples of work for metabolic equivalents.

climbed ($p = 0.01$). Examples of leisure activities associated with less than 4 METs are baking, slow ballroom dancing, golfing with a cart, playing a musical instrument, and walking at a speed of approximately 2 to 3 mph. Activities that require more than 4 METs include moderate cycling, climbing hills, ice skating, rollerblading, skiing, singles tennis, and jogging. At activity levels less than 4 METs, specific questions to establish risk gradients are less reliable (Fig. 42-1). Furthermore, a clinical questionnaire only estimates functional capacity and does not provide as objective a measurement as exercise treadmill testing or arm ergometry (10).

LABORATORY TESTING

There have been many studies addressing the utility of routine laboratory testing for surgical patients (31,35,55,64). Laboratory testing results in a new diagnosis in 0.7% of patients (61). Twenty percent of patients have abnormalities on screening studies. Forty percent have studies ordered for a recognizable indication. It is important to recognize that, statistically, 5% of normal patients on a given test will fall outside the reference range, since normal is defined by 2 standard deviations from the mean (18). Thus, with a 20-element chemistry profile, 64% of patients in a healthy population will have at least one abnormality. The next important question is, how do these abnormal results influence surgical risk? In many studies that have looked at the issue, the answer is a resounding *very little!* The chance of finding a significant laboratory abnormality that will affect the surgical outcome is less than 1%. Most clinicians are now using selective testing in their approach to preoperative assessment of patients (35) (Table 42-1).

The complete blood count is important in orthopedic patients, because patients on nonsteroidal anti-inflammatory agents may develop an iron deficiency anemia due to indo-

lent gastrointestinal bleeding. Patients with inflammatory arthritis can have anemia of chronic disease. Both situations can cause severe anemia (hemoglobin less than 8 g/dL) that will impact surgical risk. A hematocrit less than 28% has been shown to impact cardiovascular risk (10). Hip replacement and hip revision arthroplasty can be associated with significant blood loss, so it is important to have a baseline value. Studies on the preoperative value of the white blood cell count have demonstrated an abnormality rate in the range of 0% to 9.5%. Severe abnormalities are uncommon (less than 0.7%). In orthopedic patients with rheumatoid arthritis (RA), leukopenia may develop from the use of drugs such as methotrexate, infliximab, and nonsteroidal anti-inflammatory agents or in the setting of splenomegaly (Felty syndrome). Leukocytosis caused by steroid use is also possible, but it is uncommon in patients on low-dose corticosteroids (less than the equivalent of 7.5 mg of prednisone every day) for inflammatory arthritis. Abnormal platelet counts are seen in 0% to 11.8% rheumatoid patients. Severe abnormalities contributing to an increased risk of bleeding are uncommon. In the postoperative period, patients who have undergone hip arthroplasty occasionally have thrombocytopenia caused by consumptive coagulopathy. Low molecular weight heparins and unfractionated heparin can also cause thrombocytopenia, so a baseline platelet count can be important, so it is reasonable to obtain one.

Chemistry studies to assess renal function, hepatic enzyme abnormalities, serum glucose levels, and electrolyte abnormalities also are of limited usefulness as screens for asymptomatic disease. However, renal function can be adversely affected in older patients who have congestive heart failure CHF), diabetes mellitus, or hypertension or who are taking nonsteroidal anti-inflammatory agents or cox-2 inhibitors. Therefore, it is important to obtain a baseline BUN, creatinine, and urine analysis prior to hip replacement surgery. Infrequently, liver enzyme abnormalities (2 to 3 times upper

TABLE 42-1
PREOPERATIVE TESTING SCHEDULE

Preoperative Condition	HCT	PT	PTT	Na, K	Creat, BUN	Glucose	X-ray	EKG	Urine Pregnancy Test	T/SS
Procedure with blood loss	X									X
Procedure without blood loss										
40–49								X[a]		
50–64								X		
65 and over					X			X		
Cardiovascular disease										
Hypertension										
Mild										
Moderate to severe							X	X		
Congestive heart failure	X						X	X		
Ischemic heart disease	X							X		
Vascular disease										
Carotid disease								X		
Abdominal aorta disease								X		
Peripheral vascular disease								X		
Pulmonary disease							X	X		
Hepatic disease	X	X								
Renal disease	X			X	X					
Suspected pregnancy									X	
Diabetes				X	X	X		X		
Use of diuretics				X	X					
Use of digoxin				X	X			X		
Use of steroids				X		X				
Use of Tegretol				X						
Use of Coumadin		X								
Use of heparin			X							

BUN, blood urea nitrogen; Creat, creatinine; HCT, hematocrit; K, potassium; Na, sodium; PT, prothrombin time; PTT, partial thromboplastin time; T/S, type and screen units of red blood cells.
[a] Males.

limits or normal) result from use of medications (statins, acetaminophen, etc.) yet do not impact surgical outcomes. In contrast, hepatitis secondary to acute viral disease and alcohol can have adverse effects on morbidity and mortality in the perioperative period. A thorough history will identify those patients who should have liver enzyme tests done preoperatively. Although the prevalence of type II diabetes is approaching 8% in the adult population, identifying it for the first time preoperatively has not been shown to impact surgical outcome. The existence of diabetes as a chronic disease has significant impact on outcomes and will be addressed in another section of this chapter.

Coagulation studies are not helpful in identifying asymptomatic patients who will have bleeding problems. The history and physical examination are most important in assessing hemostasis. Determination of bleeding time, prothrombin time, and partial thromboplastin time is of little utility in predicting postoperative hemorrhage in a patient with no history of hemostatic disease. Nonsteroidal anti-inflammatory medications inhibit platelet aggregation, potentially prolonging bleeding.

Urinalysis is not very helpful in identifying patients at risk for infectious complications. It is difficult to demonstrate that treating a patient for asymptomatic bacteriuria will diminish the risk of hip infection. Asymptomatic bacteriuria can be found in 25% to 50% of elderly patients, and, in general, treatment does not lead to lasting cures. However, it is advisable to treat asymptomatic bacteriuria preoperatively, because many patients will have urologic instrumentation in the perioperative period, along with postoperative catheter placement or intermittent catheterization.

Chest x-ray abnormalities are very common in patients over 60 years of age (35,59), but the influence of a preoperative abnormality on the outcome of hip surgery is small (54). Although chronic obstructive lung disease and abnormalities consistent with heart failure may influence management decisions, the history and physical examination remain more important in assessing pulmonary or cardiac risk than the radiograph.

An abnormal preoperative electrocardiogram (EKG) probably deserves the most attention. Up to 52.7% of patients may have an abnormality on routine EKG. Goldman (21) has demonstrated the poor predictive value of ST-segment and T-wave changes in predicting cardiac events. Detecting a "silent" myocardial infarction (MI) based on EKG is a rare event (0.3%), but it may have some validity in risk stratification. Patients with a recent MI may be at higher risk for a perioperative MI. Bifascicular block rarely progresses to complete heart block during surgery and is not an indication for temporary pacemaker placement. Left bundle branch block (LBBB) can be a marker of left ventricular systolic dysfunction, and assessment of LV function by echocardiography should be done in patients with LBBB identified on EKG.

There are other reasons to perform preoperative laboratory testing. Often, the institution where surgery is being performed will have baseline requirements that are mandated by the hospital, surgical center, or the medical or anesthesia staff. Medicolegal issues and the fear of omission are major reasons for testing. Presently, the standards of care promoted by textbooks, physician organizations, and the current literature on laboratory testing include a selective testing approach (see Table 42-1).

In summary, laboratory testing should be selective rather than routine in patients undergoing surgery. It is difficult to find significant abnormalities that will influence management decisions regarding surgery.

CLASSIFICATION OF RISK

The American Society of Anesthesiology (ASA) has adopted Dripps' stratification system (9) (Table 42-2) to predict perioperative mortality. This system was originally designed to classify patients for a research protocol, but it was found to have predictive value for clinical outcomes.

Because there is some subjectivity in the ASA scale, other authors have sought more objective criteria for surgical risk stratification. Goldman et al. (22) and Detsky et al. (8) used multivariate analysis to stratify risk. The index of Goldman et al. was based on data collected on 1001 consecutive patients admitted to their institution for a variety of nonthoracic surgeries. They developed a multivariate point system that has been validated at other institutions as a predictor of cardiac complication following nonthoracic surgery.

Detsky et al. (8) modified the risk index by looking at the timing of MI, current or previous pulmonary edema, Canadian Cardiovascular Society angina classification, and institution-specific complication rates for types of surgical procedures (Table 42-3). Using Detsky's criteria, a specific cardiac risk can be assigned to the individual by plotting the summed points on a normogram. The exact calculation is not as important as the recognition that criteria have been established and validated to allow the clinician to preoperatively estimate cardiac risk. There are limitations to applying multivariate analysis for predicting risk in a patient; many additional factors influence outcome.

TABLE 42-3
DETSKY'S MODIFIED MULTIFACTORIAL INDEX

Status	Points
Coronary artery disease	
MI within 6 months	10
MI after 6 months	5
CSS angina class 3	10
CSS angina class 4	20
Unstable angina within 3 months	10
Alveolar pulmonary edema	
Within 6 months	10
Ever	5
Valvular disease	
Suspected hemodynamically significant aortic stenosis	20
EKG	
Nonsinus or sinus rhythm, with frequent PACs on preoperative test	5
More than 5 PVCs on EKG	5
Poor medical status	5
Age >70	5
Emergency operation	10
Total maximum points	**125**

CSS, carotid sinus stimulation; MI, myocardial infarction; PAC, premature atrial contraction; PVC, premature ventricular contraction. Reproduced from Detsky AS, Abrams HB, McLaughlin JR, et al. Predicting cardiac complications in patients undergoing non-cardiac surgery. *J Gen Intern Med.* 1986;1:212.

The variables (or clinical parameters) of these indexes offer the clinician a structure for assessment. This information can be offered to the patient, anesthesiologist, and surgeon to maximize surgical outcome. Following are some specific risk categories of patients undergoing hip replacement.

CARDIOVASCULAR RISK

The patient undergoing hip replacement often has limited functional capacity because of age or arthritis, making cardiovascular fitness assessment difficult.

TABLE 42-2
PREOPERATIVE ASSESSMENT CLASSIFICATION

ASA status	Examples of Preoperative Patients
Class 1: No disease	Healthy 25-year-old
Class 2: Mild to moderate systemic disease	65-year-old with well-controlled DM type 2
Class 3: Severe systemic disease	70-year-old with CHF and rest angina
Class 4: Life-threatening systemic disease	30-year-old with DM type 1 in ketoacidosis
Class 5: Morbidly ill	70-year-old with angina and mesenteric ischemia
E is added to each class if surgery is an emergency.	

ASA, American Society of Anesthesiology; DM, diabetes mellitus; CHF, congestive heart failure. Reproduced from Dripps RD. New classification of physical status. *Anesthesiology* 1963;24:111.

Stable angina has been shown not to be a risk factor for noncardiac surgery by several authors (8,22). Patients with unstable angina, angina at low levels of activity, or dyspnea at low levels of activity should be considered at high risk, and cardiovascular evaluation should be performed before proceeding. Recent coronary artery bypass grafting within 5 years of proposed surgery confers a low risk of perioperative cardiac complication (10).

Noninvasive pharmacologic stress tests using dipyridamole (33,36), adenosine thallium (11,56), or dobutamine echocardiography (33,34) have been helpful in assessing patients undergoing vascular or noncardiac surgery. Dipyridamole increases intracoronary adenosine, leading to vasodilatation of the coronary circulation. This creates intracoronary steals in areas of fixed coronary obstruction, leading to a relative decrease in perfusion that can be detected with thallium, and more recently on echocardiography, as segmental wall motion abnormalities. These techniques have limitations, particularly in determining whom to screen and then what to do with the information obtained (33,56). All of the modalities available have good sensitivity and specificity for detection of coronary disease, but they do not give an ischemic threshold.

Eagle et al. (11) validated a clinical index in conjunction with pharmacologic stress testing. Patients were classified into low-, intermediate-, and high-risk groups based on the presence of five risk factors: age over 70, angina, prior MI, prior CHF, and diabetes mellitus. Risk factor number correlated with postoperative cardiac events. In patients with no risk factor, 1 patient out of 29 had a cardiac event. In patients with more than two risk factors, 50% had an event. These factors put patients into risk categories correctly 71% of the time. If a patient anticipating hip surgery has risk factors for coronary events, as identified by Eagle, yet functional capacity cannot be assessed because of arthritis or age, it is advisable to perform a pharmacologic stress test.

It has been shown that there is a correlation between the degree of abnormality on thallium imaging and risk (33,34). An abnormal thallium test with fixed defects, or an abnormal test with reversible ischemia in one coronary territory, is not an indication for catheterization or revascularization. These patients can be treated medically and have an acceptable cardiac risk. Patients with global ischemia or with two or more significant areas of myocardium at risk should be studied with coronary arteriography before proceeding with hip replacement. As in all risk assessment, the risk of hip surgery and revascularization (angioplasty, vascular stent, atherectomy, or coronary artery bypass grafts) must be weighed against the benefit of the hip surgery itself (36,70).

An algorithm published by the ACC/AHA task force is widely used and referenced (Figure 42-2) (10).

RECENT MYOCARDIAL INFARCTION

Unstable angina and a recent MI (less than 6 months previously) remain the strongest predictors of perioperative myocardial ischemia. Thus it has been customary to wait until 6 months after an MI before proceeding with elective orthopedic surgery. This practice is based on the work of Tahran et al. (60) in the early 1970s and was validated by Goldman et al. (22) in 1977 and then by Steen et al. (55). Tahran et al. (60) studied 38,877 patients who had undergone anesthesia and found 422 with prior infarction. Of these 422, 37% had another infarction if they had surgery within 3 months of the prior infarction, 16% if the surgery was within 3 to 6 months, and 5% if the surgery was after 6 months. Tahran obtained statistically similar results again 6 years later. Rao et al. (51) used invasive hemodynamic monitoring in patients with a recent MI and demonstrated a 5.7% risk of MI when surgery followed the MI by 3 months or less and a 2.3% risk when the surgery was within 3 to 6 months of the MI.

Because of increased knowledge about acute coronary syndromes, improved hemodynamic monitoring, and availability of a larger array of cardiac medications, some have questioned the convention of waiting 6 months. Others have suggested that the location of the ischemic event has a bearing on perioperative risk; for example, an uncomplicated inferior wall MI is less risky than an anterior or lateral wall MI. Patients with a recent MI should be adequately evaluated and risk stratified preoperatively for residual ischemia and left ventricular dysfunction. If a recent stress test does not indicate residual myocardium risk, the likelihood of reinfarction after noncardiac surgery is low. Although there are no adequate clinical trials on which to base firm recommendations, it appears reasonable to wait 4 to 6 weeks after an MI before performing elective surgery (10).

Mortality from a perioperative MI remains high (25 to 50%) in one series due to the atypical presentation of perioperative myocardial ischemia (58). Only 50% of patients have typical chest pain, and many have atypical symptoms, such as arrhythmia, confusion, hypotension, or CHF, making the diagnosis more challenging.

PRE-EXISTING CONGESTIVE HEART FAILURE

CHF can be the consequence of many forms of cardiac disease (myocardial ischemia, aortic or mitral valvular disease, arrhythmias) and noncardiac disease (hypertension, anemia, hemochromatosis). The underlying disease and cardiac function should be optimally managed before surgery. Patients who have a history of CHF have a 6% risk of recurrent CHF and a 5% mortality (22). Those patients with an S_3 gallop, jugular venous distention, or rales have a 20% mortality. It is important to identify the cause and to reverse the CHF, if possible. Echocardiography to assess left ventricular function and the presence of significant valvular disease can be helpful preoperatively. Patients with severe impairment of left ventricular function (ejection fraction [EF] less than 25%) are at increased risk for CHF and death. Invasive monitoring is at the discretion of the anesthesiologist. Beta-blockers, angiotensin-converting enzyme (ACE) inhibitors, and angiotensin receptor blockers (ARBs) have been shown to improve survival and improve quality of life. Patients with CHF should receive ACE inhibitors or ARBs and beta-blockers preoperatively (6,47) and through the postoperative period.

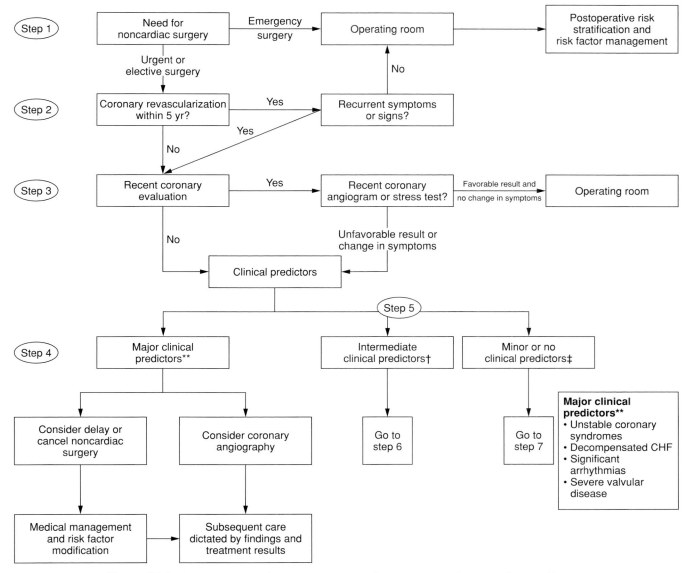

Figure 42-2 Stepwise approach to preoperative cardiac assessment. Steps are discussed in text. Subsequent care may include cancellation or delay of surgery, coronary revascularization followed by noncardiac surgery, or intensified care. (Reproduced from Eagle, KA, Berger, PB, Calkins, H, et al. ACC/AHA guideline update for perioperative cardiovascular evaluation for noncardiac surgery: executive summary: a report of the American College of Cardiology/American Heart Association Task Force on Practice Guidelines (Committee to Update the 1996 Guidelines on Perioperative Cardiovascular Evaluation for Noncardiac Surgery). *J Am Coll Cardiol.* 2002; 39:542.)

VALVULAR DISEASE

Patients with significant aortic stenosis and mitral stenosis are at greatest risk for perioperative morbidity, because these lesions tend to cause a fixed cardiac output, which in turn makes patients intolerant of increased preload (excessive intravenous fluids intraoperatively) or decreased afterload (vasodilation with spinal or epidural anesthesia). Perioperative CHF, dysrhythmias, and death occur as a consequence. Calcific aortic stenosis is becoming increasingly common in our elderly population, and recognizing and evaluat-

ing it preoperatively is critical due to the risks associated with this fixed obstructive lesion. Patients with mitral stenosis fortunately are rare in the United States. Those who have can experience significant problems with tachyarrhythmias in particular, which can compromise ventricular filling and lead to CHF. Because many anesthetic agents are afterload-reducing agents, regurgitant valves such as mitral insufficiency and aortic insufficiency do well if cardiac output is preserved. These patients should be treated for prophylaxis of bacterial endocarditis, particularly if the genitourinary tract will be manipulated by a Foley catheter in the perioperative period.

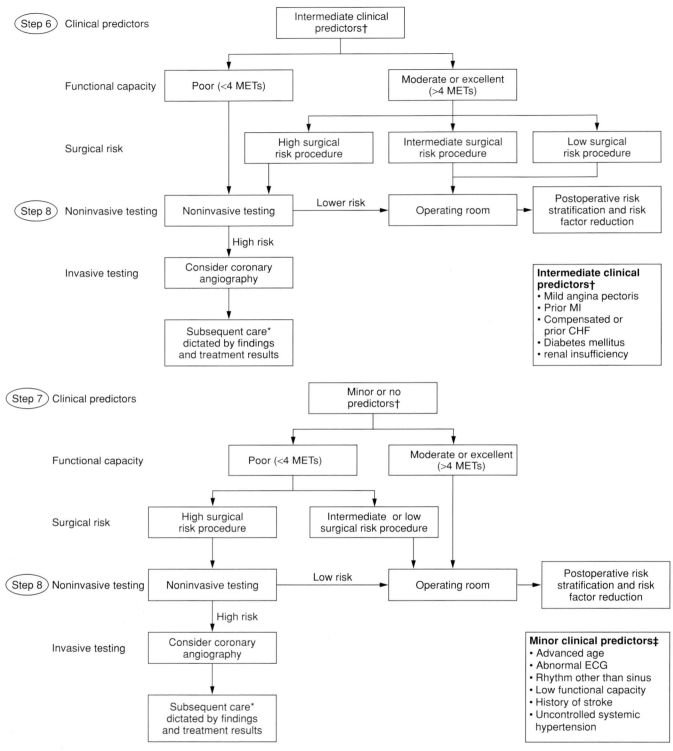

Figure 42-2 (continued)

Patients with *mechanical valves* who receive Coumadin should have it stopped 3 to 5 days in advance of surgery, and they should be converted to low molecular weight heparin in the outpatient setting. This medication should be held on the evening prior to surgery, but it can be resumed within 24 hours following hip replacement. Coumadin can be restarted the postoperative evening, since it will generally take 3 days to resume its complete anticoagulant effect. These patients should also receive subacute bacterial endocarditis (SBE) prophylaxis preoperatively.

Patients with atrial fibrillation with controlled ventricular rates generally pose no special problems. If not previously done, the underlying cause of the atrial fibrillation (coronary artery disease [CAD], pulmonary hypertension, valvular disease) needs to be identified and assessed. The internist or cardiologist needs to optimize those conditions. With the widespread use of warfarin in the treatment of atrial fibrillation to prevent stroke, Coumadin must be managed (see Table 42-6). In patients with nonvalvular atrial fibrillation, it is generally appropriate to stop Coumadin 3 to 5 days in advance of surgery and to resume it on the evening of surgery. Patients who have had embolic stokes, including those who have had valve replacements, should be converted to low molecular weight heparin as an outpatient preoperatively.

Patients who have significant ventricular arrhythmias are maintained on their usual medication. If they have ectopy with normal left ventricular function and no hemodynamic compromise, their arrhythmias are not treated. A cardiologist should assess patients with implantable defibrillators so that their defibrillators can be "turned off" during the surgical procedure to avoid spontaneous activation by operating room equipment.

PREOPERATIVE BETA-BLOCKER USE

Beta-blocker use has risen substantially in the last 2 decades. There have been substantial improvements in outcome for surgical procedures, particularly a decrease in mortality following coronary artery bypass graft (CABG). Expert opinion has recommended the use of pre-op beta-blockers in noncardiac surgery in high-risk patients in order to increase survival and decrease morbidity (2,16,37,38). Patients with known CAD, age greater than 70, history of CHF, history of stroke, renal disease, and diabetes can benefit. Two randomized, placebo-controlled trials of beta-blocker administration have been performed (37,47). One trial demonstrated reduced perioperative cardiac events, and the other demonstrated improved 6-month survival with perioperative beta-blocker usage. Patients who have had a prior MI or have reversible ischemia will benefit most from the use of beta-blockers. In addition, patients with more than two major risks for CAD (hyperlipidemia, hypertension, tobacco consumption, diabetes mellitus) should be given preoperative beta-blockers to reduce heart rate to 60 to 80 beats per minute (10).

REVASCULARIZATION

In Washington State, a retrospective study was done on hospital records of patients who had undergone surgery from 1987 to 1993. The authors compared patients with CAD who had noncardiac surgery and had recently undergone percutaneous angioplasty with those who had not undergone angioplasty. Patients with revascularization by percutaneous transluminal coronary angioplasty (PTCA) more than 90 days before surgery had a lower incidence of perioperative cardiac complications. Undergoing the procedure fewer than 90 days earlier did not confer a benefit (26). There are limited data regarding the now common use of vascular stents with PTCA for reducing perioperative cardiac events. As with PTCA, only retrospec-

tive data are available on the CABG procedure to support a positive benefit (reduced cardiac death and incident of MI) in noncardiac surgery (29).

PULMONARY ASSESSMENT

Pulmonary complications after surgery remain a leading cause of surgical morbidity (61). Unlike with cardiac evaluation, there are no proven pulmonary risk stratification indices. A history and a physical examination, along with a review of daily activity and medications, are the best means of evaluating the risk of pulmonary complications. In patients undergoing hip surgery, there are small changes in vital capacity and functional residual capacity caused by positioning, but these rarely affect oxygenation or ventilation intraoperatively. Postoperatively, an ileus can compromise pulmonary function, resulting in atelectasis. Atelectasis, aspiration, pneumonia, pulmonary edema, pleural effusion, and pulmonary embolism remain the major problems seen in this period (49).

Patients with restrictive lung disease secondary to pleural or pulmonary parenchymal disease do well in general, because respiratory drive is preserved. Patients with morbid obesity or skeletal or neuromuscular disorders that result in restrictive lung disease are at risk for pulmonary complications.

Chronic obstructive lung disease and asthma are the most common respiratory diseases encountered by medical consultants. When patients have reversible airway disease, it is preferable to avoid surgery when there is a major flare-up and to proceed when they are optimally managed medically. Theophylline preparations and all inhalers should be continued through the perioperative period.

Patients with chronic obstructive lung disease should refrain from smoking several weeks in advance of surgery and should be on an adequate medical regimen (49), which may include a variety of medications, such as oral theophylline, antibiotics, a beta$_2$-agonist inhaler, an anticholinergic inhaler, a steroid inhaler, and cromolyn sodium. Data to support aggressive preoperative treatment in these patients in an attempt to reduce postoperative complications are limited and dated.

There is no specific level of forced expiratory volume in 1 second (FEV$_1$) or other spirometric measurement to predict complications. Some authors have suggested that an FEV$_1$ of 1.2 to 2 liters is predictive of risk (5,19,61). A more useful predictor of pulmonary risk is the maximum voluntary minute ventilation, which is a measure of respiratory drive. Patients who have values below 50% of predicted are at risk for pulmonary complications. Of interest is the fact that there have been no studies to define a lower limit of FEV$_1$ at which surgery should not be performed. Williams and Brenowitz (68) studied 16 patients with severe chronic obstructive pulmonary disease (COPD) and found a 19% incidence of major pulmonary complications. On arterial blood gasses, the PCO_2 is a better predictor of risk than the PO_2. Patients with PCO_2 above 45 mm are at risk for increased pulmonary complications.

In summary, a patient's functional capacity is assessed through a history and a physical examination. If the patient is not limited in routine daily activities, and if no pulmonary disease exists, no further evaluation is necessary. Patients who have pre-existing airway disease should stop smoking and should use bronchodilators (oral theophylline, beta$_2$-agonist, and anticholinergic inhalers) and inhaled corticosteroids on a continuous basis pre- and postoperatively. Antibiotics should be used if there is evidence of bacterial infection of the airway (i.e., an abnormal chest x-ray or a change in sputum). Pre- and postoperative respiratory therapy, instruction in the use of incentive spirometry, coughing, and deep breathing exercises should be implemented (15). Early ambulation after surgery should also be encouraged.

HYPERTENSION

Little has been published on hypertension as it relates to pre-operative assessment and surgical risk, even though there are probably 55 million people who have hypertension in this country. In most such studies, the patients had mild hypertension. The standard has been that surgery in patients with diastolic pressure above 110 mm or systolic hypertension above 200 mm should be postponed until the blood pressure is adequately controlled. This was based on data from studies performed in the 1950s, 1960s, and early 1970s, on poor autoregulation of the central nervous system and renal blood flow, on the risk of myocardial ischemia, and on arrhythmias. Since those early days, it is difficult to find patients with this severe degree of hypertension who have undergone surgical treatment (50). In patients with mild to moderate hypertension, there appears to be no significant perioperative risk. Any reported morbidity has resulted from exacerbation of underlying hypertension (23).

Interestingly enough, preoperative control of blood pressure does not predict the degree of perioperative difficulties. Twenty-five percent of patients develop an exaggeration of blood pressure independent of their preoperative blood pressure (20). Wide intraoperative blood pressure swings in the uncontrolled hypertensive patient accounts for the morbidity and mortality. There are three periods in which we see hypertensive episodes: at induction of anesthesia (associated with hemodynamic instability and myocardial ischemia), in the immediate postoperative period (usually secondary to pain or hypoxia), and between days 3 and 5 (when worsening postoperative hypertension is associated with mobilization of third-space fluid; these patients respond to diuretics).

Patients with hypertension often have concomitant risk factors for surgery such as ischemic heart disease, renal disease, CHF, cerebrovascular disease, or prior MI. When these factors are also considered, the risk can be more accurately assessed.

Patients should be given their hypertension medication preoperatively, and it should be resumed as soon as possible postoperatively (see Table 42-6). If they are unable to take their medication orally, many agents can be given intravenously, but the substituted intravenous agent should be in the same class as the oral medication, if possible. It is important to avoid abrupt withdrawal of some antihypertensive agents, which can lead to rebound hypertension (e.g., central-acting agents such as clonidine [4] and beta-blockers [20]). Most antihypertensive agents have beneficial effects on the hemodynamic instability that occurs with anesthesia. Only

the diuretic class should be withheld prior to the surgery, but this remains controversial (see Table 42-6). The use of diuretics reduces plasma volume and alters potassium metabolism, resulting in intravascular and cellular potassium depletion. Resulting hypokalemia can potentiate the effects of muscle relaxant, increase cardiac atrial and ventricular arrhythmias, and increase the risk of a paralytic ileus. Many clinicians stop diuretics a few days before surgery to decrease the risk of hypovolemia and/or hypokalemia. All patients on diuretics should have preoperative laboratory evaluation, with correction of potassium to greater than 4.0.

Aggressive attempts to lower blood pressure within 48 hours of surgery can have detrimental effects on hemodynamic stability and should be avoided.

Beta-blocker usage preoperatively should be considered in all patients with hypertension or other cardiovascular risk factors (2,37).

DIABETES MELLITUS

Diabetes mellitus affects approximately 8% of the population. Type I diabetes (insulin-dependent diabetes) is a state of insulin deficiency associated with ketoacidosis; it is commonly seen in the young but can present as late as the third decade of life. Type II diabetes entails a relative resistance to endogenous insulin and is not associated with ketoacidosis. This type is more common in the adult patient presenting for arthroplasty, who is usually older and overweight. Type II diabetes is managed by diet, oral hypoglycemic agents, insulin, or a combination of the three. Complications in the form of end-organ damage are normal for both types (Table 42-4).

The clinician's approach to these patients is to assess the end-organ damage. A physical exam is done, with special attention to the existence of retinopathy (which often indicates the presence of nephropathy), the presence of vascular bruits and diminished pulses (suggestive of vascular disease), and an orthostatic blood pressure change of greater than 15 mm Hg

TABLE 42-4
COMPLICATIONS OF DIABETES

Organ System	Impact
Coronary arteries	Angina, myocardial infarction, silent ischemia
Vascular disease	Coronary artery disease, peripheral artery insufficiency, carotid disease, stroke
Kidneys	Proteinuria, decreased glomerular filtration, acidosis, hyperkalemia, prolongation of drug metabolism with decreased renal clearance
Peripheral neuropathy	Decreased nociception with increased risk for infection; impacts rehabilitation postoperatively
Autonomic neuropathy	Orthostatic hypotension, perioperative swings in blood pressure, delayed gastric emptying, urinary retention with increased risk for infection

without pulse increase or the presence of peripheral neuropathy (implying the existence of autonomic neuropathy).

An EKG is a preoperative requirement for all diabetics. The finding of a loss of RR variation on a resting EKG may indicate autonomic neuropathy. The presence of Q waves may identify an old transmural MI. Many times the patient may be unaware of previous myocardial ischemia. The incidence of silent ischemia is higher in the diabetic population than in the general population. Disappointingly, current screening tests and exercise and pharmacologic stress tests have poor predictive value for silent ischemia. The clinician should be aware of this and have a high index of suspicion and a low threshold for obtaining an EKG on postoperative days 1 through 5. In patients with established diabetes, CAD is 4 times more prevalent than in age-matched controls, and it may account for an increase in perioperative ischemia and MI (28). Patients with type II diabetes are so-called CAD risk equivalents, with a 10-year risk of coronary disease approaching 20% (25).

Assessment should include a physical exam (with attention to the volume status of the patient) and laboratory tests for serum electrolytes, blood urea nitrogen, and creatinine. A urinalysis for protein is also essential. Knowledge of the presence of renal dysfunction is necessary when choosing perioperative medication such as antibiotics or radiocontrast dyes. Patients with nephropathy have a higher prevalence of cardiovascular disease as well. Because asymptomatic bacteriuria is common, a urine culture should be obtained prior to arthroplasty.

The presence of autonomic neuropathy may complicate the postoperative course with blood pressure and pulse variations. Diabetics may also have profound hypoglycemia without symptoms. Postoperative nausea with gastroparesis is frequent in diabetic patients and is successfully treated with intravenous metoclopramide, 10 to 30 mg every 6 to 8 hours. It is a good first-line medication, for it has antiemetic effects besides improving gastric emptying.

GLUCOSE MANAGEMENT

The goal of management is to keep blood glucose levels at or below 240 mg/dL while avoiding perioperative hypoglycemia (see Table 42-6). This level is chosen due to poor wound healing in patients with poorly controlled diabetes. This is support by in vitro studies (39), but the impact in orthopedic patients undergoing joint replacement has not been studied. Abnormalities in leukocyte phagocytosis and antibody response to Gram-positive organisms may be impaired when serum glucose exceeds 250 mg/dL. Poor control may also predispose the patient to postoperative Gram-negative sepsis (41). A study in postoperative cardiothoracic patients suggests that tight control of glucose with an insulin pump can improve surgical outcomes by reducing infection rates (17). This has yet to be studied in orthopedic patients.

Diabetes type II patients on diet and oral agents should have their medications, including sulfonylureas, metformin, and thiazolidinedione (glitizone), withheld the day of surgery. The blood glucose should be checked the morning of surgery, or preoperatively, and then every 4 to 6 hours intra- and postoperatively. Human synthetic regular insulin can be administered on a sliding scale for any blood glucose over 250 mg/dL (see Table 42-6). Intravenous solutions of 5% dextrose should be administered to avoid starvation ketosis. On the morning after surgery, an American Diabetes Association (ADA) diet can be started, along with the oral hypoglycemic if the patient is taking food well.

The type II diabetic patient on insulin can be managed in a fashion similar to that outlined above. True 24-hour-acting insulins such as Lantus (insulin glargine) can be given on the evening before surgery or the morning of surgery to maintain a steady basal dose of insulin. In patients on intermediate-acting insulin preparations, half the dose can be administered on the morning of surgery, and short-acting insulin can be used every 4 to 6 hours as needed. It is important to remember that the insulin resistance of the type II diabetic creates a need for a larger dose of regular insulin per glucose decrement than is necessary with type I diabetes. The commonly used Novolin and Humulin 70/30 are combination insulins (70% NPH and 30% regular), so if insulin is used on the morning of surgery, the clinician calculates one half of 70% of the total usual dose of these combination insulins.

Many insulin management protocols for diabetes type I have been suggested. European clinicians utilized intraoperative infusion of premixed insulin—10% dextrose solution or a variable continuous insulin infusion (1). However, practice in the United States has favored a reduced dose of long-acting insulin given subcutaneously, with frequent monitoring and administration of short-acting insulin as needed. There are no comparative studies of these regimens that have evaluated glycemic control and perioperative complications for orthopedic surgery.

Good control of blood glucose should begin weeks before surgery. The type I diabetic, with the guidance of the physician, should strive to attain stable blood glucose (100 to 150 mg/dL) for at least 7 days prior to the operation. Dietary adherence in conjunction with control of glucose should replete hepatic glycogen stores, reducing the risk of intraoperative hypoglycemia. Because of insulin deficiency, type I diabetics are at risk for perioperative hyperglycemia and ketoacidosis.

The well-controlled type I diabetic can be managed with a half dose of the morning NPH or Lente and frequent serum glucose monitoring (every 4 hours), with sliding-scale coverage with short-acting insulin. Patients on long-acting insulin such as Lantus can be given their usual dose on the evening before surgery or on the morning of surgery, then can be covered with sliding-scale insulin A sliding scale with short-acting insulin should be utilized throughout the first 24 postoperative hours. The following morning, the patient should be returned to the standard insulin dose only if able to consume a full ADA diet.

For type I diabetics who demonstrate a wide variation in preoperative glucose levels or a history of poor control (i.e., the brittle diabetic), an insulin drip is most appropriate. The NPH or Lente should be reduced to 80% of the patient's standard dose the night before surgery to avoid morning hypoglycemia. When the patient arrives at the preoperative area, a blood glucose should be measured and an intravenous 5% or 10% dextrose solution begun at 100 mL per hour. Administration of dextrose avoids potential starvation ketosis. Through a separate line, an insulin infusion can be instituted by mixing 100 units of regular insulin in 500 mL of normal saline (1 U per 5 mL). The infusion is started at 2 U/hr (10 mL/hr), and the blood glucose level must be monitored hourly, with the infusion increased or decreased by 5 mL to maintain a blood glucose level between 150 and 240 mg/dL.

The continuous infusion can be maintained for the first 24 postoperative hours. The morning after surgery, two thirds of the patient's usual morning insulin should be administered subcutaneously, and the insulin infusion can be stopped 3 hours later. Coverage with a sliding scale of regular insulin is then appropriate.

For the type I diabetic managed on a continuous ambulatory subcutaneous infusion, such as with an insulin pump, the pump may be stopped at the time of presentation for surgery, an intravenous 5% dextrose solution can be started, and the insulin drip used as described. It is critical that insulin-dependent diabetic patients receive insulin continuously to minimize the risk of ketoacidosis.

CEREBRAL VASCULAR DISEASE

Patients who have asymptomatic carotid stenosis have a 1% to 2% risk of stroke after anesthesia. Patients with previous but now stable cerebral vascular disease (i.e., the last event was more than 1 year prior to surgery) are at low risk (less than 1%) for perioperative events. An asymptomatic carotid bruit with significant stenosis (greater than 70% on Doppler) is a controversial area in preoperative management (12,40). Recently published data suggest that patients with asymptomatic carotid disease should undergo surgical treatment if the stenosis is greater than 75% (12,40). This refutes the consensus from many studies in the 1970s and 1980s that medical therapy is preferable. The prior recommendations were based on risk–benefit analysis. Because the annual risk of stroke from asymptomatic carotid stenosis (greater than 50% occlusion on Doppler) is 1% to 2%, morbidity from medical therapy was lower than morbidity associated with carotid endarterectomy (CEA), in which complication rates varied from 2% to 21% (45,62). As surgical skills and postoperative care improve, the benefit may outweigh the risk, and CEA may be considered.

Most of the studies of prophylactic CEA have been done on patients undergoing cardiac and vascular surgeries, and the results are mixed. There have been no studies done on prophylactic CEA preceding total hip arthroplasty. Thus, given our current knowledge and the small risk of stroke in the asymptomatic patient, it appears to be acceptable to proceed with hip surgery before addressing the asymptomatic carotid stenosis.

Patients who have had recent transient ischemic attacks (TIAs) are at increased risk for stroke, particularly within 6 weeks of the event (66); most strokes occur within the first year after a TIA. These symptomatic patients should be thoroughly investigated for the cause of the TIA prior to any surgery. If the patient has hemodynamically significant carotid stenosis (greater than 75%), a CEA should be performed prior to elective hip surgery (44). If the stenosis is noncritical (less than 70% occlusion), CEA may not be necessary, and elective total hip arthroplasty can be scheduled. However, it seems prudent to wait at least 4 to 6 weeks after the event (27), based on the timing used to schedule a CEA after a stroke or TIA.

RHEUMATOID ARTHRITIS

Patients with rheumatoid arthritis (RA) commonly are candidates for total joint replacement as well as other surgeries. RA is associated with anatomic and physiologic changes that must be evaluated prior to general anesthesia, including cervical spine disease, anemia, and pleural and pulmonary involvement.

Studies have shown that 30% to 40% of RA patients admitted to the hospital have radiographic evidence of cervical spine subluxation (57), which commonly involves the first and second cervical vertebrae. Between 2% and 5% have demonstrable long-tract findings (63). Subluxation of a diseased atlantoaxial joint during endotracheal intubation may compromise the respiratory center of the medulla. A careful history for symptoms of pain in the C1, C2 nerve root during routine daily activity is necessary. Dynamic flexion and extension radiographs can identify this problem. If there is any question, a computed tomography (CT) scan of the upper cervical spine is obtained. Furthermore, a small subset of these patients (2% to 3% of adults with RA) may have involvement of the temporal mandibular joint, making intubation difficult (57).

Lung disease in RA patients has many manifestations. Pleuritis, interstitial fibrosis, and pleura-based nodules can result in restrictive lung disease manifested by exertional dyspnea. In addition, the interstitial fibrosis may inhibit alveolar–capillary gas exchange, lowering resting Pao_2. A history of exertional dyspnea or rales should be evaluated by a chest radiograph and spirometry, with or without carbon monoxide diffusion capacity. Although intervention to modify the pulmonary disease uncovered by this assessment is unlikely to reverse existing disease, it is important to have this baseline information to help in the assessment of postoperative hypoxemia and dyspnea.

Heart disease in RA patients may include pericarditis, myocarditis, noninfective vegetation on the valves, conduction defects, and, rarely, coronary arteritis. A history, a physical, and an EKG are sufficient screening for RA patients, following the guidelines set down previously. If a murmur exists, antibiotic prophylaxis is necessary. Anemia of chronic inflammatory disease is often found in this patient population, and preoperatively a complete blood count should always be obtained.

The use of corticosteroids is common in this patient population and should be managed as outlined later.

Ankylosing spondylitis involves the cervical and thoracic spine and results in a restrictive lung disease. This can increase the risk of postoperative pulmonary complications. Rigidity of the cervical spine makes intubation difficult.

Similarly, patients with *juvenile rheumatoid arthritis* may also have extensive ankylosis of the cervical spine, making hyperextension for visualization of the vocal cord difficult for the anesthesiologist.

Gout arthropathy commonly flares in the postoperative patient with a history of gouty arthropathy. Management is complicated by the fact that these patients are commonly on anticoagulants, which contraindicates the use of nonsteroidal anti-inflammatory drugs. Colchicine is the drug of choice but is limited by gastrointestinal distress. Colchicine 0.6 mg can be given by mouth every hour until pain is relieved or diarrhea occurs (but without exceeding six doses over 24 hours).

Immunosuppressive drugs that have disease-modifying activity (e.g., methotrexate) should be held during the week of surgery.

CHRONIC GLUCOCORTICOIDS

Many of the comorbid conditions (e.g. asthma, COPD, RA, and inflammatory bowel disease) in patients who present for total hip arthroplasty require chronic glucocorticoids. Some patients may have been on steroids within the 12 months preceding surgery for nonchronic conditions (e.g., dermatitis). Theoretically, these patients may have hypothalamic–pituitary–adrenal axis suppression and are at risk for adrenal insufficiency intra- and postoperatively. Anecdotal reports in the 1950s, 1960s, and 1970s documented adrenal insufficiency in the chronic steroid user during the perioperative period, sometimes with fatal outcomes. Consensus is difficult because the studies were heterogeneous in design, with small patient numbers, different steroid preparations, and different durations of use. They often had poorly defined endpoints. The symptoms of adrenal insufficiency can be very subtle, including anorexia, low-grade fever, mild to moderate hypotension, malaise, myalgias, and arthralgias. These symptoms may be overlooked because of their common occurrence in the postoperative period.

The most common test performed to assess adrenal reserve is the synthetic adrenocorticotropic hormone (ACTH; Cortrosyn) stimulation test. This test is the simplest to perform and has been validated by Jasani et al. (30) as a means to predict adrenal response in surgery. The test can be done at any time of day with rare side effects. It is common in our practice to do an ACTH simulation test preop to avoid the excessive use of glucocorticoids in the perioperative period.

A baseline serum cortisol is drawn, followed by intravenous administration of 250 μg of synthetic ACTH. Thirty-minute and 60-minute cortisol levels are obtained. A positive adrenal response from a baseline serum cortisol of 6 to 25 μg/dL is a rise greater than 7 μg/dL from baseline or over 20 μg/dL at 60 minutes. These issues remain controversial: How much glucocorticoid steroid is needed for suppression? What is the minimum duration of steroid use to demonstrate suppression? And once steroids are stopped, how long are the adrenals suppressed?

Graber et al. (24), in 1965, tried to answer these questions when they studied the hypothalamic–pituitary–adrenal axis response after cessation of steroids. They discovered that the equivalent of 7.5 mg of prednisone (Table 42-5) daily for 7 days or more was sufficient for suppression of this axis. They found that the hypothalamic output of corticotropin-releasing hormone returned first, followed by pituitary ACTH and finally adrenal production of cortisol. Adrenal response became appropriate 9 months, on average, after the cessation of steroids. Based on these data, some clinicians conservatively recommend that any patient who has received the equivalent of 7.5 mg of prednisone daily for 5 days be given stress steroids for up to 1 year after stopping the steroids. Because there is wide variation in individual responses to these steroids, this approach has led to excessive use of steroids. Thus, when time permits in the preoperative period, it is prudent to perform the ACTH stimulation test.

The literature is filled with regimens of steroid coverage and taper, but no comparative studies have been done. The following protocol, based on physiologic adrenal response, is widely used. A functional adrenal gland produces the equivalent of 250 to 300 mg of cortisol in 24 hours when challenged. The goal of replacement is to equal this output with equivalent exogenous steroid (see Table 42-5). A suggested regimen is 100 mg intravenous hydrocortisone 30 to 60 minutes prior to the procedure, followed by 100 mg intravenously every 8 hours for two more doses. Patients who are not on chronic steroids or who use less than physiologic doses (less than 7.5 mg/day prednisone) do not need to be tapered. Patients on chronic steroids above this dose should receive on the first postoperative day 50 mg intravenous hydrocortisone every 8 hours for three doses and on the second postoperative 25 mg every 8 hours for three doses. On the third postoperative day, the patients are returned to the standard daily dose. Monitoring of patient volume (input and output), blood pressure, glucose, and electrolytes is necessary. Some clinicians favor the use of a histamine (H_2) antagonist to avoid theoretical steroid- or stress-induced gastric ulcers.

OBESITY

Because excessive weight results in damage to lower extremity joints and in accelerated underlying arthritis, obesity is a common comorbid condition seen in adults undergoing total hip arthroplasty. One must be aware of the medical problems related to obesity and anticipate potential perioperative problems. The anecdotal consensus is that obesity imparts an increase in complications in the perioperative period (e.g., increased atelectasis, wound dehiscence, higher rate of wound infection), yet there are very few studies to document these beliefs.

Obesity imparts perioperative risk by its association with other medical conditions. It is associated with hypertension, hyperlipidemia, atherosclerotic vascular disease, left ventricular hypertrophy, changes in pulmonary function, diabetes mellitus, cholelithiasis, and gout. The clinician's responsibility is to recognize these associations and assess the patient accordingly.

TABLE 42-5
STEROID EQUIVALENTS

Steroids	Glucocorticoid Potency	Equivalent Dose (mg)
Short-acting		
Cortisol (hydrocortisone)	1	20
Cortisone	0.8	25
Prednisone	4	5
Prednisolone	4	5
Methylprednisolone	5	4
Intermediate-acting		
Triamcinolone	5	4
Long-acting		
Dexamethasone	30	0.75
Betamethasone	25	0.60

TABLE 42-6
STOPPING AND STARTING MEDICATION

Medication	Recommendation	Comment
Insulin	Half dose of NPH or Lente, sliding scale	IV fluid D5W ~2 mL/kg/hr (see text)
Oral hypoglycemic	Discontinue 1–2 days preop	Chlorpropamide long acting, stop 3 days preop
Levothyroxine	Give equal dose PO or IV day of surgery	Long-acting hormone
Propylthiouracil	Continue through morning of surgery, check level (see text)	If NPO is prolonged, administer IV beta-blocker labetalol 10 mg q 15 min, propranolol 1–2 mg q 1 hr
Estrogens		
Oral contraceptives	Stop 3 weeks preop	Increased risk of thrombosis
Replacement therapy	Stop equine 1 week preop	Transdermal may decrease thrombogenic risk
	Stop estradiol 3 weeks preop	Equine estrogen 0.625 mgs. q day = transdermal estradiol q 3 days
Cardiac		
Digoxin	Continue	Check level
Antiarrhythmic agents		
Quinidine	For SVT, hold day of surgery, substitute IV verapamil	For VT, may substitute lidocaine
Procainamide	For SVT, hold day of surgery, IV available	
Amiodarone	Hold	T_{fi} 30–60 days, hold and resume when PO
Nitrates	Continue	Change from PO to transdermal equivalents?
Calcium channel blockers	Continue	Anesthetic complication
Diuretics	Consider discontinuing	Check K^+ level, assess fluid status
Beta-blockers	Continue	May substitute IV propranolol, metoprolol, or labetalol
Pulmonary	Continue all meds	If on theophylline, check level (see text)
Antihypertensives		
Diuretics	(See above)	
Beta-blockers	(See above)	
Calcium channel blockers	Continue	Anesthetic complication
ACE inhibitors	Continue	Check K^+ level, IV enalaprilat available
Central-acting agents	Continue, associated with withdrawal	I.e.: methyldopa, reserpine, are long-acting; clonidine withdrawal increases BP and tachycardia
Peripheral-acting agents	Continue	Prazosin, hydralazine
Periop urgencies	IV labetalol 10 mg q 10 min, methyldopa 250 mg q 4 hr, nifedipine 10 mg SL (see text)	
Neurologics/Psychotropics		
Monoamime oxidase inhibitor	May be continued with caution	Recent studies of chronic users show low complication rate; caution with narcotics
Antidepressants		
Tricyclics	Hold day of surgery	Resume postop
SSRIs	Hold day of surgery	Resume postop
Phenytoin	Continue through morning of surgery, check level	Resume postop PO or through NG tube; IV available, but has potential for cardiac toxicity
Anticoagulation with warfarin		
Prosthetic mitral valve	Stop warfarin 3 days prior to surgery, begin IV heparin with a PTT goal of 50–70 sec.; start warfarin postop, evening of surgery	Resume heparin 6–12 hr postop until INR 2.5–3.5
Prosthetic aortic valve	Stop warfarin 3 days prior to surgery, begin IV heparin with a PTT goal of 50–70 sec.; start warfarin postop, evening of surgery	No heparin necessary postop
Nonvalvular atrial fibrillation	Stop warfarin 3 days prior to surgery; start warfarin postop, evening of surgery	No preop heparin necessary

Modified from Cygan R, Waitzkin H. Stopping and restarting medications in the perioperative period. *J Geriatr Med.* 1987;2:270; and from Guarnieri KM, Mekeon BP. *Perioperative Medicine.* New York: McGraw-Hill; 1994:479.
PO, by mouth; NPO, nothing by mouth; IV, intravenous; SL, sublingual; q, every; preop, preoperative; postop, postoperative; periop, perioperative; D5W, 5% dextrose in water; SVT, supraventricular tachycardia; VT, ventricular tachycardia. ACE, angiotensin-converting enzyme; BP, blood pressure; SSRI, selective serotonin reuptake inhibitor; PTT, partial thromboplastin time; INR, international normalized ratio.

Changes in pulmonary dynamics have the greatest potential impact on outcome during and after surgery. Obesity can result in increased minute ventilation, decreased compliance of the chest wall, and an increase in the energy expenditure of breathing (all to maintain a normal PO_2 and a reduced PCO_2). Abnormalities can occur in spirometric measurements, with a decrease in expiratory reserve volume (ERV) and functional residual capacity (FRC). Respiratory rate increases to maintain minute ventilation. Shallow breathing is common, and it produces overventilation of the upper lung fields and underventilation of the lower lung fields. Perfusion is unchanged, and so ventilation–perfusion mismatches are common.

Preoperative assessment should include a careful history, physical exam, and laboratory test to screen for the comorbidities of obesity. Special attention should be paid to respiratory symptoms, functional abilities in day-to-day life, and sleep disturbance. A chest x-ray, EKG, and complete blood count are appropriate in all morbidly obese patients (greater than 100% above ideal body weight) regardless of symptoms.

It would be reasonable to expect a higher incidence of postoperative atelectasis and pneumonia given these functional changes. Yet in a study of consecutive cholecystectomy patients, no difference was found in the incidence of atelectasis (46). Other studies in abdominal surgery showed no difference in postoperative pneumonia between obese and nonobese patients (49). In addition, a larger gastric volume and the frequent presence of a hiatal hernia theoretically make postoperative aspiration more likely. Data in the orthopedic literature documenting these complication rates are scant.

THYROID DISEASE

Because total hip arthroplasty is almost exclusively an elective procedure, surgery should be delayed until evaluation and treatment are begun for the hypothyroid or hyperthyroid state.

The hypothyroid condition, both treated and untreated, is common in the population undergoing hip replacement. Hypothyroidism is seen in patients with Hashimoto thyroiditis or hypofunctional goiter and in those who had previous thyroid surgery or iodine-131 radiation therapy. Patients maintained on L-thyroxine are at low risk for complications, even if the patient is mildly under- or overreplaced. The preoperative assessment in these patients should include evaluation of the thyroid status. On physical exam, the reflexes can be most helpful (i.e., hyper-reflexia in hyperthyroidism and a delayed return of the reflex response in hypothyroidism). If there is any question about the patient's thyroid status or no laboratory assessment has been done within 1 year of proposed surgery, then a highly sensitive thyroid-stimulating hormone (TSH) study should be done. A TSH level less than 0.5 μU/dL suggests a hyperthyroid state, whereas a TSH level greater than 5.0 μU/dL indicates a hypothyroid condition.

In the rare instance when hip replacement cannot be delayed in the profoundly hypothyroid patient, 300 to 500 μg intravenous L-thyroxine along with 100 mg intravenous hydrocortisone should be administered preoperatively. This should be followed with 100 mg hydrocortisone, intravenously or by mouth, daily for 1 week. L-thyroxine 25 or 50 μg should be given by mouth daily postoperatively (Table 42-6).

Hyperthyroid patients maintained on propylthiouracil (PTU) or methimazole in a euthyroid state are at no greater risk for surgery. The medication can be administered by mouth or via the nasogastric tube perioperatively. A TSH test should be performed preoperatively. The thyrotoxic patient should have surgery delayed. If surgery is urgent, the severely hyperthyroid patient should receive 1 g oral PTU and 300 mg intravenous hydrocortisone followed by 5 drops of saturated solution of potassium iodine (SSKI) (50 mg of iodide per drop) orally three times a day or 1 g sodium iodine intravenously three times a day. To manage the tachycardia and hypertension associated with thyrotoxicosis, 1 mg/min propranolol is given intravenously or 20 to 40 mg are given orally every 6 hours. Intravenous esmolol or labetalol may be substituted.

CONCLUSION

A patient presenting for total hip arthroplasty commonly has numerous comorbid conditions that can impact the immediate surgical success and long-term recovery of the patient. Although a consultant should not be asked to clear a patient for surgery and general anesthesia, he or she can be asked to preoperatively assess the patient. The objective is to identify treatable comorbid conditions, comorbid conditions that are not reversible and may adversely impact the surgical outcome, and occult conditions that can be corrected. Thus, patients are evaluated so that they may be in an optimal medical condition to undergo the proposed surgery.

REFERENCES

1. Alberti KG, Thomas DJB. The management of diabetes during surgery *Br J Anaesth.* 1979;51:693–708.
2. Auerbach AD, Goldman L. Beta blockers and reduction of cardiac events in non cardiac surgery: scientific review. *JAMA.* 2002;287:1435–1444.
3. Barnes RW, Marszalek PB, Rittgers SE. Asymptomatic carotid disease in preoperative patients. *Stroke.* 1980;11:136.
4. Brodsky JB, Bravo JJ. Acute postoperative clonidine withdrawal syndrome. *Anesthesiology.* 1976;44:519.
5. Celli BR. What is the value of preoperative pulmonary function testing. *Med Clin North Am.* 1993;77:309–325.
6. Cleland JGF. Beta blockers for heart failure: why, which, when and where. *Med Clin North Am.* 2003;87:339–371.
7. Cygan R, Waitzkin H. Stopping and restarting medications in the perioperative period. *J Geriatr Med.* 1987;2:270.
8. Detsky AS, Abrams HB, McLaughlin JR, et al. Predicting cardiac complications in patients undergoing non-cardiac surgery. *J Gen Intern Med.* 1986;1:211–219.
9. Dripps RD. New classification of physical status. *Anesthesiology.* 24;111:1963.
10. Eagle, KA, Berger, PB, Calkins, H, et al. ACC/AHA guideline update for perioperative cardiovascular evaluation for noncardiac surgery: executive summary: a report of the American College of Cardiology/American Heart Association Task Force on Practice Guidelines (Committee to Update the 1996 Guidelines on Perioperative Cardiovascular Evaluation for Noncardiac Surgery). *J Am Coll Cardiol.* 2002;39:542.

11. Eagle KA, Coley CM, Newell JB, et al. Combining clinical and thallium data optimizes preoperative assessment of cardiac risk before major vascular surgery. *Ann Intern Med.* 1989;110: 859–866.

12. Executive Committee for the Asymptomatic Carotid Atherosclerosis Study. Endarterectomy for asymptomatic carotid artery stenosis. *JAMA.* 1995;273:1421–1428.

13. Felson DT, Anderson JJ, Naimark A, et al. Obesity and knee osteoarthritis. The Framingham study. *Ann Intern Med.* 1988;109: 18–24.

14. Ferguson GG. Extracranial carotid artery surgery. *Clin Neurosurg.* 1982;29:543–574.

15. Ford GT, Guenter CA. Toward prevention of postoperative pulmonary complications. *Am Rev Respir Dis.* 1984;130:4–5.

16. Ferguson B, Coombs LP, Peterson ED, Preoperative-blocker use and mortality and morbidity following CABG surgery in North America. *JAMA.* 2002;287:2221–2227.

17. Furnary AP, Zerr KJ, Grunkemeier GL, et al. Continuous intravenous insulin infusion reduces the incidence of deep sternal wound infection in diabetic patients after cardiac surgical procedures. *Ann Thorac Surg.* 1999;67:352–360.

18. Galen RS, Gambino SR. *Beyond Normality: The Predictive Value and Efficiency of Medical Diagnosis.* New York: Wiley; 1975.

19. Gass GD, Olsen GN. Preoperative pulmonary function testing to predict postoperative morbidity and mortality. *Chest.* 1986;89: 127–135.

20. Goldman L. Noncardiac surgery in patients receiving propranolol: case reports and a recommended approach. *Arch Intern Med.* 1981;141;193.

21. Goldman L. Cardiac risks and complications of noncardiac surgery. *Ann Intern Med.* 1983;98:504–513.

22. Goldman L, Caldera DL, Nussbaum SR, et al. Multifactorial index of cardiac risk in noncardiac surgical procedures. *N Engl J Med.* 1977;297:845–850.

23. Goldman L, Caldera DL. Risks of general anesthesia and elective operation in the hypertensive patient. *Anesthesiology.* 1979;50: 285–292.

24. Graber AL, Ney RI, Nicholson WE, et al. Natural history of pituitary adrenal recovery following long-term suppression with corticosteroids. *J Clin Endocr Metab.* 1965;25:11.

25. Grundy SM,Cleeman JI, Bairey et al. Implications of recent trials for the National Cholesterol Education Program Adult Treatment Panel III guidelines. *Circulation.* 2004;110:763.

26. Guarnieri KM, Mekeon BP. *Perioperative Medicine.* New York: McGraw-Hill; 1994:479.

27. Harrison MJG, Marshall J. The finding of thrombus at carotid endarterectomy and its relationship to the timing of surgery. *Br J Surg.* 1977;64:511–512.

28. Hollenberg M, Mangan DT, et al. Predictors of postoperative myocardial ischemia in patients undergoing noncardiac surgery. Study of Perioperative Ischemia Research Group. *JAMA.* 1992;268: 205–209.

29. Hassan SA, Hlatky MA, Boothroyd DB, et al. Outcomes of noncardiac surgery after coronary bypass surgery or coronary angioplasty in the Bypass Angioplasty Revascularization Investigation (BARI). *Am J Med.* 2001;110:260–266.

30. Jasani MK, Freeman PA, Boyle JA, et al. Studies of the rise in plasma 11-hydroxycorticosteroid (11-OHCS) in corticosteroid-treated patients with rheumatoid arthritis during surgery: correlations with the functional integrity of the hypothalmo-pituitary-adrenal axis. *Q J Med.* 1968;37:407.

31. Kaplan EB, Sheiner LB, Boeckman AJ, et al. The usefulness of preoperative laboratory screening. *JAMA.* 1985;253:3576–3581.

32. Lane RT, Sawada SG, Segar DS, et al. Dobutamine stress echocardiography for assessment of cardiac risk before noncardiac surgery. *Am J Cardiol.* 1991;68:976–977.

33. Lette J, Waters D, Lapointe J, et al. Usefulness of the severity and extent of reversible perfusion defects during thallium-dipyridamole imaging for cardiac risk assessment before noncardiac surgery. *Am J Cardiol.* 1989;64:276–281.

34. London MJ, Tubau JF, Wong MG, et al. The natural history of segmental wall motion abnormalities in patients undergoing noncardiac surgery. *Anesthesiology.* 1990;73:644–655.

35. Macpherson DS. Preoperative laboratory testing: should any tests be routine before surgery? *Med Clin North Am.* 1993:77: 289–308.

36. Mangaro DT, Goldman L. Current concepts: preoperative assessment of patients with known or suspected coronary disease. *N Engl J Med.* 1995;333:1750–1756.

37. Mangano DT, Layug EL, Wallace A, et al. Effect of atenolol on mortality and cardiovascular morbidity after noncardiac surgery. Multicenter Study of Perioperative Ischemia Research Group [published erratum appears in *N Engl J Med.* 1997;336:1039]. *N Engl J Med.* 1996;335:1713–1720.

38. Marx GF, Mateo CV, Orkin LR. *Anesthesiology.* 1973;39:54.

39. McMurry J. Wound healing with diabetes mellitus. *Surg Clin North Am.* 1984;64:769–778.

40. Moore WS, Barnet HJM, Beebe HG, et al. Guidelines for carotid endarterectomy. *Stroke.* 1995;26:188–201.

41. Myers J, Do D, Herbert W, et al. A nomogram to predict exercise capacity from a specific activity questionnaire and clinical data. *Am J Cardiol.* 1994;73:591–596.

42. National Institutes of Health. Health implications of obesity. *NIH Consensus Statement.* 1985;5(9):1–7.

43. Nolan CM, Beaty HN, Bagdade. Further characterization of the impaired bactericidal function of granulocytes in patients with poorly controlled diabetes. *Diabetes.* 1978;27:889–894.

44. North American Symptomatic Carotid Endarterectomy Trial collaborators. Beneficial effects of carotid endarterectomy in symptomatic patients with high grade stenosis. *N Engl J Med.* 1991;325: 445–453.

45. Nunn DB. Carotid endarterectomy in patients with territorial transient ischemic attacks. *J Vasc Surg.* 1988;8:447–452.

46. Poe Rh, Kally MC, Dass T, et al. Can postoperative pulmonary complications after elective cholecystectomy be predicted? *Am J Med Sci.* 1988;295:29–34.

47. Poldermans D, Boersma E, Bax JJ, et al. The effect of bisoprolol on perioperative mortality and myocardial infarction in high-risk patients undergoing vascular surgery. Dutch Echocardiographic Cardiac Risk Evaluation Applying Stress Echocardiography Study Group. *N Engl J Med.* 1999;341:1789–1794.

48. Poole-Wilson PA. ACE inhibitors and ARBs in chronic heart failure: the established, the expected and the pragmatic. *Med Clin North Am.* 2003;87:373–389.

49. Presley AP, Alexander-Williams J. Postoperative chest infection. *Br J Surg.* 1974;61:448.

50. Prys-Roberts C. Hypertension and anesthesia: fifty years on. *Anesthesiology.* 1979;50:281.

51. Rao TL, Jacobs KH, El Etr AA. Reinfarction following anesthesia in patients with myocardial infarction. *Anesthesiology.* 1983;59: 499–505.

52. Reilly DF, McNeely MJ, Doerner D, et al. Self-reported exercise tolerance and the risk of serious perioperative complications. *Arch Intern Med.* 1999;159:2185–2192.

53. Reul GL, Morris GC, Howell JF, et al. Current concept in coronary artery surgery: a critical analysis of 1287 patients. *Ann Thorac Surg.* 1972;14:243.

54. Rucker L, Frye EB, Staten MA. Usefulness of screening chest roentgenograms in preoperative patients *JAMA.* 1983;250: 3209–3211.

55. Sander DP, Mckinney FW, Harris WH. Clinical evaluation and cost effectiveness of preoperative laboratory assessment on patients undergoing total hip arthroplasty. *Orthopedics.* 1989;12: 1449–1453.

56. Seeger JM, Rosenthal GR, Self SB, et al. Does routine stress thallium cardiac scanning reduce postoperative cardiac complications? *Ann Surg.* 1994;219:654–663.

57. Sledge CB. Introduction to surgical management. In: Kelly W, ed. *Textbook of Rheumatology.* Philadelphia: WB Saunders; 1985:1745.

58. Steen PA, Tinker JH, Tarhan S. Myocardial re-infarction after anesthesia and surgery. *JAMA.* 1978;239:2566–2570.

59. Tae TGT, Mushlin AI. The utility of routine chest radiographs. *Ann Intern Med.* 1986;104:663–170.

60. Tahran S, Moffitt EA, Taylor WF, et al. Myocardial infarction after general anesthesia. *JAMA.* 1972;220:1451–1454.

61. Tisi GM. Preoperative evaluation of pulmonary function. *Am Rev Respir Dis.* 1979;119:293–310.

62. Toole JF, Yuson CP, Janeway R, et al. Transient ischmic attacks: a prospective study of 225 patients. *Neurology.* 1988;18:746–753.

63. Tsahakis PJ, et al. Surgical care of the patient with rheumatoid arthritis. In: Kelly W, ed. *Textbook of Rheumatology.* Philadelphia: WB Saunders; 1985:1823.

64. Turnbull JM, Buck C. The value of preoperative screening investigations in otherwise healthy individuals. *Arch Intern Med.* 1987;147:1101–1105.

65. Wallace A, Layug B, Tateo I, et al. Prophylactic atenolol reduces postoperative myocardial ischemia. McSPI Research Group. *Anesthesiology.* 1998;88:7–17.

66. Warner MA, Divertie MB, Tinker JH. Preoperative cessation of smoking and pulmonary complications in coronary artery bypass patients. *Anesthesiology.* 1984;60:380–383.

67. Whisnant JP, Sandok BA, Sundt TM. Carotid endarterectomy for unilateral carotid system transient cerebral ischemia. *Mayo Clin Proc.* 1983;56:171–175.

68. Willians CD, Brenowitz JB. Prohibitive lung function and major surgical procedures. *Am J Surg.* 1976;132:763–766.

69. Wilson ME, Williams NB, Baskett PJF, et al. Assessment of fitness for surgical procedures and the variability of anesthetists' judgements. *Br Med J.* 1980;1:509–513.

70. Zeldin RA. Assessing cardiac risk in patients who undergo noncardiac surgical procedures. *Can J Surg.* 1984;27:402–404.

Anesthesia

43

Nigel E. Sharrock

Patients undergoing total hip replacement (THR) pose a number of specific challenges intraoperatively for anesthesiologists. Anesthetic care has been shown to affect perioperative mortality (63), transfusion requirements (31,75), deep vein thrombosis (DVT) (13,34,39), pulmonary embolism (PE) (63), and the quality of cement fixation (54). Complex airway and positioning challenges are seen in patients with ankylosing spondylitis and advanced rheumatoid arthritis (RA). Finally, life-threatening events may occur during insertion of cemented femoral components (17,47). An understanding of these issues is important to provide optimal anesthetic care.

RHEUMATOID ARTHRITIS

Patients with juvenile rheumatoid arthritis (JRA) and patients with severe adult-onset RA are often impossible to intubate using conventional laryngoscopic techniques. Patients with JRA tend to have hypoplastic mandibles with limited jaw opening, and they may have arthritis of the temporomandibular joints limiting jaw opening. There may be limited extension if the neck has been surgically fused or if ankylosis of the cervical spine has occurred as a result of the arthritic process (36,59,72).

These patients must be assessed preoperatively to determine whether oral intubation might be difficult. If difficulty is anticipated, it is advisable to use a spinal or epidural whenever possible to avoid airway difficulty. If a general anesthetic is required (e.g., for a long revision hip replacement) fiberoptic-assisted intubation should be performed. Laryngeal mask airways are being used in some centers in this situation (18).

Rheumatoid arthritis can involve the cervical spine in several ways. Degeneration of the transverse ligament may lead to subluxation at C1-2 with impingement of the spinal cord by the odontoid. In severe cases, there may also be vertical migration of the odontoid compressing the medulla. The spinal cord compromise is usually worse in flexion and reduced in extension. Subaxial disease at C4-5 may lead to cervical radiculopathy or compression of the cord in extension. Finally, patients may have ankylosis of the cervical spine as a result of the arthritis or surgical fusion (36,59,72).

Care in positioning these patients is mandatory. Excessive flexion or extension may lead to spinal cord compression. Thus, the degree of cervical spine disease should be defined preoperatively and the neck stabilized intraoperatively in a neutral position. Particular attention must be taken during intubation and while turning patients, especially if they are under general anesthesia (GA). One virtue of regional anesthesia is that patients preserve muscle tone in the neck, limiting the likelihood of uncontrolled movement of the neck.

Patients with advanced RA may have painful or stiff joints and are often osteoporotic. For this reason, they must be positioned with care. It may not be easy to flex at the hip and knees to perform regional anesthesia, so it is often easier to perform epidural anesthesia at upper rather than lower lumbar interspaces. Positioning the arms in the lateral decubitus position is important. An axillary roll must be adequate to minimize pressure on the shoulder (which may be arthritic). This is best achieved with an inflatable adjustable axillary roll (see Patient Positioning). In addition, elbows and shoulders may have limited range of motion so should be positioned in a neutral comfortable position throughout surgery.

Patients with RA may have associated diseases that affect anesthetic management and surgical outcome. Cardiac valvular disease and pericardial effusions can limit cardiac output. Restrictive lung disease can predispose to postoperative lung dysfunction. Patients with angiopathy are apt to have exaggeration of Raynaud's disease if they become cold during surgery. Laryngeal pathology may predispose to edema with intubation, and to subsequent acute upper airway compromise upon extubation (81).

These patients are often metabolically compromised from the disease as a result of treatment with steroids, nonsteroidal anti-inflammatory drugs (NSAIDs), and tumor necrosis factor alpha blockers such as Remicade® and methotrexate. They frequently are osteoporotic, anemic, and lymphopenic and prone to perioperative infection, delayed recovery, and poor outcome.

Arterial line placement may be complicated by both deformity and an inability to extend the wrist. Placing central lines may also be difficult as a result of deformity of the neck. Nevertheless, in patients with advanced rheumatoid disease, it is preferable to monitor hemodynamic function to avoid fluid overload. Should these patients develop respiratory compromise after surgery, they are difficult to manage, as emergency intubation may be impossible.

ANKYLOSING SPONDYLITIS

Ankylosing spondylitis results in ankylosis of the spine and is often associated with hip and shoulder arthritis. Apart from the technical problems posed by the arthritis, the anesthetic management may be complicated by associated heart and lung disease.

The majority of patients with ankylosing spondylitis requiring THR have fusion of the neck. It is typically fused in flexion, often with some degree of rotation, making conventional laryngoscopy impossible. Thus, if general anesthesia is required, elective sedated fiberoptic-assisted intubation should be performed. A 6- or 7-mm armored tube can be used over the bronchoscope, and endotracheal intubation performed.

Many patients can have THR performed under regional anesthesia, which avoids the complexities of airway management. If the neck is not completely fused, it is usually possible to insert an epidural or spinal anesthetic between the lower lumbar interspaces. Alternatively, a caudal anesthetic can be performed. One of the problems with caudal anesthesia is that cephalad spread is inadequate, so blood pressure does not fall sufficiently and patients are not comfortable lying in the lateral decubitus position. Nevertheless, it is usually worthwhile trying to establish a regional anesthetic in these patients.

The spine is rigid and apt to fracture, which can result in paraplegia or quadriplegia (23). Thus, care in turning and positioning is vital, especially under anesthesia. Many also have shoulder arthritis, so an appropriate axillary roll is important.

Restrictive lung disease is not uncommon, but it is usually not a limiting factor after THR. On the other hand, patients with advanced ankylosing spondylitis often have aortic valve regurgitation, aortic dilatation, and bundle branch block, which may progress to heart failure. Perioperative management is aided by monitoring central venous or pulmonary artery pressures in this setting. Neck deformity may complicate insertion of these catheters.

PATIENT POSITIONING

Total hip replacement in the supine position poses few positioning problems. Patients in the lateral decubitus position, on the other hand, have to be positioned carefully to avoid problems. First, an appropriately sized axillary roll should be inserted to relieve pressure on the shoulder itself and prevent compression of the dependent axillary artery, vein, and brachial plexus. Pain in the dependent shoulder is a particular problem in patients with broad shoulders undergoing long surgical procedures under regional anesthesia. The best technique to relieve pressure on the dependent shoulder is by using an inflatable axillary roll or Shoulder Float (OR Comfort, NJ). This can be placed beneath the chest wall and inflated until there is little pressure beneath the shoulder (this can be assessed by passing ones hand beneath the shoulder, Fig. 43-1C). The Shoulder Float was demonstrated to provide better decompression of the shoulder and less pressure on the chest wall than a liter bag of saline (25). With this device properly placed, patients are easier to manage during regional anesthesia than with nonadjustable axillary rolls.

In the lateral decubitus position, there is a tendency for the head to deviate laterally. This was prospectively studied and the angle of deviation averaged 14° (ranged from 3° to 30°) using a standard axillary roll. If an adjustable inflatable device was used, the neck angulation could be significantly decreased (Fig. 43-1). This is probably most important in patients with neck arthritis, rheumatoid arthritis, or ankylosing spondylitis.

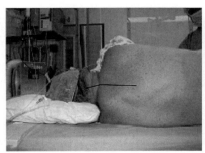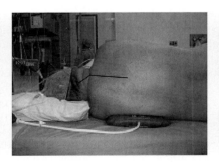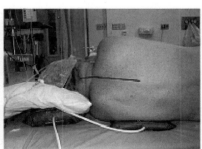

A,B   **C**

Figure 43-1   Inflation of a Shoulder Float decompresses the dependent shoulder **(A, B)**. Inflating another Shoulder Float beneath the head eliminates angulation of the neck **(C)**.

In the lateral decubitus position, particular care should be taken to prevent pressure over nerves in the lower extremity. Padding should be placed beneath the head of the fibula of the dependent leg to decrease the likelihood of peroneal nerve injury. If patients are stabilized by posts, care must be taken to avoid pressure over the femoral triangle, especially in long procedures. Pressure over the femoral triangle may compress the femoral vein or artery, predisposing to a compartment syndrome of the thigh (73). Direct compression of the femoral nerve may lead to neuropathy with quadriceps weakness after surgery.

Elderly patients with spinal stenosis should be positioned carefully as the nerve roots may become compressed in extension. Finally, the ulnar nerves and brachial plexus should be protected by careful attention to positioning of both upper extremities.

INTRAOPERATIVE MONITORING

Standard intraoperative monitoring includes pulse oximetry, electrocardiography, and noninvasive blood pressure monitoring. Patients undergoing GA require end-tidal CO_2 and temperature monitoring.

It is advisable to use arterial line monitoring with hypotensive anesthesia. Central venous pressure monitoring is also helpful to optimize fluid management.

Pulmonary artery catheters are useful in the following situations. In patients undergoing one staged bilateral cemented THR, pulmonary artery lines can detect underlying pulmonary hypertension or significant increases in pulmonary artery pressure from pulmonary emboli during the first operation. If the pulmonary artery pressure increases above 35 to 40 mm Hg systolic on the first hip replacement, it is inadvisable to proceed with the second side, as further embolism may lead to acute respiratory insufficiency.

Pulmonary artery catheters are also helpful during long-stem cemented THR, as these patients are at risk for acute pulmonary embolism and hypotension during surgery (47). Acute increases in pulmonary artery pressure can be detected, and acute hypotension treated, with epinephrine injected through the distal port of the pulmonary artery catheter (Fig. 43-2). By injecting it into the pulmonary circulation, it gains access to the coronary circulation more rapidly, restoring cardiac contractility. Patients undergoing prolonged revision THR also benefit from pulmonary artery monitoring, as it facilitates fluid balance. Management of patients with a history of congestive heart failure, severe valvular heart disease, or pulmonary hypertension are also aided by pulmonary artery monitoring, especially if excessive blood loss is expected.

Patients undergoing revision THR are at increased risk of developing sciatic palsy after surgery. Sciatic function can be assessed using GA, but not with regional anesthesia as it blunts or eliminates sensory evoked potentials.

HYPOTENSIVE ANESTHESIA

Hypotensive anesthesia reduces intraoperative blood loss (69,75). Studies have demonstrated a two- to fourfold reduction in intraoperative blood loss if mean arterial pressure (MAP) is reduced to 50 mm Hg during surgery (4,75,78). If

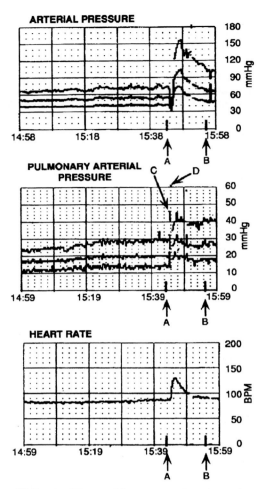

Figure 43-2 An 85-year-old woman undergoing primary THR, after placement of a Richard's screw with a long side plate. She had a history of chronic obstructive lung disease and osteoporosis. Pulmonary and radial artery pressures were stable until a 200-mm cemented femoral component was inserted (*point A*). One minute after impaction of the femoral component, pulmonary artery pressure increased acutely (*point C*) and arterial pressure decreased to 30 mm Hg. Epinephrine 25 mcg was injected through the distal port of the pulmonary artery catheter (*point D*). This resulted in a rapid restoration of arterial pressure, a transient tachycardia, and stabilization of the pulmonary artery pressure. The hip was relocated at *point B*, which resulted in no change in pulmonary artery pressure.

MAP is maintained at 60 mm Hg rather than 50 mm Hg, blood loss is about 40% greater (69). The relationship between intraoperative blood loss and MAP is shown in Figure 43-3 from a number of publications using spinal or epidural anesthesia. Blood loss during hypotensive anesthesia is related to MAP rather than to cardiac output or central venous pressure (67). Postoperative wound drainage is not increased after hypotensive anesthesia. Consequently, most studies have shown a 50% reduction in in-hospital transfusion using hypotensive anesthesia. Using hypotensive epidural anesthesia at the Hospital for Special Surgery, 6% of patients received homologous blood (7,15), compared to 29% in the United States (7) and 48% in Europe (57) using other anesthetic techniques (presumably normotension).

By reducing intraoperative blood loss, surgical exposure is enhanced, thereby reducing surgical time. Furthermore, the

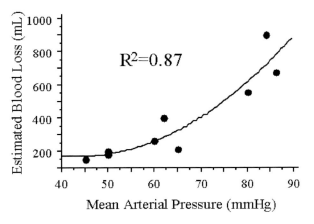

Figure 43-3   Mean intraoperative blood loss during primary unilateral total hip replacement in published articles when mean arterial pressure during surgery was recorded.

dry surface facilitates penetration of cement into cancellous bone. In a matched-pair study comparing the radiographic appearance of cemented cups, hypotensive anesthesia was associated with improved cement fixation (54). For this reason, it is possible that hypotensive anesthesia may influence long-term outcome of cemented hip arthroplasty by improving the quality of the cement–bone interface.

Hypotensive anesthesia may have other advantages. First, intraoperative blood loss is reduced (35), so that less fluid is used, making fluid overload unlikely. The reduced blood loss limits dilution and consumption of coagulation factors and subsequent postoperative rebound hypercoagulability. This may lessen the risk of DVT (34).

TECHNIQUES

Hypotensive anesthesia can be induced using either general or regional anesthesia. With GA, hypotension is achieved using deep inhalation anesthesia (which acts to dilate the arterial system and depress cardiac contractility) or with vasodilators (38). The literature suggests that blood loss is reduced to a similar degree whether hypotension is induced with vasodilators alone or by a combination of vasodilatation and cardiac depression (75). The vasodilators act on both venous and arterial vessels. One advantage of vasodilation is that it maintains cardiac output better than with deep inhalation anesthesia. Whether this has any effect on DVT rates or outcome is unknown.

An array of vasodilators has been used including intravenous infusions of sodium nitroprusside, nitroglycerine, or adenosine. Other agents include hydralazine, calcium channel blockers, and ACE inhibitors. Beta-blockers may be used to control heart rate. Labetalol is a useful agent that combines beta blockade with arterial dilatation.

HYPOTENSIVE EPIDURAL ANESTHESIA

This technique was developed to combine the virtues of epidural anesthesia (avoidance of airway problem and reduced

rate of DVT) with the benefits of induced hypotension. The technique has been described in detail (71).

Briefly, it entails injecting 20 to 25 mL local anesthetic at an upper lumbar interspace (L1-T11) to provide an extensive epidural block. This produces analgesia to T4 or above and a near complete sympathectomy (including the cardiac sympathetics). The sympathectomy results in a reduction in arterial pressure. Concurrently, a low-dose epinephrine intravenous infusion is used to stabilize the circulation. The initial dose is 2 mcg/min but the dose is adjusted, in combination with intravenous fluid, to allow the MAP to fall to 50 mm Hg while maintaining a stable heart rate. If a central venous pressure (CVP) catheter is inserted, fluid management is simplified by infusing fluid to preserve CVP in a normal range (1 to 5 mm Hg).

With this technique, arterial pressure can be reduced while maintaining heart rate, CVP, stroke volume, and cardiac output in the normal range (2,65) (Fig. 43-4). In addition, if necessary, patients can be kept awake to monitor brain function. This may be helpful in patients with neurologic impairment to document preservation of cognitive function intraoperatively.

This technique can be used in the majority of high-risk cases: patients with hypertension (68), advanced age, ischemic heart disease, or poor cardiac function (61). In-hospital mortality using this technique at the Hospital for Special Surgery is 0.1%, which demonstrates that it is not associated with adverse outcome (63). The technique should be used with caution in patients with valvular heart disease or severe carotid occlusive disease.

REGIONAL ANESTHESIA

Regional anesthesia is considered the ideal technique for THR, as it avoids many of the complex airway problems, reduces blood loss (31,40) and transfusion requirements, and is associated with a lower rate of DVT and pulmonary embolism (39,63) than GA (56). A variety of regional anesthetic techniques can be used.

Spinal anesthesia provides intense rapid onset anesthesia. Bupivacaine provides at least 3 hours of surgical anesthesia. With larger doses, higher sensory levels can be achieved, facilitating induced hypotension. If epinephrine infusions are used during spinal anesthesia, most of the benefits of epidural hypotensive anesthesia can be achieved, including a low intraoperative blood loss and DVT rate (13). Continuous spinal anesthesia is used in some centers but offers little advantage over continuous epidural and may increase the risk of adverse neurologic outcome.

More recently, the technique of combined spinal epidural anesthesia has been developed (77). A small gauge spinal needle is inserted through an epidural needle. The virtues are the rapid onset of spinal anesthesia, decreased risk of local anesthetic toxicity, with the flexibility of having an epidural catheter in place.

Any of the three techniques can be used and the advantages of one over another are minor. Epidural catheter techniques offer flexibility to extend or prolong the anesthetic or to provide postoperative analgesia. On the other hand, for straightforward primary THR, spinal anesthesia using small gauge pencil-point needles provides an excellent anesthetic, provided neurological complications are avoided (1).

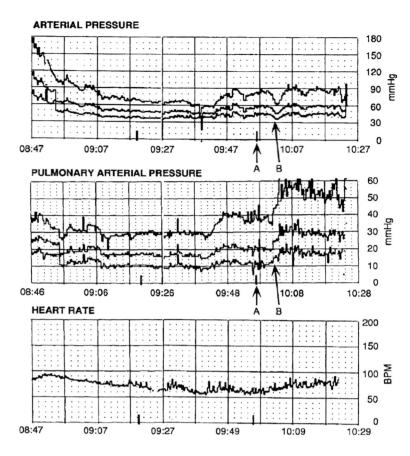

Figure 43-4 An 80-year-old man with hypertension and a preoperative low cardiac output (2.3 L/min/m²). Slight pulmonary hypertension preoperatively (40/18 mm Hg at 8:46). Surgery began at 9:20, the femoral cemented component is impacted at 9:56 (*point A*). Note there is no change in either pulmonary or radial arterial pressures following impaction. Five minutes later, the hip was relocated (*point B*), resulting in an acute increase in pulmonary artery pressure (38 to 55 mm Hg systolic) and decrease in arterial pressure (80 to 60 mm Hg systolic). Note the persistent elevation of the pulmonary artery pressure thereafter.

Regional anesthesia techniques can be combined with GA. After placement of an epidural catheter, patients can be intubated or a laryngeal mask airway inserted. If patients are ventilated, some of the advantages of regional anesthesia over GA are lost (16). On the other hand, in prolonged procedures, such as complex revision surgery, a combined technique makes it easier to manage patients, particularly by eliminating the problem from the dependent shoulder.

Sedation is an important part of management during regional anesthesia. With midazolam, amnesia can be secured. In longer cases, intravenous infusions of propofol or thiopental can provide a stable sedated state. Oxygen supplementation should be provided via nasal cannulae or face mask, and patients must be monitored with pulse oximetry.

EPIDURAL HEMATOMA

One of the limitations of the use of regional anesthesia has been the more widespread use of low-molecular-weight heparin (LMWH) to prevent DVT (55). Although rare, isolated cases of epidural hematoma have been reported in association with LMWH (26). This has lead to guidelines relating to the use of regional anesthesia in patients who are receiving anticoagulation (6,27). Although there is no doubt that epidural hematomas may develop following spinal or epidural anesthesia in patients who have received LMWH, it is the author's belief that the risk of hematoma developing following withdrawal of a catheter is minimal. Nevertheless, the guideline recommends caution using epidural analgesia in patients receiving LMWH and other anticoagulants for liability reasons. It would appear that a prudent approach would be to not administer LMWH until the epidural catheter has been removed. If postoperative epidural analgesia is considered beneficial, some other form of thromboprophylaxis should be used. The risk of epidural hematoma is minimal with patients taking aspirin (28).

APPROACHES TO BLOOD LOSS

Total hip replacement, especially prolonged revision THR, is associated with significant blood loss. Anesthetic management should be directed toward reducing bleeding and transfusion requirements while maintaining circulatory stability.

Blood loss can be minimized by using regional anesthesia or induced hypotension. Other techniques to reduce transfusions include autologous predonation of blood, use of cell saver intraoperatively, and tolerating a low postoperative hematocrit. In primary THR, a combination of predonation of one unit of blood and induced hypotension should almost eliminate the need for homologous donation (15,35).

In revision THR, more than one unit of autologous blood is usually needed. With induced hypotension, intraoperative cell salvage is not effective, because the blood loss is so small. Without induced hypotension, intraoperative cell salvage may be helpful. Other modalities, such as hemodilution of intraoperative use of antifibrinolytic agents such as aprotinin, may be used in selected cases (30,44).

Managing intraoperative blood loss is an important part of anesthetic care. In cases in which excessive blood loss is expected, hemodynamic monitoring is indicated. This facilitates preservation of blood volume and intraoperative cardiac output. Intraoperative low output states in THR may predispose to DVT formation. On the other hand, excessive fluid administration may increase the likelihood of postoperative lung dysfunction. If excessive blood loss occurs, monitoring hemodynamic state postoperatively for 12 to 24 hours may be helpful to prevent pulmonary edema from developing.

INTRAOPERATIVE HYPOTENSIVE EPISODES

Soon after methyl methacrylate was introduced as an agent to cement components during THR, episodes of intraoperative hypotension, often resulting in cardiac arrest and death, occurred. It was initially assumed that this was a result of toxic effects of methylmethacrylate monomer on the circulation. However, repeated studies demonstrated that the levels of methylmethacrylate in the blood were too low to account for the circulatory collapse (32). It has subsequently been shown that these hypotensive episodes are precipitated by intraoperative pulmonary emboli that acutely increase pulmonary artery pressure, leading to acute hypotension (11,47,83). If cardiac arrest occurs, these patients are very difficult to resuscitate. Optimal management requires an understanding of the timing and pathogenesis of intraoperative embolization.

Although hypotension may occur occasionally during insertion of the cup, the major episodes occur with insertion of a cemented femoral component. The following evidence demonstrates that these episodes are a result of embolization of bone marrow contents mixed with thrombi into the pulmonary circulation.

First, studies of patients who die acutely have fat and bone marrow emboli (mixed with fresh thrombi) in the lung. A similar pathologic picture has been observed after implantation of cemented femoral components in dogs (10,11). Second, echocardiographic imaging of the right heart during THR demonstrates showers of emboli during reaming of the

femur and more extensive echogenic masses after insertion of the cemented component (12,20,83) (Fig. 43-5). Finally, acute rises of pulmonary artery pressure have been demonstrated after impaction of cemented femoral components or after relocation of the hip (41,64) (see Figs. 43-2 and 43-4). On occasion, the acute rise in pulmonary artery pressure immediately precedes the acute hypotension (Fig. 43-2).

It has become clear that the degree of embolization depends on the degree of pressurization and the extent of violation of the femur (83). If a cement plug is firmly seated above the isthmus of the femur and the femur is well cleaned out with pulse lavage (9), the prosthesis can be inserted with significant pressurization without significant hemodynamic change. On the other hand, if a long-stem cemented prosthesis is inserted, or cement is pressurized into the distal femur, a larger amount of bone marrow will be forced into the circulation, leading to acute circulatory changes (47). Patients with poor cardiac function or pulmonary hypertension are most at risk to develop circulatory collapse from a bone marrow embolus (17).

Surgical approaches to prevent the acute hypotension include well-fitting cement plugs, pulse lavage of the femur, judicious use of pressurization when inserting long-stem cemented components, venting the femur (51), and inserting noncemented rather than cemented femoral components. Anesthetic techniques include preserving blood volume, maintaining a normal or high cardiac output, and having central venous access through which to administer epinephrine if the arterial pressure begins to fall. Finally, in high-risk cases, as mentioned earlier, injection of epinephrine through the distal port of a pulmonary artery catheter may hasten return of the circulation as it stimulates the heart, promoting transfer of the embolic material through the heart and into the lungs (47).

Once an embolic event has been identified, patients are easier to manage with pulmonary artery monitoring and serial measurement of arterial blood gases. To minimize pulmonary hypertension and optimize PaO_2, fluid management can be adjusted, cardiac output maintained, venodilators infused, and supplemental oxygen administered. The pulmonary hypertension often resolves within an hour, or it may persist for several days. If patients do not experience a cardiac arrest,

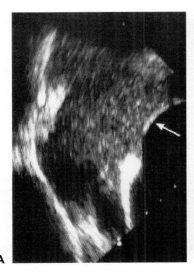 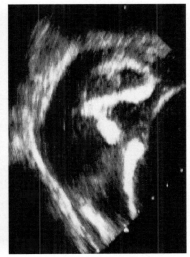

Figure 43-5 Right atrium during echocardiography. **A:** Multiple small emboli in the right atrium. **B:** A large embolus 7 cm in length, which is probably a cast of the femoral vein. (Reprinted from Christie J, Burnett R, Potts HR, et al. Echocardiography of transatrial embolism during cemented and uncemented hemiarthroplasty of the hip. *J Bone Joint Surg Br.* 1994;76B:409–412, with permission.)

A   **B**

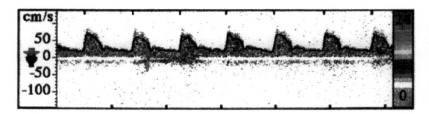

Figure 43-6 A recording of a transcranial Doppler from the middle cerebral artery during total hip arthroplasty. Note the embolic signals depicted in red. (Reprinted from Edmonds CR, Barbut D, Hager D, et al. Intraoperative cerebral arterial embolization during total hip arthroplasty. *Anesthesiology.* 2000;93:315–318, with permission.) See Color Plate.

the prognosis is excellent. Hypoxia is seldom seen acutely (20) but may develop postoperatively. Presumably, this is caused by progressive endothelial injury and pulmonary edema in association with sustained pulmonary hypertension.

In the 1970s, acute hypotension was common. Nowadays, with improved surgical techniques, acute hypotension is uncommon with primary THR but may occur with complex cases.

In rare cases, embolic material can cross to the left heart via a patent foramen ovale and lead to stroke or myocardial infarction (48,49). This may be more likely to occur during controlled ventilation (33) and with the development of acute pulmonary hypertension. Patent foramen ovale is present in about 20% of the population (33), so it is surprising that more patients do not develop fat emboli to the brain during or after THR. If someone is known to have an atrial septal defect, THR should be performed with caution in view of the risk of paradoxical embolism.

Small emboli may also traverse the pulmonary circulation (11), enter the arterial system and embolize to the brain (19). In a prospective series of patients undergoing THR under regional anesthesia, emboli in the middle cerebral artery were detected in 40% of patients using transcranial Doppler. These occurred following impaction of the cemented component or following relocation of the hip. It is unknown whether these emboli contribute to postoperative cognitive effects (82) (Fig. 43-6).

INTRAOPERATIVE FACTORS IN DEEP VEIN THROMBOSIS

Deep vein thrombosis develops during THR (8), with the period of peak thrombogenesis beginning during surgery on the femur (64). This is felt to occur with twisting and kinking

of the femoral vein, leading to obstruction of the femoral vein (52,79). Surgery on the femur releases bone marrow contents (containing thromboplastin) into the obstructed venous system. Finally, tissue injury around the twisted femoral vein may disrupt the endothelium, providing a further nidus for DVT. Thus all three factors of Virchow's triad occur promoting femoral venous thrombosis during insertion of the femoral component.

Anesthesiologists can modify this process. First, it is known that epidural and spinal anesthesia are associated with lower rates of DVT than general anesthesia (53). It is likely that this is because of enhanced blood flow to the leg during and immediately after surgery with regional anesthesia (2,14). Studies of blood flow during epidural anesthesia have shown that skeletal muscle blood flow is significantly increased if low-dose epinephrine (LDE) is used (2). This may account for the low DVT rate (10%) noted with hypotensive epidural anesthesia using LDE infusion (35,70).

Femoral venous occlusion has been documented during surgery by studying acute changes in pulmonary artery oxygen tension (s_vO_2). When an obstructed femoral vein is released, a bolus of desaturated blood enters the central circulation and is detected as an acute fall in s_vO_2 (64) (Fig. 43-7). When epinephrine is used, s_vO_2 tends to be higher and the decline in s_vO_2 less than when other agents are used (3). Therefore, it is hypothesized that during surgery the increased skeletal muscle blood flow tends to flush out the femoral vein sufficiently to retard DVT formation. Low oxygen tension in venous blood also promotes venous thrombosis (37). Thus, maintaining an adequate arterial oxygen tension and high blood flow in the leg acts to prevent DVT. Other mechanisms to prevent vasoconstriction or to maintain blood flow to the legs during surgery include maintenance of blood volume, preservation of temperature, and avoidance of alpha agents (arterial vasoconstrictors).

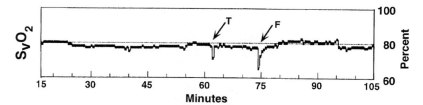

Figure 43-7 Pulmonary artery oxygen saturation during total hip replacement is recorded on a disposable transducer (American Edwards, Baxter Healthcare Corp., Irvine, CA). Note the acute fall in pulmonary artery oxygen saturation after relocation of the hip at minute 62 after trial reduction (T) with 8 minutes of potential venous occlusion and minute 74 following final reduction (F) with 12 minutes of potential venous occlusion. (Reprinted from Sharrock NE, Go G, Harpel PC, et al. Thrombogenesis during total hip replacement. *Clin Orthop.* 1995;319:16–27, with permission.)

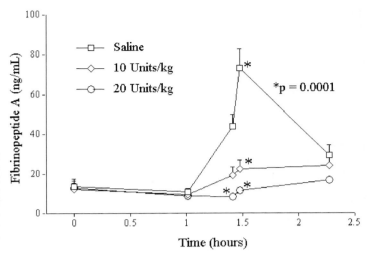

Figure 43-8 Blood levels of fibrinopeptide A (FPA) during hybrid total hip replacement. Note the increase in FPA in the saline group and the significant suppression in both 10 U/kg and 20 U/kg groups during insertion of the femoral component. (Values are mean ±SD). *p = 0.0001 compared to 10 and 20 U/kg. (Reprinted from Sharrock NE, McCabe JP, Go G, et al. Dose response of intravenous heparin on markers of thrombosis during primary total hip replacement. *Anesthesiology.* 1999;90:981–987, with permission.)

Finally, as DVT begins during surgery on the femur, it would seem logical to administer anticoagulants during this phase of surgery. Studies using 10 to 20 units/kg of heparin intravenously immediately after insertion of the cup (prior to surgery on the femur) have demonstrated a suppression of thrombogenesis (66) (Fig. 43-8). The rate of occurrence of DVT with intraoperative heparin is 8%, with a proximal DVT rate of less than 2% (29). This is lower than using perioperative LMWH (21).

Intraoperative approaches to DVT prophylaxis should not be considered sufficient. They should be combined with other perioperative modalities such as knee-high stockings, leg elevation, foot flexion/extension exercises immediately after surgery, and early ambulation. Aspirin, 650 mg daily, or Coumadin for 4 to 6 weeks should be started the night of surgery (58).

Rates of DVT with hypotensive epidural anesthesia are about 10% with surgery lasting less than 70 minutes and intraoperative blood loss of about 200 to 250 mL (70). Examination of the literature has demonstrated a relationship between DVT rate and intraoperative blood loss (71) (Fig. 43-9). Studies with DVT rates of 50% have intraoperative blood losses of 1000 mL or more, and lower rates of 10% to 15% are associated with lower blood losses (200 mL). Whether reducing blood loss minimizes the risk of DVT via altered coagulation mechanism (34,45), or whether it is merely a covariable from other factors such as surgical duration, surgical technique (22,51) or vasoconstriction, is unknown.

TEMPERATURE CONTROL

Hypothermia tends to develop during THR (5). Factors include prepping a patient with cold solutions, leaving patients uncovered in a cold atmosphere, and infusion of cold fluids intravenously. Hypothermia leads to peripheral vasoconstriction and a possibility of increased intraoperative blood loss (60), and it predisposes patients to shivering in the immediate postoperative period. Intraoperative hypothermia can be reduced with hot air blankets and by warming intravenous fluids. These

modalities are particularly important during revision or one-stage bilateral THR.

INTENSIVE POSTOPERATIVE SURVEILLANCE

Improved postoperative surveillance of selected patients probably contributed in part to a reduction in mortality observed following total joint arthroplasty at the Hospital for Special Surgery after 1986 (63). Certain groups of patients appear to benefit from overnight surveillance in a special care environment where ventilation, heart rate, cardiac rhythm, and pulmonary artery pressure can be monitored. They include patients undergoing one-stage bilateral THR or long-stem-cemented revision THR, and those who develop circulatory changes from insertion of the femoral prosthesis. In addition, high-risk patients can benefit from additional surveillance.

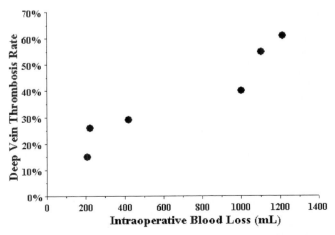

Figure 43-9 The mean intraoperative blood loss and rate of deep vein thrombosis after THA derived from six published articles (24,39,42,62,70,76). This relationship has been examined using simple linear regression.

POSTOPERATIVE PAIN CONTROL

Pain following THR is not as severe as following total knee replacement and is usually managed with oral analgesics within 24 to 48 hours. Many modes of analgesia have been utilized including intramuscular narcotics, intravenous patient controlled analgesia (PCA), intrathecal narcotics (morphine 0.1 to 0.3 mg), epidural analgesia, and more recently, lumbar plexus (psoas compartment) block (74). The techniques depend upon the availability of a pain service, facility performing regional anesthesia, perioperative use of anticoagulants (e.g., LMWH), and nursing practices.

Although pain relief does not appear to be a problem following THR, it is becoming more relevant with the pressure to discharge patients earlier. Narcotics result in nausea, vomiting, postural hypotension, and adverse cognitive effects, which may delay rehabilitation. Techniques which limit narcotic use, such as nonsteroidal anti-inflammatory agents (especially COX2 inhibitors) or regional blockade with epidural analgesia or lumbar plexus block, may enable more rapid ambulation and discharge. To obtain the optimal benefit from epidural analgesia or lumbar plexus block, aggressive physical therapy and early feeding is probably needed (43).

CONCLUSION

In the 1970s, the mortality rates following THR were about 1.3% to 1.5%; in the mid 1980s, 0.4% to 0.7% (50,63); in Great Britain in 1991, 0.31% (46,80); and at the Hospital for Special Surgery, 0.1% since 1987 (63). This reduction in mortality has been brought about by a combination of improved surgical and anesthetic techniques as well as by improvements in supportive care. The relevant anesthetic improvements include the use of regional anesthesia, intraoperative hypotension, improved monitoring and use of invasive monitoring, and postoperative surveillance in selected cases. To optimally care for patients undergoing THR, an understanding of these approaches is necessary.

REFERENCES

1. Auroy Y, Benhamou D, Bargues L, et al. Major complications of regional anesthesia in France: the SOS Regional Anesthesia Hotline Service. *Anesthesiology.* 2002;97:1274–1280.
2. Bading B, Blank S, Sculco TP, et al. Augmentation of calf blood flow by epinephrine infusion during lumbar epidural anesthesia. *Anesth Analg.* 1994;78:1119–1124.
3. Bading B, Mineo R, Sharrock NE. Arterial and mixed oxygen tension during hypotensive epidural anesthesia with either epinephrine (EPI) or norepinephrine (NEPI) infusion. *Reg Anesth.* 1993;18:10.
4. Barbier-Böhm G, Desmonts JM, Couderc E, et al. Comparative effects of induced hypotension and normovolaemic haemodilution on blood loss in total hip arthroplasty. *Br J Anaesth.* 1980;52:1039–1042.
5. Bennett J, Ramachandra V, Webster J, et al. Prevention of hypothermia during hip surgery: effect of passive compared with active skin surface warming. *Br J Anaesth.* 1994;73:180–183.
6. Bergqvist D, Wu CL, Neal JM. Anticoagulation and neuraxial regional anesthesia: perspectives. *Reg Anesth Pain Med.* 2003;28:163–166.
7. Bierbaum BE, Callaghan JJ, Galante JO, et al. An analysis of blood management in patients having a total hip or knee arthroplasty. *J Bone Joint Surg Am.* 1999;81A:2–10.
8. Binns M, Pho R. Femoral vein occlusion during hip arthroplasty. *Clin Orthop Relat Res.* 1990;255:168–172.
9. Byrick RJ, Bell RS, Kay JC, et al. High-volume, high-pressure pulsatile lavage during cemented arthroplasty. *J Bone Joint Surg Am.* 1989;71A:1331–1336.
10. Byrick R, Kay J, Mullen J. Pulmonary marrow embolism: a dog model simulating dual component cemented arthroplasty. *Can J Anaesth.* 1987;34:336–342.
11. Byrick RJ, Mullen JB, Mazer CD, et al. Transpulmonary systemic fat embolism. Studies in mongrel dogs after cemented arthroplasty. *Am J Respir Crit Care Med.* 1994;150:1416–1422.
12. Christie J, Burnett R, Potts HR, et al. Echocardiography of transatrial embolism during cemented and uncemented hemiarthroplasty of the hip. *J Bone Joint Surg Br.* 1994;76B:409–412.
13. Davis FM, Laurenson VG, Gillespie WJ, et al. Deep vein thrombosis after total hip replacement. *J Bone Joint Surg Br.* 1989;71B:181–185.
14. Davis FM, Laurenson VG, Gillespie WJ, et al. Leg blood flow during total hip replacement under spinal or general anaesthesia. *Anaesth Intensive Care.* 1989;17:136–142.
15. DiGiovanni CW, Restrepo A, Della Valle AG, et al. The safety and efficacy of intraoperative heparin in total hip arthroplasty. *Clin Orthop Relat Res.* 2000;379:178–185.
16. Donadoni R, Baele G, Devulder J, et al. Coagulation and fibrinolytic parameters in patients undergoing total hip replacement: influence of the anaesthetic technique. *Acta Anaesthesiol Scand.* 1989;33:588–592.
17. Duncan JA. Intra-operative collapse or death related to the use acrylic cement in hip surgery. *Anaesthesia.* 1989;44:149–153.
18. Dyer RA, Llewellyn RL, James MFM. Total i.v. anaesthesia with propofol and the laryngeal mask for orthopaedic surgery. *Br J Anaesth.* 1995;74:123–128.
19. Edmonds CR, Barbut D, Hager D, et al. Intraoperative cerebral arterial embolization during total hip arthroplasty. *Anesthesiology.* 2000;93:315–318.
20. Ereth MH, Weber JG, Abel MD, et al. Cemented versus noncemented total hip arthroplasty: embolism, hemodynamics, and intrapulmonary shunting. *Mayo Clin Proc.* 1992;67:1066–1074.
21. Eriksson BI, Wille-Jorgensen P, Kalebo P, et al. A comparison of recombinant hirudin with a low-molecular-weight heparin to prevent thromboembolic complications after total hip replacement [see comments]. *N Engl J Med.* 1997;337:1329–1335.
22. Fedi S, Gori AM, Falciani M, et al. Procedure-dependence and tissue factor-independence of hypercoagulability during orthopaedic surgery. *Thromb Haemost.* 1999;81:874–878.
23. Fox MW, Onofrio BM, Kilgore JE. Neurological complications of ankylosing spondylitis. *J Neurosurg.* 1993;78:871–878.
24. Fredin HO, Rosberg B, Arborelius M Jr, et al. On thromboembolism after total hip replacement in epidural analgesia: A controlled study of dextran 70 and low-dose heparin combined with dihydroergotamine. *Br J Surg.* 1984;71:58–60.
25. Gonzalez Della Valle A, Salonia-Ruzo P, Peterson MG, et al. Inflatable pillows as axillary support devices during surgery performed in the lateral decubitus position under epidural anesthesia. *Anesth Analg.* 2001;93:1338–1343.
26. Horlocker TT, Wedel DJ. Neuraxial block and low-molecular-weight heparin: balancing perioperative analgesia and thromboprophylaxis. *Reg Anesth Pain Manag.* 1998;23:164–177.
27. Horlocker TT, Wedel DJ, Benzon H, et al. Regional anesthesia in the anticoagulated patient: Defining the risks (the second ASRA Consensus Conference on Neuraxial Anesthesia and Anticoagulation). *Reg Anesth Pain Med.* 2003;28:172–197.
28. Horlocker TT, Wedel DJ, Schroeder DR, et al. Preoperative antiplatelet therapy does not increase the risk of spinal hematoma associated with regional anesthesia. *Anesth Analg.* 1995;80:303–309.
29. Huo MH, Salvati EA, Sharrock NE, et al. Intraoperative heparin thromboembolic prophylaxis in primary total hip arthroplasty. A prospective, randomized, controlled, clinical trial. *Clin Orthop Relat Res.* 1992;274:35–46.
30. Janssens M, Joris J, David JL, et al. High-dose aprotinin reduces blood loss in patients undergoing total hip replacement surgery. *Anesthesiology.* 1994;80:23–29.
31. Keith I. Anaesthesia and blood loss in total hip replacement. *Anaesthesia.* 1977;32:444–450.

32. Kim KJ, Chen da G, Chung N, et al. Direct myocardial depressant effect of methylmethacrylate monomer: mechanical and electrophysiologic actions in vitro. *Anesthesiology.* 2003;98:1186–1194.
33. Konstadt SN, Louie EK, Black S, et al. Intraoperative detection of patent foramen ovale by transesophageal echocardiography. *Anesthesiology.* 1991;74:212–216.
34. Lieberman JR, Geerts WH. Prevention of venous thromboembolism after total hip and knee arthroplasty. *J Bone Joint Surg Am.* 1994;76A:1239–1250.
35. Lieberman JR, Huo MH, Hanway J, et al. The prevalence of deep venous thrombosis after total hip arthroplasty with hypotensive epidural anesthesia. *J Bone Joint Surg Am.* 1994;76A:341–348.
36. Macarthur A, Kleiman S. Rheumatoid cervical joint disease: a challenge to the anaesthetist. *Can J Anaesth.* 1993;40:154–159.
37. Malone PC, Morris CJ. The sequestration and margination of platelets and leucocytes in veins during conditions of hypokinetic and anaemic hypoxia: Potential significance in clinical postoperative venous thrombosis. *J Pathol.* 1978;125:119–129.
38. Miller EDJ, Van Aken H. Deliberate hypotension. In: Miller RD, ed. *Anesthesia.* 5th ed. New York: Churchill Livingstone; 2000:1470–1490.
39. Modig J, Borg T, Karlström G, et al. Thromboembolism after total hip replacement: role of epidural and general anesthesia. *Anesth Analg.* 1983;62:174–180.
40. Modig J, Karlström G. Intra- and post-operative blood loss and haemodynamics in total hip replacement when performed under lumbar epidural versus general anaesthesia. *Eur J Anaesth.* 1987;4:345–355.
41. Modig J, Malmberg P. Pulmonary and circulatory reactions during total hip replacement surgery. *Acta Anaesth Scand.* 1975;19:219–237.
42. Modig J, Maripuu E, Sahlstedt B. Thromboembolism following total hip replacement: a prospective investigation of 94 patients with emphasis on the efficacy of lumbar epidural anesthesia in prophylaxis. *Reg Anesth.* 1986;11:72–79.
43. Moiniche S, Hjortso NC, Hansen BL, et al. The effect of balanced analgesia on early convalescence after major orthopaedic surgery. *Acta Anaesth Scand.* 1994;38:328–335.
44. Murkin JM, Shannon NA, Bourne RB, et al. Aprotinin decreases blood loss in patients undergoing revision or bilateral total hip arthroplasty. *Anesth Analg.* 1995;80:343–348.
45. Murray DJ, Pennel BJ, Weinstein SL, et al. Packed red cells in acute blood loss: dilutional coagulopathy as a cause of surgical bleeding. *Anesth Analg.* 1995;80:336–342.
46. Murray DW, Carr AJ, Bulstrode CJK. Pharmacological thromboprophylaxis and total hip replacement [editorial]. *J Bone Joint Surg Br.* 1995;77B:3–5.
47. Patterson BM, Healy JH, Cornell CN, et al. Cardiac arrest during hip arthroplasty with a cemented long-stem component. *J Bone Joint Surg Am.* 1991;73A:271–277.
48. Pell AC, Christie J, Keating JF, et al. The detection of fat embolism by transoesophageal echocardiography during reamed intramedullary nailing. A study of 24 patients with femoral and tibial fractures. *J Bone Joint Surg Br.* 1993;75:921–925.
49. Pell ACH, Hughes D, John K, et al. Brief report: fulminating fat embolism syndrome caused by paradoxical embolism through a patent foramen ovale. *N Engl J Med.* 1993;329:926–929.
50. Peterson MGE, Hollenberg JP, Szatrowski TP, et al. Geographic variations in the rates of elective total hip and knee arthroplasties among Medicare beneficiaries in the United States. *J Bone Joint Surg Am.* 1992;74A:1530–1539.
51. Pitto RP, Hamer H, Fabiani R, et al. Prophylaxis against fat and bone-marrow embolism during total hip arthroplasty reduces the incidence of postoperative deep-vein thrombosis: a controlled, randomized clinical trial. *J Bone Joint Surg Am.* 2002;84A:39–48.
52. Planès A, Vochelle N, Fagola M. Total hip replacement and deep vein thrombosis. *J Bone Joint Surg Br.* 1990;72B:9–13.
53. Prins MH, Hirsh J. A comparison of general anesthesia and regional anesthesia as a risk factor for deep vein thrombosis following total hip surgery: a critical review. *Thromb Haemost.* 1990;64:497–500.
54. Ranawat CS, Beaver WB, Sharrock NE, et al. Effect of hypotensive epidural anaesthesia on acetabular cement-bone fixation in total hip arthroplasty. *J Bone Joint Surg Br.* 1991;73B:779–782.
55. Renck H. Neurological complications of central nerve blocks. *Acta Anaesth Scand.* 1995;39:859–868.
56. Rodgers A, Walker N, Schug S, et al. Reduction of postoperative mortality and morbidity with epidural or spinal anaesthesia: results from overview of randomised trials. *BMJ.* 2000;321:1493.
57. Rosencher N, Kerkkamp HE, Macheras G, et al. Orthopedic Surgery Transfusion Hemoglobin European Overview (OSTHEO) study: blood management in elective knee and hip arthroplasty in Europe. *Transfusion.* 2003;43:459–469.
58. Salvati EA, Pellegrini VD Jr, Sharrock NE, et al. Recent advances in venous thromboembolic prophylaxis during and after total hip replacement. *J Bone Joint Surg Am.* 2000;82A:252–270.
59. Santavirta S, Slätis P, Kankaanpää U, et al. Treatment of the cervical spine in rheumatoid arthritis. *J Bone Joint Surg Br.* 1988;70B:658–667.
60. Schmied H, Kurz A, Sessler DI, et al. Hypothermia increases blood loss and allogeneic transfusion requirements during hip surgery. *Anesthesiology.* 1995;83:A1115.
61. Sharrock NE, Bading B, Mineo R, et al. Deliberate hypotensive epidural anesthesia for patients with normal and low cardiac output. *Anesth Analg.* 1994;79:899–904.
62. Sharrock NE, Brien WW, Salvati EA, et al. The effect of intravenous fixed-dose heparin during total hip arthroplasty on the incidence of deep-vein thrombosis. A randomized, double-blind trial in patients operated on with epidural anesthesia and controlled hypotension. *J Bone Joint Surg Am.* 1990;72A:1456–1461.
63. Sharrock NE, Cazan MG, Hargett MJL, et al. Changes in mortality after total hip and knee arthroplasty over a ten-year period. *Anesth Analg.* 1995;80:242–248.
64. Sharrock NE, Go G, Harpel PC, et al. Thrombogenesis during total hip replacement. *Clin Orthop Relat Res.* 1995;319:16–27.
65. Sharrock NE, Go G, Mineo R, et al. The hemodynamic and fibrinolytic response to low dose epinephrine and phenylephrine infusions during total hip replacement under epidural anesthesia. *Thromb Haemost.* 1992;68:436–441.
66. Sharrock NE, McCabe JP, Go G, et al. Dose response of intravenous heparin on markers of thrombosis during primary total hip replacement. *Anesthesiology.* 1999;90:981–987.
67. Sharrock NE, Mineo R, Go G. The effect of cardiac output on intraoperative blood loss during total hip arthroplasty. *Reg Anesth.* 1993;18:24–29.
68. Sharrock NE, Mineo R, Urquhart B. Haemodynamic effects and outcome analysis of hypotensive extradural anaesthesia in controlled hypertensive patients undergoing total hip arthroplasty. *Br J Anaesth.* 1991;67:17–25.
69. Sharrock NE, Mineo R, Urquhart B, et al. The effect of two levels of hypotension on intraoperative blood loss during total hip arthroplasty. *Anesth Analg.* 1993;76:580–584.
70. Sharrock NE, Ranawat CS, Urquhart B, et al. Factors influencing deep vein thrombosis following total hip arthroplasty. *Anesth Analg.* 1993;76:765–771.
71. Sharrock NE, Salvati EA. Hypotensive epidural anesthesia for total hip arthroplasty. *Acta Orthop Scand.* 1996;67:91–107.
72. Skues MA, Welchew EA. Anaesthesia and rheumatoid arthritis. Review article. *Anaesthesia.* 1993;48:989–997.
73. Smith JW, Pellicci PM, Sharrock NE, et al. Complications after total hip replacement: the contralateral limb. *J Bone Joint Surg Am.* 1989;71A:528–535.
74. Stevens RD, Van Gessel E, Flory N, et al. Lumbar plexus block reduces pain and blood loss associated with total hip arthroplasty. *Anesthesiology.* 2000;93:115–121.
75. Thompson GE, Miller RD, Stevens WC, et al. Hypotensive anesthesia for total hip arthroplasty: a study of blood loss and organ function (brain, heart, liver, and kidney). *Anesthesiology.* 1978;48:91–96.
76. Thorburn J, Louden JR, Vallance R. Spinal and general anaesthesia in total hip replacement: frequency of deep vein thrombosis. *Br J Anaesth.* 1980;52:1117–1120.
77. Urmey WF, Stanton J, Peterson M, et al. Combined spinal-epidural anesthesia for outpatient surgery. Dose-response characteristics of

intrathecal isobaric lidocaine using a 27-gauge Whitacre spinal needle. *Anesthesiology.* 1995;83:528–534.

78. Vazeery AK, Lunde O. Controlled hypotension in hip joint surgery: an assessment of surgical haemorrhage during sodium nitroprusside infusion. *Acta Orthop Scand.* 1979;50:433–441.

79. Warwick D, Martin AG, Glew D, et al. Measurement of femoral vein blood flow during total hip replacement. Duplex ultrasound imaging with and without the use of a foot pump. *J Bone Joint Surg Br.* 1994;76B:918–921.

80. Warwick D, Williams MH, Bannister GC. Death and thromboembolic disease after total hip replacement. A series of 1162 cases with no routine chemical prophylaxis. *J Bone Joint Surg Br.* 1995;77B:6–10.

81. Wattenmaker I, Concepcion M, Hibberd P, et al. Upper-airway obstruction and perioperative management of the airway in patients managed with posterior operations on the cervical spine for rheumatoid arthritis. *J Bone Joint Surg Am.* 1994;76A:360–365.

82. Williams-Russo P, Sharrock NE, Mattis S, et al. Cognitive effects after epidural vs general anesthesia in older adults. A randomized trial. *JAMA.* 1995;274:44–50.

83. Woo R, Minster GJ, Fitzgerald RH Jr, et al. Pulmonary fat embolism in revision hip arthroplasty. *Clin Orthop Relat Res.* 1995;319:41–53.

Blood Conservation in Hip Surgery

Bernard N. Stulberg   Joseph Thomas

Blood transfusion has been widely accepted as a standard of care in the treatment of perioperative anemia as a result of acute blood loss. Blood utilization has steadily increased in the United States at the rate of 6% per year since 1994 (49). In fact, by 2001, approximately 15 million units of packed red blood cells (PRBCs) were collected, with 14 million of these units being transfused to 4.9 million patients (49). The number of transfusions is expected to continue to increase as the volume of patients requiring major orthopedic, cardiac, and other complex surgical procedures increases.

Historically, a significant percentage of patients undergoing total hip replacement (THR) required PRBC transfusion. Even with advancements in orthopedic surgery, most estimates of perioperative blood loss for THR suggest decreases of hemoglobin between 4 and 5 g/dL (approximately 4 to 5 units of blood). Considering the demographics of the orthopedic surgery population, these losses are significant and can result in serious morbidity if not managed appropriately. Over the last several years, profound changes have occurred in perioperative blood management. The skyrocketing costs of blood, severe national blood shortages, and the growing knowledge of deleterious transfusion effects have patients and physicians alike searching for transfusion alternatives. It is estimated that 3 million units of PRBCs are transfused annually in the United States for elective surgeries alone. Without doubt, a significant portion of this is utilized in major orthopedic procedures. Although PRBC transfusion is still a necessity in

orthopedic management, there are several strategies and technological advancements that can have a significant impact on blood utilization.

Total hip arthroplasty (THA) has evolved dramatically over the last 3 decades; so too have concepts to address blood loss associated with THA. This chapter focuses on the concept of "blood management strategies," a concept that suggests a number of different preventative and treatment strategies that can be brought to bear to address the specific needs of each patient undergoing THA. While the focus of these strategies will be on the operation of THA, identifying the risk of blood loss anemia can be important in any hip operation.

The premise of any blood management strategy is that each patient, each surgeon, and each operative intervention experiences different risks of requiring transfusion, that those risks can be identified, and that a strategy can be implemented to address those risks for each patient. The benefit of such a strategy is to minimize the negative consequences of anemia and its treatment during the perioperative period.

In the section "Historical Perspective," we discuss approaches that have led to the possibility of strategy development, the rationale for developing patient-specific strategies, and the value to the patient and health care environment of developing patient-specific strategies. In "The Physiology of Blood Loss Anemia," we discuss the physiology of blood loss anemia in the hip patient and the data that suggest that a need exists to develop preventative and therapeutic strategies. In "Intervention Strategies," we enumerate and discuss the benefits and risks of the various pre-, intra- and postoperative treatment interventions that can be applied as part of the management strategy for a particular patient. We address the advantages, disadvantages, risks, usage, and cost of accepted and emerging technologies. In "Intervention Strategies," we suggest how individual surgeons and hospital environments can develop strategies that work to the benefit of the THA patient.

HISTORICAL PERSPECTIVE

The history of blood management in hip surgery has tended to mirror the history of blood management in other surgical specialties. Appropriate perioperative fluid and electrolyte balance is accompanied by the maintenance of the patient's hemoglobin at or above 10 g/dL (or accompanying hematocrit at 30%). With the increasing use of blood, along with growing concern about contamination of the available blood supply in the 1980s, increased effort was placed on identifying alternative strategies for dealing with blood loss and blood transfusion. As discussed in "Intervention Strategies," many of these strategies evolved from predictive strategies to estimate the need for blood, from autologous transfusion programs, and from blood order programs intended to discourage the indiscriminant use of blood transfusion and the corresponding wastage of blood and overuse of blood products. As recombinant products began to approach the marketplace, a business case developed for generating improved information about blood loss and the need for blood transfusion. Better information began to emerge as to the patient, hospital, and health system costs of minimizing blood transfusions. For the orthopedic population (and, more specifically, the total hip replacement population), this information began to improve as multicenter studies focused on product development (the erythropoietin products) began to identify specific populations at risk for transfusion and demonstrate the ability to influence this need by altered perioperative management strategies and drug interventions (20).

The arrival of Auto Immune Deficiency Syndrome (AIDS) in the early 1980s had two significant effects on blood management approaches in elective surgical populations. First, it impacted the availability of blood for use in elective surgery, as blood banks began to increase their screening vigilance. Second, it made patients and health care practitioners want to increase the safety of the blood used for transfusion and to minimize the use of homologous transfusions. A number of different options began to emerge. For the orthopedic population, significant interest and effort was directed toward the development of autologous transfusion programs and approaches that would allow for the use of salvaged blood (such as intra-operative salvage ["cell saver"] and postoperative salvage ["reinfusion drains"]). In the late 1980s there was also encouraging information coming from other medical areas that suggested that recombinant erythropoietin products could be used to increase hemoglobin levels in patients with renal disease, in patients undergoing chemotherapy for cancer, and in the AIDS population. The manufacturer of this product (Procrit, Orthobiotech, Bridgewater, NJ) began investigating its application in the elective surgery population, specifically the noncardiac, nonvascular surgery population. The manufacturer found the elective THA population and elective total knee arthroplasty (TKA) population particularly worthy of study, and several very important multicenter studies were performed to establish the potential applicability of this product (29). It was these studies that began to identify the specific patient populations at risk for transfusion following THA and TKA (and thus the indications for products such as Procrit) and to define its usefulness in relationship to other potential strategies.

It became clear that blood usage was related to a number of different aspects of THA and TKA. Most significantly related to

the use of blood was the patient's own preoperative hemoglobin. Many studies began to identify patients with starting hemoglobin (Hb) levels of 10 to 13g/dL as at greatest risk for needing transfusion postsurgery. In addition, the type of surgical procedure (and thus the degree of blood lost during surgery) would identify the risk of needing transfusion for a particular patient. This information was coupled with information that suggested that the "transfusion trigger"—the level of Hb at which it would be appropriate to transfuse a patient—also had a substantial influence on the amount of blood transfused. Historically based "transfusion triggers," such as the so-called 10/30 rule, were not necessary for most patients, and the decision to transfuse could be individualized (with most patients tolerating postoperative hemoglobin of 8.0 g/dL, and some patients even lower). Thus the ability to *know* a particular patient's Hb preoperatively, the ability to judge the degree of expected blood loss perioperatively, and the ability to judge the need for transfusion based on hemodynamic stability allowed the development of a *patient-specific* blood management strategy.

There is also increasing pressure from health care entities (hospitals and hospital systems) to address the appropriate use of transfusions and the development of patient-specific blood management strategies. Emerging clinical data suggest that there is a lower risk of infection, a greater level of patient energy and more rapid recovery, and an improved sense of well-being if patient anemia is managed effectively and if homologous transfusion can be avoided (38). This will result in a decreased hospital length of stay (LOS) and a decreased use of blood products and the resources to obtain and preserve them. Properly organized blood management strategies in a hospital environment will optimize the use of the blood bank, improve patient safety as it relates to transfusions, and avoid the costs and risks that can be associated with the acquisition and storage of autologous blood units. Indeed, in a community hospital setting in our own health care system, the initiation of a patient-specific strategy for THA and TKA has resulted in a first-year *decrease* in autologous donation of 117 units and a decrease in the overall transfusion rate from 40% to 20% of patients, with equal success in blood utilization in both THA and TKA. For 226 patients, the overall savings to the hospital was more than $50,000 (J. Thomas, unpublished data) (67). The coming years will see increased effort expended by hospitals and physicians to organize patient-specific programs to achieve the benefits of improved patient safety, improved patient outcome, and decreased hospital system costs.

THE PHYSIOLOGY OF BLOOD LOSS ANEMIA

Blood Transfusion Therapy

It was nearly 200 years ago that Blundell, a renowned obstetrician of the time, hypothesized that the most appropriate way to treat hemorrhage was to replace the blood volume with allogeneic blood from a live donor (1,2,25). Unfortunately, due to logistical problems (clotting, ABO incompatibility, etc.), most patients did not respond as expected. It was not until the early part of the 20th century that transfusion became a common practice, following the discovery of blood groups and effective ways to preserve and store the blood components safely for a period of time. Today, the process of collecting, processing, storing, and administering blood is no small chore. It is a multi-billion dollar industry that involves tens of thousands of professionals to oversee and improve the process. However, the final product is very impressive. Whole blood collected has now been separated to provide packed red cells, plasma, platelets, and dozens of other products that will be used in various pharmaceutical preparations. This chapter focuses primarily on the use of PRBCs.

Autologous Red Blood Cells

The unit of PRBCs to be administered usually contains the red cells from 450 mL of blood, along with enough plasma and anticoagulant to give a hematocrit of about 60%. The total volume of each unit of red cells varies but is often between 300 and 350 mL (200 mL of which is pure PRBCs). The additives in the anticoagulant extend the storage time of the red cell concentrate to 42 days. However, the longer red cells are stored, the less effective they are in their capacity as oxygen carriers. Unfortunately, most of the blood that is administered in a hospital is near its expiration date, often well over 3 to 4 weeks old. Several studies have shown that the dangerous effects of transfusion increase with red cell age, including reactions (63), lack of O_2 carrying capacity (42,64,68), microvascular occlusion (13,17,61), and immunomodulation (6,13,31,32,47). Red cell transfusions are indicated for the treatment of symptomatic anemia or the prevention of anemia in the presence of active bleeding or anticipated bleeding, such as surgery. However, the question of when PRBC transfusion is physiologically necessary is a complicated one and has become the topic of much controversy.

"Transfusion Trigger"

For decades, physicians used the 10/30 rule as the transfusion trigger, based on the rationale that O_2 carrying capacity needed to be maintained in case of unexpected (or expected) blood loss. The transfusion trigger had little or no scientific backing, and it was established and supported at a time when the risks of transfusion were considered to be negligible. Now that identifiable risks are associated in a dose-dependant manner with blood product transfusion, it is crucial for clinicians to transfuse only when there is a clear clinical indication. Every candidate for transfusion needs to be considered individually based on comorbidities, oxygen delivery (DO_2), oxygen consumption (VO_2), and acute blood loss (or risk thereof). There is no alternative to good clinical judgment in making the decision to transfuse a patient. In particular, this decision requires an adequate understanding of the physiology of O_2 transport, determinants that affect DO_2 and VO_2, and compensatory mechanisms in the perioperative surgical patient.

In the perioperative setting, anemia is mostly attributed to blood loss intra- and postoperatively. Acute blood loss can be classified as mild (up to 20% blood volume), moderate (20% to 40% blood volume), and severe (over 40% blood volume). There are several factors that need to be considered before initiating transfusion therapy.

Perioperative Blood Loss

There is extensive variation in the literature in regard to perioperative blood loss estimates and hemoglobin loss in THA. It has been reported that average blood loss during a hospital stay for THA is 1000 to 1500 mL (58). An estimated drop in hemoglobin of 5 g/dL or more in postoperative hip arthroplasty has also been reported in the literature (3,39). The human body has extensive compensatory mechanisms that allow it to tolerate significant losses of volume and of its oxygen carrier, hemoglobin (31). Within minutes of significant blood loss, baroreceptor reflexes mediate the initial compensatory response. Heart rate and ventilations are increased, both contributing to an increase in cardiac output, the latter by increasing right heart filling. Hyperventilation also is responsible for a fall in PCO_2 and a rise in arterial pH, both of which will increase arterial hemoglobin saturation. Shortly thereafter, vasoactive hormones, catecholamines, and angiotensin II are released to increase blood pressure and redistribute blood flow in an appropriate manner. Also important in this compensatory mechanism for acute blood loss is the redistribution of water, from the extravascular to intravascular space, and mobilization of albumin to increase oncotic pressure. Physiologically, this illustrates how healthy patients can tolerate large-volume, acute blood loss. In fact, when patients appear hemodynamically compromised in the presence of acute blood loss, it is more often in response to hypovolemia and inadequate intravascular volume than to insufficient O_2 delivery. Over recent years, this point has been made much clearer with the numerous re-evaluations of the transfusion trigger guidelines by nationally and internationally recognized medical groups (62,63).

Although there are some slight variations, most of these transfusion guidelines agree on the following: physiological and hemodynamic parameters should be assessed on an individual basis before a transfusion decision is reached. Transfusion of a clinically stable, nonbleeding patient with a hemoglobin level above 7 to 8 g/dL should be avoided in most cases.

Weiskopf (70) reported that acute isovolemic reduction of hemoglobin concentration to 5.0 g/dL did not produce evidence of inadequate DO_2 or VO_2 in conscious, healthy, resting humans. In the Jehovah's Witness population, who refuse blood on religious grounds, hemoglobin levels as low as 5 g/dL have been tolerated without an increase in mortality. While the hip surgical population discussed in this chapter does not likely fit into this category, it is important to recognize that in the presence of acute blood loss patients can often tolerate hemoglobin levels much lower than originally thought. It is important to understand that if blood volume is restored, acute blood loss anemia can be managed successfully without transfusion in many patients.

There is a need for caution in the patient with significant comorbidities, especially when these are cardiopulmonary in nature. They could possibly impair the body's natural compensatory mechanisms and inhibit its ability to enhance O_2 transport. In patients with coronary artery disease, an increase in myocardial oxygen demand secondary to increased workload may lead to inadequate perfusion of the myocardium. The increase in systemic O_2 demands may be insufficiently met in patients with congestive heart failure and could lead to multiorgan decompensation, depending on the severity of the anemia and other factors.

Patients with pulmonary disease may be unable to support the need for increased alveolar capillary O_2 diffusion and hyperventilation. An increase in the CO_2 level will also result in an increase in pH, both of which reduce hemoglobin's affinity for oxygen.

Although an appropriate transfusion trigger is still unclear in patients with significant comorbidities, this population is unlikely to tolerate hemoglobin levels below 7.0 g/dL. Therefore, the general consensus encourages the maintenance of hemoglobin levels above 7.0 to 8.0 g/dL in patients with cardiopulmonary comorbidities.

INTERVENTION STRATEGIES

Predicting Transfusion Risk

In a patient-specific blood management program, an appropriate strategy is based on an estimation of transfusion risk. There has been a significant body of work (15,37,51,52) that has attempted to address transfusion risk for both the total hip and total knee population. The development of a patient-specific strategy suggests that the surgeon, or the environment in which he or she practices, make an assessment of the need for transfusion for each patient.

There are both patient-specific and surgeon- or surgery-specific data that make that strategy development possible. As discussed in this section, there are some simple data collection approaches that can start that data acquisition process. The patient-specific factors are preoperative hemoglobin/hematocrit (Hb/Hct), blood volume (calculated from height and weight information), and general health status, as measured, for example, by the ASA rating (to establish a safe transfusion trigger). Multiple orthopedic studies (6,18,22,65) have shown that the preoperative Hb/Hct levels are the most powerful predictors of need for transfusion, with patients with Hb <13.0 g/dL being at greatest risk. Our own experience suggests that the hemoglobin level is in this range in at least one third of the female patients undergoing elective hip surgery (B. N. Stulberg, personal data). Surgeon-specific variables relate to the anticipated blood loss (anticipated EBL) associated with the planned operation by the particular surgeon. Thus, the type of operation (e.g., primary versus revision, fracture fixation versus arthroplasty), the particular surgeon's approach (both surgical approach and experience with the operative intervention), and the type of anesthesia (controlled hypotensive anesthesia versus alternatives) will influence the anticipated EBL. A simple data-tracking form can allow a surgeon or a hospital environment to acquire these data over a specific time period.

Several predictive approaches have been suggested over the past decade. Nuttal et al. (52) noted that by using predictive approaches they could lower the transfusion requirements from over 3.14 units per THA patient (cross-matched) to 1.23 units per patient transfused. This led to a more appropriate blood-ordering schedule among surgeons at their institution (52). Nelson et al. (51) using patient-derived data, and Cohen and Brecher (15), using mathematical modeling, arrived at nomograms that could help predict transfusion needs for the THA population and the predicted preoperative autologous donation (PAD) needs for both THA and TKA patients. Using these nomograms allows a surgeon to determine a patient's needs based on the anticipated EBL and a reasonable transfusion trigger. Keating et al. (37) developed nomograms for TKA and bilateral TKA that are similar to the nomogram developed by Nelson et al. (51).

The availability of intervention opportunities also played a role in the generation of substantial statistically valid clinical data related to blood usage in patients undergoing THA and TKA. Several large multicenter studies demonstrated that preoperative hemoglobin was a statistically powerful predictor of the need for a transfusion. The landmark studies of Faris et al. (22), de Andrade et al. (18), and Goodnough (28) found confirmation in the large multicenter experience reported by Bierbaum et al. (6). In a broad sweep study of transfusion experience in THA and TKA surgery, the authors evaluated the transfusion experience of 9482 patients. They identified several important features of blood management approaches in use prior to 1999: (a) the need for transfusion was directly related to the preoperative hemoglobin, with 29% of patients with hemoglobin between 10 and 13 g/dL requiring transfusion versus 8% of patients with Hb greater than 14 g/dL; (b) a large percentage of patients who participated in PAD did not receive transfusions, and this wastage varied by surgical procedure; and (c) despite PAD, a substantial percentage of patients required allogeneic transfusion, again associated with preoperative Hb/Hct and the type of operative intervention (6).

Preoperative Options

Allogeneic Blood Transfusion

Concerns about the quality, availability, and cost of the blood supply have fueled efforts to minimize the need for allogeneic blood transfusion. Transfusion of banked blood, however, has reached new levels of safety and should be relied on should the situation require it. That said, there are many reasons why it will prove beneficial to the surgeon performing hip surgery to apply techniques to *minimize* the use of allogeneic transfusion. Transfusion of allogeneic blood and its byproducts continues to be associated with a number of risks, even if they are small. Current estimates are 1:1,000,000 for HIV, 1:100,000 for hepatitis B, and 1:500 to 1:5000 for hepatitis C. These risks continue to decrease. Other associated risks include the risk of transfusion reactions (fatal and nonfatal hemolytic reactions) and alloimmunization. Of concern is the influence of transfusion on immunomodulation, where increased infection rates have been reported (6,9,12,31,32,47). The exact mechanism and true significance of periprosthetic infection are not yet understood (63). Current estimates suggest that it is likely that allogeneic blood will be required in the perioperative period for some patients. Although a number of options for minimizing the need are outlined below, patients should be made aware that surgeons are concerned not to overly utilize allogeneic blood but that, if needed, it can be used safely. Revision THA, bilateral THA, removal of THA for infection, and surgery in the elderly, including fracture repair, are the surgical interventions in which use of allogeneic transfusions is most likely.

In our hospital system, one unit of allogeneic blood costs approximately $220, excluding the processing costs, which are estimated to double that cost.

Erythropoietin Alfa (EA) plus Oral Iron (Fe) Supplementation

Erythropoietin is the main regulator of erythropoiesis. It is a glycoprotein hormone that is synthesized in the kidney and secreted by the renal cortical interstitial cells as a direct response to tissue hypoxia. Erythropoietin stimulates the recruitment and differentiation of the progenitor cells and ultimately aids in the synthesis of hemoglobin. Erythropoietin alpha (Procrit) (r-HuEPO) is a recombinant product identical in amino acid sequence and biological activity to naturally occurring erythropoietin. Clinically it has been used for the treatment of anemia for over 15 years and has indications for use in patients with chronic renal failure, nonmyeloid malignancies, and HIV infection plus anemia; in critical care patients; and in patients undergoing elective noncardiac, nonvascular surgery. In the elective surgical population, it is indicated for preoperatively determined hemoglobin levels from 10 to 13 g/dL. Two different dosing regimens are available. The two dosing regimens are 300 IU/kg/day (approximately 20,000 IU/day) subcutaneously for 15 days perioperatively (10 days preop, surgery day, and 4 days postop) and 600 IU/kg/week (approximately 40,000 IU/week) subcutaneously starting 21 days prior to the surgery (preoperative days 21, 14, and 7), with the fourth dose given in the recovery room following surgery. The weekly dosing schedule is more commonly used. It is absolutely imperative to utilize iron supplementation when administering an erythropoietic agent such as Procrit. It has been well demonstrated in the literature that even in iron replete patients a functional iron deficiency can take place when r-HuEPO is being administered (16,23,57).

A functional iron deficiency occurs when iron stores are insufficient to mobilize adequate iron for accelerated erythropoiesis associated with r-HuEPO administration even though iron levels appear "normal." The use of 200 to 450 mg of elemental iron every day is encouraged. Some patients encounter difficulties in tolerating oral forms of iron supplementation. Side effects are usually related to GI symptoms such as cramps, nausea, and diarrhea and may require alteration of the dosage or a switch to an alternative product. Patients should be encouraged to take iron with a source of vitamin C, which will increase absorption. Coffee, tea, vitamin E, and dairy products are known to reduce absorption. Parenteral iron supplementation may be more effective in providing iron when patients are intolerant of oral iron or when baseline ferritin is below 100 ng/mL (41).

A number of reports in the orthopedic literature have confirmed the ability of Procrit (r-HuEPO) to increase preoperative (baseline) hemoglobin and decrease the need for perioperative allogeneic blood transfusion (11,23,20). Stowell et al. demonstrated a more predictable avoidance of allogeneic transfusion with Procrit compared preoperative autologous donation in 470 patients undergoing THA and TKA. Use of Procrit was associated with a presurgical rise in hemoglobin of 1.3 g/dL, whereas an overall decrease in presurgical hemoglobin occurred in the PAD group (65). In prospective, randomized studies, there has been no significant safety issues related to the use of Procrit (r-HuEPO) in the orthopedic patient. Specifically, there were no differences in thrombotic/vascular events, blood pressure changes, pain, bruising, and injection site reactions in treated versus placebo populations (6,18,24).

Advantages of the erythropoietin approach include its ease of administration, its effectiveness in raising presurgical hemoglobin, and the absence of major side effects. Disadvantage include the injection approach, the logistics of organizing administration of the drug, and the cost of the drug.

Procrit pricing varies regionally, and the decision whether to reimburse for Medicare patients has been left to the states (although all states now cover administration to Medicare patients). Procrit treatment is reimbursed under Part A of the Medicare program but has not as yet proven financially profitable for the orthopedist. The cost of the treatment is approximately $1600 ($400 per injection), which is reimbursed. There is some suggestion that hospitals that organize to administer Procrit (such as in cancer centers) can make this a profitable undertaking in the elective surgical population. Given that transfusions of two units or less of allogeneic blood are not reimbursed as part of the diagnostic-related groups (DRGs), hospitals may find it worthwhile to organize programs to offer this approach to minimizing transfusion.

Preoperative Autologous Donation

In the elective surgery setting, in interventions where significant blood loss is anticipated, such as major joint reconstruction, preoperative autologous blood donation (PAD) represents an attractive alternative to allogeneic blood transfusion. PAD involves the collection and storage of a patient's blood in the preoperative period to be used in the event that transfusion becomes necessary. This process gained popularity in the 1980s and 1990s because of public fears of transfusion-transmitted HIV. However, as the safety of the blood supply improves and health care costs continue to skyrocket, it is becoming more difficult to justify the costly and often unnecessary process of autologous blood collection.

Under normal circumstances, predonated blood can be stored for 35 days when mixed with adenine citrate phosphate dextrose. The recommended interval between donations of each autologous unit is 5 to 7 days, and the last unit should be donated no less than 3 days prior to surgery. There are several requirements that need to be met prior to donation. Contraindications include these:

- Hct, <34%
- Infection (or patient on antibiotics)
- Unstable angina
- Severe aortic stenosis
- Uncontrolled hypertension
- Weight <50 kg (patient can donate smaller volumes)

PAD has several benefits. It often gives the patient and physician peace of mind and the satisfaction that attempts have been made to avoid receiving donor blood. PAD virtually eliminates the risks of viral transmission and immunologically mediated hemolytic, febrile, or allergic reactions. In addition, it may decrease the risk of transfusion-related immunomodulation, which has been associated with an increased infection rate postoperatively. Multiple studies report reductions in allogenic blood usage when PAD is utilized (55,72).

However, in the past decade vast limitations and disadvantages have been associated with PAD, which have caused most physicians and institutions to reduce or eliminate its utilization.

There are various risks still associated with PAD, such as bacterial contamination and clerical error resulting in transfusion of the wrong unit of blood. Clerical error remains the leading cause of mortality related to transfusion medicine (72). Several other disadvantages exist, especially with regard to the cost-effectiveness of PAD. Nearly half of the PAD collected in the United States every year is discarded. Leftover blood cannot be used for other patients because most autologous donors do not meet the stringent health requirements for allogeneic blood donation. In 1999, approximately 300,000 units of PAD were wasted, at an estimated cost of $180 million (10). Most reports in the medical literature have not found PAD to be cost-effective (7,19). Another consideration is the erythropoietic response to PAD. It is assumed that a patient will rapidly replace RBCs that have been drawn off for PAD purposes prior to the surgery. However, the medical literature appears to disagree (15,27,69). Although the erythropoetic response greatly depends on the time frame for phlebotomy, somewhat of a Catch-22 exists. The longer before surgery the blood is drawn off, the more time the patient will be able to replace phlebotomized RBCs, but the longer blood is stored, the more severe the storage lesion (hemolysis, loss of flexibility, lack of oxygen-delivery capability). If blood is drawn off closer to the surgical procedure, the RBC storage lesion will not be as severe, but the patient will not have had time to replace lost RBCs and will be anemic entering the procedure.

PAD remains a tool to reduce allogeneic transfusion in the elective surgical population. However, as other tools emerge, it is becoming more difficult to justify PAD on the grounds of efficacy and cost-effectiveness. An institution with a large orthopedic program that frequently encourages PAD would most likely benefit from a concerted effort to utilize PAD more judiciously by means of hospital-established, evidence-based guidelines. This may include avoiding PAD in patients who have minimal risk of receiving an allogeneic transfusion (e.g., patients who are receiving a primary total joint replacements and whose Hb >14.0 g/dL) but considering its usage, concurrently with erythropoietin alfa (28,44), in cases that will involve major blood loss (e.g., revisions, bilateral total joint replacements).

Preoperative Options

It is estimated that two thirds of transfusions performed in the United States are related to surgical procedures. Thus surgeons need to be particularly attuned to the steps they can take to minimize the loss of blood in the perioperative period. Elective surgical procedures provide opportunities to plan strategies that can be employed intraoperatively but require cooperation from and collaboration with other health care professionals. Perioperative strategies include modifications of surgical and anesthetic techniques; blood salvage strategies, including acute normovolemic hemodilution, intraoperative cell salvage, and postoperative cell salvage; and the use of hemostatic agents.

Surgical Technique

There is presently great interest in the use of minimally invasive surgical techniques to improve the speed of recovery from THA and other hip surgery without affecting the outcome of the intervention. While atraumatic surgical technique has been an educational and technical goal of all surgical training, this new wave of enthusiasm for less invasive interventions brings with it the promise of less blood loss. There is no literature available at this time to suggest that this has occurred. Whether standard or smaller incision techniques are employed, the hip surgeon should be vigilant in handling tissues to minimize the loss of blood. Irrespective of this handling, however, there is the inherent loss of blood associated with the various techniques of arthroplasty. The increasing use of uncemented components for total hip arthroplasty ensures that a certain amount of bleeding will occur around the components postoperatively, and surgical techniques will have little impact on that bleeding. The published expected EBL for a primary THA is in the range of 4 g/dL, with current information suggesting that the use of uncemented components is associated with an additional 1 g/dL drop in hemoglobin (3,39). The current enthusiasm for resurfacing THA also poses challenges for blood management, as the exposure required for proper placement of components is likely to be greater, not less, than that required for THA. In special situations, such as the Jehovah's Witness population, the surgeon may choose to use cemented fixation interfaces to decrease overall blood loss. There is current interest in the use of electrocautery techniques and collagen shrinking (Tissue Link, TissueLink, Dover, NH) to diminish blood loss at the time of intervention (43). Data from early investigations suggest that EBL can be diminished, but the ability to decrease transfusion rates is not proven. As the surgical blood loss can vary widely by surgeon and patient, proof of the effectiveness of this approach may require individual assessment of the approach for each surgeon's practice (39).

Acute Normovolemic Hemodilution

Acute normovolemic hemodilution (ANH) is performed by drawing off two or more units of fresh whole blood prior to the initiation of the planned hip surgical intervention. The volume removed is replaced with an appropriate volume of colloid to maintain adequate tissue perfusion and oxygenation. The blood is kept in the operating theater and reinfused near the end of the operative intervention. It is anticipated that the blood lost intraoperatively is of lower hemoglobin, and the blood reinfused is fresh whole blood. This technique avoids the potential for clerical error in acquiring and transporting autologous blood for the patient and provides fresh RBCs with effective O_2-carrying capacity perioperatively. The advantage of this strategy is its ability to provide an effective product with minimal risk of error in the acquisition and transport of the patient's own blood. There is little risk of clerical error, and the product is completely safe for the patient. The disadvantages relate to the need for coordination of efforts among the various health care providers, the need for additional time prior to surgery to obtain the required number of units, and its limited use in patients with significant comorbidities. When combined with intraoperative cell salvage techniques, however, the added coordination efforts are minimal. Its use is primarily in those patients who are likely to experience EBL of greater than 2 units.

Experience with this technique in primary and revision THA has been reported (45,53,59).

Hypotensive Anesthesia

Controlled hypotensive anesthesia has been shown to be an effective option for controlling intraoperative blood loss during hip arthroplasty. Sharrock et al. (60) demonstrated that a drop in mean arterial pressure of 10 mm Hg (from 60 to 50 mm) reduced mean intraoperative blood loss from 263 mL to 179 mL ($p = 0.004$) in primary THA patients. Ranawat et al. (53) demonstrated that cemented interfaces improved when these hypotensive techniques were employed instead of conventional normotensive techniques. This institution (Hospital for Special Surgery) has extensive experience with hypotensive anesthesia, and the starting mean arterial pressure used there may be lower than less experienced groups would find acceptable or comfortable. Extensive collaboration with and interest by the anesthesiology team is required if this technique is to be employed. Aggressive intraoperative monitoring (with either an arterial line or a Swan-Ganz catheter) is required.

Intraoperative Blood Salvage

Intraoperative blood salvage requires the use of special equipment and personnel able to operate it. The salvage devices use cell-washing techniques and provide concentrated RBCs for reinfusion intraoperatively and in the early postoperative period. The technique cannot completely remove bacteria or malignant cells and therefore should not be used in surgery where contamination might be present. It has the advantage of providing immediately available blood to the patient in situations where blood loss is extensive. Extensive blood loss and subsequent reinfusion of salvaged blood can result in depletion of clotting factors, and the surgical team (including anesthesiologists) should be prepared to administer fresh-frozen plasma if appropriate. This technique has been demonstrated to be useful and cost-effective when operative interventions are prolonged (e.g., in revision THA) and when EBL greater than two units is anticipated (8,71). Estimated costs for its use vary by hospital setting and can range from $800 to $1500 per operative intervention. Newer devices allow capture of lost blood in amounts of 50 mL or less and may permit this technique to be used effectively for less extensive interventions (29).

Postoperative Blood Salvage

A number of different devices are available to allow for the reinfusion of blood lost after the wound is closed (ConstaVac, Stryker, Kalamazoo MI; Hemovac Autotransfusion System, Zimmer, Warsaw, IN; Autovac, Boehringer Lavs, Norristown, PA; Socoltrans, Smith Nephew Richards, Memphis, TN; HandyVac, Leo Pharmaceutical, Ballerup, Denmark) (21). One system (OrthoPAT, Zimmer, Warsaw, IN) involves the washing of retrieved blood and can be used intra- and postoperatively. Other systems that collect blood from surgical drains involve some degree of filtration. Blood collected through drains will be diluted, hemolyzed to some extent, and devoid of clotting factors. The volume of blood that can be reinfused is thus limited, and most of these systems can be used safely only up to 4 hours after the surgical procedure. The routine use of these systems after THA is controversial for several reasons. There is controversy over the routine use of drains in THA. A number of authors have demonstrated that transfusion rates diminish with the use of drains and that Hg/Hct decreases are less when drains are not used (4,56). In addition, the risk of complications and the cost of these reinfusion systems may not be justified in situations where blood transfusion might not be required, such as in primary THA or other limited hip surgical interventions. In a careful study of the value of the OrthoPAT system, Clark et al. demonstrated that the risk reduction for allogeneic transfusion was greatest in those operative interventions with the greatest potential for blood loss—total hip revision and bilateral THA. In unilateral THA, they demonstrated that the intervention would be 2.03 times less likely to require banked blood when the OrthoPAT was used ($N = 131$ hips). Without PAD, the incidence of banked blood transfusion in primary THA was 26%, and the incidence in revision THA was 51.5% (14). The costs of these systems vary, with the OrthoPAT system being the most expensive. In our hospital, the OrthoPAT system costs $500, with a $30 additional expense for tubing and setup. The comparable cost for two units of PAD in our institution is $1386.

Antifibrinolytics

The three agents potentially useful in the perioperative period (26,49,57) are desmopressin, aprotinin, and tranexamic acid. Their use remains controversial as they are expensive, they may increase the risk of postoperative thromboembolism, their effectiveness is open to question, and they may sensitize patients so that their application may not be repeatable. The reported results in orthopedic populations are limited and somewhat conflicting. Several good reviews of their potential have been written and are useful for those who wish to pursue their evaluation more thoroughly (66).

Desmopressin is a synthetic analog of vasopressin. Within 30 minutes of infusion, it results in release of factor VIII and von Willebrand factor from the vascular endothelium (35), leading to an increase in thrombogenicity and decreased blood loss in patients with known deficiency syndromes. Its effect is less well understood in hemostatically normal patients. An early report of its use in TKA and THA showed no difference from the control (35). It is used rarely at this time.

Aprotinin is a naturally occurring proteinase inhibitor. It inhibits serine proteases such as plasmin, trypsin, and kallikrein. Thus it has the ability to regulate fibrinolysis, modulate the intrinsic coagulation pathway, and stabilize platelet function, and it exhibits anti-inflammatory properties. It has been used with success in cardiac surgery. Early reports of its use in hip surgery suggested mixed results. Janssens et al. reported that high-dose aprotinin reduced EBL in 40 patients undergoing THA from 1943 to 1446 mL ($p < 0.05$) and reduced transfusion requirements from 3.4 to 1.8 units (34). A subsequent report from Hayes et al. (30) showed no effect. A recent multicenter report (46) demonstrated aprotinin to be a safe and effective hemostatic agent in unilateral THA. The researchers performed a placebo-controlled, randomized, double-blind trial comparing three dosing regimens. Seventy-three patients received placebo; 76 received a "low-dose" regimen of aprotinin (500,000 kallikrein inhibitor units [KIU]), with no subsequent dosing; 75 received a "medium-dose" regimen consisting of a 1,000,000-KIU loading dose followed by infusion with

250,000 KIU/hour; and 75 received a "high-dose" regimen consisting of a 2,000,000-KIU loading dose followed by infusion with 500,000 KIU/hour. Thromboprophylaxis was achieved through the administration of warfarin for all patients. The study results demonstrated a significant reduction in blood transfusion (47% transfusion in the placebo group versus 28% in the low-dose group, 27% in the high-dose group, and 40% in the medium-dose group). Intraoperative loss and need for allogeneic transfusion were reduced. There was no difference in postoperative thromboembolic events among the groups. Tenholder and Cushner suggested that, while expensive, antifibrinolytics can be effective and safe for many patients undergoing THA and TKA (66). They commended aprotinin in particular because orthopedic surgeons have had the greatest experience with it, and they recommended its use in situations where blood loss would be substantial and allogeneic transfusion likely. As it is a naturally occurring protein, hypersensitivity reactions are possible, and repeated use must be done with care (66). We have had limited experience with this drug but have found it useful in certain high-risk situations (with the Jehovah's Witness population).

Tranexamic acid blocks the lysine-binding sites of plasminogen, preventing it from forming fibrin, and thus it is an inhibitor of fibrinolysis. To date, most reports of its use have been from outside the United States, where it has been shown to be effective in reducing perioperative blood loss and the need for transfusion. This has been shown for both TKA and THA populations (5,33). The optimum timing of administration has not been confirmed, and several different approaches to the timing of infusion have been reported (66). A recent report by Yamasaki et al. (73) suggested a significant decrease in postoperative blood loss occurred (particularly in the first 4 hours) when 1000 mg of tranexamic acid was infused just before the skin incision. Intraoperative blood loss was similar in the treated and control groups. Continued investigation of this drug is warranted.

Hemostatic Agents

Topical agents include thrombin, collagen, and fibrin glue. There is little literature to confirm their effectiveness in THA or other hip surgery. In one study, fibrin glue, which is made from concentrated fibrinogen and clotting factors, was shown to reduce mean postoperative blood loss in TKA, with blood loss decreasing from 878 to 360 mL in treated patients (40). This study was of 58 patients undergoing primary TKA, and the study material was sprayed on the operative wound prior to closure.

Postoperative Options

Postoperative Procrit

There are occasional situations where Procrit may be useful in the postoperative recovery phase. Such a situation might arise if the recovery of a Jehovah's Witness patient was slowed by significant acute blood loss anemia. The dosing regime is usually 10,000 IU subcutaneously every other day. Procrit is given in combination with iron therapy and can be discontinued when a significant erythropoietic response has begun and the anemia is beginning to resolve.

Special Concerns

Jehovah's Witness

The patient who is a Jehovah's Witness has specific religious parameters that will not allow him or her to accept transfusion as part of an operative intervention. Although centers are evolving that pay specific attention to the needs of these patients, one must be mindful that patients have a right to influence decisions about their care. Some Jehovah's Witness patients will allow the use of cell-salvage techniques, whereas others (approximately 10% in our experience) will not. Procrit and other drug therapies (such as aprotinin) are usually acceptable. Approach modifications, including cementation of interfaces, use of closed cell salvage techniques, modification of transfusion triggers, modification of postsurgical protocols, and other such accommodations, may be necessary. These modifications should be thoroughly discussed and agreed on by patient and health care team before intervention is begun.

Prophylactic Anticoagulation for Venous Thromboembolic Disease

The surgeon and health care team must be recognize that all of the strategies above represent only one aspect of successful perioperative management of the hip surgical patient. Most adult hip surgical interventions present some risk of postoperative thromboembolism (VTED). It is the standard of care to provide some prophylaxis for venous thromboembolism. This is a highly controversial area, and the surgeon will make a choice appropriate for his or her environment. This choice will influence blood loss following hip surgery. Each choice represents a balancing of risks and benefits, and these should be discussed with the patient. All studies addressing the use of blood conservation techniques must specifically control for the anticoagulation approach used.

DEVELOPING STRATEGIES

The establishment of a patient-specific blood management strategy begins with the identification of the individual patient's Hb/Hct. A fingerstick evaluation (Hemoccu) can be used to obtain a general idea of the Hb. This is a screening study only. An Hb of 14 or greater usually requires no additional evaluation, as the patient either may not require transfusion or will proceed with autodonation. In either situation, there will be additional serum hemoglobin obtained prior to surgical intervention (either as part of preadmission testing or as prelude to autodonation).

If a patient's Hb is between 10 and 13 g/dL by the fingerstick method, the patient is sent for a formal blood evaluation. If the level is confirmed, the patient may be a candidate for Procrit or other recombinant therapy approaches (see "Intervention Strategies"). An Hb level below 10 g/dL suggests an anemia that needs further explanation. Formal evaluation by the patient's internist or hematologist will be in order before proceeding with elective THA. The level should be corrected if possible prior to proceeding.

As an individual physician or group, it is difficult but possible (and desirable) to institute a blood management

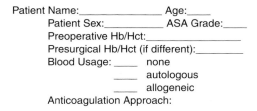

Patient Name:_____ Age:_____
Patient Sex:_____ ASA Grade:_____
Preoperative Hb/Hct:_____
Presurgical Hb/Hct (if different):_____
Blood Usage: _____ none
_____ autologous
_____ allogeneic
Anticoagulation Approach:

Figure 44-1 A simple tool to document surgeon-specific blood usage.

strategy. It is important for each surgeon to understand his or her own influence on a patient's blood loss experience. The surgeon's technique and approach to THA (primary or revision) has a direct impact on the blood lost during surgery. The surgeon must understand that influence on blood lost to be able to predict for a particular patient the depth of fall of Hb and thus the need for subsequent transfusion. This will influence the decision to use preoperative interventions, intraoperative reinfusion approaches, and postoperative strategies. Keeping track of one's own experience through use of a blood evaluation sheet (Fig. 44-1) can aid in assessing that influence.

As mentioned, several nomograms have been developed to determine the likely need for transfusion. These nomograms include in their calculations such items as the patient's starting Hb or Hct, the calculated blood volume, the expected blood loss, and the anticipated transfusion trigger. While somewhat "unwieldy" to use in a busy clinical setting, they do provide some basis for predicting a patient's specific risk of transfusion. They thus allow the surgeon and patient to participate in making decisions about appropriate interventions for addressing the anticipated blood loss.

The development of a hospital-based program requires a commitment from a number of sources. The hospital administration itself must recognize the need for such a strategy,

must help identify the resources available within the hospital (and system) to address the need, must provide educational support for staff and patients to underscore the significance of the effort to improve patient safety and patient outcomes, and must provide consistent feedback to all those involved to ensure that such programs remain meaningful and functional. Figure 44-2 presents an algorithm that can be used to systematically approach patient-specific blood management strategies. The outline in Figure 44-3 suggests some of the decision points that can be addressed in developing a hospital-wide program.

SUMMARY

Blood management in THA arthroplasty should be everyone's business. The current level of understanding of blood management in THA suggests that substantial improvement in patient outcome and significant savings in hospital and patient resources can be achieved through the continued application of evolving principles. Blood management strategies seek to identify the patient's risk for transfusion in relationship to the operative intervention and to offer ways of optimizing the patient's early postoperative Hb as part of a strategy to return the patient to full activity postoperatively. Surgical techniques that minimize blood loss and perioperative programs that individualize choices for blood management will promote the effective use of blood and blood products at a time when prudent use is warranted. If properly focused in a hospital-based or health care system–based program, blood management will result in improved resource utilization, improved patient safety, and cost-efficient use of transfusion products. Individual patient strategies will ensure that each patient has been given the chance to experience a safe and effective recovery from THA and other operative interventions about the hip joint.

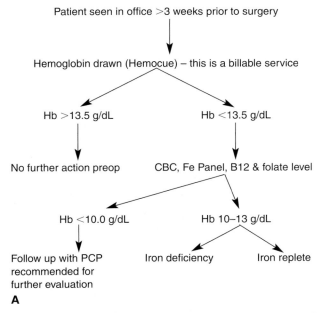

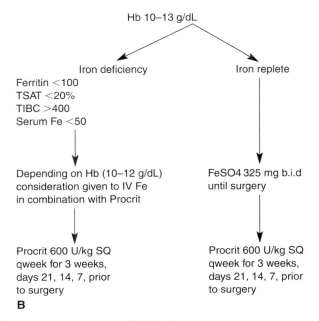

Figure 44-2 **A,B:** Suggested algorithms for determining a patient-specific blood management strategy.

1. Preoperative phase
  a. Evaluation approximately 1 month prior to surgery (Hb). Can be done in the M.D.'s office or elsewhere.
  b. Patients with Hb 10–13 g/dL are put on P.O. FeSO4 and sent to an outpatient area to receive Procrit 40,000 U SQ qweek $\times$ 3 injections.
  c. Hb can be expected to rise 1.5–2.0 g/dL preop.

2. Intraoperative phase
  a. Hypotensive anesthesia
  b. Intraoperative cell salvage
  c. Local treatment: TissueLink, platelet gel
  d. Fibrinolytics: transexamic acid, aprotinin
  e. Drain/no drain/reinfusion drain

3. Postoperative
  a. Setting lower transfusion trigger. National Orthopaedic guidelines:
    i. Non-cardiac: Hb >7.0 g/dL acceptable if patient asymptomatic.
    ii. Cardiac: Hb >8.0 g/dL acceptable if patient asymptomatic.
  b. Use of IV Fe s/p acute blood loss will rapidly support erythropoiesis.

Figure 44-3 Elements of a multi-modality approach to patient-specific blood management.

REFERENCES

1. American College of Physicians. Practice strategies for elective red blood cell transfusion. *Ann Intern Med.* 1992;116:403–406.
2. American Society of Anesthesiologists. Practice guidelines for blood component therapy: a report by the American Society of Anesthesiologists Task Force on Blood Component Therapy. *Anesthesiology.* 1996;84:732–747.
3. An HS, Mikhail WE, Jackson WT, et al. Effects of hypotensive anesthesia, nonsteroidal anti-inflammatory drugs and polymethylmethacrylate on bleeding in total hip arthroplasty patients. *J Arthrop.* 1991;6:245–250.
4. Ayers DC, Murray DG, Duerr DM. Blood salvage after total hip arthroplasty. *J Bone Joint Surg.* 1995;7A:1347–1351.
5. Benoni G, Carlsson A, Petersson C, et al. Does tranexamic acid reduce blood loss in knee arthroplasty? *Am J Knee Surg.* 1995;8: 88–92.
6. Bierbaum BE, Callaghan JJ, Galante JO, et al. An analysis of blood management in patients having a total hip or knee arthroplasty. *J Bone Joint Surg.* 1999;81A:2–10.
7. Birkmeyer JD, Goodnough LT, AuBuchon JP, et al. The cost-effectiveness of preoperative autologous blood donation for total hip and knee replacement. *Transfusion.* 1993;33:544–551.
8. Blais RE, Hadjipavlou AG, Shulman G. Efficacy of autotransfusion in spine surgery: comparison of autotransfusion alone and with hemodilution and apheresis. *Spine.* 1996;21:2795–2800.
9. Blumberg N, Heal JM. Immunomodulation by blood transfusion: an evolving scientific and clinical challenge. *Am J Med.* 1996;101: 299–308.
10. Brecher ME, Goodnough LT. The rise and fall of preoperative autologous blood donation. *Transfusion.* 2001;41:1459–1464.
11. Canadian Orthopaedic Perioperative Erythropoietin Study Group. Effectiveness of perioperative recombinant human erythropoietin in elective hip replacement. *Lancet.* 1993;341:1227–1232.
12. Carson JL. Should patients in intensive care units receive erythropoietin? *JAMA.* 2002;288:2884–2886.
13. Carson JL, Altman DG, Duff A, et al. Risk of bacterial infection associated with allogeneic blood transfusion among patients undergoing hip fracture repair. *Transfusion.* 1999;39:694–700.
14. Clark CR, Spratt KF, Blondin M, Craig S, Fink L: Perioperative blood management in total joint arthroplasty. *J. Arthroplasty,* 2006;21(1):23–25.
15. Cohen JA, Brecher ME. Preoperative autologous blood donation: benefit or detriment? A mathematical analysis. *Transfusion.* 1995; 35:640–644.
16. Cook JD, Skikne BS. Effect of enhanced erythropoiesis on iron absorption. *J Lab Clin Med.* 1992;120:746–751.
17. Corwin HL, Gettinger A, Rodriguez RM, et al. Efficacy of recombinant human erythropoietin in the critically ill patient: a randomized, double-blind, placebo-controlled trial. *Crit Care Med.* 1999;27:2346–2350.
18. de Andrade JR, Frei D, Guilfoyle M. Integrated analysis of thrombotic/vascular event occurrence in epoetin alfa treated patients undergoing major, elective orthopaedic surgery. *Orthopedics.* 1999;22[1 Suppl]:S113–118.
19. Etchason J, Petz L, Keeler E, et al. The cost-effectiveness of preoperative autologous blood donations. *N Engl J Med.* 1995;332:719–724.
20. Faris PM, Ritter MA, Abels RJ. The effects of recombinant human erythropoietin on perioperative transfusion requirements in patients having a major orthopaedic operation. The American Erythropoietin Study Group. *J Bone Joint Surg.* 1996;78A:62–72.
21. Faris PM, Ritter MA, Keating EM, et al. Unwashed filtered shed blood collected after knee and hip arthroplasties: a source of autologous red blood cells. *J Bone Joint Surg.* 1991;73A:1169–1178.
22. Faris PM, Spence RK, Larholt KM, et al. The predictive power of baseline hemoglobin for transfusion risk in surgery patients. *Orthopedics.* 1999;22[1 Suppl]:S135–140.
23. Feagan BG, Wong CJ, Kirkley A, et al. Erythropoietin with iron supplementation to prevent allogenic blood transfusion in total hip joint arthroplasty. *Ann Intern Med.* 2000;133:845–854.
24. Goldberg M, McCutchen J, Jove M, et al. A safety and efficacy comparison study of two dosing regimens of epoetin alfa in patients undergoing major orthopaedic surgery. *Am J Orthop.* 1996;25:544–552.
25. Goodnough LT, Brecher ME, Kanter MH, et al. Transfusion medicine, I: blood transfusion. *N Engl J Med.* 1999;340:438–447.
26. Goodnough LT, Brecher ME, Kanter MH, et al. Transfusion medicine, II: blood conservation. *N Engl J Med.* 1999;340:525–533.
27. Goodnough LT. Brittenham GM. Limitations of erythropoietic response to serial phlebotomy: implications for autologous blood donor programs. *J Lab Clin Med.* 1990;115:28–35.
28. Goodnough LT, Rudnick S, Price TH, et al. Increased collection of autologous blood preoperatively with recombinant human erythropoietin therapy. *N Eng J Med.* 1989;321:1163–1167.
29. Guerra JJ, Cuckler JM. Cost-effectiveness of intraoperative autotransfusion in total hip arthroplasty surgery. *Clin Orthop.* 1995;315:212–222.
30. Hayes A, Murphy DB, McCarroll M. The efficacy of single-dose aprotinin 2 million KIU in reducing blood loss and its impact on the incidence of deep venous thrombosis in patients undergoing total hip replacement surgery. *J Clin Anesth.* 1996;8:357–360.
31. Hebert PC, Qun Hu L, Biro GP. Review of physiological mechanisms in response to anemia. *Can Med Assoc J.* 1997;156:S27–40.
32. Hill GE, Frawley WH, Griffith KE, et al. Allogenic blood transfusion increases the risk of postoperative bacterial infection: a meta-analysis. *J Trauma.* 2003;54:908–914.
33. Hippapala ST, Strid LF, Wennerstrand MI, et al. Tranexamic acid radically decreases blood loss and transfusions associated with total knee arthroplasties. *Anesth Analg.* 1997;84:839–844.
34. Janssens M, Joris J, David JL, et al. High-dose aprotinin reduces blood loss in patient undergoing total hip replacement surgery. *Anesthesiology.* 1994;80:23–29.

35. Karnezis TA, Stulberg SD, Wixson RL, et al. The effects of desmopressin on patients who had total joint arthroplasty: a double-blind randomized trial. *J Bone Joint Surg.* 1994;76A:1545–1550.

36. Keating EM. Personal communication. Closed Meeting of the Knee Society; New York; 2005.

37. Keating EM, Meding JB, Faris PM, et al. Predictors of transfusion risk in orthopaedic surgery. *Clin Orthop.* 1998;No. 357:50–59.

38. Keating EM, Ranawat CS, Cats-Baril W. Assessment of postoperative vigor in patients undergoing elective total joint arthroplasty: a concise patient- and caregiver-based instrument. *Orthopedics.* 1999;22[Suppl 1]:119–128.

39. Lemos MJ, Healy WL. Blood transfusion in orthopaedic operations. Current concepts review. *J Bone Joint Surg.* 1996;78A:1260–1270.

40. Levy O, Martinowitz U, Oran A, et al. The use of fibrin tissue adhesive to reduce blood loss and the need for transfusion after total knee arthroplasty: a prospective, randomized, multicenter study. *J Bone Joint Surg.* 1999;81A:1580–1588.

41. Macdougall IC, Tucker B, Thompson J, et al. A randomized controlled study of iron supplementation in patients treated with erythropoietin. *Kidney Int.* 1996;50:1694–1699.

42. Marik PE, Sibbaldd WJ. Effect of stored blood transfusion on O_2 delivery in patients with sepsis. *JAMA.* 1993;269:3024–3029.

43. Marulanda GA, Ragland PS, Seyler TM, et al. Reductions in blood loss with use of a bipolar sealer for hemostasis in primary total knee arthroplasty. *Surg Technol Int.* 2005;14:281–286.

44. Mercuriali F, Zanella A, Barosi G, et al. Use of erythropoietin to increase the volume of autologous blood donated by orthopaedic patients. *Transfusion.* 1993;33:55–60.

45. Monk T, Goodnough L. Acute normovolemic hemodilution. *Clin Orthop.* 1998;No. 357:74–81.

46. Murkin JM, Haig GM, Beer KJ, et al. Aprotinin decreases exposure to allogeneic blood during primary unilateral total hip replacement" *J Bone Joint Surg.* 2000;82A:675–684.

47. Murphy P, Heal JM, Blumberg N. Infection of suspected infection after hip replacement surgery with autologous or homologous blood transfusions. *Transfusion.* 1991;31:212–217.

48. Muylle L. The role of cytokines in blood transfusion reactions. *Blood Rev.* 1995;9:77–83.

49. National Blood Data Resource Center. FAQs. December 15, 2005. http://www.nbdrc.org/faqs.htm.

50. National Institutes of Health. Consensus Conference. Perioperative red blood cell transfusion. *JAMA.* 1988;260:2700–2703.

51. Nelson CL, Fontenot MD, Flahiff C, et al. An algorithm to optimize perioperative blood management in surgery. *Clin Orthop.* 1998;No. 357:36–42.

52. Nuttall GA, Santrach PJ, Oliver WC Jr, et al. The predictors of red cell transfusions in total hip arthroplasties. *Transfusion.* 1996;36:144–149.

53. Oishi CS, D'Lima DD, Morris BA, et al. Hemodilution with other blood reinfusion techniques in total hip arthroplasty. *Clin Orthop.* 1997;No. 339:132–139.

54. Ranawat CS, Beaver WB, Sharrock NE, et al. Effect of hypotensive epidural anesthesia on acetabular cement-bone fixation in total hip arthroplasty. *J Bone Joint Surg.* 1991;73B:779–782.

55. Renner SW, Howanitz PJ, Bachner P. Preoperative autologous blood donation in 612 hospitals. *Arch Pathol Lab Med.* 1992;116:613–619.

56. Ritter MA, Keating EM, Faris PM. Closed wound drainage in total hip or total knee replacement: a prospective, randomized study. *J Bone Joint Surg.* 1994;76A:35–38.

57. Rutherford CJ, Schneider TJ, Dempsey H, et al. Efficacy of different dosing regimens for recombinant human erythropoietin in a simulated perisurgical setting: the importance of iron availability in optimizing response. *Am J Med.* 1994;96:139–145.

58. Sculco P. Global blood management in orthopaedic surgery. *Clin Orthop.* 1998;No. 357:43.

59. Shander A, Rijhwani T. Acute normovolemic hemodilution. *Transfusion.* 2004;44:26S–34S.

60. Sharrock NE, Mineo R, Urquhart B, et al. The effect of two levels of hypotension on intraoperative blood loss during total hip arthroplasty performed under lumbar epidural anesthesia. *Anesth Analg.* 1993;76:580–584.

61. Simchon S. Influence of reduced red cell deformability on regional blood flow. *Am J Physiol.* 1987;253:898–903.

62. Spence RK. Anemia in the patient undergoing surgery and the transfusion decision: a review. *Clin Orthop.* 1998;No. 357:19–29.

63. Spence RK. Current concepts and issues in blood management. *Orthopedics.* 2004;27(suppl):S643–651.

64. Spiess, BD. Blood transfusion: the silent epidemic. *Ann Thorac Surg.* 2001;72:S1832–1837.

65. Stowell CP, Chandler H, Jove M, et al. An open-label, randomized study to compare the safety and efficacy of perioperative epoetin alfa with preoperative autologous blood donation in total joint arthroplasty. *Orthopedics.* 1999;22(suppl):S105–112.

66. Tenholder M, Cushner F. Intraoperative blood management in joint replacement surgery. *Orthopedics.* 2004;27(suppl):S663–668.

67. Thomas, J. Annual report of the advanced bloodless medicine and surgery: orthopaedic blood utilization 2003/2004. Unpublished data.

68. Walsh TS, McArdle F, McLellan SA, et al. Does the storage time of transfused red blood cells influence regional or global indexes of tissue oxygenation in anemic critically ill patients? *Crit Care Med.* 2004;32:364–371.

69. Wasman J, Goodnough LT. Autologous blood donation for elective surgery: effect of physician transfusion behavior. *JAMA.* 1987;258:3135–3137.

70. Weiskopf RB, Viele MK, Feiner J, et al. Human cardiovascular and metabolic response to acute, severe isovolemic anemia. *JAMA.* 1998;279:217–221.

71. Wilson WJ. Intraoperative autologous transfusion in revision total hip arthroplasty. *J Bone Joint Surg.* 1989;71A:8–14.

72. Woolson ST, Watt JM. Use of autologous blood in total hip replacement. *J Bone Joint Surg.* 1991;73A:76–80.

73. Yamasaki S, Masuhara K, Fuji Takeshi. Tranexamic acid reduces postoperative blood loss in cementless total hip arthroplasty. *J Bone Joint Surg.* 2005;87A:766–770.

Venous Thromboembolism Following Total Hip Arthroplasty

45

Brian T. Feeley   *Jay R. Lieberman*

Total hip arthroplasty is an extremely successful orthopaedic procedure that consistently improves the quality of life of patients. However, there remains a significant risk of morbidity and mortality from venous thromboembolic disease. Despite well-designed clinical studies analyzing the safety and efficacy of a variety of modalities of prophylaxis against thromboembolic disease, an ideal prophylactic agent has yet to be identified. Additional areas that require further study include the appropriate duration of prophylaxis, the influence of different modalities of anesthesia on the rate of deep vein thrombosis, and the treatment of calf vein thrombosis.

Although most surgeons agree that deep vein thrombosis prophylaxis is necessary after total hip arthroplasty, there is no general consensus regarding the best prophylactic regimen. In general, surgeons tend to balance the efficacy versus the safety of the various prophylactic agents available. Surgeons are particularly concerned about bleeding because of its potential impact on hematoma formation, reoperation, and prolonged hospital stays. Our recommendation is that surgeons select a prophylaxis regimen that can be used in an effective and safe manner in their particular practice setting. The purpose of this chapter is to review the literature regarding diagnosis and treatment of venous thromboembolic disease after total hip arthroplasty.

PATHOGENESIS

The formation of thrombi is associated with Virchow's triad of venous stasis, endothelial injury, and hypercoagulabilty. This triad has been found to occur during the perioperative period in total hip arthroplasty. Venous stasis results from positioning of the limb during the procedure, localized postoperative swelling, and reduced mobility after the operation (20,30,33). Occlusion of the femoral vein during dislocation of the hip joint and insertion of the hip prosthesis has been demonstrated with the use of intraoperative venography (20,99,137). In addition, a dramatic reduction in the venous capacitance of the lower extremity and in venous outflow has been demonstrated during hip arthroplasty (97).

Deep vein thrombosis usually develops in areas of decreased flow, often at a valve cusp or the soleal vein. The majority of calf thrombi are small and clinically insignificant. Proximal vein thrombi may be nonocclusive and asymptomatic, and some of

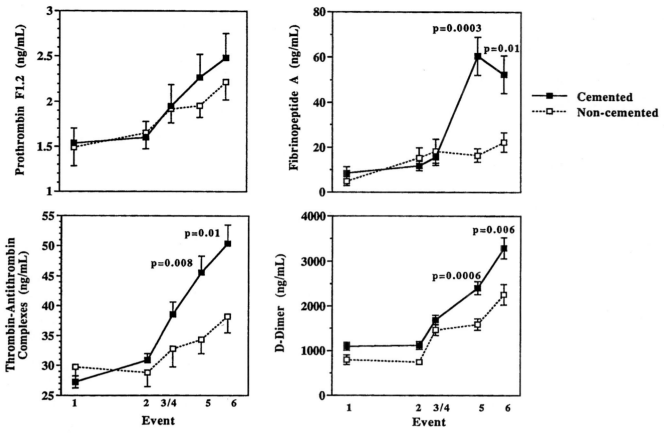

Figure 45-1 The graphs show the changes in prothrombin F1.2, thrombin–antithrombin complexes, fibrinopeptide A, and D-dimer during total hip arthroplasty with a cemented femoral component. There was no change in the level of any of these four markers after insertion of a cementless acetabular component (*second data point*). However, the levels increased with the insertion of the cemented femoral components (*data points 4 and 5*). (From Sharrock NE, Go G, Harpel PC, et al. Thrombogenesis during total hip arthroplasty. *Clin Orthop*. 1995;319:1–12, with permission.)

these will resolve without adverse effects. However, there is a strong association with proximal deep vein thrombosis and pulmonary embolism. Even nonocclusive silent proximal thrombi may result in a symptomatic or fatal pulmonary embolism (80,88,101).

Thrombosis of the veins in the calf is generally an asymptomatic, self-limiting process that resolves spontaneously. There is a low risk of embolization and chronic venous insufficiency. However, unsuppressed thrombi of the calf have the potential to propagate proximally, which leads to a substantial risk of pulmonary embolism.

Injury to the endothelium may occur as a result of positioning and manipulation of the extremity as well as from thermal injury from bone cement (20,112,136). The trauma associated with a total hip arthroplasty can result in sustained activation of tissue thromboplastin factor and other clotting factors, which subsequently localize at sites of vascular injury and areas of venous stasis (24,139). Furthermore, blood loss during the surgery results in a reduction of antithrombin (AT) III and inhibition of the endogenous fibrinolytic system, which allows thrombus growth and propagation (38,51,59,156).

Sharrock and colleagues studied circulating markers of thrombin generation and fibrinolysis during different stages in hip arthroplasty to define exactly when the thrombogenic stimulus reached its peak (130). The procedures were performed under hypotensive epidural anesthesia. They analyzed the production of multiple markers of thrombin generation including prothrombin F1.2, thrombin–antithrombin complexes, fibrinopeptide A, and D-dimer at the following time points: (a) before epidural injection; (b) after insertion of acetabular components; (c) 90 seconds after trial reduction (after femoral reaming); (d) after insertion of a cemented or cementless prosthesis; (e) 90 seconds after final reduction of the hip; (f) and 10 minutes later (Fig. 45-1). The prothrombin F1.2, thrombin–antithrombin, fibrinopeptide A, and D-dimer levels were markedly increased during insertion of the femoral component, but minimally changed by osteotomy of the femoral neck or insertion of an acetabular component. Interestingly, the authors also found the levels of fibrinopeptide A and D-dimer were always significantly greater after insertion of a cemented femoral component compared to a noncemented component. The authors concluded that cementation of a femoral component was associated with global interosseous pressurization and release of thrombo-plastin in bone marrow or fat, which would lead to the pro-nounced increases of thrombin–antithrombin complexes, fibrinopeptide A, and D-dimer when compared to a cement-less prosthesis.

This study confirmed that the period of maximal throm-bogenesis is during the insertion of a femoral component during a total hip arthroplasty. Femoral neck osteotomy and insertion of the acetabular component did not stimulate a significant thrombogenic response. The changes in the thrombogenic markers were more pronounced after inser-tion of a cemented femoral prosthesis compared to a nonce-mented prosthesis. In addition, there was moderate sup-pression of the intraoperative thrombogenesis markers in patients who received 1000 units of heparin just prior to implantation of the femoral component, suggesting that serious consideration be given to selecting modes of pro-phylaxis that can be effective in the perioperative period (130).

EPIDEMIOLOGY

There are many risk factors for the development of deep vein thrombosis (Table 45-1) (64). However, even without under-lying risk factors, patients who undergo total hip arthroplasty are at the highest risk for the development of venous throm-boembolism (29,88). Without either mechanical or pharma-cologic prophylaxis, deep vein thrombosis will develop in 40% to 60% of these patients. Proximal deep vein thrombosis will develop in 15% to 25%, and a fatal pulmonary embolism in 0.5% to 2% (6,29,35,72,80,87,88,152,158). Pulmonary embolism is the most common cause of death after total hip arthroplasty when thromboprophylaxis is not used (134).

TABLE 45-1

RISK FACTORS FOR VENOUS THROMBOEMBOLIC DISEASE

Clinical risk factors
    Advanced age
    Fractures of the pelvis, hip, femur, or tibia
    Paralysis or prolonged immobility
    Prior venous thromboembolic disease
    Surgery—operations involving the abdomen, pelvis,
        lower-extremities, and abdomen
    Obesity
    Congestive heart failure
    Myocardial infarction
    Stroke
Hemostatic abnormalities (hypercoagulable states)
    Antithrombin III deficiency
    Protein C deficiency
    Protein S deficiency
    Dysfibrinogenemia
    Lupus anticoagulant and antiphospholipid antibodies
    Myeloproliferative disorders
    Heparin-induced thrombocytopenia
Disorders of plasminogen and plasminogen activation

Genetic diseases leading to thrombophilic states such as factor V Leiden mutation, antiphospholipid antibody syn-drome, and protein C and S deficiency confer additional risk of venous thromboembolism in the patient undergoing total hip arthroplasty but are often undiagnosed until a major embolic episode. Few studies have examined the rate of deep vein thrombosis in patients with underlying genetic risk fac-tors for venous thromboembolism. Wahlander et al. exam-ined 1600 consecutive patients undergoing total hip arthro-plasty (146). In the patient population, there was a 5.5% incidence of factor V Leiden mutation, and a 2.9% incidence of prothrombin gene mutation. Despite similar prophylactic treatment in all patients, there was a significantly higher rate of deep vein thrombosis and pulmonary embolism in patients with either the factor V Leiden or prothrombin mutation com-pared to age-matched control patients. However, the authors did not recommend routine preoperative blood screening for these gene mutations since the overall risk of pulmonary embolism remained low even in these patients (146).

Lowe et al. (92) examined 375 patients undergoing total hip arthroplasty in multiple centers in Europe for risk factors that lead to increased risk of deep vein thrombosis. They deter-mined that factor V Leiden deficiency was a major risk factor for the development of postoperative venous thromboembolism. However, due to its low overall incidence in the population, they did not recommend preoperative screening for factor V Leiden mutation. Woolson et al. (157) examined 36 patients with heterozygosity for factor V Leiden and found 6 patients with a deep vein thrombosis after total hip arthroplasty, com-pared to 4 out of 43 control patients. This difference was not significant. Since the overall rate of thrombophilic disorders is low and the rate of venous thromboembolism following total hip arthroplasty is not markedly increased in patients with these disorders, routine preoperative screening is not recom-mended at this time.

With shorter hospital stays, the occurrence of deep vein thrombosis increasingly occurs after hospital discharge. White et al. examined over 19,000 hip and knee arthroplasties from 1991 to 1993 in California (151) and determined that although the rate of symptomatic deep vein thrombosis was low (2.8%), a majority (76%) occurred after hospital discharge. Most patients (88%) received either warfarin or low-molecular-weight heparin for chemoprophylaxis, and the average duration of prophylaxis was 4 weeks with warfarin, but not reported for low-molecular-weight heparin. The average time until diagnosis of a symptomatic deep venous thrombosis was 17 days after total hip arthroplasty and 7 days after total knee replacement. This suggests a slower development of deep vein thrombosis following total hip arthroplasty and that perhaps the duration of prophylaxis should be different for these procedures.

Oishi et al. (101) screened 273 consecutive total hip and knee arthroplasty patients with duplex ultrasonography to assess the clinical course of distal deep vein thrombosis. Forty-one patients (15%) developed a distal vein thrombosis. The prevalence of distal vein thrombosis was significantly lower in total hip arthroplasty compared to total knee arthroplasty (9% compared to 23%, respectively). Patients with a positive duplex scan had serial duplex scans on postoperative days 7 and 14. Of the 41 patients with a distal vein thrombosis, 7 (17%) had evidence of propagation by postoperative day 14. Pellegrini et al. (108) reported that 4 of 23 patients (17%) with an untreated calf thrombosis developed a symptomatic pulmonary embolism. Therefore, patients with a distal deep vein thrombosis after total hip arthroplasty are at increased risk of proximal clot propagation and should be anticoagulated or followed closely with serial duplex scans to delineate proximal clot migration.

DIAGNOSIS

The clinical signs of a deep vein thrombosis include pain and tenderness in the calf or thigh, unilateral swelling, erythema, a positive Homan's sign, low-grade fever, and tachycardia. However, in more than 50% of patients, the diagnosis is not apparent by physical exam (8,83,122,143).

Laboratory Tests

Multiple laboratory tests have been developed for the diagnosis of deep vein thrombosis, although their clinical use is currently limited. Routine laboratory studies including complete blood count and serum chemistries are not helpful in the diagnosis of either deep vein thrombosis or pulmonary embolism. Coagulation studies have proven more promising in the diagnosis of deep vein thrombosis. Selective tests for D-dimer have recently been used in the diagnosis of deep vein thrombosis (8,26,103,111,150). Wells et al. (150) demonstrated that in patients who were thought to be clinically unlikely to have a deep vein thrombosis, a negative D-dimer test was effective in ruling out the presence of a clot. Schutgens and colleagues examined 812 patients for suspected deep vein thrombosis (126). The likelihood of a deep vein thrombosis was determined clinically and the patients were graded based on probability of a deep vein thrombosis. One out of 176 patients with low probability score and a negative D-dimer test developed a deep vein thrombosis during follow-up exams. Furthermore, in patients with a high probability score and a negative D-dimer, only 3 out of 39 patients (7.7%) developed a deep vein thrombosis. Thus, although a positive D-dimer test cannot definitively diagnose a deep vein thrombosis, the absence of a positive D-dimer test, especially in patients with low clinical probability, can effectively rule out a deep vein thrombosis. Although no laboratory test to date has been developed that can diagnose the presence of a venous thromboembolism, the D-dimer test is gaining acceptance in ruling out the presence of a deep vein thrombosis or pulmonary embolism (11,103).

Screening Considerations

There has been a continuing trend toward a decrease in the length of hospital stay following primary and total hip arthroplasty (10,54). Due to concerns with compliance and bleeding, as well difficulties with outpatient monitoring, some surgeons have been reluctant to continue postoperative prophylaxis following discharge from the hospital. Postoperative screening has therefore received increased attention because even the most effective forms of prophylaxis are associated with venous thromboembolic events and pulmonary emboli following discharge (6,139). However, despite the improvement in imaging modalities, screening studies appear to be most effective in detection of symptomatic venous thromboemboli (25,145).

Multiple imaging modalities are currently available for the detection of venous thromboemboli. The proper choice in screening options must be made based on the ability to detect proximal deep vein thrombi, as it is well accepted that they are the major source of pulmonary emboli. Safety, cost, reproducibility, and patient comfort all must be factored into the decision as to what screening tool to use. At present, the modalities that can be considered for screening after total hip arthroplasty are contrast venography, venous ultrasonography, Doppler sonography, iodine-125-fibrinogen scanning, and impedance plethysmography.

Contrast venography has classically been described as the gold standard test for the diagnosis of deep vein thrombosis. Contrast venography allows for accurate visualization of the deep venous system of the entire lower extremity, including the proximal deep veins and distal calf veins (83,77,117). However, contrast venography has fallen out of favor as a routine screening tool for multiple reasons. It routinely detects small thrombi of questionable importance, it is an invasive study with associated pain, hypersensitivity reactions are relatively common, and thrombi can occur secondary to the venography itself (1,18,74). Furthermore, it is not cost-effective as a routine screening test (122).

Venous ultrasonography is a noninvasive diagnostic imaging technique that gives a two-dimensional cross-sectional representation of tissue and a direct visualization of the thrombus (Fig. 45-2). Ultrasound has emerged as the clinical choice for diagnosis of symptomatic venous thrombosis after hip arthroplasty (19,145). Venous ultrasonography is painless, and it is able to reliably detect thrombi in the proximal veins of symptomatic patients and with interoperator variability (67,68,83). However, the efficacy of ultrasound as a screening tool remains controversial because of concerns related to the ability to accurately detect proximal thrombi in asymptomatic patients (22,40,58,83,154,155).

Robinson et al. (118) performed a prospective randomized study on over 1000 patients to determine the efficacy of duplex ultrasonography as a screening tool following total hip arthroplasty. Patients were treated with warfarin following the procedure and were randomized to either the screening group or the control group that received a sham screening procedure. In the screening group, 13 of 518 patients (2.5%) were found to have an asymptomatic deep venous thrombosis, and 4 patients subsequently developed a symptomatic proximal deep venous thrombosis. In the placebo group, 3 patients developed symptomatic proximal deep venous thrombosis, and 2 had a nonfatal pulmonary embolism. There was no significant difference in the rate of clot formation between the groups, and there was no significant reduction in the rate of pulmonary embolism in the screening group. The authors concluded that use of screening compression ultrasonography at hospital discharge does not seem to be justified in this setting. Another potential problem with using ultrasound as a screening tool is it remains highly dependent on the skill of the operator (56). Thus, it is important that an institution perform a prospective analysis comparing ultrasonography with venography before the former is used to diagnose asymptomatic proximal thrombi.

Impedance plethysmography and ^{125}I-fibrinogen scanning are not used alone as screening devices as they have limited ability to detect proximal thrombi after total hip arthroplasty (36).

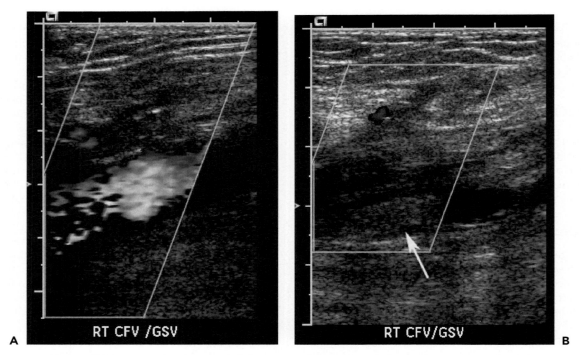

Figure 45-2 A Doppler ultrasound of the common femoral vein. **A:** Patent flow is seen as demonstrated by the bright color flow through the vein. **B:** A thrombus has formed (*arrow*) limiting the flow of blood through the common femoral vein.

The timing of postoperative screening for deep vein thrombosis after total hip arthroplasty remains controversial. Some surgeons prefer to perform screening prior to discharge, and anticoagulation prophylaxis is discontinued if the screening test is negative. Verato and associates performed a prospective study where patients were screened at postoperative day 5 following total hip arthroplasty for venous thromboemboli with ultrasound. Patients received warfarin prophylaxis beginning the evening of the surgery. Nine out of 202 patients had a positive ultrasound and continued therapy. Of the 193 negative patients, only 2 (1%) developed a subsequent deep vein thrombosis, as noted by ultrasound on postoperative day 15 (145). However, with shorter hospital stays after total hip arthroplasty, this may no longer be a safe mechanism to protect patients from venous thromboemboli after hip arthroplasty. In general, it appears to be safer and more cost-effective to continue prophylaxis after discharge than to develop and maintain a screening program.

PROPHYLAXIS FOLLOWING TOTAL HIP ARTHOPLASTY

Both pharmacologic and mechanical approaches have been used to decrease the risk of venous thromboembolism after total hip arthroplasty. The pharmacologic approaches have included warfarin, heparin, low-molecular-weight heparin, fondaparinux, aspirin, and dextran. Mechanical approaches have included compression stockings, sequential intermittent pneumatic compression boots, and intermittent plantar compression.

Pharmacologic Methods

Warfarin

Warfarin exerts its anticoagulant effect by blocking a vitamin K hydroxylase in the liver, inhibiting the transformation of vitamin K. The production of vitamin K–dependent clotting factors II, VII, IX, and X are subsequently inhibited (71) (Fig. 45-3). Warfarin has been successfully used for over 40 years as a prophylaxis agent following hip surgery (3,9,35,47,127,156). Warfarin has been shown to decrease the prevalence of deep vein thrombosis by approximately 60% and proximal venous thrombosis by 70% when compared with no prophylaxis (29).

The senior author assessed the efficacy of low-dose warfarin prophylaxis in 1299 patients treated at the UCLA Medical Center following primary or revision total hip arthroplasty performed between 1987 and 1993. Twelve symptomatic pulmonary emboli were diagnosed postoperatively (1.1%). Patients with a prior history of symptomatic venous thromboembolic disease had a significantly increased risk of developing a symptomatic pulmonary embolism after total hip arthroplasty. The incidence of a major bleeding event was 2.3% (32 patients). There was significantly increased risk of developing a postoperative hematoma if the patient's prothrombin time exceeded 17 seconds. The average duration of low-dose warfarin prophylaxis was 15 days. However, there were 616 patients who received an average of 11 days of prophylaxis and only 2 (0.4%) of these patients developed a symptomatic pulmonary embolism. We presently use 2 weeks of low-dose warfarin prophylaxis when this mode of prophylaxis is selected after total hip arthroplasty (90). The target international normalized ratio (INR) value is 2.0.

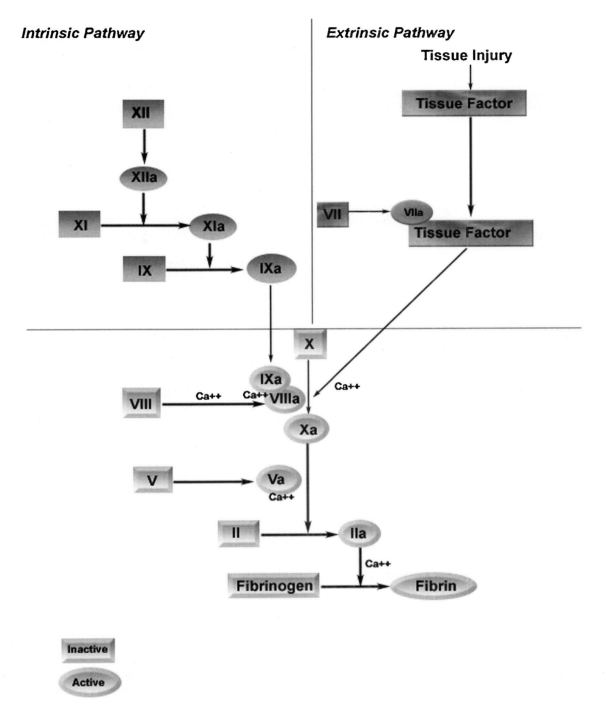

Figure 45-3   The coagulation cascade: intrinsic and extrinsic pathways.

Warfarin has been shown to be effective in decreasing the prevalence of deep vein thrombosis when compared to no prophylaxis (29). Warfarin is administered orally and is less expensive than other anticoagulants (4). However, there are several drawbacks associated with the use of warfarin. Warfarin has been associated with a 1% to 5% occurrence of major postoperative bleeding (4,86,90,105). In addition, warfarin also interacts with other medications due to its metabolism in the cytochrome P450 system in the liver. The combination of warfarin and nonsteroidal anti-inflammatory agents has been shown to increase the risk of hemorrhagic peptic ulcer by nearly 13-fold in an elderly patient population (135). Because protein C and protein S synthesis is also vitamin K dependent, warfarin has a delayed onset of action. In the study by Lieberman et al. (90), the average patient did not reach the target level of anticoagulation (prothrombin time 14 to 17 seconds) until the third postoperative day. Fifty percent of the patients reached the target level of anticoagulation by postoperative day 3, 69% by postoperative day 4, 85% by postoperative day 5, and 92% by postoperative day 6. However, two of the patients developed an in-hospital symptomatic pulmonary embolism on postoperative days 0 and 3, respectively (90). Therefore, when using warfarin prophylaxis, the patients may be left relatively unprotected during the period of greatest risk for the development of thrombosis.

A number of number of studies have compared the use of warfarin to other postoperative treatment modalities in recent years. Freedman et al. performed a meta-analysis of all randomized, controlled trials from 1966 to 1998 that compared the use of one prophylactic agent to another in patients undergoing total hip arthroplasty (52). Fifty-two studies with 10,929 patients were reviewed. Warfarin had the lowest rate of proximal deep vein thrombosis (6.3%), as well as the lowest rate of symptomatic pulmonary embolism (0.16%). There was not an increase in risk of major bleeding episodes postoperatively in patients taking warfarin compared to placebo (52).

Warfarin prophylaxis is usually initiated with a 5-mg dose either the evening before or 10-mg dose the evening of the operation. Subsequent doses are determined by measurement of the prothrombin time or INR. Traditionally, when using the low-dose warfarin protocol, the target prothrombin time was between 1.3 and 1.5 times the control value. However, the anticoagulant effect associated with a particular prothrombin time has varied considerably among different laboratories, depending on the thromboplastin sensitivity (27). To correct this problem, most institutions use the INR), which represents the prothrombin time ratio that would have been obtained if the international reference thromboplastin had been used instead of the local reagent. The INR is defined as the observed prothrombin time ratio raised to the power of the international sensitivity index of the specific thromboplastin used. Current literature supports an INR between 1.8 and 2.5 for prophylaxis after total joint arthroplasty (88).

The warfarin dose is adjusted each day based on the previous INR. There is no consensus on a standard dosing guide for warfarin based on the previous INR. Anderson and colleagues developed a nomogram to properly dose warfarin in the postoperative period following hip arthroplasty (5). Their nomogram was as effective as physician directed therapy in achieving a therapeutic range, maintaining patients in a therapeutic range, and limiting thrombus formation.

Warfarin remains a safe and effective agent for prophylaxis following hip arthroplasty. Although it appears to be not quite as effective as low-molecular-weight heparin in preventing venous thromboembolic disease, there is a decreased risk of bleeding complications. More randomized clinical trials are needed to fully compare warfarin to other treatment modalities.

Heparin

Standard unfractionated heparin is a heterogeneous mixture of glycosaminoglycans. The major anticoagulant effect of heparin is due to the high binding affinity of a unique pentasaccharide and antithrombin III (AT III). The interaction of heparin with AT III accelerates the ability of heparin to inhibit thrombin, factor IX, and factor Xa. A minimum 18-saccharide chain length is required for tertiary complex formation (12,70,73).

Standard low-dose heparin (5000 units administered subcutaneously twice daily) is not recommended after operations on the hip because of its relatively low efficacy in the prevention of proximal deep vein thrombosis (66,87,113,137).

Adjusted-dose heparin has been employed to limit coagulation on the premise that it would be more likely than fixed dose heparin to overcome the hypercoagulable state after total hip arthroplasty (37,87,113,137). The anticoagulant effects of heparin are usually monitored by the activated partial thromboplastin time (aPTT), which is sensitive to the inhibitory effects of heparin on thrombin, factor IX, and factor Xa (12). The first dose of heparin is given 1 to 2 hours preoperatively or within 12 hours after the procedure. Subsequent doses are given every 8 to 12 hours and are adjusted to achieve an aPTT of 1 to 5 seconds more than the upper limit of normal for the hospital laboratory. The blood sample to measure the aPTT time must be drawn 4 to 6 hours after the morning dose of the heparin (88).

In a comparison of adjusted-dose heparin with fixed low-dose heparin, both Leyvraz et al. (87) and Taberner et al. (138) reported that adjusted-dose heparin was more effective and was not associated with increased bleeding. Although adjusted-dose heparin provides effective prophylaxis after total hip arthroplasty, it requires daily laboratory monitoring of the aPTT. Therefore, at the present time it is rarely used as a primary agent for chemoprophylaxis following total hip arthroplasty.

Low-Molecular-Weight Heparin

Low-molecular-weight fractions of commercial heparin are prepared by either chemical or enzymatic depolymerization. The low-molecular-weight heparins are relatively homogeneous in size, with molecular weights between 1000 and 10,000 daltons. They act by enhancing the activity of AT III, although, because of their small size, their primary effect is mediated through the inhibition of factor Xa. Since a minimum chain length of 18 saccharides is required for tertiary complex formation (heparin–AT III–thrombin), low-molecular-weight heparins are able to inhibit factor Xa but not thrombin (Fig. 45-4) (12,70,73).

The low-molecular-weight heparins offer several advantages to standard heparin. There is significantly less bleeding than standard heparin because inhibition of platelet function is reduced, and there is less microvascular permeability than with standard heparin (73). The pharmacokinetics provide additional advantages: the low-molecular-weight heparins have improved bioavailability (90% compared to 30% to 40% for standard heparin); reduced binding to plasma proteins, vascular endothelium, and circulating cells; and a prolonged circulating half-life compared to standard heparin. These properties result in a more predictable antithrombotic effect with little interindividual variation. There are multiple clinical advantages as well. The same dose can be used for all patients (usually a fixed dose based on the body weight in kilograms of the patient), and there is no need for laboratory monitoring. Prophylactic doses of low-molecular-weight heparins do not increase the aPTT or the rate of bleeding (73). The low-molecular-weight heparins are metabolized in the renal system and therefore should be used with caution in patients with renal insufficiency.

The low-molecular-weight heparins as a class of drugs have been shown to safely and reliably reduce the risk of proximal and distal deep vein thrombosis by at least 70% compared to placebo (29,75,98,99,135). Turpie et al. compared the efficacy and safety of enoxaparin with those of placebo after total hip arthroplasty (142). The overall rate of thrombosis was much higher in the placebo group (21 out of 50 patients, 42%) compared to the enoxaparin group (6 out of 50 patients,

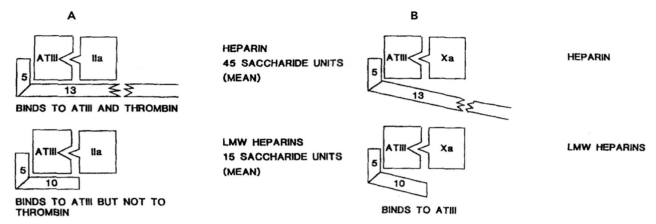

Figure 45-4   A: Inactivation of thrombin. Heparins must bind AT III via the high-affinity pentasaccharide, and thrombin through an additional 13 saccharide units to inactivate thrombin. Low-molecular-weight heparins that do not contain 18 saccharide units bind to AT III but not to thrombin. **B:** Inactivation of factor Xa. Heparins bind to AT III via the high-affinity pentasaccharide to inactivate factor Xa. Both standard heparin and low-molecular-weight heparins can inactivate factor Xa. (From Hirsh J, Levine MN. Low molecular weight heparin. *Blood.* 1992;79:2, with permission.)

12%). In addition, the proximal clot rate was only 4% in the enoxaparin group compared to 20% in the placebo group.

Multiple studies have compared low-molecular-weight heparins to unfractionated heparin (85,113). Both Eriksson et al. (44) and Colwell et al. (32) reported a greater efficacy with low-molecular-weight heparins compared with unfractionated heparin, without an increase in the rate of bleeding. Furthermore, in two meta-analyses, by Nurmohamed et al. (99) and Leizorovicz et al. (84), noted a decreased overall rate of thrombus formation and decreased bleeding when comparing the low-molecular-weight heparins to unfractionated heparin following total hip arthroplasty.

Colwell et al. (31) performed a multicenter randomized trial comparing the efficacy of adjusted-dose warfarin to low-molecular-weight heparin in preventing formation of symptomatic deep venous thrombosis and pulmonary emboli. Patients were analyzed during and after hospitalization. During hospitalization, 4 (0.3%) of the patients who received low-molecular-weight heparin had venous thromboembolic disease compared with 17 (1.1%) of those who received warfarin ($p = 0.0083$). However, at 3 months following discharge, 51 (3.4%) of those managed with low-molecular-weight heparin and 39 (2.6%) of those managed with warfarin had venous thromboembolic disease ($p > 0.05$). There were 26 major bleeding episodes: 18 in the low-molecular-weight heparin group and 8 in the adjusted-dose warfarin group ($p = 0.55$). The risk of a major bleeding episode was related to the timing of the first dose of low-molecular-weight heparin: 14 of the 18 patients in this group had their first dose within 12 hours following surgery. The authors concluded that low-molecular-weight heparin was more effective in the immediate postoperative period in decreasing the risk of symptomatic venous thromboembolism formation than adjusted-dose warfarin, but there was no difference in the rate of deep venous thrombosis following discharge.

Despite the clinical advantages of low-molecular-weight heparins over unfractionated heparins and warfarin, there are significant adverse reactions that limit the efficacy of low-molecular-weight heparins. Most importantly, there is an increased risk of postoperative bleeding episodes with the use of low-

molecular-weight heparins. Multiple studies have demonstrated that postoperative bleeding was associated with administration of enoxaparin within 12 hours following surgery. Geerts et al. found that 5 out of 129 patients receiving enoxaparin 12 hours following total hip arthroplasty had a major bleeding event, compared to only 1 out of 136 receiving adjusted-dose heparin ($p < 0.05$) (57). Similarly, Colwell et al. found an increased rate of major bleeding episodes comparing enoxaparin to warfarin following total hip arthroplasty (18 out of 1516 treated with enoxaparin; and 8 out of 1495 treated with warfarin, $p < 0.05$) (31). In general, it is recommended that enoxaprin be administered a minimum of 12 hours after surgery.

In the North American Fragmin Trial, patients undergoing total hip arthroplasty were randomized to receive dalteparin either preoperatively or a half-dose 4 hours postoperatively, or warfarin the evening of the surgery. During the trial, there were no major bleeding episodes in either the preoperative or postoperative dalteparin group. There was, however, an increased risk of minor bleeding in both the preoperative and postoperative dalteparin group compared to the warfarin group (17.6% in the preoperative group; 20.0% in the postoperative group; 8.9% in the warfarin group, $p < 0.05$ vs. both). There was a significantly reduced incidence of total deep vein thrombosis as well as proximal deep vein thrombosis in the dalteparin groups compared to the warfarin groups (78). Evidence from the North American Fragmin Trial suggest that some low-molecular-weight heparins such as dalteparin may be able to be given in the immediate postoperative period following surgery (4 hours), thus leaving the patient unprotected for a shorter period of time. An analysis of the randomized trials comparing low-molecular-weight heparins to warfarin therapy demonstrated that low-molecular-weight heparins were more effective in reducing overall asymptomatic deep venous thrombosis rates, but with generally higher bleeding rates (31,49,78,79,96,124).

Because of the differences in the compositions, dosing profiles, and activities of the various low-molecular-weight heparins, additional studies will be required to determine if there is a clinically relevant difference between one low-molecular-weight heparin and another. Cost considerations are also a

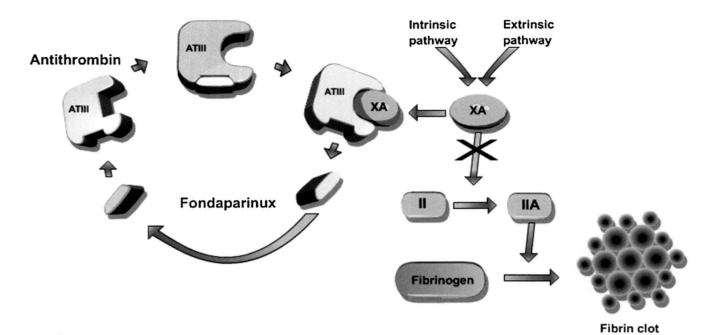

Figure 45-5 Mechanism of action of fondaparinux. Fondaparinux binds to antithrombin III (AT III), causing a confirmational change in the binding site for Factor Xa (Xa). Factor Xa selectively binds to ATIII-Fondaparinux and is subsequently degraded, thus decreasing the formation of factor IIa and clot formation. (Adapted from Turpie AG, Gallus AS, Hoek JA. A synthetic pentasaccharide for the prevention of deep-vein thrombosis after total hip replacement. *N Engl J Med.* 2001;344:619–25, with permission.)

relevant factor in considering the use of these agents in the orthopaedic community. Overall, however, the low-molecular-weight heparins are safe effective agents in limiting the incidence of thromboembolic disease following total hip arthroplasty.

Fondaparinux

Fondaparinux is a new entirely synthetic agent that acts as a specific inhibitor of factor Xa, with no direct inhibition of thrombin (109,110,147) (Fig. 45-5). The antithrombotic activity of fondaparinux is due to antithrombin-III mediated selective inhibition of factor Xa. Synthesis of factor Xa occurs at the junction of the intrinsic and extrinsic pathways. Fondaparinux selectively binds to AT III, causing an irreversible conformational change at the binding site for factor Xa. The conformational change enhances the neutralization activity of AT III for factor Xa. Neutralization of factor Xa interrupts the coagulation cascade and inhibits thrombin formation and clot development (Fig. 45-5). Fondaparinux has no influence on platelet activity and does not enhance fibrinolytic activity. Previous dose–range studies have suggested that daily postoperative injections of 2.5 mg fondaparinux could significantly reduce the risk of venous thromboembolism following total hip replacement (141).

Fondaparinux has been compared to enoxaparin, a low-molecular-weight heparin, in multiple studies (140–142). Turpie et al. (140) performed a randomized, double-blind prospective trial in 2275 consecutive patients undergoing elective total hip arthroplasty. Patients received their first dose of fondaparinux 6 hours following the surgery, and their first dose of low-molecular-weight heparin 12 hours following the surgery. Patients in both groups were continued on antithrombotic therapy for an average of 7 days. In the fondaparinux group, 44 out of 784 patients had a deep venous thrombus formation (5.6%). The low-molecular-weight heparin group performed similarly, with 65 out of 796 patients with overall deep venous thrombus formation (8.2%, $p = 0.099$). There was no difference between groups in proximal thrombus formation (fondaparinux 1.7%, low-molecular-weight heparin 1.2%), or in symptomatic pulmonary embolism group (fondaparinux 0.4%, low-molecular-weight heparin 0.1%).

Side effects from fondaparinux appear to be limited. The most common major adverse effect was bleeding. The risk of a major bleeding episode was increased significantly if the first dose of fondaparinux was administered within 6 hours of the surgery. Thrombocytopenia was another common adverse effect, with moderate thrombocytopenia (50,000 to 100,000 platelets/mL) occurring in 2.9% of patients, and severe thrombocytopenia (less than 50,000 platelets/mL) occurring in 0.2% of patients. Since fondaparinux is metabolized in the kidney and excreted in the urine, severe renal impairment is a contraindication for its use. Periodic hematocrit, platelet counts, and serum creatine levels are recommended for patients who are administered fondaparinux.

At this point, fondaparinux appears to be as safe and effective as the low-molecular-weight heparins in chemoprophylaxis following total hip replacement. However, more studies will need to be performed as fondaparinux becomes more widely used in the orthopaedic community.

Aspirin

Aspirin inhibits platelet aggregation by inhibiting thromboxane A2, thereby decreasing thrombus formation. Historically, aspirin has been used as a chemoprophylactic agent following total hip arthroplasty to prevent thromboembolic disease.

Although aspirin does lower the risk thrombotic complications following total hip arthroplasty, it is not as effective as either low-molecular-weight heparins or warfarin in preventing symptomatic thrombotic disease.

As part of a larger randomized multicenter study, The Pulmonary Embolism Prevention (PEP) Trial examined 4088 patients undergoing elective arthroplasty (115). The patients were randomized to 35 days of aspirin ($n = 2047$) or placebo ($n = 2041$). There were 22 venous thromboemboli in the aspirin group (1.1%), compared to 26 in the placebo group (1.3%). There were 8 pulmonary emboli in each group (0.4%) ($p < 0.05$). In addition, 16 patients required evacuation of a hematoma in the aspirin group (0.8%), compared to 8 in the placebo group (0.4%). The authors concluded that aspirin did not reduce the risk of deep vein thrombosis following elective hip arthroplasty procedures. However, the PEP trial had significant limitations with its methodology, including numerous protocol violations in their placebo group (32% of the patients received aspirin or another NSAID during the study period, and 35% received low-molecular-weight heparin), thus limiting conclusions that can be made regarding the efficacy of aspirin as a prophylactic agent following total hip arthroplasty.

Freedman et al. performed a meta-analysis comparing agents for risk of deep venous thrombosis (52). Eight studies assessing aspirin as an agent for chemoprophylaxis were identified. In the meta-analysis, aspirin therapy was associated with a 19.7% risk of distal deep vein thrombosis, a 11.4% risk of proximal deep vein thrombosis, and a 1.3% risk of pulmonary embolism (52). In contrast, the reduction with warfarin was 17.1%, 6.3%, and 0.16%, respectively; and 9.6%, 7.7%, and 0.36% with low-molecular-weight heparins, respectively. In summary, aspirin appears to lower the risk of thrombotic complications following total hip arthroplasty but is outperformed by warfarin and low-molecular-weight heparins. However, there are orthopaedic surgeons that still prefer aspirin prophylaxis because of its convenience and safety profile. It is our hope that aspirin will be evaluated in a randomized clinical trial to confirm its efficacy.

Dextran

Dextran has moderate efficacy in the reduction of deep vein thrombosis after total joint procedures. However, the use of dextran is limited because of concerns about volume overloading, hypersensitivity reactions, bleeding, cost, and the availability of alternatives that offer better protection (50,53,63,65,66,91).

Mechanical Methods

Intermittent pneumatic compression

Intermittent pneumatic compression (IPC) boots reduce stasis in the lower extremity by increasing the velocity of venous blood flow and by enhancing local endogenous fibrinolytic activity (2,150). Recent studies have demonstrated no statistical difference in systemic levels of tissue plasminogen activator or plasminogen activator inhibitor 1 with or without the use of IPC boots, suggesting that there is no difference in systemic fibrinolysis (94). The use of these devices is appealing because they do not require laboratory monitoring, there is no potential for bleeding, and they are generally well tolerated by patients.

A number of randomized prospective studies have demonstrated pneumatic compression boots to be effective in reducing the overall rate of deep vein thrombosis, but there is concern about their efficacy with respect to proximal clot formation (7,44). In a randomized, prospective trial, Woolson and Watt (156) studied the efficacy of IPC alone (76 hips), IPC and aspirin (72 hips), and IPC and low-dose warfarin (67 hips). Patients were screened at the time of discharge with either venography on the operated limb or bilateral venous ultrasonography (156). The frequency of proximal deep vein thrombosis was 12% (9 patients) in the IPC group alone, 10% (7 patients) in the IPC and aspirin group, and 9% (6 patients) in the IPC and warfarin group. Although the proximal thrombus rates were similar in all three groups, a significant difference might have been noted if a larger patient population had been analyzed (156).

Lachiewicz and colleagues (81) prospectively studied 330 patients following hip arthroplasty with either aspirin or IPC. Duplex ultrasonography and pulmonary angiograms were performed at 7 to 14 days following surgery. Although there was no difference in the rate of proximal or distal deep venous thrombosis, there was a significantly decreased risk of pulmonary embolism in the IPC group. Although these data are promising, it could be argued that IPC needs to be compared to a more effective prophylactic agent to better assess its clinical utility in preventing symptomatic thromboembolic disease.

Hooker et al. (76) recently performed a prospective study on 425 patients who underwent 502 total hip arthroplasties (324 primary and 178 revisions). The patients were managed intraoperatively and postoperatively with elastic compression stockings and IPC boots alone. Venous duplex ultrasound was performed at 6 days and the patients were subsequently followed for 1 year for the development of thrombi. They determined that IPC alone led to a low prevalence of deep vein thrombosis (4.6%) and symptomatic pulmonary embolism (0.1%), as well as a low rate of wound hematoma formation (1.0%). However, 19 of the 23 clots that formed in the patients treated with IPC were proximal clots, suggesting that IPC has limited efficacy in preventing proximal clot formation.

In three randomized trials comparing the efficacy of warfarin to IPC, a significant difference in proximal clot rates was noted (7,48,106). The proximal clot rates in patients treated with warfarin ranged from 0% to 5%, compared to 5% to 14% proximal clot rates in patients treated with IPC alone following total hip arthroplasty.

Based on the data from the aforementioned randomized trials and the prospective study by Hooker et al., there is concern that IPC devices may have limited effectiveness in the prevention of proximal clot formation. The other major disadvantages associated with IPC are compliance and the inability to provide monitored prophylaxis after hospital discharge. Given the risk of development of a symptomatic pulmonary embolism from a proximal venous thrombus, further investigation is required before pneumatic compression boots can be recommended as a sole means of prophylaxis after total hip arthroplasty.

Intermittent Plantar Compression

Intermittent plantar compression in the foot is another form of mechanical prophylaxis. Phlebographic studies have identified a large plantar venous system that is rapidly emptied with compression of the plantar arch during weight bearing. A pneumatic device ("foot pump") has been developed that fits onto the foot and mimics the hemodynamic effects that occur during normal walking. This device is supposed to increase venous return while not having the risk of bleeding associated with pharmacologic prophylaxis and the discomfort associated with intermittent compression devices of the leg (46,55,123).

Studies comparing intermittent plantar compression to either placebo or a fixed dose of heparin have demonstrated decreased overall thrombosis rates in patients who had intermittent plantar compression as prophylaxis (46,123). Warwick et al. performed a prospective comparison of a foot pump and low-molecular-weight heparin on 290 consecutive patients. Deep vein thrombosis was documented on postoperative day 6, 7, or 8 with venography. Deep vein thrombosis was detected in 24 out of 147 (18%) patients using the foot pumps, compared to 18 out of 143 (13%) using enoxaparin ($p < 0.05$) (148). One patient using the foot pumps had a nonfatal pulmonary embolism, compared to none of the patients treated with enoxaparin.

At this time, intermittent plantar compression cannot be recommended as the sole means of prophylaxis until larger randomized prospective trials are performed comparing this mechanical device to low-dose warfarin or low-molecular-weight heparins. It may serve as an effective adjunctive agent when combined with other pharmacologic agents but this has not been tested in randomized trials.

Compression stockings alone do not reduce the risk of thromboembolism acceptably and, therefore, should not be considered as the sole option for patients who have had a hip arthroplasty (29,98).

INFLUENCE OF ANESTHESIA ON THE RATE OF THROMBOSIS

Multiple studies have documented a decreased rate of deep vein thrombosis in patients who had a total hip arthroplasty performed under spinal or epidural anesthesia compared to patients who have general anesthesia (41,89,116,127,134). Patients in these studies did not receive thromboembolic prophylaxis. It is hypothesized that the decrease in the formation of thrombi associated with regional anesthesia is due to the sympathetic blockade, with subsequent vasodilatation and an increased blood flow to the lower extremities that occurs with this anesthetic technique. Total hip arthroplasty generally results in a hypercoagulable state secondary to systemic activation of the coagulation cascade (Fig. 45-6). Blood loss has been reported to be decreased with the use of epidural anesthesia alone or a combination of epidural and general anesthesia compared to anesthesia alone (39). It has been hypothesized that if loss of blood and transfusion requirements could be minimized, the formation of clots might be decreased (62,89,132–134).

Sharrock and associates (129,131–134) attempted to test this hypothesis by the use of hypotensive anesthesia in patients undergoing a total hip arthroplasty. In a series of studies, these authors demonstrated extremely low rates of proximal clots. Blood loss and transfusion requirements in

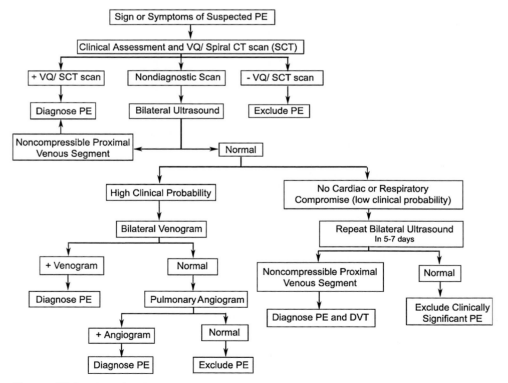

Figure 45-6 Algorithm for diagnosis of a pulmonary embolism. PE, pulmonary embolism; VQ, ventilation-perfusion; CT, computed tomography; DVT, deep vein thrombosis.

these patients were remarkably low compared with those in other studies. The major limitations of hypotensive anesthesia include the need for considerable anesthetic expertise and routine invasive hemodynamic monitoring. These factors may limit the use of hypotensive epidural anesthesia in some centers (89).

There is strong evidence that without prophylaxis, patients who have regional anesthesia have a lower overall rate of deep vein thrombosis than those who have general anesthesia. However, it has not been determined whether regional anesthesia further reduces the formation of thrombi in patients who also receive effective prophylaxis. To date, a prospective, randomized trial has not been performed to answer this important question.

DURATION OF THROMBOPROPHYLAXIS

The optimal duration of thromboprophylaxis following elective total hip arthroplasty remains controversial. There is a perceived risk of increased bleeding episodes as well as wound complications in patients who are treated with prolonged oral or subcutaneous anticoagulant therapy. Although the initial stimulants for thrombus formation occur during the perioperative period, clinically detectable clot formation most likely develops later in the postoperative course. Caprini et al. performed a study to determine when the onset of clot formation occurred in patients who were on warfarin therapy after total hip arthroplasty (28). Nineteen of 125 patients developed a deep venous thrombosis as diagnosed by duplex ultrasonography. Of the 19 patients, 6 (31%) developed a thrombosis at 1 week, and 13 (69%) developed a thrombosis at 1 month after total hip arthroplasty. Late venous thrombosis was much more likely to occur when the target INR did not consistently reach therapeutic range of 2.0 to 3.0.

A prospective, randomized controlled study was performed to determine the effect of prolonged oral anticoagulation on the rate of venous thromboembolism following hip arthroplasty (114). Patients were randomized to discontinue warfarin at the time of hospital discharge (an average of 5 days) or at 4 weeks after the surgery. In the patients treated with warfarin only to the time of hospital discharge, there was a 5.1% incidence of ultrasound confirmed venous thrombosis. Only 1 patient out of 184 (0.5%) developed a deep vein thrombosis in the prolonged treatment group, a difference that was statistically significant compared to the inpatient group. One patient in the extended treatment group did have a major bleeding episode, although the INR was found to be supratherapeutic (5.9). The authors concluded that extending the duration of warfarin treatment safely improved the outcomes of patients who received a total hip arthroplasty.

Heit and colleagues (69) performed a randomized, double-blind, placebo-controlled study on the effectiveness of extended duration low-molecular-weight heparin therapy following total hip or knee replacement. The authors randomized 1195 patients to short-term (4 to 10 days) or extended duration (6 weeks) of ardeparin therapy. Following hospital discharge, there was no difference in the rates of duplex ultrasound documented deep vein thrombosis (1.5% in the extended treatment group, 2.0% in the placebo group, $p > 0.2$). In addition, there was no difference in the rates of major or minor bleeding (2 cases in the extended treatment group, 3 cases in the placebo group, $p > 0.2$). The authors concluded that extended duration of prophylaxis with ardeparin did not significantly reduce the cumulative incidence of symptomatic venous thromboembolism or death after total hip or knee arthroplasty.

The Enoxaparin Clinical Trial Group performed a randomized study to assess the efficacy of enoxaparin treatment following total hip arthroplasty for either 7 days or 3 weeks. The 435 patients were randomized to either short-term enoxaparin followed by placebo, or extended duration enoxaparin treatment. There was a significantly higher incidence of patients with venous thromboembolism in the short-term treatment group compared to the extended treatment group (26.6% vs. 8.0%, $p < 0.05$). The authors concluded that prolongation of enoxaparin thromboprophylaxis following hip replacement for a total of 4 weeks provided therapeutic benefit without a compromise in patient safety (34).

Eikelboom et al. (43) performed a meta-analysis of randomized studies to determine the effects of extended-duration prophylaxis against venous thromboembolism after total hip or knee arthroplasty. Nine studies were reviewed: eight with low-molecular-weight heparin, and one with unfractionated heparin. Extended duration treatment (30 to 42 days) significantly reduced the frequency of symptomatic venous thromboembolism (1.3% vs. 3.3%) as well as asymptomatic venous thromboembolism (9.6% vs. 19.6%). Extended duration therapy had no increase in the rate of major bleeding episodes, although there was an increase in minor bleeding episodes (3.7% vs. 2.5%) that was clinically significant.

Although there is evidence that extending postoperative anticoagulant prophylaxis beyond the hospital course after total hip replacement provides additional safety over short-term chemoprophylaxis, this has not gained widespread acceptance in clinical practice. There have been only two studies assessing the influence of extended prophylaxis in patients using oral anticoagulants. Heit et al. (69) noted no difference in symptomatic clot formation when comparing 4 to 10 days of prophylaxis versus 6 weeks of prophylaxis. Prandoni et al. (114) did find a reduction in clot formation when patients received prolonged warfarin prophylaxis. However, the patients in the control group received an average of only 5 days of warfarin prophylaxis and only 66% (116 of 176) of the patients reached the target level of prophylaxis.

A major problem in determining whether or not prophylaxis should be prolonged is that most of the studies have not assessed symptomatic venous thrombosis or pulmonary embolism as an end point. In addition, the comparison would be more valuable if 2 weeks of prophylaxis was compared to 28 or 35 days rather than stopping prophylaxis at the time of discharge. There are still concerns regarding out-of-hospital monitoring, adverse effects, cost-effectiveness, and patient compliance. In our institution, 2 weeks of postoperative chemoprophylaxis has been safe and effective, and this duration of prophylaxis is supported by most randomized trials in the literature (6,14,17,34,42,88,93,153). However, further studies assessing symptomatic deep venous thrombosis rates are necessary to determine the optimal duration of treatment for each treatment modality. It seems that the ultimate goal should be to risk-stratify patients based on the risk for development of venous thromboembolic disease. In the future, genetic testing may help clinicians identify patients that need prolonged chemoprophylaxis.

DIAGNOSIS OF PULMONARY EMBOLISM

Patients who undergo total hip arthroplasty are at high risk for developing a pulmonary embolism or proximal vein thrombosis. The classic signs of pulmonary embolism include pleuritic chest pain, tachycardia, tachypnea, dyspnea, and a pleurtic rub. Electrocardiogram can be helpful in the diagnosis of pulmonary embolism as it can show tachycardia and a right ventricular strain pattern. The surgeon must maintain a high index of suspicion, as the clinical findings are often nonspecific and subtle.

The primary method of diagnosis of pulmonary embolism is with imaging studies. When a pulmonary embolism is suspected, a ventilation/perfusion (VQ) scan or a pulmonary angiogram, may be used to diagnose a pulmonary embolism. A ventilation/perfusion scan is the appropriate initial study to obtain in many institutions unless the patient has an abnormal chest radiograph. However, due to the high percentage of indeterminate studies (73% of all studies performed) (144) and lack of intraobserver agreement inherent in ventilation/perfusion scans (21), spiral CT scan is becoming the first-line imaging study for diagnosis of pulmonary emboli (125). The major disadvantage of spiral CT scans is the higher number of clinically irrelevant peripheral emboli that can be detected. If the ventilation/perfusion scan demonstrates a high probability of pulmonary embolism, then the patient should be started on either unfractionated heparin therapy or low-molecular-weight heparin and transferred to a monitored setting. If the patient has a low probability of pulmonary embolism following ventilation/perfusion scan, then a duplex scan should be obtained to rule out proximal thrombosis. If a proximal clot is present, then the patient requires heparinization. If the patient has a moderate probability scan and a negative ultrasound, and there is a high index of suspicion, a pulmonary angiogram should be obtained to confirm the diagnosis of pulmonary embolism (107,120).

TREATMENT OF PROXIMAL THROMBUS FORMATION AND PULMONARY EMBOLISM

The objectives of treating a proximal venous thrombus are to prevent a fatal pulmonary embolism, reduce the morbidity from the thromboembolic process, prevent recurrence, and minimize the risk of postphlebitic complications. Treatment of a proximal clot or pulmonary embolism begins with intravenous heparin or low-molecular-weight heparin. Heparin has an immediate effect on the intrinsic cascade of the coagulation system. The first dose of unfractionated heparin is usually a bolus of 5000 USP units followed by a starting infusion of 30,000 USP units/day. However, when pulmonary embolism is diagnosed in the early postoperative period, the initial bolus dose should be eliminated to avoid the risk of major bleeding episodes (82). The first aPTT is obtained 4 to 6 hours after the initial bolus dose and is used to properly titrate the rate of heparin infusion. The goal is to maintain an aPTT

between 1.5 and 2 times the laboratory value. During the heparin therapy, the patient should be monitored closely for complications associated with heparin use. Gastrointestinal prophylaxis with pepcid to limit the risk of ulcer bleeding should be administered. The hematocrit and platelets should be monitored daily as well, as heparin-induced-thrombocytopenia is a well-recognized complication of heparin therapy. Lawson, et al. (82), determined that there was a significantly higher risk of other postoperative complications including gastrointestinal bleeding, hematoma formation, loosening of the prosthesis, and early revision arthroplasty in patients who receive heparin therapy in the early postoperative period for treatment of a suspected pulmonary embolism. Therefore, the decision whether or not to administer intravenous heparin in a patient with a unconfirmed diagnosis of pulmonary embolism should be based on the clinician's index of suspicion.

Until recently, intravenous heparin has been the mainstay for early therapy for an acute pulmonary embolism or proximal thrombus. Studies have now been performed to compare low-molecular-weight heparin to intravenous heparin in the acute treatment of pulmonary embolism. In a study by Findik et al., there was no difference in mortality or repeat pulmonary emboli in patients treated with enoxaparin or heparin (45). Simmoneau et al. prospectively randomized 612 patients with acute pulmonary embolism to either intravenous heparin or low-molecular-weight heparin, followed by oral anticoagulation therapy. At two time points (8 days and 90 days), there was no difference in the rates of recurrent thromboembolism, major bleeding, or death. The authors concluded that low-molecular-weight heparin therapy was as safe and effective as intravenous heparin. Although some studies suggest low-molecular-weight heparins may still be better suited to treat smaller or asymptomatic pulmonary emboli (60), there is accumulating evidence that treatment of acute pulmonary emboli with low-molecular-weight heparins is quite reasonable. Currently, a dose of 2 mg/kg of low-molecular-weight heparin is given twice a day. The patient is treated with the low-molecular-weight heparin and warfarin until the INR reaches 2.0 for two consecutive days.

The purpose of heparin therapy is to prevent extension of the clots and recurrence of the pulmonary embolism. Warfarin therapy is initiated at the same time as the heparin therapy. Once the INR reaches 2.0 to 3.0 for two consecutive days, the heparin therapy may be discontinued. If a patient develops a clot within the first 10 days after total hip arthroplasty, we recommend keeping the INR at 2.0 to reduce the risk of hematoma formation. Although there is no firm guideline, warfarin therapy is usually continued for 6 months. Contraindications for long-term warfarin therapy include pregnancy, liver insufficiency, noncompliance, alcoholism, uncontrolled hypertension, active bleeding, and inability to comply with monitoring (119).

There is general agreement that proximal deep vein thrombosis should be treated with anticoagulation, but the treatment of isolated calf deep vein thrombosis following total hip arthroplasty remains controversial. It has been well documented that patients with an isolated calf vein thrombosis are at risk for proximal extension (101,108,119). Oishi et al. documented a 17% rate of proximal clot propagation after total joint arthroplasty. In addition, patients with untreated deep calf vein thrombosis are at increased risk of developing post-phlebitic syndrome (101).

There are a number of alternatives to intravenous heparin therapy for patients who develop isolated calf vein thrombosis following total hip arthroplasty. Pellegrini et al. reported that none of the 55 patients with a calf vein thrombosis treated with low-dose warfarin developed a symptomatic pulmonary embolism (108). The INR was maintained between 2.0 and 3.0 in this study. The duration of anticoagulation therapy remains controversial, and recommendations range from 6 weeks to 3 months (119). Oishi et al. recommended that duplex scan be repeated 2 weeks after total hip arthroplasty. No thrombus propagation occurred if proximal extension had not occurred by 2 weeks after joint arthroplasty (101). To date, there have been no randomized trials assessing the efficacy of anticoagulation compared to serial screening for calf deep vein thrombosis. Based on the available data we recommend either continuing warfarin prophylaxis for 6 weeks if a calf thrombus is diagnosed or repeating the duplex ultrasound each week for at least 2 weeks to be certain that there has been no proximal clot propagation.

A vena cava filter is usually not necessary for routine prophylaxis after hip arthroplasty. A vena cava filter is appropriate in scenarios where the patient is diagnosed with a proximal clot or pulmonary embolism and is unable to receive anticoagulation on a long-term outpatient basis.

PROPHYLAXIS FOR THE HIGH-RISK PATIENT

Patients with a history of symptomatic pulmonary embolism or deep vein thrombosis are at increased risk for developing venous thromboembolic disease after total hip arthroplasty. In our study at UCLA, there was a significantly increased risk of developing a symptomatic pulmonary embolism if the patient had a prior symptomatic pulmonary embolism or symptomatic deep vein thrombosis (88). Adjustments in routine prophylaxis regimens should be considered for such patients.

The senior authors' protocol is to obtain a preoperative duplex ultrasonography study prior to total hip arthroplasty in patients with a history of venous thromboembolic disease. This allows one to delineate an abnormal scan preoperatively so that patients do not receive prolonged prophylaxis (i.e., 6 months) unnecessarily. The preoperative scan should be compared with any scan that is obtained postoperatively. Consideration should be given to combining warfarin prophylaxis with a low-molecular-weight heparin until the INR level reaches 2.0. Another option is to start the warfarin the evening prior to surgery. In addition, we recommend extending the duration of prophylaxis for 6 weeks for these high-risk patients. Although there has been no randomized study in the literature to support this regimen, our data suggest that these patients require more aggressive prophylaxis. A consultation with a hematologist may be helpful when treating patients with a prior deep venous thrombosis.

Patients on chronic warfarin prophylaxis because of a history of atrial fibrillation or a mechanical heart valve need to have an alteration in their prophylaxis regimen. In general, we recommend consultation with the patients' internist or cardiologist to determine the thromboembolic risk. The warfarin

prophylaxis is usually stopped 5 days prior to the operative procedure. The thromboprophylactic regimen instituted will depend on the risk for clot development. In many cases a low-molecular-weight heparin will be administered to the patient after the warfarin is stopped and this agent will be administered until 12 to 24 hours prior to the surgical procedure. Postoperatively, patients are usually administered both warfarin and low-molecular-weight heparin, as well as mechanical devices. The low-molecular-weight heparin is discontinued when the INR reaches 2.0. Although the efficacy of this protocol has not been confirmed via experimental trials, it has been effective in the senior author's practice. When altering the patient's prophylaxis regimen because of a prior history of thromboembolic disease or chronic warfarin prophylaxis, it is important to explain to the patient that there is an increased risk of postoperative bleeding because of the aggressive prophylaxis regimen.

COST-EFFECTIVENESS OF THROMBOPROPHYLAXIS

Multiple studies in the orthopaedic literature have demonstrated that failure to use prophylaxis is expensive, whereas the routine use of preventive measures is cost-effective (4,14–16,96,100,102). Efficacious prophylaxis against deep vein thrombosis not only reduces symptomatic thromboembolic complications and save lives but may also save health care dollars.

Salzman and Davies performed the first cost-effectiveness study of thromboembolic prophylaxis following hip arthroplasty (121). They estimated that aspirin, dextran, heparin, and warfarin reduced the rate of thrombosis and the cost of care of these patients compared to no prophylaxis. Oster et al. also concluded that each of six possible methods of prophylaxis reduced the rate of death and the cost per patient, with the most efficacious options resulting in the greatest cost savings (102).

Paiement et al. (104) calculated that routine in-hospital use of warfarin would save the lives of 16 of every 1000 patients who had a hip arthroplasty and would also decrease the cost of care of these patients by $170,000. According to their theoretical analysis, a combination of low-dose warfarin therapy for 12 weeks after the procedure would result in an extremely low rate of pulmonary embolism (less than 1 in 1000 patients). In addition, a routine ultrasonography before discharge would result in charges of $50,000 for every life that was saved. However, hospital stay was longer at the time the study was published.

Despite its higher cost per dose, studies have suggested that low-molecular-weight heparins may be cost-effective compared to low-dose warfarin (13,15,95,100). Botteman et al. (23) performed a short- and long-term cost-effective analysis of low-molecular-weight heparin and warfarin. They determined that low-molecular-weight heparin resulted in a $133 reduction per patient in the short term, and an $89 reduction per patient over the life span of the patient. They concluded that low-molecular-weight heparin significantly reduced the economic burden of patients and health care providers following total hip arthroplasty.

Recent studies have compared the new agent fondaparinux to enoxaparin and found that fondaparinux is more cost-effective than enoxaparin following total hip arthroplasty (61). Gordois and colleagues found a minimal cost-effective benefit of fondaparinux in Great Britain (61). The £27 reduction was due both to the lower cost of the drug and the lower incidence of thromboembolic events.

Any cost-effectiveness analysis has potential limitations, including uncertainty about many of the assumptions used in the analysis, and the possibility of bias if the study is funded by industry. However, these studies encourage consideration of a variety of factors when selecting a mode of prophylaxis rather than just the frequency of deep vein thrombosis and the acquisition cost of the prophylaxis agent used. They also allow comparison of one intervention with other diagnostic, therapeutic, or preventive considerations that are competing for constrained health care resources.

RECOMMENDATIONS

Total hip arthroplasty is an extremely successful procedure for eliminating pain and dysfunction in patients with hip disease. However, without postoperative chemoprophylaxis, patients are at high risk for venous thromboembolic disease and pulmonary embolism. The most effective prophylactic agents for patients include low-molecular-weight heparin, warfarin, and fondaparinux. Although none of these agents are ideal, they have been demonstrated in controlled trials to be safe and effective in reducing the risk of thrombotic events following total hip arthroplasty. The selection of a particular mode of therapy depends on the experience of the surgeon and the individual factors of the patient. Although the ideal duration of prophylaxis is unknown, a minimum of 10 to 14 days of prophylaxis is safe and effective. Routine screening is not necessary unless patients have a known risk factor for thromboembolic disease. The goal in the future is to risk-stratify patients based on genetic screening to determine the most appropriate agent and duration of prophylaxis.

REFERENCES

1. Albrechtsson U, Olsson CG. Thrombotic side-effects of lower-limb phlebography. *Lancet.* 1976;1:723–724.
2. Allenby F, Boardman L, Pflug JJ, et al. Effects of external pneumatic intermittent compression on fibrinolysis in man. *Lancet.* 1973;2:1412–1414.
3. Amstutz HC, Friscia DA, Dorey F, et al. Warfarin prophylaxis to precent mortality from pulmonary embolism after total hip replacement. *J Bone Joint Surg.* 1989;71A:321–326.
4. Anderson DR, O'Brien BJ, Levine MN, et al. Efficacy and cost of low-molecular-weight heparin compared with standard heparin for the prevention of deep vein thrombosis after total hip arthroplasty. *Ann Intern Med* 1993;119:1105–1112.
5. Anderson DR, Wilson SJ, Blundell J, et al. Comparison of a nomogram and physician-adjusted dosage of warfarin for prophylaxis against deep-vein thrombosis after arthroplasty. *J Bone Joint Surg Am.* 2002;84A:1992–1997.
6. Arcelus JI, Caprini JA, Traverso CI. Venous thromboembolism after hospital discharge. *Semin Thromb Hemost.* 1993;19(suppl 1):142–146.
7. Bailey JP, Kruger MP, Solano FX, et al. Prospective randomized trial of sequential compression devices vs. low-dose warfarin for deep venous thrombosis prophylaxis in total hip arthroplasty. *J Arthroplasty.* 1991;6(suppl):S29–S35.
8. Baker WF Jr. Diagnosis of deep venous thrombosis and pulmonary embolism. *Med Clin North Am.* 1998;82:459–476.
9. Balderston RA, Graham TS, Booth RE, et al. The prevention of pulmonary embolism in total hip arthroplasty. *J Arthroplasty.* 1989;4:217–221.
10. Barrack RL, Sawhney J, Hsu J, Cofield RH. Cost analysis of revision total hip arthroplasty. A 5-year followup study. *Clin Orthop.* 1999;369:175–178.
11. Bates SM, Kearon C, Crowther M, et al. A diagnostic strategy involving a quantitative latex D-dimer assay reliably excludes deep venous thrombosis. *Ann Intern Med* 2003;138:787–794.
12. Becker RC, Ansell J. Antithrombotic therapy. An abbreviated reference for clinicians. *Arch Intern Med.* 1995;155:149–161.
13. Bell GK, Goldhaber SZ. Cost implications of low molecular weight heparins as prophylaxis following total hip and knee replacement. *Vasc Med.* 2001;6:23–29.
14. Bergqvist D. Enoxaparin: a pharmacoeconomic review of its use in the prevention and treatment of venous thromboembolism and in acute coronary syndromes. *Pharmacoeconomics.* 2002;20:225–243.
15. Bergqvist D, Jonsson B. Cost-effectiveness of prolonged out-of-hospital prophylaxis with low-molecular-weight heparin following total hip replacement. *Haemostasis.* 2000;30(suppl 2):130–135;discussion 128–129.
16. Bergqvist D, Matzsch T. Cost/benefit aspects on thromboprophylaxis. *Haemostasis.* 1993;23(suppl 1):15–19.
17. Bergqvist D, Matzsch T, Burmark US, et al. Low molecular weight heparin given the evening before surgery compared with conventional low-dose heparin in prevention of thrombosis. *Br J Surg.* 1988;75:888–891.
18. Bettmann MA, Paulin S. Leg phlebography: the incidence, nature and modication of undesirable side effects. *Radiology.* 1977;122:101–104.
19. Beuhler KO, D'Lima DD, Colwell CW Jr, et al. Venous thromboembolic disease after hybrid hip arthroplasty with negative duplex screening. *Clin Orthop.* 1999:168–177.
20. Binns M, Pho R. Femoral vein occlusion during hip arthroplasty. *Clin Orthop.* 1990;255:168–172.
21. Blachere H, Latrabe V, Montaudon M, et al. Pulmonary embolism revealed on helical CT angiography: comparison with ventilation-perfusion radionuclide lung scanning. *AJR Am J Roentgenol.* 2000;174:1041–1047.
22. Borris LC, Chrstiansen HM, Lassen MR, et al. Comparison of real-time B-mode ultrasonography and bilateral ascending phlebography for detection of postoperative deep vein thrombosis following elective hip surgery. *Thromb Haemost.* 1989;61:363–365.
23. Botteman MF, Caprini J, Stephens JM, et al. Results of an economic model to assess the cost-effectiveness of enoxaparin, a low-molecular-weight heparin, versus warfarin for the prophylaxis of deep vein thrombosis and associated long-term complications in total hip replacement surgery in the United States. *Clin Ther.* 2002;24:1960–1986;discussion 1938.
24. Bredbacka S, Andreen M, Blomback M, et al. Activation of cascade systems by hip arthroplasty. No difference between fixation with and without cement. *Acta Orthop Scand.* 1987:213–235.
25. Brothers TE, Frank CE, Frank B, et al. Is duplex venous surveillance worthwhile after arthroplasty? *J Surg Res.* 1997;67:72–78.
26. Brotman DJ, Segal JB, Jani JT, et al. Limitations of D-dimer testing in unselected inpatients with suspected venous thromboembolism. *Am J Med.* 2003;114:276–282.
27. Bussey HI, Force RW, Bianco TM, et al. Reliance on prothrombin time ratios causes significant errors in anticoagulations therapy. *Arch Intern Med.* 1992;152:278–282.
28. Caprini JA, Arcelus JI, Motykie G, et al. The influence of oral anticoagulation therapy on deep vein thrombosis rates four weeks after total hip replacement. *J Vasc Surg.* 1999;30:813–820.
29. Clagett GP, Anderson FAJ, Levine MN, et al. Prevention of venous thromboembolism. *Chest.* 1992;102(suppl):S391–S407.
30. Clark C, Cotton LT. Blood flow in deep veins of the legs. Recording technique and evaluation of methods to increase flow during operation. *Br J Surg.* 1968;55:211–214.
31. Colwell CW Jr, Collis DK, Paulson R, et al. Comparison of enoxaparin and warfarin for the prevention of venous thromboembolic disease after total hip arthroplasty. Evaluation during hospitalization and three months after discharge. *J Bone Joint Surg Am.* 1999;81:932–940.

32. Colwell CW Jr, Spiro TE, Trowbridge AA, et al. Use of enoxaparin, a low-molecular-weight heparin, and unfractionated heparin for the prevention of deep venous thrombosis after elective hip replacement. A clinical trial comparing efficacy and safety. Enoxaparin Clinical Trial Group. *J Bone Joint Surg Am.* 1994;76:3–14.

33. Comerota AJ, Stewart GJ. Operative venous dilation and its relation to postoperative deep venous thrombosis. In: Goldhaber SZ, ed. *Prevention of Venous Thromboembolism.* New York: Mercel Dekker; 1993:25–49.

34. Comp PC, Spiro TE, Friedman RJ, et al. Prolonged enoxaparin therapy to prevent venous thromboembolism after primary hip or knee replacement. Enoxaparin Clinical Trial Group. *J Bone Joint Surg Am.* 2001;83A:336–345.

35. Coventry MB, Noland DR, Beckenbaugh RD. "Delayed" prophylactic anticoagulation: a study of results and complications in 2,012 total hip arthroplasties. *J Bone Joint Surg Am.* 1973;55A: 1487–1492.

36. Cruickshank MK, Levine MN, Hirsh J, et al. An evaluation of impedance plethysmography and 125I-fibrinogen leg scanning in patients following hip surgery. *Thromb Haemost.* 1989;62: 830–834.

37. Dachavanne M, Ville D, Berruyer M, et al. Randomized trial of a low molecular weight heparin (Kabi 2165) versus adjusted-dose subcutaneous standard heparin in the prophylaxis of deep-vein thrombosis after elective hip surgery. *Haemostasis.* 1989;29:5–12.

38. D'Angelo A, Kluft C, Verheijen J, et al. Fibrinolytic shut down after surgery: impairment of the balance between tissue-type plasminogen activator and its specific inhibitor. *Eur J Clin Invest.* 1985;15:308–312.

39. Dauphin A, Raymer KE, Stanton EB, et al. Comparison of general anesthesia with and without lumbar epidural for total hip arthroplasty: effects of epidural block on hip arthroplasty. *J Clin Anesth.* 1997;9:200–203.

40. Davidson BL, Elliot CG, Lensing AW, et al. Low accuracy of color Dopploer ultrasound in the detection of proximal leg vein thrombosis in asymptomatic high-risk patients. *Ann Intern Med* 1992;117:735–738.

41. Davis FM, Laurenson VG, Gillespie WJ, et al. Deep vein thrombosis after total hip replacement. A comparison between spinal and general anesthesia. *J Bone Joint Surg Am.* 1989;71B:181–185.

42. Douketis JD, Eikelboom JW, Quinlan DJ, et al. Short-duration prophylaxis against venous thromboembolism after total hip or knee replacement: a meta-analysis of prospective studies investigating symptomatic outcomes. *Arch Intern Med.* 2002;162: 1465–1471.

43. Eikelboom JW, Quinlan DJ, Douketis J. Extended duration prophylaxis against venous thromboembolism after total hip or knee replacement: a meta-analysis of the randomised trials. *Lancet.* 2001;358:9–15.

44. Eriksson BI, Kalebo P, Anthmyr BA, et al. Prevention of deep-vein thrombosis and pulmonary embolism after total hip replacement. Comparison of low-molecular weight heparin and unfractionated heparin. *J Bone Joint Surg Am.* 1991;73A:484–493.

45. Findik S, Erkan ML, Selcuk MB, et al. Low-molecular-weight heparin versus unfractionated heparin in the treatment of patients with acute pulmonary thromboembolism. *Respiration.* 2002;69:440–444.

46. Fordyce MJF, Ling RSM. A venous foot pump reduces thrombosis after total hip replacement. *J Bone Joint Surg.* 1992;74B:45–49.

47. Francis CW, Davidson BL, Berkowitz SD, et al. Ximelagatran versus warfarin for the prevention of venous thromboembolism after total knee arthroplasty. A randomized, double-blind trial. *Ann Intern Med* 2002;137:648–655.

48. Francis CW, Pellegrini VD, Marder VJ, et al. Comparison of warfarin and external pneumatic compression in prevention of venous thrombosis after total hip replacement. *JAMA.* 1992;267: 2911–2915.

49. Francis CW, Pellegrini VD Jr, Totterman S, et al. Prevention of deep-vein thrombosis after total hip arthroplasty. Comparison of warfarin and dalteparin. *J Bone Joint Surg Am.* 1997;79:1365–1372.

50. Fredin H, Bergqvist D, Cederholm C, et al. Thromboprophylaxis in hip arthroplasty. Dextran with graded compression or preoperative dextran compared in 150 patients. *Acta Orthop Scand.* 1989;60:678–681.

51. Fredin H, Nilsson B, Rosberg B, et al. Pre- and postoperative levels of antithrombin III with special reference to thromboembolism after total hip replacement. *Thromb Haemost.* 1983;49: 158–161.

52. Freedman KB, Brookenthal KR, Fitzgerald RH Jr, et al. A meta-analysis of thromboembolic prophylaxis following elective total hip arthroplasty. *J Bone Joint Surg Am.* 2000;82A:929–938.

53. Gallus A, Raman K, Darby T. Venous thrombosis after elective hip replacement: the influence of preventive intermittent calf compression or preoperative dextran compared in 150 patients. *Acta Orthop Scand.* 1989;60:678–681.

54. Ganz SB, Wilson PDJ, Cioppa-Mosca J, et al. The day of discharge after total hip arthroplasty and the achievement of rehabilitation functional milestones: 11-year trends. *J Arthroplasty.* 2003;4:453–457.

55. Gardner AMN, Fox RH. The venous footpump: influence on tissue perfusion and prevention of venous thrombosis. *Ann Rheum Dis.* 1992;51:1173–1178.

56. Garino JP, Lotke PA, Kitziger KJ, et al. Deep venous thrombosis after total joint arthroplasty. The role of compression ultrasonography and the importance of the experience of the technician. *J Bone Joint Surg Am.* 1996;78:1359–1365.

57. Geerts WH, Jay RM, Code KI, et al. A comparison of low-dose heparin with low-molecular-weight heparin as prophylaxis against venous thromboembolism after major trauma. *N Engl J Med.* 1996;335:701–707.

58. Ginsberg JS, Caco CC, Brill-Edwards P, et al. Venous thrombosis in patients who have undergone major hip or knee surgery: detection with compression US and impedance plethysmography. *Radiology.* 1991;181:651–654.

59. Gitel SN, Salvati EA, Wessler S, et al. The effect of total hip replacement and general surgery on antithrombin III in relation to venous thrombosis. *J Bone Joint Surg.* 1979;61A:653–656.

60. Goldhaber SZ. Optimizing anticoagulant therapy in the management of pulmonary embolism. *Semin Thromb Hemost.* 1999; 25(suppl 3):129–133.

61. Gordois A, Posnett J, Borris L, et al. The cost-effectiveness of fondaparinux compared with enoxaparin as prophylaxis against thromboembolism following major orthopedic surgery. *J Thromb Haemost.* 2003;1:2167–2174.

62. Gray DH, Mackie CEF. The effect of blood transfusin on the incidence of deep vein thrombosis. *Aust N Z Orthop.* 1989;242: 212–231.

63. Group TDES. Low-molecular-weight heparin (enoxaparin) vs. dextran 70: the prevention of post-operative deep vein thrombosis after total hip replacement. *Arch Intern Med.* 1991;151: 1621–1624.

64. Hansson PO, Eriksson H, Welin L, et al. Smoking and abdominal obesity: risk factors for venous thromboembolism among middle-aged men: "the study of men born in 1913." *Arch Intern Med.* 1999;159:1886–1890.

65. Harris WH, Athanasoulis C, Waltman AC, et al. Prophylaxis of deep-vein thrombosis after total hip replacement. Dextran and external pneumatic compression compared with 1.2 or 0.3 gram of aspirin daily. *J Bone Joint Surg.* 1985;67A:57–62.

66. Harris WH, Salzman EW, Athanasoulis C, et al. Comparison of warfarin, low-molecular-weight dextran, aspirin, and subcutaneous heparin in prevention of venous thromboembolism following total hip replacement. *J Bone Joint Surg Am.* 1974;56: 1552–1562.

67. Heijboer H, Buller HR, Lensing AW, et al. A comparison of real-time compression ultrasonography with impedance plethysmography for the diagnosis of deep-vein thrombosis in symptomatic outpatients. *N Engl J Med.* 1993;329:1365–1369.

68. Heijboer H, ten Cate JW, Buller HR. Diagnosis of venous thrombosis. *Semin Thromb Hemost.* 1991;17:259–268.

69. Heit JA, Elliott CG, Trowbridge AA, et al. Ardeparin sodium for extended out-of-hospital prophylaxis against venous thromboembolism after total hip or knee replacement. A randomized, double-blind, placebo-controlled trial. *Ann Intern Med.* 2000; 132:853–861.

70. Hirsh J, Dalen JE, Deykin D, et al. Heparin: mechanism of action, pharmacokinetics, dosing considerations, monitoring, efficacy and safety. *Chest.* 1992;102(suppl):S337–S351.

71. Hirsh J, Dalen JE, Deykin D, et al. Oral anticoagulants. Mechanisms of action, clinical effectiveness, and optimal therapeutic range. *Chest.* 1992;102(suppl):S312-S326.
72. Hirsh J, Levin M. Prevention of venous thrombosis in patients undergoing major orthopaedic surgical procedures. *Br J Clin Pract.* 1989;65(suppl):2–8.
73. Hirsh J, Levine MN. Low molecular weight heparin. *Blood.* 1992;79:1-17.
74. Hoek JA, Lensing AW, ten Cate JW, et al. The clinical utility of objective diagnostic tests for diagnosing deep vein thrombosis of the leg. *Br J Clin Pract.* 1989;65(suppl):26–35.
75. Hoek JA, Nurmohamed MT, Hamelynck KJ, et al. Prevention of deep vein thrombosis following total hip replacement by low molecular weight heparinoid. *Thromb Haemost.* 1992;67:28–32.
76. Hooker JA, Lachiewicz PF, Kelley SS. Efficacy of prophylaxis against thromboembolism with intermittent pneumatic compression after primary and revision total hip arthroplasty. *J Bone Joint Surg Am.* 1999;81:690–696.
77. Hull RD, Hirsh J, Carter CJ, et al. Diagnostic efficacy of impedance plethysmography for clinically suspected deep-vein thrombosis. *Ann Intern Med.* 1985;102:21–28.
78. Hull RD, Pineo GF, Francis C, et al. Low-molecular-weight heparin prophylaxis using dalteparin extended out-of-hospital vs in-hospital warfarin/out-of-hospital placebo in hip arthroplasty patients: a double-blind, randomized comparison. North American Fragmin Trial Investigators. *Arch Intern Med.* 2000;160:2208–2215.
79. Hull RD, Raskob GE, Pineo G, et al. A comparison of subcutaneous low-molecular-weight heparin with warfarin sodium for prophylaxis against deep-vein thrombosis after hip or knee implantation. *N Engl J Med.* 1993;329:1370–1376.
80. Kakkar VV, Howe CT, Flanc C, et al. Natural history of postoperative deep-vein thrombosis. *Lancet.* 1969;2:230–232.
81. Lachiewicz PF, Klein JA, Holleman JB Jr, et al. Pneumatic compression or aspirin prophylaxis against thromboembolism in total hip arthroplasty. *J South Orthop Assoc.* 1996;5:272–280.
82. Lawton RL, Morrey BF. The use of heparin in patients in whom a pulmonary embolism is suspected after total hip arthroplasty. *J Bone Joint Surg.* 1999;81:1063–1072.
83. Leclerc JR, Illescas F, Jarzem P. Diagnosis of deep vein thrombosis. In: Leclerc JR, ed. *Venous Thromboembolic Disorders.* Philadelphia: Lea & Febiger: 1991:176–228.
84. Leizorovicz A, Haugh MC, Chapuis FR, et al. Low molecular weight heparin in prevention of perioperative thrombosis. *BMJ.* 1992;305:913–920.
85. Levine MN, Hirsh J, Gent M, et al. Prevention of deep vein thrombosis after elective hip surgery. A randomized trail comparing low molecular weight heparin with standard unfractionated heparin. *Ann Intern Med.* 1991;114:545–551.
86. Levine MN, Hirsh J, Landefeld S, et al. Hemorrhagic complications of anticoagulant treatment. *Chest.* 1992;102(suppl):S352–S363.
87. Leyvraz PE, Bachmann F, Hoek JA, et al. prevention of deep vein thrombosis after hip replacement: randomized comparision between unfractionated heparin and low molecular weight heparin. *BMJ.* 1991;303:543–548.
88. Lieberman JR, Geerts WH. Prevention of venous thromboembolism after total hip and knee arthroplasty. *J Bone Joint Surg Am.* 1994;76:1239–1250.
89. Lieberman JR, Huo MM, Hanway J, et al. The prevalence of deep venous thrombosis after total hip arthroplasty with hypotensive epidural anesthesia. *J Bone Joint Surg Am.* 1994;76:341–834.
90. Lieberman JR, Wollaeger J, Dorey F, et al. The efficacy of low dose warfarin prophylaxis in preventing pulmonary embolism following total hip arthroplasty. *J Bone Joint Surg.* 1997;79A:319–325.
91. Ljungstromg KG, Renck H, Stranberg K, et al. Adverse reactions to dextran in Sweden 1970–1979. *Acta Chir Scand.* 1983;149:253–262.
92. Lowe GD, Haverkate F, Thompson SG, et al. Prediction of deep vein thrombosis after elective hip replacement surgery by preoperative clinical and haemostatic variables: the ECAT DVT Study. European Concerted Action on Thrombosis. *Thromb Haemost.* 1999;81:879–886.
93. Lowe GD, Sandercock PA, Rosendaal FR. Prevention of venous thromboembolism after major orthopaedic surgery: is fondaparinus an advance? *Lancet.* 2003;362:504–505.
94. Macaulay W, Westrich G, Sharrock N, et al. Effect of pneumatic compression on fibrinolysis after total hip arthroplasty. *Clin Orthop.* 2002;399:168–176.
95. Matzsch T. Thromboprophylaxis with low-molecular-weight heparin: economic considerations. *Haemostasis.* 2000;30(suppl 2):141–145;discussion 128–129.
96. Menzin J, Colditz GA, Regan MM, et al. Cost-effectiveness of enoxaparin vs low-dose warfarin in the prevention of deep-vein thrombosis after total hip replacement surgery. *Arch Intern Med.* 1995;155:757–764.
97. Menzin J, Richner R, Huse D, et al. Prevention of deep-vein thrombosis following total hip replacement surgery with enoxaparin versus unfractionated heparin: a pharmacoeconomic evaluation. *Ann Pharmacother.* 1994;28:271–275.
98. Mohr DN, Silverstein MD, Murtaugh PA, et al. Prophylactic agents for venous thrombosis in elective hip surgery. Meta-analysis of studies using venographic assessment. *Arch Intern Med.* 1983;153:2221–2228.
99. Nurmohamed MT, Rosendaal FR, Buller HR, et al. Low-molecular-weight heparin versus standard heparin in general and orthopaedic surgery: a meta-analysis. *Lancet.* 1992;340:152–156.
100. O'Brien BJ, Anderson DR, Goeree R. Cost effectiveness of enoxaparin versus warfarin prophylaxis against deep-vein thrombosis after total hip replacement. *Can Med Assn J.* 1994;150:1083–1090.
101. Oishi CS, Grady-Benson JC, Otis SM, et al. The clinical course of distal deep venous thrombosis after total hip and total knee arthroplasty, as determined with duplex ultrasonography. *J Bone Joint Surg Am.* 1994;76:1658–1663.
102. Oster G, Tuden RL, Colditz GA. A cost-effectiveness analysis of prophylaxis against deep-vein thrombosis in major orthopaedic surgery. *JAMA.* 1987;257:203–208.
103. Oswald CT, Menon V, Stouffer GA. The use of D-dimer in emergency room patients with suspected deep vein thrombosis: a test whose time has come. *J Thromb Haemost.* 2003;1:635–636.
104. Paiement G, Wessinger SJ, Harris WH. Cost-effectiveness of prophylaxis in total hip replacement. *Am J Surg.* 1991;161:519–524.
105. Paiement G, Wessinger SJ, Hughes R, et al. Routine use of adjusted low-dose warfarin to prevent venous thromboembolism after total hip replacement. *J Bone Joint Surg.* 1993;75A: 893–898.
106. Paiement G, Wessinger SJ, Waltman AC, et al. Low-dose warfarin versus external pneumatic compression for prophylaxis against venous thromboembolism following total hip replacement. *J Arthroplasty.* 1987;2:23–26.
107. Patterson BM, Healey JH, Cornell CN, et al. Cardiac arrest during hip arthroplasty with a cemented long-stem component. A report of seven cases. *J Bone Joint Surg Am.* 1991;73:271–277.
108. Pellegrini VD Jr, Clement D, Lush-Ehmann C, et al. The John Charnley Award. Natural history of thromboembolic disease after total hip arthroplasty. *Clin Orthop.* 1996;333:27–40.
109. Petitou M, Duchaussoy P, Herbert JM, et al. The synthetic pentasaccharide fondaparinux: first in the class of antithrombotic agents that selectively inhibit coagulation factor Xa. *Semin Thromb Hemost.* 2002;28:393–402.
110. Petitou M, Lormeau JC, Choay J. Chemical synthesis of glycosaminoglycans: new approaches to antithrombotic drugs. *Nature.* 1991;350:30–33.
111. Philbrick JT, Heim S. The d-dimer test for deep venous thrombosis: gold standards and bias in negative predictive value. *Clin Chem.* 2003;49:570–574.
112. Planes A, Vochelle N, Fagola M. Total hip replacement and deep vein thrombosis. A venographic and necropsy study. *J Bone Joint Surg.* 1990;72B:9–13.
113. Planes A, Vochelle N, Mazas F, et al. Prevention of postoperative venous thrombosis a randomized trial comparing unfractionated heparin with low molecular weight heparin in patients undergoing total hip replacement. *Thromb Haemost.* 1988;60:407–410.
114. Prandoni P, Bruchi O, Sabbion P, et al. Prolonged thromboprophylaxis with oral anticoagulations after total hip arthroplasty: a prospective controlled randomized study. *Arch Intern Med.* 2002;162:1966–1971.
115. Prevention of pulmonary embolism and deep vein thrombosis with low dose aspirin: Pulmonary Embolism Prevention (PEP) trial. *Lancet.* 2000;355:1295–1302.

116. Prins MH, Hirsh J. A comparison of general anesthesia and regional anesthesia as a risk factor for deep vein thrombosis following hip surgery: a critical review. *Thromb Haemost.* 1990;64: 497–500.

117. Rabinov K, Paulin S. Roentgen diagnosis of venous thormbosis in the leg. *Arch Surg* 1972;104:134–144.

118. Robinson KS, Anderson DR, Gross M, et al. Accuracy of screening compression ultrasonography and clinical examination for the diagnosis of deep vein thrombosis after total hip or knee arthroplasty. *Can J Surg.* 1998;41:368–373.

119. Robitalle D, Leclerc JR, Bravo G. Treatment of venous thromboembolism. In: Leclerc JR, ed. Venous thromboembolic disorders. Philadelphia: Lea & Febiger, 1991:267–302.

120. Rosenthal I, Herba MK, Leclerc JR. Diagnosis of pulmonary embolism. In: Leclerc JR, ed. Venous thromboembolic disorders. Philadelphia: Lea & Febiger, 1991:229–266.

121. Salzman EW, Davies GC. Prophylaxis of venous thromboembolism: analysis of cost effectiveness. *Ann Surg.* 1980;191:207–218.

122. Sandler DA, Martin JF, Duncan JS, et al. Diagnosis of deep-vein thrombosis: comparison of clinical evaluation, ultrasound, plethysmography, and venoscan with X-ray venogram. *Lancet.* 1984;2:716–719.

123. Santori FS, Vitullo A, Stopponi M, et al. Prophylaxis against deep-vein thrombosis in total hip repalcement. Comparison of heparin and foot impulse pump. *J Bone Joint Surg.* 1994;76B: 579–583.

124. Sarasin FP, Bounameaux H. Out of hospital antithrombotic prophylaxis after total hip replacement: low-molecular-weight heparin, warfarin, aspirin or nothing? A cost-effectiveness analysis. *Thromb Haemost.* 2002;87:586–592.

125. Schoepf UJ, Costello P. CT angiography for diagnosis of pulmonary embolism: state of the art. *Radiology.* 2004;230:329–327.

126. Schutgens RE, Ackermark P, Haas FJ, et al. Combination of a normal D-dimer concentration and a non-high pretest clinical probability score is a safe strategy to exclude deep venous thrombosis. *Circulation* . 2003;107:593–597.

127. Sculco TP, Ranawat CS. The use of spinal anesthesia for total hip replacement arthroplasty. *J Bone Joint Surg.* 1975;57A:173–177.

128. Seagroatt V, Tan HS, Goldacre M, et al. Elective total hip replacement: incidence, emergency readmission rate, and postoperative mortality. *BMJ.* 1991;303:1431–1435.

129. Sharrock NE, Brien WW, Salvati EA, et al. The effect of intravenous fixed-dose heparin during total hip arthroplasty on the incidence of deep-vein thrombosis. A randomized, double-blind trial in patients operated on with epidural anesthesia and controlled hypotension. *J Bone Joint Surg Am.* 1990;72:1456–1461.

130. Sharrock NE, Go G, Harpel PC, et al. The John Charnley Award. Thrombogenesis during total hip arthroplasty. *Clin Orthop.* 1995;319:16–27.

131. Sharrock N, Go G, Mineo R, et al. The hemodynamic and fibrinolytic response to low dose epinephrine and phenylephrine infusions during total hip replacement under epidural anesthesia. *Anesth Analg.* 1992;76:765–771.

132. Sharrock NE, Mineo R, Urquhart B. Hemodynamic effects and outcome analysis of hypotensive extradural anesthesia in controlled hypertensive patients undergoing total hip arthroplasty. *Br J Anaesth.* 1991;67:17–25.

133. Sharrock N, Mineo R, Urquhart B. Hemodynamic response to low-dose epinephrine infusion during hypotensive epidural anesthesia for total hip replacement. *Reg Anesth.* 1990;15:295–299.

134. Sharrock NE, Ranawat CS, Urquhart B, et al. Factors influencing deep vein thrombosis following total hip arthroplasty under epidural anesthesia. *Anesth Analg.* 1993;76:765–771.

135. Shorr RI, Ray WA, Daugherty JR, et al. Concurrent use of nonsteroidal anti-inflammatory drugs and oral anticoagulants places elderly persons at high risk for hemorrhagic peptic ulcer disease. *Arch Intern Med.* 1993;153:1665–1670.

136. Simonneau G, Leizorovicz A. Prophylactic treatment of postoperative thrombosis: a meta-analysis of the results from trials assessing various methods used in patients undergoing major orthopaedic (hip and knee) surgery. *Clin Trials Meta-Anal.* 1993;28:177–191.

137. Stamatakis JD, Kakkar VV, Sagar S, et al. Femoral vein thrombosis and total hip replacement. *BMJ.* 1977;2:223–225.

138. Taberner DA, Poller L, Thomson JM, et al. Randomized study of adjusted vs. fixed low dose heparin prophylaxis of deep vein thrombosis in hip surgery. *Br J Surg.* 1989;76:933–935.

139. Trowbridge A, Boese CK, Woodruff B, et al. Incidence of posthospitalization proximal deep venous thrombosis after total hip arthroplasty. *Clin Orthop.* 1994;299:203–208.

140. Turpie AG, Bauer KA, Ericksson BI, et al. Postoperative fondaparinux versus postoperative enoxaparin for prevention of venous thromboembolism after elective hip-replacement surgery: a randomised double-blind trial. *Lancet.* 2002;359: 1721–1726.

141. Turpie AG, Gallus AS, Hoek JA. A synthetic pentasaccharide for the prevention of deep-vein thrombosis after total hip replacement. *N Engl J Med.* 2001;344:619–625.

142. Turpie AG, Levine MN, Hirsh J, et al. A randomized controlled trial of a low-molecular weight heparin (enoxaparin) to repvent deep-vein thrombosis in patients undergoing elective hip surgery. *N Engl J Med.* 1986;315:925–929.

143. Vaccaro P, Van Aman M, Miller S, et al. Shortcomings of physical examination and impedance plethysmography in the diagnosis of lower extremity deep venous thrombosis. *Angiology.* 1987;38: 232–235.

144. Value of the ventilation/perfusion scan in acute pulmonary embolism. Results of the prospective investigation of pulmonary embolism diagnosis (PIOPED). The PIOPED Investigators. *JAMA.*1990;263:2753–2759.

145. Verlato F, Bruchi O, Prandoni P, et al. The value of ultrasound screening for proximal vein thrombosis after total hip arthroplasty: a prospective cohort study. *Thromb Haemost.* 2001;86: 534–537.

146. Wahlander K, Larson G, Lindahl TL, et al. Factor V Leiden (G1691A) and prothrombin gene G20210A mutations as potential risk factors for venous thromboembolism after total hip or total knee replacement surgery. *Thromb Haemost.* 2002;87: 580–585.

147. Walenga JM, Bara L, Petitou M, et al. The inhibition of the generation of thrombin and the antithrombotic effect of a pentasaccharide with sole anti-factor Xa activity. *Thromb Res.* 1988;51: 23–33.

148. Warwick D, Harrison J, Glew D, et al. Comparison of the use of a foot pump with the use of low-molecular-weight heparin for the prevention of deep-vein thrombosis after total hip replacement. A prospective, randomized trial. *J Bone Joint Surg Am.* 1998;80: 1158–1166.

149. Weitz JI, Michelsen J, Gold K, et al. Effects of intermittent pneumatic calf compression on postoperative thrombin and plasmin activity. *Thromb Haemost.* 1986;56:198–201.

150. Wells PS, Anderson DR, Rodger M, et al. Evaluation of D-dimer in the diagnosis of suspected deep-vein thrombosis. *N Engl J Med.* 2003;349:1227–1235.

151. White RH, Romano PS, Zhou H, et al. Incidence and time course of thromboembolic outcomes following total hip or knee arthroplasty. *Arch Intern Med.* 1998;158:1525–1531.

152. Wolf LD, Hozack WJ, Rothman RH. Pulmonary embolism in total joint arthroplasty. *Clin Orthop.* 1993;288:219–233.

153. Wong NN. Fondaparinux: a synthetic selective factor-Xa inhibitor. *Heart Dis.* 2003;5:295–302.

154. Woolson ST, McCrory DW, Walter JF, et al. B-mode ultrasound scanning in the detection of proximal venous thrombosis after total hip replacement. *J Bone Joint Surg.* 1990;72A:983–987.

155. Woolson ST, Pottorff G. Venous ultrasonography in the detection of proximal vein thrombosis after total knee arthroplasty. *Clin Orthop.* 1991;73:131–135.

156. Woolson ST, Watt JM. Intermittent pneumatic compression to prevent proximal deep venous thrombosis during and after total hip replacement. A prospective, randomized study of compression alone, compression and aspirin, and compression and low-dose warfarin. *J Bone Joint Surg.* 1991;73A:507–512.

157. Woolson ST, Zehnder JL, Maloney WJ. Factor V Leiden and the risk of proximal venous thrombosis after total hip arthroplasty. *J Arthroplasty.* 1998;13:207–210.

158. Wroblewski BM, Siney PD, White R. Fatal pulmonary embolism after total hip arthroplasty. Seasonal variation. *Clin Orthop.* 1992;276:222–224.

Nursing Care of the Hip Replacement Patient

46

Regina M. Barden   *Michaelene Abran*

More than 260,000 hip replacements are performed in the United States annually. As the number of surgeries has increased over the past decade, the demands on the staff caring for this cohort of patients have also increased. Patients are coming into physicians' offices with much more knowledge and information on hip replacement surgery as a result of access to information on the Internet, direct consumer marketing, and information provided by the media. This has generally led to increased patient expectations regarding the surgery, recovery, and ultimate outcome of the procedure.

Because of the ability of surgeons to do hip replacements and send patients home quickly, even on the day of surgery, some major alterations have taken place in how nurses and other health care professionals on the joint replacement team need to coordinate patient care in order to provide a safe environment and optimize the outcome of the surgery.

The role of the nurse in the care of the hip replacement patient is to educate, provide safe and competent care, and coordinate the care provided by the multidisciplinary team. Nurses need to accomplish these goals while adhering to staff regulations intended to get patients independent and ready for discharge in a shorter and shorter time frame. This has created the challenge of meeting the high expectations of patients while maintaining nursing staff satisfaction.

As the mandate continues for decreasing length of stay while maintaining a high quality of care, greater importance is placed on streamlining patient care preoperatively, postoperatively, and after discharge.

The nursing role can vary throughout the perioperative phase. A clinical specialist, nurse practitioner, nurse clinician, or physician assistant is often the professional the patient first meets on the initial evaluation in the physician's office. This person is a critical link in providing the continuity of care required for the patient throughout the perioperative phase. While the patient is hospitalized, nurses in admitting, surgery, and recovery and on the postoperative unit will have critical roles to play in providing necessary care. Following discharge from the hospital, home care nurses may also play a vital roll. As hospital stays have become shorter, and fewer patients are qualifying for admission to rehabilitation centers, the role of the home health provider in monitoring the patient for early postoperative complications has become critical.

PATIENT EDUCATION

Patient education begins when the patient is first informed by the physician that he or she is a candidate for joint replacement surgery. The patient must be informed of the preoperative requirements, the mechanics of the surgical procedure, including implant alternatives and choices; the postoperative plan of care; and expectations after discharge. To optimize implant longevity, patients should be made aware of recommendations regarding lifestyle changes, possibly including modification of job responsibilities and recreational activities.

The importance of preoperative education has been shown to decrease anxiety, length of stay, and postoperative pain. Educational interventions can help alleviate patient fears and ultimately improve surgical outcomes (2).

Educating patients and families for hip replacement surgery requires a coordinated approach. It is essential to identify potential learning barriers that the patient may be faced with, such as anxiety and fear, learning or reading disabilities, hearing or vision impairment, and cultural or language differences. Not only are preoperative classes an efficient and effective way to teach multiple patients at one time, but patients often find it beneficial to be able to listen to the questions being asked by other patients. Such classes also provide an opportunity for patients to network with each other, which may help alleviate many of their fears and concerns about surgery. Some programs also include a tour of the unit. Formal preoperative classes allow for a multidisciplinary approach to preparing the patient for surgery and may be provided by any combination of hospital-based nurses, office nurses, therapists, social workers, and physicians.

- **Nursing.** The nurse can provide information on the risks and benefits of surgery and explain how the procedure is done, showing the normal anatomy of the hip and how it changes with arthritis. The nurse can also describe what to expect during the perioperative period. The use of anatomic models, Power Point presentations, and video can be effective for this form of education.
- **Physical therapy.** The physical therapist will focus on the techniques and protocols that will be used to help the patient gain functional independence. The therapist may demonstrate the use of assistive devices such as crutches or a walker and specific exercises that the patient may be able to practice preoperatively. The postoperative goal of the eventual safe return of the patient to his or her own home or environment is stressed, along with the necessary hip precautions.
- **Occupational therapy.** The occupational therapist will focus on activities of daily living following discharge from the hospital, including personal hygiene and dressing. The therapist will discuss the need for assistive devices, along with recommended home and job modifications. Included in the teaching will be postop hip precautions and reinforcement of behaviors that protect a patient's hip from dislocating.
- **Social work/discharge planning.** These health care professionals will be responsible for making the appropriate referral for the patient to a home care agency, rehabilitation unit, or skilled nursing facility. Appropriate discussion of support systems, psychosocial issues, and home needs can help calm patient and family concerns regarding the necessary care and support the patient will require after discharge. Ideally, planning for the postdischarge phase should be initiated in the preoperative phase and continued throughout the course of hospitalization. Insurance and financial concerns can be addressed at this time.

It has been shown that patients retain less than 50% of medical information immediately after listening to and speaking with a health care provider (13). Therefore, other types of educational material, such as videos, teaching websites, and custom or standardized teaching books or pamphlets that patients can take home for additional review can be very useful. Family members should be encouraged to participate in classes or individual teaching sessions to gain a better understanding of how they can be a support for the patient. A contact phone number and contact person for the patient to call with additional questions or concerns can make the patient feel more comfortable and well cared for as the day of surgery approaches.

An alternative to group or classroom-style teaching is to provide patient and family education on a one-on-one basis. This can be done by a nurse working within a physician's practice, and it provides the health care professional a better opportunity to get to know the patient and the specific physical and psychosocial issues that may affect the patient's surgical experience. The educational information can be individualized and made understandable for each patient. One-on-one education is especially useful for patients who require a translator. This teaching format provides an atmosphere that can be much more comfortable for the patient and family, offers a more intimate way for the patient to communicate with the health care provider, and allows the provider to address individual concerns more easily.

The ultimate goal is to have the patient come into surgery with an appropriate understanding of the risks and benefits of surgery, understand what to expect after surgery, know what he or she can do to optimize the outcome, and also have appropriate expectations regarding the procedure. Health care professionals need to help guide the patient in making the decision to undergo surgery while maintaining realistic expectations. The only way to accomplish this is with good communication between the physician, the multidisciplinary health care professionals, and the patient.

PREPARING THE PATIENT FOR SURGERY

Prior to the patient's admittance for surgery, the following areas should be addressed.

- **Preoperative medical clearance.** This clearance should be completed for each patient as a way to identify any medical issues that could adversely affect the patient undergoing this elective procedure.
- **Anesthesia clearance.** Meeting with an anesthesiologist may be indicated for a patient with a previous adverse experience with anesthesia, complex medical issues, or abnormalities with their lumbar or cervical spine that may alter recommended anesthesia techniques or agents.
- **Dental clearance.** This clearance is indicated for patients who have any dental issues or who have not recently had their routine checkup.
- **Pain management.** Evaluation by a pain specialist is helpful for patients coming in for surgery who are opioid sensitive or opioid tolerant. These patients can be difficult to manage postoperatively, and it is useful to discuss these issues and have a perioperative pain management plan in place prior to surgery.
- **Blood management.** As per a physician's protocol, it is necessary to discuss the various blood replacement options. These may include the storing of autologous blood or direct donor blood and the use of a cell saver device. In the anemic population, patients may be identified for erythropoietin therapy.

■ **Insurance authorization.** This is mandatory for coverage of the procedure and hospitalization. The number of hospital days allowed will be indicated. Patients need to be made aware of the number of in-patient hospital days their insurance will allow for their surgery, along with what types of services and facilities are covered after discharge. This information can help the patients develop realistic expectations regarding their hospital stay and posthospital treatments.

■ **Discharge planning.** An assessment of the patient's preoperative functional level, home environment, and available support system is important to help determine what the patient's posthospital needs may be. Discussing the patient's expected level of function and when and where the patient may need assistance may decrease the patient's anxiety regarding discharge to home. This information should be shared with the social service or discharge planner who will be caring for the patient when hospitalized.

As hospital lengths of stays are becoming shorter, it is extremely important that medical, psychosocial, economic, and environmental issues be addressed prior to admission (27). This process is often coordinated by the nurse case manager. The position of RN case manager can be developed to follow elective surgery patients. This person should have clinical expertise in issues specific to hip replacement surgery as well as interdisciplinary team building, problem solving, communication, and relationship skills, along with a strong commitment to collaborative practice (16). The role of a multidisciplinary team manager is to coordinate patient-focused care across a continuum from preadmission through postdischarge. A nurse who knows the patient and the patient's medical and social issues prior to surgery can share this information with the necessary health care providers on the team, which allows for improved planning and individualization of patient care.

Prehabilitation

Hip replacement surgery can place a significant stress on a person's functional capacity. There is evidence that suggests that measures of functional capacity before orthopedic surgery may affect postoperative functional capacity (13,14). Patients with greater fitness preoperatively will have faster rehabilitation after major surgery (14,15).

The prehabilitation process is a way to help prepare patients for the stressors associated with surgery by improving their functional capacity before the surgical event. The goal of this process is to help the patients become stronger physically and thus better able to withstand the stress of surgery, decreasing the length of time required to regain independence postoperatively and enabling them to return to an independent living level more quickly (10).

These programs should be individualized for each patient. Not all patients may be candidates for prehabilitation. Contraindications for prehabilitation may include severe medical conditions, acute trauma, or such debilitation from the patient's orthopedic condition as to make exercise impossible (10). Some of the key components of a prehabilitation program include warm-up, cardiovascular conditioning, strength training, and flexibility exercises. Consultation with a physical therapist is advantageous for patients who are candidates for prehabilitation.

Management of Critical Pathways

A critical pathway is a tool used to coordinate nursing practice and patient care objectives during the perioperative period. It should include a structured approach to routine patient assessment, testing, medications, pain management, wound care, nutrition, activity progress, psychosocial issues, and discharge planning. It can be used as a bedside tool to guide and manage patient progress during the postoperative course.

The use of a pathway allows health care professionals to determine if a patient's recovery is progressing as expected. Variances from the pathway can be documented, and the patient can be returned to the pathway in a timely manner.

Pathways are developed and maintained through a multidisciplinary approach. Regular meetings of pathway members may include a physician, an RN case manager, physician assistant, a staff nurse, a physical therapist, an anesthesiologist, a pain management RN, a physical therapist, an occupational therapist, utilization management and social services personnel. These meetings provide an opportunity to discuss pathway compliance issues, problems with current order sets, and recommended changes for improvement of patient care.

Based on critical pathways, standardized order sets can be developed. This fosters consistency of care among joint replacement patients at a particular institution while still allowing for variations in the practices of individual surgeons. An example of a critical pathway for hip replacement patients can be found in Chapter 57. A challenge for the pathway system is the variation of lengths of stay that are being developed among the individual surgeons. Because of these altered lengths of stay, it can be difficult for institutions to adhere to one pathway for all patients undergoing hip replacement surgery. The development of surgeon-specific pathways for one procedure can make it a less effective tool in the management of hip replacement patients.

SURGERY DAY

In general, patients are usually admitted approximately 2 hours prior to the procedure. Certain medical conditions may require the admission of a patient 1 or more days prior to surgery. The patient is prepared and escorted to the preoperative holding area. In preparing the patient for surgery, the preoperative nurse should focus on decreasing patient anxiety by providing reassurance and answering additional questions the patient may have in a calm and reassuring manner. The nurse initiates correct site verification procedures, including a review of the consent and the medical record number and confirmation of the availability of blood products requested. The nurse will have the patient state his or her name and date of birth, the procedure to be done, and the correct site. Correct site identification is based on the fourth goal developed by the Joint Commission on Accreditation of Healthcare Organization (JCAHO). Nurses involved in caring for patients undergoing surgery need to help establish and implement a policy and procedure that is consistently followed (4).

A thorough preoperative nursing assessment should include a chart review to check for the presence of the medical history and physical exam, laboratory reports, chest x-ray and other necessary imaging studies, ECG results, and current medications. Vital signs, allergies, and previous surgeries are reviewed. The nurse should assess the patient's mental status and identify any communication barriers. Following this review, the nurse can individualize patient care based on the needs of the patient throughout the surgical experience.

Once the preparation is complete, the patient is taken to the operating room.

Following completion of surgery, the patient will be transferred to the postanesthesia care unit (PACU).

THE PACU

Here the nurse will closely monitor the patient's cardiac, respiratory, and neurovascular status. Pain control is addressed, and the surgical dressing and drain are checked for excessive bleeding. Vital signs are checked every 15 minutes. The patient stays in the recovery room until the general and/or regional anesthesia has been reversed. The time the patient remains in the PACU will depend on the anesthetic agents used and the patient's individual response.

THE ORTHOPEDIC UNIT

The orthopedic inpatient care unit is the place where patients progress to increasing independence for eventual discharge to home, rehabilitation, or a skilled care unit. The inpatient unit may have a number of different staff members to care for the patient: nurses, assistive personnel or techs, physical and occupational therapists, and discharge planners or social workers.

The nurse is the main caregiver for the patient in this environment, assessing the patient's vital signs, surgical wounds, diet progress, intake and output, surgical drains, pain control status, use of orthotics, and educational needs. The nurse administers and monitors responses to all patient medications ordered by the physician. To assist the nurse, there are usually staff members known as nursing assistants. The nurse is able to delegate certain tasks to nursing assistants while maintaining ultimate responsibility for all patient care. Duties typically delegated include the taking of vital signs, activities

of daily living, toileting, ambulation of patients, measuring of drain output, and feeding of patients when necessary. Any information or data gathered by a nursing assistant needs to be interpreted by the nurse, who has the appropriate knowledge. Some hospitals or medical centers specially train nursing assistants to do other tasks, like performing electrocardiographs or drawing blood.

Care issues extend from the PACU to arrival in the postop care unit. Immediate concerns include medical stability, neurovascular status assessment, and adequate pain control management. The nurse meets the patient in the patient's room and completes an initial assessment. This assessment includes a set of vital signs as well as an evaluation of the mental, cardiovascular, respiratory, integumentary, GI, and neurovascular status, with particular attention to the operative extremity. Patient equipment that is in use is checked at this time, including any infusion pumps for intravenous fluids or pain medications, urinary Foley catheters, surgical drains, and immobilizers, braces, or splints that may be in place.

Positioning

Appropriate positioning of the postoperative total hip patient is essential. Improper positioning may result in dislocation of the hip prosthesis. Patients typically arrive on the floor with their legs abducted by means of an abductor pillow, a blanket, or a regular pillow placed between their legs (Fig. 46-1). To decrease the risk of dislocation, keeping the legs abducted and in neutral alignment is recommended while the patient is in bed. This decreases the risk of dislocation. When it is necessary to turn a patient, the abductor device is kept between the patient's legs (Fig. 46-1). The patient is then turned onto his or her side. Depending on surgeon preference, this may be the surgical side or the nonsurgical side. Because it is essential to maintain appropriate positioning, movement in bed is difficult for the postsurgical hip patient. Often an overhead bed trapeze is helpful for assisting the patient while in bed and for mobilizing the patient in and out of bed.

If a patient has a history of recurrent dislocation or is at higher risk for dislocation due to the complexity of the surgery, the physician may require the patient to wear a hip

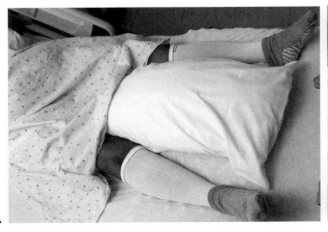 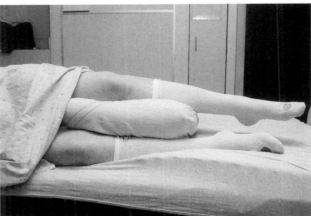

A   **B**

Figure 46-1   **A:** A pillow used to maintain hip abduction. **B:** A patient turned to the nonoperative side after surgery with a pillow between legs to maintain abduction.

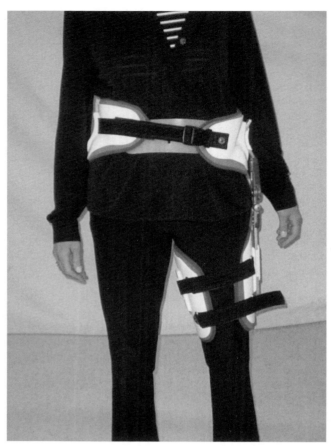

Figure 46-2 A hip abduction orthosis used to limit mobility in the unstable hip patient.

abductor orthosis (Fig. 46-2). This device is customized for each patient to limit hip mobility during the early postoperative period, when tissue healing is taking place.

Position restrictions for the hip replacement patient are surgeon dependent and may include limiting flexion to less than 90° and prohibiting adduction past neutral (Fig. 46-3).

Skin Integrity

The patient's skin is assessed postoperatively and on a daily basis for pressure ulcers. Pressure ulcers acquired in the hospital can increase a patient's length of stay and increase the risk of other complications such as sepsis. Pressure sores are most likely to develop on the heels and coccyx in the hip replacement patient. If a patient is at increased risk for decubitus ulcers, the nurse should utilize prophylactic measures to prevent them from developing, such as elevation of the heel off the mattress and frequent position changes. The Braden assessment tool is a commonly used screening method to determine a patient's risk of developing a pressure ulcer. It has six subscales that look at a patient's degree of sensory perception, physical activity, skin moisture, nutritional intake, exposure to friction and sheer, and ability to change or control body position (6). The nurse numerically grades each subscale, and the resulting score can indicate a patient's risk of developing pressure ulcers.

Neurovascular Status

Hip replacement surgery carries the risk of neurologic and vascular injury. Although most of these injuries are diagnosed in the immediate postoperative period, they may develop later secondary to indwelling epidurals, positioning, excessive swelling, or bleeding.

Nursing assessment of a patient's neurovascular status (NVS) begins in the PACU and continues throughout the patient's hospitalization. Prompt and accurate assessments are necessary for quality orthopedic care. NVS assessments are usually done every 4 hours for 24 hours and then every 8 hours for the remainder of the hospital stay. The initial assessment includes motor function, sensory changes, temperature, color, capillary refill, peripheral pulses, and excessive pain (1). The findings on the surgical extremity are compared to those for the nonsurgical leg. It is the responsibility of the nurse to perform an accurate neurovascular assessment, document the data, and communicate the findings to the physician and other members of the health care team to help prevent or promptly detect potential complications.

Thromboembolic events are among the more common complications following hip replacement surgery (17). Signs of a deep vein thrombosis (DVT) may include calf pain, a positive Homan sign, leg swelling, redness, and warmth over the area (23). Clinical diagnosis can be nonspecific. Patients may have a DVT without having symptoms, and symptoms of a DVT may be present and objective signs not present (17). Another complication that can develop as a result of a DVT is a pulmonary embolism (PE), where the clot travels to the pulmonary circulation. The symptoms a patient may experience as a result of a PE include shortness of breath and chest pain (usually worse on inspiration). The patient may appear anxious, apprehensive, and confused. On physical exam, the nurse should assess for signs of hypoxia, tachypnea, dyspnea, and tachycardia. The patient may exhibit signs of a fever, diaphoresis, hemoptysis, and possible cardiac arrhythmias (17). This is a medical emergency, and a spiral CT chest scan or ventilation perfusion scan is usually done to diagnose this complication.

Most surgeons will place their patients on a thromboembolic prophylactic protocol after surgery to prevent the development of pulmonary emboli, which can be potentially fatal. The protocol may consist of the use of pharmacologic measures such as warfarin, aspirin, low molecular weight heparin, or unfractionated heparin. Mechanical devices that can be used to decrease the incidence of DVT include intermittent sequential compression devices, foot pumps, and antiembolic stockings (Fig. 46-4). Along with early ambulation, the nurse should encourage the patient to perform foot and ankle pumps and exercises at least 10 times an hour while awake to increase circulation and prevent venous stasis.

Pulmonary Care

In order to prevent pulmonary complications in the postoperative period, the nurse begins working on pulmonary toilet upon arrival on the floor. Patients are encouraged to work on coughing and deep breathing and use incentive spirometry on an hourly basis while awake. Lung sounds are assessed by nursing every shift or more frequently as needed.

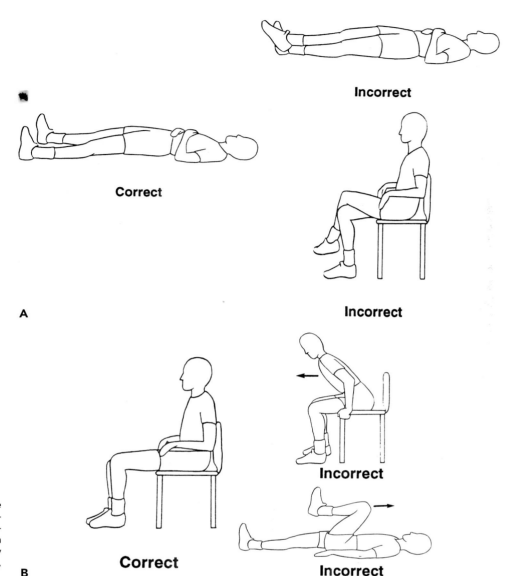

Figure 46-3 Hip precautions are reviewed with patients to help prevent hip dislocation. **A:** No adduction past neutral. **B:** No flexion greater than 90°. (Photos courtesy of Rush University Medical Center, Department of Physical Therapy.)

Wound Care/Drains

The surgical dressing is usually removed the first day after the procedure. Frequent assessments are done to evaluate for excessive drainage. If the patient has excessive drainage, the dressing should be reinforced and the physician notified.

Wounds need to be monitored for signs and symptoms of infection. Erythema, excessive warmth, and chronic drainage need to be reported to the physician.

Wound drains are often placed by the surgeon at the end of the procedure and are left in for approximately 24 to 48 hours after surgery. A standard drain and collection system is shown in (Fig. 46-5). Nursing is responsible for emptying the drainage and recording the amount of drainage collected. Some surgeons opt to use an autotransfusion device in more complex cases (Fig. 46-6). This type of drain allows for the collection of postoperative blood and reinfusion of the blood back to the patient within a certain time period. Usually this process takes place in the first 6 hours after surgery. Postoperative autotransfusion

may elevate the patient's blood count to a level that will decrease the need for homologous transfusion. Patient vital signs are monitored per the institution's policy, which often follows the same protocol used for standard transfusions.

Fluid Management

Nursing is responsible for maintaining accurate intake and output (I&O) records during the postoperative period. This responsibility includes monitoring urine output and the output from any drain in place. Many of hip surgery patients will have a Foley catheter in place for 24 to 48 hours after surgery. Once the Foley is removed, nursing will need to assess for urinary retention. Patients will remain on intravenous (IV) fluids until they are able to tolerate oral fluids. It is not uncommon for hip surgery patients to experience orthostatic hypotension as a result of perioperative blood loss, use of regional anesthesia, and immobility. The need for supplemental hydration may be necessary.

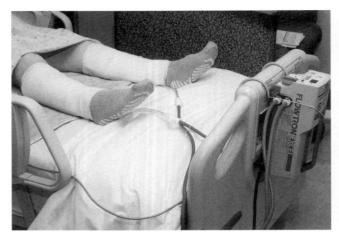

Figure 46-4 Intermittent sequential compression device used to help decrease the risk of deep vein thrombosis.

Pain Management

Effective pain management is a necessary requirement for promoting good surgical outcomes and high patient satisfaction (11). The demand for increased efficiency in patient mobilization and decreased hospital stay has increased the need for aggressive pain management in the hip replacement patient. It is a patient's right to expect adequate management of pain. National standards have been devised for pain management by regulatory groups such as JCAHO (8). The nurse plays a crucial role in the assessment of pain, the administration of pain interventions, and the evaluation of the effects of these interventions. Good assessment skills and recommendations of medications and the routing and timing of medications are important for adequate pain management.

Upon arrival at the inpatient unit, the nurse will complete an assessment of pain. It is important to reassure patients that pain medications are needed and are an important part of the recovery process. Each patient needs to be aware that the initial steps toward recovery will be easier with good pain control. The goal is to ensure both adequate pain relief and maintenance of an alert mental status and adequate respiratory

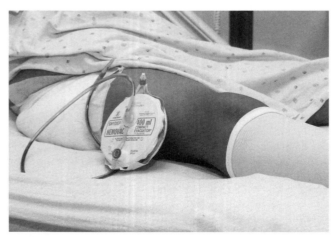

Figure 46-5 Postoperative standard drainage collection system.

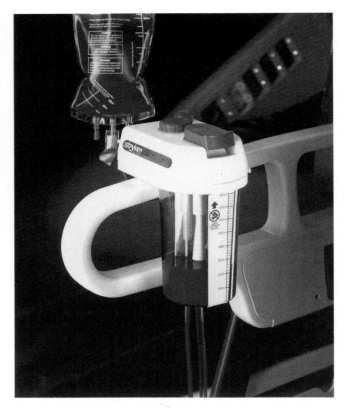

Figure 46-6 Autotransfusion blood collection device. (Photo courtesy of Stryker, Inc.)

function. There are different methods for assessing the level of pain experienced by a patient. No matter which method is used, it should be individualized to the particular patient's perception of pain. Both verbal and nonverbal pain scales are available. A common visual analog scale consists of a 10-cm line that the patient uses to rate the pain being experienced on a scale of 0 to 10, with 0 being no pain at all and 10 being the worst imaginable pain (5,24). It is important to educate the patient and staff on the use of this scale (20,21). The scale allows patients to place their own conceptual framework around what the worst imaginable pain means to them. Another scale, known as the "Wong Baker Face Scale," is a gradient of facial expressions from a happy face to a sad, sobbing face. Each face on the scale corresponds to a numeric value for pain (25). This method is useful for cognitively impaired patients or for patients with low literacy, and it is used so patients can correlate their feeling of pain with a particular expression and thus communicate their level of discomfort (19). Typically, a hospital has a standard of pain assessment that is followed throughout the institution for all patient populations

Common methods used to control pain after hip replacement surgery include epidural analgesia and patient-controlled analgesic (PCA) pumps. The use of these can be dictated by physician preference, patient choice, or procedural limitation. These two methods can provide immediate pain medication by delivering medication on patient demand or by continuous infusion. The combination of on-demand and continuous infusion is also used. An epidural provides pain control by an infusion of prescribed pain medication into the epidural space. It is set with specific dose limits over specified periods of time to ensure that the patient has the smallest possible risk of respiratory depression. The epidural may or may not allow the patient to press a button during periods of increased pain to self-administer an additional bolus of epidural medication over the baseline continual infusion. The self-administration capability should also have time and dose limitations that can be set for patient safety. In the case of PCA pumps, pain medication is delivered intravenously upon patient demand. The patient typically presses the button of the PCA machine, causing it to deliver a preset dose of pain medication through the IV line. Dose and time limits are set to avoid overdose and respiratory depression.

In both of the above-mentioned methods of pain medication delivery, the key is to give patients the ability to access pain medication immediately and hopefully obtain relief without having to wait for the nurse to prepare and administer pain medications. In some instances, the physician preference is for the use of intramuscular (IM) pain medications; however, their analgesic effect is not as immediate as with the PCA or epidural, and they often result in greater patient discomfort.

Typically, after the first 24 hours postop, the patient is progressed from parenteral to oral analgesics. For the patient to participate in activities such as physical therapy, adequate pain control must be maintained throughout the hospital stay. Attention should be given to ensuring that the patient is premedicated with oral pain meds in anticipation of physical therapy, allowing enough time for the medications to take effect. The types of oral analgesics commonly used include oxycodone, hydrocodone, tramadol, and acetaminophen. More recently, the use of anti-inflammatory medications perioperatively has been recommended (7,18).

Another means of enhancing postsurgical pain control is thermal therapy. The use of heat or cold therapy is often recommended for this patient population. Swelling of the surgical area can be a major discomfort factor, but it can be treated with the application of ice. Thermal therapy can also be beneficial for the patient who complains of muscular aches related to surgical positioning or hospital mattresses.

The use of complementary and alternative medicine, such as relaxation methods, massage therapy, music therapy, deep breathing, and meditation, has increased over the past decade as an intervention that may help change a patient's perception of pain. The most effective approach to managing pain is a multimodal approach encompassing pharmacologic and nonpharmacologic strategies (22).

GI Status

Immediately following surgery, patients are maintained on intravenous fluids and progressed from clear liquids to solids over the first 24-hour period. Progression of diet is dependent on the nursing assessment for presence of bowel sounds. Stool softeners may be initiated as soon as the patient tolerates oral medication.

Since pain control is a priority in the hip replacement patient, and the use of pain medications is necessary to achieve that goal, the side effect of nausea often has to be managed. Many times the patient at rest in bed will have no nausea until he or she begins moving. Because of this, depending on physician preference, prophylactic antiemetics may be given to the postsurgical hip patient for a finite period of time immediately after surgery. There are many antiemetics on the market. These medications come in all forms—IM, IV, oral, or rectal suppositories—and their effectiveness may vary from patient to patient. It is typically easiest for the patient if nausea can be controlled pre-emptively. If the patient is treated on a prophylactic basis for nausea, oral antiemetics are often the most cost-effective. Some oral agents can exacerbate patient symptoms, necessitating the use of other methods.

The complication of paralytic ileus needs to be considered in patients who have continuous nausea and vomiting along with diminished bowel sounds.

Patient Mobility

Starting the evening of surgery, the patient may be encouraged to dangle on the side of the bed or to get to a chair under the supervision of the nurse. This is dependent on each surgeon's protocol. It is important that pertinent information concerning specific issues or restrictions be relayed to the nurse either verbally or through written orders. When getting a patient out of bed after total hip arthroplasty, it is usually easiest to get the patient out of bed on the nonsurgical side. Weight-bearing orders are per physician protocol. Most hip replacement patients require the use of some sort of assistive device, such as crutches or a walker, for the first few weeks after surgery. This is usually dependent on the surgical approach and the method of implant fixation.

Physical and occupational therapy will normally begin the first day after surgery.

The goals of therapy are to promote patient safety and functional independence prior to discharge from the hospital. The physical therapist will evaluate the patient in regards to muscle strength, joint range of motion, and functional ability to perform bed mobility, transfers, gait, and stairs. It is important to obtain a history on the patient's preoperative level of activity, functional ability, number of stairs, and support system available. Goals are established based on where the patient will be going after discharge. Once the goals are established, the therapy sessions will focus on helping the patient achieve the level of functional ability needed in order to be discharged safely. The occupational therapist will focus on the resumption of activities of daily living such as personal hygiene activities, dressing, car transfers, cooking, and doing the laundry. The patient will be instructed on the proper use of assistive devices such as the reacher, sock donner, raised toilet seat, long-handled sponge, and shoehorn.

Preparing for Discharge

By the second day after surgery, although medical stability and wound observation remain priorities, the focus now includes increasing the patient's mobilization, strength, and endurance in order to prepare for discharge. Activities are incorporated into the patient's routine to foster a return to independence. The patient is encouraged to assist with the activities of daily living as much as can be tolerated. This includes bathing and getting up to the bathroom. For toileting in particular, a bedside commode may be helpful for those patients who are unable to ambulate to the bathroom, as it assists in reinforcing methods of getting in and out of bed.

Also, a bedside commode can be raised or lowered based on the patient's height and thus can help the patient obey the precaution not to flex the hip over 90°. Once the patient can ambulate to the bathroom, a raised toilet seat is recommended, especially for taller patients.

The length of stay for the hip replacement patient has decreased steadily over the last decade. It is not uncommon for patients to be discharged within 3 days of their surgery. This makes it vital for the discharge planning to be started prior to admission of the patient for surgery. The discharge planner will work closely with the nurse case manager, staff nurse, physical therapist, occupational therapist, and physician to help anticipate the discharge needs and coordinate assistance for the patient. Options for patients after the acute hospital setting include discharge to home, transfer to an acute rehabilitation center, and transfer to a subacute or skilled nursing facility. Patients are ready for discharge home when they exhibit safety with transfers in and out of bed and while ambulating with their assistive devices on level surfaces. Patients need to be safe on stairs (if required at home). It is ideal for patients to be afebrile at the time of discharge. With shorter hospital stays, more patients are being discharged with low-grade postoperative temperatures. Patients should be instructed to check temperatures at home and report to their physician if a high temperature persists or increases. Wounds should be dry or have minimal drainage without erythema at the time of discharge. Once a patient is discharged to home, he or she will usually have home services arranged by the discharge planner. These may include a visiting nurse 1 to 2 times per week and a physical therapist 3 times per week. Occupational therapy may also be consulted for a home visit to assess the patient's home environment, make appropriate recommendations to aide the patient with safety, and offer guidance with activities of daily living.

If a patient does not meet the requirements for discharge to home, the patient should be evaluated for transfer to an acute or subacute facility. Which facility will accept the patient will depend on the patient's medical comorbidities, home environment, support system, and insurance coverage. Patients requiring transfer to one of these facilities are usually there for an additional 5 to 10 days.

Discharge Instructions

This is the time to review and reinforce key concepts. Answering patient and family questions will decrease patient anxiety about leaving the hospital. Prior to discharge, the patient and family should be educated both verbally and in writing in the following areas.

■ **Wound care.** Caring for the wound is surgeon dependent. The patient should be instructed on dressing changes, any specific care of the surgery site required, and bathing restrictions. Signs and symptoms of infection should be addressed, along with when to notify the physician.
■ **Medications.** The discharge medications, the reasons for use, and the administration schedule should be discussed. Special attention should be given to the thromboembolic prescription, including adverse reactions and dietary restrictions. If the patient will be discharged on a low molecular heparin, the patient or caregiver needs to be instructed on

giving the injection. It is important to discuss the continued need for pain medication after discharge. Patients should be made aware that increased pain and swelling is not uncommon once home in their own environment due to an increase in their activity level.
■ **Diet.** Patients are instructed to resume their normal diet as tolerated. They need to be made aware of restrictions as they pertain to prescribed medication. As constipation continues to be a concern with the use of narcotic pain medications, patients should be encourage to drink an adequate volume of fluids and eat foods high in fiber.
■ **Activities.** After discharge, patients should continue to exercise as instructed by the therapist. Encouraging patients to increase their activity level will improve strength and endurance. Reinforcement of hip precautions to prevent dislocation should be dictated by surgeon preference. A discussion of the signs and symptoms of hip dislocation should include severe hip pain, shortening of the limb, and abnormal leg rotation. The physician should be notified if any of these symptoms are present. Continued use of assistive devices is recommended until the physician indicates differently. Driving is dependent on the physician's direction. This limitation is secondary to leg weakness and the use of narcotic medication.
■ **Other Complications.** The patient should be aware of the signs and symptoms of DVT and PE. When to contact the physician for problems such as an elevated temperature, increased pain and swelling in the leg, and increased wound drainage, as well as what is a medical emergency, should be reviewed.

POSTDISCHARGE RECOVERY

Once the patient is discharged home from the hospital or rehabilitation setting, the patient will begin to resume his or her normal preoperative routine. Home care services may continue for the next few weeks, depending on the physical progress of the patient. Usually patients will transition from home therapy to outpatient therapy as they become more independent. Depending on individual patient requirements, physical therapy can last for 6 to 12 weeks after surgery.

It is important for patients to realize that continuation of their exercises after completion of formal physical therapy is crucial for an optimal surgical outcome. Complete recovery may take 4 to 6 months after surgery.

Follow-Up

The patient will return for the initial postoperative evaluation approximately 3 to 6 weeks after surgery. At this visit, the patient is assessed for wound healing, joint mobility, muscle strength, pain control, swelling, and patient function. By this point, the patient has completed or is close to completing the prophylactic anticoagulation therapy. X-rays are obtained to evaluate component fixation and position.

By 6 weeks after surgery, the patient has progressed to more independent ambulation and is or will soon be off assistive devices. Continued follow-up visits are per individual physician protocols. The patient needs to be made aware that the hip prosthesis is a mechanical part that needs lifelong monitoring.

Return to Work

The time frame for the resumption of work is usually occupation dependent. Patients with a more sedentary job may be able to return to work much sooner than patients returning to a more active and physical job. Job modification or career change counseling may be indicated for a patient whose job places excessive physical demands on the joint replacement.

Activity

Activity precautions, including any specific motion precautions, are usually lifted at 6 weeks after surgery. The lifting of these restrictions allows the patient to become more independent in dressing and daily activities. Patients can gradually resume low-impact activities as their physical strength allows. These would include activities like walking, swimming, bike riding, dancing, and golfing. Most patients also resume driving by this time. Activity restrictions are physician dependent and often include higher impact activities such as jogging, jumping, contact sports, singles tennis, and racquetball.

Sexual Activity

Sexual activity is a normal part of many patients' lives. A successful THA has been shown to improve sexual function for many patients (26). Resuming sexual activity after hip surgery is a topic that should be addressed with all patients as part of the standard discharge teaching process. It is a topic that is not often discussed by the treating physician (9). It is easier if the health care provider introduces the subject, as many patients feel uncomfortable and will leave without asking questions. Most physicians allow patients to resume sexual activity between 1 and 3 months after surgery (9). It is important to discuss with patients hip precautions and recommended safe positions. Providing the patient with an information sheet explaining recommended positions for the patient and partner may be helpful (3,9).

Long-Term Infection Prevention

To help prevent the development of a hematogenous joint infection, the patient should be educated as to the importance of obtaining immediate medical care if he or she develops symptoms of a bacterial infection, such as dental abscesses or a skin, bladder, or sinus infection. A review of the individual physician's long-term antibiotic prophylaxis regimen should be discussed with the patient prior to discharge and on an ongoing basis at follow-up visits. For example, the patient might need for prophylactic antibiotic therapy prior to a dental procedure and other invasive procedures where bacteria may be introduced in the bloodstream.

SUMMARY

Total hip replacement surgery is a remarkable success story, as demonstrated by the increasing number of surgeries performed and the studies showing excellent long-term results. It is a procedure that generally provides a decrease in pain and improved mobility, resulting in better function and improved quality of life for patients.

Perioperative patient education remains of utmost importance. Patients who have a clear understanding of the perioperative process will feel more in control of their recovery and ultimately will be more involved in their recovery process. Nursing plays a critical role in continually educating patients throughout the surgical experience by introducing new concepts and reinforcing previously taught information.

Early conditioning through prehabilitation can make a patient better prepared for surgery physically, psychologically, and psychosocially and can be very beneficial in expediting the path to recovery.

Optimal patient outcomes are often related to the preparation and care patients receive perioperatively. Good communication among the patient, physician, and health care team will help patients develop and maintain realistic expectations and can ultimately improve the outcome of surgery.

Nursing needs to be proactive in anticipating what the physical, emotional, and safety needs of patients may be given the trend toward less invasive surgery and shorter hospital stays. While a nurse is just one member of the multidisciplinary team caring for a hip replacement patient, he or she often serves as the hub of information for the patient and all other team members. At every point in the surgery process, the nurse is a crucial link to information, care, positive outcome, and high patient satisfaction.

REFERENCES

1. Altizer L. Neurovascular assessment. *Orthop Nurs.* 2002;21(4): 48–50.
2. Altizer L. Patient education for total hip or knee replacement. *Orthop Nurs.* 2004;23(4):283–292.
3. Arthritis Foundation. *A Guide to Intimacy with Arthritis.* Atlanta: Arthritis Foundation; 1998. Brochure.
4. Beyea SC. The national patient safety goals and their implications for perioperative nurses. *AORN J.* 2003;77:1241–1245.
5. Bodian CA, Freedman G, Hossain S, et al. The visual analog scale for pain: clinical significance in postoperative patients. *Anesthesiology.* 2001;95:1356–1361.
6. Bryant RA, Pieper B. Mechanical forces: pressure, shear, and friction. In *Nursing Management.* 2nd ed. St. Louis: CV Mosby; 2002:221–264.
7. Buvanendran A, Kroin JS, Tuman, KJ, et al. Effects of perioperative administration of a selective cyclooxygenase 2 inhibitor on pain management and recovery of function after knee replacement. *JAMA.* 2003;18:2411–2418.
8. Curtiss CP. JCAHO: meeting the standards for pain management. *Orthop Nurs.* 2001;20(2):27–30.
9. Dahm DL, Jacofsky D, Lewallen DG. Surgeons rarely discuss sexual activity with patients after THA: a survey of members of the American Association of Hip and Knee Surgeons. *Clin Orthop.* 2004;428:237–240.
10. Ditmyer MM, Topp R, Pifer M. Prehabilitation in preparation for orthopaedic surgery. *Orthop Nurs.* 2002;21(5):43–52.
11. Ekman EF, Koman LA. Acute pain following musculoskeletal injuries and orthopaedic surgery. *J Bone Joint Surg.* 2004;86:1316–1327.
12. Forin P, Clarke A, Joseph L, et al. Outcomes of total hip and knee replacement. *Arthritis Rheum.* 1999;42:1722–1728.
13. Geier KA. Improving outcomes in elective orthopaedic surgery: a guide for nurses and total joint arthroplasty patients. *Orthop Nurs.* 2000;19(suppl):3–34.
14. Gilbey HJ, Ackland TR, Wang AW, et al. Exercise improves early functional recovery after total hip arthroplasty. *Clin Orthop Relat Res.* 2003;No. 408:193–200.
15. Huo MH, Brown BS. What's new in hip arthroplasty. *J Bone Joint Surg.* 2003;85A:1852–1864.
16. Lopez-Bushnell K, Gary G, Mitchell P, et al. Joint replacement and case management in indigent hospitalized patients. *Orthop Nurs.* 2004;23(2):113–117.

17. Maher AB, Salmond SW, Pellino TA. Complications of orthopaedic disorders and orthopaedic surgery. In *Orthopaedic Nursing.* 3rd ed. WB Saunders; 2002:239–245.
18. Mallory TH, Lombardi AV, Fada RA, et al. Pain Management for joint arthroplasty: preemptive analgesia. *J Arthroplasty.* 2002;17:129–133.
19. McCaffery M, Pasero C. *Pain: Clinical Manual.* 2nd ed. St. Louis: CV Mosby; 1999:95.
20. McCaffrey M, Pasero C. Teaching patients to use a numerical pain-rating scale. *Am J Nurs.* 1999;99(12):22–24.
21. McCaffery M, Pasero C. Using the 0–10 pain rating scale: nine common problems solved. *Am J Nurs.* 2001;101(10):81–82.
22. Pellino TA, Gordon DB, Engelke ZK, et al. Use of nonpharmaco-logic interventions for pain and anxiety after total hip and total knee arthroplasty. *Orthop Nurs.* 2005;24(3):182–189.
23. Schoen, DC. *Core Curriculum for Orthopaedic Nursing.* 4th ed. Pitman, NJ: Anthony J. Janotti, Inc; 2001:175–176.
24. Serlin RC, Mendoza TR, Nakamura Y, et al. When is cancer pain mild, moderate or severe?: grading pain severity by its interference with function. *Pain.* 1995;61:277–284.
25. Smeltzer SC. Pain Management. In *Brunner and Suddarth's Testbook of Medical Surgical Nursing.* 9th ed. Philadelphia: Lippincott Williams & Wilkins; 2000:175–201.
26. Stern SH, Fuchs MD, Ganz SB, et al: Sexual function after total hip arthroplasty. *Clin Orthop.* 1991;269:228–235.
27. Wammack L, Mabrey J. Outcomes assessment of total hip and total knee arthroplasty: critical pathways, variance analysis, and continuous quality improvement. *Clin Nurse Spec.* 1998;12: 122–129.

Surgical Approaches

47

William A. McGann

SUPERFICIAL LANDMARKS

The bony landmarks of the pelvis and femur provide initial guidance to the incisions and orientation of the pelvis for the various approaches to the hip. Anteriorly, the prominent anterior–superior iliac spine (ASIS) marks the anterior limit of the iliac crest and serves as an attachment for the sartorius muscle and the inguinal ligament. The two ASISs define the transverse, coronal, and sagittal orientation of the pelvis. The coronal plane of the pelvis is defined by the tangential plane to the symphysis pubis and the ASISs.

Posteriorly, the iliac crest ends at the posterior–superior iliac spine (PSIS), which is defined by a superficial skin dimple. The bony ischial tuberosity is easily palpated beneath the lower edge of the gluteus maximus.

Laterally, the greater trochanter is most easily defined at its posterior–superior corner, or tubercle. The gluteus medius is tendinous at its posterior border and can be defined close to its insertion into the greater trochanteric tubercle. The anterior aspect of the greater trochanter blends with the tendon of the gluteus medius and is softer and less distinct to palpation. The trochanteric ridge marks the distal extent of the greater trochanter and may be palpable at its junction with the vastus muscle of the thigh. Anterolaterally, the tensor fascia muscle sheath can be defined by oblique palpation at the lateral hip (diagonal). Anteriorly, the longitudinally oriented rectus femoris tendon and muscle can usually be palpated just below the inguinal ligament and ASIS near its origin on the anterior–inferior iliac spine (AIIS). Near to the midline, the bony pubic tubercle can be palpated just lateral to the midline at the point of insertion of the inguinal ligament. Further medial, the adductor longus is easily identified as the most palpable tendon of the adductor group. The femoral artery can be palpated below the inguinal ligament in the femoral triangle at a point midway between the ASIS and symphysis pubis.

VASCULAR ANATOMY

The superior gluteal artery is the largest branch from the internal iliac artery and exits the pelvis through the greater sciatic notch in a position superior to the piriformis muscle. A superficial division supplies the gluteus maximus, and a deep branch supplies the gluteus medius, gluteus minimus, and tensor fascia muscles. Small branches of the superior and inferior arteries communicate between the deep side of the maximus and the superficial side of the medius and are at risk during dissection between these two muscles in a variety of hip approaches. The deep portion of the superior gluteal artery courses deep to the gluteus medius and runs along the proximal border of the gluteus minimus to anastomose at the ASIS with the ascending branch of the lateral circumflex and the deep iliac circumflex artery. An inferior division of the deep branch extends across the gluteus minimus toward the trochanter where it anastomoses with branches of the lateral circumflex artery.

The obturator artery branches from the internal iliac artery and is closely approximated to the lateral wall of the pelvis on the obturator fascia. The artery lies between the obturator nerve and vein. The close proximity of these neurovascular structures to the inner wall of the acetabulum places them at risk to injury from penetration through the acetabulum, such as from screw placement during hip replacement, or fracture fixation. The obturator artery penetrates the obturator membrane and exits the pelvis through the obturator foramen. After exiting the foramen, the obturator artery divides into anterior and posterior branches. The anterior branch anastomoses with the posterior branch and the medial circumflex artery and supplies the obturator externus, pectineus, adductors, and gracilis muscles. The posterior branch anastomoses with the anterior branch and also branches to the inferior gluteal supply. An acetabular branch penetrates the acetabular fossa beneath the transverse acetabular ligament to enter into the ligamentum teres to provide one of the three major sources of blood to the femoral head.

The inferior gluteal artery branches from the internal iliac artery and exits the pelvis inferior to the piriformis to supply the gluteus maximus. Posterior branches of the inferior gluteal artery pass along the lower border of the piriformis across the sciatic nerve. The sciatic nerve receives a branch from this artery and is named the arteria comitans nervi ischiadici. The inferior gluteal artery continues in a distal direction to provide arterial branches to the short rotator muscle. In fracture work, these muscular branches may be important to maintain adequate circulation to bone fragments.

The femoral artery is defined proximally at the level of the inguinal ligament and distally at the adductor hiatus of the thigh. The femoral triangle is bounded proximally by the inguinal ligament, medially by the adductor longus, laterally by the sartorius, and at the floor by the iliacus, psoas major, pectineus, and adductor brevis. The saphenous nerve accompanies the femoral artery and vein within the adductor canal. The profunda femoris artery arises from the femoral artery and branches into medial and lateral circumflex, perforators, and muscular branches.

The medial circumflex divides into an ascending branch that supplies surrounding muscles and anastomoses with the obturator artery. A transverse branch supplies some of the adductors. A posterior branch divides into superficial, lateral, and deep branches superficially to anastomose with the inferior and superior gluteal arteries, the lateral femoral circumflex artery, and the first perforating artery. This communication is termed the cruciate anastomosis. The cruciate anastomosis represents an extensive collateral blood supply system to the lower limb. The posterior deep branch passes along the quadratus femoris muscle and anastomoses proximally with branches of the gluteal arteries. An acetabular branch of the posterior deep branch may accompany the obturator branch to the acetabular fossa.

The lateral circumflex artery arises from the profunda branch and divides into three branches: ascending, transverse, and descending. The ascending branch courses on the border of the rectus femoris muscle beneath the tensor fascia lata to anastomose with the superior gluteal circulation. This branch is important in anterior and anterolateral approaches. The transverse branch is important in lateral approaches and runs laterally to penetrate and lie within the vastus lateralis just distal to the trochanteric ridge. The transverse branch may anastomose with the medial circumflex and first perforator arteries.

MUSCULAR ANATOMY

The anterior group of thigh muscles includes the sartorius, tensor fascia lata, and quadriceps. The quadriceps muscle group consists of the four anterior thigh muscles: rectus femoris, vastus lateralis, vastus intermedius, and vastus medialis. The rectus femoris is the only quadriceps that crosses both the hip and the knee joints. The two origins of the rectus include a direct head that arises from the AIIS, and an indirect head that blends with the superior acetabular labrum. The vastus lateralis is the largest of the quadriceps group.

Posteriorly, the massive gluteus maximus muscle arises from the posterior gluteal line, iliac crest, and a portion of the posterior surface of the sacrum and coccyx, the tendinous aspect of the sacrospinous and sacrotuberous ligaments, and the underside of the gluteus aponeurosis. About three fourths of the gluteus maximus tendon blends with the tendon of the tensor fascia muscle to form the tethering band of the iliotibial tract. The iliotibial tract crosses both the hip and knee joints and is thickened between the iliac crest tubercle and the tibia. This band overlies the trochanteric bursa against the greater trochanter to assist in stabilizing the pelvis and abduction of the hip. One fourth of the gluteus maximus tendon inserts directly into the proximal femur to function as the prime decelerator of the hip during gait.

The gluteus medius arises from both the external surface of the ilium and the underside of the tensor fascia. The extensive origin of the gluteus medius serves as a powerful anchor for the muscle and maximizes the abductor function by directing tension laterally along the iliac crest through the fascia lata and iliotibial tract. Although it is a prime abductor, its anterior insertion into the greater trochanter also makes it an internal rotator of the hip. Hip reconstructions that increase the tension of the gluteus medius may also cause internal rotation as a result. Its fibers are oriented in an oblique fashion and can be differentiated from the gluteus maximus and minimus by this characteristic during difficult surgical dissections through this region (see Fig. 47-46).

The gluteus minimus lies beneath the gluteus medius and contributes about one fifth of the abductor power to the hip. The muscle arises from the ilium between the anterior and inferior gluteal lines. The muscle becomes tendinous over the anterior capsule and inserts partially into the capsule and the anterior portion of the greater trochanter.

The piriformis muscle and tendon exits through the greater sciatic notch in a downward oblique direction as it inserts into the piriformis fossa of the greater trochanter. Its location defines the superior- and inferior-located neurovascular structures that exit through the sciatic notch. The sciatic nerve runs deep to the piriformis, and thus the muscle is not a protector of the nerve during deep posterior exposure of the hip and posterior acetabulum.

The obturator internus tendon exits the lesser sciatic notch from its origin on the inner wall of the pelvis and inserts caudad to the piriformis tendon on the greater trochanter. It is often conjoined with the piriformis tendon. When released, it can be seen to be multipennate on its deep surface, unlike any other short rotator. The small fleshy muscles of the gamelli lie superior and inferior to the obturator internus tendon.

The obturator externus muscle arises from the outer bone and membrane of the obturator foramen and inserts inferior to the obturator internus tendon. The iliopsoas is a combination of the intrapelvic muscles: the iliacus and the psoas major. They function together to flex and externally rotate the femur.

NEUROANATOMY

The hip and pelvis are innervated by the lumbosacral plexus. The lumbosacral plexus is formed from the lumbar plexus and the sacral plexus in the abdomen. The lumbar plexus lies in the abdomen and divides into anterior and posterior branches. The main anterior division becomes the obturator nerve, and the posterior division becomes the femoral nerve. The sacral plexus is formed in the pelvis and receives connections from the fourth and fifth lumbar nerve roots known as the lumbosacral trunk. The posterior branches supply the muscles of the buttock and also form the peroneal portion of the sciatic nerve. The anterior branches contribute major supply to the tibial portion of the sciatic nerve. The tibial portion of the sciatic supplies the muscles of the thigh, calf, and foot.

The superior and inferior gluteal nerves arise from posterior divisions of the lumbosacral plexus. The superior gluteal nerve passes through the greater sciatic notch, above the piriformis. It then courses deep to the gluteus medius. The inferior gluteal nerve passes through the notch with the sciatic nerve to the lower edge of the piriformis to enter into the gluteus maximus.

The posterior femoral cutaneous nerve (lesser sciatic nerve) arises from the sacral plexus and travels deep to the piriformis to supply skin of the lower buttock and posterior thigh.

ANTERIOR APPROACH

The anterior approach, also known as the iliofemoral or Smith-Petersen approach, dissects the interval between the sartorius and rectus femoris muscles (femoral nerve innervated), and the tensor fascia and gluteus minimus and medius muscles (superior gluteal innervated), and thus is a true internervous approach. The approach is lateral to the sensory lateral femoral cutaneous nerve, which penetrates the sartorial fascia roughly 1 inch (range 2 to 5 cm) below the ASIS. The nerve commonly penetrates the fascia adjacent to the superficial circumflex iliac artery.

The original description of the approach describes excellent exposure of the superior portion of the hip capsule and acetabulum, emphasizing the supra-articular exposure of the hip joint for open reductions of congenital hip dislocations. It was also suggested to be of possible value for acetabular exposure for hip arthrodesis (57,58). This approach evolved to include exposure for hip fractures (49). The extended exposure provides excellent access to the inner and outer tables of the ilium, the anterior hip, and the acetabulum but severely limits posterior acetabular visualization.

The extensive exposure of the ilium and acetabulum afforded by this approach is a result of the extensive stripping of the abductors off the ilium. The extent of subperiosteal dissection of the gluteus medius and tensor fascia muscle groups off of the ilium depends upon the demands of exposure for each operation. Extensive release of the abductors results in a high incidence of residual weakness of the abductors and formation of heterotopic bone. The approach is most useful where extensive exposure of the anterior column is necessary, such as in the case of pelvic osteotomy or pelvic fracture. The patient position in this approach is considered ideal for hip arthrodesis since accurate positioning of the limb can be ascertained by intraoperative reference to the pelvis via the ASIS and pubic symphysis landmarks. The approach avoids major disturbance to the femoral head blood supply, as contrasted to the posterior approach, and therefore can be useful in cases of avascular necrosis, or internal fixation in the pediatric age group.

The position of the patient for the anterior approach is supine, but it may be modified by elevating the affected side slightly upward with a sandbag. If the support is placed near to the midline, the soft tissues of the posterior and lateral hip will fall posteriorly and aid in the retraction of soft tissues.

The incision is carried along the iliac crest border about 2 to 3 cm lateral to the iliac crest beginning at the junction of the middle and anterior thirds of the crest. The fascial incision should leave a small remnant of the fascia next to the bone for later reapproximation (Fig. 47-1A). At the ASIS, the incision is carried distally toward the knee, slightly lateralward along the anterior border of the tensor fascia lata muscle sheath. The anterior border of the tensor fascia muscle is usually palpable near its origin close to the ASIS. Rotation of the hip externally helps to define the lateral border of the sartorius as it extends from the ASIS obliquely toward the medial aspect of the knee. Blunt dissection carried down to the fascia through subcutaneous tissue helps to identify the lateral femoral cutaneous nerve, which penetrates the fascia to become superficial approximately 1 inch (range 2 to 5 cm) below the inguinal ligament. The nerve exits the fascia close to the penetration of the superficial circumflex iliac artery. The nerve should be retracted medially to allow deeper dissection. The lateral femoral cutaneous nerve branches to innervate the lateral and posterior surfaces of the thigh, to the level of the greater trochanter proximally (Fig. 47-2). It is important to keep the dissection lateral to the main nerve trunk because damage to this nerve can lead to anesthesia of the lateral thigh, or a painful neuroma. Care should also be taken to avoid pressure on this nerve from self-retaining retractors. Alternatively, the anterior fascial envelope of the tensor fascia muscle can be split to avoid the encounter with the nerve. As the sheath of the tensor is opened, the dissection is carried over the anterior border of the tensor muscle, preserving the medial fascia of the tensor and thus protecting the lateral femoral cutaneous nerve from injury (Fig. 47-3) (42).

The deep dissection in this approach releases the abductors from the ilium. Beginning at the ASIS, the tensor fascia lata muscle origin can be dissected laterally off of the lateral wing of the ilium. The amount of muscle elevated from the lateral iliac wing can be increased as needed to improve the degree of proximal surgical exposure. The major ascending branch of the lateral circumflex artery, which is located between the gluteus medius muscle and rectus femoris tendon, should be identified and ligated (Fig. 47-4). The rectus femoris can then be divided to completely expose the anterior hip capsule (Fig. 47-5). The tendons may be tagged for later reattachment. It may not be necessary to divide the reflected and direct heads of the rectus muscle.

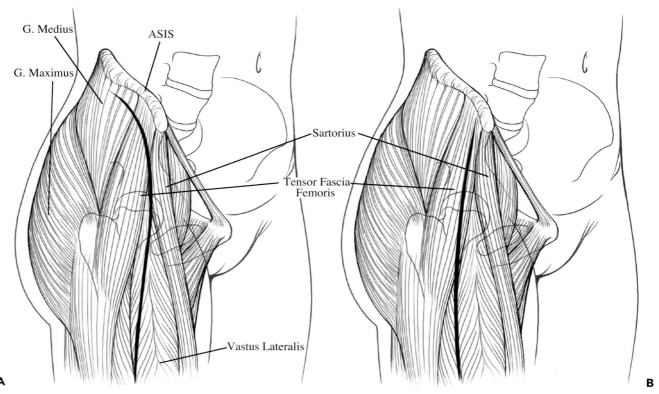

G. Medius

G. Maximus

ASIS

Sartorius

Tensor Fascia Femoris

Vastus Lateralis

A

B

Figure 47-1 **A:** Anterior approach: Smith-Petersen incision. The distal incision splits between the tensor and the sartorius muscles. Note the iliac incision preserves a cuff of tissue to reapproximate the abductors. **B:** Anterior approach modification: Hueter. The dissection mimics the distal portion of the Smith-Petersen approach. The tensor sheath is entered to avoid the sometimes difficult dissection between tensor and sartorius and also to minimize the risk of injury to the lateral femoral circumflex nerve.

The approach allows limited access to the medial pelvic structures. To gain further access to the anterior column of the acetabulum and somewhat limited exposure to the quadrangular space of the acetabulum on the medial wall of the pelvis, the inguinal ligament and sartorius origin can be released from the ASIS (Fig. 47-6). Further dissection along the anterior column can be extended as far as the iliopectineal eminence. The iliopsoas muscle is located medially overlying a portion of the hip capsule, and an extension of capsular iliacus can be seen to insert onto the anterior hip capsule.

It is possible to carry the dissection medially to the inner pelvis. After release of the inguinal ligament from the ASIS, the subperiosteal elevation of a portion of the iliopsoas can be extended into the true pelvis to the level of the greater sciatic notch. The inguinal ligament can later be reattached with sutures placed through drill holes on the ASIS. It is important to isolate the fatty compartment containing branches of the lateral circumflex artery located inferior to the hip capsule and above the iliopsoas tendon.

With the superior, anterior, medial, and inferior hip capsule exposed, a capsulotomy can now be performed and, if indicated, the hip prepared for dislocation. The acetabulum and anterior aspect of the head and neck are exposed by release of the capsule from the anterior border of the acetabulum. Any anterior acetabular osteophytes and a portion of the

AIIS may be osteotomized to facilitate the anterior hip dislocation. Following the capsulotomy or capsulectomy of the hip, dislocation of the hip can be achieved by external rotation, adduction, and flexion of the femur.

A modification of the anterior approach described by Hueter provides limited access to the anterior hip for procedures such as biopsy, synovectomy, labral excision, or arthrotomy. This approach is essentially a limited Smith-Petersen approach and utilizes only the distal portion of the classic approach (Fig. 47-1B). A straight incision is described that extends from the ASIS toward the lateral border of the patella. The tensor muscle sheath is entered to avoid injury to the lateral femoral cutaneous nerve. The muscle should be released from its sheath proximally to the level of the iliac crest for maximal exposure. The deep muscle fascia of the tensor is then incised overlying the rectus femoris. The ascending circumflex vessel is ligated. Capsulectomy can be performed for an arthrotomy or arthroplasty. Access is quite limited at the superior lip of the hip and to the acetabulum. The proximal incision can be extended to a Smith-Petersen approach.

A pitfall to the anterior approach is the poor definition of the starting point between tensor and sartorius muscles. If the dissection is carried medial to the sartorius, damage to the femoral nerve and the lateral femoral cutaneous sensory branch may occur. For this reason, it is best to attempt to

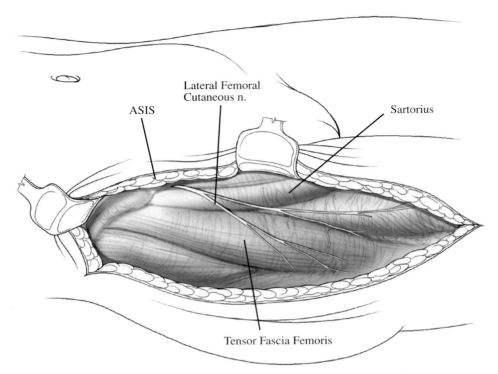

Figure 47-2 Lateral femoral cutaneous nerve. Branches of the lateral femoral cutaneous nerve may interfere with the anterior approach as they extend across the line of deep dissection between the tensor and sartorius muscles.

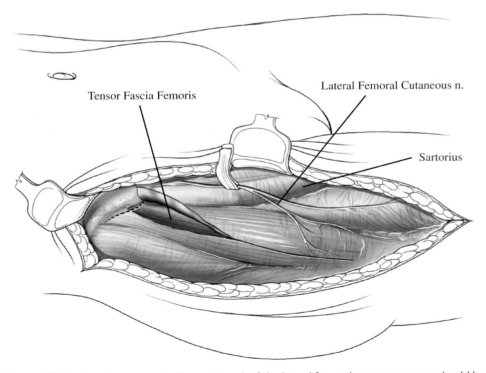

Figure 47-3 Anterior approach. The main trunk of the lateral femoral cutaneous nerve should be identified and retracted medially. The technique of splitting the tensor sheath to minimize the risk of nerve injury is shown.

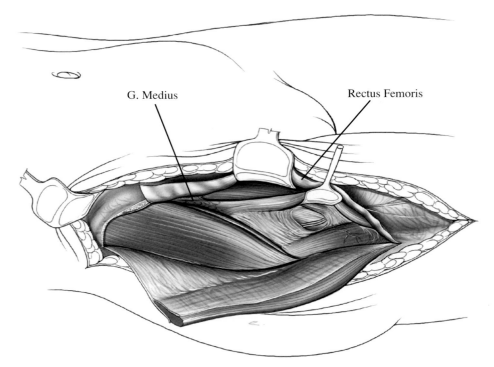

G. Medius

Rectus Femoris

Figure 47-4   Anterior approach. The tensor has been released from its origin to expose the gluteus medius. The ascending branch of the lateral femoral circumflex can be found in the deep tissue between the gluteus medius and the rectus femoris (deep retractor).

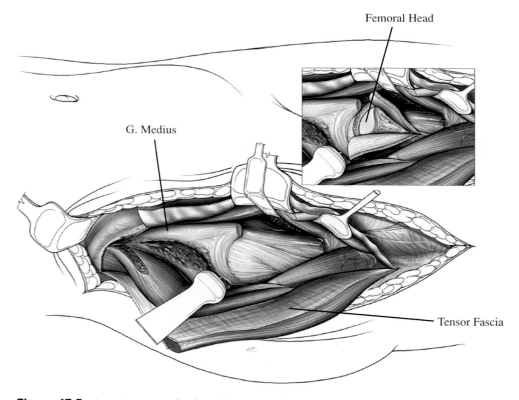

Femoral Head

G. Medius

Tensor Fascia

Figure 47-5   Anterior approach, deep dissection. The rectus femoris tendon has been released near its origin to allow further exposure of the medial hip capsule. In the proximal wound, a portion of the gluteus medius and gluteus minimus has been released to improve the exposure of the superior hip capsule. The capsulotomy can then be performed to expose the anterior hip (*inset*).

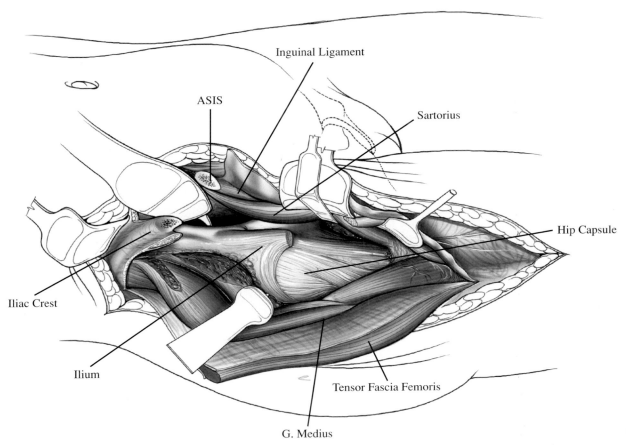

Inguinal Ligament

ASIS

Sartorius

Hip Capsule

Iliac Crest

Ilium

Tensor Fascia Femoris

G. Medius

Figure 47-6 Anterior approach, extensive exposure. The exposure to the anterior column and medial acetabular wall can be accomplished by further dissection. The ASIS has been released and the sartorius and inguinal ligament retracted medially. The iliopsoas can be dissected posteriorly to expose a portion of the acetabular wall to the level of the sciatic notch.

identify the anterior border of the tensor fascia muscle more distally and carry the dissection between sartorius and tensor from distal to proximal near the level of the ASIS. In this way, the sartorius will be the first muscle encountered on the medial aspect of the incision, and the tensor will be found immediately lateral. To visually differentiate this interval, the sartorius muscle can be noted to be muscular at its origin, and the tensor fascia lata to be tendinous at its origin.

ANTEROLATERAL APPROACH

The anterolateral approach provides limited exposure to the anterior hip for a variety of procedures. It has limited use in reconstructive procedures because of limitations in the exposure of the proximal femur for prosthetic insertion. It is an excellent approach for anterior hip arthrotomy, biopsy, and fracture reduction because of its limited dissection of the major muscle groups. The anterolateral approach dissects between the gluteus medius muscle and tensor fascia muscle, both of which are innervated by the superior gluteal nerve. It is therefore not a true internervous approach. It does not allow as extensive an access to the anterior column as the anterior approach provides. The upper femur is accessible by

dissection of the vastus muscle groups from the proximal femur. The advantage of the anterolateral approach over the anterior or Smith-Petersen approach is that it is less invasive of the abductors.

The approach was popularized by Watson-Jones in his description of fracture fixation to provide better exposure of the hip without the extensive dissection that is characteristic of the anterior approach (66). He felt that the only advantage to the Smith-Petersen technique was in the recognition of malaligned femoral nails. Watson-Jones then developed the anterolateral approach to expose the head of the femur, the fracture, and the entire length of the femoral neck and upper shaft of the femur in one field of view to facilitate accurate internal fixation. The approach is useful for cases of total or partial hip replacement, femoral neck fracture, hip arthrotomy, and femoral neck biopsy. The approach can be performed without disturbance of the blood supply to the femoral head.

The Harris lateral approach is somewhat similar to the anterolateral approach (26). It can be performed with or without a trochanteric osteotomy. The exposure is more extensive than the technique of Watson-Jones and is useful for pelvic osteotomies and hip reconstruction. Harris described a curvilinear incision with the apex directed posteriorly at the level of the

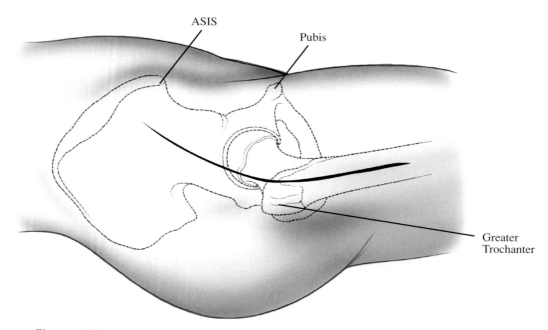

ASIS

Pubis

Greater
Trochanter

Figure 47-7 Anterolateral approach. The typical curvilinear incision for the anterolateral approach. For hip arthroplasty where greater exposure is needed, the apex of the incision may be placed more posterior to the level of the posterior edge of the greater trochanter.

posterior trochanter. The anterior interval between medius and tensor can then be developed to expose the anterior surface of the hip. The exposure is facilitated by a transverse incision in the fascia lata. This allows better exposure of the acetabulum over the anterior aspect of the femur. Extensive release of the entire capsule and short external rotators allows good visualization of the proximal femur for reconstructive procedures. The approach can be expanded if needed by adding a trochanteric osteotomy at any time in the procedure.

The patient can be positioned in a variety of ways for the anterolateral approach. Commonly, the patient is inclined upward from the supine position using a bump near the midline as described in the anterior approach. A long curvilinear incision is made, apexed posteriorly at the tip of the greater trochanter extending to the posterior third of the trochanter and then distally along the axis of the femoral shaft (Fig. 47-7) (66). The fascia is divided along the line of the skin incision (Fig. 47-8). The anterior border of the gluteus medius is readily identified. The original description described a partial release of the anterior fibers of the gluteus medius from the trochanteric insertion. Beginning at the trochanteric ridge (also known as the vastus ridge), at the insertion point of the anterior fibers of the gluteus medius, dissection is carried proximally up the anterior border of the gluteus medius muscle while separating the tensor muscle in an anterior direction. Within approximately the first 3 cm of dissection a minor vascular branch of the superior gluteal trunk is encountered extending into the tensor fascia muscle from the gluteus medius (Fig. 47-9). This small branch can be ligated or cauterized. The second branch more proximally contains a neurovascular bundle and limits the extent of proximal dissection in the anterolateral approach

(Fig. 47-10). This second neurovascular branch should be preserved, as it contributes significant nerve supply from the superior gluteal nerve to the tensor muscle. A marking suture placed in the muscle may help to prevent inadvertent splitting of the muscle and subsequent nerve damage. With the tensor fascia muscle retracted medial and anterior, and the gluteus medius retracted posterior and lateral, exposure of the deeply located gluteus minimus is accomplished (Fig. 47-11). External rotation and abduction of the femur aids in this exposure. Flexion of the hip relaxes the gluteus medius fibers and also reduces tension in the tissue flap that contains the femoral nerve and vessels. Dissection in a medial direction on the hip capsule to the border of the gluteus minimus exposes the anterior capsule of the hip as far as the anterior acetabular rim. The direct head of the rectus tendon can be easily palpated along the anteromedial border of the hip capsule. To gain exposure of the anterior column, a blunt cobra retractor can be placed beneath the rectus tendon by blunt dissection of anterior soft tissue slightly inferior to the axis of the femoral head, over the brim of the anterior column (Fig. 47-12). An index finger can be safely passed over the anterior column in a posterior direction into the pelvis. Rotation of the digit anteriorly identifies the tight tendon of the direct head of the rectus femoris which extends from its origin on the AIIS into the thigh. The blunt rectus retractor can then be safely substituted for the digit over the anterior column and beneath the direct head of the rectus tendon for excellent exposure of the anteromedial hip capsule. It is important not to dissect in an inferior direction along the anterior column below the level of the femoral head, and medial because vascular injury can result to either the femoral vessels in a medial direction or to the femoral circumflex

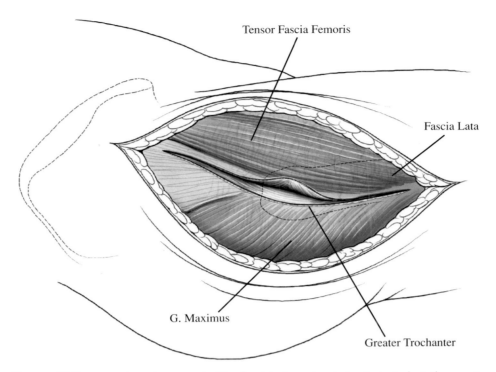

Tensor Fascia Femoris

Fascia Lata

G. Maximus

Greater Trochanter

Figure 47-8 Anterolateral approach. The fascial dissection is best started at the greater trochanter, where the bursae will help to identify the plane of dissection superficial to the gluteus medius.

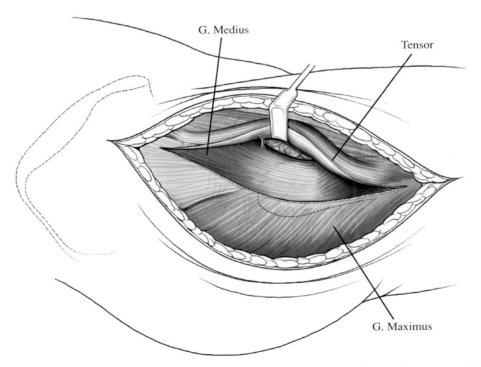

G. Medius

Tensor

G. Maximus

Figure 47-9 Anterolateral approach. The first branch is encountered a few centimeters proximal to the insertion of the gluteus medius. This connection is sacrificed to allow deeper exposure.

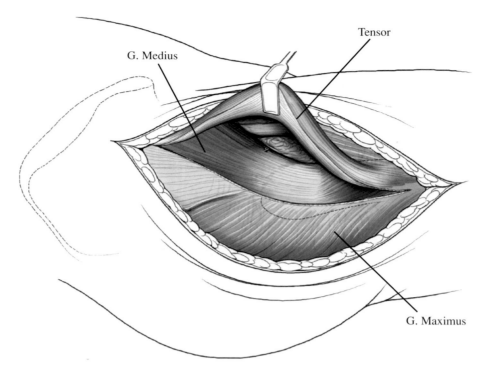

G. Medius

Tensor

G. Maximus

Figure 47-10 Anterolateral approach. The tensor is retracted anteriorly, and the anterior border of the gluteus medius is easily seen. The minor vascular bundle is ligated between the tensor and the medius, but the proximal neurovascular bundle is preserved.

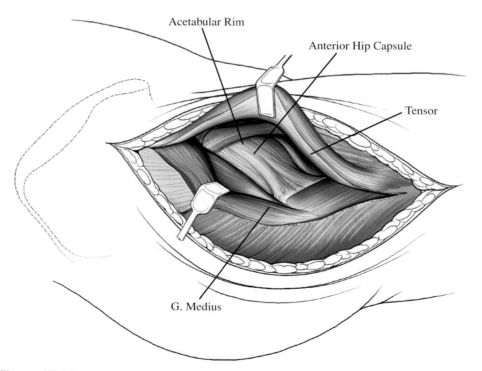

Acetabular Rim

Anterior Hip Capsule

Tensor

G. Medius

Figure 47-11 Anterolateral approach. The deep retraction of the gluteus medius posteriorly exposes the gluteus minimus tendon. Flexion and external rotation of the hip improves the exposure to the anterior hip capsule. The rectus still covers the anterior acetabular rim.

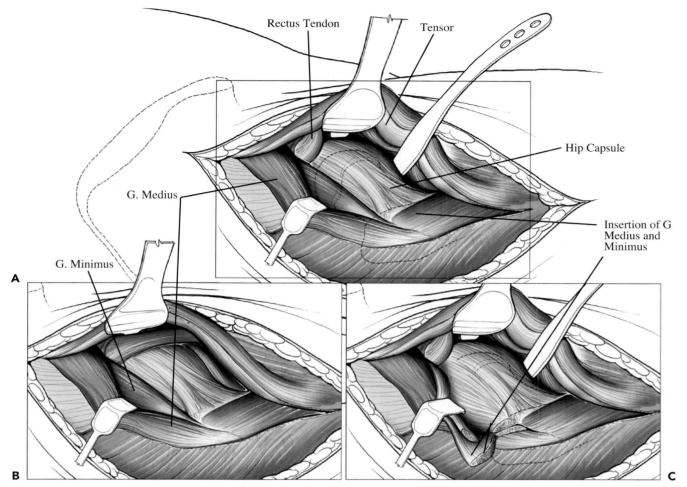

Figure 47-12 Anterolateral approach. **A:** For limited exposure of the hip, the rectus retractor may be placed above the rectus tendon. **B:** The blunt rectus retractor is placed beneath the tendon and inside the pelvis to complete the medial exposure. A blunt inferior cobra retractor protects the vascular structures inferior to the hip capsule. **C:** Improvement in the exposure of the superior capsule is obtained by the partial release of the gluteus medius and minimus from the anterior trochanter.

vessels inferiorly (Fig. 47-13). Alternatively, the rectus tendon can be released and later reattached. To improve the distal wound exposure of the femoral neck and shaft, a portion of the vastus lateralis muscle origin can either be split or be released from the vastus lateralis ridge and intertrochanteric line. As described by Muller, exposure of more superior capsule of the hip can also be accomplished by a partial release of the fibers of the gluteus medius from the distal trochanter (51). He described the dissection of the medius fibers proximally to the level of the bursa that exists between the gluteus minimus and the greater trochanter. To gain additional exposure of the superior hip, either a trochanteric osteotomy or more extensive release of the anterior fibers of the gluteus medius can be performed. The detailed technique of the transtrochanteric or the direct lateral approach can be followed. The gluteus medius fibers can be safely split a distance of approximately 3 cm proximal to the level of the superior acetabular rim. More extensive proximal dissection risks injury to the superior gluteal neurovascular branches.

Additional relaxation of the posterior fascia lata flap can be accomplished by a transverse cut in the gluteus maximus fascia and fascia lata just distal to the musculotendinous junction as described by Harris. A modified incision described by Burwell curves the Watson-Jones incision posterior instead of anterior (9). This modification reportedly allows easier dislocation of the hip by relaxation of the posterior fascia lata on the trochanter, as in the technique described by Harris.

The anterior, inferior, and limited superior hip capsule are well exposed at this stage of the procedure. The capsule is incised along the upper border of the neck, dissected from the anterior intertrochanteric line, and retracted as a triangular flap to expose the femoral neck. After capsular incision or excision, the hip is then dislocated anteriorly by externally rotating the femur. Further femoral neck exposure distally can be facilitated by subperiosteal elevation of the vastus muscle from the proximal femur.

A key point to anterior hip exposure is the avoidance of any neurovascular injury caused by placement of anterior

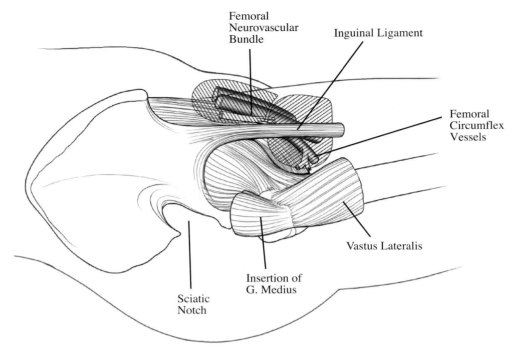

Figure 47-13 Potential neurovascular injury—anterior and inferior hip retraction. Danger zones exist for substantial injury in the anterior–inferior and inferior region of the hip. Retractors placed over the anterior column below the axis of the hip center may injure the femoral nerve or artery. The inferior hip capsule is in close proximity to the circumflex vessels; thus it is best to bluntly dissect the inferior tissue directly from the inferior capsule and retract it caudally during the capsulotomy.

retractors over the anterior column. If a retractor is placed beneath the direct head of the rectus and over the anterior column of the acetabulum, a blunt retractor should be utilized. The tip of the retractor will tend to lie in an anteroinferior quadrant of the hip and is at risk for neurovascular injury if the tip of the retractor is too long or sharp. Alternatively, a retractor can be placed superficial to the direct rectus origin in the superior and anterior quadrant of the hip overlying the anterior column. This may be helpful in cases of weak or absent bone of the anterior column, where a retractor may not function safely or efficiently. Alternatively, a sharp cobra retractor may be safely placed over the AIIS if the tip of the retractor is directed properly. There is less risk of neurovascular injury in this area if one is careful to place the tip adjacent to the inner wall of the acetabulum or ilium and avoid penetrating the tip directly medial into soft tissue. Excessive retraction should be avoided to minimize risk to the femoral neurovascular structures located in the inferior and medial wound.

Dissection in the inferior direction to expose the inferior capsule is also a critical vascular region. Within the inferior extracapsular tissue, dissection may easily encounter the lateral circumflex artery and vein in the inferior wound and lead to profuse bleeding. Dissection of the soft tissues off the inferior hip capsule should be performed carefully between the fat and capsular tissues to avoid vascular injury. A Key or Cobb elevator works well for this task, followed by careful retraction with a blunt cobra to safely expose the inferior capsule.

DIRECT LATERAL APPROACH

The direct lateral approach to the hip provides access to the hip joint through the anterior hip capsule directly through the anterior portion of the abductors. It can provide excellent access to both the anterior hip and upper femur, with a similar exposure to the anterolateral approach. With modifications of the approach, the direct lateral method can be quite versatile, even in cases that require extensive exposure, such as total joint revision. The direct lateral approach was first described and named the transgluteal approach by Bauer in 1979 (5) and was popularized by Hardinge in 1982 (24). The approach is useful in cases of femoral neck fracture, proximal femoral osteotomy, slipped capital femoral epiphysis, synovectomy, and partial or total hip replacement.

The advantage of the direct lateral approach for arthroplasty is the preservation of the posterior soft tissue of the hip. This factor should reduce the risk of a posterior hip dislocation that is seen most commonly with the posterior approach. However, this advantage is at the expense of abductor disruption on the trochanter, which leads to a higher risk of a postoperative limp (10,18). This may be a suitable compromise for the patient at high risk for dislocation, such as the elderly and neurologically compromised patient undergoing total hip or endoprosthetic replacement. Additionally, the femoral head blood supply can be preserved using this approach.

The direct lateral approach and its modifications differ from the standard lateral approach that uses a trochanteric osteotomy via the preservation of soft tissue continuity

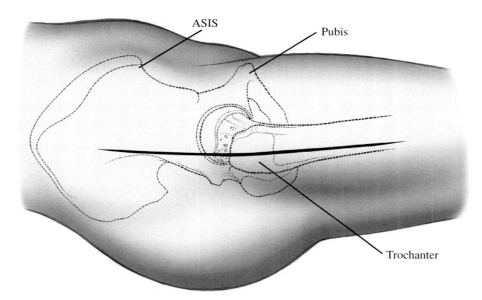

Figure 47-14 Incision for direct lateral approach. The midincision overlies the greater trochanter. The proximal half of the incision may be curved slightly posterior to improve the exposure to the proximal femur.

between the gluteus medius and vastus lateralis muscle groups. This connection helps to offset the forces of the abductors by distributing the tension into the vastus fascia. In modified forms, the direct lateral approach may contain a fragment of trochanteric bone within this connection. The direct lateral approach is not a true internervous approach because a portion of the gluteus medius muscle is divided.

The patient may be placed in either the supine, semilateral, or lateral position. The lateral position has a reported advantage of better visualization and better retraction of posterior tissues (18) (Fig. 47-14).

In the description by Hardinge, the skin incision for the direct lateral approach is centralized over the greater trochanter 8 cm long and runs parallel to the anterior border of the femoral shaft (Fig. 47-14). The proximal incision extends 5 cm posterior, ending at a point even with the ASIS. The deep incision into fascia lata is made directly overlying the greater trochanter, and the margins are retracted in an anterior and posterior direction. With the hip in extension, the fibers of the gluteus medius are divided a short distance proximally (Fig. 47-15). The dissection is carried distally into the vastus lateralis, and the entire muscle and tendinous

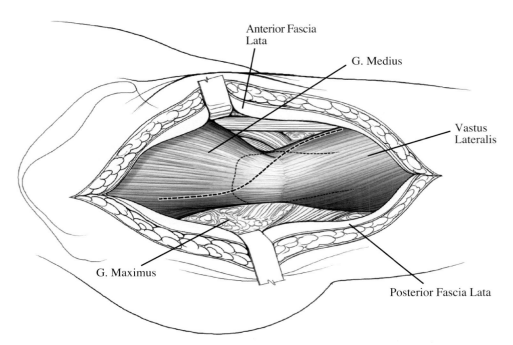

Figure 47-15 Deep incision, direct lateral (Hardinge). The incision releases the majority of the insertion of the gluteus medius and minimizes the release of the vastus lateralis.

attachment is elevated off of the trochanter sharply. An anterior flap is created consisting of muscles and tendons of the gluteus medius and vastus lateralis. The gluteus minimus is also dissected from the bone and is included with the anterior tissue flap. The thigh is abducted, and retractors are placed to expose the anterior hip capsule. Capsulotomy can then be performed, and the hip is dislocated anteriorly by an external rotation force to the femur.

There are modifications of the direct lateral approach in the manner and extent of the dissection of the soft tissue structures (Fig. 47-16). A modification of the direction in the split of the gluteus medius and vastus lateralis fibers has been described by Frndak and Mallory that preserves more of the superior gluteus medius than the Hardinge description but releases more of the vastus lateralis (19). Frndak and Mallory described their approach with a more anterior incision compared to the Hardinge incision. The direction of the split in the gluteus medius is determined by palpation of the femur over the femoral neck, by which incision splitting centers directly over the femoral neck. The vastus lateralis is dissected more distally than in the Hardinge method. The hip is dislocated after the superior and anterior capsule is either incised or excised. After the femoral neck is resected, the acetabulum is exposed by placing the lower extremity in the fully extended position with the proximal femur retracted posterior to the acetabulum.

Other authors have described a more extensive dissection in the proximal and distal directions using the direct lateral approach. Elevation of the incision distally through the vastus lateralis is preferable to proximal dissection of the gluteus medius. This will minimize traction or injury to the inferior branch of the superior gluteal nerve that is located in the proximal wound (3,6).

Most of the problems reported with the direct lateral approach are those associated with the loss of abductor function. Weakness may result from injury to the nerve supply, but it is most often due to a disruption of the tendinous attachments of the abductors. Studies of the separation of the gluteus medius attachment have detected some degree of separation in about half of the patients, but a significant limp was associated with separations of more than 2.5 cm (3,6,35,46,52,62).

The proximal extent of the wound of the direct approach is a muscle-splitting approach and is limited by the potential for nerve damage. The proximal dissection through the gluteus medius places the superior gluteal nerve at risk. The main branch of the superior gluteal nerve has been measured within the muscle to a distance of between 4.5 and 4.9 cm above the level of the superior acetabular rim, and safe dissection is assured if 4 cm above the acetabulum, or 5 cm above the tip of the trochanter is not exceeded (18,25,31). Patients who are short statured or who have branching of the nerve within that zone are at higher risk for nerve injury (35). Excessive retraction of the gluteus medius flap should be avoided to minimize risk to the nerve. A significantly higher incidence of limp and heterotopic ossification has been reported with the direct lateral approach, as compared to the posterolateral approach (10,18).

Historically, a type of lateral approach was also described by McFarland. The approach released the insertion of the gluteus medius and the gluteus minimus from the trochanter (44). This extensive release is problematic because of the difficulty in healing the tendon back to bone. Clinical problems of abductor weakness and limp caused by avulsion of the gluteus medius tendon can be expected with this type of approach.

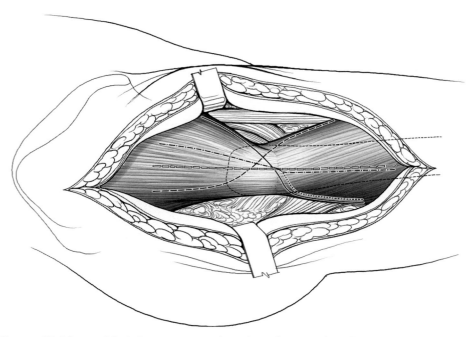

Figure 47-16 Modified deep incisions, direct lateral approaches. From posterior–proximal: (1) Hardinge, (2) Stracathro, (3) Bauer: includes two choices for the distal incision—straight for exposure of only the hip, and posterior (*dotted*) for added exposure of the proximal femur, (4) Frndak/Mallory (*solid line*).

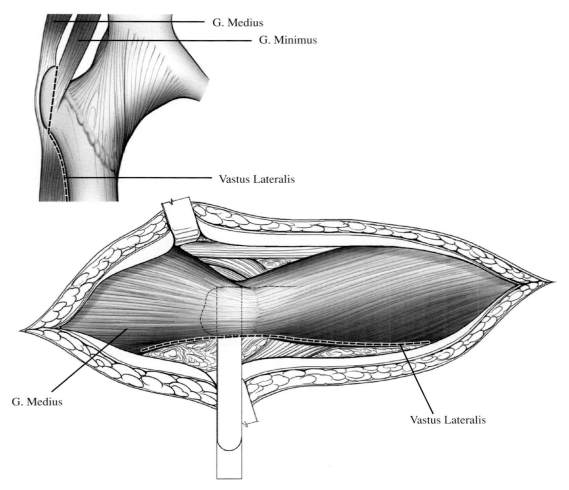

G. Medius

G. Minimus

Vastus Lateralis

G. Medius

Vastus Lateralis

Figure 47-17 Direct approach with trochanteric slide. The technique of maintaining all of the attachments of the gluteus medius, trochanter, and vastus lateralis is shown. A posterior incision to the muscle preserves the innervation of the vastus. The cut into the trochanter may be made deeper to include the gluteus minimus with the slide.

Trochanteric Slide Modification

A modification of the direct lateral approach, termed the trochanteric slide, has been described by Dall which alters the method of dissection of the abductors from the trochanter (16). In this description, a fragment of anterior trochanteric bone is removed in continuity with the gluteus medius, trochanteric connective tissue, and vastus (21).

The trochanteric slide approach is reported to be useful in both revision total hip replacement surgery and difficult primary hip arthroplasty. In the case of total hip revision where femoral component subsidence has occurred, the trochanter may be difficult to advance back to its bed using a conventional transtrochanteric osteotomy. The technique allows for some adjustment in the location of the reattachment of the trochanteric bone. However, there are limits as to how far the trochanteric fragment can be displaced and reattached (14,50).

The osteotomy for the trochanteric slide begins just anterior to the tendinous insertion of the gluteus medius into the greater trochanter. The osteotomy is placed lateral to the inser-

tion of the gluteus minimus and leaves the minimus attached to the anterior tubercle of the greater trochanter (Fig. 47-17). Alternatively, a thicker segment of greater trochanter may be created to include the gluteus minimus insertion (12). The bony fragment with attached tendon and muscle can then be held by a self-retaining retractor (Fig. 47-18). Exposure of the anterior–superior capsule is completed. The short rotators can then be released from the posterior attachment for additional mobility of the femur.

Dislocation of the hip is accomplished with the hip in flexion, adduction, and external rotation with the leg placed anteriorly. Occasionally, release of the iliopsoas tendon may be required to permit dislocation. A curved retractor placed beneath the proximal femur helps to elevate the proximal femur from the wound. A blunt Hohman retractor placed posterolaterally along the proximal femoral diaphysis provides access to the proximal femur and anterior and lateral aspects of the femoral shaft. According to its advocates, the trochanteric slide approach provides adequate exposure even for revision surgery where access to the medullary canal is necessary.

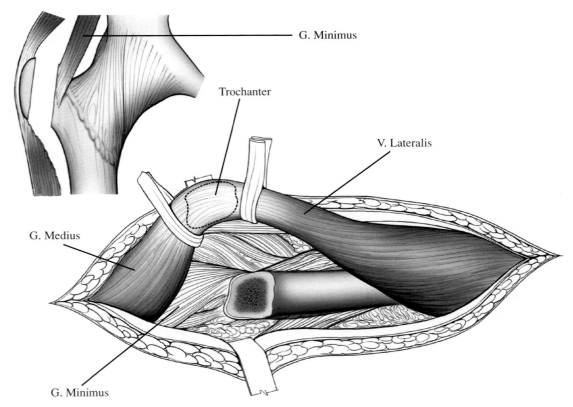

G. Minimus

Trochanter

V. Lateralis

G. Medius

G. Minimus

Figure 47-18   Trochanteric slide. The soft tissue is retracted anteriorly and may be held with self-retractors. The anterior capsule can then be dissected for the exposure to the hip.

Closure is accomplished by suturing the gluteus minimus tendon near to its original location. Trochanteric wires may be placed circumferentially about the lesser trochanter and through the trochanteric fragment. Reattachment of the bony fragment can be problematic in cases of poor-quality bone, or in destruction of the trochanteric bed caused by a fracture, or in a low femoral neck osteotomy (3). This may necessitate the creation of a smaller bone fragment at the time of the exposure.

In cases where the reconstruction has lengthened the leg, the trochanteric fragment in the trochanteric slide technique may not return to its original bed. Mobilization to a limited extent by elevating the undersurface of the abductor from the ilium has been described to facilitate trochanteric advancement. Alternatively, the trochanteric fragment can be excised from the overlying soft tissue, while preserving the continuity of the gluteus medius and the vastus lateralis (21).

Extensile Modification

An extensile modification to the direct lateral approach has been described that involves a more extensive elevation of the vastus lateralis and intermedius from the femur. As with all of the direct lateral techniques, the extensile description maintains soft tissue continuity of the abductors and the vastus. The extensile exposure has been reported to be useful for revision arthroplasty.

The incision for the extensile approach is described as curvilinear from a posterior position 10 to 15 cm superior to the greater trochanter, and carried distally across the greater trochanter. In revision hip replacement, the incision is extended distally along the lateral thigh to the level of the implanted prosthesis or cement plug. The fascia lata and gluteus maximus fascia are incised along the original incision line. The vastus lateralis is then released proximally off of the trochanteric ridge and dissected from the femur and lateral intermuscular septum. The perforating vessels are ligated. The vastus lateralis and vastus intermedius is reflected as a unit. The gluteus medius and minimus tendon is elevated proximally, from the anterior trochanter (Fig. 47-19). The anterior capsule can then be exposed and a capsulectomy is performed. The posterior portion of the gluteus medius is preserved, similar to the direct lateral approach. Alternatively, if the gluteus medius tendon appears atrophic, an oscillating saw can be used to create an osteotomy in the coronal plane of the trochanter. A 4- or 5-mm-thick section of bone is released from the anterior trochanter (Fig. 47-20). The authors describe a more secure closure when such a fragment of bone is utilized. In cases of external rotation contracture, the hip can be rotated internally for the short rotators to be divided, and a posterior capsulectomy can be performed. Access to both the acetabulum and femur are sufficient for revision arthroplasty of both the acetabulum and femur. To improve visualization of the femur for cement removal, 7-mm portals may be placed in the anterior

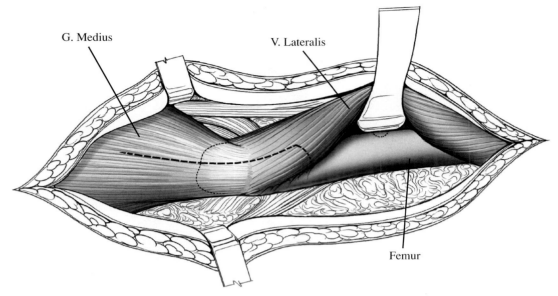

Figure 47-19 Extensile modification of the direct lateral approach. Incision is shown to release the gluteus medius and minimus from the anterior trochanter to allow exposure of the anterior hip capsule.

femoral cortex to illuminate and provide direct visualization of the intermedullary canal. The closure is accomplished by reattachment of the entire anterior and posterior flaps. If an anterior trochanteric fragment has been taken, reattachment of the bone through drill holes is recommended (31).

TRANSTROCHANTERIC APPROACH

The transtrochanteric approach offers broad simultaneous exposure of the femoral shaft and acetabulum and allows for consistent orientation of components and the unobstructed

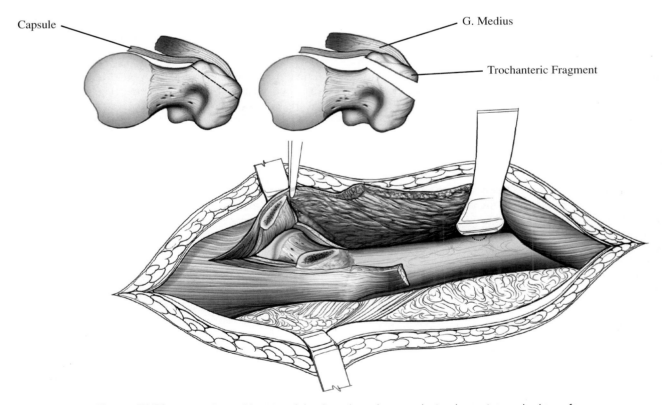

Figure 47-20 Extensile modification of the direct lateral approach. An alternative method to soft tissue release is shown. A fragment of bone is released from the anterior greater trochanter which preserves muscular and capsular attachments. A capsulotomy is then performed.

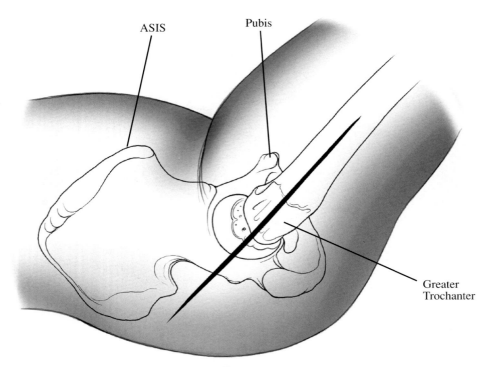

Figure 47-21   Transtrochanteric incision. The hip is flexed to 45°, which allows a straight skin incision that is aligned with the fibers of the gluteus maximus muscle. With the hip extended, this incision mimics the shape of a posterolateral incision.

technique of insertion of cement for total hip components. This advantage may be important in difficult primary total hip arthroplasties, but especially in revision arthroplasty. In the case of revision arthroplasty, soft tissue contracture and scarring can interfere with exposure or removal of existing components, as well as the insertion of new components. In addition, the transtrochanteric approach also allows for advancement and potential lateralization of the abductor mechanism to improve soft tissue tension about the hip, and also to improve abductor function by improving mechanical efficiency of the hip. Other indications for this approach include cases of femoral shortening (to restore abductor tension), major acetabular reconstruction to gain adequate exposure, and whenever exposure is needed in a complex case (27). Prior to total joint replacement, the technique was advocated for exposure in both arthroplasty and arthrodesis of the hip (36). The option of a trochanteric osteotomy was mentioned by Langenbeck in the 1870s to facilitate exposure of the hip following a gunshot wound. The transtrochanteric osteotomy can be anatomically divided into intracapsular and extracapsular techniques.

Intracapsular Transtrochanteric Osteotomy

The intracapsular technique of the transtrochanteric lateral approach was improved and popularized for primary hip replacement by the successful work of Sir John Charnley and his innovations in low-friction arthroplasty of the hip. The improvement in the technique of wire fixation of the trochanter reduced the incidence of trochanteric nonunion and was partially responsible for the successful results

reported using the Charnley hip replacement. The trochanteric osteotomy can be incorporated with a variety of approaches to the hip including the anterolateral and posterolateral approaches (40).

The approach begins with the patient in the supine position and the hip flexed to 45°. An incision is centered at the vastus lateralis ridge of the trochanter (Fig. 47-21). Although the incision is straight, with the hip in extension the proximal limb of the incision is seen to be angulated posteriorly. The fascial incision is made in line with the skin incision, just posterior to the tensor fascia lata muscle. It is helpful to preserve a 5-mm band of dense fascia lata just posterior to the tensor muscle to provide a secure closure. Adduction of the hip helps to add tension to the tensor fascia lata during the incision. Additional exposure can be easily and safely obtained by simply extending the distal and proximal limbs of the incision to provide anterior and posterior relaxation of the tissues. Few approaches offer such an extensile means of additional exposure.

The Charnley technique next describes the release of a small arcuate of gluteus medius connective tissue from the anterior border of the greater trochanter to gain access to the anterior hip capsule. A right angle retractor is placed over the anterior border of the gluteus medius with the femur in abduction to expose the anterior hip capsule (Fig. 47-22). Fatty tissue is dissected off of the anterior capsule along the axis of the femoral neck as far medial as the anterior column of the acetabulum. The vastus lateralis is released from the vastus ridge and elevated off the proximal femur a short distance of 2 to 3 cm. Cauterization or ligation of the lateral trochanteric artery is required, as it courses from the anterior

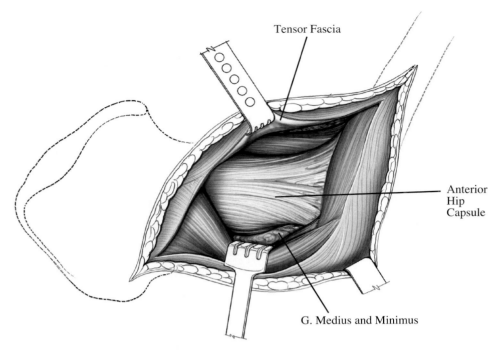

Tensor Fascia

Anterior
Hip
Capsule

G. Medius and Minimus

Figure 47-22 Anterior capsule exposure. With the self-retractor placed anterior and posterior, and the rake retractor placed on the gluteus medius, the anterior hip capsule is exposed after dissection of the anterior soft tissue. Abduction of the femur facilitates this exposure.

vastus muscle. The anterior capsule is then entered sharply with a longitudinal incision. This capsular incision is placed along the midaxis of the femoral neck. This was later modified to a more distal location along the lower border of the neck to preserve additional trochanteric capsule. Through this incision, an angle clamp is placed intracapsularly and passed superior to the femoral neck, penetrating the posterior–superior capsule medial to the greater trochanter (Fig. 47-23). This clamp is used to pass the Gigli hand saw deep to the posterior–superior tubercle of the trochanter. Internal rotation and adduction of the femur facilitates the trochanteric cut. This maneuver will minimize the chance of creating an undersized trochanteric fragment that can result by cutting too superficially into the posterior trochanter (Figs. 47-24 and 47-25). The saw cut exits at the level of the vastus ridge. While retracting the trochanteric fragment proximally, care is taken to place the angled retractor onto the iliotrochanteric capsule. Vigorous retraction on the trochanter bone can fragment the trochanter and make its reattachment difficult. With the trochanter retracted proximally, and the femur adducted, hemostasis can be accomplished. Branches requiring cauterization include the posterior circumflex artery on both the femoral and the trochanteric fragment, the trochanteric branch near the anterior bed of the trochanter (a branch of the lateral circumflex), and a branch of the anterior circumflex along the anterior capsule of the femur. The hip can be internally rotated to safely complete the posterior capsulotomy to the level of the acetabular labrum by cutting upward in a direction away from the sciatic nerve, which lies directly posterior (Fig. 47-26). A bone hook can then be delivered onto the posterior femoral neck. Using traction on the femoral head with the femur in moderate adduction and external rotation,

the hip can be dislocated in a lateral and anterior direction. The femoral head can then be osteotomized through the femoral neck at the desired level. A horizontal self-retaining retractor is placed between the femoral neck and the iliotrochanteric soft tissue. This retractor creates tension on the superior and inferior segments of retained capsule termed the iliotrochanteric and pubofemoral capsule. Excessive force on the retractor should be avoided to minimize the risk of stripping these important capsular attachments. The anterior–posterior capsule retractor helps to expose the acetabulum (Fig. 47-27). It is important to carefully place the posterior teeth of the anterior–posterior retractor in the segment of preserved posterior capsule so that the sciatic nerve is not injured. If there is inadequate posterior capsule, the anterior–posterior retractor should be excluded. The piriformis is usually still attached to the trochanteric fragment and Charnley routinely released it to prevent excessive tension on the trochanteric fragment and also to prevent piriformis irritation to the sciatic nerve. Excellent exposure of the acetabulum is obtained. The horizontal and vertical retractors can then be removed for excellent exposure of the proximal femur and medullary canal.

The Charnley transtrochanteric lateral technique incorporates a capsulotomy rather than a capsulectomy and retains a strong inferior capsular attachment between the inferior acetabulum and femur, and superiorly between the ilium and the trochanter. When the trochanter is advanced and reattached, the iliotrochanteric capsule is tensioned to improve static stability of the hip. Advancement and lateralization also aids in the dynamic function of the abductors. Charnley considered these preserved attachments to be critical to the stability of the arthroplasty.

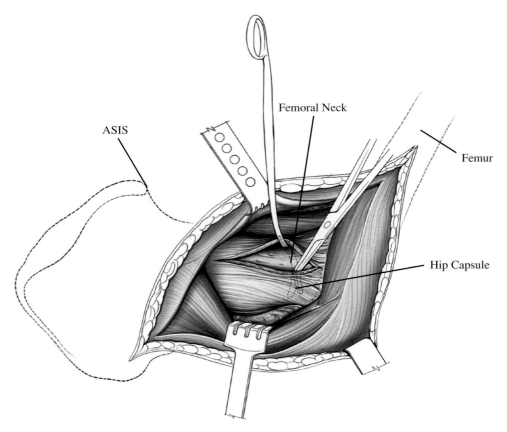

ASIS

Femoral Neck

Femur

Hip Capsule

Figure 47-23   Passage of the intracapsular clamp. The clamp is placed between the femoral neck and the superior hip capsule. The initial placement of a curved retractor inferiorly assures proper intra-articular access.

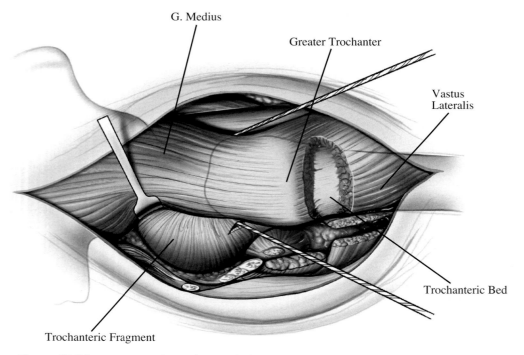

G. Medius

Greater Trochanter

Vastus Lateralis

Trochanteric Bed

Trochanteric Fragment

Figure 47-24   Positioning the Gigli saw, which is positioned for the trochanteric osteotomy. The saw exits the posterior capsule and begins the cut posterior to the trochanteric tubercle. This step assures an adequately large fragment of trochanteric bone. The femur is adducted slightly to facilitate this important step.

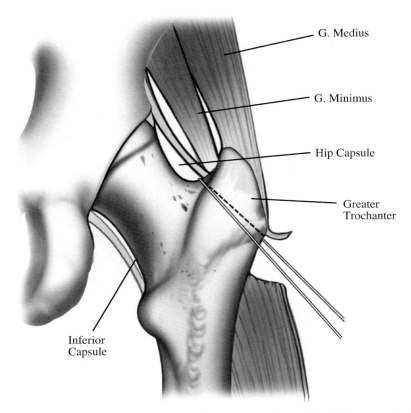

G. Medius

G. Minimus

Hip Capsule

Greater
Trochanter

Inferior
Capsule

Figure 47-25   The direction of the Gigli cut. The proper position of the Gigli saw at the femoral neck sulcus. Note that the saw is deep to the superior hip capsule. The initial cut is made in a more distal direction, and as the cut proceeds the saw is directed more lateral. This maneuver also assures an adequate trochanteric fragment.

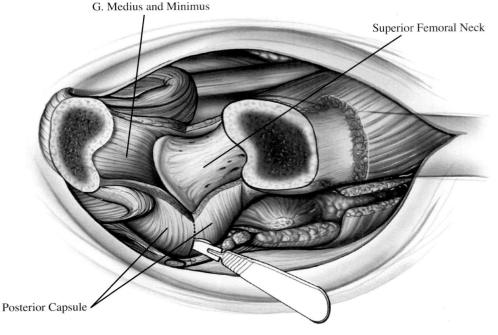

G. Medius and Minimus

Superior Femoral Neck

Posterior Capsule

Figure 47-26   Completion of the posterior capsulotomy. The retracted trochanter fragment exposes the posterior capsule for the cut to be finalized under direct vision. Internal rotation of the femur is helpful. The cut should always be made in a direction away from the sciatic nerve.

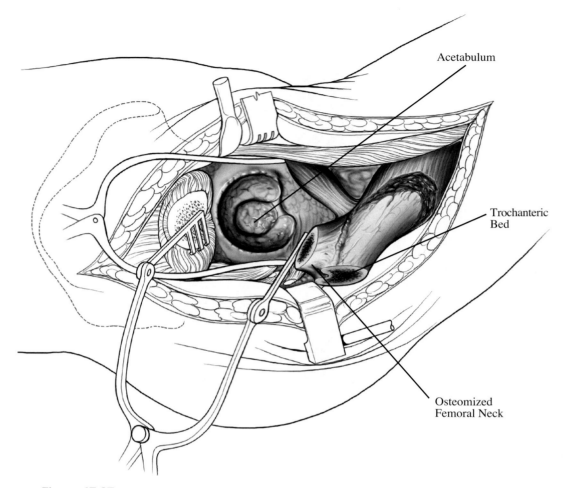

Acetabulum

Trochanteric
Bed

Osteomized
Femoral Neck

Figure 47-27 Acetabular exposure. The horizontal and vertical retractors provide the sustained retraction for excellent exposure of the acetabulum. Alternatively, a large cobra retractor may be placed inferiorly with its tip placed beneath the acetabular teardrop, to retract the femur downward.

Extracapsular Transtrochanteric Approach

The extracapsular trochanteric osteotomy technique, as advocated by Harris, sacrifices the hip capsule and preserves the insertions of the gluteus minimus and medius muscles on the trochanter. The extracapsular trochanteric osteotomy may be useful in primary and revision arthroplasty, hip osteotomies, trauma, and tumor cases, where wide exposure is needed as in reconstructive cases with severe contractures, deformities, or leg length inequality. In revision hip arthroplasty, the trochanteric osteotomy can facilitate exposure of the proximal femur and may decrease the risk of femoral cortex perforation during cement removal (29). By sacrificing the iliotrochanteric segment of hip capsule, the trochanteric fragment is free to be advanced as needed along the femoral shaft. Release of this static tether to the trochanter may also minimize excessive tension to the trochanteric reattachment and improve the rate of bony union. The patient can be positioned in a lateral or semilateral position. The semilateral position, which tilts the pelvis posteriorly about 30° from the vertical, is more versatile, especially when counterincisions along the iliac crest are needed to gain access to the pelvis.

The extracapsular technique has been described through either an anterolateral or posterolateral incision. After exposure is made of the trochanter, the extracapsular interval is identified. The interval is easily located with the hip in extension between the superior hip capsule and the gluteus minimus tendon. Palpation and visualization of the tendon are carried out by placement of the left index finger on a left hip (the right index finger on a right hip) a distance of one phalanx anterior to the distal anterior border of the trochanter, one phalanx turned 90° proximal again, and the gluteus minimus tendon border is usually palpable (Figs. 47-28 and 47-29). Visualization of the tendon by flexing and externally rotating the hip may be needed to confirm the medial edge of the tendon beneath the front edge of the gluteus medius. A blunt elevator (e.g., Cushing, Joker) can then be placed beneath the minimus tendon in the extracapsular interval and advanced superiorly over the top of the capsule. The vastus muscle is released sharply from the trochanteric ridge (Figs. 47-30 and

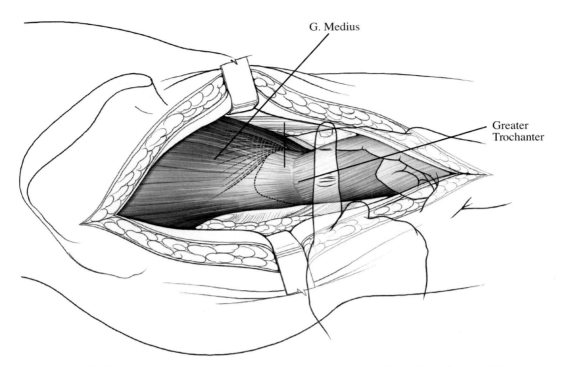

G. Medius

Greater
Trochanter

Figure 47-28 Extracapsular exposure. Initial reference to the insertion of the gluteus minimus (*vertical line*) begins at the anterior insertion of the gluteus medius.

47-31). Medially, the vastus muscle arises in a V-shaped pattern along the intertrochanteric line and should be incised along this origin (Fig. 47-32). In a posterior wound, with the hip in slight internal rotation, a Key elevator is used to elevate the soft tissue from the posterior rotator tendons. This maneuver ensures that the sciatic nerve is not adherent to the osteotomy site. It is very important at this step to confirm the location of the sciatic nerve. The sciatic nerve is usually palpable along the body of the ischium about midway between the posterior border of the acetabulum and the ischial tubercle (Fig. 47-33). Having exposed the anterior and posterior limits of the trochanter, a wide osteotome can then be directed toward the blunt elevator, held in the sulcus of the femoral neck (Fig. 47-34). If the osteotomy is initiated more proximal to the vastus ridge, a portion of the remaining anterior fibers of the gluteus medius will remain attached to the distal trochanteric bed of the femur. These fibers are released sharply to allow the trochanteric fragment to be retracted proximally.

The advantage of this technique of trochanteric osteotomy is in the control of the size of the trochanter as determined by the entry point and direction of the osteotome. This method is most applicable in revision arthroplasty surgery to minimize the deleterious effects of a steeply inclined osteotomy. A steeply inclined osteotomy violates the proximal medullary canal and bone stock of the trochanteric bed, which may be further affected by extrusion of methyl methacrylate cement in the case of a cemented prosthetic stem. These factors may contribute to an increase in the risk of a nonunion. A more horizontal osteotomy preserves an adequate trochanteric bed for

the trochanteric fragment to be reattached. This modified cut is made by starting the osteotome proximal to the vastus lateralis ridge and directing the osteotome in a more transverse plane toward the femoral axis (Figs. 47-35 and 47-36). The smaller fragment may be mobilized as needed to be transferred distally onto the lateral trochanteric bone or femoral shaft (Fig. 47-37) (29). Complications in the creation of a small trochanteric fragment may include fragmentation, fracture, or damage from the trochanteric wires which may lead to nonunion. Alternatively, such as in cases of small trochanteric anatomy, a larger fragment may be taken by entering the osteotome more distal to the vastus ridge at a steeper angle to maximize its size.

Regardless of the size of the osteotomy, fragmentation of the trochanter must be avoided. To avoid fragmentation, it is critical not to lever the osteotome in any distal–proximal fashion. However, the osteotome can be manipulated very carefully in an anterior–posterior fashion in the plane of the osteotomy to assist in the cut. A useful technique to minimize bony fragmentation is to stage the cuts of the osteotomy. Directing a narrow half-inch osteotome along the anticipated anterior and posterior trochanteric cut before advancing to the larger, wider osteotome helps to minimize the fragmentation at the margins of the trochanter (Fig. 47-38). This method is also useful in the case of a femoral component that is not to be revised and that fills the trochanteric bed. By the creation of a horseshoe-shaped osteotomy of the trochanter, an adequate fragment of trochanteric bone can be obtained without damaging the retained femoral component.

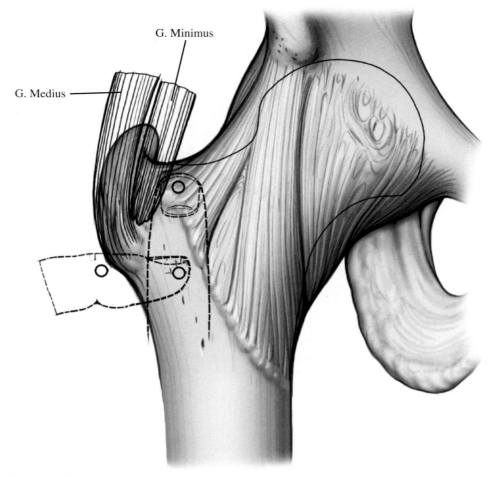

G. Minimus

G. Medius

Figure 47-29 Extracapsular exposure, gluteus minimus. This maneuver determines the starting point for placement of the retractor beneath the gluteus minimus. A distance of a phalanx beginning at the anterior insertion of the gluteus medius and then the same distance superiorly usually allows palpation of the tendon edge. This can be confirmed by direct visualization after retraction of the anterior border of the gluteus medius and abduction and external rotation of the femur.

Once the osteotomy is completed, the hip is placed in adduction to enlarge the field of view. Sharp dissection of the remaining gluteus minimus that may be attached to the femur helps to free up the trochanter fragment. The remaining superior hip capsule is readily exposed from its underside for excision or incision to allow the freedom to dislocate the hip. The hip is dislocated by femoral adduction and external rotation across the table. It is important to place the knee in flexion at this point in order to minimize traction to the sciatic nerve. Elevation of the femur at the knee with the use of a soft bolster assists in flexing the knee, particularly in short-statured individuals whose femur is so short as to not drape over the far side of the table and allow flexion of the knee (Fig. 47-39). The bolster may also assist in the exposure of the acetabulum by lowering the proximal femur in the wound. After dislocation, the femoral neck can be osteotomized, or the femoral prosthesis can be removed from the canal as in the case of a revision. Self-retaining retractors can be placed between the femur and the trochanter, and cobra retractors can be placed anterior to the acetabulum and inferior to gain excellent exposure of the acetabulum.

In revision hip surgery, exposure of the femoral canal is greatly facilitated by a technique known as "skeletonization" of the proximal femur (Fig. 47-40). This technique elevates soft tissue attachments to the proximal femur and can be incorporated in any of the transtrochanteric techniques. The stripping of structures may include the vastus musculature from the proximal femur over the lateral and anterior surfaces, the upper portion of the adductors, the linea aspera posteriorly, and, if necessary, the iliopsoas tendon. The most effective exposure usually results from the release of the structures that insert onto the linea aspera. The proximal femur is effectively "delivered" upward out of the wound. Skeletonization exposes the femoral shaft and can greatly facilitate the estimation of the direction of the medullary canal during revision surgery. In addition, the periosteal dissection of the soft tissues from the femoral shaft allows fractures or perforations to be detected that may result from errors in intramedullary cement removal or component insertion.

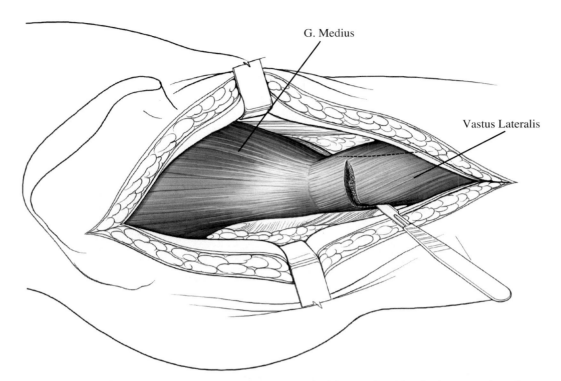

Figure 47-30 Extracapsular exposure, vastus lateralis. The initial incision in the vastus is an L shape. The incision may begin a short distance distal to the vastus ridge (0.5 to 1.0 cm) to preserve a proximal cuff of tissue to be used for closure.

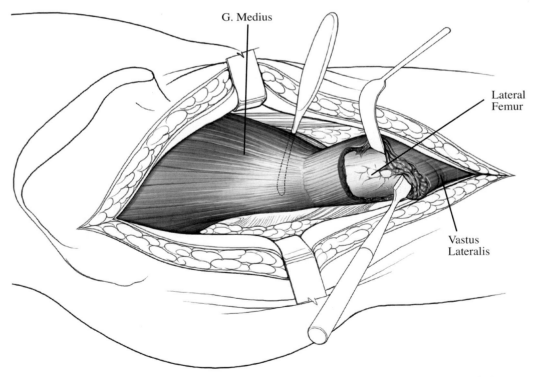

Figure 47-31 Exposure, lateral femur. The release of the vastus is performed as needed to expose the lateral femur. The anterior angled retractor should be carefully controlled to avoid injury to the femoral nerve that is located deep to the retractor. The blunt retractor superiorly lies beneath the minimus and above the capsule.

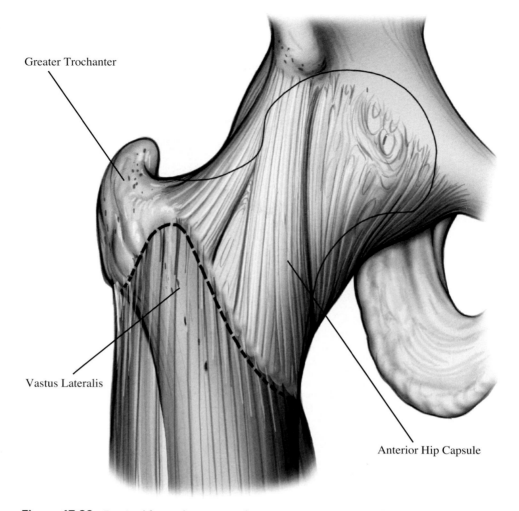

Greater Trochanter

Vastus Lateralis

Anterior Hip Capsule

Figure 47-32 Proximal femoral exposure. The proper anatomic incision line to release the vastus origin from the anterior proximal femur is shown. Note the V shape at its attachment to the intertrochanteric ridge.

Disadvantages of the trochanteric osteotomy mainly relate to the problem of nonunion. A nonunion may be painful for the patient, and if there is migration of the trochanter a limp will usually result. Trochanteric migration with resulting abductor weakness may also increase the risk for dislocation. Minor problems of trochanteric osteotomy include bursitis caused by wire irritation and wire fragmentation with potential migration into the articulation or soft tissues.

Biplane Modification (Chevron)

A biplane (chevron) modification of the straight trochanteric osteotomy has been reported to minimize the complications of the straight osteotomy (Fig. 47-41). The biplane modification is reported to provide improved inherent stability in both anterior–posterior and rotational planes, better surface contact to maximize healing, easier anatomic replacement of the trochanter, and improved postoperative management (67).

The improved stability with this type of osteotomy is reported to allow postoperative management to be the same as for nonosteotomized patients (7).

The technique of the biplane osteotomy begins with a careful outline of the superior, anterior, and posterior borders of the trochanter. Anterior and posterior limbs of equal size are planned. The angle of the anterior limb is cut 30° to the parasagittal plane, and the second limb is cut 120° to 130° from the first osteotomy. The cuts are ideally made using an oscillating saw. The remainder of the approach follows the techniques of the transtrochanteric approach described above.

Extended Proximal Femoral Osteotomy

A more extensive trochanteric osteotomy has been described to include a portion of the proximal femur for special circumstances in hip surgery. The so-called extended proximal femoral osteotomy (EPFO) and extended trochanteric

(*text continues on page* 712)

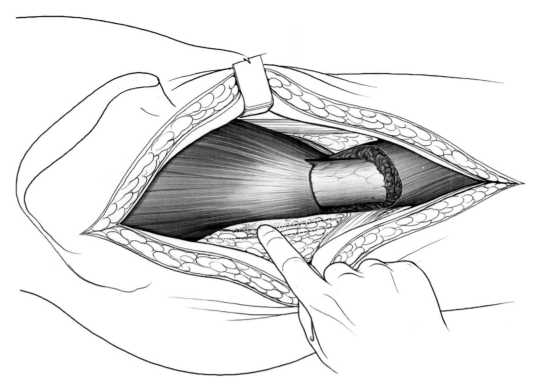

Figure 47-33 Location of the sciatic nerve. Prior to trochanteric osteotomy, it is important to locate the sciatic nerve. Usually, the nerve is readily palpable in the fatty tissue between the acetabular rim and the ischial tuberosity. Rarely, the nerve may be extremely close to the dissection, and this requires extra care to avoid injury.

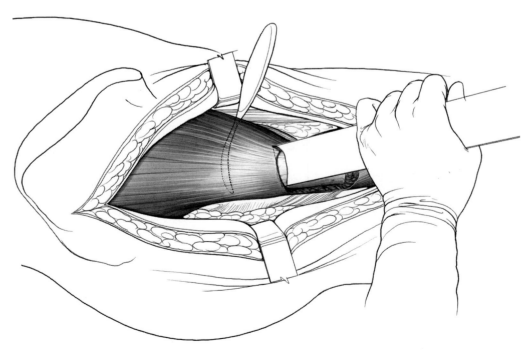

Figure 47-34 Standard, straight osteotomy. A wide osteotome is positioned near the vastus ridge and directed to the blunt retractor. This assures that the abductors will be included with the trochanteric fragment.

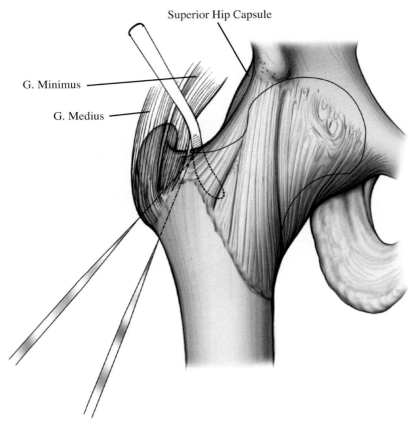

Figure 47-35 Variations on the trochanteric osteotomy. The entry point, and the direction, can be varied to allow different sized trochanteric fragments to be made. The target for the cut remains the retractor located in the sulcus.

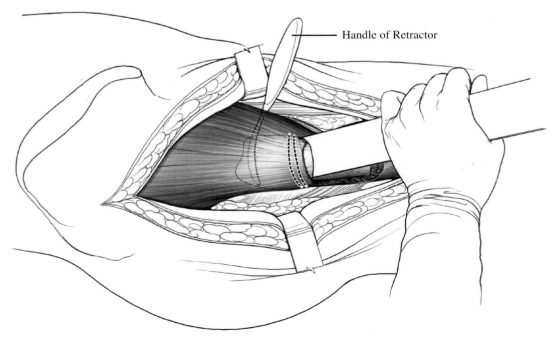

Figure 47-36 Starting position of the osteotome. The starting position may vary to preserve the femoral bone and capsule. Cuts that are initiated proximal to the vastus ridge require some sacrifice of the gluteus medius insertion.

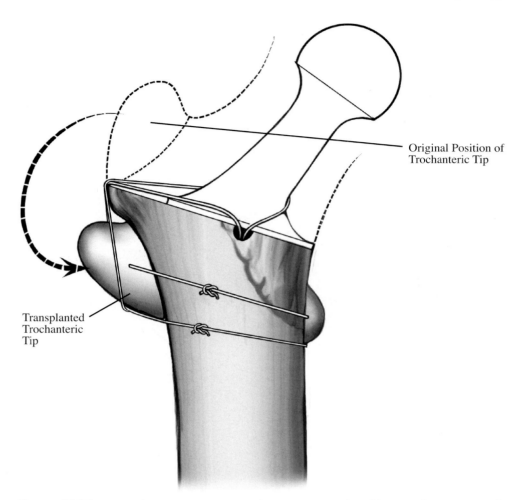

Original Position of
Trochanteric Tip

Transplanted
Trochanteric
Tip

Figure 47-37 Proximal osteotomy cut. It may be necessary or desirable to perform a proximal trochanteric osteotomy to preserve the proximal femoral bone stock. Occasionally, the trochanteric bed will be sacrificed and require this technique as shown. (Adapted from Harris WH. Revision surgery for failed, nonseptic total hip arthroplasty. *CORR.* 1982;170:8.)

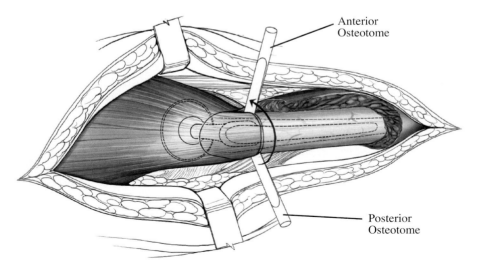

Anterior
Osteotome

Posterior
Osteotome

Figure 47-38 Anterior and posterior osteotomies. To minimize the risk of fragmentation of the trochanter, smaller osteotomes can be used along the anterior and posterior cortex to gradually osteotomize the trochanter. This is especially helpful for cases with femoral prostheses that extend into the bed of the greater trochanter.

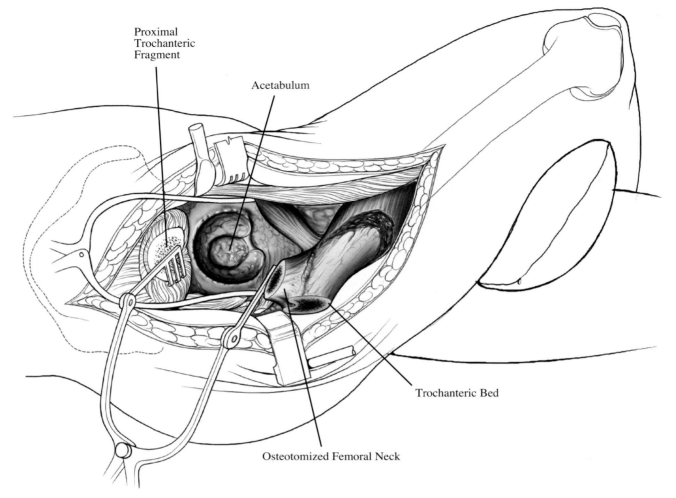

Proximal
Trochanteric
Fragment

Acetabulum

Trochanteric Bed

Osteotomized Femoral Neck

Figure 47-39 Acetabular exposure. A bolster placed beneath the distal femur will help to depress the proximal femur during acetabular exposure. This should be removed to expose the proximal femur.

osteotomy (ETO) have been advocated in revision hip surgery to improve the technique of cement removal and femoral component extraction (12,53,68). Both techniques osteotomize the bony cortex of the proximal femur to varying amounts and elevate the vastus musculature from the cortex. The distal extent of the ETO is described as 3 to 10 cm distal to the vastus ridge, whereas the EPFO is described to end 8 to 16 cm distal to the tip of the trochanter. The length of the trochanteric fragment can be varied according to the need for exposure of the proximal femoral canal with either method. The EPFO technique also preserves the attachment of the vastus lateralis fascia to the vastus ridge to offset the pull from the abductors. In contrast to the EPFO method, the ETO method releases the vastus lateralis attachment to the bony vastus ridge. The advantages of the EPFO over the standard trochanteric osteotomy are the improved exposure of the medullary canal and improved distal access to areas requiring distal cement removal or bone ingrowth disruption. The proximal femur is opened through the femoral cortex as a one third semicircumferential segment and levered with an ante-

rior hinge to expose the medullary contents. The tissue segment includes the gluteus medius, greater trochanter, anterolateral femoral diaphysis, and vastus lateralis. This wide exposure is accomplished with the preservation of soft tissue attachments to the bone to assist bony union. In addition, the soft tissue tension can be adjusted (68).

The indication for the ETO includes cases where additional exposure or access is needed. In cases of revision, the technique may be useful for the well-bonded or extensively cemented long stem, or for a cementless stem with considerable bony or firm fibrous ingrowth that exists in the distal part of the prosthesis. It may be useful for additional exposure, where proximal bone deformities either hamper distal cement removal or interfere with straight reaming of the femoral canal for reimplantation. This technique can also be substituted for a transtrochanteric osteotomy when there is a substantially deficient trochanteric bed.

The osteotomy can be used with either a posterior approach, an anterolateral approach, or a trochanteric slide approach. The proximal osteotomy is carried out prior to

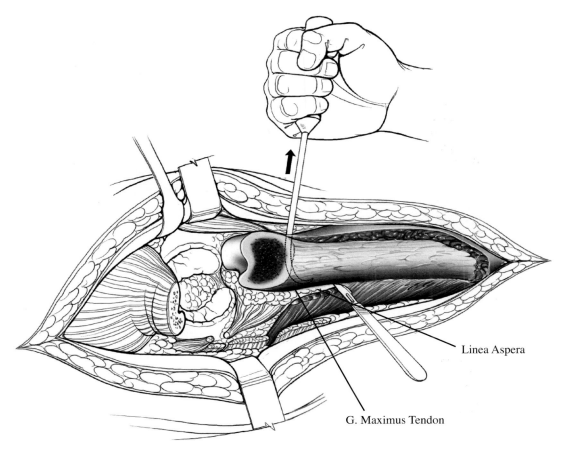

Linea Aspera

G. Maximus Tendon

Figure 47-40 Technique of skeletonization. For added exposure of the femoral shaft and medullary canal, skeletonization is necessary. Tension applied to soft tissue allows safe release of the linea aspera and hip capsule using careful sharp technique against bone. The bolster should be removed from under the distal femur.

dislocation of the hip if there is any difficulty with dislocation due to bony overgrowth, subsidence, or stiffness. The short external rotators are incised from the trochanter, and a portion of the gluteus maximus is released from the femur. Capsulectomy is performed in a complete fashion. The vastus lateralis is then elevated from the lateral intermuscular septum, but the fascia is left intact on the vastus lateralis ridge. The osteotomy extends in a line from the quadrate tubercle at the base of the greater trochanter distally to a point of the maximal exposure required for the procedure. The posterior osteotomy line is begun just anterior to the linea aspera. A one third partial circumference osteotomy of the posterolateral femoral shaft is performed (Fig. 47-42). A high-speed burr can be directed from posterolateral to anterior to create this segment if the medullary canal is not excessively compromised by a prosthetic stem. The osteotomy can be completed by connecting the burr holes with an osteotome. An oscillating saw is usually needed to complete the final proximal–anterior osteotomy. By careful elevation of the fragment of bone and muscle, exposure of the medullary contents is accomplished. At closure, to help add tension to the abductors, a portion of the distal fragment can be removed to allow advancement of the bony osteotomy fragment. The bone is reattached using circumferential wires or cables. A pitfall to this technique is damage to the sciatic nerve, and thus it is important to palpate

and protect the sciatic nerve while completing the posterior extent of the osteotomy. Occasionally, for safety reasons, complete exposure of the nerve may be necessary, especially if extensive scar tissue is present.

Alternatively, Wagner has described an extended osteotomy performed through the femoral muscle mass (Fig. 47-42). His technique creates a similar anterolateral bony fragment but creates the anterior hinge by maneuvering a thin osteotome longitudinally through the vastus musculature in multiple locations along the proposed anterior osteotomy (11). The cortical and trochanteric myo-osseous flap is then hinged along the anterior osteotomy from the posterior in a similar fashion to the EPFO method. In contrast to the ETO and EPFO methods, the Wagner method preserves virtually all of the soft tissue attachments to the bony fragment to preserve the bone circulation.

Extensile Triradiate Approach

An extensile triradiate approach has been described for use in difficult primary and revision procedures, complex acetabular fractures, and major structural allograft reconstruction in total hip replacement (45,61). This approach provides complete anterior and posterior exposure of the hip capsule and can be most helpful for anterior column defects, pelvic dehiscence,

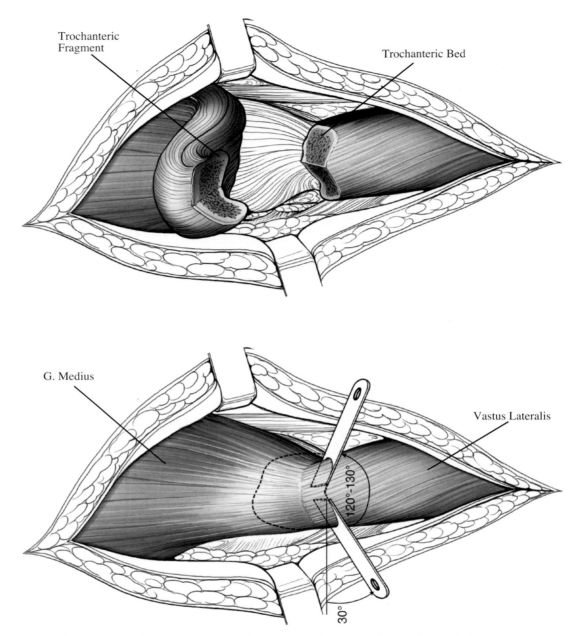

Figure 47-41   Chevron osteotomy. The technique is illustrated using the oscillating saw. This method will minimize the chance of fragmenting the trochanteric bone.

intrapelvic prostheses, obesity, and tumor reconstruction (39). In addition, a major advantage of this approach is the ability to identify and protect the femoral nerve and vascular structures, which are at particular risk in certain congenital dysplastic cases and in anterior column reconstructions.

The approach begins with a triradiate-shaped incision that is apexed to the tip of the greater trochanter (Fig. 47-43). To minimize circulatory compromise of the skin, it is important to maintain the vascular connections from the fascia to the subcutaneous tissue, and also to maintain the superior flap angle at least 120°. The approach extends anteriorly along the anterior border of the tensor muscle, preserving its blood supply from the superior gluteal artery. The sartorius and rectus

femoris muscles may be detached at their origins to expose the anterior column. The gluteus medius and minimus muscles can next be elevated from the iliac crest. A trochanteric osteotomy can then be performed with release of the short rotators, and the gluteus maximus muscle split along its fibers to create access to the ilium, hip capsule, and posterior column. It is critical to avoid tension or injury to the superior gluteal neurovascular bundles that tether the superior triradiate flap.

The inner surface of the acetabulum, iliac wing, and superior pubic ramus can be exposed by extending the approach in an ilioinguinal direction to the level of the symphysis pubis. Intrapelvic prostheses can be safely removed through the

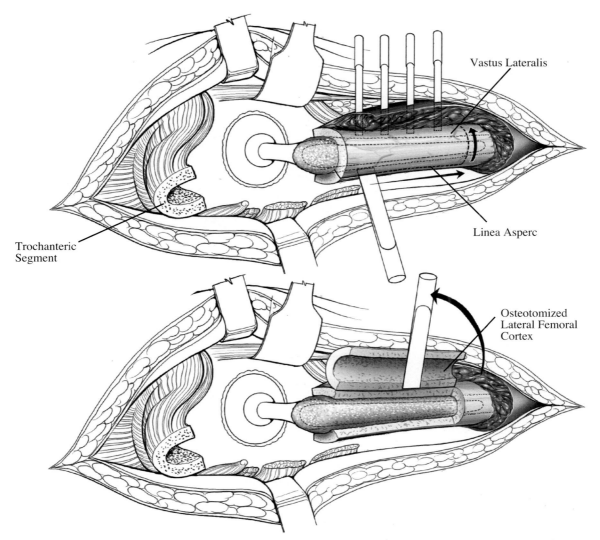

Figure 47-42 Extended proximal femoral osteotomy. The greater trochanter may be included with the distal fragment of femoral shaft. The posterior osteotomy is performed along drill holes just lateral to the linea aspera. Alternatively, the muscle may remain attached to the fragment, and the anterior osteotomy carefully performed using narrow osteotomes placed through the vastus muscle.

approach by virtue of the control and access to the major vessels in the pelvis.

POSTERIOR AND POSTEROLATERAL APPROACHES

Posterior Approach

The approach described by Moore is considered to be the classic posterior approach to the hip. Austen Moore from South Carolina described this so-called Southern approach. This approach is excellent for exposure of the posterior capsule, posterior acetabular wall, ischium and posterior trochanter, and upper femur and allows limited exposure of the acetabulum after excision of the femoral head. Because of its limited exposure to the acetabulum, it is most suitable for isolated

femoral procedures, such as endoprosthetic arthroplasties, rather than acetabular reconstructions. Inferiorly, the medial circumflex vessels are at risk for injury and subsequent disruption of the femoral head blood supply; thus, this approach is generally restricted to reconstructive cases where the femoral head is sacrificed.

The patient can be positioned either in a lateral manner for reconstructions or prone for fracture work of the posterior acetabulum and column. The Moore incision extends from the PSIS to the posterior border of the trochanter and then extends 10 to 13 cm distally along the axis of the femoral shaft. This incision is similar to the Osborne incision, except that the Osborne incision is extended only 5 cm on its distal limb. Both of these posterior incisions—the Moore and the Osborne—split the fibers of the gluteus maximus. These two incisions differ slightly from the posterolateral approach because their distal limbs are located along the posterior

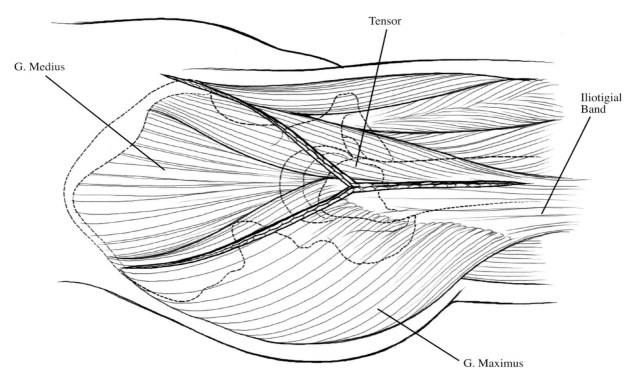

Figure 47-43 Triradiate incision. The three limbs of the approach are shown. The angle of the two superior incisions may be widened to minimize the risk of vascular disturbance to the flap.

border of the greater trochanter. The incisions for the postero-lateral approaches are located more centrally, or anterior on the trochanter. In addition, the proximal portion of the incision is more caudad than in the posterolateral approaches and thus splits the gluteus maximus fibers. The posterolateral approaches described as Kocher, Kocher–Langenbeck, and modifications described by Gibson, Marcy and Fletcher, and Harris all approach the hip cephalad to the gluteus maximus muscle, rather than splitting its fibers.

After the fibers of the gluteus maximus have been split, the deep dissection is carried out. The short rotators, which include the piriformis, superior gemellus, obturator internus, inferior gemellus, and quadratus femoris, may be released. The capsule can then be incised in a T or H fashion. The hip is then ready to dislocate by a combination of flexion and internal rotation of the hip.

A modified posterior approach described by Iyer preserves the original soft tissue attachments of the posterior hip. However, the Iyer technique splits a portion of the gluteus medius, and a portion of the greater trochanter is osteotomized and reattached (34). This modified approach allows excellent exposure of both the acetabulum and femoral shaft that is similar to the exposure achieved with a posterolateral approach. The technique is applicable to both revision arthroplasty and complex primary arthroplasty. For revision surgery, Shaw described a modification that preserved soft tissue distal to the osteotomy to maintain continuity with the trochanteric fragment (55). Advantages to this approach are the excellent exposure of the hip with preservation of the attachments of the gluteus medius and trochanter.

Posterolateral Approach

The posterolateral approach developed from a combination of the posterior approach described by Langenbeck in 1873 and a distal limb approach described by Kocher in 1887. Langenbeck described his approach in the treatment of infectious complications of gunshot wounds. He proposed several advantages over other approaches, including the relative ease and speed of the approach, and the preservation of muscle attachments to the trochanter that resulted in much less bleeding. The original Langenbeck incision was referred to as early as 1867, and its advantages were presented by Langenbeck in 1873 at the Congress of the German Society of Surgery (64). The Langenbeck incision extended from the PSIS to the trochanter tip with the hip held at 45°. Kocher modified the approach by shifting the approach to the anterior aspect of the trochanter and added a distal extension in line with the femur. Kocher's approach was designed to improve the exposure of the acetabulum for the treatment of tuberculosis (17,38). Gibson modified the approach to improve the exposure of the hip, by adding the release of the two main abductors of the hip, the gluteus medius and minimus muscles (20). Marcy and Fletcher described their approach for the insertion of endoprostheses as a modification of the Gibson approach that preserved both the gluteus medius and minimus insertions into the trochanter (41). The names Kocher and

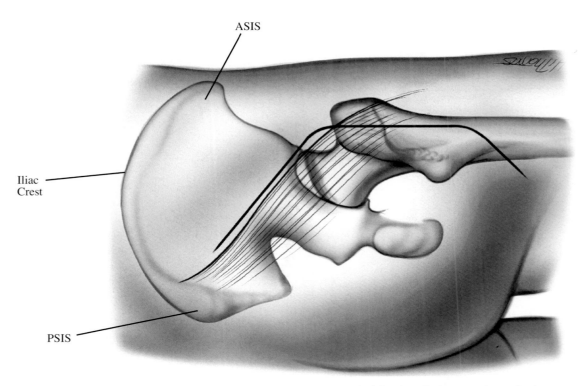

ASIS

Iliac
Crest

PSIS

Figure 47-44   Modified posterolateral incision. The proximal of the three limbs extends proximal to the superior border of the gluteus maximus. The middle limb is placed slightly anterior to the middle of the greater trochanter but posterior to the tensor muscle. The distal limb is made at a 45° angle to assist the mobility of the posterior flap.

Langenbeck were combined and the approach was popularized by Judet and LeGrange who described the combined incision for exposure of pelvic fractures in 1958. A further modification of the Kocher incision was described by Harris who added an additional third limb from the distal end of the incision which was carried in a posterior direction at an angle of 45° (Figs. 47-44 and 47-45) (27). This modification improves the exposure of both the acetabulum and femur by relieving tension from the skin, subcutaneous fat, fascia lata, and gluteus maximus. The modification is particularly helpful in the exposure of large or oversized individuals by improving posterior retraction of the posterior flap. The posterolateral and modified posterolateral approaches allow excellent exposure of the hip and acetabulum and posterior pelvic structures for procedures such as total joint arthroplasty, fixation of acetabular and posterior column pelvic fractures, and tumor excision (Fig. 47-46). The exposure provides primary access of the superior retroacetabular surface along the entire posterior column to the ischium and limited indirect access to the lateral surface of the anterior column and the medial aspect of the posterior column and the quadrangular space.

In revision arthroplasty surgery, the posterolateral approach can often provide good exposure of the femur and acetabulum without the need for trochanteric osteotomy. This approach may be indicated for exposure in cases of loose acetabular sockets with intact femoral components, loose cemented femoral components that do not require difficult cement removal, and cementless stems that can be

removed by simple access to the upper femur. To avoid scratching a retained femoral component during acetabular exposure, the femoral head or Morse-taper surface should be protected with a cover while the femur is retracted anteriorly. If exposure is found to be inadequate, the approach can be modified by adding a trochanteric osteotomy at any stage of the exposure.

The patient is positioned in the lateral or semilateral position for both the posterior and posterolateral approaches. For fracture work, the posterolateral approach may be best performed with the patient in the prone position, particularly if indirect access is needed to the quadrangular space of the pelvis. The lower limb is best draped free to allow rotational control of the femur and to help expose the posterior rotators and hip capsule.

The skin incision for the modified Kocher–Langenbeck approach runs along the upper border of the gluteus maximus, which is determined at the skin level by angulating posteriorly 2 cm proximal to the tip of the trochanter toward the posterior spine. To avoid splitting of the gluteus maximus fibers, the incision in the fascia can be initiated in the distal wound and then advanced to the proximal limb while the underside of the fascia and upper border of the gluteus maximus muscle are being palpated.

The middle component of the incision should be carried from the midline of the trochanter, or slightly anterior, to facilitate posterior exposure of the hip. The anterior limit of the middle limb is the posterior border of the tensor muscle.

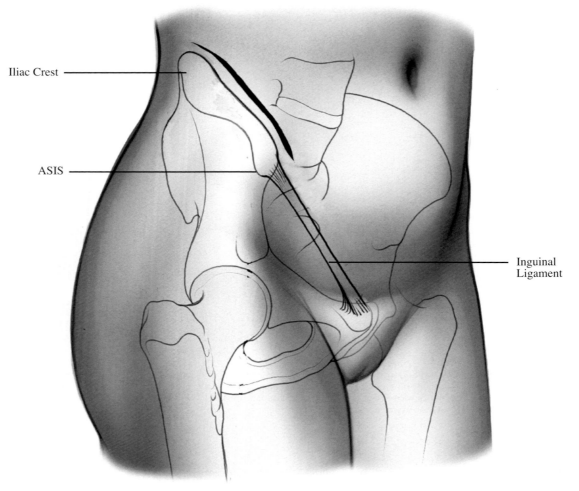

Iliac Crest

ASIS

Inguinal
Ligament

Figure 47-45 Counterincision to the posterolateral approach. This incision is parallel to the posterolateral incision and is made along the iliac crest, or slightly medial to it. It stops at the ASIS but can be continued distally for extensive exposure of the anterior column (see text).

The posterolateral incision and its modifications provide the initial approach to the deeper dissection and exposure of the hip described below. The skin and subcutaneous tissue are incised down to the deep fascia, observing for the posterior border of the tensor muscle envelope, which is often visible or indicated by small perforating vessels at its posterior margin. If the muscle is encountered, the subcutaneous tissue can be undermined from the fascia lata in a posterior direction to preserve a margin of fascial tissue. The proximal limb of the posterolateral approach can be carried through the upper muscular tissue of the gluteus maximus or can be carried slightly more proximal to run along the upper border of the muscle, preserving all of the muscle of the gluteus maximus as described previously. A digit can be placed beneath the fascia and the underside of the gluteus maximus palpated with the index finger. The border is readily palpable, and the extent of the proximal incision can be directed above the muscular edge as a true internervous plane (Fig. 47-47). It is sometimes necessary to bluntly dissect some of the origin of the gluteus medius attaching to the undersurface of the fascia that blends

with the gluteus maximus. When creating the split of the maximus in the posterior limb of the Kocher–Langenbeck approach, careful attention near the proximal end of the incision will avoid tearing of the communicating vascular anastomosis. This vessel represents a communicator between inferior and superior gluteal vascular bundles and is visible leading from the proximal body of the gluteus medius muscle and entering into the gluteus maximus.

After the fascia has been incised, anterior–posterior retraction of the fascia is accomplished with a self-retaining retractor such as a Charnley retractor. The posterior portion of the retractor should be placed near the musculotendinous border of the gluteus maximus, with care taken to avoid too deep a placement near the sciatic nerve.

To help relieve tension of the gluteus maximus during arthroplasty, particularly during internal rotation of the femur to access the femoral canal, a portion of the gluteus maximus tendon insertion into the femur can be safely released (Fig. 47-48). An angle retractor helps facilitate exposure of the tendon by retracting the vastus lateralis muscular sheath. It is

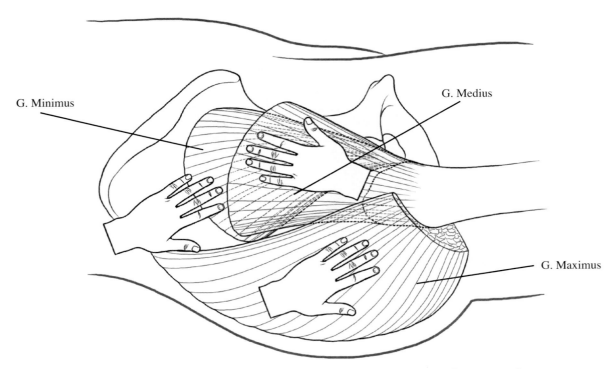

G. Minimus

G. Medius

G. Maximus

Figure 47-46   Differentiation of gluteus maximus, medius, and minimus. In difficult cases of exposure, particularly those with pre-existing surgery, it can be useful to orient the layers according to the muscle fiber directions. These mimic the direction of the fanned fingers as shown. The gluteus medius fibers run in a more parallel direction to the femoral shaft, or more proximal and anterior in its anterior half. The gluteus maximus and minimus are aligned together but are crosswise to the medius.

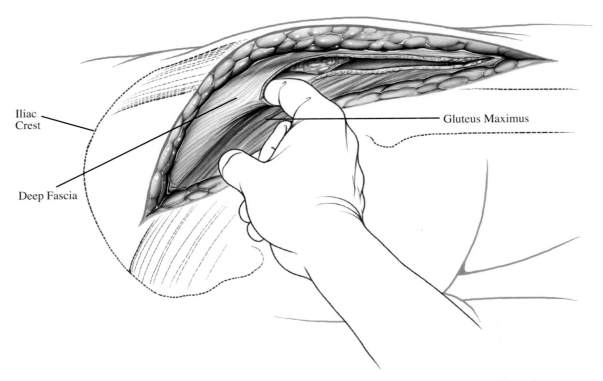

Iliac
Crest

Deep Fascia

Gluteus Maximus

Figure 47-47   Posterolateral approach, proximal limb. To steer the deep fascial incision above the border of the gluteus maximus, the digit may be used to palpate its edge. This is best performed after the distal limb has been incised.

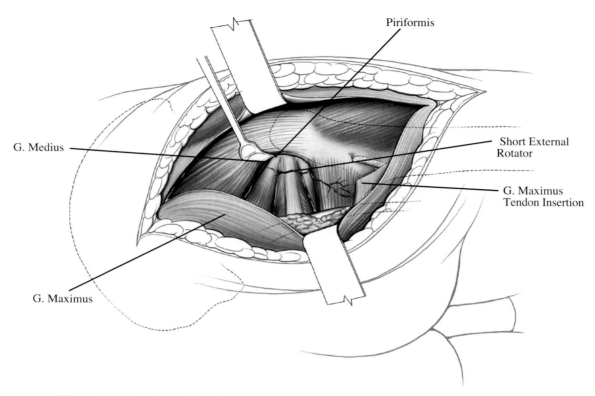

Piriformis

G. Medius

Short External
Rotator

G. Maximus
Tendon Insertion

G. Maximus

Figure 47-48   Release of the gluteus maximus insertion. Some or all of the femoral insertion may be performed as shown. It is important to leave a stump to reapproximate the tendon. Careful knife technique will usually preserve the anastomotic vessel located immediately subjacent to the tendon. It should be reattached using nonabsorbable material in a figure-eight fashion.

important to leave at least a 1.5-cm stump of the tendon on the femur for subsequent reattachment. Immediately beneath the tendon is a large vascular communicating anastomosis leading to the perforators that can usually be preserved by careful incision. The trochanteric bursae may be preserved, or it may be excised if it is thickened or inflamed.

The posterior approach can now be made to the hip joint. With the knee flexed to 90°, the hip is internally rotated 30°, and extended. Extension of the hip relaxes the gluteus maximus to facilitate the broad access to the posterior structures, as well as to provide relaxation of the sciatic nerve. The veil of thin fascial tissue can then be incised along the posterior border of the gluteus medius, preserving all of the gluteus medius attachment to the trochanter. Blunt dissection performed with an elevator or a sponge cleanly displaces fatty tissue overlying the short rotators of the hip. It is important to dissect close to the posterior border of the trochanter to avoid unnecessary bleeding from the deeper branches lying against the posterior acetabular wall. Several vascular branches are visible overlying the short rotators. The vessels are branches of the inferior gluteal artery, which borders the lower edge of the piriformis tendon, the medial circumflex branches found at the upper border of the quadratus femoris, and distal communicating branches that extend to the first perforator. These communications are known as cruciate anastomoses. This network of vessels provides a large collateral blood supply to the hip and can provide an important source of blood supply to the lower limb. After cauterization of the small vessels, the piriformis

tendon can usually be visibly identified, but it is more often palpable by the thumb placed over the posterior border of the gluteus minimus and short rotator muscles (Figs. 47-49 and 47-50). The piriformis tendon can be released near its insertion to expose the underlying posterior capsular insertion of the gluteus minimus. Incise the thin fascial envelope of the gluteus minimus near its capsular insertion, and with the use of an elevator, the gluteus minimus muscle can be freed from the superior hip capsule to help the exposure and also to avoid tearing the muscle during retraction. A Lane lever or suitably narrow cobra retractor can then be placed beneath the gluteus minimus to expose the superior hip capsule (Fig. 47-51).

The obturator internus tendon is often visible just caudad to the muscle belly of the superior gemellus and can be released sharply. The short rotators should be divided 2 cm from the edge of the trochanter if the anastomotic blood supply from the circumflex to gluteal arteries are to be preserved such as in a nonreconstructive case. A tag suture in the tendon of the obturator internus can be utilized as a protector of the sciatic nerve because it courses deep to the nerve. The obturator internus is an important landmark for acetabular fracture work as well as for sciatic nerve protection. Protection of the sciatic nerve can be more critical in cases that involve greater dissection such as in periacetabular osteotomies and acetabular and pelvic fractures involving the posterior column. Except in rare instances, the piriformis lies anatomically superficial to the sciatic nerve when reflected toward the midline and cannot be used as a protector. Next, the obturator externus is

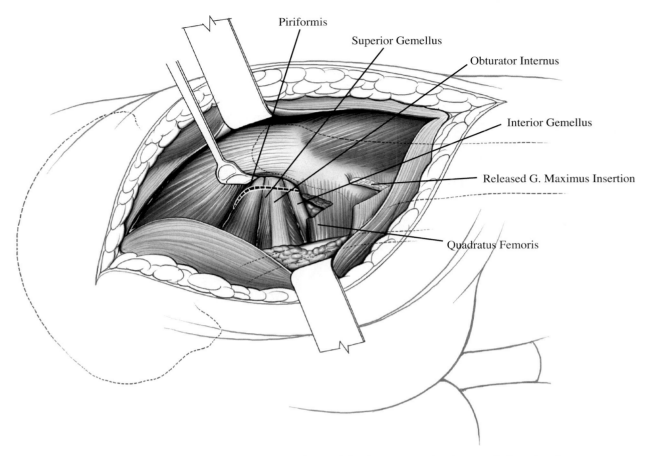

Piriformis

Superior Gemellus

Obturator Internus

Interior Gemellus

Released G. Maximus Insertion

Quadratus Femoris

Figure 47-49   Incision of short rotators. Release of the short rotators begins superiorly at the pir-iformis tendon and extends through the superior gemellus muscle, obturator internus tendon, infe-rior gemellus, and quadratus femoris. The vascular anastomosis of the medial circumflex artery is encountered at the underside of the quadratus femoris.

identified deeply at the posterior–inferior border of the femoral neck as it inserts into the lower portion of the greater trochanter. The obturator externus can be hooked with a right angle clamp, delivered out of the wound, and released sharply at its insertion. The obturator externus is too difficult to reat-tach and can be safely sacrificed. A blunt cobra can then be placed inferior to the hip capsule and levered caudad to broadly expose the inferior capsule (Fig. 47-51). The extensive exposure now visualizes the superior, posterior, and inferior hip capsule. A hip capsulotomy or capsulectomy can be safely carried out under full visualization of the capsule.

A modified capsulotomy may be performed to preserve a portion of the capsule for repair that will provide stability to the hip (Fig. 47-52). This repair provides a static barrier to posterior hip dislocation, which is a known complication of the posterior approach after arthroplasty. A special incision is required for the capsulotomy. The author's technique pre-serves two limbs of posterior capsule to be later reapproxi-mated after the arthroplasty. This method preserves a trochanteric limb, which extends into the superior portion of the hip and trochanter, and an acetabular limb, which extends down to the inferior and posterior acetabulum. This check-rein will tighten as in the normal hip, with the hip in flexion

and internal rotation. This tensioning of the capsule improves the posterior stability of the hip, limiting the tendency of pos-terior dislocation after the posterolateral approach. The limbs of capsule are overlapped and therefore tightened slightly to add tension to the sling with the hip internally rotated 25° to 30° and flexed 90°. Such a static repair can be combined with a dynamic repair of the piriformis and obturator internus ten-dons to the trochanteric limb of the capsule to improve stabil-ity of the hip and maintain proprioceptive function.

The sciatic nerve should be routinely palpated at some point during the deeper approach to be aware of an occasional variation in its location toward the lateral portion of the wound. The nerve can be easily palpated by moving a digit from the posterior wall of the acetabulum across the ischium, toward the ischial tuberosity. Approximately midway, the nerve will be palpable as the digit rides over the nerve located against the body of the ischium. The majority of sciatic nerves are confidently palpated without the need for direct exposure of the nerve.

In cases of arthroplasty, it is appropriate to measure leg length just prior to dislocation of the hip. This can be done with a Steinman pin (one eighth inch) placed into the ilium about 1 inch above the acetabulum, or with a simple pen

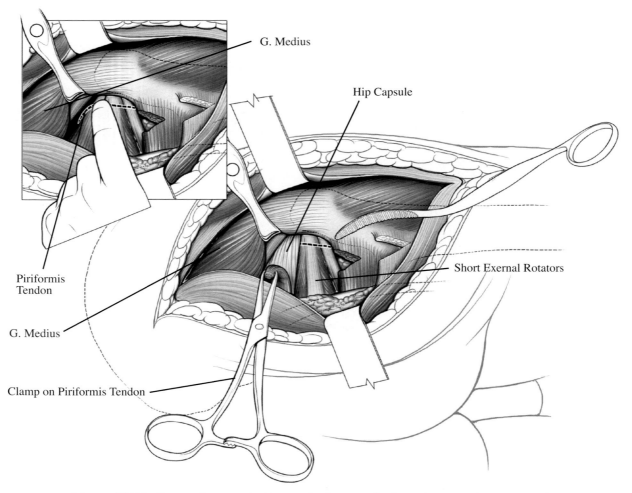

G. Medius

Hip Capsule

Piriformis
Tendon

G. Medius

Short Exernal Rotators

Clamp on Piriformis Tendon

Figure 47-50 Entry to the posterior hip capsule. Occasionally, the piriformis tendon may be diffi-cult to see beneath the gluteus medius muscle. It is frequently palpable just deep to the posterior tubercle of the greater trochanter. An angled retractor facilitates its exposure (*inset*). A window to the hip capsule is created by the release of the piriformis tendon. The posterior border of the min-imus muscle is visible and provides the point of insertion of a superior retractor.

mark on the drape or skin and the trochanter. After assembly of the trial prosthesis, a second measurement can be taken and compared with this reference measurement. It is impor-tant to reference the leg in the same position of flexion and rotation to maintain accuracy.

The hip is then dislocated by a combination of internal rotation, flexion, and adduction. An in situ osteotomy of the femoral neck may be required to safely dislocate the femoral head. This situation may include cases of severe femoral osteoporosis combined with protrusio of the hip, severe anky-losis of the hip, an ipsilateral total knee replacement whereby excess torque may fracture the supracondylar area, or conver-sion of a hip fusion. In this special circumstance, it is possible to osteotomize the femoral neck at the subcapital level in situ using an osteotome or a reciprocating saw (Fig. 47-53). This will allow the femur to be retracted anteriorly without the need for a trochanteric osteotomy. The femoral head and neck can then be pulled from the acetabulum directly or, in severe cases, they may need to be sectioned in situ and extracted in fragments.

Exposure of the dislocated femoral head can be facilitated by the use of an appropriately broad retractor with the tibia held upward and the femur internally rotated. It is important to maintain the knee at about 90° because excessive flexion may place unwanted tension on the femoral nerve. In the case of an arthroplasty, the femoral neck will need to be osteotomized. The remaining quadratus muscle can be sharply released from the posterior femoral neck to expose the poste-rior femoral neck from the head of the femur to the lesser trochanter. An osteotomy guide can then be positioned for the femoral neck osteotomy. When the trochanter is being pre-served, the transverse neck osteotomy must not create a notch defect in the trochanter that could lead to a fracture of the trochanter. The second cut is in a sagittal plane and longitudi-nal to the axis of the femoral shaft; it begins over the superior femoral neck and extends to the end of the first osteotomy. This second cut is angled in the plane of the trochanter, which is typically retroverted 25° or 30°. It is important not to leave prominent anterior femoral neck bone that could impinge on the acetabulum during flexion and internal rotation. The

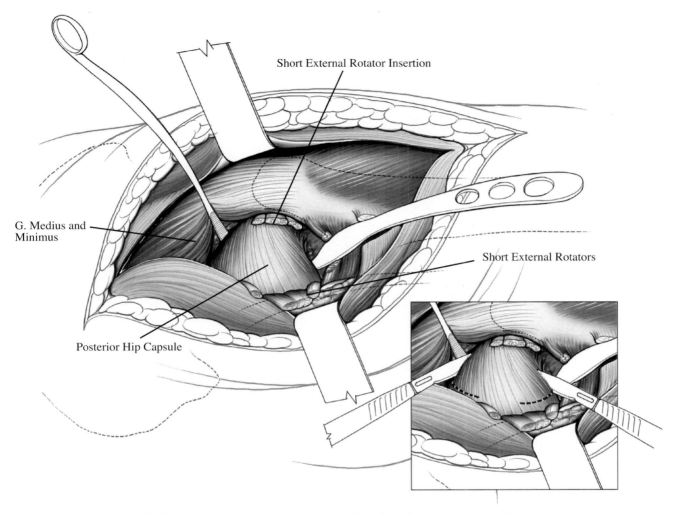

Short External Rotator Insertion

G. Medius and Minimus

Short External Rotators

Posterior Hip Capsule

Figure 47-51 Posterior capsule exposure. Blunt cobra-shaped retractors are helpful to retract the gluteus minimus superiorly, and the obturator externus and quadratus inferiorly. The capsulotomy incisions can be made along the superior and inferior capsule in-line and beneath each of the retractors (*inset*). The surgeon should cut away from the sciatic nerve when the posterior incisions are made. Alternatively, a posterior capsulectomy can be performed.

femoral head is grasped with a wide clamp and rotated outward as the remaining anterior capsule is sharply incised from the femoral head and neck fragment. During incision of the hip capsule in the deep wound, the knife should always point anterior, away from the sciatic nerve.

The acetabulum is now ready for exposure. The femur, minus the femoral head, is rotated externally back to a neutral position, and the hip is flexed 30° or 40° and adducted slightly. The knee is flexed to 45° to relax the sciatic nerve. Knee flexion at this stage of acetabular exposure is critical to minimize the risk of sciatic palsy. Because the hip is in flexion the sciatic nerve is vulnerable to traction injury if the knee is extended. This point is particularly important in short-statured individuals who have less excursion of the sciatic nerve before injury ensues. However, flexion of the knee to more than 45° may limit the exposure by tension created in the rectus femoris. To expose the acetabulum, a long cobra may be carefully placed over the anterior column of the

acetabulum to retract the femur anteriorly. This cobra should be placed equatorial or slightly cephalad. If the cobra is placed caudad over the anterior rim or column, there is a higher risk of neurovascular damage caused by the cobra penetrating into the vascular sheath and femoral nerve. The cobra should to be levered against the femoral neck and not the trochanter to avoid a fracture of the trochanter. Once the femur is displaced by the cobra, the soft tissue can easily be visualized below the inferior capsule, and branches of the medial circumflex can be electrocauterized. Larger veins may sometimes exist, and these should be ligated. A small blunt cobra retractor can then be placed below the acetabular teardrop, inferior to the transverse acetabular ligament in an extracapsular position to help expose the acetabulum. The tip of the blunt cobra can safely penetrate the obturator membrane if the cobra is placed in a direct inferior position (i.e., 6 o'clock). A large, deep retractor that is smooth at its edge, such as a Richardson design, should be placed against the posterior acetabular lip.

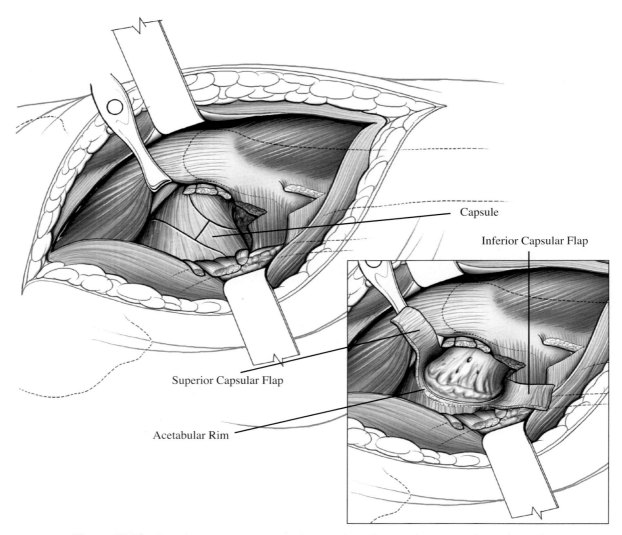

Capsule

Inferior Capsular Flap

Superior Capsular Flap

Acetabular Rim

Figure 47-52 Capsulotomy: posterior capsule static sling. The capsulotomy may be performed in an H pattern to preserve some capsule for hip stability. The superior limb should preserve as much of its trochanteric insertion, and the inferior limb should preserve the posterior–inferior attachment of the capsule to the acetabulum.

This retractor will adequately protect the sciatic nerve and structures posterior to the acetabulum and provide excellent acetabular exposure. It is dangerous to place any retractors into the greater sciatic notch for risk of vascular or sciatic nerve injury.

Occasionally, the exposure at this stage is limited, and several steps may be taken to improve it. The first step is to sharply release the remaining anterior–superior capsule at the edge of the acetabular rim. This release can be done under direct vision and safely extended to the anterior edge of the acetabulum in the area of the AIIS. The second place to check for tension is the anterior–inferior capsule, which may also be tight and can be released toward the lower anterior portion of the acetabulum. It is important not to dissect beyond the capsule into the inferior soft tissues where circumflex vessels are located. A third step is to prop the foot in an upward direction with the knee flexed in order to internally rotate the femur and deliver the trochanter out of the field. These three steps

will ensure adequate acetabular exposure in the majority of cases. If exposure is still inadequate at this point, a trochanteric osteotomy will be necessary. If necessary, limited exposure of the ilium can be obtained after trochanteric osteotomy by subperiosteal dissection of the gluteus muscle off of the superior acetabular as far anteriorly as the AIIS. Extreme caution is necessary at the proximal extent of this dissection so as to avoid major vascular injury to the inferior gluteal vessels emerging from the greater sciatic notch.

In situations that require access to the inner pelvis, a counterincision can be made and added to a posterolateral approach (Fig. 47-45). A counterincision may be indicated for cases such as pelvic osteotomy and difficult revisions that necessitate inner pelvic exposure to minimize vascular injury, such as in severe protrusio or cases requiring removal of cementoma from within the pelvic area. The second incision provides excellent access to the quadrangular space of the acetabulum and can facilitate osteotomy of the ilium by protecting vital intrapelvic structures.

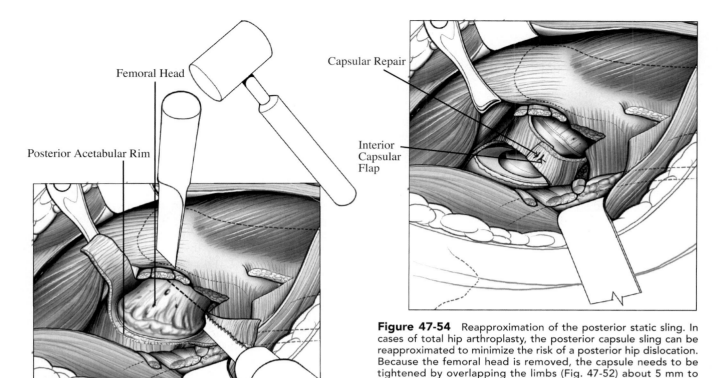

Figure 47-53 In situ femoral neck osteotomy. An initial osteotomy may be needed in a subcapital fashion to allow the extraction of the femoral head. An osteotome may be used on soft bone, but a reciprocating saw is safe and more effective in cases of hard bone.

Figure 47-54 Reapproximation of the posterior static sling. In cases of total hip arthroplasty, the posterior capsule sling can be reapproximated to minimize the risk of a posterior hip dislocation. Because the femoral head is removed, the capsule needs to be tightened by overlapping the limbs (Fig. 47-52) about 5 mm to restore the tension in the capsule. The capsule sling should tension in about 20° to 30° of internal rotation with the hip in 90° of flexion. The limbs should be reattached using heavy, nonabsorbable suture in a mattress fashion. The piriformis and obturator internus tendons may be reattached to the superior sling near their insertions for additional dynamic stability.

The counterincision begins at the superior margin of the iliac crest at the ASIS and extends proximally as far as necessary. When combined with a posterolateral approach, these incisions allow inner pelvic exposure without disrupting the abductors of the hip. Anterior column exposure can be extended inferiorly and medially along the superior pubic ramus by releasing the inguinal ligament or combining the counterincision with an ilioinguinal approach for further exposure of the superior pubic ramus. In addition, it is possible to harvest bone graft from the inner table of the ilium through this counterincision without affecting the major abductors of the hip.

Closure of the posterolateral approach following arthroplasty is accomplished by first reattaching the static posterior capsule limbs, followed by reattachment of the obturator internis and the piriformis (Fig. 47-54). If the offset of the hip has been altered and the trochanter lateralized, then it is usually not possible to reattach the short rotators. Usually the obturator internis has such a short excursion that adequate reattachment is usually not possible. The gluteus maximus tendon can

be reapproximated with several figure-eight sutures, taking care to avoid injuring the anastamotic vessels on its underside.

ILIOINGUINAL, EXTENDED ILIOFEMORAL, AND COMBINED APPROACHES

Ilioinguinal Approach

The ilioinguinal approach is a modification of the Smith-Petersen iliofemoral approach. It was modified by Judet and Letournel in order to gain access to the anterior aspect of the pelvis and the acetabulum where exposure is needed distal to the iliopectineal eminence. Exposure proximal to the iliopectineal eminence is adequate using the classic iliofemoral approach. The ilioinguinal approach allows access to the inner ilium, the inner surface of the true pelvis and sacroiliac joint, the quadrilateral plate to the spinous process and obturator foramen, the anterior column to the superior pubic ramus, and the symphysis pubis. The outer aspect of the ilium can also be exposed by the release of the abductors, but this exposure is at the expense of bone circulation, which may be detrimental, especially in fracture work. Heterotopic ossification is not considered a major risk with this approach if the abductors are not released. This approach does not allow direct access to the hip joint unless there is acetabular bone disruption, such as a fracture.

Indications for this approach include fractures, reconstructions, tumors, and periacetabular osteotomies. Pelvic fractures of the anterior wall or anterior column, and T-type acetabular fractures can be readily exposed and successfully fixed using this approach.

The patient is positioned supine for the approach, with the affected side elevated between 0° and 30°. Alternatively, a bolster may be placed beneath the sacrum to elevate the pelvis from the table and thus facilitate maneuverability of the pelvis and soft tissue. Extending the drapes to beyond the opposite iliac crest and upper abdomen facilitates orientation and exposure for this approach. A Foley catheter is desirable to decompress the bladder and allow proper retraction of deep tissues for improved exposure.

The incision can be considered to be a combination of two limbs: one medial and the other lateral (Fig. 47-55). The medial limb extends from 2 or 3 cm above the symphysis pubis toward the ASIS, and the lateral limb extends posteriorly from the ASIS to beyond the gluteus medius tubercle of the iliac crest. The incision may be placed more caudad to the iliac crest to avoid late incisional pain caused by irritation from tight garments.

The deeper exposure is initiated at the lateral limb by elevation of the external oblique from the iliac crest (Fig. 47-56). It is important to extend the dissection far enough posteriorly into the external oblique, which becomes muscular as it inserts into the iliac crest. Subperiosteal dissection of the iliacus muscle medially toward the iliac fossa is carried posteromedially to the level of the capsule of the sacroiliac joint.

In the medial limb, the external oblique fascia is incised parallel and just proximal to the inguinal ligament as far medial as the external inguinal ring (Fig. 47-57). In males the spermatic cord is isolated, whereas in females the round ligament is isolated. The inguinal canal is then opened by dissecting the lower flap of the external oblique aponeurosis. The ilioinguinal nerve is visible as it penetrates the internal oblique musculature. The internal oblique and transverse abdominis fascia are incised adjacent to the conjoined tendon and beneath the spermatic cord. The internal oblique and transverse abdominis can then be mobilized from the inguinal ligament. The inferior epigastric artery crosses the floor of the inguinal canal at the medial border of the deep inguinal ring and requires ligation. In the lateral portion of the dissection, the lateral femoral cutaneous nerve can be identified as it penetrates 1 to 3 cm medial to the ASIS. This nerve may be either preserved or transected. The transversalis fascia can then be incised while preserving an inferior flap of a few millimeters for later reapproximation. (This fascia covers the lymphatic and vascular compartments.) Medially, the transversalis fascia can be dissected off the inguinal ligament and the rectus abdominis fascia. Further exposure of the symphysis can be carried out by release of additional rectus fascia to include the contralateral rectus tendon.

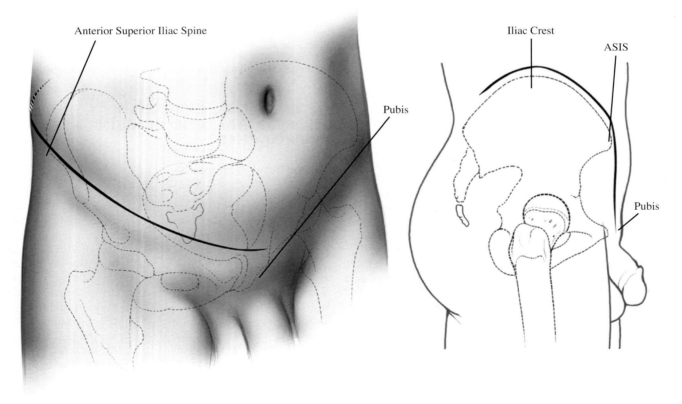

Figure 47-55 Ilioinguinal approach. The medial limb of the incision extends from the ASIS to a few centimeters above the symphysis pubis. The lateral limb extends along the iliac crest, but the skin incision may be placed distal to the crest to minimize the risk of incisional pain.

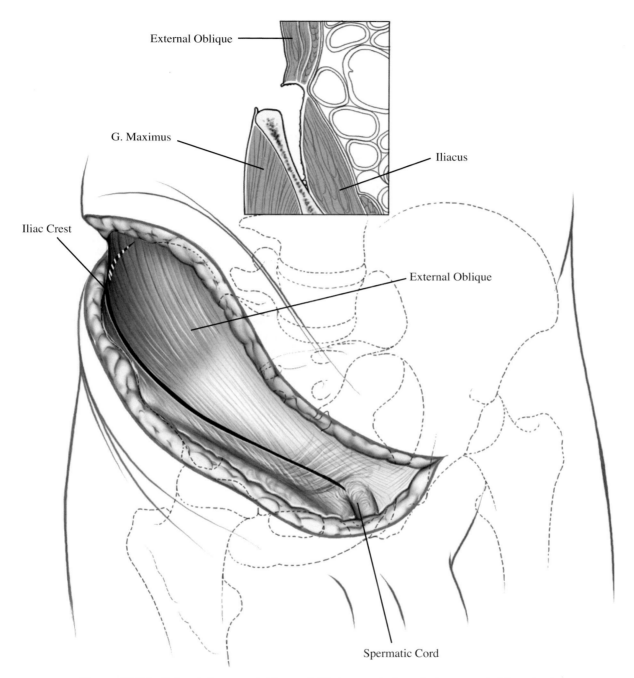

External Oblique

G. Maximus

Iliacus

Iliac Crest

External Oblique

Spermatic Cord

Figure 47-56 Ilioinguinal approach. The medial limb extends through the external oblique fascia to the level of the external inguinal ring. The posterior limb is extended deeply along the iliac crest (*inset*).

In the deep wound, the tissue adjacent to the iliopsoas compartment can now be incised. Adjacent to the femoral nerve can be found the iliopectineal fascia, which is a continuation of the investing fascia of the iliopsoas (Fig. 47-58). The iliopectineal fascia is the key to access from the false to the true pelvis and also aids in separating the muscular from the vascular compartment. Medial to the iliopectineal fascia are the external iliac vessels and the lymphatics. At the proximal border of the iliopectineal fascia, a small vascular leash can be identified and released to allow better exposure of the deeper structures. A Penrose drain can be used to surround and retract the iliopsoas and femoral nerve. Medial retraction of the iliopsoas allows deeper visualization of the ilium to the level of the sacroiliac joint (Fig. 47-59). The pelvis can now be visualized between these three mobile tissue envelopes: the iliopsoas with femoral nerve, the external iliac vessel sheath, and the spermatic cord (or round ligament). Flexion and external rotation of the hip relaxes the iliopsoas

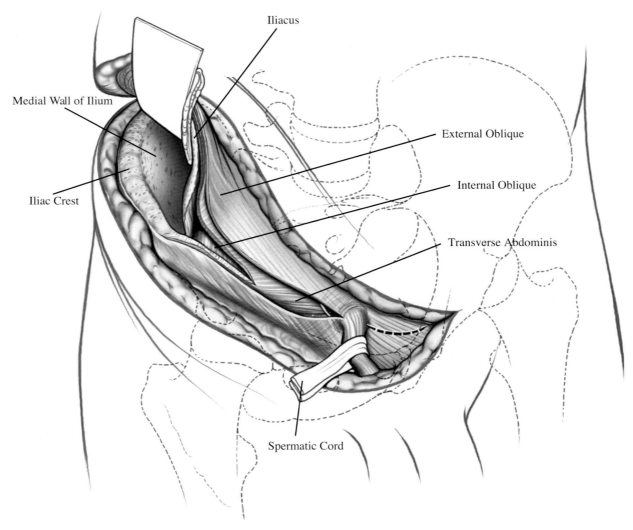

Iliacus

Medial Wall of Ilium

External Oblique

Internal Oblique

Iliac Crest

Transverse Abdominis

Spermatic Cord

Figure 47-57 Ilioinguinal approach. The transverse abdominis and internal oblique are incised beneath the spermatic cord, adjacent to the conjoined tendon. Further exposure medially is performed by release of the rectus tendon.

and facilitates maneuverability to aid in exposure of the pelvic brim from the sacroiliac joint to as far as the lateral aspect of the superior pubic ramus. Lateral retraction of the external iliac vessels with medial retraction of the spermatic cord exposes the superior pubic ramus. Lateral retraction of the spermatic cord exposes the pubic symphysis (Fig. 47-60).

The symphysis pubis, pubic tubercle, and superior pubic ramus can be further exposed by dissecting medially, releasing the inguinal ligament and conjoined tendon from beneath the spermatic cord. If further dissection of the pubis is necessary, the rectus fascia can be sharply released from the pubis and joined with the more lateral release of the conjoined tendon and inguinal ligament. The retropubic space can be identified by release and retraction of the ipsilateral rectus head. Blunt dissection of the vascular sheath can be carried out to elevate the sheath from the superior pubic ramus and allow complete exposure of the superior ramus. Aberrant vascular branches connecting the obturator with the external iliac system should be identified (see the Vascular Anatomy section). Deeply, the

obturator neurovascular branches can be identified deep to the rim of the superior ramus. A vascular anastomosis usually occurs between the external iliac and the obturator arteries and runs over the ramus. However, occasionally an anomaly may occur whereby the obturator artery arises solely from the external iliac artery, in which case the branch should be preserved.

Closure is accomplished by reapproximation of the external oblique, reattachment of the rectus abdominis, and fascia of the internal oblique and transverse abdominis to the inguinal ligament and the roof of the external oblique overlying the spermatic cord.

Extended Iliofemoral Approach

The extended iliofemoral approach was developed by Emil Letournel in 1975 to gain access to the whole outer aspect of the ilium. This approach exposes both the anterior and posterior columns simultaneously. Complete exposure of the iliac

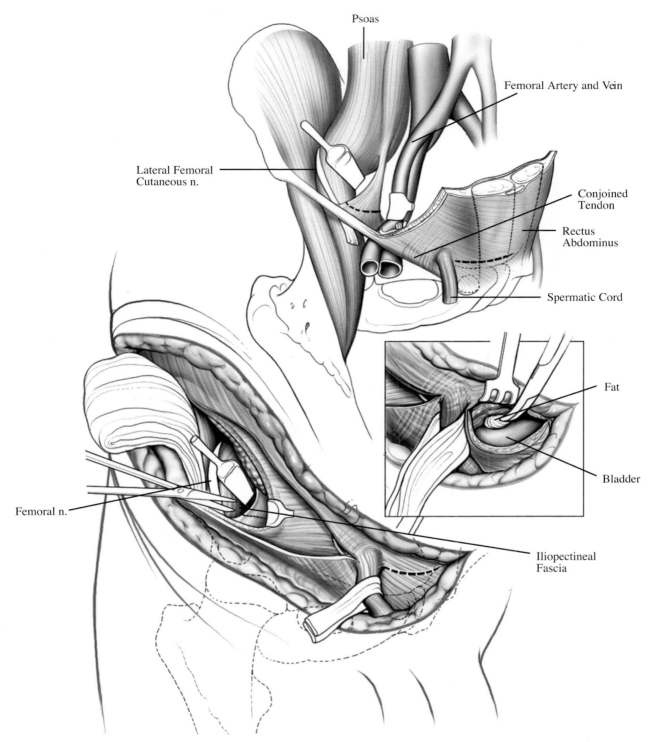

Psoas

Femoral Artery and Vein

Lateral Femoral
Cutaneous n.

Conjoined
Tendon

Rectus
Abdominus

Spermatic Cord

Fat

Bladder

Femoral n.

Iliopectineal
Fascia

Figure 47-58 Ilioinguinal approach. The iliopectineal fascia is identified adjacent to the femoral nerve. This key landmark separates the muscular from the vascular compartments.

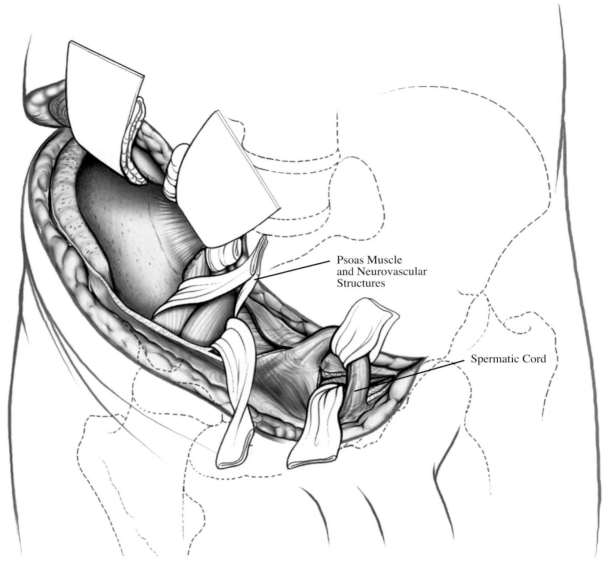

Psoas Muscle
and Neurovascular
Structures

Spermatic Cord

Figure 47-59 Ilioinguinal approach. The medial retraction of the iliopsoas muscle allows visualization of the iliac fossa to the sacroiliac joint. Flexion and external rotation of the hip improves this exposure.

crest to the ischial tuberosity is accomplished. However, exposure to the internal iliac fossa is accessible only indirectly by digital palpation and not direct visualization. This approach allows access to the ischial tuberosity, iliac spine, and the posterior column; to the outer aspect of the ilium; and anteriorly to the border of the iliopectineal area. A hip capsulotomy allows intra-articular exposure. The indication for this approach is for certain acetabular fractures to gain simultaneous access to both the anterior and posterior columns. It is usually done for pelvic fractures with complete exposure of the posterior column. It is a true internervous approach that separates the tensor muscle (superior gluteal nerve innervated) from the femoral innervated group.

The patient is positioned on a fracture table, or fluoro table, in the lateral position to allow for mobility and to ade-

quately access both anterior and posterior. The limb is draped free, and the hip should be extended and the knee flexed to protect the sciatic nerve against tension. The skin incision extends from the PSIS to the ASIS and distally down the anterior thigh toward the lateral border of the patella. The abductors are released from the iliac wing. It is important to extend the dissection in a posterior direction to include the PSIS for adequate mobility of the tissue flap. The approach enters the tensor sheath, unlike the classic Smith-Petersen, to avoid exposure and potential injury to the lateral femoral cutaneous nerve. The approach should enter the tensor sheath distally from 10 to 15 cm distal to the ASIS. The tensor sheath should be entered and incised in a proximal direction to the ASIS. The distal incision can then join with the remaining proximal incision at the iliac crest. Release of the tensor from

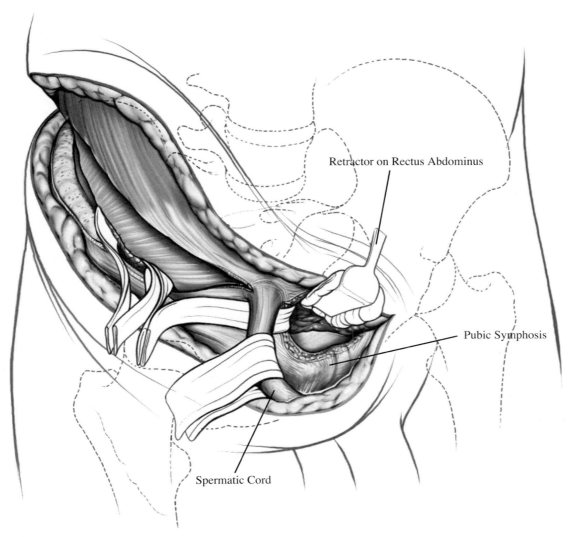

Retractor on Rectus Abdominus

Pubic Symphosis

Spermatic Cord

Figure 47-60 Ilioinguinal approach. The lateral retraction of the spermatic cord exposes the pubic symphysis.

the crest will expose the circumflex iliac artery that extends around the iliac spine. The deep dissection is extended by entering the floor of the tensor sheath with the tensor muscle retracted laterally. An incision through the sheath exposes the rectus femoris muscle and minor branches of the lateral femoral circumflex artery. The ascending branch from the lateral circumflex artery is at a deeper level. The rectus can then be retracted medially to allow proximal dissection to the indirect head of the rectus femoris. The indirect head can then be released near the insertion into the AIIS to allow the exposure to extend over the superior hip capsule. Deep to the rectus tendon, the main ascending branch of the lateral femoral circumflex is encountered and is ligated. The surface of the vastus lateralis muscle can be traced to its origin at the vastus lateralis tubercle. The muscular fibers of the gluteus minimus can be seen to extend further distally than its tendon's insertion on the greater trochanter. The insertions of the gluteus minimus and medius may be released from the

anterior greater trochanter for additional exposure. A dense tendinous portion of the gluteus medius is located more posteriorly overlying the greater trochanter and may also be released and later reapproximated. There may be a significant problem with abductor function after such extensive release from the greater trochanter. If adequate exposure can be accomplished without sharp release of the abductors (gluteus minimus and gluteus medius), it should be considered. Further posterior release may be undertaken for complete exposure by release of the tendinous insertion of the gluteus maximus and short external rotators of the hip. This will allow near-circumferential exposure of the hip joint and the entire posterior column. A hip arthrotomy can be performed at any stage in the exposure, whereas a complete capsulotomy will allow distraction of the hip to visualize the acetabular roof in cases of acetabular fracture.

To gain additional anterior exposure, the sartorius and inguinal ligament may be released with the direct head of the rectus femoris. This allows access to the inner aspect of the ilium after elevation of the iliopsoas. This extension devascularizes bone, however, and thus may not be indicated, especially in fracture cases.

Combined Approaches

The combination of approaches allows access to the hip and acetabulum, anterior and posterior columns, and where fractures are comminuted and excellent access is needed. The main indication for a combined approach is when simultaneous access to both anterior and posterior columns is needed. Although extensile exposures of the hip and pelvis can provide extensive pelvic and hip exposures, they involve soft tissue stripping from bone. This stripping may lead to complications such as heterotopic bone or devascularization of bone. The combined approaches were popularized as an alternative to the use of the extensile approaches such as the extended iliofemoral and triradiate approaches to avoid such complications.

REFERENCES

1. Alonso JE, Davila R, Bradley E. Extended iliofemoral versus triradiate approaches in management of associated acetabular fractures. *CORR.* 1994;305:81.
2. Amstutz HA. *Hip Arthroplasty.* New York: Churchill Livingstone; 1991.
3. Baker AS, Bitounis VC. Abductor function after total hip replacement. *J Bone Joint Surg.* 1989;71B:47.
4. Bauer R, Kerschbaumer F, Poisel S. *Atlas of Hip Surgery.* New York: Thieme; 1996.
5. Bauer RF, Kerschgaumer F, Poisel S, et al. The transgluteal approach to the hip joint. *Arch Orthop Trauma.* 1979;95:47.
6. Berman AT, Salter FL, Koenig T. Revision total hip replacement without trochanteric osteotomy. *Orthopedics.* 1987;10:755.
7. Berry DJ, Muller ME. Chevron osteotomy and single wire reattachment of the greater trochanter in primary and revision total hip arthroplasty. *CORR.* 1993;294:155.
8. Brackett EG. A study of approaches. *Boston Med J.* 1912;166:235.
9. Burwell HN, Scott D. A lateral intermuscular approach to the hip joint for replacement of the femoral head by a prosthesis. *J Bone Joint Surg.* 1954;36B:104.
10. Callaghan JJ, Dysart SH, Savory CG. The uncemented porous-coated anatomic total hip prosthesis. *J Bone Joint Surg.* 1988; 70A:337.
11. Cameron HU. *The Technique of Total Hip Arthroplasty.* St. Louis: Mosby Year Book; 1992.
12. Cameron HU. Use of a distal trochanteric osteotomy in hip revision. *Contemp Orthop.* 1991;23:235.
13. Carlson DC, Robinson HJ. Surgical approaches for primary total hip arthroplasty. *CORR.* 1987;222:161.
14. Charnley J. *Low Friction Arthroplasty of the Hip.* New York: Springer-Verlag; 1979.
15. Chapman MW. *Operative Orthopedics.* Philadelphia: JB Lippincott; 1993.
16. Dall D. Exposure of the hip by anterior osteotomy of the greater trochanter. *J Bone Joint Surg.* 1986;30B:382.
17. Dumont F. Die Resektion des Huftgelenkes nach Kocher. *Correspondenz-Blatt fuer Schweizer Aerzte.* 1887;17:225.
18. Foster DE, Hunter JR. The direct lateral approach to the hip for arthroplasty. *Orthopedics.* 1987;10:274.
19. Frndak PA, Mallory TH, Lombardi AV. Translateral approach to the hip. The abductor muscle split. *CORR.* 1993;295:131.
20. Gibson A. Posterior exposure of the hip joint. *J Bone Joint Surg.* 1950;32B:183.
21. Glassman AH, Engh CA, Bobyn JD. A technique of extensile exposure for total hip arthroplasty. *J Arthroplasty.* 1987;2:11.
22. Gray H, Goss CM. *Gray's Anatomy.* Philadelphia: Lea and Febiger; 1973.
23. Gruebel Lee DM. *Disorders of the Hip.* Philadelphia: JB Lippincott; 1993.
24. Hardinge K. The direct lateral approach to the hip. *J Bone Joint Surg.* 1982;64B:17.
25. Hardy AE, Synek V. Hip abductor function after the Hardinge approach: brief report. *J Bone Joint Surg.* 1988;70B:673.
26. Harris WH. A new lateral approach to the hip joint. *J Bone Joint Surg.* 1967;49A:891.
27. Harris WH. Advances in surgical technique for total hip replacement. *CORR.* 1980;146:188.
28. Harris WH. Extensive exposure of the hip joint. *CORR.* 1973;91:58.
29. Harris WH. Revision surgery for failed, nonseptic total hip arthroplasty. *CORR.* 1982;170:8.
30. Harty M, Joyce J. Surgical approaches to the hip and femur. *J Bone Joint Surg.* 1963;45A:175.
31. Head WC, Mallory TH, Berklacich FM, et al. Extensile exposure of the hip for revision arthroplasty. *J Arthroplasty.* 1987;2:265.
32. Henry AK. *Exposures of long bones and other surgical methods.* Bristol, England: John Wright and Sons; 1927.
33. Hoppenfeld S, de Boer P. *Surgical exposures in orthopaedics.* Philadelphia: JB Lippincott; 1984.
34. Iyer KM. A new posterior approach to the hip joint. *Injury.* 1981;13:76.
35. Jacobs Lg, Buxton RA. The course of the superior gluteal nerve in the lateral approach to the hip. *J Bone Joint Surg.* 1989;71A:1239.
36. Jergesen F, Abbott LC. A comprehensive exposure of the hip joint. *J Bone Joint Surg.* 1955;37A:798.
37. Kasser JR. *Orthopedic Knowledge Update 5.* Rosemont, IL: American Academy of Orthopaedic Surgeons; 1996.
38. Kocher T. *Textbook of Operative Surgery.* 4th ed. London: HJ Stiles; Edinburgh: Adam and Charles Black; 1903.
39. Krackow K, Steinman H, Cohn BT, et al. Clinical experience with a triradiate exposure of the hip for difficult total hip arthroplasty. *J Arthroplasty.* 1988;3:267.
40. Light TR, Keggi KJ. Anterior approach to hip arthroplasty. *CORR.* 1980;152:255.
41. Marcy GH, Fletcher RS. Modification of the posterolateral approach to the hip for insertion of femoral head prosthesis. *J Bone Joint Surg.* 1954;36A:142.
42. Masquelet AC. *An Atlas of Surgical Exposures of the Lower Extremity.* Philadelphia: JB Lippincott; 1993.
43. Matta J, Letournel E, Browner B. Surgical management of acetabular fractures. *Instruct Course Lect.* 1986;35:382.
44. McFarland B, Osborne G. Approach to the hip. A suggested improvement on Kocher's method. *J Bone Joint Surg.* 1954;36B:364.
45. Mears DC, Rubash HE. *Pelvic and Acetabular Fractures.* Thorofare, NJ: Slack; 1986.
46. Minns RJ, Crawford RJ, Porter ML, et al. Muscle strength following total hip arthroplasty. *J Arthroplasty.* 1993;8:625.
47. Moore AT. Metal hip joint: a new self-locking vitallium prosthesis. *South Med J.* 1952;45:1015.
48. Moore KL. *Clinically Oriented Anatomy.* Baltimore: Williams & Wilkins; 1985.
49. Morrey BF. *Reconstructive Surgery of the Joints.* New York: Churchill Livingstone; 1991.
50. Mostardi RE, Askew MJ, Gradisar IA Jr, et al. Comparison of functional outcome of total hip arthroplasties involving four surgical approaches. *J Arthroplasty.* 1988;3:279.
51. Muller ME. Total hip prostheses. *CORR.* 1970;72:46.
52. Nazarian S, Tisserand Ph, Brunet C, et al. Anatomic basis of the transgluteal approach to the hip. *Surg Radiol Anat.* 1987;9:27.
53. Peters PC, Head WC, Emerson RH Jr. An extended trochanteric osteotomy for revision total hip replacement. *J Bone Joint Surg.* 1993;75B:158.
54. Poss R. Intertrochanteric osteotomy in osteoarthritis of the hip. *Instruct Course Lect.* 1986;35:129.
55. Shaw JA. Experience with a modified posterior approach to the hip joint. *J Arthroplasty.* 1991;6:11.
56. Smith-Peterson MN. A new supra-articular subperiosteal approach to the hip joint. *Am J Orthop Surg.* 1917;15:592.
57. Smith-Peterson MN. Approach to and exposure of the hip joint for mold arthroplasty. *J Bone Joint Surg.* 1949;31A:40.
58. Smith-Peterson MN, Cave EF, Vangorder GW. Intracapsular fractures of the neck of the femur. *Arch Surg.* 1931;23:715.

59. Sochart DH, Paul AS, Kurdy NM. A new osteotome for performing chevron trochanteric osteotomy. *Acta Orthop Scand.* 1995;5: 445.

60. Steinberg M. *The Hip and Its Disorders.* Philadelphia: WB Saunders; 1991.

61. Stiehl J. Acetabular allograft reconstruction in total hip arthroplasty. Part 2: Surgical approach. *Orthop Rev.* 1991;20:425.

62. Syensson O, Skold S, Blomgren G. Intergrity of the gluteus medius after the transgluteal approach in total hip arthroplasty. *J Arthroplasty.* 1990;5:57.

63. Turner RH, Scheller AD. *Revision Total Hip Arthroplasty.* New York: Grune and Stratton; 1982.

64. vonLangenbeck B. Congress of German Society for Surgery, 4th session, 1873, printed: Arch Surgery: Ueber die Schussverletzungen des Huftgelenks. *Klin Chir.* 1874;16:263.

65. Waldrop JT, Ebraheim NA, Yeasting RA, et al. The location of the sacroiliac joint on the outer table of the posterior ilium. *J Orthop Trauma.* 1993;7:510.

66. Watson-Jones R. Fractures of the neck of the femur. *Br J Surg.* 1935;23:787.

67. Wroblewski BM, Shelley P. Reattachment of the greater trochanter after hip replacement. *J Bone Joint Surg.* 1985;67B:736.

68. Younger TI, Bradford MS, Magnus RE, et al. Extended proximal femoral osteotomy. *J Arthroplasty.* 1995;10:329.

Alternatives to Arthroplasty

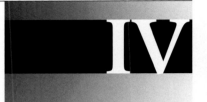

Arthroscopy

48

Joseph C. McCarthy   Jo-Ann Lee

The applications of arthroscopy have enjoyed exponential growth in modern orthopaedic practice as techniques and clinical applications have developed that allow minimally invasive diagnostic and therapeutic procedures, particularly for the knee and shoulder. Arthroscopic management of hip pain and hip disorders has not received similar attention. The concept of hip arthroscopy was first introduced in 1931 by Burman (4), but it did not resurface in the North American literature until 1977, when Gross (25) reported his experience with arthroscopy of congenitally dislocated hips. Sporadic reports of clinical application of arthroscopic techniques in the hip joint continued to appear in the literature through the early 1980s. In 1980, Vakilif and Warren (56) reported arthroscopic removal of entrapped cement following total hip arthroplasty, and Holgersson et al. (29), in 1981, reported the use of hip arthroscopy in the evaluation and treatment of juvenile chronic arthritis.

The theoretical advantages of hip arthroscopy include the ability to thoroughly inspect the hip joint, potentially to remove offending tissues, to treat a myriad of problems that previously were either undiagnosed or managed with open arthrotomy, and finally to document and stage the changes within the joint, all with a minimally invasive procedure and a shortened rehabilitation period. The relatively slow development of arthroscopy of the hip in North American centers, however, is understandable. The femoral head is deeply recessed in the bony acetabulum, and it is convex in shape unlike the more planar surface of the knee. The ability to distend the hip joint is less than that of the knee, and the fibrocapsular and muscular envelope is thicker. Additionally, the relative proximity of the sciatic nerve, the lateral femoral cutaneous nerve, and the femoral neurovascular structures place them at some risk (7,12,34).

Nevertheless, diagnostic and therapeutic applications of hip arthroscopy have developed over the last 10 years, and recent innovations in technique have allowed thoughtful advancement. Eriksson et al. (15) recognized and quantitated hip capsule distention and distraction forces necessary to allow adequate visualization of the femur and the acetabulum. Johnson (33) articulated techniques of needle positioning, anatomic landmarks, and cannula placement, and Glick et al. (22) contributed their experience with the lateral decubitus positioning and peritrochanteric portal placement. Adaptation of arthroscopy equipment and instruments specifically for the hip joint has led to safe visualization and instrumentation of the hip joint.

INDICATIONS

Current accepted indications for hip arthroscopy include management of labral tears, removal of loose bodies, resection or staging of chondral lesions, synovial biopsy, subtotal synovectomy, synovial chondromatosis, osteoarthritis, osteochondritis dissecans, investigation of the hip joint for unresolved mechanical hip pain, and the treatment of septic arthritis or pyarthrosis (13,17,18,22,24,28,30–33,41,42, 49,60).

More recent applications include arthroscopy post total hip arthroplasty for removal of loose screws or intra-articular third bodies; removal of bullets, shrapnel, or foreign bodies; treatment of chondral lesions in association with osteonecrosis or slipped capital femoral epiphysis; and crystalline arthropathy (gout etc.) (6,36,39,40,43,44,46). Removal of an impinging osteophyte on the femoral neck, and extra-articular procedures such as iliotibial band or iliopsoas resection have been reported, but no outcome studies are available on those procedures to date.

EVALUATION OF HIP PAIN

Hip pain, particularly in the young adult, is often mechanical and may arise from a number of structures in and about the hip joint. Most patients will demonstrate dissipation of hip pain and clinical response to conservative measures given time and compliance. When a patient's hip pain persists, is reproducible on physical examination and does not respond to appropriate conservative measures including rest, ambulatory support, nonsteroidal anti-inflammatory drugs, or physical therapy, hip arthroscopy may be of significant value (37,42).

The majority of conditions that cause pain in the region of the hip joint can be diagnosed from a comprehensive history, physical examination, and plain radiographs. These conditions include clinical entities such as iliotibial band tendonitis, greater trochanteric bursitis, inguinal or femoral hernia, hip fractures and dislocations, osteonecrosis, osteoarthritis, and calcified intra-articular loose bodies. For clinical entities such as iliopsoas tendonitis, inflammatory arthritis, early avascular necrosis, occult fractures, psoas abscess, tumor, upper lumbar radiculopathy, and vascular abnormalities, more sophisticated radiographic techniques, including computed tomography (CT), magnetic resonance imaging (MRI), or radioisotope studies, may facilitate diagnosis of persistent hip pain (14,48,50).

Despite vigorous investigation, a subset of patients have persistent symptoms despite negative or equivocal radiographic studies. Arthroscopy can lead to a definitive diagnosis in as many as 40% of these cases (41). Unexpected focal degenerative arthritis, chondromalacia, chondral flap tears, nonossified loose bodies, synovitis, labral lesions, and synovial chondromatosis have all been diagnosed in these circumstances.

Labral Tears

A torn acetabular labrum, like loose bodies, may present with catching, locking, pain, or a click in the hip joint. Although labral tears have been recognized in the orthopedic literature for some time, recently there has been increased attention to this clinical entity (10,17,31,44,45). Altenburg (1) was the first to suggest that a torn acetabular labrum may predispose a patient to subsequent degenerative changes. Cartlidge and Scott (8) and Ueo and Hamabuchi (55) independently implicated labral tears and degeneration in the subsequent development of coxarthrosis.

Labral tears may present without a prior history of trauma. Some tears are considered congenital, and they have been associated with acetabular dysplasia, slipped capital femoral epiphysis, and Legg–Calvé–Perthes disease (26). In these cases, radiographs may reveal a cystic indentation in the lateral roof of the acetabulum. Harris et al. (27) described an intra-articular labrum and labral tears in patients undergoing total hip arthroplasty for end-stage degenerative changes.

The acetabular labrum is similar to the meniscus of the knee. Both contain avascular regions that preclude healing after injury. Minimal injury to the acetabular labrum, when subjected to repetitive motion and stress from the articulation of the femoral head, may progress. Reciprocal injury to corresponding chondral surfaces of the femoral head can occur as

well. Furthermore, the duration of symptoms and severity of labral injury found at arthroscopy have been statistically correlated (44).

Fitzgerald (17) showed that the majority of labral injuries documented (45 out of 49, or 92%) occurred at the anterior marginal attachment of the acetabulum. McCarthy et al. (44), in a series of 58 consecutive patients who were noted to have labral tears, also found that 96% occurred in the anterior quadrant. Ikeda et al. (31), however, looked at a younger patient population and noted an 86% incidence of posterosuperior labral injuries and tears.

Treatment of acetabular labral tears usually involves judicious debridement of the unstable labral segment. Because of the excellent visualization provided by the arthroscope and the minimally invasive nature of the procedure, arthroscopic management of these lesions can be quite useful.

Chondral Lesions

Anterior acetabular chondral injuries frequently are seen with anterior labral tears. These most frequently are initiated at the labrochondral junction and represent the "watershed lesion" (Fig. 48-1). It cannot be overemphasized that the extent of chondral damage has the most direct relationship to surgical outcome (16,46). Acetabular cysts also have been shown in association with labral tears and chondral injuries, especially in those with advanced dysplasia and degenerative joint disease. In these situations the cyst is most often the result of, not the cause of, the patient's mechanical symptoms (45). Therefore, similar to the treatment of a Baker's cyst in the knee, treatment should be directed at the intra-articular chondral abnormality. McCarthy et al. (45) in a series of 456 arthroscopies found chondral lesions were most frequently found in the anterior quadrant. In that study 73% of patients

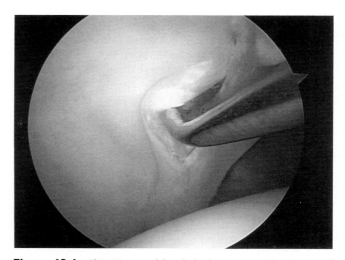

Figure 48-1 This 40-year-old male had progressive hip pain and catching episodes. Hip arthroscopy demonstrated a watershed lesion in the anterior socket. Follow-up: After surgery, the patient's pain was much improved. There was occasional aching in the groin, especially with hyperextension or sudden pivoting movements for the first 3 months after surgery, and after that time he noted a dramatic improvement. There were no further buckling or locking episodes. The patient has returned to work and exercise.

with fraying or a tear of the labrum had chondral lesions, most of which (94%) were located in the anterior acetabulum adjacent to the labral tear. Chondral lesions in the anterior acetabulum only occurred in 6% of patients that did not have a labral tear. The severity of the chondral lesions (grade III or IV) was also greater in patients with labral tears or fraying than those with a normal labrum ($p = 0.0144$). The severity of chondral lesions increased from 46% to 75% ($p = 0.0021$) when fraying of the labrum was present.

In approximately one third of patients (37%), the articular surface appeared normal with no evidence of softening of fissuring, whereas another one third (37%) had evidence of serious cartilage damage, consisting of large areas of fissuring (grade III; 11%) or full-thickness erosion (grade IV; 26%) (Fig. 48-2). The severity of cartilage damage varied with anatomic location, the most severe involvement being observed anteriorly (average Outerbridge score 2.88 of a possible 4), with less severe degenerative changes posteriorly (average score 2.17; $p <0.0001$), and laterally (average score 2.12; $p <0.0001$). Overall, 41% of anterior lesions involved exposure of subchondral bone (Outerbridge IV), compared with only 12% of posterior lesions ($p = 0.0001$) and 6% of lateral lesions ($p = 0.0001$). Chondral injuries may occur in association with a multitude of hip conditions including labral tears, loose bodies, posterior dislocation, osteonecrosis, slipped capital femoral epiphysis, dysplasia, and degenerative arthritis. The difficulty in diagnosing these lesions as well, as their effect on outcome, provides a convincing rationale for arthroscopic hip surgery.

Loose Bodies

The clinical presentation of locking or catching with activity can be associated with intra-articular loose bodies. Many conditions may lead to retained material that can become trapped

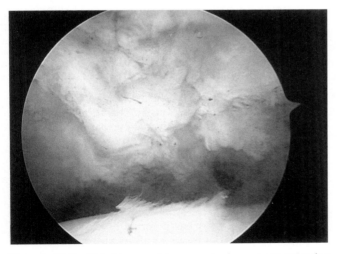

Figure 48-2 This 46-year-old woman had recurrent episodes locking and catching of the hip. She underwent hip arthroscopy which revealed a torn labrum, grade III chondromalcic wear of the anterior femoral head, and grade IV wear of the anterior and superior socket with a large chondral flap. Postoperatively the locking and catching stopped, but she continued to have severe groin pain with most activity. One year postoperatively she underwent total hip arthroplasty.

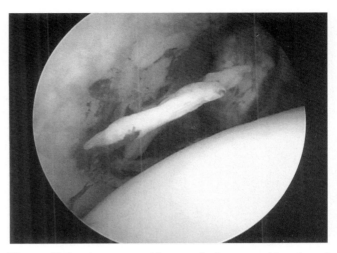

Figure 48-3 This 34-year-old woman had recurrent hip pain and catching. Arthroscopy revealed two large loose bodies within the fovea of the joint. Follow-up: After arthroscopic surgery, there were no further locking episodes. The patient has returned to full-time work without the use of any support devices.

in the acetabular fossa and cause pain. Arthroscopy is the least traumatic method of removing loose or foreign bodies from the joint.

Osteochondral fragment removal after trauma, dislocation, loose bodies associated with osteochondritis dissecans, and free-floating or pedunculated intra-articular bodies associated with synovial chondromatosis have all been removed with the arthroscope (23,36,49,60). Diagnosis of loose bodies is often based on history and physical findings, as plain radiographic diagnosis may be difficult, with overlying phleboliths, bowel gas, bony shadows, and the relatively small size of a calcified loose body (Fig. 48-3).

A number of authors have reported experience using the arthroscope to remove foreign material from the hip joint (5,23,35,49,59,60). As with arthroscopy in other joints, debris such as retained cement, wires, and projectiles may be visualized and removed.

Synovitis

Inflammatory arthritides of the hip are often difficult to diagnose. Because of recent advances in histopathologic diagnosis and rheumatologic management of inflammatory arthritis, histologic examination of synovial tissue may be helpful prior to initiating therapy. Arthroscopy allows minimally invasive synovial biopsy. Additional information including the extent of the synovitis and the state of the articular surfaces can be simultaneously ascertained (Fig. 48-4).

Arthroscopic synovectomy can be useful in the management of inflammatory conditions, but a total synovectomy is difficult if not impossible with current techniques (15,20,29, 30,36,51,60). Traditional open synovectomy requires dislocation of the femoral head from the acetabulum, with the inherent risk of avascular necrosis and a prolonged rehabilitation period. Janssens et al. (32) described arthroscopic synovectomy as an adjunct to diagnosis and treatment of pigmented villonodular synovitis. As the techniques for hip arthroscopy

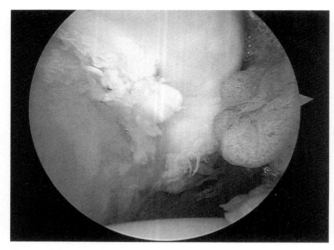

Figure 48-4 This 56-year-old man had unremitting inguinal pain and catching. Hip arthroscopy demonstrated synovitis impinging between the femoral head and acetabulum which was resected. He had grade II chondral lesion with a small flap and a torn anterior labrum. He underwent resection of the labral tear and chondroplasty. At 1-year follow-up he has no rest or weight bearing pain or catching.

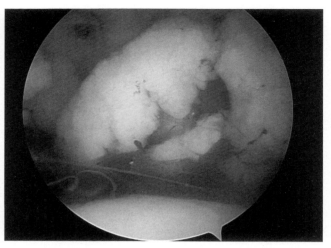

Figure 48-5 A 32-year-old woman presented with hip pain that had been worsening over a 5-year period with freqent locking episodes and a limp. She was being treated by a chiropractor for back injury and psoas muscle strain. Prior to her appointment she had a CT scan which showed synovial chondromatosis. At arthroscopy she had a frayed anterior labrum, and grade II chondromalacic changes of the anterior and superior socket as well as the anterior femoral head. She had over 40 loose bodies removed and a partial synovectomy. After surgery, the patient's buckling episodes did not recur and there was marked improvement in comfort. The patient is ambulatory without support.

improve, the role of early arthroscopic intervention in inflammatory arthritis will expand.

Synovial Chondromatosis

Synovial chondromatosis is a metaplastic synovial condition that results in the production of numerous loose bodies. Although benign, this tumorous entity may be recurrent. The loose bodies when nonossified can make diagnosis of this disease extremely difficult.

Symptoms of synovial chondromatosis may include the onset of dull aching pain, catching or locking sensations, and mild restriction of motion. McCarthy has reported an 80% false-negative rate for radiological investigations including plain radiography, bone scintography, CT, plain MRI, and arthrography in evaluating intractable hip pain (42). Diagnostic yield may be increased with gadolinium-enhanced MRI, which may demonstrate multiple intra-articular filling defects, and is recommended in the evaluation of patients whose relatively normal initial studies fail to adequately explain the disabling hip symptoms (48). Clinical history and examination therefore remain invaluable in directing the appropriate management of patients with synovial chondromatosis.

Treatment modalities have traditionally focused on removal of loose bodies, lavage, and synovectomy. Surgical removal of loose bodies and synovectomy may relieve symptoms and prevent hip joint degeneration, the sequelae of which can be especially devastating in the younger patient population commonly affected by the condition.

The role of hip arthroscopy in the treatment of synovial chondromatosis involves removal of loose bodies and subtotal synovectomy. Arthroscopy of the hip avoids the considerable surgical exposure and prolonged rehabilitation associated with open hip arthrotomy and synovectomy.

Arthroscopic treatment in the author's experience of 28 cases to date has consisted of clarification of diagnosis, removal of between 5 and 300 loose bodies (especially those clustered within the fovea), treatment of articular damage, and synovectomy (Fig. 48-5). There has been a 14% recurrence rate over a 12-year period in this series where a second arthroscopy was performed without intercedent scarring. In addition, arthroscopy, in contrast to open arthrotomy, has been performed without the attendant risks of osteonecrosis, heterotopic bone, deep vein thrombophlebitis, neurovascular injury, or infection.

Avascular Necrosis of the Femoral Head

The role of hip arthroscopy in avascular necrosis of the femoral head remains controversial. This theoretical debate centers around whether the increased pressure from joint distention will further exacerbate the avascular status of the femoral head. Villar has reported possible progression following hip arthroscopy (58). Others have found arthroscopy helpful in staging the articular surface changes for possible osteotomy or bone grafting, and they have not observed progression attributable to the arthroscopic procedure (30,40).

McCarthy et al. (40) has reported on a series of seven patients with mechanical symptoms in early-stage avascular necrosis that underwent hip arthroscopy. All patients had debridement of labral pathology and chondral flaps, and one patient had a concomitant core decompression (Fig. 48-6). At average 2-year follow-up, six of the seven patients were relieved of mechanical symptoms and experienced significant pain reduction. One patient with a grade IV chondral lesion of the femoral head went on to require total hip arthroplasty.

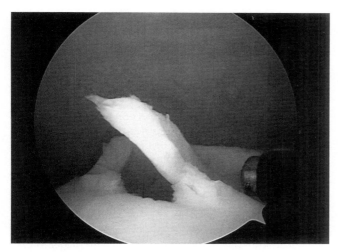

Figure 48-6 A 44-year-old man presented 1-year post core decompression of his right hip for pain and catching. An arthrogram MRI showed a torn labrum and no collapse of the femoral head. At surgery the anterior labrum was torn and he had grade IV changes of the anterior femoral head and grade III changes of the anterior acetabulum. Six months after surgery his pain had returned and he chose to undergo total hip arthroplasty.

Intra-Articular Foreign Bodies

Intra-articular foreign bodies such as bullet fragments can affect the hip with or without an associated fracture. The senior author has removed bullets from two different patients that migrated into the joint years after the initial trauma. In another patient following attempted removal of a femoral intramedullary rod, a metallic fragment had migrated into the joint, embedding itself, like a piece of glass, into the superior lateral aspect of the acetabulum. At surgery the femoral head had already been scratched by this metallic shard. All these objects were successfully removed endoscopically.

Crystalline Diseases

Crystalline diseases such as gout or pseudogout can produce extreme hip joint pain and may or may not be accompanied by an elevated or normal serum uric acid level. Joint fluid analysis with polarized light microscopic verification confirms the diagnosis. At arthroscopy, high concentrations of crystals diffusely distributed throughout the synovium as well as embedded within the articular cartilage of the acetabulum (44). Arthroscopic treatment consists of copious lavage, mechanical removal of crystals, and synovial biopsy if necessary. Crystalline diseases often coexist with other pathology which ultimately leads to the diagnosis.

Post Total Hip Arthroplasty

Most patients with painful total hip arthroplasty can be diagnosed by conventional means: clinical (leg length discrepancy, abductor weakness, etc.), radiographic (component loosening, malposition, trochanteric nonunion, etc.), or by special studies (e.g., bone scan, aspiration arthrogram for subtle loosening or sepsis). When unexplained symptoms persist despite appropriate conservative treatment, arthroscopy can be beneficial. The

senior author has arthroscopically evaluated a series of eight patients post total hip arthroplasty with unremitting pain and negative laboratory and radiographic workups. Two cases of joint sepsis were lavaged and debrided arthroscopically in addition to intravenous antibiotics without recurrent sepsis at 2-year follow up. Intra-articular metal fragments and a loose acetabular screw were successfully removed via arthroscopic means in two different patients. Three cases had hip arthroscopy for persistent and debilitating pain despite negative radiographics and aspiration arthrogram. Findings included a loose acetabular component; corrosion at the interface of a metal on metal articulation; and in two, dense scar tissue impingement at the head cup interface and synovitis. Arthroscopy is not a substitute for open hip debridement and/or resection arthroplasty. However, it is of value in difficult cases to improve diagnostic accuracy while reducing hospital costs and patient morbidity.

Osteoarthritis

The pain from mild to moderate osteoarthritic changes of the femoral head or acetabulum may far exceed the conventional radiographic evidence of degenerative wear, usually characterized with joint space narrowing, osteophyte formation, subchondral sclerosis, and cystic changes. The absence of these finding on plain radiographs does not exclude osteoarthritis (41). Asymmetric, focal chondral degenerative changes, particularly in the anterosuperior aspect of the femoral head or acetabulum, may appear normal on anteroposterior pelvic radiographs. Arthroscopic examination will identify the exact extent and location of chondral degeneration and exclude other pathology. Detailed knowledge of the wear pattern, along with accurate staging of the lesions, is useful when subsequent surgical procedures such as osteotomy or arthroplasty are considered.

Arthroscopic lavage can give significant pain relief in patients with moderately advanced osteoarthritic changes, but this relief of symptoms is often temporary if other mechanical etiologic sources of pain are not identified and addressed (15,57). Debridement and chondral abrasion may have a role in the management of osteoarthritis that is not advanced enough to justify more aggressive surgical options such as joint replacement (28). This is particularly applicable in young patients in whom the surgeon may wish to avoid or delay total joint arthroplasty.

Septic Arthritis

Arthroscopic management of pyarthrosis in other joints, particularly the knee, is well established. The basic principle is decompression of the joint space, removal of necrotic debris, and copious lavage of the joint. Villar (57) and others (3,54,57) have reported successful application of hip arthroscopy in the treatment of isolated infections. In addition to joint decompression, material can be obtained for microbiologic analysis, and the destructive chondral changes can be assessed and documented.

OPERATIVE TECHNIQUE

Hip arthroscopy requires exacting technique, careful preoperative positioning, and a thorough appreciation of the anatomic relationships about the hip joint. Accurate portal placement is essential for optimal visualization and operative access. Positioning of the patient is a matter of surgical preference, but the femoral head must be distracted from the acetabulum to allow a complete view of the articular surfaces. Finally, the surgeon must be cognizant of the cross-sectional relationships of the tissue planes and neurovascular structures around the hip and their relative proximity to the portals used to visualize the joint.

Distraction

Distraction is necessary to visualize the intra-articular structures of the hip (15,20,22,41). The actual force required to distract the femoral head from the acetabulum varies considerably from individual to individual, and it has been reported to range from 25 lb (approximately 112 N) to 200 lb (approximately 900 N). This upper range was necessary only in unanesthetized adult volunteers, and it is clearly excessive for any extended period.

To reduce the distraction force required, patients are anesthetized, usually with general anesthesia and skeletal muscle relaxation, and the resting negative intra-articular pressure is released, which can be achieved by joint capsule puncture with a spinal needle and injection of saline solution. By releasing the vacuum within the joint with arthrocentesis and injection of saline, the force necessary to distract the joint is lessened. Eriksson et al. (15) estimated that as much as half of

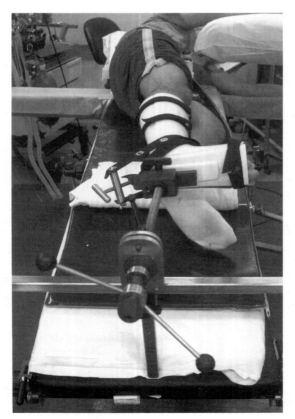

Figure 48-7 Patient in the lateral decubitus position. The leg is supported in the hip distraction apparatus. Note the perineal post assists with lateralization of the proximal femur.

the total resistance to hip distraction in nonanesthetized patients was related to the negative pressure and resultant vacuum effect. The relative contribution of the vacuum force within the hip joint is greater with adequate muscle relaxation. There is considerable individual variation in the other restraints to joint distraction, namely, the intra- and extra-articular soft tissues.

In many cases, the peripheral aspect of the hip can be examined without traction. If the hip is flexed (45°) and externally rotated (30°), the anterior capsule becomes relatively patulent and can be distended with saline, making portal entry and visualization of the femoral neck relatively easy. The traction force can then be increased as necessary to allow inspection of the central joint compartment, between the femoral head and acetabulum. In most patients, distraction can be performed with 50 lb (225 N) or less. Most important, every effort should be made to limit the periods of distraction with higher forces.

Distraction can be achieved with a standard fracture table or with other specialized limb distractors (Fig. 48-7). One important caveat is that a lateral force as well as a distal distraction force should be applied. The resultant vector force is parallel to the femoral neck, which is more effective in distracting the femoral head from the bony acetabulum. A fluoroscopic image intensifier is used in the anteroposterior plane to determine the relative distraction of the femoral head from the acetabulum.

Patient Positioning

Supine Position

The supine position is a familiar position to many surgeons. The setup is similar to that used for fixation of hip fractures, utilizing a fracture distraction table and image intensifier. Axial traction is placed on the extremity, and the hip joint is inspected in the anteroposterior and lateral planes with the image intensifier to assess the degree of joint distraction and for orientation purposes, recognizing that less force will be necessary to distract the hip after arthrocentesis. The distraction table should allow some method for quantitation of force applied to the limb. Additionally, the perineal post support is placed laterally to effect a lateral force on the hip. After initial distraction of the hip, flexion and internal rotation of the limb allow relaxation of the anterior aspect of the capsule, which facilitates arthrocentesis. An unscrubbed assistant can be quite helpful with variances of traction and limb position.

Lateral Position

The lateral position as popularized by Glick et al. (21,22) has several advantages for visualization of the hip joint. The patient is placed in the lateral decubitus position, which allows direct access to the joint along the superior, anterior, or posterior femoral neck. A fracture table or a specialized lateral hip distractor with a tensometer can be used (Fig. 48-8).

Compared to the supine position in which the anterolateral portal is often utilized, the lateral position provides comfortable access to the hip joint via the paratrochanteric approaches (Fig. 48-9). Because the hip capsule is thinner laterally along the neck and the muscle envelope is not as developed, the arthroscope can be inserted with ease. The trochanter acts as a constant anatomic landmark, and the femoral neck can be used as a palpable structure with the trocar to assist with

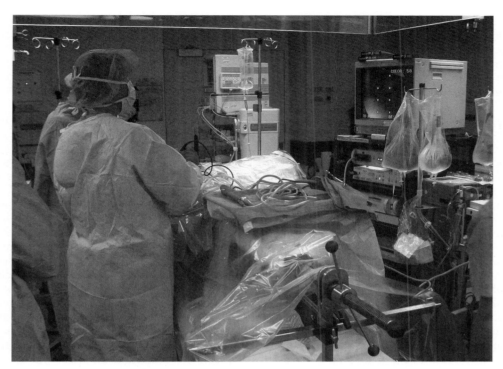

Figure 48-8 The patient is having a right hip arthroscopy in lateral decubitus position with the right foot in a specialized hip distractor (Innomed, Savanah, GA). The surgeon stands behind the patient with the video equipment and power equipment positioned in the front of the patient.

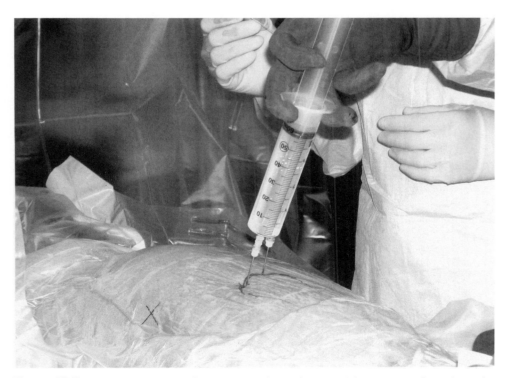

Figure 48-9 Two long spinal needles are inserted into the joint. Saline is injected to relieve the negative intra-articular pressure and to serve as directional guides for trocar placement.

orientation during instrument placement. Additionally, because a considerable amount of the pathology addressed in the hip with hip arthroscopy occurs in the anterior aspect of the joint, a paratrochanteric portal allows visualization of the anterior aspect of the joint with a 30° scope instead of the 70° scope often necessary with the anterolateral portal.

Instrumentation

The depth of the hip joint requires specially designed extra-long arthroscopic instruments passed through cannulae long enough to protect soft tissues surrounding the hip. A specially designed guide wire is then passed through the center of a spinal needle, and once positioned in the joint, a blunt cannulated trocar is inserted for controlled penetration of the hip capsule. Once the portals have been established, the hip is distended with fluid using an arthroscopic pump to maintain constant pressure. A standard 30° scope can visualize most of the joint by varying the angle and exchanging portals. Extra-length curved shaver blades allow for operative arthroscopy around the femoral head. Long suction punches and long graspers are needed to resect and aspirate tissue and loose bodies (Fig. 48-10). Thermal devices are useful in debriding the torn labral and chondral flaps or inflamed synovial tissue folds. High-frequency thermal energy or lasers can be used for cutting and coagulation as well as ablation and capsular shrinkage. Initially inserted long spinal needles (6-inch, 16-gauge) allow release of the negative pressure vacuum phenomenon created with joint distraction and act a guide for ideal portal placement. Confirmation of hip joint access can be performed with placement of preliminary anterior and posterior paratrochanteric portal spinal needles. Sterile saline is injected into one needle with egress of fluid out the other needle, confirming that both needles are intra-articular.

Utilizing the inserted spinal needles as a directional guide, a blunt trocar with metallic cannula or sheath is inserted to the level of the hip capsule after a small stab skin incision is made. The diameter of the working cannulas is 4 mm, and this mates well with the outer diameter of the corresponding nerve hook and/or shavers required to perform arthroscopic surgery. Because the cannulas are telescoping, the smallest one has an inner diameter of 2 mm, and the larger ones have inner diameters of 7 and 10 mm. Each of these larger cannulas can be inserted over the working cannula to facilitate removal of large loose bodies or alligator forceps without loss of the primary portal. The blunt trocar is exchanged with a sharp trocar for controlled penetration of the hip capsule. The trocar is removed and the arthroscope is inserted through the cannula into the hip joint with attached irrigation fluid infusion pump, to allow visual confirmation of hip joint entry. A similar technique is performed for the other portal, which can be utilized as an outflow to gravitation or assembled into the infusion pump to allow improved hip joint distraction.

All arthroscopic instrumentation should be passed through sturdy metallic sheaths or cannulas long enough to traverse soft tissues surrounding the hip once a portal is made. Retained cannulas prevent loss of joint capsular distention and loss of visualization through multiple perforations in the hip capsule. They also reduce the risk of instrumentation breakage, further trauma to periarticular soft tissue, and neurovascular injury. In addition, retained cannulas allow for an easy interchange of instrumentation between portals to allow better visualization and instrumentation access to the hip joint.

Most of the intra-articular structures in the hip joint can be visualized by varying the angle of the arthroscope and the portals utilized (38,41). Both 30° and 70° arthroscopes should be available to allow improved visualization. Furthermore, specialized arthroscopic working instrumentation, such as

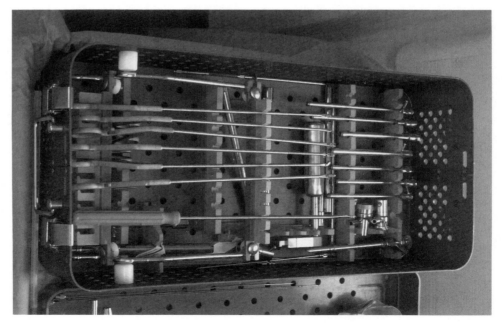

Figure 48-10 Extra-long arthroscopic instrumentation is used to access the hip joint. **A:** The arthroscope and instrument sheaths are accompanied by sharp and blunt trocars. **B:** Standard mechanical shavers will pass through the long cannulas. Flexible cannulas can be used to allow introduction of curved tipped shavers.

shavers, burrs, drills, and loose body retrievers, need to be of appropriate length and diameter to traverse the soft tissue envelope of the hip and allow manipulation within the hip joint.

Portal Placement

Portal placement requires palpation, identification, and marking of the anatomic landmarks including the femoral pulse and neurovascular bundle. There are five portals commonly utilized including the direct anterior, the anterior paratrochanteric or anterolateral, the proximal trochanteric, the posterior paratrochanteric or posterolateral, and the direct posterior portal. The nomenclature and definitions regarding these portals or approaches is not consistent in the literature. When placing anterior portals, caution must be taken to avoid the lateral femoral cutaneous nerve and the femoral neurovascular bundle. External rotation of the foot should be avoided using a posterior portal. The supine position requires three operating portals for the majority of cases. The senior author prefers two main paratrochanteric portals (anterior and superior) that allow visualization of the entire joint for 95% of cases.

Anterior (Anterolateral) Portal

The anterior portal allows visualization of the anterior femoral neck, the anterior aspect of the joint, the superior retinacular fold, and the ligamentum teres (12). To achieve adequate visualization of the anterior labrum or the anterior acetabulum a 70° arthroscope is required.

The portal is placed at the intersection of perpendicular lines drawn laterally from the superior aspect of the symphysis pubis, and inferiorly from the anterior superior iliac spine. A spinal needle is directed from this point medially and superiorly at 45° in each plane. When the joint capsule is entered, the joint is distended with normal saline. At this point, the amount of joint distraction can be assessed with the image intensifier. A blunt-tipped trocar is advanced in the direction of the spinal needle, down to the joint capsule, which will give the tactile sensation of a firm but not solid structure. The blunt trocar is exchanged for the sharp trocar, which is advanced through the thick anterior capsule. The anterior portal places the arthroscope close to the lateral femoral cutaneous nerve, which may result in a partial or complete neuropraxia. If the scope is placed inferior to the neck, the ascending branch of the lateral femoral circumflex artery is as risk. The femoral neurovascular bundle is 3 to 4 cm medial to the insertion site for the anterior portal (12). The localization of the femoral pulse distal to the inguinal ligament can help prevent inadvertent injury to these structures.

Anterior Paratrochanteric Portal

The greater trochanter serves as the reference for each of the paratrochanteric portals. The anterior paratrochanteric portal is placed 2 cm anterior and 1 cm proximal to the anterosuperior corner of the greater trochanter. In the same manner as described for the anterior portal, the joint is entered with the trocar at approximately the intertrochanteric line. The capsule is relatively thin at its insertion on the anterior femoral neck. However, because of the relative obliquity of the trocar to the joint capsule and the anteversion of the femoral neck, an arthroscope directed too anterior and inserted too deeply risks injury to the femoral neurovascular bundle (11).

This portal allows visualization of the femoral head, the anterior neck, and the anterior intrinsic capsular folds (12). The synovial tissues beneath the zona orbicularis and the anterior labrum can be easily seen and addressed from this portal as well.

Proximal Trochanteric Portal

This portal is relatively safe and is often used as an instrumentation portal to triangulate with other optical portals (38,41). The superior tip of the trochanter is palpated, and the spinal needle is inserted just proximal to the trochanter, and it is then advanced medially and slightly superiorly, directly toward the superior dome of the acetabulum. As with the anterior paratrochanteric portal, if the trocar is aimed too anterior, there is risk of injury to the femoral neurovascular structures.

In addition to serving as a primary portal for instrumentation, the arthroscope is placed in the proximal trochanteric portal for excellent visualization of the fovea, the femoral head, and the acetabular labrum (34).

Posterior Paratrochanteric Portal

This portal corresponds directly with the anterior paratrochanteric portal. The entry site is 2 to 3 cm posterior to the tip of the greater trochanter at the level of the anterior paratrochanteric portal. The trocar is advanced with the femur in a neutral or slightly internally rotated position, as external rotation of the hip places the posterior margin of the greater trochanter precariously close to the sciatic nerve.

Despite the potential hazard with this portal, it affords an excellent view of the posterior aspect of the femoral head, the posterior labrum, the posterior capsule, the ligament of Weitbrecht, and the inferior edge of the ischiofemoral ligament.

Posterior Portal

This portal should be used only in conjunction with a small skin incision, dissecting down to the posterior capsule, and identifying the sciatic nerve and the superior gluteal vessels (12). A miniarthrotomy is made at the posterior margin of the capsule and the arthroscope is inserted. This approach is far less traumatic than a formal arthrotomy, and, with the aid of the arthroscope, the posterior joint may be visualized and the pathology addressed without dislocation of the hip joint. Several authors have removed foreign bodies via this approach (23,47,59).

CLINICAL PRESENTATION

Intractable hip pain of intra-articular etiology can present in a variety of ways in the adult. Patients can have pain referable to the anterior groin, anterior thigh, buttock, greater trochanter, and medial knee. Furthermore, mechanical symptoms of persistent clicking, catching, locking, giving way, and restricted range of motion can indicate an intra-articular etiology. Symptoms are usually preceded by a traumatic event, either a fall or a twisting injury, and can present in a variety of age groups depending on the etiology. In addition, symptoms are generally exacerbated with activity and improved with rest.

Patients who are candidates for hip arthroscopy must have reproducible symptoms and physical findings that are functionally limiting. Furthermore, an adequate trial of conservative treatment including rest, use of nonsteroidal anti-inflammatory drugs, ambulatory support, and physical therapy, must be pursued before treatment with hip arthroscopy is entertained. In order to determine which patients would benefit from hip arthroscopy, McCarthy et al. retrospectively reviewed 94 consecutive patients with intractable hip pain who underwent hip arthroscopy (41). They demonstrated significant associations between preoperative clinical presentation and arthroscopic operative findings. The presence of loose bodies within the hip joint, whether ossified or not, correlated with locking episodes ($r = 0.845$, $p = 0.00$) and anterior inguinal pain ($r = 1$, $p = 0.00$). Acetabular labral tears detected arthroscopically correlated significantly with symptoms of anterior inguinal pain ($r = 1$, $p = 0.00$), painful clicking episodes ($r = 0.809$, $p = 0.00$), transient locking ($r = 0.370$, $p = 0.00$), or giving way ($r = 0.320$, $p = 0.0024$), and with the physical findings of a positive Thomas extension test ($r = 0.676$, $p = 0.00$). The findings of a chondral defect of the femoral head or acetabulum statistically correlated with anterior inguinal pain ($r = 1$, $p = 0.00$), but with no other specific findings. In addition, Fitzgerald (13), in a retrospective review of acetabular labral tears, noted 44 of 55 patients (80%) to demonstrate a palpable or audible click, with 48 of 55 patients (87%) reporting groin pain. However, only 48 patients were treated surgically and only 12 underwent arthroscopic confirmation.

RADIOLOGIC EVALUATION

Radiologic workup of intractable pain referable to the hip can include plain radiographs, arthrography, bone scintigraphy, CT, and MRI. Plain radiographs may demonstrate loose bodies or degenerative arthritis, but overall they have a very poor diagnostic yield for intra-articular pathology including the early stages of degenerative joint disease. Arthrography may increase diagnostic yield, and Fitzgerald (17) noted hip arthrography to be positive in 44 of 50 patients (88%) with a suspected acetabular labral tear. However, only 12 patients out of a total of 55 (22%) underwent hip arthroscopy, with no mention of arthrographic correlation to intraoperative findings. Furthermore, bone scintigraphy has a low specificity for intra-articular abnormalities such as loose bodies, labral tears, and chondral defects.

Edwards et al. (14) noted a poor diagnostic yield by MRI in patients with intractable hip pain. They prospectively studied 23 patients who underwent MRI followed by hip arthroscopy within a 3-week period. MRI poorly identified those patients with chondral softening, fibrillation, or partial-thickness defects less than 1 cm, and it gave a less reliable demonstration of osteochondral loose bodies and labral tears, which, they noted, were readily identified and treated with hip arthroscopy. The addition of contrast agents in both CT and MRI may increase the diagnostic yield of intra-articular hip pathology.

Despite a normal radiologic workup, there are many patients who continue to remain symptomatic. In the same study noted previously, McCarthy et al. (44) noted an 80% false-negative rate for all radiologic investigations (plain radiography, bone scintigraphy, CT, MRI, and arthrography) evaluating intractable hip pain. When they excluded those diagnoses that were evident on plain films (e.g., loose bodies, and stages III and IV degenerative joint disease), accurate diagnosis of unremitting hip pain by any radiologic modality was accomplished only 4% of the time. The most commonly overlooked cause of pain was acetabular labral lesions, for which there is currently no reliable radiologic means of diagnosis. In their group of 94 patients with intractable hip pain, 52 (55%) had acetabular labral injuries, all of which were well visualized and debrided at arthroscopy.

CASE EXAMPLES

Case 1 (Fig. 48-11): A 25-year-old female hockey player presented with a 3-year history of left hip pain worsening over time. She denied a history of trauma. She had to cut back on a great

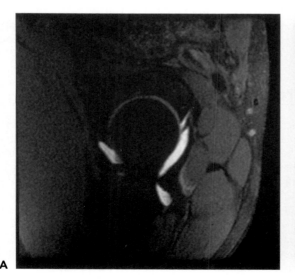
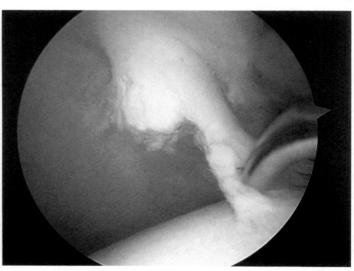

A   B

Figure 48-11   Case 1. **A:** Sagittal MRI of the hip demonstrated a torn anterior acetabular labrum.
B: Hip arthroscopy demonstrated an unstable anterior labral tear that was mechanically debrided back to a stable rim. Postoperatively, there was symptomatic relief of the patient's mechanical hip pain.

deal of her training because of a painful catching sensation in the anterior groin region of the left hip. Her symptoms were unresponsive to exercise modification, rest, and nonsteroidal medication, and she is now taking time off from skating.

Physical examination revealed a full active and passive range of motion. The McCarthy test reproduced the patient's pain and catching sensation, and a palpable click could be appreciated in the left groin. Plain radiographs were significant only for mild acetabular dysplasia. An MRI ordered prior to referral showed no evidence of a labral tear and no loose bodies or other pathologic changes.

At hip arthroscopy, the anterior labrum was enlarged and torn with an unstable labral flap that protruded into the joint space. The chondral surfaces were intact. The synovium juxtaposed to the labral tear was mildly inflamed. The labral tear was mechanically debrided back to a stable edge. The patient has since returned to active sports participation and remains pain free at over 1-year follow-up.

Case 2 (Fig. 48-12): This 57-year-old woman presented with a 6-month history of worsening left hip pain. The pain began after she was ballroom dancing and wrenched her leg. Radiographs at that time demonstrated no fracture and minimal degenerative changes. Her pain persisted despite the use of anti-inflammatory medication and physical therapy. Plain radiographs showed some subchondral cysts above the left acetabular dome. An MRI study revealed an intraosseous ganglia in the anterior superior acetabulum. Bone scan showed mild increased activity corresponding to the ganglia seen on the MRI. An MRI arthrogram showed extension of the ganglion into the anterior labrum. Her groin pain progressed and was made worse by getting up from a chair, climbing stairs, and getting out of a car. She could not extend her leg backward. She experienced a clicking sensation that made her fear the leg would buckle.

On physical examination, she walked with a shortened stance on the left. She had groin pain with a palpable click with the McCarthy test. A resisted straight leg raise also repro-

duced her pain. Left hip motion was 115° of flexion, 0° of extension, 40° of abduction, 10° of internal rotation, and 40° of external rotation with pain.

At hip arthroscopy, she had a torn anterior labrum as well as fraying of the superior labrum and grade III changes in the socket and on the anterior aspect of the femoral head. Postoperatively, her catching episodes resolved, she could get in and out of the car and climb stairs with ease. She has resumed ballroom dancing and is pleased with her progress at 3-year follow-up.

Case 3 (Fig. 48-13): A 40-year-old male presented with left hip anterior hip pain for 11 months with no history of trauma. His pain progressed despite rest and anti-inflammatory medications. Rotation and sudden movements would cause a sharp catching in the groin. He was unable to run or play squash or soccer because the leg would buckle. On exam he had full range of motion and a normal gait. He did have a palpable click with the McCarthy test but no pain. Resisted straight-leg raising reproduced his groin pain. He had an arthrogram MRI of the hip, which revealed a torn anterior labrum.

Hip arthroscopy revealed a frayed and torn anterior and diffuse grade II chondromalacia changes of the socket. He also had 4+ synovitis with crystals visible in the joint fluid and imbedded in the acetabular cartilage. Postoperatively, he had no rest or weight bearing pain and his buckling episodes disappeared. He was being treated with indocin for gout, which was discontinued when his uric acid level was 5.7 at 6 weeks postoperatively. At 6 months postoperatively, he remains asymptomatic.

Case 4 (Fig. 48-14): A 67-year-old woman was evaluated 3 years following a revision left total hip replacement. Three 16-gauge wires had been used to reapproximate a trochanteric osteotomy. There was migration of a trochanteric wire fragment adjacent to the articulation. She complained of deep aching pain with hip rotation and demonstrated a positive Trendelenburg sign. There was no evidence of buckling,

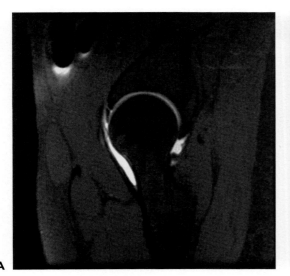

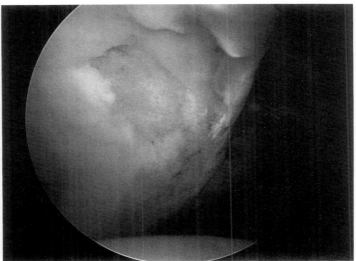

A   B

Figure 48-12   Case 2. **A:** Arthrogram MRI demonstrating anterior acetabular labral tear and preservation of the articular cartilage and joint space. **B:** At arthroscopy, the anterior labrum was torn with grade III changes of the anterior socket.

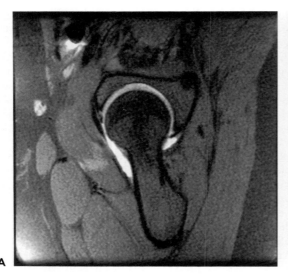
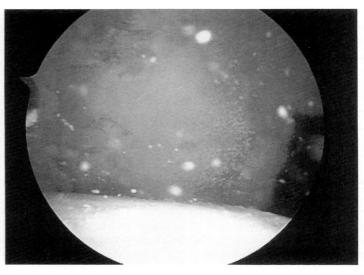

Figure 48-13 Case 3. **A:** An arthrogram MRI showed an anterior labral tear. **B:** Arthroscopy findings: a torn anterior labrum, diffuse grade II changes of the socket and crystals in the joint fluid and imbedded in the acetabular cartilage were found at hip arthroscopy.

grinding, or locking of the joint. Given her intractable pain, the proximity of the migrated wire to the femoral head interface, and the senior author's expertise in arthroscopy of the hip joint, the patient consented to removal, though preferring arthroscopy to open arthrotomy. The Luque wire was indeed within the joint pseudocapsule, in proximity to the femoral head–polyethylene articulation. The wire was approximately 1.5 inches long. In addition two porous beads were present within the joint. All three metal fragments were successfully removed via arthroscopy. Five years later she presented with recurrent symptoms, and an additional wire fragment had migrated near the joint. At arthroscopy the fragment was removed. After each surgery she was fully weight bearing with a cane at the 1-week postoperative visit and did not require analgesics.

RISKS, COMPLICATIONS, AND CONTRAINDICATIONS

The risks associated with hip arthroscopy are variable depending on the surgeon's experience and the surgical approach. Comprehensive knowledge of anatomy and landmarks are crucial to preventing damage to neurovascular structures. Rodeo et al. (52) reviewed the neurologic complications resulting from arthroscopy. Most were caused by traction injuries or by direct trauma to cutaneous nerves such as the lateral femoral cutaneous nerve. Transient neuropraxia to both the pudendal and the sciatic nerve have been documented (41,53). Pressure necrosis of the foot, scrotum, or perineum are other potential complications related to the

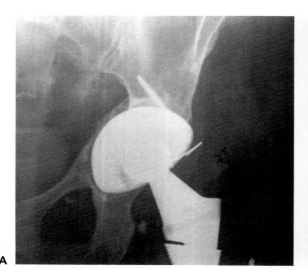
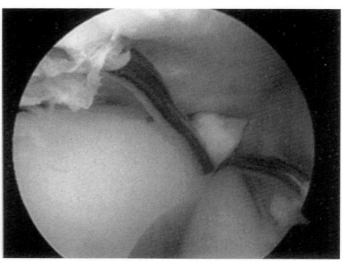

Figure 48-14 Case 4. **A:** Radiographs showed broken trochanteric wire near the joint articulation post total hip arthroplasty. **B:** Arthroscopic photo of wire within the joint pseudocapsule, in proximity to the femoral head–polyethylene articulation.

traction apparatus. Avoidance of these complications is possible if close attention is paid to the force and duration of traction. Intermittent release of the traction is important, and the use of a well-padded perineal post is essential.

Complications related to the intra-articular manipulation of instruments include scuffing of the articular surfaces and breakage of arthroscopic instrumentation (9,41,53). Scuffing and fluid extravasation are the most frequently reported complications but rarely cause permanent damage (2). Broken instruments can result and may require further surgery. For this reason, all arthroscopic instrumentation should be passed through sturdy metallic sheaths to prevent multiple attempts at hip joint penetrance and perforations of the hip capsule. Perforation of the labrum upon entry to the joint is a serious complication that can be avoided by using the image intensifier to confirm instrument placement. Scuffing of the femoral head can occur to varying extent with or without distraction.

Other potential complications include infection and a theoretical risk of accelerating avascular necrosis of the femoral head (41,53). Postoperative infection has not been reported and is probably as rare as it is with arthroscopic procedures of other joints, caused by the large volume of irrigating solution utilized.

In the author's experience of over 1500 hip arthroscopies, there is a 5% complication rate. There have been no infections or pulmonary embolism. One patient, with factor V Leiden deficiency, developed a deep vein thrombosis 1-month postarthroscopy. There have been no instruments broken within the joint. There have been no cases of avascular necrosis to date, and 6% of patients have had MRI studies postarthroscopy. There has been no associated muscle or vessel damage and no permanent damage to the sciatic, peroneal, or pudendal nerves. Less than 2% of patients have experienced transient peroneal hyperthesias that have been associated with difficult distraction and the length of the case, such as in synovial chondromatosis. There have been two cases of neuropraxia to the lateral femoral cutaneous nerve. Mild chondral scuffing has occurred in 3% of patients, which has also been associated with difficult distraction such as mild protrusio or associated degenerative joint disease.

Avoiding complications involves judicious patient selection. Candidates for hip arthroscopy should include only those patients with mechanical symptoms (catching, locking, or buckling) that have failed to respond to conservative therapy. Physical exam findings can include any or all of the following: a positive McCarthy sign (with both hips fully flexed, the patient's pain is reproduced by extending the affected hip, first in external rotation, then in internal rotation) (43); inguinal pain with flexion, adduction, and internal rotation of the hip; and anterior inguinal pain with ipsilateral resisted straight leg-raising. Gadolinium enhanced MRI imaging is much more sensitive for detecting labral tears than traditional MRI. McCarthy et al. demonstrated 78% accuracy for anterior labral tears. It is not as reliable at detecting chondral defects or nonossified loose bodies.

The foremost disadvantage to hip arthroscopy is the length of the learning curve due to the difficulty of the procedure. Access to the hip joint is difficult because of the resistance to distraction resulting from the large muscular envelope, the strength of the iliofemoral ligament, and negative intra-articular pressure.

Relative contraindications for hip arthroscopy include morbid obesity, not only because of difficulty achieving distraction limitations but also the length of instruments necessary to access the joint. Sepsis with accompanying osteomyelitis or abscess formation requires open surgery. Osteonecrosis, moderate dysplasia, and synovitis in the absence of mechanical symptoms do not warrant arthroscopy. Joint ankylosis, dense heterotopic bone formation, or considerable protrusio limit the potential for hip distraction and may preclude arthroscopy. In the senior author's opinion advanced osteoarthritis is a contraindication.

Patient selectivity and diagnostic acumen are critical to successful outcomes. The technical challenge of hip arthroscopy involves a high learning curve. Visiting high-volume centers, attending instructional courses, and practicing in bioskills laboratories all contribute to the clinician becoming technically proficient. Meticulous attention to positioning, distraction time, and portal placement are essential. Complication rates are reported between 0.5% and 5%, most often related to distraction (2,9,19,41,52,53). Improvements in technique and instrumentation have made hip arthroscopy an efficacious way to diagnose and treat a variety of intra-articular problems.

CONCLUSION

Hip arthroscopy is an exciting evolving technique for the diagnosis and treatment of hip disease. Previously, the anatomic configuration of the hip joint, the paucity of equipment tailored to the procedure, and concerns about potential complications limited the number of cases performed. However, better understanding of appropriate portal placement and experience with short periods of traction have made it possible to visualize the intra-articular structures of the hip joint in virtually every case.

Candidates for hip arthroscopy must have reproducible symptoms and physical findings that are functionally limiting, and they must have failed an adequate trial of conservative treatment. Improvements in arthroscopic technique and instrumentation have made it possible to arthroscopically diagnose and treat a variety of intra-articular etiologies of intractable hip pain previously misdiagnosed or requiring an open procedure. However, hip arthroscopy is extremely technique sensitive, requiring a thorough knowledge of anatomic relationships to prevent potential catastrophic neurovascular complications. Anatomic cadaveric dissection and hip arthroscopic workshops are helpful in familiarizing the clinician with cross-sectional anatomy prior to performing hip arthroscopy.

Further advancements are necessary in optical equipment, manual and motorized instruments, and simple, reliable traction devices specific for this procedure. Refinements in patient selection and the increased availability of specific outcome data will help to define the role of hip arthroscopy in orthopedic practice.

REFERENCES

1. Altenberg AR. Acetabular labrum tears: a cause of hip pain and degenerative arthritis. *South Med J.* 1977;70:174–175.
2. Bartlett CS, DiFelice GS, Buly RL, et al. Cardiac arrest as a result of intraabdominal extravasation of fluid during arthroscopic removal of a loose body from the hip joint of a patient with an acetabular fracture. *J Orthop Trauma.* May 1998;12:294–299.

3. Bould M, Edwards D, Villar RN. Arthroscopic diagnosis and treatment of septic arthritis of the hip joint. *Arthroscopy*. 1993;9:707–708.

4. Burman M. Arthroscopy or the direct visualization of joints. *J Bone Joint Surg*. 1931;4:669–695.

5. Byrd JW. Hip arthroscopy for posttraumatic loose fragments in the young active adult: three case reports. *Clin J Sport Med*. 1996;6:129–133; discussion 133–124.

6. Byrd JW, Jones KS. Prospective analysis of hip arthroscopy with 2-year follow-up. *Arthroscopy*. 2000;16:578–587.

7. Byrd JW, Pappas JN, Pedley MJ. Hip arthroscopy: an anatomic study of portal placement and relationship to the extra-articular structures. *Arthroscopy*. 1995;11:418–423.

8. Cartlidge IJ, Scott JH. The inturned acetabular labrum in osteoarthrosis of the hip. *J R Coll Surg Edinburgh*. 1982;27:339–344.

9. Clarke MT, Arora A, Villar RN. Hip arthroscopy: complications in 1054 cases. *Clin Orthop*. 2003;406:84–88.

10. Dameron T. Bucket-handle tear of the acetabular labrum accompanying posterior dislocation of the hip. *J Bone Joint Surg Am*. 1959;41:131–134.

11. Dorfmann H, Boyer T. Hip arthroscopy utilizing the supine position [comment]. *Arthroscopy*. 1996;12:264–267.

12. Dvorak M, Duncan CP, Day B. Arthroscopic anatomy of the hip. *Arthroscopy*. 1990;6:264–273.

13. Edwards D, Villar R. Arthroscopy of the hip joint. *Practitioner*. 1992;236(1519):924, 926, 929.

14. Edwards DJ, Lomas D, Villar RN. Diagnosis of the painful hip by magnetic resonance imaging and arthroscopy. *J Bone Joint Surg Br*. 1995;77:374–376.

15. Eriksson E, Arvidsson I, Arvidsson H. Diagnostic and operative arthroscopy of the hip. *Orthopedics*. 1986;9:169–176.

16. Farjo LA, Glick JM, Sampson TG. Hip arthroscopy for acetabular labral tears. *Arthroscopy*. 1999;15:132–137.

17. Fitzgerald RH Jr. Acetabular labrum tears. Diagnosis and treatment. *Clin Orthop*. 1995;311:60–68.

18. Frich LH, Lauritzen J, Juhl M. Arthroscopy in diagnosis and treatment of hip disorders. *Orthopedics*. 1989;12:389–392.

19. Funke EL, Munzinger U. Complications in hip arthroscopy. *Arthroscopy*. 1996;12:156–159.

20. Glick J. *Operative Arthroscopy*. New York: Raven Press; 1991.

21. Glick JM. Hip arthroscopy using the lateral approach. *Instr Course Lect*. 1988;37:223–231.

22. Glick JM, Sampson TG, Gordon RB, et al. Hip arthroscopy by the lateral approach. *Arthroscopy*. 1987;3:4–12.

23. Goldman A, Minkoff J, Price A, et al. A posterior arthroscopic approach to bullet extraction from the hip. *J Trauma*. Nov 1987;27:1294–1300.

24. Gondolph-Zink B, Puhl W, Noack W. Semiarthroscopic synovectomy of the hip. *Int Orthop*. 1988;12:31–35.

25. Gross R. Arthroscopy in hip disorders in children. *Orthop Rev*. 1977;6:43–49.

26. Harris WH. Etiology of osteoarthritis of the hip. *Clin Orthop*. 1986;213:20–33.

27. Harris WH, Bourne RB, Oh I. Intra-articular acetabular labrum: a possible etiological factor in certain cases of osteoarthritis of the hip. *J Bone Joint Surg Am*. 1979;61:510–514.

28. Hawkins RB. Arthroscopy of the hip. *Clin Orthop*. 1989;249:44–47.

29. Holgersson S, Brattstrom H, Mogensen B, et al. Arthroscopy of the hip in juvenile chronic arthritis. *J Pediatr Orthop*. 1981;1:273–278.

30. Ide T, Akamatsu N, Nakajima I. Arthroscopic surgery of the hip joint. *Arthroscopy*. 1991;7:204–211.

31. Ikeda T, Awaya G, Suzuki S, et al. Torn acetabular labrum in young patients. Arthroscopic diagnosis and management. *J Bone Joint Surg Br*. 1988;70:13–16.

32. Janssens X, Van Meirhaeghe J, Verdonk R, et al. Diagnostic arthroscopy of the hip joint in pigmented villonodular synovitis. *Arthroscopy*. 1987;3:283–287.

33. Johnson L. *Arthroscopic Surgery Principles and Practice*. St Louis: CV Mosby; 1986.

34. Keene GS, Villar RN. Arthroscopic anatomy of the hip: an in vivo study. *Arthroscopy*. 1994;10:392–399.

35. Keene GS, Villar RN. Arthroscopic loose body retrieval following traumatic hip dislocation. *Injury*. 1994;25:507–510.

36. Krebs VE. The role of hip arthroscopy in the treatment of synovial disorders and loose bodies. *Clin Orthop*. 2003:406:48–59.

37. Margheritini F, Villar RN. The efficacy of arthroscopy in the treatment of hip osteoarthritis. *Chir Organi Mov*. 1999;84:257–261.

38. Mason JB, McCarthy JC, O'Donnell J, et al. Hip arthroscopy: surgical approach, positioning, and distraction. *Clin Orthop*. 2003;406:29–37.

39. McCarthy J, Barsoum W, Puri L, et al. The role of hip arthroscopy in the elite athlete. *Clin Orthop*. 2003;406:71–74.

40. McCarthy J, Puri L, Barsoum W, et al. Articular cartilage changes in avascular necrosis: an arthroscopic evaluation. *Clin Orthop*. 2003;406:64–70.

41. McCarthy JC. Hip arthroscopy: applications and technique. *J Am Acad Orthop Surg*. 1995;3:115–122.

42. McCarthy JC, Busconi B. The role of hip arthroscopy in the diagnosis and treatment of hip disease. *Orthopedics*. 1995;18:753–756.

43. McCarthy JC, Lee JA. Acetabular dysplasia: a paradigm of arthroscopic examination of chondral injuries. *Clin Orthop*. 2002;405:122–128.

44. McCarthy JC, Noble PC, Schuck MR, et al. Acetabular and labral pathology. In: MCCarthy JC, ed. *Early Hip Disorders: Advances in Detection and Minimally Invasive Treatment*. New York: Springer-Verlag; 2003:113–134.

45. McCarthy JC, Noble PC, Schuck MR, et al. The Otto E. Aufranc Award: the role of labral lesions to development of early degenerative hip disease. *Clin Orthop*. 2001;393:25–37.

46. McCarthy JC, Noble PC, Schuck MR, et al. The watershed labral lesion: its relationship to early arthritis of the hip. *J Arthroplasty*. 2001;16(8 suppl 1):81–87.

47. Meyer NJ, Thiel B, Ninomiya JT. Retrieval of an intact, intraarticular bullet by hip arthroscopy using the lateral approach. *J Orthop Trauma*. 2002;16:51–53.

48. Newberg AH, Newman JS. Imaging the painful hip. *Clin Orthop*. 2003;406:19–28.

49. Okada Y, Awaya G, Ikeda T, et al. Arthroscopic surgery for synovial chondromatosis of the hip. *J Bone Joint Surg Br*. 1989;71:198–199.

50. Palmer WE. MR Arthrography of the Hip. *Semin Musculoskelet Radiol*. 1998;2:349–362.

51. Parisien JS. Arthroscopy of the hip. Present status. *Bull Hosp Joint Dis Orthop Inst*. 1985;45:127–132.

52. Rodeo SA, Forster RA, Weiland AJ. Neurological complications due to arthroscopy. *J Bone Joint Surg Am*. 1993;75:917–926.

53. Sampson TG. Complications of hip arthroscopy. *Clin Sports Med*. 2001;20:831–835.

54. Stutz G, Kuster MS, Kleinstuck F, et al. Arthroscopic management of septic arthritis: stages of infection and results. *Knee Surg Sports Traumatol Arthrosc*. 2000;8:270–274.

55. Ueo T, Hamabuchi M. Hip pain caused by cystic deformation of the labrum acetabulare. *Arthritis Rheum*. 1984;27:947–950.

56. Vakilif S, Warren R. Entrapped foreign body within the acetabular cup in THR. *Clin Orthop*. 1980;150:159–162.

57. Villar R. Arthroscopic debridement of the hip: a minimally invasive approach to osteoarthritis. *J Bone Joint Surg Br*. 1991;73(suppl 1):170–171.

58. Villar RN. Arthroscopy. *BMJ*. 1994;308(6920):51–53.

59. Williams MS, Hutcheson RL, Miller AR. A new technique for removal of intraarticular bullet fragments from the femoral head. *Bull Hosp Joint Dis*. 1997;56:107–110.

60. Witwity T, Uhlmann RD, Fischer J. Arthroscopic management of chondromatosis of the hip joint. *Arthroscopy*. 1988;4:55–56.

Resection Arthroplasty

49

Thomas A. McDonald   *Steven F. Schutzer*

HISTORICAL PERSPECTIVES

Resection arthroplasty is one of the oldest surgical procedures described for the treatment of pathologic conditions of the hip joint. Between the early 1800s and the present, however, resection of the femoral head and neck has been transformed from a primary procedure (for septic hips, coxarthrosis, and ankylosing spondylitis) to a salvage procedure largely for the management of infected total hip arthroplasties (THAs) or wound breakdown secondary to neurologic impairment.

This operation was described by Schmalz in 1817, and later by White in 1821; both had removed the femoral head from patients with tuberculosis of the hip joint (47,65). Barton in 1827 created a pseudarthrosis after femoral osteotomy for an ankylosed hip (4). Subsequently, Fock in 1861 and Blenke in 1899 reported using resection arthroplasty for infection of the hip joint and severe unilateral osteoarthritis (9,18).

The operation is often referred to as the "Girdlestone procedure" after Mr. G. R. Girdlestone, who in 1923 advocated resection of the femoral head and neck and a portion of the lateral aspect of the acetabulum for the treatment of advanced tuberculosis and pyogenic infections (20–22). In 1945, Girdlestone also recommended the procedure for the treatment of unilateral hip osteoarthritis (23). The Girdlestone procedure was a modification of the method originally performed by Sir Robert Jones in 1921 for ankylosis of the hip joint, in which the greater trochanter with its muscles was attached to the stump of the femoral neck after resection of the femoral head.

Taylor in 1950 reported on 93 patients who underwent resection arthroplasty (60,61). Seventy-three patients had unilateral or bilateral osteoarthritis, 11 had ankylosing spondylitis, and 9 were infected. By his criteria, 90% of the patients had a good result. Taylor stated that this procedure adequately relieved pain, corrected deformity, and restored range of motion to the hip. Furthermore, he felt that with proper postoperative management, hip stability was maintained.

Instability of the hip secondary to resection of the femoral head and shortening of the limb, however, has been reported and is a major cause of postoperative morbidity. To improve stability, some have advocated performing a proximal femoral osteotomy in addition to the resection arthroplasty. Lorenz in 1919 and Schanz in 1922 described a resection arthroplasty combined with an abduction osteotomy for nonunions of femoral neck fractures and osteoarthritis secondary to coxa vara (55). Hackenbroch in 1935 reported a similar operation in which a 30° subtrochanteric osteotomy was performed in hopes of improving the postoperative instability (26).

In 1949, J. S. Batchelor described removal of the femoral head in 50 hips, with an addition of angulation osteotomy in 32 patients to improve stability. The osteotomy was often performed as a secondary procedure 3 to 5 weeks after the primary resection. Seventy-eight percent of the patients had a satisfactory result (6,7).

Gruca in 1950 reported on 224 hips that underwent resection arthroplasty and a complex "dynamic" osteotomy of the proximal femur. The operation was indicated for quiescent tuberculosis, congenital hip dislocation in the adult, ankylosing spondylitis, and intra-articular pseudarthrosis. Ninety percent of the patients had satisfactory outcomes as characterized by a stable, painless joint with range of motion varying between 40% and 100% of normal (25).

A one-stage resection-angulation osteotomy later was popularized by Milch. In his series of 64 cases, a Moore–Blount blade plate was used for internal fixation of the osteotomized fragments. Approximately 92% of the patients had pain relief, and 82% had improved range of motion (37,38).

In a study comparing arthrodesis, cup arthroplasty, osteotomy, and resection arthroplasty with or without osteotomy, Shepard concluded that patients had more predictable long-term favorable results with combined resection and angulation osteotomy (56). In addition, in comparing resection of the femoral head with and without osteotomy, there was greater pain relief with resection alone, whereas more stability was achieved with concurrent osteotomy (41,56).

Parr et al., in a review of 41 patients, also compared patients who had a resection arthroplasty with or without an angulation osteotomy. Although the number of patients was small, the overall hip score was better in patients with the osteotomy (47). Adding to the controversy, Murray et al., in a review of 32 patients found that resection arthroplasty alone resulted in 90% patient satisfaction with regard to relief of pain, range of motion, and muscle strength and concluded that an osteotomy was not necessary for improved function (43,44).

This issue has never been totally resolved. Yet the controversy over whether to perform a concurrent or a second-stage osteotomy after resection of the femoral head and neck has now been clearly overshadowed by the development of the cup arthroplasty, femoral endoprosthesis, and THA. With these innovations, the Girdlestone procedure fell into relative obscurity and is currently recommended almost exclusively for the treatment of infected hip arthroplasty and occasionally for severe proximal femoral bone loss associated with failed THA.

INDICATIONS AND CONTRAINDICATIONS

The indications for resection arthroplasty have changed dramatically during the past century and are summarized in Table 49-1. Initially it was used to eradicate tuberculosis or other pyogenic infections of the hip joint (Figs. 49-1 through 49-5). In the first half of the 20th century, the effectiveness of

TABLE 49-1
INDICATIONS FOR RESECTION ARTHROPLASTY

Primary Procedure
1. Septic, osteomyelytic hip
2. Ankylosing spondylitis
3. Osteoarthritis
4. Rheumatoid spondylitis
5. Femoral neck nonunions
6. Infected fractures treated with internal fixation
7. Severe acetabuli protrusio
8. Severe spastic disorders
9. Tumor
10. Charcot joint

Salvage Procedure
1. Infected total joints, endoprosthesis
2. Extensive bone loss

resection arthroplasty in controlling infection, relieving pain, and returning satisfactory function broadened its application to other deformities of the hip joint such as osteoarthritis, ankylosing spondylitis, rheumatoid spondylitis, nonunions of the femoral neck, infected fractures treated with internal fixation, bilateral neglected congenital hip dislocation, and for severe protrusio (2,4–7,9,20–23,40,53,56,60,61).

The original technique described by Girdlestone and others has been modified. Today, the level of the femoral neck resection is proximal to the intertrochanteric line to preserve as much femoral neck length as possible, and the superolateral acetabular margin is usually not resected.

With the increasing number of hip arthroplasty procedures being performed, the concept of the "pseudoarthrosis test," described by Charnley, may need to be reintroduced. Charnley accepted patients for THA only if their symptoms were of such severity that, if their arthroplasty failed, a pseudarthrosis would not make them any worse.

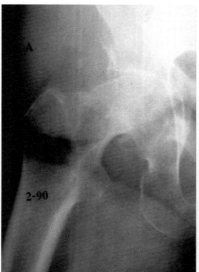
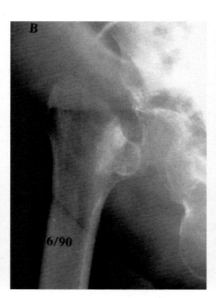
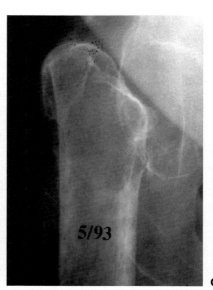

Figure 49-1 **A:** Radiograph of a patient with a septic hip and concurrent femora neck fracture, who underwent a resection arthroplasty. **B:** Proximal migration of the femur noted on 4-month postoperative radiograph. **C:** At 3-years postoperatively, bone has remodeled with smooth sclerotic surfaces and there is no sign of infection.

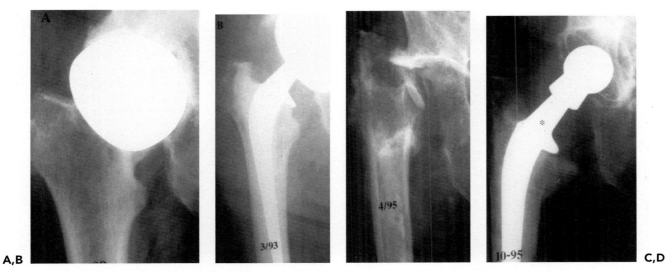

Figure 49-2   A: Serial radiographs of a patient with a cup arthroplasty, who developed progressive acetabular sclerosis with pain. **B:** A successful cemented THA was performed, with a press-fit acetabular component. **C:** Two years later, the patient developed a *Staphylococcus aureus* infection and required a resection arthroplasty. Note that the level of resection was at the intertrochanteric line. **D:** Six months later, the patient had a successful reimplantation with a cemented calcar THA.

Contraindications to pseudarthrosis are not clearly defined. However, obesity is a severe impediment not only to the operation but more importantly to the postoperative rehabilitation. Taylor stated that the use of the upper extremities and prolonged external support is an absolute necessity (60). Severe bone loss also affects the outcome of the procedure because of resultant increased instability in these situations.

THE ROLE OF RESECTION ARTHROPLASTY IN INFECTED THA

Infection after THA is a serious complication, and several treatment strategies have been proposed over the years. Options include chronic antibiotic suppression, irrigation and debridement with component retention, one-stage exchange

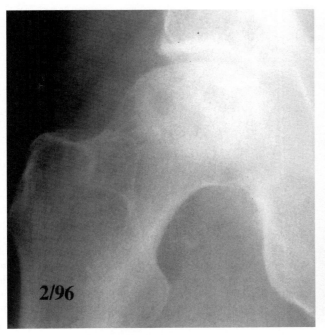
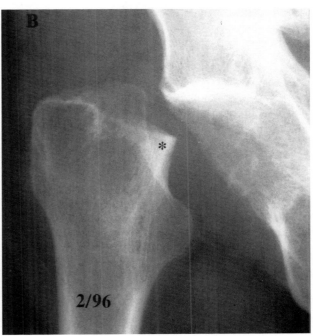

Figure 49-3   Radiograph demonstrating the hip of a patient with end-stage renal failure. The patient had documented stage II avascular necrosis and then developed a septic hip. **A:** Note the cystic sclerotic changes within the femora head. **B:** A resection arthroplasty was performed. The *asterisk* denotes the level of resection in the femoral neck proximal to the intertrochanteric line.

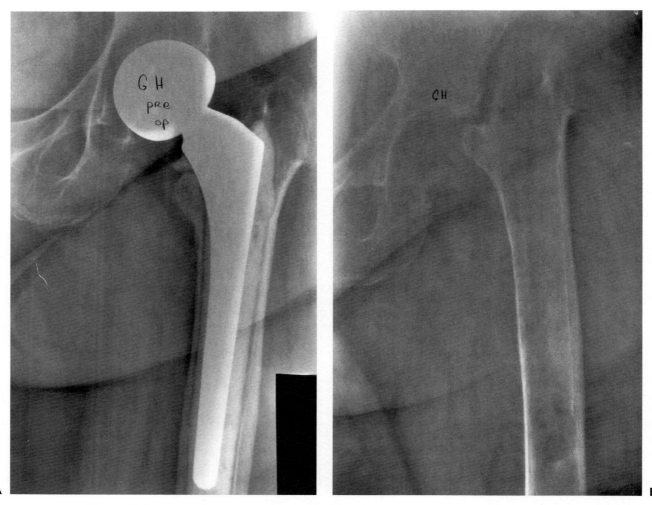

Figure 49-4 This 72-year-old woman with septic loosening and osteopenic bone underwent bipolar replacement for a femoal neck fracture. **A:** Six months later, she presented with a *Staphylococcus epidermidis* infection. **B.** Resection arthroplasty was performed (removing all cement).

arthroplasty, two-stage exchange arthroplasty, one-stage or two-stage arthrodesis, and permanent resection.

Because of differences in patient comorbidities as well as bacterial organism virulence, the outcome of these different modalities has varied widely. Pagnano et al. (46) reported a combined series success rate of 82.7% for one-stage direct exchange with antibiotic impregnated cement, whereas exchange procedures using bone cement not containing antibiotics had a much lower success rate (58%). The highest success rate, however, was attained with two-stage procedures using antibiotic beads or spacers in the interim, and antibiotic-impregnated cement at the time of reimplantation. With this technique, 93.4% of 227 patients had successful outcome (46).

Two-stage exchange is currently the most popular approach to the treatment of infected THA in the United States. In between stages, depot administration of antibiotic is possible using an interval spacer. The use of an antibiotic-loaded implant has several purposes: (a) maintaining soft tissue tension and limb length, (b) facilitation of patient mobilization, and (c) easier subsequent revision. One option for this interval spacer is a temporary functional spacer known as PROSTALAC (prosthesis of antibiotic-loaded acrylic cement; DePuy Orthopaedics, Inc., a Johnson and Johnson Company, Warsaw, IN). Some aspects of the system reported as potential disadvantages include the use of special molds, the specified cost, and the involvement of a metal-on-polyethylene articulation. In situations where the PROSTALAC system is not available, other techniques of molding antibiotic-impregnated cement into the shape of an appropriately sized unipolar hemiarthroplasty prosthetic spacer have been described (31). Pearle and Sculco described the use of a Teflon mold to cast the shape of an antibiotic-loaded cemented hemiarthroplasty (ANTILOCH) (49). Barrack recommended using a Rush pin (Berivon; Meridian, MS) as an endoskeleton to create an antibiotic-impregnated methyl methacrylate spacer. This technique has the advantage of low cost while maintaining the ability to match a wide variety of lengths and offsets (5).

The decision to reimplant or leave a patient with resection arthroplasty can be difficult and is dependent upon a variety of host and microbiologic issues. Relevant factors in the decision include the acuteness or chronicity of the infection, the

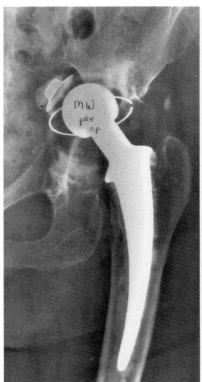
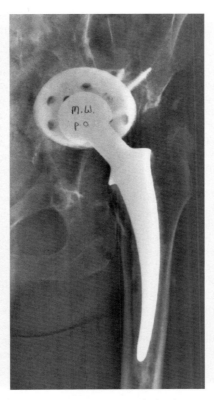
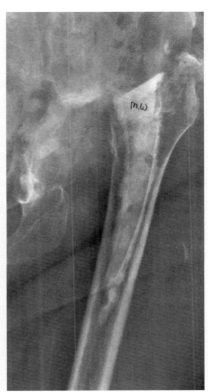

A,B

C

Figure 49-5 Example of a patient with aseptic acetabular loosening and nonreconstructible acetabulum who underwent resection arthroplasty. **A:** This 70-year-old woman had rheumatoid arthritis with diffuse upper and lower extremity involvement. She presented with acetabular component loosening 12 years after primary THA. **B:** Her uncemented acetabular component reconstruction became unstable. **C:** Resection arthroplasty with acetabular bone grafting was performed rather than attempt a further reconstruction because of the poor bone stock and low demands of the patient. No attempt was made to remove the femoral canal cement because of the osteopenic bone.

type of infecting organisms (56, 70) and their antibiotic sensitivities, patient health factors including immunocompromise and compliance, presence of recurrent infection or failed reimplantation, and the presence of substantial bone loss.

In patients with recurrent infections after a previous two-stage exchange arthroplasty, resection arthroplasty may be the only remaining option. Several reports have documented the poor prognosis in this population with regards to function and rate of recurrence (46,64). Similarly, for elderly patients who are not capable of independent mobilization or have a limited life expectancy, patients who are severely immuno-compromised or who are intravenous drug abusers, resection arthroplasty may still be the best solution.

Severe bone stock deficiency has, in the past, been considered a contraindication to reimplantation (33,52). However, function after a resection arthroplasty is also related to the level of resection of the proximal femur, with worse results seen in patients with extensive femoral bone deficiency (24). This perhaps makes reconstruction in these patients, when possible, seem a more desirable option. The challenge of utilizing various techniques to restore bone in these complex cases, however, can be daunting. Reactivation and recurrence of infection is not uncommon. Not surprisingly, two-stage

reimplantation has been shown to provide functionally superior results to Girdlestone arthroplasty alone (17).

The eradication of infection using a two-stage procedure has been reported to be in the range of 60% to 100% (12). Garvin and Hansen's (19) thorough review of the literature showed that a two-stage exchange arthroplasty technique with the use of local antibiotic therapy via antibiotic-impregnated beads has an average of 91% successful results, and they concluded that this is the preferred treatment for infected THA.

Given the problems with soft tissue and bone stock deficiencies, complications with two-stage exchange arthroplasties are common. Charleton's review of 44 patients with a minimum 2- to 9-year follow-up documented an 11.4% dislocation rate, 39% persistent limp, and 41% rate of postoperative medical complication. Other reports have documented the rate of dislocation after one and two-stage reimplantations to be in the range of 3.8% to 18% (12).

Traditional resection arthroplasty still has a role as a salvage procedure for infected total hip replacements not amenable to one-stage and two-stage reimplantation. Patients must expect, however, significant leg-length discrepancies, 3 to 6 cm, for example (10); the dependency on walking aids for ambulation; and a high probability of some persistent pain.

SURGICAL TECHNIQUE

Primary Resection Arthroplasty

In his original report on acute pyogenic arthritis of the hip, Girdlestone recommended a lateral approach to the hip through a transverse incision (21). Two parallel transverse deep incisions are made resecting the gluteal muscle down to the ileum just above the acetabulum. The greater trochanter is resected, and then the femoral neck is osteotomized at the intertrochanteric line. The superolateral acetabular rim is also resected. All cartilage, diseased bone, and soft tissue are debrided. The skin is sutured to the edges of the wound. The wound is packed with gauze wicks and rubber drains to enhance drainage. This procedure was effective in the treatment of acute tuberculosis and pyogenic infections of the hip. If the hip was ankylosed in the presence of infection, only soft tissue was resected, without removal of the femoral head and neck, thus maintaining some stability of the joint.

This surgical technique has been modified over the years so that less radical dissection is performed (23,45,59,60). The greater trochanter and associated abductor muscled are left intact, thus preserving greater stability and function of the hip postoperatively. This also allows for possible later total hip reconstruction—something not possible with the classic Girdlestone procedure.

An anterior (Smith-Peterson), anterolateral, or posterolateral approach to the hip can be used to perform the procedure. The capsule is either incised or excised, or created into a flap for later interposition. Once adequate exposure of the acetabulum and femoral neck is achieved, the femoral neck is osteotomized at the level of the intertrochanteric line or proximal to it, and the femoral head and neck are removed. In a retrospective review of 48 resection arthroplasties, Grauer et al. studied the impact of the anatomic level of resection of the femoral neck and demonstrated that the more proximal resection correlated with a better clinical score (24). Ballard et al., however, demonstrated no specific trend based on the level of resection (3).

All osteophytes should be removed from the posterior superior and lateral walls of the acetabulum. Some surgeons have advocated removing a large portion of the lateral lip of the acetabulum, to allow the surface of the acetabulum to be parallel to the intertrochanteric line of the proximal femur. Girdlestone, Taylor, and Scott also emphasized the need to resect the acetabular rim to prevent bony impingement between the upper end of the femur and the pelvis (20–23,57,60). Parr et al. achieved good results, however, without resecting a portion of the acetabulum (47). Today, if secondary total hip replacement is a consideration, it is preferable not to resect acetabular bone stock.

The cartilage of the acetabulum is then removed with reamers or large curettes to expose bleeding cancellous bone. A complete synovectomy, removal of any bony exostoses, irrigation, and closure over suction drains completes the operation.

Management of the hip joint capsule has also been controversial. Nelson advocated anterior capsular interposition in a noninfected hip to prevent bone-to-bone apposition and felt that this was essential for the development of a pseudarthrosis (45). Murray et al. achieved satisfactory results, however, without soft tissue interposition (44).

Two modifications of this procedure have been described. To reduce the tendency toward external rotation caused by the iliopsoas muscle, (a) the lesser trochanter can be osteotomized and transferred to the anterolateral aspect of the femur, or (b) the lesser trochanter can be simply excised (58). This will allow the limb to rest in a more neutral position. This technique, however, may compromise late reconstruction; if this is anticipated, lesser trochanter osteotomy should be avoided.

Combining a proximal femoral abduction osteotomy with the Girdlestone resection has been recommended to enhance hip stability postoperatively (7,25,37,38). The Milch resection-angulation osteotomy was popularized as an adjunct to the Girdlestone procedure. The level of this osteotomy, usually the lower end of the ischial tuberosity, is marked on the femur. The femur is then externally rotated until it abuts against the pelvic wall, then it is adducted until it lies parallel with the pelvic inclination. A Moore–Blount blade plate or Synthes blade plate is inserted into the upper portion of the femur to form an angle equal to the calculated postosteotomy angle. A 30° closing wedge osteotomy at the subtrochanteric level is performed. The distal fragment is abducted and then internally rotated 20° to 25° and secured to the blade plate. The osteotomy provides two parallel surfaces, enhancing hip stability and maintaining hip mobility. When the osteotomy is used to compensate for limb-length discrepancy, up to 5 cm can be corrected. Because of the significant femoral canal incongruity created by this procedure, it can substantially compromise future hip reconstruction.

Secondary (Salvage) Resection Arthroplasty

When the Girdlestone resection arthroplasty is used for the removal of an infected THA or femoral endoprosthesis, the goal of the procedure is to facilitate removal of the implant, cement, and all infected tissue (42,65). Differences exist between the primary and secondary procedures in regard to the amount of femoral neck and acetabulum resected. As a definitive procedure, the femoral neck may be resected at the level of the intertrochanteric line. If this is the first of a staged procedure, as much bone stock as possible should be preserved to assist in the second-stage reimplantation. All bony exostoses, acetabular osteophytes, and loose cement should be removed. Muller routinely resected the lateral lip of the acetabular roof during his resection arthroplasties for infected hip prosthesis (42), but again this is unnecessary in most cases. In debilitated patients with poor acetabular bone stock, resection arthroplasty may be the definitive procedure (Fig. 49-5).

Modifications of the Girdlestone procedure have been introduced to facilitate implant and cement removal. Standard trochanteric osteotomy, cortical window, or lateral guttering of the femur are all methods that have been described to facilitate removal of cement. The advantages of standard trochanteric osteotomy included easier access for femoral and acetabular implant and cement removal, and therefore a decreased risk of femoral fracture. The disadvantages include (a) difficulties in securely reattaching the trochanter to the lateral cortex, (b) high rate of trochanteric nonunion, (c) potential for late dislocation, and (d) limp, should nonunion occur. Today, the extended proximal femoral osteotomy is widely used and facilitates cement removal (39).

After resection arthroplasty for infection, the hip is usually closed over drains, and the patient is treated with intravenous antibiotics sensitive to the cultured organism. The type of antibiotic, duration of treatment, and interval before reimplantation are based on the virulence of the organism, the quality of the soft tissues and bone stock, and the overall health status of the patient. With time, soft tissue healing may impart enough stability to the hip so that the patient is satisfied with the resection arthroplasty alone.

POSTOPERATIVE MANAGEMENT

Postoperative care is directed toward the establishment of a stable fibrous pseudoarthrosis between the femur and pelvis and maximized leg lengths. The early reports of resection arthroplasty advocated placement in skeletal traction of 10 lb to 30 lb in neutral to slight internal rotation for 6 weeks. Active and gentle assisted range-of-motion exercises of the hip and knee was begun 3 weeks after the operation. For patients not undergoing secondary total hip replacement, traction was then followed by 4 to 6 months of minimal weight bearing in an ischial weight-bearing caliper with the use of crutches. At 6 to 8 months after surgery, the patient was allowed to progressively bear weight.

This prolonged convalescence in traction and with external support was recommended to reduce the amount of limb shortening inherent to the procedure, as well as to avoid external rotation contracture of the limb. Several large studies have demonstrated no subjective or objective difference when traction or calipers were not used postoperatively. Shortening is a natural consequence of this procedure, with leg-length discrepancy between 2.5 and 5 cm. A shoe lift can compensate for the differences in length. Most patients will require the assistance of external support in the form of a cane or crutch forever. All patients have a significant abduction lurch, with a piston-type gait. Addition of an abduction osteotomy has not improved these results (6,7,25,37,38).

FUNCTIONAL OUTCOME

In assessing the outcome of this particular procedure, the goals must be considered. Resection arthroplasty has three goals: pain relief, restoration of function, and eradication of infection. Whether the resection arthroplasty is a primary or a salvage operation, the goals are the same. Interpretation and comparison of the results between studies is difficult. Studies regarding the satisfaction achieved after resection arthroplasty are conflicting (Tables 49-2 and 49-3), because few studies apply both a subjective and an objective hip score to determine the effectiveness of the Girdlestone procedure. When resection arthroplasty is used as a primary procedure, the reported results are dramatically different from those obtained when it is a salvage procedure for an infected arthroplasty. Generally, the latter has demonstrated inferior results.

Primary Arthroplasty

When interpreting and comparing results, it is important to distinguish between primary Girdlestone pseudarthrosis and resection arthroplasty following aseptic failure of a total hip arthroplasty.

Reports of primary resection arthroplasties have demonstrated similar results in regard to pain relief, restoration of function, control of infection, and overall patient satisfaction (6,7,25,29,37,38,60,67). Bilateral resection arthroplasties, unilateral resection with contralateral hip disease, and infection tend to have worse results. Most studies report substantial (from 80% to 100%) pain reduction after resection arthroplasty (44,62). Eradication of pyogenic or tuberculous infection is

TABLE 49-2

PRIMARY RESECTION ARTHROPLASTY OF THE HIP: REVIEW OF THE LITERATURE[a]

Authors	Number	Diagnosis	Function	% Pain Relief	% Eradication of Infection	% Satisfaction
Batchelor	50	Multiple	All walk with aid			78
Gruca	224	Multiple				98
Milch	56	Multiple	Unilateral > bilateral Secondary >1°	92		
Taylor	93	Multiple				90
Shepard	70	Multiple	>30 mobility index 70%/56%	78		70 unilateral 26 bilateral
Murray	32	Multiple	88% walk Prefer support LLD 1.3 cm	94		
Collis	76	Femoral neck fx. OA/infection	100% ambul + external support	74	93	
Parr	38	Multiple	Ave Iowa-70	80	83	
Haw	40	Multiple	25% indep. 25% cane 50% bilateral	72	100	77 No radiographic correlation
Tuli	30	Tuberculous	90% squat/sit Ave. 3.5 cm LLD	98	90	53% G/30% F 17% P

[a]Modified from Ballard et al. Resection arthroplasty of the hip. *Journal of Arthroplasty* 1995;10:772–779.

TABLE 49-3

RESECTION ARTHROPLASTY FOR SEPTIC TOTAL HIP: REVIEW OF THE LITERATURE[a]

Authors	Number	Diagnosis	Function	% Pain Relief	% Eradication of Infection	% Satisfaction
Clegg	30	Septic THA	10% improvment All + external support	90	80	
Mallory	10	Septic THA	All + external support	30	100	100 No radiograph correlation
Campbell	52	Septic THA	70% bil. support	44	73 No correlation with retained cement	40% before implant 88% then before pseudoarthrosis
Petty	21	Septic THA	Ave Iowa-49	33	76 No correlation with retained cement	14
Hamblen	55	Septic THA	43% dbl. support	87	80	Best result in 30%
Bitter	14	Septic THA	86% indep. ambul.		86	7
McElwaine	22	Septic THA		100	86 No correlation with retained cement	33
Bourne	33	Septic THA	85% + support HHS-60 LLD-4 cm	91	97	79
Canner	33				82	60
Kantor	41	Septic THA	83% comm. amb LLD-6.1 cm	7	33 without cement 59 with cement	Best results with Healed wound and HO
Marchetti	104	Septic/aseptic	55% G/E after asept 45% B after septic LLD-3–5 cm	73	87	72
Pazzaglia	15	SSeptic/aseptic	Iowa-66 LLD-4.2 cm		100	
Grauer	48	Multiple	51% poor LLD-3–11 cm	33	97	
Ballard	46	Multiple	95% indep. ambul. LLD-5.4 cm 84% Iowa > 70	77	98	72
Ahlgren	27	Septic THA	81% ambul.		71 No correlation with retained cement	97

[a]Modified from Ballard et al. Resection arthroplasty of the hip. *Journal of Arthroplasty* 1995;10:772–779.

equally successful, occurring in up to 90% of cases (15,29, 47,62).

Functional results in these reports are similar. Most of the patients remain ambulatory but rely on use of external support of either a crutch or a cane, because of fatigue, instability, or pain. Easy fatigability is common since the energy required and the oxygen consumed with use of crutches or walker (up to 240% of normal) are similar to patients with an above-knee amputation (30).

Reports containing specific functional hip scores after primary resection arthroplasty have been infrequent. Parr et al. reported an average Iowa hip score of 70, and Haw and Gray, using the Lazensky grading system, demonstrated an overall average of 3.8 (which corresponds to a good rating) (29,47). Shepard reported deterioration of clinical outcome with time. Seventy percent of the hips had a mobility index greater than 30 (in the satisfactory range) at less than 3 years, which decreased to 56% after 5 years (56).

In several studies, the overall satisfaction rate ranged from 70% to 90%, using subjective criteria. All patients tend to have a limb-length disparity, ranging from 2.5 to 5 cm, and an abductor lurch. The amount of shortening was not influenced by traction postoperatively or by the use of calipers. Shortening, instability, and abductor lurch did not necessarily constitute failure. Elimination of infection, achievement of acceptable motion, and reduction in pain were the appropriate goals of this procedure, which were achieved in the majority of patients over time.

Secondary (Salvage) Resection Arthroplasty

Results from resection arthroplasty for septic and aseptic loosening of THA have been quite variable (Table 49-3). Clegg reported that only 10% of the patients improved in regard to their walking ability (13). Campbell et al. reviewed 52 patients, 70% of whom were still dependent on double support for ambulation (11). Grauer et al. demonstrated poor function in 51% of their patient population (24). Petty and Goldsmith showed that the overall Iowa hip score was 49, and a study by Bourne et al. revealed that 85% required walking aides at all times and the Harris hip score was only 60 points (10,50).

A study by Marchetti et al. also revealed a clear difference between the results of resection arthroplasty after septic and aseptic loosening. No poor results occurred in the aseptic loosening group, and 55% of hips were graded as excellent to good. In contrast, poor functional results were seen in 45% of the septic hips treated by resection arthroplasty (35). In a retrospective study, Pazzaglia et al. reviewed patients that had a total hip prosthesis reimplanted compared with those left with a resection arthroplasty. Using the Iowa hip rating scale, they showed that the reimplanted group was rated significantly higher for function, gait, and absence of deformity (48).

More encouraging results have been reported by other authors. Ahlgren et al., Ballard et al., and Kantor et al. reported more than 80% of the patients remained community ambulators with some form of external support (1,3,30). Ballard et al. also reported an Iowa hip rating greater than 70 in 84% of their patients (3).

When all of the retrospective studies are combined, only 62.5% of patients reported significant relief of pain. One of the reasons for residual pain is impingement of the proximal femur against the pelvic wall. Several studies have addressed the level of femoral resection and its impact on outcome. Kantor et al. and Ballard et al. demonstrated no correlation between level of resection and final outcome (3,30) (Fig. 49-3).

Controversy concerning the need for complete cement removal in all cases of resection arthroplasty remains. However, in septic cases, a compelling argument can be made for removal of all cement from the femur. Clegg reported 20% infection recurrence and advocated complete cement removal through a lateral guttering of the femur if necessary (13). Kantor et al. demonstrated that 59% of the hips with persistent infection had retained cement, as opposed to 33% that did not (30). Studies by Petty et al., McElwaine and Colville, and Ballard et al. reported no correlation of retained cement with clinical outcome (3,36,50). They recommend removing as much cement as possible without compromising the integrity of the proximal femur.

The reported patient satisfaction after resection arthroplasty for failed THA is variable. Petty and Goldsmith had only 3 of 21 patients satisfied, and Bitter and Petty, only 1 of 14 (8,50). McElwaine and Colville, in 22 patients, reported only 33% satisfaction, although 100% pain relief and 86% control of infection were achieved (36). Patient expectations may be influenced by having had a successful THA prior to failure. Some studies, however, do report a reasonable outcome following secondary resection arthroplasty: Ahlgren et al., Ballard et al., Bourne et al., Mallory et al., and Marchetti et al. have all reported satisfactory outcomes in greater than 70% of hips (1,3,10,34,35). The small number of patients in each series, the variables in the procedure itself, and the variables in the outcome tools utilized to assess results may account for these substantial discrepancies.

COMPLICATIONS

Following primary resection arthroplasty and secondary salvage resection arthroplasty for the treatment of chronic deep infection, the major postoperative complication is recurrence of infection. Recurrence rates of 10% to 20% have been reported. This may reflect the virulence of the bacteria, incomplete debridements, retained cement or hardware, or a compromised host. Whether an antibiotic-impregnated polymethyl methacrylate spacer is implanted to enhance eradication of bacteria during resection arthroplasty is dependent on a variety of factors, including surgeon preference. For intractable infections with persistent draining sinuses and larger dead spaces after Girdlestone pseudarthrosis, Collins et al. also used a vastus lateralis flap to fill the space and provide vascularity to the wound (14).

Painful bony impingement can be avoided through proper surgical technique. If a true Girdlestone procedure is being carried out, strict adherence to the surgical protocol may yield better results. Surgeons may, however, opt for retaining as much femoral neck length as possible and leaving the acetabulum intact if reimplantation is being considered. With severe proximal bone loss from osteolysis, stress shielding, or infection, femoral–pelvic impingement is less a problem, but significant shortening and instability are universal and difficult to control.

Other complications are directly related to removal of a septic or aseptic hip prosthesis especially if these implants are well fixed and stable. Hamblen performed 17 trochanteric osteotomies to facilitate removal of the implant and cement; 15 ended in nonunion (27,28). Other complications, such as perforation of the femoral cortex and femoral fracture, have been reported after aggressive removal of cement. The latter are probably the most common complications because of the thin femoral cortices, osteoporotic bone, and intramedullary cement present in the revision setting. In the presence of a fully coated ingrown stem, extraction is difficult and sometimes impossible without significant injury to the host bone.

SUMMARY

The procedure originally described as the Girdlestone resection arthroplasty has evolved over the last century. Initially used for primary tuberculosis and other pyogenic infections of the hip, it later was applied to treatment of osteoarthritis, ankylosing spondylitis, and femoral neck nonunions. The procedure is not technically demanding, but attention to detail is mandatory in creating a proper pseudarthrosis.

However, the development of femoral endoprostheses and THAs to treat these conditions has changed the role of resection arthroplasty, which is currently used as a salvage procedure for septic and aseptic loosening with severe proximal bone loss. The goals remain the same: to relieve pain, restore motion and function, eradicate infection, and maximize function. Appropriate preoperative counseling, as Charnley advocated, with the "pseudarthrosis test" is still advisable and should occur prior to THA, revision arthroplasty, reimplantation, and Girdlestone procedures.

When the procedure is done correctly and for the proper indications, one can expect adequate pain relief, control of infection, and improvement of hip motion. Functional results may vary depending on patient demands and expectations, as well as the general health status of the patient. Most patients can anticipate remaining an independent ambulator with some form of external support for assistance. Patients should expect a limb-length discrepancy, abductor lurch, hip instability, and early fatigue with walking. These side effects can be minimized with the use of a cane, crutch, and shoe lift.

Resection arthroplasty has a prominent place in orthopedic history. Although its role has become diminished since the advent of THA, it is still a valuable procedure when trying to attain the goals of eradication of infection, preserving motion at the hip, and providing a moderate amount of pain relief. The indications for resection arthroplasty have become quite narrow and focused, but it remains a useful and important procedure in the approach to complex problems of the hip.

REFERENCES

1. Ahlgren SA, Gudmundsson G, Bartholdsson E. Function after removal of a septic hip prostheses. *Acta Orthop Scand.* 1980;51: 541–545.
2. Albinana J, Gonzalez-Moran G. Painful spastic hip dislocation: proximal femoral resection. *Iowa Orthop J.* 2002;22:61–65.
3. Ballard WT, Lowery DA, Brand RA. Resection arthroplasty of the hip. *J Arthroplasty.* 1995;10:772–779.
4. Barton JR. On the treatment of ankylosis by the formation of artificial joints: new operation. *North Am Med Surg J.* 1827;4:279.
5. Barrack RL. Rush pin technique for temporary antibiotic-impregnated cement prosthesis for infected total hip arthroplasty. *J Arthroplasty.* 2002;17:600–603.
6. Batchelor JS. Excision of the femoral head and neck in cases of anklyosis and osteoarthritis of the hips. *Proc R Soc Med.* 1945;38: 689–690.
7. Batchelor JS. Pseudoarthosis for ankylosis and arthritis of the hip. *J Bone Joint Surg.* 1949;31B:135.
8. Bittar EA, Petty W. Girdlestone arthroplasty for infected total hip arthroplasty. *Clin Orthop.* 1982;170:83–87.
9. Blenke A. Ein Beitragzur Lehre der Kontrakfuren und Ankylosen im Huftgelenk und deren Behandlung bes auf blutigem Wege. *Z Orthop Chir.* 1899;6:279.
10. Bourne RB, Hunter GA, Rorabeck CH, et al. A six year follow-up of infected total hip replacements managed by Girdlestone arthroplasty. *J Bone Joint Surg.* 1984;66N:340–343.
11. Campbell A, Fitzgerald B, Fischer WD, et al. Girdlestone pseudoarthrosis for failed total hip replacement. *J Bone Joint Surg.* 1978;60B:441.
12. Charlton WP, Hozack WJ, Teloken MA, et al. Complications associated with reimplantation after girdlestone arthroplasty. *Clin Orthop.* 2003;407:119–126.
13. Clegg J. The results of the pseudoarthrosis after removal of an infected total hip prosthesis. *J Bone Joint Surg.* 1977;59B:298–301.
14. Collins DN, Garvin KL, Nelson CL. The use of the vastus lateralis flap in patients with intractable infection after resection arthroplasty following the use of a hip implant. *J Bone Joint Surg.* 1987;69:510–516.
15. Collis DK, Johnston RC. Complete femoral head and neck resection: clinical follow-up study. *J Bone Joint Surg.* 1971;53A: 396–397.
16. Duncan CP, Beauchamp CP. A temporary antibiotic loaded joint replacement system for management of complex infections involving the hip. *Orthop Clin North Am.* 1993;24:751–759.
17. Duncan CP, Masri BA. The role of antibiotic-loaded cement in the treatment of an infection after a hip replacement. *Instr Course Lect.* 1995;44:305–313.
18. Fock C. Bemerkungen und Erfahrungen uber die Resktion im Huftgelenk. *Langenbeck Arch Klin Chir.* 1861;1:172.
19. Garvin KL, Hanssen AD. Current concepts review: infection after total hip arthroplasty. *J Bone Joint Surg.* 1995;77A:1576–1588.
20. Girdlestone GR. Acute pyogenic arthritis of the hip. *Clin Orthop.* 1982;170:3–7.
21. Girdlestone GR. Acute pyogenic arthritis of the hip. *Lancet.* 1943;1:419–421.
22. Girdlestone GR. Arthrodesis and other operations for tuberculosis of the hip. In: *The Robert Jones Birthday Volume. A Collection of Surgical Essays.* London: Oxford University Press; 1928:347.
23. Girdlestone GR. Pseudoarthrosis: discussion on the treatment of unilateral osteoarthritis of the hip. *Proc R Soc Med.* 1945;38:363.
24. Grauer JD, Amstutz HC, O'Carroll PF, et al. Resection arthroplasty of the hip. *J Bone Joint Surg.* 1989;71A:669–678.
25. Gruca A. The treatment of quiescent tuberculosis of the hip joint by excision and dynamic osteotomy. *J Bone Joint Surg.* 1950;32B; 174–182.
26. Hackenbroch M. Das malum Coxae senile. *Chirurgie.* 1935;7:857.
27. Hamblen DL. Diagnosis of infection and the role of permenant excision arthroplasty. *Orthop Clin North Am.* 1993;4:743–749.
28. Hamblen DL, Fisher WD. Excision arthroplasty as a salvage procedure. In: Ling RSM, ed. *Complications of Total Hip Replacement.* Edinburgh: Churchill Livingstone; 1984:272.
29. Haw CS, Gray DH. Excision arthroplasty of the hip. *J Bone Joint Surg.* 1976;58B:44–47.
30. Kantor GS, Stream JA, Dorr LD, et al. Resection arthroplasty following infected total hip replacement arthroplasty. *J Arthroplasty.* 1986;1:83–89.
31. Koo KH, Yang JW, Cho SH, et al. Impregnation of vancomycin, gentamicin, and cefotaxime in a cement spacer for two-stage cement reconstruction in infected total hip arthroplasty. *J Arthroplasty.* 2001;16:882–892.
32. Leunig M, Chosa E, Speck MK, et al. A cement spacer for two-stage revision of infected implants of the hip joint. *Int Orthop.* 1998;22: 209–214.
33. Lieberman JR, Callaway GH, Salvati EA, et al. Treatment of the infected total hip arthroplasty with a two-stage reimplantation protocol. *Clin Orthop.* 1994;301:205–212.
34. Mallory TH. Excision arthroplasty with delayed wound closure for infected total hip replacement. *Clin Orthop.* 1978;137:106–111.
35. Marchetti PG, Toni A, Baldini N, et al. Clinical evaluation of 104 hip resection arthroplasties after removal of a total hip prosthesis. *J Arthroplasty.* 1987;2:37–41.
36. McElwaine JP, Colville J. Excision arthroplasty for infected total hip replacements. *J Bone Joint Surg.* 1984;66B:168–171.
37. Milch H. Surgical treatment of the stiff, painful hip. The resection angulation osteotomy. *Clin Orthop.* 1963;31:48–57.
38. Milch H. The resection-angulation operation for hip joint deformities. *J Bone Joint Surg.* 1955;37A:699–717.
39. Miner TM, Momberger NG, Chong D, et al. The extended trochanteric osteotomy in revision hip arthroplasty: a critical review of 166 cases at mean 3-year, 9-month follow-up. *J Arthroplasty.* 2001;16(8 suppl 1):188–194.
40. Morley DC, Schmidt RH. Protrusio acetabuli prosthetica. *Orthop Rev.* 1986;15:135–140.
41. Muller KH. Resection of the femoral head and neck and resection-angulation osteotomy. In: Tronzo RG, ed. *Surgery of the Hip Joint.* Philadelphia: Lea and Febiger; 1973:644–656.
42. Muller ME. Preservation of septic total hip replacement versus Girdlestone operation. In: *The Hip: Proceedings of the Second Open Scientific Meeting of the Hip Society.* St. Louis: CV Mosby; 1974:308.
43. Murray WR. Treatment of the infected total hip arthroplasty. *Instr Course Lect.* 1986;35:229–233.
44. Murray WR, Lucus DB, Inman VT. Femoral head and neck resection. *J Bone Joint Surg.* 1964;46A:1184–1197.
45. Nelson CL. Femoral head and neck excision arthroplasty. *Orthop Clin North Am.* 1971;2:127–137.
46. Pagnano MW, Trousdale RT, Hanssen AD. Outcome after reinfection following reimplantation hip arthroplasty. *Clin Orthop.* 1997;338:192–204.
47. Parr PL, Croft C, Enneking W. Resection of the head and neck of the femur with and without angulation osteotomy. *J Bone Joint Surg.* 1971;53A:935–944.
48. Pazzaglia UE, Ghiselli F, Ceffa R, et al. Evaluation of reimplant total hip prostheses and resection arthroplasty. *Orthopaedics.* 1988;11:1141–1145.
49. Pearle AD, Sculco TP. Technique for fabrication of an antibiotic-loaded cement hemiarthroplasty (ANTILOCH) prosthesis for infected total hip arthroplasty. *Am J Orthop.* 2002;31:425–427.

50. Petty W, Goldsmith S. Resection arthroplasty following total hip arthoplasty. *J Bone Joint Surg.* 1980;62A:889–896.

51. Phelan DM, Osmon DR, Keating MR, et al. Delayed reimplantation arthroplasty for candidal prosthetic joint infection: a report of 4 cases and review of the literature. *Clin Infect Dis.* 2002;34:930–938.

52. Salvati EA, Chekofsky KM, Brause BD, et al. Reimplantation in infection: a 12-year experience. *Clin Orthop.* 1982;170:62–75.

53. Sanchez-Sotelo J, Trousdale RT, Berry DJ, et al. Surgical treatment of developmental dysplasia of the hip in adults. I: Nonarthroplasty options. *J Am Acad Orthop Surg.* 2002;10:321–333.

54. Schoellner C, Fuerderer S, Rompe JD, et al. Individual bone cement spacers (IBCS) for septic hip revision-preliminary report. *Arch Orthop Trauma Surg.* 2003;123:254–259.

55. Schroder J, Saris D, Besselaar PP, et al. Comparison of the results of the Girdlestone pseudarthrosis with reimplantation of a total hip replacement. *Int Orthop.* 1998;22:215–218.

56. Shepard MM. A further review of the results of operations on the hip joint. *J Bone Joint Surg.* 1960;42B:177–204.

57. Scott JC. Pseudoarthrosis of the hip. *Clin Orthop.* 1963;31:31–38.

58. Somerville EW. Girdlestone pseudoarthrosis of the hip. In: Rob C, Smith R, eds. *Operative Surgery. Orthopaedics.* Part 1. Philadelphia: JB Lippincott; 1969:256–260.

59. Stienberg ME, Steinberg DR. Girdlestone pseudoarthrosis. In: Tronzo RG, ed. *Surgery of the Hip Joint.* Vol 2. 2nd ed. New York: Springer-Verlag; 1984:421–432.

60. Taylor RG. Pseudoarthrosis of the hip joint. *J Bone Joint Surg.* 1950;32B:161–165.

61. Taylor RG. Pseudoarthosis of the hip joint. In: *Proceedings of the Ninth Congress of International Society of Orthopaedic Surgery and Traumatology.* Brussels: International Society of Orthopaedic Surgery and Traumatology; 1963:152–157.

62. Tuli SM, Mukherjee SK. Excision arthroplasty for tuberculous and pyogenic arthritis of the hip. *J Bone Joint Surg.* 1981;63B: 29–32.

63. Weil Y, Mattan Y, Liebergall M, et al. Brucella prosthetic joint infection: a report of 3 cases and a review of the literature. *Clin Infect Dis.* 2003;36:e81–86.

64. Went P, Krismer M, Frischhut B. Recurrence of Infection after revision of infected hip arthroplasties. *J Bone Joint Surg.* 1995;77B:307–309.

65. White A. Obituary. *Lancet.* 1849;1:324.

66. Younger AS, Duncan CP, Masri BA, et al. The outcome of two-stage arthroplasty using a custom-made interval spacer to treat the infected hip. *J Arthroplasty.* 1997;12:615–623.

67. Younger AS, Duncan CP, Masri BA. Treatment of infection associated with segmental bone loss in the proximal part of the femur in two stages with use of an antibiotic-loaded interval prosthesis. *J Bone Joint Surg Am.* 1998;80:60–69.

Arthrodesis

John J. Callaghan

To date, total hip arthroplasty has not been perfected to the point of adequately meeting the needs of the young active patient over a normal life span. Therefore, hip arthrodesis must remain a viable alternative for such a patient with unilateral hip disease. Unfortunately, hip arthrodesis is nearly extinct in North America, with limited patient acceptance and few orthopedic surgeons with enthusiasm for or experienced in performing the procedure. However, studies have shown hip arthrodesis to be compatible with a functional and productive life (16,53).

Although hip arthrodesis was commonly performed for debilitating hip arthritis until the 1930s, it was abandoned, largely for procedures that allowed hip mobility as well as pain relief. In the 1930s, the cup arthroplasty procedure served as an alternative to arthrodesis, relieving pain and obtaining or maintaining motion in patients afflicted with hip arthritis. Thirty years later, total hip arthroplasty became the most popular procedure for advanced hip arthritis. In the middle 1970s, resurfacing procedures were advocated as an alternative to conventional cemented total hip replacement in younger patients. At present, noncemented total hip arthroplasty, at least on the acetabular side of the construct, is performed in younger patients with end-stage hip arthritis. All of these procedures have demonstrated inferior long-term results in younger patients when compared with the results in older patients, especially on the acetabular side of the construct

(9,25,41,51,58). This is at least in part related to the inevitable generation of particulate wear debris at the bearing surface of the total hip arthroplasty. With the life expectancy of patients in their teenage years or twenties reaching up into the seventies and early eighties, and with a better understanding of the limitations of total hip arthroplasty in the young, hip arthrodesis has resurfaced as a viable consideration for young active patients with disabling arthritis.

HISTORICAL PERSPECTIVE

Hip arthrodesis was first attempted by Lagrane of France in 1886 (21). It was performed on a 16-year-old girl with dislocation and unspecified arthritis of the hip. The dislocated head was restored to the acetabulum and fixed with wires, resulting in the first pseudarthrosis. Albee is the father of hip arthrodesis in the United States (2), initially describing intraarticular arthrodesis in 1908 and extra-articular arthrodesis in 1915 (Figs. 50-1 and 50-2). Brittain popularized extra-articular arthrodesis with intertrochanteric osteotomy and ischial femoral bone grafting in 1941 (Fig. 50-3) (15). However, these concepts had been developed previously by DeBeule (1909) (21), Maragliano (1921), Calvé (1931), and Trumble (1922) (60). Although the use of internal fixation to obtain hip fusion was popularized by Van Nes (1922), Watson-Jones championed transarticular nail arthrodesis (1939) (Fig. 50-4) (61). Onji et al. (1965) described intramedullary arthrodesis (Fig. 50-5) (3,43). Davis (1954) described the use of a muscle-pedicle iliac bone graft to augment hip fusion (Fig. 50-6) (46). The principles of the now popular cobra-head plate arthrodesis described by Schneider in 1966 (50) (Fig. 50-7) came from Charnley's central dislocation and internal compression fixation technique (1953) (Fig. 50-8) (20). The concept was to enhance the union rate by applying compression across the two bones to be united and displacing the femoral head medially, to lower the hip joint reaction forces by shortening the lever arm. Subtrochanteric and intertrochanteric osteotomy was also developed to decrease hip joint forces, thus promoting fusion.

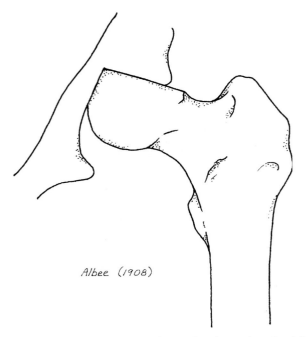

Figure 50-1   The intra-articular arthrodesis described by Albee (2).

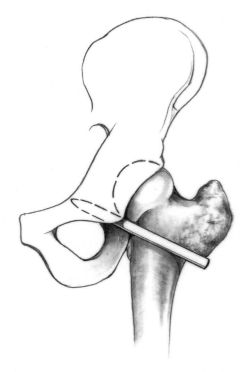

Figure 50-3   The extra-articular arthrodesis with subtrochanteric osteotomy described by Brittain (15).

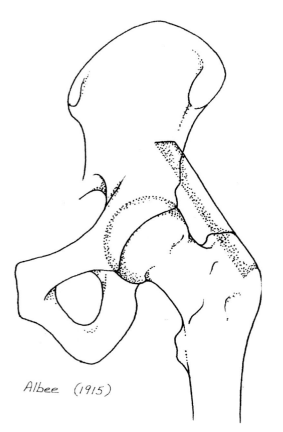

Figure 50-2   The extra-articular arthrodesis described by Albee (2).

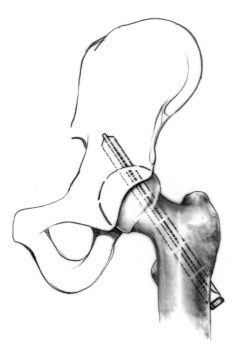

Figure 50-4   The transarticular nail arthrodesis described by Watson-Jones (61).

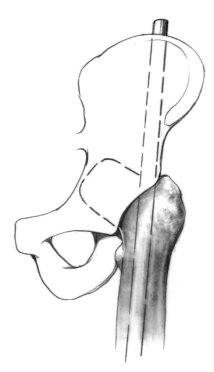

Figure 50-5   The intramedullary arthrodesis described by Onji et al. (43).

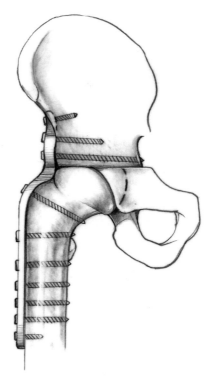

Figure 50-7   The cobra-head plate arthrodesis with pelvic osteotomy described by Schneider (50).

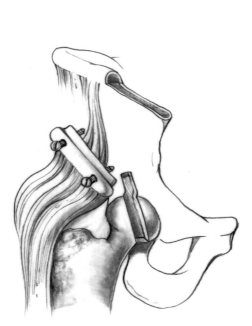

Figure 50-6   The iliac bone graft augmentation described by Davis.

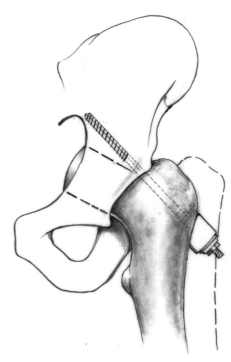

Figure 50-8   The central dislocation and internal compression arthrodesis described by Charnley (20).

LONG-TERM RESULTS OF HIP ARTHRODESIS

Most reports of hip arthrodesis focus on a specific technique and concentrate on the ability to obtain fusion (4,6,7,8,10, 11,14,15,19–24,31–33,35–37,39,40,42–44,46,47,49,50,52, 54–56,59–62). Reports by Sponseller et al. (53) and Callaghan et al. (16) highlight the long-term results of hip arthrodesis, averaging 38 and 35 years of follow-up, respectively. These studies demonstrate the long-term durability of the procedure. After hip arthrodesis, patients worked for an average of 33 and 28 years, respectively, many at jobs requiring manual labor, including farming. Although back and ipsilateral knee pain occurred in up to 60% of patients at final follow-up, it did not generally present until at least 20 years after the procedure, and it was usually not debilitating. However, many ipsilateral knees demonstrated ligamentous laxity, especially in the anteroposterior direction (mostly in posterior translation). Contralateral hip pain was less common at final follow-up. Although most patients had continued to live productive lives, many (65%) were uncertain whether they would have undergone the procedure again. Some patients had trouble with daily activities, including the inability to put on socks and shoes and the inability to sit in chairs for extended periods of time. A small minority of patients reported problems with sexual intercourse. Female patients were able to deliver vaginally. A small number of patients had their arthrodesis converted to total hip arthroplasty because of disabling back or ipsilateral knee pain (Table 50-1).

ARTHRODESIS POSITION

Gait analysis has demonstrated that compensation for absent hip motion is accomplished by increased transverse and sagittal rotation of the pelvis, increased motion in the sound hip, and increased flexion of the knee throughout the stance phase of gait on the fused side (1,27,29,45).

Various positions of fusion have been recommended over the years. Many early writings recommended the hip of a short limb be fused in some abduction to increase the functional length (distance from the umbilicus to the medial malleolus) of the patient's limb (61). Stinchfield and Cavallaro (56) found better gait in patients fused in slight adduction. Sponseller et al. (53) discovered more knee varus deformity in patients fused in abduction. Callaghan et al. (16) found that patients fused in abduction had more ipsilateral knee and low back pain than patients fused in adduction. Patients fused in slight adduction had the lowest incidence of low back and ipsilateral knee pain in that series. Internal rotation should be avoided to prevent interference with the opposite foot during gait, and slight external rotation (10° to 15°) aids in application of footwear when flexing the knee.

Although scientific data concerning the optimal position of hip flexion are lacking, it is recommended that there be 20° to 30° of flexion, with slightly higher values in patients who will spend much of their time sitting. Thus, the recommended position of fusion is in neutral or slight adduction (5°), flexion of 25° to 30°, and external rotation of 10°. Abduction and internal rotation should be avoided. It should be noted that, in children, Fulkerson (24) has demonstrated a drifting of the arthrodesis into adduction over long-term follow-up; therefore, in children, no more than minimal adduction should be attempted.

INDICATIONS AND CONTRAINDICATIONS

Although any patient with isolated hip arthritis and greater than 30 years of life expectancy may be a candidate for hip arthrodesis, the optimal candidate is a laborer under age 30 or 35 years. In this day and age, with the many unrealistic expectations of society, we believe that only optimal candidates should be considered for hip arthrodesis. The patient should be intent on returning to the work force in the capacity as previously. Although some studies have demonstrated improvement in back pain after arthrodesis, we can recommend this procedure only in patients who are free of low back, ipsilateral knee, and contralateral hip pain and who are without degenerative radiographic changes in these areas. For patients with idiopathic or steroid- or alcohol-induced aseptic necrosis who have had radiographic changes of aseptic necrosis for more than a year, it is prudent to obtain an MRI of the opposite hip before considering arthrodesis. Patients with pain or radiographic abnormality in the ipsilateral knee, contralateral hip, or low back should not be considered for the procedure. These are considered absolute contraindications. In addition, ipsilateral knee instability is a contraindication for the procedure. Although patients with neurologic deficiencies (e.g., cerebral palsy) were previously considered candidates, a better alternative procedure would probably be a Girdlestone with intermuscular opposition or total hip arthroplasty.

Patients must appear psychologically stable and motivated to return to work. Any patient who is not intent on returning to work after the procedure is not considered a good candidate for hip arthrodesis. We give all potential candidates for the procedure and their families our articles on the long-term results of hip arthrodesis, and before surgery is scheduled we have them contact patients who have had an arthrodesis. In addition, patients who are taller than 72 inches are warned of the difficulty they may encounter when sitting in crowded circumstances such as movie theaters and auditoriums.

TABLE 50-1
LONG-TERM RESULTS OF HIP ARTHRODESIS

	Sponseller et al. (53)	Callaghan et al. (16)
Length of follow-up (y)	38	35
Average age when hip was fused (y)	14	25.3
Average age at follow-up (y)	52	62.1
Low back pain (% of patients)	57	61
Pain in the ipsilateral knee (% of patients)	45	57
Conversion to arthroplasty (% of patients)	13	21
Pain in the contralateral hip (% of patients)	17	28

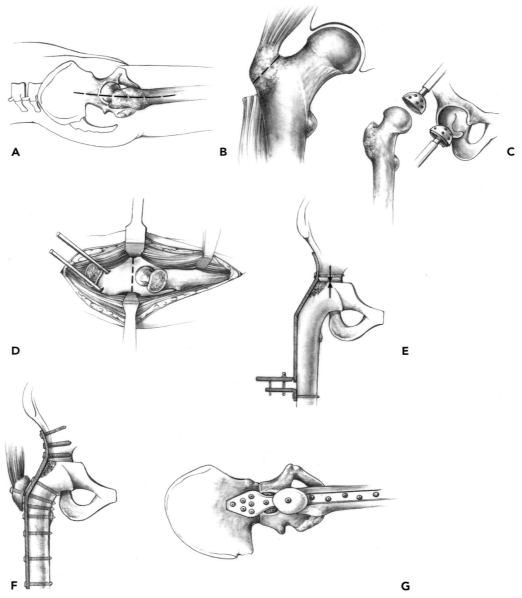

Figure 50-9 **A:** An incision for the application of the cobra-head plate. **B:** A greater trochanteric osteotomy to expose the hip joint. **C:** Application of a concave reamer on the femoral head and of a convex reamer in the acetabulum to allow optimal fit between the femoral head and the acetabulum. **D:** Pelvic osteotomy demonstrated from the lateral view. **E:** Initial iliac screw and AO tensioner applied to cobra-head plate. Anteroposterior **(F)** and lateral **(G)** views of the greater trochanter reattached through a cobra-head plate. (Figures are reprinted from *Clin Orthop.*) (42).

OPERATIVE TECHNIQUE

Whatever technique the surgeon utilizes for hip fusion, it should maximize bony contact, provide rigid internal fixation, provide compression at the fusion site, minimize shortening, and facilitate future conversion to total hip arthroplasty. Although, as previously described, there are many techniques for obtaining hip fusion, the use of a cobra-head plate is currently the most popular method (42,50). We prefer supine positioning of the patient, with a bump under the involved

hip. In the past, an electrocardiogram sticker was placed on the contralateral anterior superior iliac spine to define the landmark of the opposite hemipelvis, but we currently prep the opposite leg and pelvis.

A midlateral incision is made 8 cm above and proceeding 8 cm distal to the greater trochanter, in the interval between the tensor fascia lata and the gluteus maximus muscle (Fig. 50-9A). The anterior and posterior borders of the gluteus medius are identified, and a trochanteric osteotomy is performed, avoiding the medial femoral circumflex vessels to

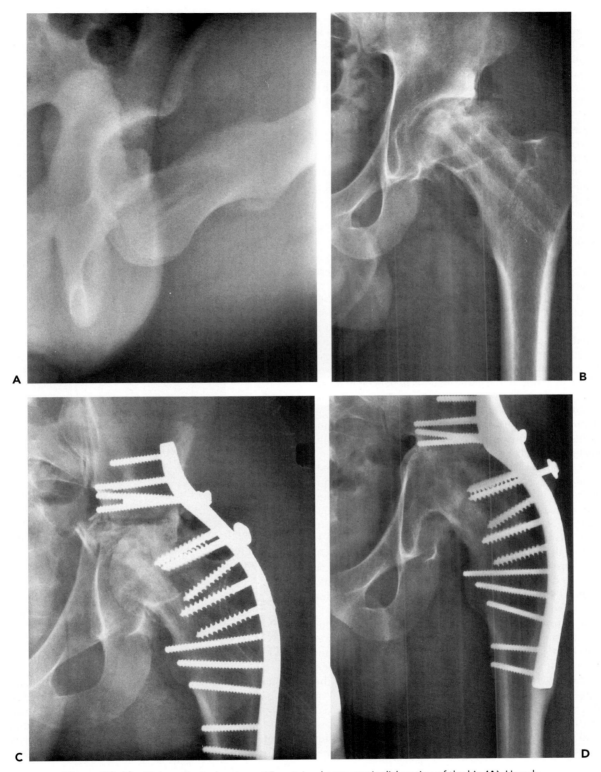

Figure 50-10   Male patient who at age 15 sustained a traumatic dislocation of the hip (**A**). He subsequently developed aseptic necrosis of the femoral head and collapse, with secondary acetabular changes (**B**), although tibial strut grafting had been performed. Because of his disabling clinical symptoms, he elected to have a hip arthrodesis. An early postoperative radiograph (**C**) demonstrates the pelvic osteotomy, which was performed to bring the subluxated femoral head into the acetabulum. Note that all of the necrotic femoral head was not removed and that the distal end of the plate is bent medially to prevent abduction of the femur. The 4-year follow-up postoperative radiograph demonstrates fusion of the hip with the femur in slight adduction (**D**).

the femoral head, which are located in the posterolaterosu-
perior position of the femoral neck (Fig. 50-9B). The joint
capsule is incised from the acetabular insertion with a secondary longitudinal limb from the acetabulum toward the
anterosuperior surface of the femoral head and neck to
avoid damage to the medial femoral circumflex vessels that
perfuse the femoral head. The femoral head is dislocated
anteriorly.

A concave hemispherical reamer is then used to shape the
femoral head to fit the acetabulum (Fig. 50-9C). In cases of
aseptic necrosis, no attempt is made to remove all dead bone,
as this would excessively shorten the limb. Instead, the head is
reamed and 7/64-inch drill holes are placed in the necrotic
fragment. The acetabulum is exposed and reamed with convex
reamers, to the same size as the femoral head and down to
bleeding bone (usually through the subchondral cortex, unless
there is marked acetabular subchondral sclerosis). Pelvic
osteotomy is only performed in cases in which the femoral
head is subluxated, so the osteotomy provides femoral head
coverage and contact with the acetabulum (Fig. 50-9D).

After placing the limb in 5° to 10° of adduction, 10° of
external rotation, and 25° to 30° of hip flexion, the nine-hole
cobra-head plate is contoured to the femur. Hip flexion is
determined by placing a bump under the posterior femur that
provides 10° to 15° of apparent flexion (in the supine position, the natural lumbar lordosis already creates 15° of flexion). Although a long sterile goniometer is beneficial in determining these measurements, an image intensifier can also be
used to aid positioning. (The intensifier is centered on the
pelvis, with the ischial tuberosities and a portion of the femur
on the screen. Next, the beam is centered over the femur, and
the angle between pelvis and femur is readily measured.)

When contouring the plate, a distal bend is needed to prevent the plate and screws from abducting the leg. A 4.5-mm
cortical screw is initially placed through the plate and ilium,
and the AO tensioner is applied to the femur to obtain compression (Fig. 50-9E). The remaining screws are attached to
the femur through the plate, and the greater trochanter is
attached over the plate with a screw and washer (Fig. 50-9F,G).
If the opposite leg has been draped out, a Thomas test can be
performed to determine the amount of hip flexion that has
been obtained. Bone graft from the reamings is applied to any
gaps between the plate, ilium, and femoral head and neck.

Closure is routine. If fixation is stable, the patient begins
walking with touchdown weight bearing the following day. A
removable brace is used for large or potentially noncompliant
patients and for those with less than optimal fixation and
bony contact. Weight bearing is increased at 6 weeks if the
fusion appears to be progressing radiographically, and by 3 or
4 months, most patients are walking without support. A recent
series of cases in which this technique was utilized demonstrated no cases of pseudarthrosis at short-term follow-up
(42). The average Harris hip rating changed from 45 points
preoperatively to 84 points postoperatively, and a 2.6-cm average leg-length discrepancy was documented. A case using this
technique is illustrated in Figure 50-10.

A less destructive method has been described recently.
Two incisions are used: an anterior Smith-Peterson
approach is used to dislocate and débride the hip joint, and
a lateral incision is used to place a compression screw with
side plate. Two or three additional large cancellous screws

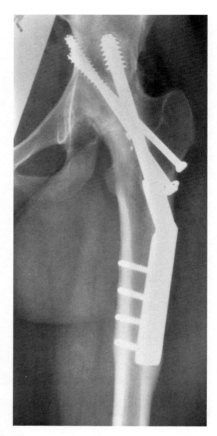

Figure 50-11   Hip arthrodesis using a two-incision technique
and a compression screw for fixation.

are placed across the joint, and a plaster cast is used if necessary (Fig. 50-11). In patients in whom a pseudarthrosis
occurs, we have used a large piece of iliac crest cortical cancellous graft (which is screwed into the anterior ileum and
femoral neck) to obtain union. These patients are casted for
2 or 3 months.

OPERATIONS AROUND HIP ARTHRODESIS AND HIP ARTHRODESIS CONVERSION TO TOTAL HIP ARTHROPLASTY

When patients develop contralateral hip or ipsilateral knee
pain after hip arthrodesis, consideration may be given to performing a total hip replacement contralateral to the hip fusion
or a total knee arthroplasty below a hip fusion. Although this
would not be our recommendation, except in very low
demand patients (with less than 5 or 10 years life expectancy),
these options have been described (26,49). In patients with
contralateral total hip arthroplasties, Garvin et al. (26) reported
a 40% loosening incidence at 7 years, and problems with knee
motion were noted at 7 years in patients with ipsilateral total
knee arthroplasty, although stable cement–bone interfaces
were seen. Liechte (34) reported a 9% loosening incidence at
1 to 8 years in patients undergoing total hip arthroplasty
opposite a fused hip.

The femur may need to be cut higher anteriorly or posteriorly, depending on the flexion at the fusion site (Fig. 50-12) (28). If any additional deformity of the proximal femur is noted with preoperative templating, subtrochanteric osteotomy or special components (usually of the congenital hip dysplasia [CDH] type) may be necessary. In addition, the lateral edge of the acetabulum and the superior lateral femoral neck should be preserved to allow optimal acetabular component coverage. After osteotomy of the fusion, the ischium, the pubis, and the inferior acetabulum should be identified. A retractor may be placed in the obturator foramen after débriding the fusion mass medial to the pulvinar fat and transverse acetabular ligament, which will allow identification of the acetabular floor and medial wall (Fig. 50-13). These landmarks will help orientate the acetabular reamers. The acetabular dome subchondral plate is usually absent because of previous surgery or bone remodeling around the fusion. Hence, care must be taken not to excessively ream into the ilium (Fig. 50-14).

Femoral preparation is routine, but excessive leg lengthening (greater than 2 or 3 cm) should be avoided to prevent sciatic nerve palsy. If the limb is not short, it is easy to gain excessive length during a conversion. Adequate bone must be removed to prevent excessive lengthening. While trochanter reattachment is routine in most cases, in patients with markedly deficient gluteus medius and minimus musculature, tenodesis of the iliotibial band into the greater trochanter (using No. 5 nonabsorbable suture through holes in the trochanter) may aid in obtaining hip stability. In all cases with deficient hip abductor muscles, we brace the patient for 6 weeks postoperatively. Late instability may require revision with a constrained socket. At initial reconstruction, the use of an acetabular shell that can later accept a constrained liner may be advisable, especially if the gluteus medius and minimus are markedly deficient.

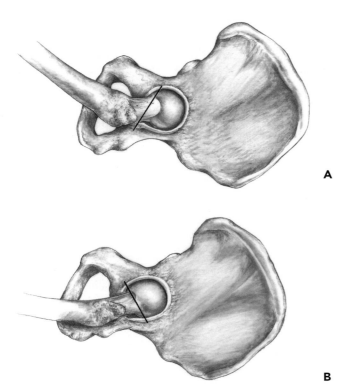

Figure 50-12 Osteotomy of the hip. Fusion in the sagittal plane during conversion to total hip arthroplasty is dependent on whether the hip was fused in flexion **(A)** (osteotomy higher on the neck anteriorly) or extension **(B)** (osteotomy lower on the neck anteriorly). (Reprinted with permission from Hardinge K, Williams D, Etienne A, et al. Conversion of fused hips to low friction arthroplasty. *J Bone Joint Surg.* 1977;59:385–392.)

In patients with disabling low back pain, ipsilateral knee pain (with end-stage degenerative changes on radiographs), and contralateral hip pain (with end-stage degenerative changes on radiographs), conversion of the arthrodesis to a total hip arthroplasty should be considered (5,13,17,28,30,38,57). This operation should be performed only for disabling pain, and it is customary to see the patient several times before deciding to perform surgery. The patient must understand the potential risk of converting a functional stable hip into a nonfunctional unstable hip. The operation should never be performed simply because the patient desires to have hip motion.

Several technical considerations should be followed when converting a hip arthrodesis to a total hip arthroplasty. A transtrochanteric approach is optimal. This allows atraumatic handling of any gluteus medius or minimus that remains and allows extensile exposure of the fusion site. In many cases, the gluteus medius and minimus may be completely replaced by fibrosis and fat. Some believe this is more common if fusion was performed in the preadolescent years (i.e., before age 12). We know of no good way to evaluate preoperatively or predict the postoperative function of these muscles. If an extra-articular fusion was performed, care must be taken to assure that the sciatic nerve or surrounding vasculature was not incorporated into the fusion mass. Certainly, all dissection should proceed (whether the fusion was intra- or extra-articular) subperiosteally on bone when identifying the acetabulum and femur at the fusion site.

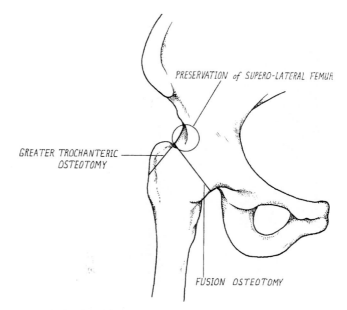

Figure 50-13 The greater trochanter and fusion site osteotomy, in the anterior projection, when converting a hip arthrodesis to a total hip arthroplasty. It is imperative to preserve the superolateral femoral neck and superolateral acetabulum to provide optimal acetabular component coverage.

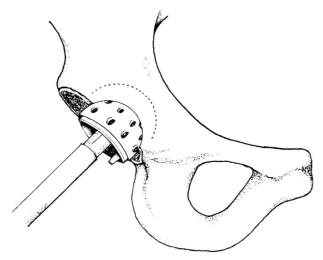

Figure 50-14 Orientation for reaming at the level of the superolateral border of the obturator foramen. A retractor in the obturator foramen can aid in orientation. Exposing the ischium and superior pubic ramus can also be helpful. There is usually no acetabular subchondral plate present, so excessive superior and medial reaming should be avoided, as illustrated. Note preservation of the superolateral femoral neck and acetabulum.

Results of hip arthrodesis conversion to total hip replacement (5,13,17,28,30,38,57) have demonstrated excellent relief of back pain, with less predictable relief of ipsilateral knee and contralateral hip pain (Fig. 50-15). However, the conversion operation allows more optimal biomechanical load transfer to these joints if they require a total joint arthroplasty at a later time. Long-term results of hip fusion conversion to total hip

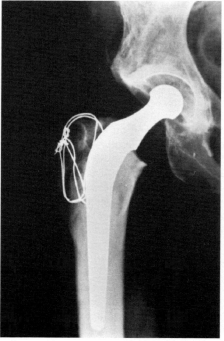

TABLE 50-2

LONG-TERM RESULTS OF THE CONVERSION FROM HIP ARTHRODESIS TO TOTAL HIP REPLACEMENT

	Hips (*N*)	Average Follow-up (years)	Revision For Aseptic Loosening (%)	Revision for Dislocation (%)
Strathy et al. (57)	80	10.4	15	1.2
Kilgus et al. (30)	41	7	15	2.5

arthroplasty have demonstrated marked improvement in patient symptoms. However, one half of the patients will require ambulatory support, and one study demonstrated a higher incidence of acetabular loosening with conversion to a total hip replacement than with primary total hip arthroplasty (Table 50-2).

SUMMARY

Hip arthrodesis can provide durable long-term pain relief and excellent long-term function for young patients who suffer from unilateral debilitating arthritis of the hip. If disabling low back, ipsilateral knee, and contralateral hip problems occur late, hip arthrodesis conversion to total hip replacement can relieve symptoms. However, hip arthrodesis is indicated only for the highly motivated, active young

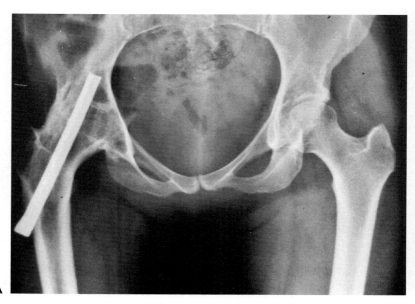

Figure 50-15 A 14-year follow-up of patient with conversion of her fusion (**A**) to total hip arthroplasty (**B**). Note inferior medial acetabular component placement.

patient. Of patients who had had a successful arthrodesis in our study, two thirds were not sure whether they would have made that decision given the option of total hip arthroplasty. Watson-Jones has put the operation in the proper perspective (61).

It is obvious that there may be caution in advising such an operation for patients who are more than 60 years old, because many of them do not want to be able to walk 10 to 20 miles, go mountaineering, climb ladders, or run and jump. They may prefer a palliative procedure such as arthroplasty or osteotomy, which gives them all they need, along with the ability to sit elegantly and comfortably.

REFERENCES

1. Ahlback S, Lindahl O. Hip arthrodesis: the connection between function and position. *Acta Orthop Scand.* 1966;37:77–87.
2. Albee FH. Arthritis deformans of the hip: a preliminary report of a new operation. *JAMA.* 1977;1:1908.
3. Altchek M. Is hip fusion ever needed today, and if so, how can it be done? *Orthop Rev.* 1975;4:23.
4. Alvie I. Arthrodesis of the hip: a method allowing weight-bearing and walking postoperatively. *Acta Orthop Scand.* 1962;32:451–456.
5. Amstutz HC, Sakai DN. Total joint replacement for ankylosed hips. *J Bone Joint Surg.* 1975;57A:619–625.
6. Arguello JM, Cardellicchio R. Arthrodesis of the hip with osteotomy and fixation with angled plate and transarticular screws: indications and limitations. *Ital J Orthop Traumatol.* 1982;8:423–430.
7. Axer A. Compression arthrodesis of the hip joint: a preliminary report. *J Bone Joint Surg.* 1961;43A:492–504.
8. Barmada R, Abraham E, Ray RD. Hip fusion utilizing the cobra-head plate. *J Bone Joint Surg.* 1976;58A:541–544.
9. Barrack RL, Mulroy RD, Harris WH. Improved cementing techniques and femoral component loosening in young patients with hip arthroplasty. *J Bone Joint Surg.* 1992;74B:385–389.
10. Beauchamp CP, Duncan CP, McGraw RW. Don't throw away the reamers: a new technique of hip arthrodesis. *J Bone Joint Surg.* 1985;67B:330.
11. Besser MI. A muscle transfer to replace absent abductors in the conversion of a fused hip to a total hip arthroplasty. *Clin Orthop.* 1982;162:173–174.
12. Blasier RB, Holmes JR. Intraoperative positioning for arthrodesis of the hip with the double beanbag technique. *J Bone Joint Surg.* 1990;72A:766–769.
13. Brewster RC, Coventry MB, Johnson EW. Conversion of the arthrodesed hip to a total hip arthroplasty. *J Bone Joint Surg.* 1975;57A:27–30.
14. Brien WW, Golz RJ, Kuschner SH, et al. Hip joint arthrodesis utilizing anterior compression plate fixation. *J Arthroplasty.* 1994;9:171–176.
15. Brittain HA. Ischiofemoral arthrodesis. *Br J Surg.* 1941-42;29:93–104.
16. Callaghan JJ, Brand RA, Pedersen DR. Hip arthrodesis: a long-term follow-up. *J Bone Joint Surg.* 1985;67A:1328–1334.
17. Cameron HU, Jung YB. Results of total hip arthroplasty without trochanteric osteotomy following hip fusion. *Orthop Rev.* 1987;16:646–650.
18. Carnesale PG. Arthrodesis of the hip: a long-term study. *Orthop Digest.* 1976;12–14.
19. Carter PJ, Wickstrom J. Arthrodesis of the hip: an assessment of results on one hundred patients. *South Med J.* 1971;64:451–458.
20. Charnley J. *Compression arthrodesis.* London: Livingstone; 1953.
21. DeBeule F. La resection de la Hanche suivie de Fixation de l'extremite superieure du femur a la tuberosite ischiatique. *J Chir (Brux).* 1909;9:173.
22. DePalma AF, Fenlin JM Jr. Arthrodesis of the hip with intramedullary fixation. *Clin Orthop.* 1966;48:191–207.
23. Duncan CP, Spangehl M, Beauchamp C, et al. Hip arthrodesis: an important option for advanced disease in the young adult. *Can J Surg.* 1995;38:39–45.
24. Fulkerson JP. Arthrodesis for disabling hip pain in children and adolescents. *Clin Orthop.* 1977;128:296–302.
25. Garcia-Cimbrele E, Munuera L. Early and late loosening of the acetabular cup after low-friction arthroplasty. *J Bone Joint Surg.* 1992;74A:1119–1129.
26. Garvin KL, Pellicci PM, Windsor RE, et al. Contralateral total hip arthroplasty or ipsilateral total knee arthroplasty in patients who have a long-standing fusion of the hip. *J Bone Joint Surg.* 1989;71A:1355–1362.
27. Gore DR, Murray MP, Sepic SB, et al. Walking patterns of men with unilateral surgical hip fusion. *J Bone Joint Surg.* 1975;57A:759–767.
28. Hardinge K, Williams D, Etienne A, et al. Conversion of fused hips to low friction arthroplasty. *J Bone Joint Surg.* 1977;59B:385–392.
29. Hauge MF. The knee in patients with hip joint ankylosis. Clinical survey and bio-mechanical aspects. *Acta Orthop Scand.* 1973;44:485–495.
30. Kilgus DJ, Amstutz HC, Wolgin MA, et al. Joint replacement for ankylosed hips. *J Bone Joint Surg.* 1990;72A:45–54.
31. Kostuik J, Alexander D. Arthrodesis for failed arthroplasty of the hip. *Clin Orthop.* 1984;188:173–182.
32. Lam SJ. Arthrodesis of the hip with special reference to early mobilization without external splintage. *J Bone Joint Surg.* 1968;50B:14–23.
33. Lange M. Arthrodesis of the hip: review of a series of more than five hundred cases. *J Int Coll Surg.* 1958;29:638–643.
34. Liechti R. *Hip Arthrodesis and Associated Problems.* Berlin: Springer; 1974.
35. Lindahl O. Determination of hip adduction especially in arthrodesis. *Acta Orthop Scand.* 1965;36:453.
36. Lindahl O. Hip joint arthrodesis: to find the best position. *Acta Orthop Scand.* 1966;37:317–327.
37. Lipscomb PR, McCaslin FE. Arthrodesis of the hip: review of 371 cases. *J Bone Joint Surg.* 1961;43A:923–938.
38. Lubahn JD, Evarts CM, Feltner JB. Conversion of ankylosed hips to total hip arthroplasty. *Clin Orthop.* 1980;153:146–152.
39. Matta JM. Hip joint arthrodesis utilizing anterior compression plate fixation [letter comment]. *J Arthroplasty.* 1994;9:665.
40. McKee GK. Arthrodesis of the hip with a lag-screw. *J Bone Joint Surg.* 1957;39B:477–486.
41. Mulroy WF, Estok DM, Harris WH. Total hip arthroplasty with use of so-called second-generation cementing techniques: a fifteen year average follow-up study. *J Bone Joint Surg.* 1995;77A:1845–1852.
42. Murrel GA, Fitch RD. Hip fusion in young adults: using a medial displacement osteotomy and cobra plate. *Clin Orthop.* 1994;300:147–154.
43. Onji Y, Kurata Y, Kido H. A new method of hip fusion using an intramedullary nail: a preliminary report. *J Bone Joint Surg.* 1965;47B:690–693.
44. Price CT, Lovell WW. Thompson arthrodesis of the hip in children. *J Bone Joint Surg.* 1980;62A:1118–1123.
45. Ralston HJ. Effects of immobilization of various body segments on the energy cost of human locomotion. In: *Proceedings of the Second International Ergonomics Conference.* Dortmund, Germany: 1964. Reprinted: *Ergonomics* 1965;Suppl:53–60.
46. Ranawat CS, Jordan LR, Wilson PD. A technique of muscle-pedicle bone graft in hip arthrodesis: a report of its use in ten cases. *J Bone Joint Surg Am.* 1971;53A:925–934.
47. Roberts CS, Fetto JF. Functional outcome of hip fusion in the young patient: follow-up study of 10 patients. *J Arthroplasty.* 1990;5: 89–96.
48. Romness DW, Morrey BF. Total knee arthroplasty in patients with prior ipsilateral hip fusion. *J Arthroplasty.* 1992;7:63–70.
49. Schneider CA, Brooks AL, Waggener M, et al. Positioning the arthrodesed hip. *Orthop Rev.* 1985;14:424–428.
50. Schneider R. Hip arthrodesis with the cobra head plate and pelvic osteotomy. *Reconstr Surg Traumatol.* 1974;14:1.
51. Schulte KR, Callaghan JJ, Kelley SS, et al. The outcome of Charnley total hip arthroplasty with cement after a minimum twenty-year follow-up. *J Bone Joint Surg.* 1993;75A:961–975.
52. Schumm HC. Extra-articular immobilization of the hip joint. *Surg Gynecol Obstet.* 1929;48:112.

53. Sponseller PD, McBeath AA, Perpich M. Hip arthrodesis in young patients: a long-term follow-up study. *J Bone Joint Surg.* 1984;66A: 853–859.

54. Steel HH, Lin PS, Betz RR, et al. Iliofemoral fusion for proximal femoral focal deficiency. *J Bone Joint Surg.* 1987;69A: 837–843.

55. Stewart MJ, Coker TP. Arthrodesis of the hip: a review of 109 patients. *Clin Orthop.* 1969;62:136–150.

56. Stinchfield FE, Cavallaro WU. Arthrodesis of the hip joint: a follow-up study. *J Bone Joint Surg.* 1950;32A:48–58.

57. Strathy GM, Fitzgerald RH Jr. Total hip arthroplasty in the ankylosed hip: a ten-year follow-up. *J Bone Joint Surg.* 1988;70A:963–966.

58. Sullivan PM, MacKenzie JR, Callaghan JJ, et al. Total hip arthroplasty with cement in patients who are less than fifty years old. *J Bone Joint Surg.* 1994;76A:863–869.

59. Thompson FR. Combined hip fusion and subtrochanteric osteotomy allowing early ambulation. *J Bone Joint Surg.* 1956;38B:13–22.

60. Trumble HC. Method of fixation of the hip joint by means of an extra-articular bone graft. *Aust N Z J Surg.* 1932;1:411.

61. Watson-Jones R. Arthrodesis of the osteoarthritic hip. *JAMA.* 1938;110:278.

62. White RB Jr. Arthrodesis of the hip. In: *The Hip: Proceedings of the Twelfth Open Scientific Meeting of the Hip Society.* St. Louis: CV Mosby; 1984:54–67.

Osteotomy: Overview

51

Robert T. Trousdale   *Dennis Wenger*

The treatment of the arthritic hip in the young patient remains a challenge for the reconstructive surgeon. Total hip arthroplasty remains a very successful operation for end-stage degenerative joint disease in the elderly patient, but historically both cemented and uncemented total hip replacements in young, active patients have been fraught with relatively high failure rates. Furthermore, young patients who present with hip pain often have conditions that are amenable to nonarthroplasty procedures. Osteotomies about the hip are most useful when there are morphological abnormalities present that can be corrected with an osteotomy in the presence of viable articular cartilage (1). Structural abnormalities about the hip joint may decrease the surface area and increase the unit load of articular cartilage to a point where it cannot function satisfactorily (10). Furthermore, impingement problems about the hip secondary to torsional abnormalities of the socket or femoral abnormalities can lead to secondary hip arthritis. Articular cartilage about the hip functions within a narrow range of tolerances. When exceeded, as in various structural abnormalities, failure of the cartilage will occur. Ewald and others have shown that when a unit load of 23 kg/inch^2 (3.5 kg/cm^2) is exceeded, articular cartilage viability and function are compromised. The primary goal of an osteotomy is either to increase the joint contact area, thereby decreasing the load about the hip to a level that is compatible with normal articular function, or to relieve an impingement problem. Osteotomy also allows one to improve joint mechanics and achieve a more functional range of motion by eliminating fixed deformities. The biological capacity of cartilage to regenerate is not fully understood and is difficult to estimate.

Patients who are best served by a hip osteotomy are those with structural abnormalities in which realignment of the hip will either increase the joint contact area, as in developmental hip dysplasia; unload a necrotic femoral head in patients with limited avascular necrosis; or relieve an impingement problem of the hip caused by torsional abnormalities of the femur and/or acetabulum (Fig. 51-1). Other less common indications for osteotomy include leg-length inequality, slipped capital femoral epiphysis, Legg–Calvé–Perthes disease (LCPD), protrusio acetabuli, epiphyseal dysplasia, and femoral neck nonunion. Contraindications include inflammatory arthritis, severe stiffness, active infection, and severe secondary arthritis. Age, weight, occupation, status of the ipsilateral knee, lumbar spine, and leg lengths should all be taken into account when considering a hip osteotomy.

PELVIC OSTEOTOMY

Pelvic osteotomies are indicated for young patients who have structural problems about the hip that can be improved with reorientation pelvic osteotomy. The most common indication for a pelvic osteotomy is classic developmental hip dysplasia. Other indications for pelvic osteotomy include retrotorsion abnormalities of the acetabulum or post-traumatic developmental hip dysplasia (9). Pelvic osteotomy for classic hip dysplasia should be limited to young patients who have symptomatic hip dysplasia without excessive proximal migration of the hip center of rotation, a reasonably well preserved hip range of motion, and no more than mild to moderate secondary degenerative changes (Fig. 51-2) (25). Prognosis is poor for patients with severe secondary arthritis (22,23). In most patients with hip dysplasia, the primary anomaly is located on the acetabular side of the joint, and hence pelvic osteotomy permits correction of this abnormality.

Many types of pelvic osteotomies have been described for the treatment of hip dysplasia. Reconstructive osteotomy is intended to restore more normal hip anatomy and biomechanics, improve symptoms, and perhaps prevent secondary arthritis. Salvage osteotomy is performed to relieve pain when the articular surface congruity cannot be restored because of marked anatomic abnormality. Previously described reconstructive procedures have included single and double innominate osteotomies and various types of triple and periacetabular osteotomies. A single Salter innominate osteotomy is beneficial for children but is often insufficient for adolescents

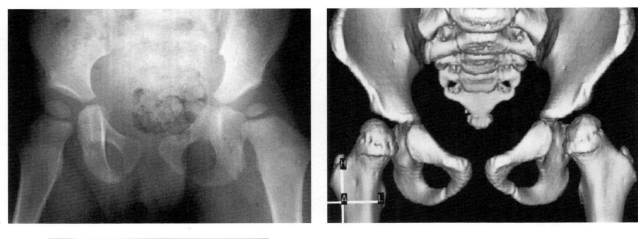

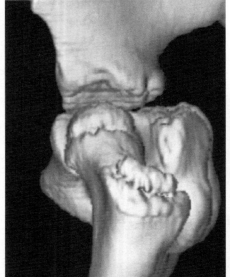

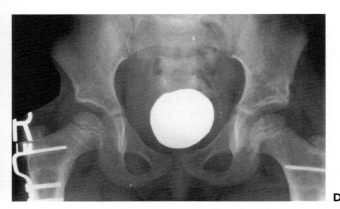

Figure 51-1 **A:** Plain radiograph of a 3-year-old girl with bilateral hip dysplasia. The degree of acetabular deficiency is difficult to determine on the plain film. **B:** Anteroposterior 3DCT image of both hips, taken at age 3.5 years, demonstrates bilateral hip dysplasia. **C:** The lateral view of the left hip demonstrates a type III (midsuperior) deficiency (21). This type of dysplasia can be seen only on the lateral view in a 3DCT. The inside of the acetabular roof can be visualized on the straight lateral 3DCT view. In a normal hip, this inner surface can barely be seen on the direct lateral view. **D:** After corrective surgery performed at age 4 years. Because the right hip had type I deficiency (21), we performed only a proximal femoral osteotomy. The more severe dysplasia in the left hip was treated with combined proximal femoral osteotomy plus Pemberton-type acetabuloplasty. The plain radiograph taken 1 year after surgery (at age 5) demonstrates nearly normal hip coverage bilaterally. This patient demonstrates our current goal for treatment of hip dysplasia, which is to produce a normal head–acetabular relationship by age 5 to 6 years in order to minimize the chance for premature arthritis in early adult life. Only with early osteotomies can very nearly normal hip morphology be achieved.

and adults. It lateralizes the hip joint, which is undesirable in the dysplastic hip. Triple osteotomies were developed in an attempt to avoid lateralization and to increase the amount of correction that is obtainable. LeCour reported his technique of triple osteotomy in 1965 and recommended division of the pubis and ischium close to the symphysis pubis (13). Correction is limited by the size of the fragment and the attached muscles and ligament to the sacrum. One year later, Hoff described a technique that allowed all three osteotomies to be performed through a single anterior incision (11). The Steele osteotomy differs from the Hoff osteotomy in that the

ischial cuts are quite far from the joint, and the Steele osteotomy is performed through three separate incisions (20). All of these various triple osteotomies can lead to a notable asymmetry of the pelvis if a substantial amount of correction is obtained. Tönnis and Sprafke, as well as Carlioz et al., described juxta-articular triple osteotomies that allow for increased correction with less resultant pelvic deformity (2,22). These techniques avoid the problems that can arise when the sacropelvic ligaments are left attached to the osteotomized fragment, which often limits the mobility of the fragment; however, they may result in the creation of a

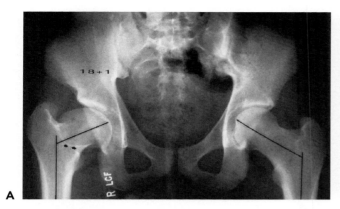
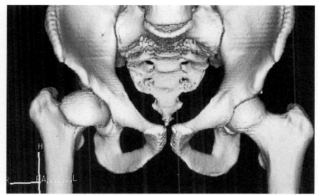
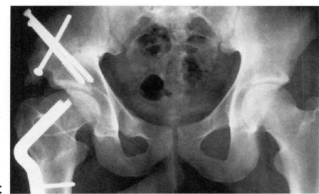

Figure 51-2 **A:** Anteroposterior pelvic radiograph in an 18-year-old man who had developed right LCPD at age 9 and was treated with a containment orthosis. He now complained of intermittent right hip pain. The film demonstrates the classic deformity of healed LCPD, with a "sagging rope" sign (*short arrows*) that extends from the inferior border of the neck medially to the superior border laterally, as well as a functional coxa vara on the right side. **B:** The anteroposterior 3DCT view of the pelvis shows a severely flattened femoral head with an externally rotated femur. The anterolateral inferior margin of the flattened femoral head exactly coincides with the shape and the site of the sagging rope sign noted on the plain radiograph. The 3DCT view of the hip combined with a 2DCT view of the distal femoral condyle demonstrated a functional retroversion of the true articulating posteromedial portion of the head (not illustrated). **C:** A valgus–flexion–(internal rotation) osteotomy and a triple innominate osteotomy (acetabulum also demonstrates dysplasia) were performed. At follow-up examination (radiograph taken 1 year and 4 months after operation), the patient was symptom free and walked with a normal gait. Anteroposterior pelvic radiograph in an 18-year-old woman with left hip pain. In infancy, she had been treated for bilateral hip dysplasia. Because of continued pain at age 18, she underwent a left proximal femoral varus derotational osteotomy in another hospital. She stated that her pain improved for a short time and then recurred.

large defect within the ischium and osteotomized acetabulum, necessitating special measures for stabilization postoperatively.

Various periacetabular osteotomies that have been described by Eppright (7), Wagner (25), and Ninomiya and Tagawa (17) provide good lateral coverage, but the amount of anterior coverage and the extent that the joint can be medialized are often limited. These osteotomies often leave the teardrop in its original position and thus become intra-articular. All of these periacetabular osteotomies are juxta-articular and may deprive the acetabular fragment of its vascular blood supply except for that derived from the capsule. The risk of avascular necrosis of the osteotomized fragment is increased if the capsule is opened for the treatment of any associated lesions of the labrum. Ninomiya and Tagawa (17) reported the results of circumferential acetabular osteotomy in 41 patients who had been followed for an average of 4 years

and 6 months. The authors concluded that in "the majority of the hips either limp or pain with exertion or both had disappeared and a satisfactory range of motion had been restored." They did not discuss the degree of coverage obtained. The Bernese periacetabular osteotomy discussed in detail in Chapter 53 has many advantages compared with other periacetabular osteotomies (8). Avoiding the pitfalls of pelvic osteotomy is important in light of the fact that these procedures are complex (5,12). The surgeon's overall experience and expertise are important factors affecting the prevalence of complications. The learning curve is long and the potential complication rate is high. Training with surgeons who routinely perform this procedure and practicing in a laboratory are recommended. Nerve dysfunction is a potential complication of pelvic osteotomy. If one does the osteotomy through an anterior exposure, the lateral femoral cutaneous nerve or some of its branches can be injured during the surgical

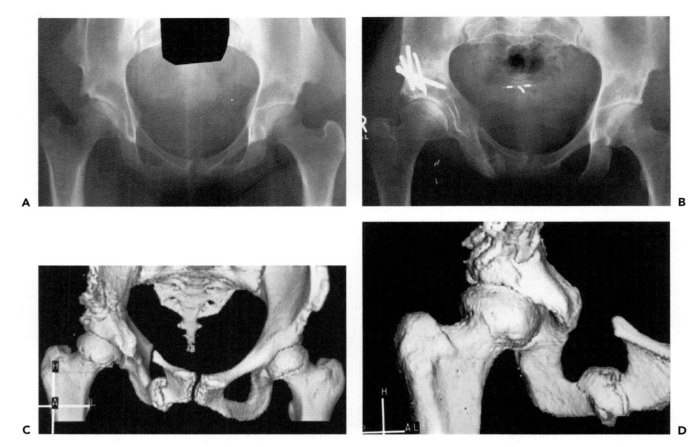

Figure 51-3 **A:** This 17-year-old girl had painful right hip dysplasia despite prior treatment with open reduction and capsulorrhaphy, varus derotational osteotomy, and Salter innominate osteotomy on the right hip and Salter innominate osteotomy on the left. **B:** Plain radiograph after right hip triple innominate osteotomy. Acetabular coverage is improved, and the pattern of the *sourcil* is normalized. However, she continued to complain of dull groin pain. **C:** An anteroposterior 3DCT view of both hips demonstrates nearly normal coverage of the femoral head on the right but also demonstrates a frank nonunion of the superior pubic ramus. The inferior ischial ramus demonstrates a hypertrophic nonunion. **D:** An oblique 3DCT view of the right hip demonstrates a marked gap in the superior pubic ramus that is the likely cause of the groin pain. One of the disadvantages of triple innominate osteotomy is lateralization of the joint as well as external rotation of the acetabular fragment, which can produce a gap in the superior pubic ramus, resulting in nonunion. Careful bone graft or medialize of the acetabular fragment can minimize the risk of this complication. This patient had continued symptoms and was treated by bone grafting plus A-O reconstruction plate fixation of the superior ramus pseudarthrosis.

approach. Femoral nerve palsies have been reported with the use of a direct anterior approach or in patients with previous surgery. Pelvic osteotomies can be performed with intraoperative electromyographic monitoring. In one series, EMG changes developed in approximately 25% of patients, but usually there was no sequela. Most vascular complications that arise during pelvic osteotomies occur with anterior approaches, and thrombosis in the femoral or iliac artery can potentially threaten the viability of the limb.

Pelvic osteotomy exiting through the posterior column or extension into the joint can occur. Intra-articular extension of a pelvic osteotomy has been reported, especially in hips with marked proximal femoral head migration or a laxed inferior capsule. Such intra-articular extension does not cause articular incongruity if it is low, but it can interrupt the blood supply to the acetabular fragment and contribute to necrosis of the osteotomized acetabular fragment. Extension of the iliac

osteotomy into the weight-bearing surface of the joint can create an incongruent joint and should be avoided. Pelvic nonunion is relatively rare in iliac osteotomies, although pubic nonunions have been reported (Fig. 51-3). Heterotopic ossification is rare with the use of modified anterior approaches that leave the abductors unviolated. Improper correction is probably the most common error after pelvic osteotomy. Proper correction should be considered, with proper medialization of the hip center of rotation, proper anteversion of the acetabular fragment, proper lateral correction, and proper anteroposterior (AP) correction (Fig. 51-4). Overcorrection of a pelvic osteotomy can lead to anterolateral impingement and/or posterior subluxation of the femoral head. The results of pelvic osteotomies for hip dysplasia have been well described in the literature, and the majority of series report marked improvements in pain, femoral head coverage, and function (4,14,16,19,24).

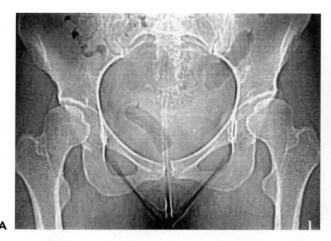

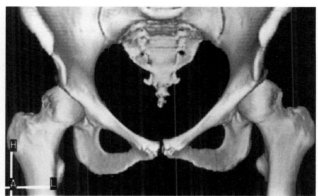

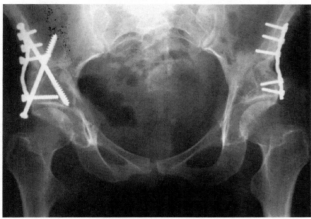

Figure 51-4 **A:** This 24-year-old woman had bilateral symptomatic hip dysplasia. Scout film for the computerized tomographic analysis demonstrates upward oblique pattern of the sourcil (original radiograph lost). **B:** Anteroposterior 3DCT view of both hips demonstrates anterolateral deficiency of the acetabulum. **C:** Plain radiograph taken 2 years after Ganz osteotomy demonstrates increased coverage and congruency.

FEMORAL OSTEOTOMY

Femoral osteotomy should be done for the rare patient with a dysplastic hip where the majority of the deformity is located on the femoral side of the joint. In most patients with dysplasia, the primary deformity lies on the acetabular side of the joint, and an acetabular osteotomy is the proper procedure, as discussed above (Fig. 51-5). In those few patients where the proximal femur is the primary site of deformity, an intertrochanteric osteotomy is a very reliable procedure. Radiographic improvement of the femoral head coverage should be seen on functional abduction views. One should assess anteroposterior head coverage to make sure anterior coverage is satisfactory before embarking on a femoral osteotomy. Patients should have at least 15° to 20° of abduction, and pain should be absent when the hip is placed in abduction. Mild anterior femoral head deficiencies can be accommodated for with slight extension of the osteotomy. Care should be taken not to extend the proximal fragment more than 15° or 20° or future hip arthroplasty may be more difficult. If varus correction of more than 25° is considered, a concurrent greater trochanteric advancement should be considered. Varus osteotomy invariably leads to shortening of the limb up to 1.5 cm, and this can be minimized by performing a straight osteotomy without significant wedge removal. Valgus osteotomy is also useful in some patients with develop-

mental hip dysplasia. It is indicated when the femoral head is elliptical, with a large inferior-medial osteophyte. Bombelli referred to this osteophyte as a "capital drop osteophyte." These hips often have a proximally migrated greater trochanter, a large periacetabular osteophyte, and increased neck shaft angles. Biomechanically a valgus producing osteotomy will open the superolateral joint space and load the medial osteophyte. It also displaces the center of rotation of the femoral head medially, favorably altering the lever arm of the hip joint. Intertrochanteric osteotomy is also a relatively attractive alternative for some carefully selected patients with avascular necrosis (6,15,18,21). The goal of the osteotomy in these patients is to move the necrotic segment away from the weight-bearing surface, bringing normal articular cartilage supported by healthy bone into the weight-bearing area. The ideal patient for an osteotomy is a young patient who has a relatively small necrotic lesion with no or minimal collapse. Patients who have large lesions or advanced disease are better served with arthrodesis or total hip arthroplasty, depending on their age and activity level. Plain radiographs and computed tomography are helpful in mapping the necrotic lesion. The size of the lesion may then be estimated on the anteroposterior and lateral radiographs. Necrotic arc angles can be obtained by taking a point in the middle of the femoral head and extending lines to the joint surface where the necrosis stops. Adding the angles on the anteroposterior and lateral

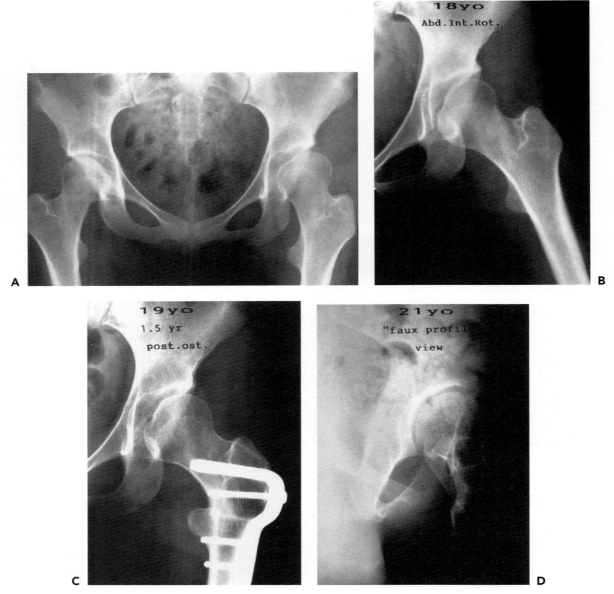

Figure 51-5   A: Preoperative plain radiograph demonstrates a typical dysplastic hip on the left. The left acetabular sourcil is represented as a short, upward oblique irregular radiodensity. The CE angle is negative. The proximal femur demonstrates coxa valga and caput valgum. **B:** Preoperative plain radiograph with the femur placed in abduction–internal rotation suggests improved coverage of the femoral head. (However, in retrospect, the oblique sourcil suggests that the primary problem is in the acetabulum, although the patient does have coxa valga.) **C:** Postoperative radiograph taken 1.5 years after proximal femoral varus osteotomy demonstrates a decreased neck–shaft angle and an improved CE angle. However, the patient continued to have hip pain. **D:** *Faux profil* view of the left hip performed at age 21 demonstrates anterolateral deficiency of the acetabulum. The smooth acetabular rim shadow is interrupted at the level of the midfemoral head.

view is helpful in patient selection. Patients who have lesions with arc angles up to 200° have been shown to be favorable candidates for a proximal femoral osteotomy. Patients who are on steroids, have ongoing systemic disease, or have large lesions with necrotic arc angles more than 200° are not considered osteotomy candidates in our clinic. An uncommon but excellent indication for valgus intertrochanteric osteotomy is a femoral neck nonunion. Pauwels has shown that femoral neck

fractures that have a high inclination angle from the horizontal have a higher risk of nonunion secondary to the large shear forces placed at the fracture site. The principle of valgus osteotomy is to convert the shear forces to compressive forces across the fracture line. The implant of choice for these osteotomies is a 110°, 120°, or 130° blade plate. The amount of correction is determined by the angulation of the nonunion. If a Pauwels angle of 60° exists, a 30° to 35° corrective osteotomy is

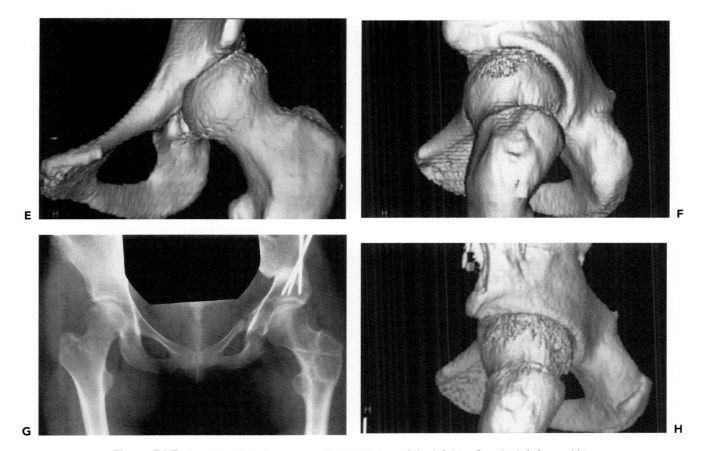

Figure 51-5 (*continued*) **E:** Anteroposterior 3DCT view of the left hip after the left femoral hip osteotomy confirms poor lateral coverage of the femoral head. **F:** A lateral 3DCT view of the left hip clarifies the anterolateral deficiency of the femoral head suggested by the *faux profil* view. **G:** Because of continued left hip pain, a triple innominate osteotomy of the left hip was performed. The radiograph demonstrates increased coverage of the femoral head and improved congruency of the hip joint. The orientation and shape of the sourcil are nearly normal. This case illustrates the need for combined femoral and acetabular osteotomy in those cases that show both femoral abnormalities and acetabular dysplasia. **H:** Lateral 3DCT view of the same hip, after triple innominate osteotomy, demonstrates markedly improved anterolateral coverage. Acetabular dysplasia can be corrected only by acetabular procedures.

performed to get the Pauwels angle to 25° to 30°. This is the angle at which the resultant forces across the hip joint are perpendicular to the fracture site. Blade position in the head as well as entry of the blade in the lateral femur is critical. These patients also have often had previous internal fixation devices, and the blade should be placed in an area of solid bone. The majority of complications seen after proximal intertrochanteric osteotomy are technical in nature. Hemorrhage, hematoma, infection, and nerve palsy are all quite rare. Inaccurate seating of the chisel and blade can be avoided by careful technique and frequent radiographic checks. Occasionally one can have perfect chisel placement, but the blade is inserted and follows a different tract. Using fluoroscopy and taking care to slow down when excessive resistance is met when inserting a blade will minimize inadvertent placement. If the blade follows a different tract, poor correction or protrusion of the blade outside the femoral neck can occur. If one places the osteotomy and chisel tract within 1.5 cm of each other, a fragmentation of this bony bridge may occur. Nonunion or loss of fixation is relatively uncommon.

CONCLUSION

Young patients with structural problems about the hip joint are often candidates for alternative procedures. Patients with classic hip dysplasia, impingement problems, torsional abnormalities of the socket, and femoral neck nonunions and selected patients with avascular necrosis are excellent candidates for osteotomies about the hip if the patients are young and there is viable articular cartilage remaining.

REFERENCES

1. Bombeli R. *Osteoarthritis of the Hip: Pathogenesis and Consequent Therapy.* Berlin: Springer-Verlag; 1976.
2. Carlioz H, Khouri N, Hulin P. Osteotomie triple juxtacotyloidienne. *Rev Chir Orthop.* 1982;68:497–501.
3. Chiari K. Medial displacement osteotomy of the pelvis. *Clin Orthop.* 1974;98:55–71.
4. Crockarell J, Trousdale RT, Cabanela ME, et al. Early experience with the periacetabular osteotomy: the Mayo Clinic experience. *Clin Orthop.* 1999;363:45–53.

5. Davey JP, Santore RF. Complications of periacetabular osteotomy. *Clin Orthop.* 1999;363:33–37.

6. Dean MT, Cabanela ME. Transtrochanteric anterior rotational osteotomy for avascular necrosis of the femoral head: long term results. *J Bone Joint Surg.* 1993;75B:597–601.

7. Eppright RH. Dial osteotomy of the acetabulum in the treatment of dysplasia of the hip. *J Bone Joint Surg.* 1975;57A:1172.

8. Ganz R, Klaue K, Vinh TS, et al. A new periacetabular osteotomy for the treatment of hip dysplasias: technique and preliminary results. *Clin Orthop.* 1988;232:26–36.

9. Giori NJ, Trousdale RT. Acetabular retroversion is associated with osteoarthritis of the hip. *Clin Orthop.* 2003;417:263–269.

10. Harris WH. Etiology of the osteoarthritis of the hip. *Clin Orthop.* 1986;213:20–33.

11. Hopf A. Hüftpfannenverlagerung durch doppelte Beckenosteotomie zur Behandlung der Hüftgelenksdysplasie und Subluxation bei Jugendlichen und Erwachsenen. *Z Orthop.* 1966;101:559.

12. Hussell JG, Rodriquez JA, Ganz R. Technical complications of the Bernese periacetabular osteotomy. *Clin Orthop.* 1999;363: 81–92.

13. LeCoeur P. Corrections des défauts d'orientation de l'articulation coxo-femorale par osteotomy de l'isthme iliaque. *Rev Chir Orthop.* 1965;51:211.

14. Matta JM, Stover MD, Siebenrock K. Periacetabular osteotomy through the Smith-Peterson approach. *Clin Orthop.* 1999;363: 21–32.

15. Mont MA, Fairbank AC, Jinnah RH, et al. Varus osteotomy for avascular necrosis of the femoral head: results of long-term follow-up. Paper presented at the annual meeting of the American Academy of Orthopaedic Surgeons; New Orleans; February 26, 1994.

16. Murphy SB, Millis MB. Periacetabular osteotomy without abductor dissection using direct anterior exposure. *Clin Orthop.* 1999;364:92–98.

17. Ninomiya S, Tagawa H. Rotational acetabular osteotomy for the dysplastic hip. *J Bone Joint Surg.* 1984;66A:430–436.

18. Scher MA, Jakim I. Intertrochanteric osteotomy and autogenous bone grafting for avascular necrosis of the femoral head. *J Bone Joint Surg.* 1993;75A:1119–1133.

19. Siebenrock KA, Scholl E, Lottenbach M, et al. Bernese periacetabular osteotomy. *Clin Orthop.* 1999;363:9–20.

20. Steel HH. Triple osteotomy of the innominate bone. *J Bone Joint Surg.* 1973;55A:343–350.

21. Sugioka Y, Hotokebuchi T, Tsutsui H. Transtrochanteric anterior rotational osteotomy for idiopathic and steroid-induced necrosis of the femoral head: indications and long-term results. *Clin Orthop.* 1992;277:111–120.

22. Tönnis D. *Congenital Dysplasia and Dislocation of the Hip in Children and Adults.* Heidelberg: Springer-Verlag; 1987.

23. Trousdale RT, Ekkernkamp A, Ganz R, et al. Periacetabular and intertrochanteric osteotomy for the treatment of osteoarthrosis in dysplastic hips. *J Bone Joint Surg.* 1995;77A:73–85.

24. Trumble SJ, Mayo KA, Mast JW. The periacetabular osteotomy: minimum 2 year follow-up in more than 100 hips. *Clin Orthop.* 1999;363:54–63.

25. Wagner H. Osteotomies for congenital hip dislocation. In: *The Hip: Proceedings of the Fourth Open Scientific Meeting of the Hip Society.* St. Louis: CV Mosby; 1976:45.

Proximal Femoral Osteotomy

52

John C. Clohisy   Perry L. Schoenecker

Primary total hip arthroplasty is an excellent surgical treatment for end-stage degenerative conditions of the hip. In the elderly patient population, total hip replacement consistently provides major pain relief, improved function, and excellent survivorship (4,18). Nevertheless, in younger, active patients the limitations of total hip arthroplasty are manifested over time by problems related to wear debris from the articulating surface. These include aseptic component loosening and periprosthetic osteolysis (4,16,22). Despite recent improvements in implant design and prosthetic materials, the limitations of total hip arthroplasty in younger patients will likely continue over the next several decades. As a result of this, the potential benefits of osteotomy or "joint preservation" surgery have become more evident over the past decade. Additionally, our understanding of hip deformities that are associated with secondary osteoarthritis continues to improve, and surgical techniques have evolved to address these pathologies (9,14,27,31,37,44). Thus, the role of alternative hip procedures in the treatment of young adult patients is likely to increase over the next decade.

The association of a pre-existing hip joint deformity and the development of secondary osteoarthritis of the hip is well documented in the literature (1,12,43). For example, Aronson (1) detected underlying deformities in 76% of patients with advanced osteoarthritis of the hip. Hip dysplasia (43%), Perthes disease (22%), and slipped capital femoral epiphysis (SCFE) (11%) were the most common abnormalities. Stulberg et al. (43) documented that 79% of patients with "idiopathic" osteoarthritis of the hip had a pistol grip deformity or acetabular dysplasia, and Harris emphasized that over 90% of patients with osteoarthritis had an underlying deformity of the joint that was present at the cessation of growth. These important studies underscore the concept that osteoarthritis of the hip is commonly associated with a pre-existing, mechanical disorder. In the mechanically compromised hip, abnormal joint loading can produce an excessive load per unit area at the articular surface and result in premature degeneration of otherwise normal articular cartilage. If left untreated, progressive degenerative articular disease ensues and secondary osteoarthritis can develop (36). Most importantly, patients with anatomic abnormalities of the hip frequently present with symptoms prior to the development of advanced joint deterioration. If these disorders are diagnosed early, corrective osteotomy surgery can be extremely beneficial (27). The goals of this type of surgery are to correct the anatomic abnormality, optimize congruency of the hip, decrease the load per unit area of articular surface, and improve the biomechanics of the joint. Clinically, an osteotomy should provide relief of symptoms and delay or prevent the progression of secondary osteoarthritis. As such, osteotomy surgery has distinct indications and goals when compared to total joint replacement surgery.

Several conditions of the hip including developmental dysplasia (DDH), Perthes deformities, SCFE, posttraumatic abnormalities (malunions and nonunions), and osteonecrosis are potentially amenable to osteotomy surgery (Table 52-1). This chapter will focus on the role of proximal femoral osteotomy in the treatment of these various hip disorders in skeletally mature patients. It should be emphasized that the success of osteotomy surgery about the hip is dependent upon careful patient selection, detailed preoperative planning, sound surgical technique, and effective postoperative rehabilitation.

TABLE 52-1

PROXIMAL FEMORAL OSTEOTOMY SURGERY RESULTS FOR SELECTED HIP CONDITIONS

Study Mean	Follow-Up (Years)	Disease	% Satisfactory	# of Hips	Mean Age (Years)	Osteotomy Type
Iwase et al. (19)	15	DDH	87%	52	25	Varus
Pellici et al. (37)	9	DDH	75%	56	35	Varus
Gotoh et al. (15)	15	DDH/OA[a]	51%	31	43	Valgus-extension
Iwase et al. (19)	15	DDH/OA[a]	38%	58	37	Valgus
Mont et al. (31)	11.5	Osteonecrosis	76%	37	32	Varus
Scher and Jakim (41)	5	Osteonecrosis	87%	45	33	Valgus-flexion[b]
Marti et al. (27)	7	Nonunion femoral neck	80%	50	53	Valgus
D'Souza et al. (10)	7	OA (variable deformity)	87%	23	38	Valgus-extension[c] Varus-extension[c]

[a]Salvage osteotomies in dyplastic hips with progressive or advanced secondary osteoarthritis.
[b]Combined with curettage and autogenous grafting of necrotic segment.
[c]Osteotomy type determined by hip deformity.

PATIENT EVALUATION

The patient history is focused on determining the etiology of symptoms, assessing the severity of disease, and providing information on the potential role of osteotomy surgery. The initial interview should elicit any history of childhood or adolescent hip disease, previous hip surgery, hip trauma, or risk factors for osteonecrosis. The duration of the problem, the character and location of pain, and activities that potentiate the symptoms should be noted. The examiner should question about episodes of snapping, popping, or locking that may suggest soft tissue pathology about the hip or a mechanical intra-articular component to the disease. Additionally, the patient should be questioned whether there is a specific "comfort position" for the involved hip, as this may provide information regarding the optimal position for joint reorientation. Care should be taken to identify any symptoms that suggest an alternative etiology of the patient's hip discomfort. Concurrent lumbar spine problems, ipsilateral knee disease, and any history suggestive of inflammatory arthritis need to be investigated. The occupation, activity level, tobacco and alcohol use, and overall medical condition should be assessed, as these are important factors to be considered when contemplating osteotomy surgery in adult patients. When discussing surgery, it is very important to determine that the patient understands the disease and the goals of treatment. The patient should be interested and willing to actively participate in a relatively involved postoperative rehabilitation program.

On examination, the general physical condition and body habitus of the patient is noted. Sitting posture and gait pattern are observed. Hip abductor function is assessed with the Trendelenburg test and side-lying abduction strength testing. Leg-length determination is made with the patient standing, noting the presence or absence of a balanced pelvis. Range of motion of the hip is carefully assessed as is the presence of pain and hip joint irritability during the motion examination.

An impingement test (combined flexion, adduction, and internal rotation) is performed to check for discomfort that may indicate labral pathology or anterior femoroacetabular impingement. Special attention is given to the hip position that mimics the femoral osteotomy. For example, a varus-extension osteotomy is mimicked by clinical abduction and flexion of the hip. It is important to determine that the patient is clinically comfortable with the hip positioned in the orientation to be achieved by the osteotomy. Additionally, the surgeon must verify that the hip has adequate range of motion to accommodate the proposed reconstruction, as a hip without satisfactory motion may respond poorly to osteotomy surgery. In general, approximately 90° of hip flexion should be present. One exception is the patient with a severe SCFE or a posttraumatic deformity in which hip flexion may be restricted from malalignment rather than degenerative changes. The neurovascular status of the extremity should also be determined, especially in patients with a history of previous hip trauma and/or surgery.

A complete radiographic examination of the involved hip is extremely important in optimizing patient selection, preoperative planning, and accurate surgical technique. At the initial visit, we obtain a full hip series including a standing anteroposterior pelvis, false profile, frog lateral, and cross-table lateral of the hip. When considering a proximal femoral osteotomy, functional radiographs are obtained to check congruency and to mimic the osteotomy. These radiographs are performed with the surgeon or assistant holding the extremity and are utilized to confirm clinical comfort in a position of radiographic congruency and to facilitate preoperative planning. An abduction functional view is performed to assess the hip for a varus-producing osteotomy. A flexion-adduction view of the hip is obtained to evaluate for a valgus-extension osteotomy. The functional radiographs should demonstrate joint congruency without hinging and ideally show an improvement or at least maintenance of the joint space. When studying osteonecrotic lesions of the femoral head, tangential views (40) with 30° of relative caudad and cephalad angulation can be obtained to better define the size and location of the osteonecrotic segment. The extent of osteonecrosis can also be estimated by the total arc of head involvement as determined by adding the sum of the osteonecrotic angle from the anteroposterior and lateral radiographs (17). If congruency or the optimal joint reorientation position is questionable with functional radiographs, a hip exam with fluoroscopy can provide additional information regarding the joint suitability for osteotomy surgery.

Adjunctive imaging tests are frequently performed to thoroughly evaluate and define the pathology present in the hip being considered for osteotomy surgery. Magnetic resonance arthrogram (32) may be indicated to assess acetabular labral disease, articular cartilage integrity, acetabular rim pathology, and femoral head and femoral neck anatomy. Alternatively, a computed tomography (CT) scan of the hip can be useful for more detailed characterization of osseous pathology about the hip and can facilitate preoperative planning (19). Sources of bony impingement, femoral head–neck junction anatomy, version of the acetabulum and osteonecrotic lesion size and location are also better defined with CT scan images. Clearly, preoperative assessment of all potential pathology enables the surgeon to develop a comprehensive surgical plan and optimize the results of the procedure.

PREOPERATIVE PLANNING

Preoperative planning optimizes surgical preparation and is an essential component of proximal femoral osteotomy surgery (5,10,29,33). Steps of the procedure are reviewed by the surgeon to facilitate the procedure and minimize intraoperative problems. A comprehensive preoperative plan should outline the details of deformity correction, guide pin placement, blade plate type, and position and osteotomy location and reduction. Changes in leg length due to the anticipated osteotomy are also addressed. Therefore, an accurate image of the expected result is created and is used as a reference for the procedure.

A varus-producing osteotomy is usually performed with a transverse osteotomy at the superior aspect of the lesser trochanter and a 90° blade plate for reduction and fixation of the osteotomy fragments (Fig. 52-1). The angle of the chisel and blade insertion dictates the amount of varus correction obtained. For example, if the blade is inserted at a 110° angle to the femoral shaft in the frontal plane, a 20° correction will be obtained when the 90° blade plate is inserted and the osteotomy is reduced. The blade length is estimated with templates, and the blade plate offset (10, 15, or 20 mm) is determined to maintain the horizontal offset between the center of the femoral head and the longitudinal axis of the femoral shaft. Specifically, offset is maintained by medial displacement of the femoral shaft for varus osteotomies and lateral displacement for valgus osteotomies. A varus osteotomy shortens the extremity, and the preoperative plan determines the amount of shortening to be produced. For valgus-producing osteotomies, an angled blade plate (110°, 120°, or 130°) is utilized. The amount of valgus correction is

determined by the angle of insertion and the blade plate angle. For example, a 30° correction is obtained by inserting a 120° blade plate at a 90° angle to the femoral shaft in the frontal plane. With reduction of the osteotomy and fixation of the plate a 30° correction is obtained. Valgus osteotomies lengthen the extremity, and resection of bone may be required to maintain equal leg lengths if the involved extremity was not short preoperatively.

In the past, proximal femoral osteotomies have been categorized as displacement or angulation procedures, but today the majority of osteotomies include displacement and angulation to achieve a multiplanar correction. In addition to alterations in the frontal plane, rotation and sagittal plane corrections should be determined as part of the preoperative plan. Flexion or extension of the osteotomy can be templated on a cross-table lateral view of the hip. A flexion intertrochanteric osteotomy refers to the technique of flexing the femoral shaft with respect to the proximal fragment. Flexion is added to the osteotomy by inserting the blade plate with anterior angulation with respect to the sagittal plane of the femur. When the osteotomy is reduced a relative apex posterior angulation is produced between the osteotomy fragments, yet with a no-wedge technique the resultant deformity is minimized. Functionally a flexion correction enhances hip flexion motion and brings the posterior femoral head articular cartilage into the weight bearing zone. The femoral shaft is reduced to the plate, creating flexion at the osteotomy site. Similarly, extension of the osteotomy is performed by posterior angulation of the blade and reduction of the distal fragment to the plate (Fig. 52-2). An extension osteotomy will reduce flexion and enhance extension of the hip. The more anterior articular cartilage of the femoral head will be delivered into the weight bearing zone. If a rotational correction is planned, the desired change in rotation is determined by the clinical exam and anterior K-wires can be used to guide the correction of the rotational deformity. The intraoperative rotation exam is critical in confirming that the intended correction has been achieved. In general, a balanced internal and external rotation of the hip will provide good clinical function.

SURGICAL TECHNIQUE

The detailed preoperative plan based upon the underlying hip disease, physical exam findings, and functional radiographs determines the type and magnitude of correction to be achieved by the proximal femoral osteotomy. The need for hip joint exploration to address labral pathology and/or osseous impingement at the time of osteotomy is also determined preoperatively. In general, a no-wedge osteotomy technique (10) is utilized to obtain correction and minimize the distortion of the proximal femur (Figs. 52-1 and 52-2). The patient is positioned supine on a radiolucent table and translated toward the surgeon's side of the table to enable frog-leg lateral fluoroscopy views of the hip during the procedure. A small bump is placed underneath the involved hip. The entire lower extremity is draped free, and a lateral approach to the proximal femur is performed (Fig. 52-3). The straight lateral incision is centered on the middle greater trochanter and

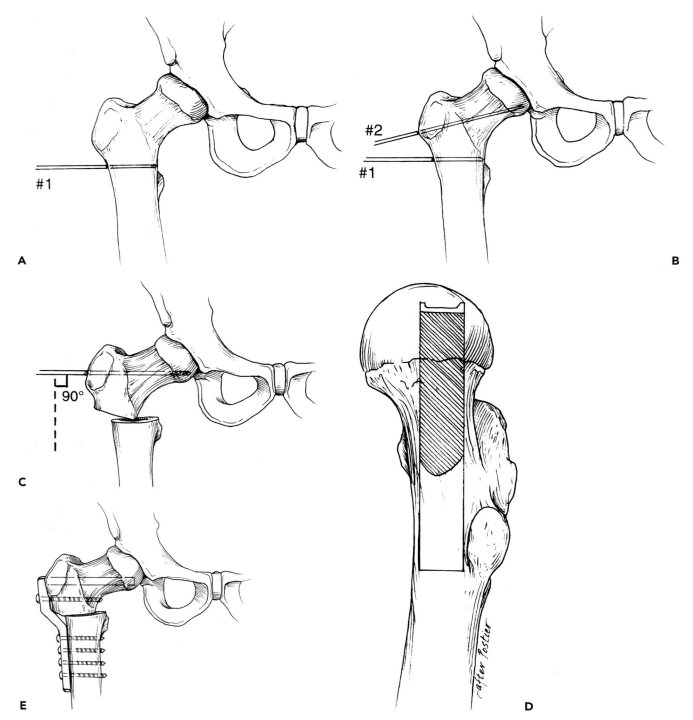

Figure 52-1 Diagram of surgical technique for no-wedge intertrochanteric proximal femoral osteotomy. **A:** Guide wire (#1) insertion for anticipated transverse intertrochanteric osteotomy position. **B:** Guide wire (#2) insertion for blade plate chisel position to obtain varus correction. **C:** Osteotomy and reduction with varus correction and medial displacement of the femoral shaft. **D:** Chisel position from the lateral view demonstrating anterior insertion site with respect to the lateral greater trochanter and a central position in the femoral neck. **E:** Osteotomy reduction and fixation with a 90° blade plate. (Reproduced and adapted from Trousdale RT. Femoral osteotomy. In Sedel L, Cabanela M, *Hip Surgery: Materials and Developments.* London: Martin Dunitz; 1998, with permission.)

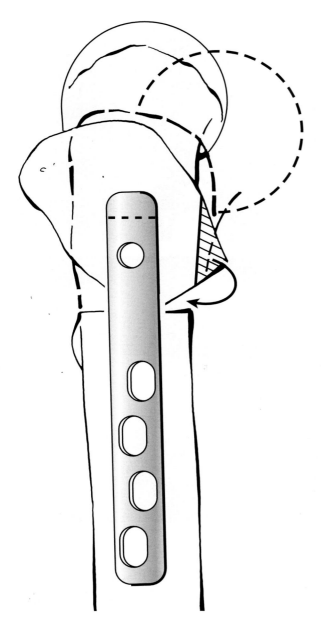

Figure 52-2 Diagram of extension osteotomy reduction with no-wedge technique. Extension proximal femoral osteotomy reduction is shown with a no-wedge technique. Note that the distal fragment is translated posteriorly and there is apex anterior correction. Most importantly, the proximal and distal fragments are aligned to minimize the proximal femoral deformity and allow femoral stem insertion at the time of subsequent arthroplasty The anterior bony wedge of the proximal fragment can be used for bone grafting. (Modified from Ganz R, MacDonald SJ. Indications and modern techniques of proximal femoral osteotomies in the adult. *Semin Arthroplasty.* 1997;8:38–50, with permission.)

proximal femur, from anterior to posterior, and extends from the tip of the greater trochanter distally 15 to 25 cm. The subcutaneous tissue and fascia lata are incised longitudinally, and the underlying vastus lateralis is released from its origin at the vastus tubercle and from the intermuscular septum posteriorly.

The vastus lateralis is then reflected anteromedially to expose the lateral proximal femur. If necessary, the anterior hip joint, femoral head, and femoral neck can be exposed via the Watson–Jones approach with detachment and anterior retraction of the anterior fibers of the gluteus medius. An anterior capsulotomy enables access to the anterior acetabular labrum, femoral head, and femoral neck. In flexion osteotomies an anterior capsulotomy should be performed to allow extension of the proximal fragment after the correction is obtained. This minimizes the risk of a postoperative flexion contracture of the hip, which can result from excessive tension of the anterior hip capsule after a flexion osteotomy. A simple capsulotomy can be accomplished without detachment of the anterior fibers of the gluteus medius.

After surgical exposure, K-wires are placed to guide the osteotomy cut and the blade insertion (Fig. 52-1). First, a K-wire is placed perpendicular to the femoral shaft at the superior aspect of the lesser trochanter. This K-wire acts as a guide for the transverse osteotomy cut and as a reference for the insertion of the second K-wire. A second K-wire is then placed along the intended path of the blade chisel but is positioned slightly superior to allow chisel insertion inferiorly. The angle of insertion for the second K-wire is determined by preoperative planning, and care is taken to position this wire centrally, from anterior to posterior, in the femoral neck. To place the blade centrally in the femoral neck it should be inserted in the anterior half of the lateral greater trochanter. In general, varus and flexion/extension osteotomies are performed with a 90° blade plate, while valgus corrections are obtained with blade plates ranging from 110° to 130°, depending upon the magnitude of correction. The position of the K-wires is checked with fluoroscopy to insure optimal blade position and osteotomy location. The lateral cortex is then drilled at the site of chisel insertion. The insertion site should provide a 1.5- to 2.0-cm bony bridge of lateral femur cortex between the blade entry point and the osteotomy site. This minimizes the risk of fracture in this location. The chisel is advanced with the second K-wire guiding the direction of insertion in the frontal plane and the central location in the femoral neck. If flexion or extension of the osteotomy is desired, this is incorporated by adjusting the anterior/posterior angulation of the chisel with respect to the femoral shaft. The chisel should be sequentially advanced and extracted to prevent incarceration in the proximal femur. Once fully seated, final blade length is determined from calibrations on the chisel. Rotation of the femur is then marked with a superficial longitudinal cut in the lateral cortex or alternatively; additional K-wires can be positioned anteriorly to assist in rotational corrections. The transverse osteotomy is made with an oscillating saw at the upper level of the lesser trochanter. The osteotomy cut is made sequentially with irrigation to prevent overheating at the osteotomy site. A 1-inch straight osteotome is then placed in the osteotomy site, and the proximal and distal fragments are mobilized by levering of the osteotome. The blade chisel is removed from the proximal fragment, the proximal fragment is stabilized with a large bone tenaculum, and the blade plate is inserted along the prepared track. The blade plate is further secured to the proximal fragment with a 4.5-mm cortical screw. The proximal and distal osteotomy fragments are again mobilized, and the osteotomy is reduced

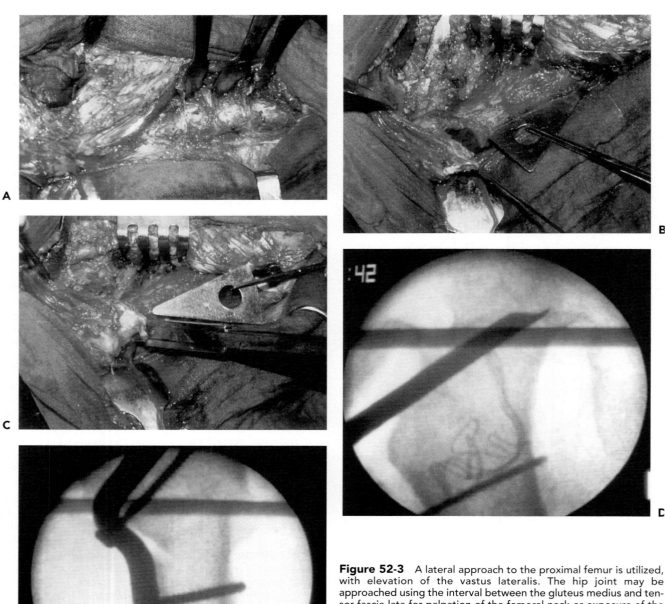

Figure 52-3 A lateral approach to the proximal femur is utilized, with elevation of the vastus lateralis. The hip joint may be approached using the interval between the gluteus medius and tensor fascia lata for palpation of the femoral neck or exposure of the anterior hip capsule **(A)**. The blade track is referenced relative to the femoral shaft using a series of metal wedges of known angulation, and appropriate anteversion of the blade is referenced using a wire placed along the anterior femoral neck, or via direct visualization **(B)**. The blade plate is inserted prior to osteotomy **(C)**, and its correct position is verified radiographically. Note the Kirschner wire at the planned level of osteotomy **(D)**. A final intraoperative radiograph confirms appropriate blade plate insertion, osteotomy, and angular correction **(E)**. See Color Plate.

by approximation of the lateral femur to the plate. The rotation line is used to facilitate the reduction, and care should be taken to align the two fragments without a major step off. The plate position is maintained with a Verbrugge clamp, and the plate fixed to the lateral femur under compression with two to four screws. A tensioning device is not necessary but can be utilized for varus osteotomies. It is important to realize that excessive tension can result in loss of the varus

osteotomy correction. Final reduction and fixation of the osteotomy is assessed with fluoroscopy in the anteroposterior and lateral planes, and hip range of motion is checked by clinical examination.

The patient is mobilized the day after surgery, and physical therapy is started for gait training with toe-touch weight bearing for 6 weeks. At 6 weeks active hip strengthening exercises are initiated with an emphasis on hip abductor strengthening, and weight bearing is progressively increased. The patient is advanced to full weight bearing at 6 to 12 weeks depending upon the details of the case. Unrestricted activity is permitted when radiographic healing of the osteotomy is evident. Hardware removal is recommended approximately 1 to 2 years after the osteotomy to facilitate future conversion to total hip arthroplasty if required.

SPECIFIC INDICATIONS

There exist several well-established indications for proximal femoral osteotomy, which will be discussed below according to disease type. First, it is important to emphasize that patient selection is critical in adult osteotomy surgery, and multiple patient-related factors need to be considered when contemplating treatment options. In general, joint preservation surgery is considered for healthy patients less than 50 years old without inflammatory or advanced degenerative disease of the hip. The patient should have significant clinical symptoms and ideally should not be obese or an active tobacco smoker, which can negatively impact bony healing. Preoperative clinical and radiographic evaluation should insure that the hip range of motion will accommodate the proposed correction, and that the reconstruction will significantly enhance the biomechanical and biologic environment of the joint. It is important to note that full rehabilitation of the hip after a proximal femoral osteotomy, especially varus-producing, may take up to 1 year. The patient should be advised of this preoperatively and be prepared for an extensive rehabilitation program postoperatively.

DDH of the hip is the most common deformity that results in hip symptoms in young adulthood and premature secondary osteoarthritis later in life (1,12,43,30). Murphy et al. have demonstrated that a center-edge angle less than 16°, an acetabular index greater than 15°, and uncovering of the femoral head of more than 31% are associated with advanced, premature secondary osteoarthritis. Thus, hip dysplasia can be an excellent indication for osteotomy surgery about the hip (27,38,45). This disorder can be characterized by a spectrum of deformities on both sides of the joint that are present to varying degrees in each case. On the acetabular side, anterolateral femoral head coverage is deficient, the acetabular sourcil is inclined superolaterally, the articular surface area is reduced, and the joint center is in a relative lateral position. On the femoral side, coxa valga is common, and excessive anteversion, femoral head deformities, and canal stenosis can also be present. Proximal femoral osteotomy may be indicated for various reasons in the surgical treatment of residual hip dysplasia. If the deformity is primarily a coxa valga with lateral joint overload, a varus proximal femoral osteotomy can be considered. However, it should be noted that residual acetabular disease is usually the more profound component of the deformity. Presently, many surgeons, including ourselves, prefer to address an acetabular deformity with reorientation of the acetabulum rather than with a femoral procedure (9,27). Nevertheless, a varus proximal femoral osteotomy can be considered in selected cases if the acetabular dysplasia is mild (15,35). In this clinical situation a varus correction can be combined with extension to better contain the femoral head anterolaterally and decrease the load per unit surface area along the anterolateral acetabular rim (Fig. 52-4). Previous studies have demonstrated good results at long-term follow-up with an isolated varus femoral osteotomy. Specifically, Iwase et al. (15) reported on 52 hips without major degenerative changes treated with a varus osteotomy and followed for an average 20 years. Using an end-point of further hip surgery or a Harris hip score less than 70 points, they reported survivorship of 89%, 87%, and 82% at 10, 15, and 20 years after surgery. Pellici et al. (35) reviewed 56 hips treated with a varus osteotomy, and at 9-year follow-up found 72% of the hips to have a good or excellent result. Importantly, better results tended to be in hips with minimal or no preoperative degenerative disease.

Cases of severe dysplasia with a combined acetabular and femoral deformity present a very challenging reconstructive

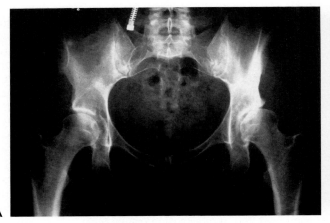 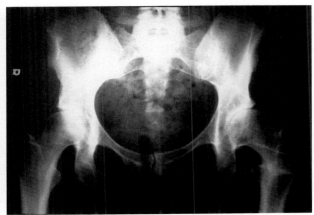

A   B

Figure 52-4 Varus-extension proximal femoral osteotomy for residual hip dysplasia. Standing anteroposterior pelvis **(A)** in a 41-year-old female with developmental hip dysplasia and activity-related left hip pain. These radiographs demonstrate acetabular dysplasia, coxa valga, and moderate secondary osteoarthritis preoperatively. This patient was treated with a varus extension proximal femoral osteotomy and had a good clinical result at 4-year follow-up **(B)**.

problem. Occasionally, severe deformities cannot be adequately corrected with an isolated acetabular procedure. In such cases, a varus proximal femoral osteotomy can be combined with an acetabular reorientation to optimize hip joint congruency and containment of the femoral head. This is an excellent indication for proximal femoral osteotomy in the dysplastic hip, because it enhances the reconstruction achieved with an acetabular procedure.

A final indication for femoral osteotomy in the dysplastic hip is in the salvage situation in which lateral subluxation and secondary osteoarthritic changes are associated with a medial capital drop osteophyte of the femoral head (located at the inferomedial margin of the femoral head) and a medial osteophyte of the acetabular floor (5,7,11,15,21,33). In this situation a valgus-extension proximal femoral osteotomy can be considered to reposition the capital drop osteophyte to articulate with the medial acetabular osteophyte and increase the weight bearing zone of the hip. This osteotomy can improve congruity, unload the anterosuperolateral joint space, and increase the weight bearing surface area. The results of this technique are less predictable due to the salvage nature of the procedure, yet symptom relief and delaying the need for replacement surgery is accomplished in the many of the patients. Gotoh et al. (11) reported survival rate of 51% at 15 years for 31 hips treated with a valgus-extension osteotomy for advanced osteoarthritis in dysplastic hips. Iwase et al. (15) studied 58 hips with progressive or end-stage osteoarthritis that were treated with a salvage valgus osteotomy. Survival rates were 66%, 38%, and 19% at 10-, 15-, and 20-year follow-up, respectively. It is important to emphasize that in the salvage situation the early results and long-term survivorship are less predictable, and careful patient selection and realistic expectations are essential for a satisfactory result.

Residual deformity from Legg–Calvé–Perthes disease has been associated with secondary osteoarthritis by several investigators (1,12,25,42). McAndrew and Weinstein reported on 37 affected hips followed for an average 48 years and found 15 (41%) had undergone hip replacement surgery at or before the sixth decade of life. Stulberg et al. (42) further clarified that aspherical congruent and aspherical incongruent hips were at risk for secondary osteoarthritis in adulthood. In addition to Legg–Calvé–Perthes disease of childhood, a "Perthes-like" deformity of the hip can also result from osteonecrosis of the femoral head associated with early treatment for DDH. These deformities are primarily on the femoral side (Fig. 52-5) but can be associated with a secondary acetabular dysplasia (Fig. 52-6). The proximal femoral deformity is most notable for coxa magna, coxa plana, coxa breva, and relative trochanteric "overgrowth." These patients require careful evaluation to discern the etiology of hip symptoms. Labral pathology, joint overload, joint incongruency, abductor fatigue, and femoroacetabular impingement must all be considered when outlining a surgical treatment strategy. In cases with primarily a femoral deformity, a valgus osteotomy can be effective in improving congruency, decreasing the load per unit area at the joint surface, lengthening the extremity, improving abductor function, and enhancing clinical hip abduction (Fig. 52-5). Abductor function is improved with the valgus osteotomy because the greater trochanter is displaced distally and laterally. In the severely deformed femur with major trochanteric overgrowth, a combined trochanteric advancement may be necessary to prevent excessive lateralization of the trochanter and enhance the distal transfer. In hips with a Perthes femoral deformity and an associated secondary acetabular dysplasia, a combined acetabular reorientation and proximal femoral osteotomy should be considered (2). With this comprehensive approach both the acetabular and femoral deformities can be addressed to optimize the hip reconstruction (Fig. 52-6).

Another cause of hip dysfunction in the young patient, and premature osteoarthritis in adulthood, is a residual deformity from a SCFE (1,12,43). The SCFE deformity most commonly involves posteromedial displacement of the epiphysis, resulting in an extension and retroversion deformity of the proximal femur. An apparent varus deformity is also present (5). These patients most commonly complain of restricted hip flexion and symptoms from anterior femoroacetabular impingement combined with an external rotation deformity of the involved lower extremity. Direct correction of this deformity can be performed at the level of the femoral neck, although the risk of osteonecrosis makes this technique less attractive. Alternatively, a transverse intertrochanteric osteotomy can adequately address the deformity with less risk of osteonecrosis (13). Specifically, a flexion and derotation osteotomy can correct the deformity and markedly improve clinical symptoms. The flexion correction should aim to place the femoral shaft perpendicular to the epiphysis in the sagittal plane. Valgus can be incorporated into the osteotomy (47) but is frequently obtained with the flexion correction alone. An anterior capsulotomy should also be performed to ensure postoperative hip extension. After capsulotomy and fixation of the osteotomy, the anterior hip joint should be inspected for residual femoroacetabular impingement. If present, the prominent anterolateral femoral head–neck can be resected. Severe SCFE deformities can require major deformity corrections (>50°), and in these cases it is important to align the proximal and distal fragments by combining anterior translation and flexion of the distal fragment. This preserved alignment facilitates future total hip arthroplasty surgery.

Osteonecrosis of the femoral head remains a challenging disorder to treat, and optimal treatment methods continue to be debated (20). The literature does support the intertrochanteric osteotomy as an effective surgical strategy for the treatment of a select subgroup of patients. It must be emphasized that these patients are carefully evaluated, and various factors must be considered when contemplating an intertrochanteric osteotomy for the diagnosis of osteonecrosis. The etiology of disease, stage of disease, size of osteonecrotic lesion, location of osteonecrotic lesion, and medical comorbidities must all be assessed. In well-selected candidates, proximal femoral osteotomy can be very effective. Scher and Jakim (39) evaluated the results of a valgus-flexion intertrochanteric osteotomy (combined with autogenous grafting of the avascular segment) in the treatment of Ficat stage III (8) osteonecrosis. They reported 87% survivorship at 5-year follow-up using further surgery or a Harris Hip score less than 70 points as an end-point for failure. Similarly, Mont et al. (28) reviewed 37 varus osteotomies (26 with a combined flexion or extension component) in the treatment of Ficat stage II and III disease. At 11.5-year follow-up they noted 76% good or excellent results. Importantly, favorable results were associated with lesions that had a combined osteonecrotic angle less than 200° (17) and were not receiving

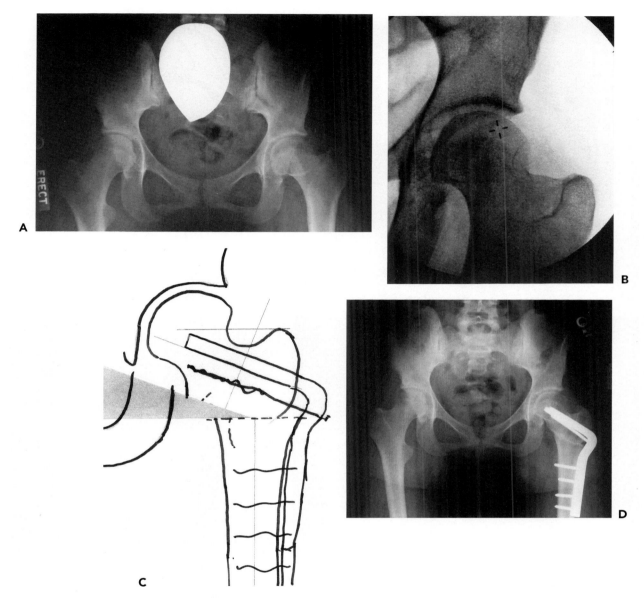

Figure 52-5 Proximal femoral valgus osteotomy for residual Perthes deformity of the proximal femur. This 19-year-old female with a history of Perthes disease presented with activity-related abductor fatigue and groin pain. The standing pelvic radiograph **(A)** depicts a Perthes deformity of the proximal femur without a secondary acetabular deformity. A functional adduction radiograph of the hip **(B)** demonstrates congruity for a valgus osteotomy. The preoperative planning sketch **(C)** for the valgus femoral osteotomy and a 4-month follow-up radiograph **(D)** with the desired correction and osteotomy healing are shown.

continuous high-dose corticosteroids. We consider patients with a subchondral fracture and/or femoral head collapse without significant joint space narrowing as potential candidates for osteotomy surgery. The ideal candidate is a compliant, healthy patient not on corticosteroids who has a lesion with a combined osteonecrotic angle on the anteroposterior and lateral radiographs of less than 200°. Anterolateral lesions that can be delivered away from the weight bearing surface of the femoral head are treated with a flexion-valgus osteotomy. This repositions the healthier posteromedial femoral head articular cartilage and subchondral bone into the weight bearing zone. Anteromedial lesions that cannot be delivered away

from the weight bearing zone with a valgus osteotomy are managed with a varus flexion osteotomy to utilize the healthy posterolateral femoral head as the primary weight bearing surface (Fig. 52-7). With flexion osteotomies an anterior capsule release is performed to allow hip extension, and the maximal flexion correction is approximately 35°, as larger corrections may not be tolerated clinically.

Selected posttraumatic deformities and nonunions of the proximal femur can be excellent indications for osteotomy surgery. For example, nonunions of the femoral neck are associated with profound clinical symptoms and can be effectively managed with osteotomy surgery in the majority of cases.

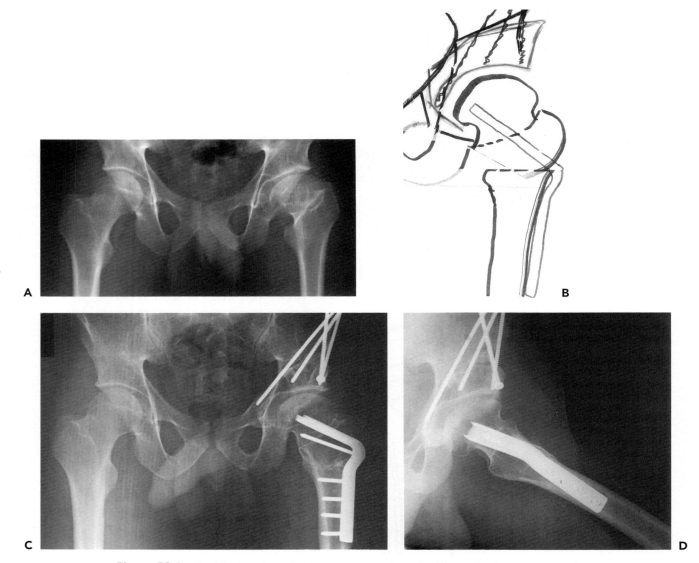

Figure 52-6 Combined periacetabular osteotomy and proximal femoral valgus osteotomy for a Perthes deformity with secondary acetabular dysplasia. Preoperative anteroposterior pelvic radiograph (**A**) of a 21-year-old male with a history of Perthes disease in childhood, leg-length discrepancy, and a 2-year history of progressive hip pain. A Perthes deformity of the proximal femur is noted, and secondary acetabular dysplasia is present. This patient was treated with a combined periacetabular osteotomy and a valgus proximal femoral osteotomy, as demonstrated in the preoperative plan (**B**). The femoral osteotomy lengthened the extremity, enhanced the congruency of the joint, improved clinical abduction, and improved abductor function. This patient had an excellent clinical result 3 years later (**C, D**). See Color Plate.

Marti et al. (23) reviewed 50 cases of femoral neck nonunion treated with Pauwels valgus-producing osteotomy (34) at an average 7.1-year follow-up. They observed 86% of the nonunions to be healed, while 14% had been converted to total hip replacements. With this technique a laterally based wedge osteotomy is performed at the intertrochanteric level, and an angled blade plate (usually 120°) is used for valgus correction and fixation. The tension and shear forces across the nonunion secondary to varus displacement are converted to a compressive force with the correction (Fig. 52-8). This results in fracture union and joint preservation in the majority of cases.

In treating proximal femoral malunions the deformity characteristics must be carefully determined and corrective osteotomy surgery planned to address the specific deformity details of each case (24). In the intertrochanteric region a transverse osteotomy at the superior aspect of the lesser trochanter and the no-wedge technique can be utilized to correct multiplanar deformities and obtain predictable healing (Fig. 52-9). An angled blade plate (110° to 130°) is employed for valgus corrections, and a 90° blade plate for varus, flexion/extension, and rotational deformities.

In addition to osteotomies designed to address the specific disorders outlined above, displacement and angulation osteotomies have also been advocated for the treatment of osteoarthritis (7,21,26,46). In general, the literature on these techniques is somewhat difficult to interpret because the

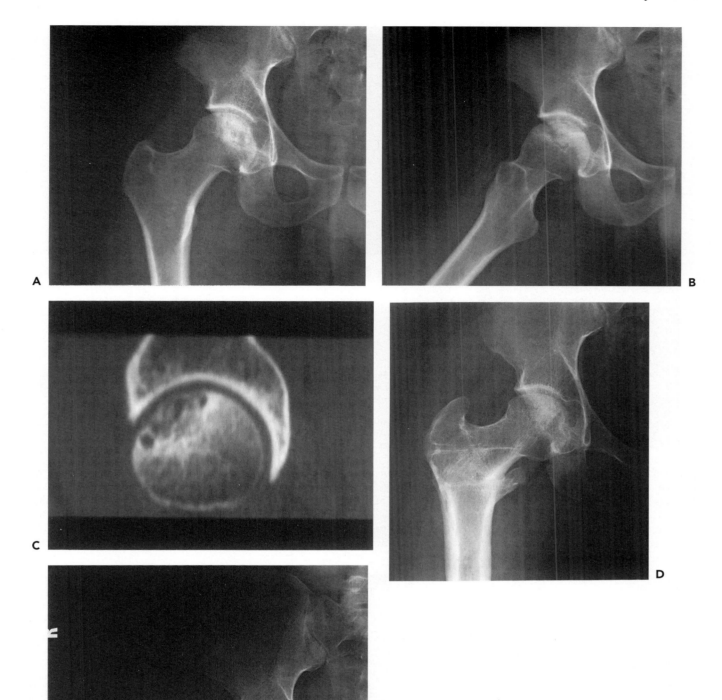

Figure 52-7   Flexion-varus proximal femoral osteotomy for osteonecrosis of the femoral head. Anteroposterior **(A)** and frog-leg lateral **(B)** radiographs of a healthy 28-year-old male with right hip pain and a history of corticosteroid treatment in the past. A sagittal CT scan image localizes this lesion to the antero-medial aspect of the femoral head, and demonstrates the poste-rior femoral head to be free of disease **(C)**. This patient had Ficat stage III osteonecrosis and was treated with a flexion varus osteotomy to displace the lesion away from the weight bearing dome of the femoral head. The healthy posterolateral femoral head articular cartilage and subchondral bone was repositioned into the weight bearing zone. At 4-year follow-up **(D, E)** the patient had an excellent clinical result.

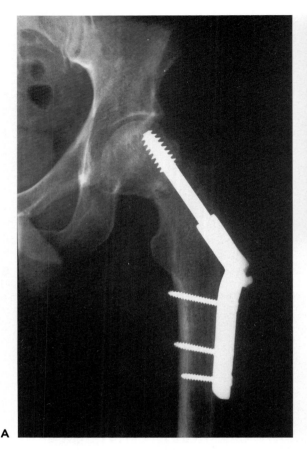

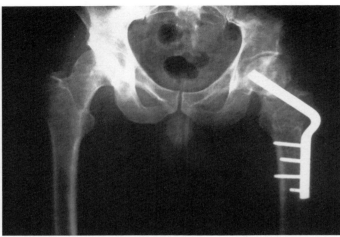

Figure 52-8   Pauwels valgus osteotomy for nonunion of the femoral neck. A varus nonunion of a femoral neck fracture in a healthy 41-year-old male laborer with severe hip pain is shown **(A)**. A Pauwels valgus femoral osteotomy was performed to transform the tension and shear forces at the nonunion site into a compressive force **(B)** that stimulates fracture healing. This patient had an excellent clinical result at 2-year follow-up.

preoperative deformities and exact details of osteotomy correction are not completely defined in some studies. Satisfactory results are reported in 46% to 67% of patients at 10- to 15-year follow-up (7,21,26,46). Today pure medial displacement osteotomies have been mostly abandoned due to unpredictable results. Nevertheless, a relatively recent study by

D'Souza et al. (7) is noteworthy in that the type of intertrochanteric osteotomy performed was based upon the biomechanical principles of Bombelli (5) and Pauwels (33). Specifically, a valgus-extension osteotomy was performed for patients with anterosuperolateral osteoarthrosis, a flattened femoral head, a capital drop osteophyte of the femoral head,

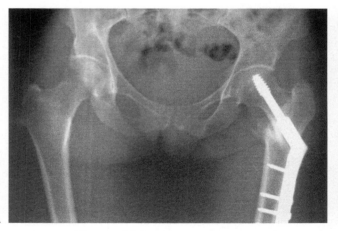

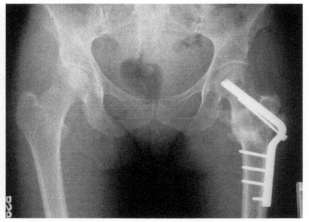

Figure 52-9   Posttraumatic deformity (malunion, valgus-flexion-derotation proximal femoral osteotomy). Standing anteroposterior pelvis **(A)** of the left hip in a 39-year-old female referred for evaluation of persistent hip pain after treatment of an intertrochanteric femoral fracture. Prior to fracture, the patient was an active, recreational runner. She presented complaining of lateral hip pain, leg-length discrepancy, and lack of internal rotation of the left hip. On examination she had a severe limp, profound abductor weakness, a 2-cm leg-length discrepancy and malrotation with −10° of internal rotation. This proximal femoral malunion was treated with a valgus-derotation femoral osteotomy **(B)**. She had an excellent clinical result and was asymptomatic at 4.5-year follow-up.

and a medial acetabular osteophyte. The goal of this technique being to shift the center of stress from anterosuperolateral to the medial joint between the femoral head and acetabular osteophyte. Alternatively, a varus-extension osteotomy was performed for anterosuperolateral osteoarthritis and a round femoral head to increase the abductor lever arm, create a more horizontal direction of the resultant force on the hip, and center the femoral head in the acetabulum. With these techniques they reported an 87% survivorship at 7 years and 67% survivorship at 12 years. Clearly, some patients with significant osteoarthritis benefit from intertrochanteric osteotomy, yet it should be emphasized that careful patient selection and surgical treatment based upon sound biomechanical principles must be followed to optimize clinical results in this group of patients.

TOTAL HIP ARTHROPLASTY AFTER PROXIMAL FEMORAL OSTEOTOMY

Proximal femoral osteotomies are performed to prevent or delay end-stage degenerative disease of the hip. Nevertheless, over several years or decades many of these patients may eventually come to total hip arthroplasty. The results of total hip arthroplasty after proximal femoral osteotomy have been evaluated by various investigators (3,6,41). Boos et al. (6) compared 74 primary total hip arthroplasties after femoral osteotomy with a diagnosis-matched group of standard hip replacements at 5- to 10-year follow-up. Importantly, the majority of these cases (74%) had removal of the osteotomy hardware performed at a separate procedure prior to replacement surgery. They concluded that perioperative complications, infection rate, and revision rates were similar in both groups. Nevertheless there was a trend toward improved survivorship in the group without previous osteotomy. The trochanteric osteotomy rate was higher and surgical times longer in cases with a previous osteotomy. Thus, previous osteotomy surgery is not necessarily associated with a higher complication rate, as reported by some authors (3,41), but does make subsequent total hip arthroplasty technically more demanding. In addition, long-term survivorship of arthroplasty after femoral osteotomy, to our knowledge, has not been documented in the literature. These findings underscore the importance of a well-executed osteotomy to minimize the difficulty of subsequent hip replacement. Most importantly, the proximal and distal fragments should be aligned without creating a major residual deformity of the proximal femur. In contrast to a wedge resection technique, the no-wedge technique enables major corrections without creating an angular deformity (Figs. 52-6 and 52-7). This facilitates femoral stem insertion at the time of arthroplasty. If malalignment does result from osteotomy surgery, subsequent arthroplasty may be compromised by suboptimal femoral stem position, suboptimal fixation, and an increased risk of intraoperative proximal femoral fracture (3,41). In severe cases of malalignment after osteotomy, a combined subtrochanteric osteotomy and replacement procedure may be required.

Retained hardware is the second major aspect of proximal femoral osteotomy surgery that can impact subsequent arthroplasty. Fixation hardware removal 1 to 2 years after osteotomy surgery minimizes future hardware-related complications. Specifically, this eliminates problems associated with hardware removal at arthroplasty, decreases the amount of soft tissue dissection and surgical time, and enables biologic remodeling of the proximal femur and healing of screw sites. Therefore, the potential benefit of routine hardware removal after proximal femoral osteotomy surgery seems to outweigh the small risk associated with these procedures.

REFERENCES

1. Aronson J. Osteoarthritis of the young adult hip: etiology and treatment. *Instr Course Lect.* 1986;35:119–128.
2. Beck M, Mast JW. The periacetabular osteotomy in Legg-Perthes-like deformities. *Semin Arthroplasty.* 1997;8:102–107.
3. Benke GJ, Baker AS, Dounis E. Total hip replacement after upper femoral osteotomy. A clinical review. *J Bone Joint Surg Br.* 1982;64:570–571.
4. Berry DJ, Harmsen WS, Cabanela ME, et al. Twenty-five-year survivorship of two thousand consecutive primary Charnley total hip replacements: factors affecting survivorship of acetabular and femoral components. *J Bone Joint Surg Am.* 2002;84A:171–177.
5. Bombelli R. *Structure and Function in Normal and Abnormal Hips: How to Rescue Mechanically Jeopardized Hips.* New York: Springer; 1993.
6. Boos N, Krushell R, Ganz R, et al. Total hip arthroplasty after previous proximal femoral osteotomy. *J Bone Joint Surg Br.* 1997;79:247–253.
7. D'Souza SR, Sadiq S, New AM, et al. Proximal femoral osteotomy as the primary operation for young adults who have osteoarthrosis of the hip. *J Bone Joint Surg Am.* 1998;80:1428–1438.
8. Ficat RP. Idiopathic bone necrosis of the femoral head. Early diagnosis and treatment. *J Bone Joint Surg Br.* 1985;67:3–9.
9. Ganz R, Klaue K, Vinh TS, et al. A new periacetabular osteotomy for the treatment of hip dysplasias. Technique and preliminary results. *Clin Orthop.* 1988;232:26–36.
10. Ganz R, MacDonald SJ. Indications and modern techniques of proximal femoral osteotomies in the adult. *Semin Arthroplasty.* 1997;8:38–50.
11. Gotoh E, Inao S, Okamoto T, et al. Valgus-extension osteotomy for advanced osteoarthritis in dysplastic hips. Results at 12 to 18 years. *J Bone Joint Surg Br.* 1997;79:609–615.
12. Harris WH. Etiology of osteoarthritis of the hip. *Clin Orthop.* 1986;213:20–33.
13. Imhauser G. [Late results of Imhauser's osteotomy for slipped capital femoral epiphysis (author's transl)]. *Z Orthop Ihre Grenzgeb.* 1977;115:716–725.
14. Ito K, Minka MA 2d, Leunig M, et al. Femoroacetabular impingement and the cam-effect. A MRI-based quantitative anatomical study of the femoral head-neck offset. *J Bone Joint Surg Br.* 2001;83:171–176.
15. Iwase T, Hasegawa Y, Kawamoto K, et al. Twenty years' followup of intertrochanteric osteotomy for treatment of the dysplastic hip. *Clin Orthop.* 1996;331:245–255.
16. Keener JD, Callaghan JJ, Goetz DD, et al. Twenty-five-year results after Charnley total hip arthroplasty in patients less than fifty years old: a concise follow-up of a previous report. *J Bone Joint Surg Am.* 2003;85A:1066–1072.
17. Kerboul M, Thomine J, Postel M, et al. The conservative surgical treatment of idiopathic aseptic necrosis of the femoral head. *J Bone Joint Surg Br.* 1974;56:291–296.
18. Klapach AS, Callaghan JJ, Goetz DD, et al. Charnley total hip arthroplasty with use of improved cementing techniques: a minimum twenty-year follow-up study. *J Bone Joint Surg Am.* 2001;83A:1840–1848.
19. Klaue K, Wallin A, Ganz R. CT evaluation of coverage and congruency of the hip prior to osteotomy. *Clin Orthop.* 1988;232:15–25.
20. Lieberman JR, Berry DJ, Mont MA, et al. Osteonecrosis of the hip: management in the 21st century. *Instr Course Lect.* 2003;52:337–355.
21. Maistrelli GL, Gerundini M, Fusco U, et al. Valgus-extension osteotomy for osteoarthritis of the hip. Indications and long-term results. *J Bone Joint Surg Br.* 1990;72:653–657.

22. Maloney WJ, Galante JO, Anderson M, et al. Fixation, polyethylene wear, and pelvic osteolysis in primary total hip replacement. *Clin Orthop.* 1999;369:157–164.
23. Marti RK, Schuller HM, Raaymakers EL. Intertrochanteric osteotomy for non-union of the femoral neck. *J Bone Joint Surg Br.* 1989;71:782–787.
24. Mast JW, Mayo KA. The intertrochanteric osteotomy for nonunion or malunion of fractures of the proximal femur. *Semin Arthroplasty.* 1997;8:51–68.
25. McAndrew MP, Weinstein SL. A long-term follow-up of Legg–Calvé–Perthes disease. *J Bone Joint Surg Am.* 1984;66:860–869.
26. Miegel RE, Harris WH. Medial-displacement intertrochanteric osteotomy in the treatment of osteoarthritis of the hip. A long-term follow-up study. *J Bone Joint Surg Am.* 1984;66:878–887.
27. Millis M, Murphy S, Poss R. Osteotomies about the hip for the prevention and treatment of osteoarthrosis. *J Bone Joint Surg Am.* 1995;77A:626–647.
28. Mont MA, Fairbank AC, Krackow KA, et al. Corrective osteotomy for osteonecrosis of the femoral head. *J Bone Joint Surg Am.* 1996;78:1032–1038.
29. Muller ME. Intertrochanteric osteotomy: indication, preoperative planning, technique. In: Schatzker J, ed. *The Intertrochanteric Osteotomy.* Berlin: Springer-Verlag; 1984:26–66.
30. Murphy SB, Ganz R, Muller ME. The prognosis in untreated dysplasia of the hip. A study of radiographic factors that predict the outcome. *J Bone Joint Surg Am.* 1995;77:985–989.
31. Notzli HP, Wyss TF, Stoecklin CH, et al. The contour of the femoral head-neck junction as a predictor for the risk of anterior impingement. *J Bone Joint Surg Br.* 2002;84:556–560.
32. Palmer WE. MR arthrography of the hip. *Semin Musculoskelet Radiol.* 1998;2:349–362.
33. Pauwels F. *Biomechanics of the Normal and Diseased Hip. Theoretical Foundation, Technique and Results of Treatment. An Atlas.* New York: Springer; 1976.
34. Pauwels, F. *Der Schenkelhalsbruch ein mechanisches Problem: Grundlagen des heilungsvorganges Prognose und kausale Therapie.* Stuttgart: Ferdinand Enke Verlag; 1935.
35. Pellicci PM, Hu S, Garvin KL, et al. Varus rotational femoral osteotomies in adults with hip dysplasia. *Clin Orthop.* 1991;272:162–166.
36. Poss R. The role of osteotomy in the treatment of osteoarthritis of the hip. *J Bone Joint Surg Am.* 1984;66:144–151.
37. Reynolds D, Lucas J, Klaue K. Retroversion of the acetabulum. A cause of hip pain. *J Bone Joint Surg Br.* 1999;81:281–288.
38. Sanchez-Sotelo J, Trousdale RT, Berry DJ, et al. Surgical treatment of developmental dysplasia of the hip in adults. I: Nonarthroplasty options. *J Am Acad Orthop Surg.* 2002;10:321–333.
39. Scher MA, Jakim I. Intertrochanteric osteotomy and autogenous bone-grafting for avascular necrosis of the femoral head. *J Bone Joint Surg Am.* 1993;75:1119–1133.
40. Schneider R. Radiologische Funktionaldiagnostic zur Planung der intertrochanteren Osteotomie. *Verh Schweiz Ges Orthop.* 1970;131.
41. Soballe K, Boll KL, Kofod S, et al. Total hip replacement after medial-displacement osteotomy of the proximal part of the femur. *J Bone Joint Surg Am.* 1989;71:692–697.
42. Stulberg SD, Cooperman DR, Wallensten R. The natural history of Legg–Calvé–Perthes disease. *J Bone Joint Surg Am.* 1981;63:1095–108.
43. Stulberg SD, Cordell LD, Harris WH, et al. Unrecognized childhood hip disease: a major cause of idiopathic osteoarthritis of the hip. In: *The Hip Proceedings of the Third Open Scientific Meeting of The Hip Society.* St. Louis: CV Mosby; 1975:212–220.
44. Tonnis D, Heinecke A. Acetabular and femoral anteversion: relationship with osteoarthritis of the hip. *J Bone Joint Surg Am.* 1999;81:1747–7170.
45. Trousdale RT, Ekkernkamp A, Ganz R, et al. Periacetabular and intertrochanteric osteotomy for the treatment of osteoarthrosis in dysplastic hips. *J Bone Joint Surg Am.* 1995;77:73–85.
46. Weisl H. Intertrochanteric osteotomy for osteoarthritis. A long-term follow-up. *J Bone Joint Surg Br.* 1980;62B:37–42.
47. Whiteside LA, Schoenecker PL. Combined valgus derotation osteotomy and cervical osteoplasty for severely slipped capital femoral epiphysis: mechanical analysis and report preliminary results using compression screw fixation and early weight bearing. *Clin Orthop.* 1978;132:88–97.

Periacetabular Osteotomy

53

Michael B. Millis   *Stephen B. Murphy*

Developmental dysplasia of the hip (DDH), comprising a spectrum of deformity, is a common cause of hip dysfunction and eventual osteoarthrosis in the adult (1,4,6,7,49,53,70) (Fig. 53-1B). In many parts of the world, including North America, central Europe, and Japan, hip dysplasia is the single largest etiology of osteoarthrosis of the adult hip (1,53). Cited rates of end-stage arthrosis secondary to dysplasia range from about 40%, in North America, to as high as 88%, in Japan (53). Historically, 50% or more of patients with dysplasia have developed osteoarthrosis by age 50 (1,81). Approximately 90% of patients with dysplasia are female. Though DDH is well recognized as a major orthopedic problem in infancy and childhood, about two thirds of our adult patients who are treated for symptomatic hip dysplasia have no history of prior diagnosis of DDH.

The anatomic components of hip dysplasia include (a) dysplasia of the acetabulum, (b) abnormalities in shape and alignment of the proximal femur, and (c) versional abnormalities of

the acetabulum, proximal femur, or both (47,50,72). In the large majority of patients with symptomatic hip dysplasia, the acetabular deformity predominates. The resulting undercoverage of the femoral head laterally and usually anteriorly has the negative long-term mechanical consequence of intolerable loading of the acetabular rim structures, frequently leading to arthrosis (4,13,27,58). Posterior and lateral deficiency unaccompanied by anterior deficiency, associated with acetabular retroversion, can occur as well, particularly in men (Fig. 53-2A–C) (15,17,38,60,67). While about 90% of symptomatic adult dysplastic hips have acetabular dysplasia with or without femoral dysplasia, about 10% have isolated femoral dysplasia with normal or nearly normal acetabular development.

Uncorrected acetabular dysplasia, once symptoms develop, tends to cause progressive symptoms and relatively early irreversible arthrosis—often as early as the third or fourth decade of life. The young and active nature of many symptomatic dysplasia patients makes joint-preserving measures, rather than joint replacement, the first choice in treatment. If appropriate joint-preserving surgery for the dysplastic hip is carried out before arthrosis is present, excellent results can be achieved. Indeed, many dysplastic hips otherwise destined for end-stage arthrosis are still functioning well decades after joint-preserving surgery (54,63,66,73,79).

RATIONALE FOR PERIACETABULAR OSTEOTOMY

The cornerstone of contemporary joint-preserving treatment for symptomatic acetabular dysplasia is realignment osteotomy of the pelvis or periacetabular region, as it has been since Salter's innovation of innominate osteotomy in the 1950s (61). Salter brilliantly hypothesized that pelvic osteotomy through the innominate bone, to reorient the oblique dysplastic acetabulum into a more normal position, would stabilize the hip. Subsequent clinical use of innominate

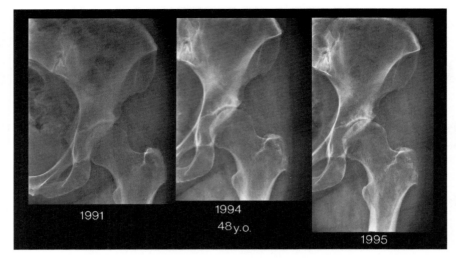

Figure 53-1 Anteroposterior (AP) radiographs of woman initially presenting with a painful dysplastic left hip at age 44. In 4 years, at age 48, she had developed end-stage arthrosis. Intervention with a reorientation osteotomy in 1991, at age 44, may have prevented or delayed secondary arthrosis. (Courtesy of Dr. R. Trousdale.)

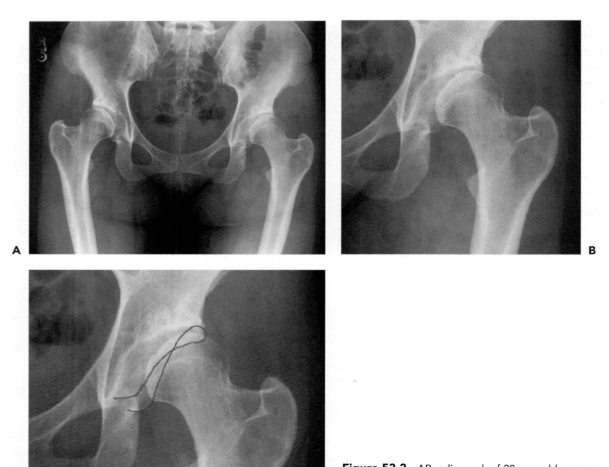

Figure 53-2 AP radiograph of 28-year-old woman with bilateral acetabular dysplasia with deficiency of coverage, mostly posterolaterally (A). The anterior and posterior rims can be seen and demonstrate better coverage anterolaterally than posterolaterally (the crossover sign) (B,C). These relatively retroverted hips require redirection that improves posterior and lateral coverage without creating anterior impingement.

osteotomy and its related procedures has led to an impressive record of nearly 50 years of improving on the natural history of acetabular dysplasia in DDH patients treated both before and after skeletal maturity.

The mechanical goal of acetabular realignment surgery is to normalize both the static and the dynamic mechanical environment of the unstable, rim-loaded dysplastic hip as much as possible (20,27,34). Surgical reorientation of the dysplastic acetabulum is a delicate act of balancing. It is important to reorient the dysplastic acetabulum in such a way as to eliminate the shear forces acting on the acetabular rim without creating femoroacetabular impingement (15,52).

The Bernese periacetabular osteotomy (PAO) (14,34, 65,66) is among the most useful of the several surgical techniques for acetabular reorientation that have evolved from Salter's innominate osteotomy. The efficiency and versatility of PAO in achieving a variety of multidirectional corrections has led to its current favored place in the armamentarium of hip joint–preserving surgeons in many parts of the world.

EVOLUTION OF ACETABULAR REDIRECTION SURGERY

All osteotomies of the pelvis that aim to improve the alignment of the dysplastic acetabulum are based on the principles of normalizing hip joint stability and reducing pathologic stress on the hyaline cartilage surface,(4,20,34), particularly the rim (27). Pelvic osteotomies employed to correct acetabular dysplasia include the following: Salter innominate osteotomy (61), double and triple innominate osteotomies (21,31,69,71), juxta-articular triple osteotomies (5,73), and PAOs (14,55,56,77).

Because the direction and magnitude of correction from Salter's osteotomy (Fig. 53-3A) are limited in the mature hip by the relative inelasticity of the mature symphysis pubis, several new osteotomies have been described to allow more extensive correction. The Sutherland double innominate osteotomy (71) (Fig. 53-3B) and the Steel triple innominate osteotomy (69) (Fig. 53-3C) improved to some extent on the degree of possible realignment. However, in both the Sutherland and Steel procedures, the degree of correction was still constrained by the tether of the sacrospinous ligaments on the large pelvic osteotomy fragment. Even more powerful corrections were sought, leading to the development of the PAOs (43) (the spherical PAO and the Bernese PAO) (14,34,55,56,65,77), which currently are the most frequently used pelvic osteotomies in the mature, prearthritic dysplastic hip.

The juxta-articular triple osteotomy of Tönnis (72,73) (Fig. 53-3D) has advantage over the Steel procedure, in that correction is not tethered by the sacrospinous ligaments, and secondary pelvic deformity is minimized. However, as in all triple osteotomies, the posterior column is disrupted.

All of the true PAOs separate the acetabulum from the remainder of the pelvis while leaving an intact posterior column, but they vary widely in their technique.

Spherical rotational osteotomy, developed independently in Europe by Wagner (77) and in Japan by Nishio and Tagawa (55), creates a spherical acetabular fragment with curved chisels in order to allow free angular correction and considerable intrinsic stability (Fig. 53-3E). This procedure is sometimes called "dial osteotomy" in the North American literature (12)

or "RAO," for "rotational acetabular osteotomy," in the Japanese literature. Significant medialization of the spherical fragment, which is desirable in correcting cases of lateralized dysplastic acetabula, is impossible without extensive modification of the spherical osteotomy bed (an additional Chiari-like osteotomy cut was described by Wagner) (77). Further, the small size of the fragment precludes robust fixation. An additional drawback of the rotational osteotomies as performed by their innovators was the reluctance of these surgeons to perform simultaneous capsulotomy out of concern for the capsular contribution to the blood supply of the small acetabular fragment.

Wagner's long-term results for more than 400 spherical osteotomies performed through a Smith-Petersen approach have been reported (79) but not published. Ninomiya, the disciple of Tagawa, has built up an impressive body of experience from performing more than 1000 rotational acetabular osteotomies using cuts similar to Wagner's but with smaller chisels and an anterolateral/posterolateral approach (55,56).

The Bernese PAO, with several variations in surgical approach, has evolved into the current preferred method for redirection of the mature dysplastic acetabulum in North America, much of Europe, and in a number of other centers around the world.

Advantages of the Bernese PAO are many (14,34). The posterior column remains intact. The quadrilateral plate is part of the acetabular fragment, allowing free adjustment of medial-lateral position of the joint. The acetabular fragment is large enough to allow quite stable fixation. The remaining blood supply to the osteotomized acetabular fragment is vigorous enough to allow simultaneous arthrotomy of the joint to treat intraarticular problems (2,18). Secondary deformity of the pelvis is minimized, facilitating subsequent vaginal childbirth (76). In addition, PAO can be performed with minimal abductor dissection, which facilitates rehabilitation (34,51).

CLINICAL AND RADIOGRAPHIC EVALUATION

Evaluation of the patient with a symptomatic hip should begin with a careful interview to ask certain key questions regarding hip function and symptoms. A directed physical examination should follow the interview, with imaging the next stage in the analytic sequence.

Common Symptoms in Hip Dysplasia

Most patients with hip dysplasia experience a period of normal or near normal hip function during childhood and adolescence. In general, more severely dysplastic hips become symptomatic sooner than less severely affected hips, although age at presentation can vary widely. An initial symptomatic period of abductor fatigue, presenting as a mild activity-related limp or intermittent ache in the region of the greater trochanter, often is noted only in retrospect, after more severe symptoms have developed.

The development of groin pain, which typically is more severe than the previous abductor symptoms, frequently leads to the initial radiographs that confirm the diagnosis of acetabular dysplasia. The groin pain may reflect overload of the tissues of the acetabular rim (27). Persistence of the abnormal

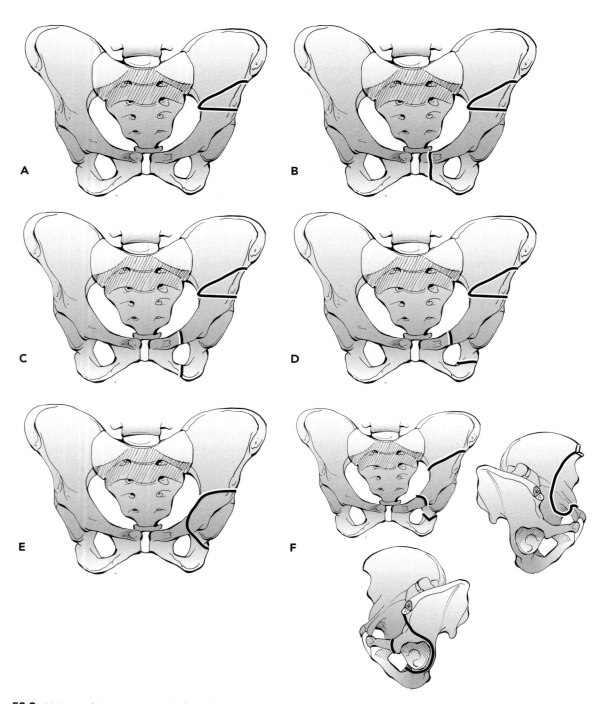

Figure 53-3 Various pelvic osteotomies. **A:** The Salter innominate osteotomy. The Salter innominate osteotomy involves a single osteotomy cut passing from the superior aspect of the sciatic notch to the anterior inferior spine area. Anterolateral redirection of the acetabulum is achieved by rotation through an axis running from the posterior aspect of the osteotomy to the symphasis pubis. The amount of correction is limited by the elasticity of the symphysis, particularly in the mature patient. **B:** The Sutherland double innominate osteotomy. The Sutherland double innominate osteotomy employs a supplemental vertical pubic osteotomy just lateral to the symphasis to supplement the innominate cut. The pubic osteotomy allows some improvement in correction over the Salter osteotomy in older patients in whom stiff symphyses is a limiting factor. **C:** The Steele triple innominate osteotomy. The Steele triple innominate osteotomy supplements the classic innominate cut with a superior pubic osteotomy just medial to the iliopectineal eminence. The inferior pubic osteotomy affords additional mobility to the acetabular fragment, but tethering of the fragment by the intact attachments of the sacrospinous ligament tend to limit major corrections and introduce a tendency to retroversion. **D:** The Tönnis triple pelvic osteotomy. Tönnis's osteotomy is a juxta-articular procedure, with the ischial osteotomy performed very close to the inferior margin of the acetabulum, passing from the posterior column area proximal to the ischial spine and extending anteriorly to the infracotyloid groove of the ischium, exiting in the inferior portion of the obturator foramen. The additional osteotomy cuts are the classic innominate osteotomy cuts passing from the greater sciatic notch to the anterior inferior spine area. The third osteotomy is of the superior pubic ramus just medial to the iliopectineal emminence. The location of the ischial osteotomy proximal to the ischial spine frees the acetabular fragment from the tethering effect of the sacrospinous ligament. The posterior column is, however, transgressed both by the innominate cut and the ischial osteotomy, breaking the pelvic ring and rendering the pelvis less stable than in the periacetabular osteotomies, which leave the posterior column intact. **E:** Spherical acetabular osteotomy. The spherical osteotomy employs special curved chisels to create broad congruous osteotomy surfaces around the periacetabular region. The relative great freedom of correction of the mobilized acetabular fragment is counterbalanced by its relatively small size, which can compromise its blood supply and complicate robust fixation. **F:** The Bernese PAO. The Bernese PAO creates a multicornered mobile acetabular fragment small enough to be mobilized for large corrections, medialized as needed, and with adequate volume and blood supply to allow both robust osteosynthesis for early function and capsulotomy for simultaneous intra-articular surgery.

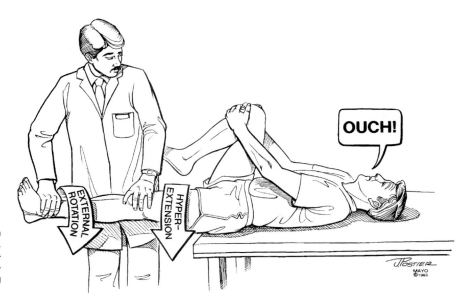

Figure 53-4 Anterior hip apprehension test employs passive extension, adduction, and external rotation to demonstrate anterior apprehension or pain, signifying anterior instability of the hip, a frequent finding in symptomatic acetabular dysplasia.

rim loading leads predictably to subacute or acute exacerbation of symptoms as the labrum stretches or tears or the rim suffers a fatigue fracture.

This symptom complex, first termed the "acetabular rim syndrome" in the classic article by Klaue et al. (27), includes the feeling that the hip catches, locks, or gives way. Patients will often describe a sense that the hip is "out of place." There is often intermittent sharp groin pain radiating down the thigh. Although these mechanical symptoms are well known to be associated with acetabular labral tears, it must be remembered that the isolated acetabular labral tear is a rare phenomenon. *The overwhelming majority of labral tears are associated with important structural hip abnormalities* (80), of which dysplasia and impingement-producing deformities are most common. Therefore, patients who are diagnosed with a labral tear always should be evaluated for hip dysplasia (10) and femoroacetabular impingement (15,25,57), since the most successful treatment of such symptomatic hips usually requires correction of the primary structural abnormality that has led to the secondary labral or rim damage.

Physical Examination of the Dysplastic Hip (16)

The physical examination should include a careful evaluation of gait and hip muscle strength and precise measurement of pain-free and painful arcs of motion.

Although no single element in clinical evaluation can guarantee an excellent result after PAO, a pain-free flexion–extension arc of more than 100° is highly suggestive of the smoothly mobile, congruous joint that seems to respond best to the procedure. Pain-free passive abduction similarly is a positive prognostic sign. The more limited the pain-free arc, the more articular damage likely to be present. A Trendelenburg sign is almost always present in the adult patient with symptomatic dysplasia, although exercise may

be needed to demonstrate it. Abductor fatigability may also be demonstrated by the "bicycle test," performed in side-lying by seeking tenderness over the exercising abductors as the up hip is moved through cycling motions. The most useful information is derived from examination of the hip in a supine position (16,36). The anterior impingement test (AIT) is a passive flexion–adduction–internal rotation maneuver, with sharp groin pain indicating a positive test. By bringing the femoral neck into contact with the anterior rim and labrum, the AIT nonspecifically can elicit pain secondary to any locally damaging condition, including dysplasia, inflammation, or impingement.

The most dramatic examination maneuver is the apprehension test (Fig. 53-4). This is performed by having the patient lie supine at the end of the examination table with the contralateral hip flexed. The examiner then carefully brings the affected hip into maximum hyperextension and external rotation. Anterior pain or apprehension with this maneuver suggests anterior instability of the hip joint.

Radiographic Evaluation of Mature Hip Dysplasia (16,72)

Initial plain radiographs include a weight-bearing orthograde anteroposterior (AP) pelvis, the *faux profil* (false profile) (Fig. 53-5) view (32), and the Von Rosen (flexion–abduction–internal rotation) view. The AP pelvis view demonstrates the position of the acetabulum relative to the pelvis, lateral coverage, lateral subluxation, the degree of secondary arthrosis, femoral development, and any joint asphericity (16).

On this AP radiograph, the positions of the anterior and posterior rims of the acetabulum can also be seen, allowing assessment of anterior and posterior coverage and acetabular anteversion or retroversion (38). If reduced femoral head–neck offset is suspected, a true lateral view of the hip taken in 15° of internal rotation can show the anterolateral area, where reduced offset is most commonly problematic

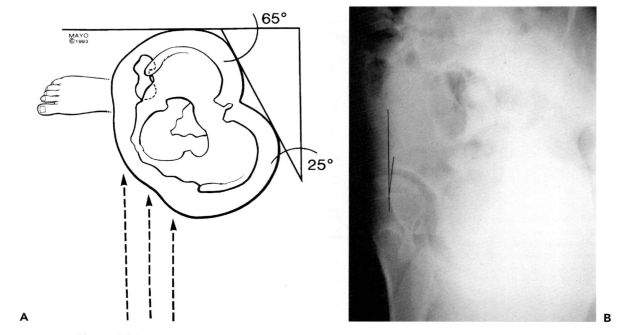

Figure 53-5 **A:** Axial view of the radiographic technique for the *faux profil* (false profile) view described by Lequesne (32). The hip being examined is the one closest to the radiographic casette. The femoral neck is perpendicular to the film. **B:** False profile view of a dysplastic right hip showed poor anterior femoral head coverage, with the anterior center-edge angle measuring only a few degrees.

(11). The lack of femoral head–neck offset can cause postoperative anterior femoroacetabular impingement as a result of increased anterior acetabular coverage (52). This potential problem can be anticipated preoperatively and managed intraoperatively. The false profile view is perhaps the most critical view of all, showing the amount of anterior coverage, cartilage interval narrowing, and subluxation (Fig. 53-5).

Of the many measurements that can made from plain radiographs of the hip, among the most convenient and useful are the lateral center-edge angle of Wiberg; the anterior center-edge angle (VCA angle) (72) quantitating anterior coverage, measured on the false profile view; and the acetabular index (72), measuring the tilt of the sourcil in the mature hip. The lower limits of normal for the lateral and anterior center-edge angles seem to have some ethnic variation, and males tend to have deeper acetabula, and hence larger center-edge angles, than females. The lower limit of normal for the lateral center-edge angle in the Caucasian female seems to be about 25°.

The area of normal subchondral sclerosis in the acetabular roof, called the "sourcil," is roughly horizontal in the normal hip, though a tilt of this sclerotic zone into either varus or valgus by 10° is accepted as being in the normal range. The lower limits of normal for the anterior center-edge angle is approximately +20°.

Functional Radiographs and MR Imaging

Hips with acetabular dysplasia that are round and freely mobile and without significant secondary arthritis respond predictably well to periacetabular osteotomy. Hips that are less ideal present greater challenges for decision making. These "borderline" hips often benefit from additional "functional"

radiographic evaluation (16,48). The most important functional radiograph is the supine AP pelvis view taken with the hips in flexion, internal rotation, and abduction. This view simulates the AP radiographic appearance of the relationship of the femoral head and acetabulum to be expected after rotation of the acetabulum in an anterior and lateral direction. Similarly, the false profile view with the hip in flexion simulates the congruence to be expected after periacetabular osteotomy (48). C-arm evaluation of the hip with "spot" images is useful on rare occasions, although the limited field of view on the image intensifier is problematic. Functional views can demonstrate hinging of the joint, which might impact negatively on the operative result. The appearance of the postoperative cartilage space interval can also be predicted. Similarly, the false profile view in flexion simulates the appearance of the joint with improved anterior coverage.

Further information in questionable hips can be obtained by examining the hip under fluoroscopy. Unlike static radiographs and magnetic resonance imaging (MRI), fluoroscopy is currently the only simple method of dynamically evaluating the joint.

MRI can be very instructive in analyzing the dysplastic hip (26,33,35,37). It can be used to assess the extent of hyaline and fibrocartilage (labral) damage. The dGEMRIC technique employs intravenous gadolinium to obtain delayed images of not only the labrum, by an indirect arthrogram effect, but also the articular cartilage itself (26). The gadolinium tends to penetrate the articular cartilage in direct proportion to the loss of glycosaminoglycan from the cartilage, allowing this type of study to offer a noninvasive measure of the degree of osteoarthrosis much more accurate than plain radiography.

This type of analysis offers the potential for making important decisions for or against joint preservation in the questionable hip with moderate arthrosis.

Radial MRI studies, with image plains rotating around the femoral neck axis, can also be very helpful, not only for assessing labral or rim damage but also for quantifying femoral head–neck offset (23,35,37).

CT Scanning (29,50)

CT is occasionally useful in sorting out versional issues. It also allows 3-D modeling, which is also of occasional use.

INDICATIONS AND CONTRAINDICATIONS FOR PERIACETABULAR OSTEOTOMY

PAO as a symptom-relieving, joint-preserving measure is indicated for most mature hips with symptomatic acetabular dysplasia if they have concentric motion and little or no secondary arthrosis. PAO is, in general, contraindicated prior to closure of the triradiate cartilage, because the osteotomy lines cross the triradiate physes and would disturb terminal acetabular growth (34).

The use of periacetabular osteotomy in an asymptomatic situation is controversial. While Murphy et al. (49) noted that dysplastic hips with lateral center-edge angles of 17° or less seem inevitably to develop arthrosis by age 60, and while there is a clear association of acetabular dysplasia with the development of osteoarthrosis (1,6,81), most surgeons prefer to perform acetabular realignment surgery in patients who have already developed symptoms.

The ideal mechanical indication for PAO is a spherically congruous mature hip with acetabular rim overload resulting from an oblique acetabulum and in which acetabular realignment can eliminate the rim overload without inducing impingement.

Decision making may be difficult when the hip is incongruous or has moderate secondary arthrosis. In these borderline situations, individual patient factors, such as patient age, size, understanding, and expectation, become quite important. In the end, both congruity and physiologic coverage are essential for normal hip function. Improving coverage at the expense of congruity is rarely, if ever, indicated.

A serious problem is choosing the wrong hip for the procedure. It is a very frustrating experience for a patient to undergo and rehabilitate from a major hip procedure, only to go on to early failure and require further surgery. Conversely, it is far more common for dysplastic hips that are amenable to joint-preserving surgery to be ignored, leaving the hip joint to wear out in a young patient. Selecting which borderline hips should be treated by joint-preserving surgery is as difficult as proper execution of the surgery itself.

Pre-existing Arthrosis

Deciding for or against joint preserving surgery for hips with a moderate degree of cartilage interval narrowing (as seen on plain radiographs or MRI) can be difficult (48). Often, anterosuperior subluxation of the femoral head can make the AP pelvis view appear to show significant cartilage loss. Anterosuperior subluxation can be identified on the false profile view. These hips will often demonstrate restoration of a normal cartilage interval once the joint is reduced and stabilized. In cases where true cartilage interval narrowing exists, the finding of an improved cartilage interval on functional radiographs (taken in flexion and abduction) is a favorable sign.

Conversely, the finding of cartilage interval narrowing that does not improve in any position suggests that realignment osteotomy is not likely to be helpful.

Joint Surface Asphericity

Aspherical hip joints present special challenges for joint-preserving surgery (15,30). These hips can present with a history consistent with physeal growth arrest, postreduction capital necrosis, or Legg–Calvé–Perthes disease. As a general rule, these hips impinge in abduction. Typically, these hips rotate concentrically in the flexion-extension plane but eventually impinge anteriorly in flexion as well. Finally, these hips also often have poor internal–external rotation. While these hips may present with a normal cartilage space interval, consideration of the asphericity is critical. Impingement in abduction will worsen with improved lateral coverage, and impingement in flexion will worsen with improved anterior coverage. Lateral impingement may be managed by osteochondroplasty of the lateral portion of the femoral head or valgus femoral osteotomy. Anterior impingement may be managed by osteochondroplasty of the anterior portion of the femoral head–neck junction (30,52). Unfortunately, preoperative functional radiographs cannot predict the behavior of the joint after osteochondroplasty. Intraoperative management of the incongruity is at least as important as the acetabular redirection procedure itself. If the incongruity is felt to be unmanageable, then acetabular redirection surgery is contraindicated.

Varus Osteotomy for Coxa Valga

Indications for or against simultaneous varus femoral intertrochanteric osteotomy remain incompletely defined (19,62). Mild or even moderate proximal femoral deformity (i.e., coxa valga, coxa vara, or versional variation) associated with acetabular dysplasia can often be left uncorrected if the acetabular redirection procedure alone can establish a stable, congruous, impingement-free femoroacetabular relationship. If, however, the intraoperative radiograph taken after the acetabular realignment reveals subluxation, incongruity, or impingement that is correctable by proximal femoral osteotomy, the proximal femoral procedure should be carried out, either under the same anesthetic or as a planned second procedure (19).

PREOPERATIVE PREPARATION

Preoperative patient education includes instruction in a partial weight-bearing gait. General anesthesia is routine, often with a supplemental epidural (useful intraoperatively for controlled hypotension to reduce blood loss) continuing for the first 2 to 3 postoperative days. Prophylactic antibiotics are given at the inception of anesthesia, and bladder catheterization is carried out. A cell saver is very useful, since the intraoperative blood loss is quite variable and not predictable.

Useful surgical equipment includes special curved Hohmann retractors, 30°-angled forked-tip Ganz acetabular chisels, long AO pelvic screws, and pelvic reduction instruments (Fig. 53-6). Power equipment, particularly a thin-bladed oscillating saw, is necessary. A radiolucent operating table is mandatory.

SURGICAL TECHNIQUE

A variety of surgical approaches may be used to perform PAO (23,39,51). Each approach has distinct advantages and disadvantages, with trade-offs between increased direct visualization and maintenance of soft-tissue integrity. The early Bernese series was performed through the classic Smith-Petersen interval (68), with extensive subperiosteal exposure of both inner and outer surfaces of the ilium (14,68). This full Smith-Petersen approach offers the advantage of extensive direct visualization of the capsule and the iliac and posterior column cuts.

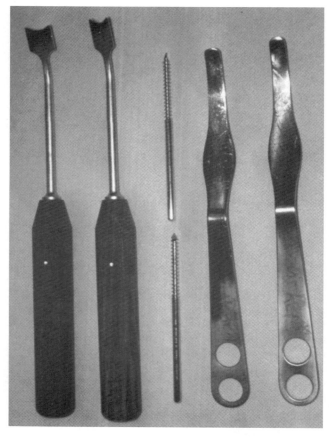

Figure 53-6 Some of the special instruments useful for performing the Bernese PAO. The 15- and 30-mm forked-tip osteotomes have an angled shaft 40 mm from their tips. They were designed by Professor Ganz specifically for this procedure. The specially curved Hohmann retractors, found in standard pelvic reduction kits, are useful for retraction of intrapelvic structures in a medial direction while performing the intrapelvic portions of the procedure. Partially threaded Schanz screws are useful for mobilizing the osteotomized acetabular fragment.

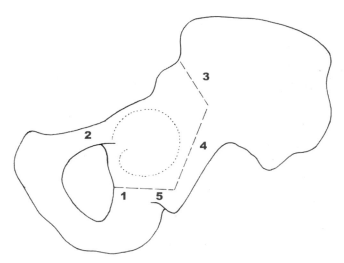

Figure 53-7 Medial view of the right hemipelvis. The various osteotomy cuts performed in the course of the Bernese PAO are numbered in the sequence usually performed. Cut no. 1 is an anterior incomplete ischial osteotomy, performed with a forked Ganz chisel from anterior to posterior to a depth of about 2 cm. The chisel is inserted carefully into the dissected interval created between the medial capsule and the psoas tendon.

Cut no. 2 is the superior pubic ramus osteotomy. It is classically performed with the hip flexed and adducted, with the soft tissues retracted to create an interval lateral to the psoas tendon and medial to the hip joint. Subperiosteal to this section around the ramus allows retractors to protect the obturator structures, while the psoas and femoral neurovascular structures are retracted medially. While a straight osteotome classically is used for the posteromedially directed osteotomy, a Gigli saw is an alternative.

Cut no. 3 is an iliac osteotomy that begins much more proximally than originally described, at or just distal to the anterior superior spine. The cut is directed vertically, in the direction of the apex of the sciatic notch, stopping 1 cm short of the iliopectineal line. The abductor origin is not disturbed during this osteotomy, with Hohmann retractors carefully protecting the soft structures both medial and lateral to the osteotomy as it is performed carefully with an oscillating saw.

Cut no. 4 is the osteotomy of the posterior column. It passes from the posterior end of the saw cut, just above the iliopectineal line, and bisects the posterior column, being directed at the ischial spine. It passes the posterior margin of the acetabulum equidistant from the posterior acetabular margin and the anterior margin of the sciatic notch as it descends toward the ischial spine. It continues to a point at least 4 cm below the iliopectineal line.

Cut no. 5 is the posterior ischial osteotomy. It begins at the inferior point of the posterior column osteotomy, at least 4 cm below the iliopectineal line to avoid entering the inferior acetabulum. This osteotomy is performed entirely within the pelvis, carefully dividing the medial cortex as the chisel is directed anteriorly, laterally, and inferiorly. Judicious use of bone spreaders and the Schanz screw often makes creation of this osteotomy with a chisel unnecessary, since a spontaneous indirect fracture often occurs with fragment manipulation.

The extensive lateral exposure gives comfort to the less experienced surgeon, but at the expense of abductor dissection and reduced vascularity to the anterior ipsilateral pelvis.

An even more extensive medial exposure can be achieved if the surgeon employs the second window of the ilioinguinal approach, which lies medial to the psoas and femoral nerve. The use of this medial window does allow direct visualization of the ischial osteotomy. We consider the potential morbidity

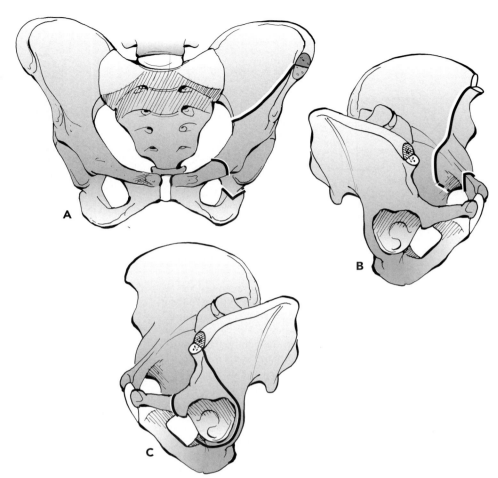

Figure 53-8 Pelvic diagrams outlining where the osteotomies are performed. Note the posterior column of the osteotomy is left intact. Once the osteotomies are complete, the fragment is rotated in the desired direction of correction, usually anteriorly and laterally. It may be medialized as desired. Fixation typically is accomplished with multiple long 4.5-mm cortical screws, although 3.5-mm screws are sometimes used if the pelvic wall is thin.

of the femoral neurovascular structures to be a relative contraindication to the routine use of the ilioinguinal approach for PAO (23,24).

Our preferred routine surgical approach for PAO, the "direct anterior approach"(34,51), is a modification of the Smith-Petersen exposure that allows the reasonably experienced surgeon adequate exposure for safe osteotomy cuts and anterior arthrotomy for articular inspection, with labral débridement or anterior neck osteoplasty if needed. The abductor origin on the iliac crest is not disturbed, allowing excellent postoperative abductor function. While PAO can be performed by the experienced surgeon without image intensifier control, limited use of the image intensifier makes the more limited surgical exposures more user-friendly (39).

OPERATIVE SEQUENCE

PAO involves an initial exposure of the surfaces to be osteotomized. An anterior arthrotomy is usual to inspect the anterior joint and rim to diagnose and treat unstable labral tears or other treatable lesions that might compromise the operative result. A series of PAO cuts are performed (Fig. 53-7). The acetabular fragment then is mobilized and redirected. A "provisional best" position for the realigned fragment is chosen. Provisional fixation is carried out with Kirschner wires.

Impingement is ruled out by inspection with motion. The optimal alignment is confirmed with an orthograde pelvis radiograph. Definitive fixation then is achieved with multiple long screws (Fig. 53-8). Final imaging confirms satisfactory realignment and osteosynthesis. Careful soft-tissue repair follows.

Exposure

Positioning is supine on a padded radiolucent table, with the ipsilateral lower extremity draped free. The operative field extends from the costal margin proximally to the anterior midline medially, distally to the midthigh, and laterally past the lateral midline (Fig. 53-9).

If an extended ilioinguinal exposure is planned, both iliac crests and abdomen are prepped into the field (10,25).

Since the medial portion of the iliofemoral exposure is sufficient for most hips (Fig. 53-2) (24,42,51), a Salter-type incision may be placed along the groin crease in thin patients and most females. A more longitudinal incision, however, favored by Professor Ganz himself, facilitates exposure and exploration of the joint. The more longitudinal incision is particularly useful in the male patient or in any muscular or obese patient.

Initially, the external oblique is reflected medially off the central portion of the iliac crest to allow subperiosteal exposure

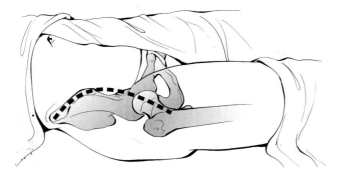

Figure 53-9 Operative position and skin incision. Patient is positioned supine on a radiolucent table, with the ipsilateral limb draped free. The operative field extends proximally to the costal margin and medially to the midline. The classic skin incision is convex anteromedially, centered just distal and lateral to the anterior superior spine. An alternative for thin patients is the bikini incision of Salter.

of the medial wall of the ilium. The origins and insertions of the abductors and tensor are left intact. The anterior superior spine is left undissected until an approximately 2 × 2 × 2 cm predrilled block of it is osteotomized, to reflect medially with the attached sartorius and inguinal ligament insertions.

The sartorius–tensor interval is entered within the envelope of the tensor, to protect the lateral femoral cutaneous nerve, which is carried medially. Within the interval, the reflected tendon of the rectus is located and is divided over a right-angle clamp. After release of the reflected tendon, the straight head of the rectus and the underlying iliocapsularis muscle can be sharply elevated in a distal and medial direction off the anterior inferior iliac spine and the hip capsule, respectively (Fig. 53-10).

The proximal structures medial to the iliac crest are mobilized from lateral to medial. These include the external oblique muscle, the inguinal ligament attached to the small osteotomy fragment of AIIS, the iliacus, and the psoas, all of which are reflected together in a medial direction from the iliac crest, the medial wall of the ilium, the iliac fossa, and the anterior capsule.

There is a nearly constant, and often quite large, perforating vessel located posteriorly on the medial iliac wall, just superficial to the iliopectineal line and just anterior to the sacroiliac joint. This vessel should be located, coagulated at its entry into the iliacus, and plugged with wax or coagulated at its entry point into the ilium.

Hip flexion and adduction allows the lateral aspect of the psoas sheath to be opened. Mobilizing the iliopsoas in an anterior and medial direction facilitates extending the subperiosteal exposure of the medial pelvic wall to the necessary depth of at least 5 cm to the iliopectineal line. The sciatic notch need not be entered, although the posterior column should be stripped subperiosteally deep enough to allow a reverse bent Hohmann retractor to be placed onto the ischial spine to retract the iliopsoas medially.

More anteriorly, working under the psoas and the femoral neurovascular structures, the superior pubic ramus is exposed to at least 1 cm medial to the iliopectineal eminence. With care, the obturator membrane is elevated from the superolateral corner of the obturator foramen, both anteriorly and posteriorly, to allow the placement of Hohmann-type retractors

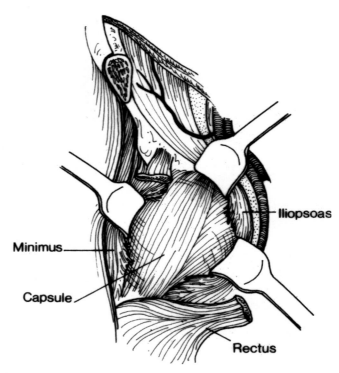

Minimus

Capsule

Iliopsoas

Rectus

Figure 53-10 Exposure of the pericapsular region employing the direct anterior approach for PAO. The abductor origin has been left undisturbed. The sartorius inguinal ligament insertion has been reflected distally and medially, along with the anterior superior spine osteotomy fragment. The rectus and iliocapsularis have been reflected distally and medially as a unit off the capsule. The iliopsoas has been reflected off the capsule as the hip is flexed and adducted. The capsule is well exposed.

under the ramus for the superior ramus osteotomy. Care is taken to mobilize the obturator vessels and nerve medially from the obturator tunnel. The most distal medial dissection is performed between the capsule and psoas to the level of the inferior femoral head. In this interval between the capsule and psoas tendon, the infracotyloid groove of the ischium can be palpated with the tip of a scissors, just proximal to the obturator externus tendon.

The capsule is seen quite well at this point.

Cut No. 1: Anterior Ischial Osteotomy

After the exposure is complete, a partial osteotomy of the anterior aspect of the ischium is performed with the special angled Ganz chisel (Fig. 53-11). Placement of this osteotomy must be just distal to the inferior capsule, to avoid damaging both the joint and the acetabular artery that enters the inferior acetabulum. This ischial osteotomy is placed within the infracotyloid groove, just above the obturator externus tendon, which in turn lies just proximal to the important medial femoral circumflex artery. Placing the osteotomy distal to the groove may not only damage the circumflex vessel but may hinder fragment rotation later in the operation.

Since the sciatic nerve lies just lateral to the ischium at this level, it is most important to avoid allowing the chisel tip to stray lateral to the lateral ischial cortex. Recognizing the feeling of the contour of the groove is most important for localizing the chisel correctly. Biplane fluoroscopic confirmation of the chisel position can be helpful for confirming that the chisel tip is seated within the groove (Fig. 53-11B,C)

The anterior-to-posterior chisel cut is extended approximately 2 cm deep. The strong medial ischial cortex must be divided, although the lateral-most cortex, which is softer, may be left intact, to be fractured indirectly later. The chisel is removed from the anterior interval.

An option at this point is to extend ischial osteotomy in a posterior direction along the medial ischial wall. This is done by inserting an angled chisel inside the pelvis, posterior to the superior pubic ramus, over the iliopectineal line, to find the posterior-most extension of the ischial osteotomy cut. The image intensifier allows proper positioning of the tip of the angled chisel between the inferior joint surface and the lesser

sciatic foramen as it scores the medial ischial cortex, working in a posterior direction toward the posterior column. The lateral cortex is not broken. This scoring is intended only to facilitate the indirect ischial fracture, which is the last step before fragment mobilization.

Arthrotomy

If arthrotomy is indicated, the anterior hip joint capsule is opened radially, just distal to the labrum (45,51). The labrum, acetabular rim, and femoral head are inspected. Labral tears (10,23), hyaline cartilage lesions, and synovial ganglia are sought and treated as needed. The possibility of femoroacetabular impingement is checked. Intra-articular pathology is best treated before acetabular rotation, when access to the

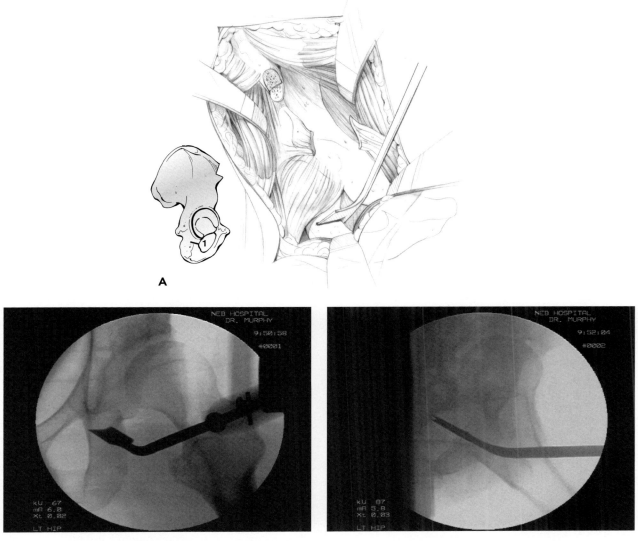

Figure 53-11 Anterior ischial osteotomy: cut no. 1. **A:** Careful development of the interval between the psoas tendon and the medial capsule allows placement of the forked Ganz chisel against the anterior ischium within the infracotyloid groove, just distal to the capsule and proximal to the obturator externis tendon. **B,C:** Confirmation of an extra-articular position may be achieved by image intensifier control.

joint is optimal. Obvious sources of impingement can be treated prior to acetabular rotation, but a final assessment for impingement after acetabular rotation is even more important (15,25,52). It is therefore useful to leave the capsulotomy open until after fragment rotation has been carried out.

Cut No. 2: Superior Pubic Ramus Osteotomy

Blunt Hohmann retractors are placed around the superior pubic ramus, and a spiked Hohmann retractor is impacted into the superior pubic ramus underneath the psoas tendon, at least 1 cm medial to the iliopectineal eminence (Fig. 53-12). With the femoral and obturator tissues thus protected, the classic osteotomy technique employs an osteotome to create the osteotomy, which must be angled from anterolaterally to posteromedially to avoid the joint and from distally and laterally to proximally and medially to facilitate later fragment mobilization. An alternative technique employs a Gigli saw, which can be passed under the superior ramus from posteriorly to anteriorly.

Cut No. 3: Iliac Osteotomy

The iliac osteotomy has been modified from its original description, to achieve more safety from intra-articular fracture by creating a larger bridge of bone between the iliac osteotomy line and the superior surface of the hip joint (Fig. 53-13). The iliac osteotomy begins much more proximally than described originally. The osteotomy line is roughly vertical in the supine

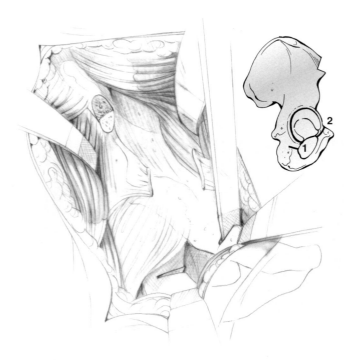

Figure 53-12   Superior pubic ramus osteotomy: cut no. 2. The superior pubic ramus osteotomy is performed at a point medial to the iliopectineal emminence, just lateral to the psoas tendon with the hip flexed and adducted. Careful protection of the soft tissues is achieved by retractors placed subperiosteally around the superior ramus into the superolateral corner of the obturator foramen.

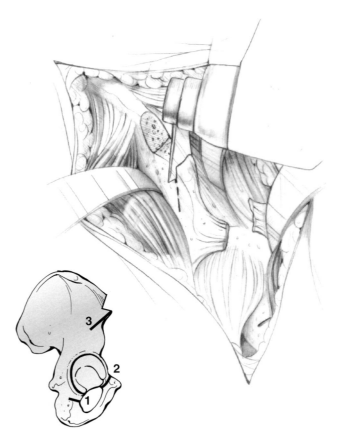

Figure 53-13   Supra-acetabular iliac osteotomy: cut no. 3. The iliac osteotmy is performed with an oscillating saw, with careful subperiosteal protection of the abductors laterally and the iliacus medially. The cut begins high on the ilium, just below the anterior superior spine. It is a vertical cut in the supine patient, directed toward the apex of the sciatic notch, stopping 1 cm short of the iliopectineal line.

patient. It begins just distal to the anterior superior spine and is directed toward the apex of the sciatic notch. The osteotomy ends posteriorly about 1 cm superficial to the iliopectineal line.

Just *prior* to performing the iliac osteotomy, a small lateral window is created along the outer iliac wall, distal to the crest, to allow the atraumatic insertion of a narrow spiked Hohmann retractor to protect the abductors and tensor. The iliacus and psoas are retracted medially, to allow insertion of the oscillating saw.

The oscillating saw is employed with saline cooling, to minimize heat-induced tissue necrosis. The saw cut ends about 1 cm above the iliopectineal line, well short of the sciatic notch. Bone wax is useful to control bleeding from the medial surface of the saw cut. Gelfoam is useful for packing the small lateral window.

Cut No. 5: Posterior Column Osteotomy

Preservation of the posterior column is essential for maintaining pelvic stability with PAO (Fig. 53-14). The placement of the posterior column osteotomy is quite important for this reason, but also because the posterior acetabulum lies quite near the osteotomy line.

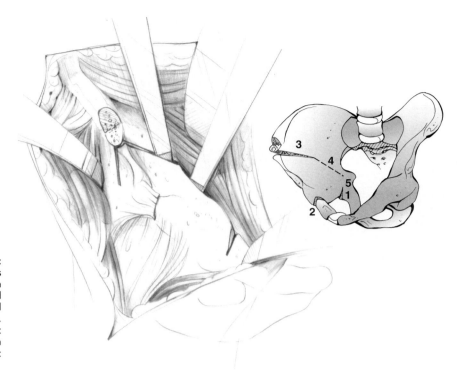

Figure 53-14 Posterior column osteotomy: cut no. 4. The posterior column osteotomy is performed from within the pelvis with a straight chisel. It begins at the posterior end of the socket, passes over the iliopectineal line, and is directed toward the ischial spine. The cut remains between the anterior aspect of the sciatic notch and the posterior margin of the acetabulum. It continues to a point at least 4 cm below the iliopectineal line.

For safety, the osteotomy line should bisect the posterior column as it is made along the medial aspect of the pelvis. A bridge of at least 1 cm should be maintained between this posterior column osteotomy and the joint in order to avoid intra-articular fracture. This osteotomy lies at an angle of about 120° with the saw cut. It is directed from the posterior end of the saw cut toward the ischial spine. This osteotomy is made with a straight chisel, with the hip in nearly full *extension*, to relax the sciatic nerve, which lies close to the posterior column as it exits the sciatic notch. The chisel should extend to, but not beyond, the lateral cortex as it passes over the iliopectineal line and descends to a point at least 4 cm into the true pelvis in the direction of the ischial spine. Pring et al. note that EMG monitoring most frequently reveals sciatic nerve irritation during this posterior column osteotomy (59).

Cut No. 5: Posterior Ischial Osteotomy

The final osteotomy, the posterior ischial osteotomy (Fig. 53-15), connects the inferior end of the posterior column osteotomy (cut no. 4) with the anterior ischial osteotomy (cut no. 1). Placing a large bone spreader onto the cortical edges of the iliac osteotomy allows the iliac osteotomy to be opened anteriorly, to extend and evert the somewhat mobile acetabular fragment. In addition, a Schanz screw may be inserted in an anteroposterior direction with a T-handled chuck into the anterior portion of the acetabular fragment. The Schanz screw and the bone spreader together allow even more aggressive eversion. This maneuver usually propagates the posterior column osteotomy into the ischial spine, allowing even further eversion. The medial wall of the true pelvis becomes somewhat more visible. One usually can detect the completing indirect ischial fracture by placing the tip of the angled Ganz

chisel along the medial pelvic wall anterior to the ischial spine at a level at least 4 cm below the iliopectineal line.

Since the remaining small ischial bony bridge is stressed by the bone spreader, minimal use of the Ganz chisel often leads to satisfying completion of the ischial osteotomy. If necessary, using the image intensifier in the oblique projection (40) or 50° caudad projection allows confident posteroanterior completion of the ischial osteotomy with the angled chisel, with

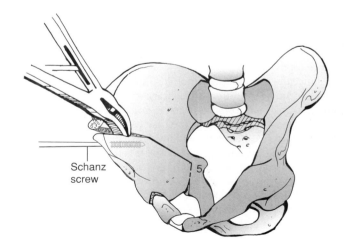

Figure 53-15 Posterior ischial osteotomy: cut no. 5. The posterior ischial osteotomy represents the division of the small remaining bridge of bone between the posterior column osteotomy and the previously made anterior ischial osteotomy. This small bridge often fractures spontaneously with fragment mobilization. Extending and everting the acetabular fragment with a bone spreader in the posterior column osteotomy often leads to an indirect fracture of the remaining bridge of bone.

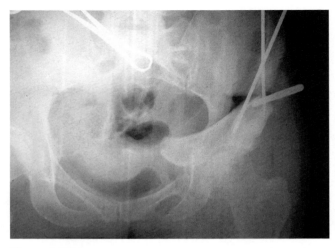

Figure 53-16 Intraoperative x-ray control. An orthograde AP radiograph of the pelvis is useful for determining that an optimum correction has been achieved. The rotated view complicates assessment. Factors to be checked include congruence, the attitude of the weight-bearing zone of the acetabulum, the location of the anterior and posterior rims, and the Shenton line.

the ischial osteotomy line now extending from the posterior column to the obturator foramen.

Fragment Mobilization/Acetabular Redirection

After completion of the bone cuts, the acetabular fragment is mobilized by using a combination of maneuvers and instruments. Internally rotating the acetabular fragment with the Schanz screw and bone spreader often completes the indirect fracture of the ischium.

Caution is needed during fragment mobilization. It is very important not to lever too aggressively on the Schanz screw before the fragment is mobile because the screw can cut out and will then be useless. Therefore, on some occasions we do not even insert the Schanz screw until the final mobilization. Also, care must be taken not to place bone spreaders on soft cancellous bone.

Once the acetabulum is mobile, the Schanz screw is inserted into the anterior portion of the fragment, if that has not been already. The anterior Schanz screw and chuck (used as a joystick), the bone spreader in the iliac osteotomy, and a Weber bone clamp placed anteromedially (just lateral to the superior pubic ramus osteotomy) can be used together to mobilize and rotate the fragment as desired in three dimensions.

Since improving anterior and lateral coverage of the femoral head is a usual goal in PAO, rotating the mobilized acetabulum in an anterior (extension) and lateral direction (adduction) is usual.

Any anterior hinging during fragment rotation implies incomplete mobilization. In this situation, the various osteotomy cuts may need to be revisited.

After fragment mobilization and rotation, it is useful for the posterosuperior corner of the acetabular fragment to be impacted in a proximal direction into the medullary canal of the proximal ilium, both to avoid any lengthening effect and to maximize intrinsic stability.

The superior pubic ramus osteotomy surfaces will displace as the fragment rotates, and with extreme corrections, a diastasis may result. In this case, local bone grafting will reduce the risk of nonunion. With extreme corrections, local grafting of the superior ramus may be needed to reduce the risk of nonunion.

Provisional fixation is achieved with multiple 3/32-inch smooth Kirschner wires drilled through the iliac crest into extra-articular locations within the acetabular fragment. Passive range of motion is assessed, and an AP radiograph of the pelvis is taken.

Selection of Optimal Acetabular Fragment Position

The exposure, osteotomy cuts, and fragment mobilization can indeed be challenging to the surgeon performing PAO. Achieving the optimal position of the mobilized acetabulum is, however, the crucial portion of the operation. In general, one wishes to choose an alignment that achieves hip stability, normalizes the mechanical environment of the acetabular rim, maintains or achieves congruity, and avoids impingement—all while minimizing loss of motion.

The degree and direction of correction are determined by the specific deformity (50), although the correction typically includes adduction and extension of the socket to improve lateral and anterior coverage.

One must avoid leaving the acetabulum in a retroverted position, because this alignment is highly associated with symptomatic arthrosis–producing impingement. The mobilized socket has a tendency to externally rotate, and at least one sixth of dysplastic acetabula are retroverted preoperatively (36,37), so residual retroversion must actively be prevented. Slight internal rotation of the acetabular fragment is often indicated to avoid retroversion.

Since many dysplastic hips have joint centers more lateral than normal, medialization of the socket is often appropriate. Lateral repositioning of the socket should be avoided.

The intraoperative AP pelvis radiograph taken after provisional fixation should reveal a horizontal weight-bearing zone, no joint center lateralization, normal acetabular version (no crossover sign), and congruous joint surfaces.

Range-of-motion examination should reveal flexion to 90° without impingement and at least 20° of abduction. If motion is more limited, then impingement must be ruled out by direct inspection and/or imaging. If more free motion is required than is present, or if the radiograph is unsatisfactory in any way, various options, including changing fragment position, must be considered.

If anterior impingement is present and is due to insufficient offset of the femoral neck, an osteoplasty of the anterior neck may be performed easily through the anterior capsulotomy.

Osteosynthesis and Fragment Trimming

When satisfactory correction has been confirmed, the Schanz screw is removed, and definitive fixation is accomplished by multiple long cortical screws between the pelvis and the acetabular fragment (Fig. 53-17). Three or four long 4.5-mm cortical screws drilled from the iliac crest into the acetabular

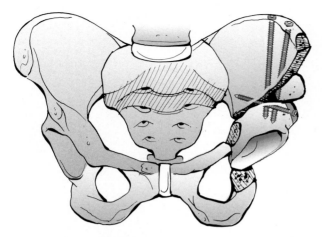

Figure 53-17 Osteosynthesis and fragment trimming. After optimal fragment position has been confirmed, provisional K-wire fixation is converted to definitive fixation with multiple long cortical screws drilled from the iliac crest into the acetabular fragment. The anteriorly protruding anterior inferior spine area is osteotomized and impacted with vascularized bone graft with its attached glutteus minimus muscle into the anterior osteotomy cleft, where it may be fixed with the most anterior iliac crest screw. A supplemental anterior to posterior "home run" screw directed from the anterior inferior spine area into the posterior column above the sciatic notch greatly enhances fragment stability.

fragment provide adequate fixation in most patients. Most PAO surgeons supplement the iliac crest screws with an anterior-to-posterior "home run screw." This supplemental screw is directed from the anterior inferior iliac spine area proximal to this joint in the acetabular fragment into the posterior column in the major pelvic fragment, above the apex of the sciatic notch. In the exceptional case, a medial reconstruction plate may augment questionable fixation in weak bone.

The prominent anterior inferior portion of the acetabular fragment routinely is trimmed, rotated, and inserted, with muscle still attached, into the anterior portion of the iliac osteotomy, where it is fixed with the most anterior of the long iliac crest screws. Further bone graft may be harvested as needed from prominent corners of the fragment for packing into the remaining osteotomy clefts.

Soft-Tissue Repair

A drill hole is made through the AIIS area to allow transosseous refixation of the straight rectus tendon. Multiple drill holes are made through the crest for transosseous repair of the iliacus. The ASIS osteotomy fragment is anatomically replaced and fixed with a short 3.5 mm screw, after which the iliac crest sutures to the iliacus are tightened.

A deep suction drain is placed within the pelvis and brought anteriorly out the sartorius-tensor interval. More superficial closure is done routinely. A compressive gauze and Ace spica bandage are applied.

POSTOPERATIVE CARE

Drains are removed after about 36 hours, and dressings changed after 48 hours. A CPM machine is employed if exten-

sive intra-articular surgery has been done. Gentle, active assisted range-of-motion exercises are begun on the first postop day. Patients are mobilized rapidly with a one-sixth body weight partial weight bearing with two crutches, usually beginning on postop day 2 or 3. No increase in weight bearing and no resistive exercises are allowed for at least 6 weeks. Anticoagulation is usual for 6 weeks. We find that PAO patients are often safer doing therapy at home without a visiting therapist, since this may decrease the likelihood of injury. Straight leg raising should be avoided for at least 6 weeks until the rectus heals.

Clinical reevaluation at 6 weeks typically shows very good abductor strength and fair hip flexor strength. If there is freedom from pain, good muscular control, and signs of satisfactory healing on radiographs at that time, weight bearing is advanced to 50% body weight with two crutches. The addition of formal therapy can be helpful at that point. Patients often progress to weight bearing as tolerated at 9 to 12 weeks from surgery, depending on symptoms, muscular recovery, and the degree of arthrosis present in the joint preoperatively. We tend to protect patients with arthrosis from full weight-bearing longer than the patients who are free of arthrosis. Activities are slowly resumed as hip function allows.

COMPLICATIONS

Since most of these procedures are performed by surgeons who have a special interest in joint-preserving surgery and hip dysplasia, major complications, while potentially serious, are fairly uncommon (9,24).

Neurapraxia

Lateral femoral cutaneous nerve dysfunction is a common minor problem, though frank meralgia paresthetica is quite rare—it occurred in only 1 out of more than 750 hips in our series. Fortunately, placing the fascial incision over the tensor, rather than between the tensor and sartorius, minimizes the incidence of this problem. Whether patients have normal sensation or poor sensation in the long run, lateral femoral cutaneous nerve dysfunction is rarely bothersome after 4 months.

Sciatic, femoral, and obturator nerve palsies have far greater significance, but all occur in less than 1% of cases.

The sciatic nerve is at risk in the proximal notch and also along the lateral side of the ischium, where the osteotome is directed during the final bone cut. Taking care to avoid excessive retraction and to avoid passing the blade of the osteotome beyond the confines of the bone reduces these risks. Maintaining the hip in a relatively extended position during the posterior column osteotomy may also reduce risk of sciatic neurapraxia, since at least one study has suggested this portion of the procedure is associated with acute neurologic monitoring changes (59). In our series, patients with previous hip surgery and males seem at relatively increased risk for sciatic neurapraxia.

Femoral nerve injury is reliably avoided by treating the femoral nerve, iliopsoas, and rectus femoris as a single unit, always staying either lateral or medial to these three structures. Dissecting between the femoral nerve and the rectus risks injury to the branches that course through that interval. In

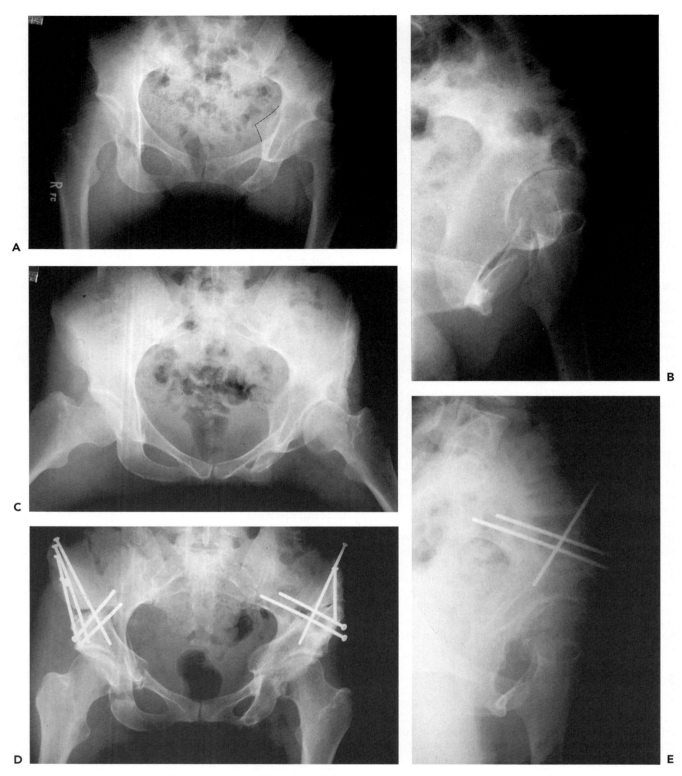

Figure 53-18   **A:** Forty-year-old female with 20-year history of left greater than right hip pain exacerbated by activity. Triple osteotomy at age 25 only temporarily relieved symptoms, which progressed greatly over last 10 years. Radiographs show retroverted, persistently dysplastic acetabulum in left hip, with large supra-acetabular cyst and anterior cartilage space narrowing. Right hip has moderate but less symptomatic acetabular dysplasia with less subluxation. **B:** False profile view shows anterior cartilage space narrowing with large anterior acetabular cyst. **C:** Von Rosen view (flexion–abduction–internal rotation) confirms excellent motion, no hinging, and restoration of excellent cartilage space in left hip. **D:** Six-month follow-up x-ray shows healed left PAO with normalized acetabular version and restored Shenton line. Cartilage space is wide. Patient was asymptomatic on left side, walking without limp. She had requested PAO on her now more symptomatic right side, which had been performed 1 week before. **E:** False profile view of left hip taken at time of right PAO, 6 months following left-sided procedure. Anterior cyst has been removed from weight-bearing zone and is healing.

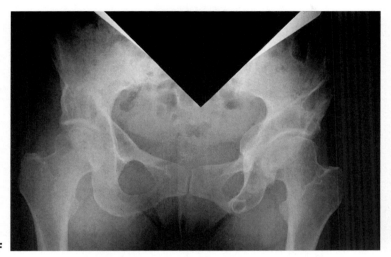

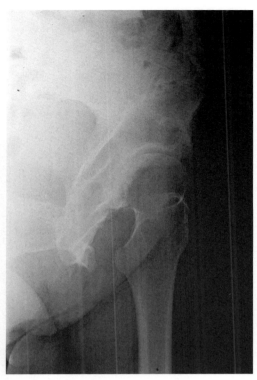

F   G

Figure 53-18 (*continued*) **F:** Standing AP radiograph 9 years following left PAO and 8.5 years following right PAO. Patient is asymptomatic bilaterally and fully active in recreational sports, including tennis and skiing. Excellent range of motion retained. Trendelenburg sign absent bilaterally. Small lateral femoral head osteophyte unchanged from 6-month postop. Cartilage space unchanged from 6-month postop. **G:** False profile view of left hip taken 9 years following PAO. Anterior cyst nearly completely healed; anterior coverage good; anterior cartilage space unchanged from 6-month postop.

addition, one should maintain the hip flexed and the knee extended while working under the psoas.

The obturator nerve can be protected by performing strict subperiosteal dissection around the superior pubic ramus and obturator tunnel.

Intra-articular Fracture

Intra-articular fracture is rare, occurring in less than 1% of cases. Revision cases and cases where arthrosis has made the periacetabular bone brittle present an increased risk for this complication. Maintaining larger than usual bone bridges between the osteotomy lines and the joint may be protective in such cases.

Nonunion

Depending on osteotomy displacement, superior pubic ramus nonunion can occur in more than 1% of procedures but is generally asymptomatic. Nonunion or delayed union of the iliac and posterior column of the osteotomy occurs rarely, but more frequently in incongruous hips, where rotational forces may be transferred to the osteotomy site during healing.

Ischial nonunion has an incidence of about 1%. It seems associated with ligamentous laxity or iatrogenic extension of the ischial osteotomy into the lesser sciatic foramen. Two of

our eight cases were symptomatic and required plating for relief.

Two delayed iliac unions were associated with the use of 3.5-mm iliac screws without a home run screw. One patient was a heavy smoker. Bone grafting and insertion of heavier screws led to rapid union in both patients.

Stress Fracture

Fourteen patients (about 2%) have had stress fractures of the inferior pubic ramus, associated in each with a very narrow medial segment of the inferior ramus. Symptoms of ischial discomfort appeared in each patient about 10 weeks after surgery, as they weaned off crutches. All have healed radiographically and clinically without treatment.

Late Labral Tears

Since the reoriented dysplastic hip joint is not normal, and even the untorn labrum in such hips may be structurally unsound (33,35,45), late labral tears can occur after PAO. These isolated tears can often be managed arthroscopically, provided that the joint shows no signs of instability or impingement. Excellent symptomatic relief has been achieved in most of the more than 30 such "secondary" arthroscopies in our series (3).

TABLE 53-1
RESULTS OF VARIOUS PAO SERIES

Author	Year	No. of Hips	Mean Age at Time of Procedure	Pre/Postop Lat Center Edge	Pre/Postop Anterior Center Edge	Pre/Postop Tönnis Angle	Follow-up	GE/F/P	Failures/THR	Risk Factors for Failure
Crockarell (Mayo)	1999	21; 4 ITO	21 y	2/24	−6/+38	24/11	Min. 2 y; mean 38 mo.	? HHS 62 pre, 86 post	1 THR	Grade 2 OA
Trumble (Mast)	1999	123; 33 ITO	33 y	6/29	3/28	23/6	Min 2 y; mean 4.3 y	83% G/E	7 THR	Grade 3 OA
Matta	1999	66; 10 ITO	34 y	−1.5/27	−.4/27.2	25/3.2	Min 27 mo. Mean 4 y	75% G/E	5 THR at mean 7.1 y	Grade 3 OA
Siebenrock	2001	71; 16 ITO	29.3 y	6/34	4/26	26/6	Min 10 y; mean 11.3 y	73% G/E	13 THR	Labral tear, grade 3 OA, malcorrection
Millis		153; 25 ITO	24.5 y	2/25	3/26	23/4	Min 5 y; mean 8.5 y	80% G/E	20 THR	Labral tear, grade 2–3 OA, incongruence

OA, osteoarthritis; THR, total hip replacement.

Vascular Disturbance

No major vascular disturbance has occurred to our knowledge in our series. The use of the ilioinguinal approach has been implicated in scattered cases of iliac and femoral thromboses around the world (23).

Mean estimated intraoperative blood loss has approximated 1200 cc, although isolated cases of more than 4000 cc blood loss have occurred without recognized major vessel disruption.

Osteonecrosis of the Acetabulum

This complication is possible if an intra-articular osteotomy injures the acetabular artery. It has not occurred in our series or in Berne.

Infection

Two cases of deep infection occurred very early in our experience, when we were using the full Smith-Petersen exposure, prior to our adopting the abductor-sparing approach. Both cases healed with multiple débridements and antibiotics. Both hips remain preserved more than 12 years after PAO.

RESULTS

Many clinical studies have published results of PAO in the past several years (Table 53-1) (8,39,40,66,75). Major radiographic corrections are nearly universal. Recent attention to avoiding overcorrection and retroversion seems likely to lead to further improvement.

Concentric hip joints that are treated before the onset of arthritis and are appropriately corrected typically function for an indefinite period of time. Failures have been associated with pre-existing arthrosis (74), incongruity (48), inadequate correction (66), and, rarely, excessive correction (66).

Siebenrock's report of the original Bernese experience revealed hip joint survivorship of 82% at an average follow-up of 11.3 years in 71 hips (66). Seventy-three percent of the patients had good to excellent results (66). Factors associated with failure included more advanced arthrosis at the time of surgery, older patient age, and inadequate correction.

Trousdale et al. reported results as a function of preoperative arthrosis (Tönnis grade) at a mean of 4 years after surgery (74). Thirty-two of 33 patients with grades 1 and 2 arthritis had good to excellent results, whereas 8 or 9 patients with advanced arthrosis had poor results.

Similarly, Murphy and Deshmukh reported on results at a mean of 5.4 years after surgery (48). Hip joint survivorship was 100% (21/21) in hips with grade 1 arthrosis, 82% (18/22) in hips with grade 2 arthrosis, 87% (7/8) in patients with grade 3 arthrosis, and 0% (0/1) in patients with grade 4 arthrosis. The grade 2 failures had unmanageable incongruity, and the grade 3 failure showed no improvement in the cartilage space interval on preoperative functional radiographs. The grade 3 hips that functioned well all had an improved cartilage space interval on functional radiographs.

The Children's Hospital–Boston series of more than 600 PAOs has reported on 154 of 188 consecutive hips with minimum 5-year follow-up (mean, 8.5 years) (39). Mean age at PAO was 25 years (9 to 54 years). Radiographic corrections were excellent, with the mean correction of CE angle from +2° to +25°, anterior CE angle from −2° to +27°, and Tönnis sourcil tilt angle from +25° to +5° postop. Failure, defined by WOMAC pain score or THR, has occurred in 26 hips to date. Univariate analyses identified three independent predictors of failure: labral tear ($p < .01$), preoperative joint incongruity (fair or poor by Yasunaga's classification; $p < .01$) (82), and Tönnis grade 3 or 4 arthrosis (72). Risk of failure at a mean of 8.5 years after surgery was more than 95% if there was a labral tear and preoperative joint congruity was only fair or poor. Conversely, if there was no labral tear and joint congruity was good or excellent, risk of failure was less than 5%. Most hips had minimal or no symptoms at follow-up, while all but two hips had been symptomatic preoperatively.

CONCLUSION

The Bernese periacetabular osteotomy has emerged as the most commonly employed acetabular redirection method in North America and much of Europe for stabilizing the congruous dysplastic mature hip. Advantages of the procedure include minimal abductor morbidity, excellent exposure of the joint, freedom to individualize acetabular position without creating significant secondary deformities, strong fixation, and preservation of pelvic stability through an intact posterior column. Results are routinely good to excellent in congruous hips properly treated prior to the onset of advanced arthrosis. The procedure can be very effective in certain aspherical hips and in certain very carefully selected hips with moderate pre-existing arthrosis, but the risk of failure remains higher.

REFERENCES

1. Aronson J. Osteoarthritis of the young adult hip: etiology and treatment. *Instr Course Lect.* 1986;35:119–128.
2. Beck M, Leunig M, Ellis T, et al. The acetabular blood supply: implications for periacetabular osteotomies. *Surg Radiol Anat.* 2003;25:361–367.
3. Belzile E, Kocher M, Kim YJ, et al. Personal communication.
4. Bombelli R. *Structure and Function in Normal and Abnormal Hips: How to Rescue Mechanically Jeopardized Hips.* 3rd ed. New York; Springer-Verlag; 1993.
5. Carlioz H, Khouri N, Hulin P. Osteotomie triple juxtacotyloidienne. *Rev Chir Orthop.* 1982;68:49–501.
6. Cooperman DR, Wallensten R, Stulberg SD. Acetabular dysplasia in the adult. *Clin Orthop.* 1983;175:79.
7. Cooperman DR, Wallensten R, Stulberg SD. Post-reduction avascular necrosis in congenital dislocation of the hip. *J Bone Joint Surg.* 1980;62A:247–258.
8. Crockarell JR, Trousdale RT, Cabanel ME, et al. Early experience and results with the periacetabular osteotomy: the Mayo Clinic experience. *Clin Orthop.* 1999;363:45–53.
9. Davey JP, Santore RF. Complications of periacetabular osteotomy. *Clin Orthop.* 1999;363:33–37.
10. Dorell JH, Catterall A. The torn acetabular labrum. *J Bone Joint Surg.* 1986;68B:400.
11. Eijer J, Leunig M, Mohamed MN, et al. Cross-table lateral radiograph for screening of anterior femoral head-neck offset in patients with femoroacetabular impingement. *Hip Int.* 2001;11: 37–41.
12. Eppright RH. Dial osteotomy of the acetabulum in the treatment of dysplasia of the hip. *J Bone Joint Surg.* 1975;57A:1172.

13. Felson DT. Risk factors for osteoarthritis: understanding joint vulnerability. *Clin Orthop.* 2004;427(suppl):S16–21.
14. Ganz R, Klaue K, Vinh TS, et al. A new periacetabular osteotomy for the treatment of hip dysplasias: technique and preliminary results. *Clin Orthop.* 1988;232:26–36.
15. Ganz R, Parvizi J, Beck M, et al. Femoroacetabular impingement: a cause for osteoarthritis of the hip. *Clin Orthop.* 2003 Dec;417:112–120.
16. Garbuz DS, Masri BA, Haddad F, et al. Clinical and radiographic assessment of the young adult with symptomatic hip dysplasia. *Clin Orthop.* 2004;418:18–22.
17. Giori NJ, Trousdale RT. Acetabular retroversion is associated with osteoarthritis of the hip. *Clin Orthop.* 2003;417:263–269.
18. Hempfing A, Leunig M, Notzli HP, et al. Acetabular blood flow during Bernese periacetabular osteotomy: an intraoperative study using laser Doppler flowmetry. *J Orthop Res.* 2003;21:1145–1150.
19. Hersche O, Casillas M, Ganz R. Indications for intertrochanteric osteotomy after periacetabular osteotomy for adult hip dysplasia. *Clin Orthop.* 1998;347:19–26.
20. Hipp J, Sagano D, Millis MB, et al. Planning acetabular redirection osteotomies based on joint contact pressures. *Clin Orthop.* 1999;364:134–143.
21. Hopf A. Huftpfannenverlagerung durch doppelte Beckenosteotomie zur Behandlung der Huftgelenksdysplasie und Subluxation bei Jugendlichen und Erwachsenen. *Z Orthop.* 1966;101:559.
22. Hsieh PH, Shih CH, Lee PC, et al. A modified periacetabular osteotomy with use of the transtrochanteric exposure. *J Bone Joint Surg.* 2003;85A:244–250.
23. Hussell JG, Mast JW, Mayo KA, et al. A comparison of different surgical approaches for periacetabular osteotomy. *Clin Orthop.* 1999;363:64–72.
24. Hussell JG, Rodriguez JA, Ganz R. Technical complications of the Bernese periacetabular osteotomy. *Clin Orthop.* 1999;363:81–92.
25. Ito K, Minka MA, Leunig M, et al. Femoroacetabular impingement and the cam effect: a MRI-based quantitative anatomical study of the femoral head-neck offset. *J Bone Joint Surg.,* 2001;83B:171–176.
26. Kim YJ, Jaramillo D, Millis MB, et al. Assessment of early osteoarthritis in hip dysplasia with delayed gadolinium-enhanced magnetic resonance imaging of cartilage. *J Bone Joint Surg.* 2003;85A:1987–1992.
27. Klaue K, Durnin C, Ganz R. The acetabular rim syndrome: a clinical presentation of dysplasia of the hip. *J Bone Joint Surg.* 1991;73B:423.
28. Klaue K, Ganz R. Pelvic osteotomies in the adult. In: Chapman MW, ed. *Operative Orthopaedics.* Philadelphia: JB Lippincott, 1993;1839–1844.
29. Klaue K, Wallin A, Ganz R. CT evaluation of coverage and congruency of the hip prior to osteotomy. *Clin Orthop.* 1988;232:15–25.
30. Lavigne M, Parvizi J, Beck M, et al. Anterior femoroacetabular impingement: techniques of joint preserving surgery *Clin Orthop.* 2004;418:61–66.
31. LeCoeur P. Corrections des defauts d'orientation de l'articulation coxo-femorale par osteotomie de l'isthme iliaque. *Rev Chir Orthop.* 1965;51:211.
32. Lequesne M, de Séze S. Le faux profil du bassin: nouvell incidence radiographique pour l'étude de la hanche: son utilité dans les dysplasies et les différentes coxopathies. *Rev Rhum Mal Osteoartic.* 1961;28:643.
33. Leunig M, Podeszwa D, Beck M, et al. Magnetic resonance arthrography of labral disorders in hips with dysplasia and impingement. *Clin Orthop.* 2004;418:74–80.
34. Leunig M, Siebenrock K, Ganz R. Rationale of periacetabular osteotomy and background work. *J Bone Joint Surg.* 2001;83A:438–448.
35. Leunig M, Werlen S, Ungersbock A, et al. Evaluation of the acetabular labrum by MR arthrography. *J Bone Joint Surg.* 1997;79B:230–234.
36. Li PL, Ganz R. Morphologic features of congenital acetabular dysplasia: one in six is retroverted. *Clin Orthop.* 2003;416:245–253.
37. Locher S, Werlen S, Leunig M, et al. MR-arthrography with radial sequences for visualization of early hip pathology not visible on plain radiographs [in German]. *Z Orthop Ihre Grenzgeh.* 2002;140:52–57.

38. Mast J, Brunner RL, Zebrack J. Recognizing acetabular version in the radiologic presentation of hip dysplasia. *Clin Orthop.* 2004;418:48–53.
39. Matheny T, Kim YJ, Matero C, et al. The Boston minimum 5 year experience with Bernese periacetabular osteotomy. Submitted for publication.
40. Matta JM, Stover MD, Siebenrock K. Periacetabular osteotomy through the Smith-Petersen approach. *Clin Orthop.* 1999:363:21–32.
41. Mayo KA, Trumble SJ, Mast JW. Results of periacetabular osteotomy in patients with previous surgery for hip dysplasia. *Clin Orthop.* 1999;363:73–80.
42. McGrory BJ, Trousdale RT, Cabanela ME, et al. Bernese periacetabular osteotomy: surgical techniques. *J Orthop Tech.* 1993;1:179–191.
43. Millis MB. Reconstructive osteotomies of the pelvis for the correction of acetabular dysplasia. In: Sledge C, ed. *Master Techniques in Orthopaedic Surgery: The Hip.* Philadelphia: Lippincott-Raven; 1998:157–182.
44. Millis MB, Kim YJ. Rationale of osteotomy and related procedures for hip preservation: A review. *Clin Orthop.* 2002;405:108–121.
45. Millis MB, Murphy SB. Die periazetabulare osteotomie mit simultaner arthrotomie uber den direkten vorderen zugang. *Orthopade.* 1998;27:751–758.
46. Millis MB, Murphy SB. Use of CT reconstruction in planning osteotomy of the hip. *Clin Orthop.* 1992;274:154–159.
47. Millis MB, Murphy SB, Poss R. Osteotomies about the hip for the prevention and treatment of osteoarthritis. *J Bone Joint Surg.* 1995;77A:626–647.
48. Murphy SB, Deshmukh R. Periacetabular osteotomy: radiographic predictors of outcome. *Clin Orthop.* 2002, 405:168–174.
49. Murphy SB, Ganz R, Muller ME. The prognosis in untreated dysplasia of the hip: a study of radiographic factors that predict the outcome. *J Bone Joint Surg.* 1995;77A:985–989.
50. Murphy SB, Kijewski PK, Millis MB, et al. Acetabular dysplasia in the adolescent and young adult. *Clin Orthop.* 1990;261:213.
51. Murphy, SB, Millis, MB. Periacetabular osteotomy without abductor dissection using the direct anterior exposure. *Clin Orthop.* 1999;364:92–98.
52. Myers SR, Eijer H, Ganz R. Anterior femoroacetabular impingement after periacetabular osteotomy. *Clin Orthop.* 1999;363:93–99.
53. Nakamura S, Ninomiya S, Nakamura T. Primary osteoarthritis of the hip joint in Japan. *Clin Orthop.* 1989;241:190–196.
54. Nakamura S, Ninomiya S, Takatori, et al. Long term outcome of rotational osteotomy: 145 hips followed for 10–23 years. *Acta Orthop Scand.* 1998;69:259–265.
55. Ninomiya S, Tagawa H. Rotational acetabular osteotomy for the dysplastic hip. *J Bone Joint Surg.* 1984;66A:430.
56. Ninomiya S. Rotational acetabular osteotomy for the severely dysplastic hip in the adolescent and adult. *Clin Orthop.* 1989;247:127–137.
57. Notzli HP, Wyss TF, Stoecklin C, et al. The contour of the femoral head-neck junction as a predictor for the risk of anterior impingement. *J Bone Joint Surg.* 2002;84B:556–560.
58. Pauwels F. *Biomechanics of the Normal and Diseased Hip.* New York: Springer-Verlag; 1976.
59. Pring ME, Trousdale RT, Cabanela ME, et al. Intraoperative electromyograpyhic monitoring during periacetabular osteotomy. *Clin Orthop.* 2002;400:158–164.
60. Reynolds D, Kucas J, Klaue K. Retroversion of the acetabulum: a cause of hip pain. *J Bone Joint Surg.* 1999;81B:281–288.
61. Salter RB. Innominate osteotomy in the treatment of congenital dislocation and subluxation in the hip. *J Bone Joint Surg.* 1961;43B:518.
62. Schatzker J. *The Intertrochanteric Osteotomy.* Berlin: Springer-Verlag; 1984.
63. Schramm M, Pitto RP, Rohm E, et al. Long-term results of spherical acetabular osteotomy. *J Bone Joint Surg.* 1999;81B:60–66.
64. Severin E. Contribution to the knowledge of congenital dislocation of the hip joint. *Acta Chir Scand.* 1941;63(suppl):84.
65. Siebenrock KA, Leunig M, Ganz R. Periacetabular osteotomy: the Bernese experience. *J Bone Joint Surg.* 2001;83:449–455.

66. Siebenrock KA, Schoeniger R, Ganz R. Anterior femoro-acetabular impingement due to acetabular retroversion: treatment by periacetabular osteotomy. *J Bone Joint Surg.* 2003;85A:278–286.

67. Siebenrock KA, Scholl E, Lottenbach M, et al. Bernese periacetabular osteotomy. *Clin Orthop.* 1999;363:9–20.

68. Smith-Petersen, MN. Approach to and exposure of the hip joint for mold arthroplasty. *J Bone Joint Surg.* 1949A;31:40–46.

69. Steel HH. Triple osteotomy of the inominate bone. *J Bone Joint Surg.* 1973;55A:343–350.

70. Stulberg SD, Harris WH. Acetabular dysplasia and development of osteoarthritis of the hip. In: *The Hip.* St. Louis: CV Mosby; 1974.

71. Sutherland DH, Greenfield R. Double innominate osteotomy. *J Bone Joint Surg.* 1977;59A:1082–1091.

72. Tönnis D. *Congenital Dysplasia and Dislocation of the Hip.* Berlin: Springer-Verlag; 1987.

73. Tönnis D, Arning A, Bloch M, et al. Triple pelvic osteotomy. *J Peditr Orthop B* 1994;3:54–67.

74. Trousdale RT, Ekkernkamp A, Ganz R. Periacetabular and intertrochanteric osteotomy for the treatment of osteoarthrosis in dysplastic hips. *J Bone Joint Surg.* 1995;77A:73–85.

75. Trumble SJ, Mayo KA, Mast J. The periacetabular osteotomy: minimum 2 year follow-up in more than 100 hips. *Clin Orthop.* 1999;363:54–63.

76. Valenzuela RG, Cabanela ME, Truesdale RT. Sexual activity, pregnancy, and childbirth after periacetabular osteotomy. *Clin Orthop.* 2004;418:146–152.

77. Wagner H. Experiences with spherical acetabular osteotomy for the correction of the dysplastic acetabulum. In: Weil UH, ed. *Acetabular Dysplasia: Skeletal Dysplasias in Childhood.* New Tork, Springer-Verlag; 1978:141–145. *Progress in Orthopaedic Surgery;* vol. 2.

78. Wagner H. Osteotomies for congenital hip dislocation. In: *The Hip: Proceedings of the Fourth Open Scientific Meeting of the Hip Society.* St. Louis: CV Mosby; 1976:45–66.

79. Wagner H. The reconstructive osteotomy: perspectives on the concept after 30 years experience with acetabular osteotomy. Paper presented at the Harvard Course on Osteotomy of the Hip and Knee; Boston; May 6, 1992.

80. Wenger DE, Kendell KR, Miner MR, et al. Acetabular labral tears rarely occur in the absence of bony abnormalities. *Clin Orthop.* 2004;426:145–150.

81. Wiberg G. Studies on dysplastic acetabula and congenital subluxations of the hip joint with special reference to the complications of osteoarthritis. *Acta Chir Scand.* 1939;58(suppl):7–38.

82. Yasunaga Y, Takahashi K, Ochi M, et al. Rotational acetabular osteotomy in patients forty-six years of age or older: comparison with younger patients. *J Bone Joint Surg.* 2003;85A:266–272.

Steel Triple Innominate and Chiari Osteotomy

54

Maurice Albright

STEEL TRIPLE INNOMINATE OSTEOTOMY

Rationale

The triple osteotomy of the innominate bone is a redirectional reconstruction obtained by circumacetabular osteotomies of the ilium, ischium, and pubis. It was first described in the English literature by Howard Steel in 1973 (30). The acetabular redirectional osteotomy was designed to realize the goal of covering the femoral head at the anatomic level of the acetabulum with articular cartilage in the older child with closed triradiate cartilage and in adolescent or adult patients (Fig. 54-1). An important aspect of the operation is that the articular surfaces of the joint be congruent or will become congruent after surgery. There is a distinct advantage to using the patient's natural acetabular cartilage to cover the femoral head.

The rationale for treatment of symptomatic acetabular dysplasia in young adults is based on two concepts. First, although there are no prospective controlled data comparing patients with and without surgical treatment, it is known that the majority of patients who develop hip arthritis in the fifth and sixth decades of life have some form of congenital or developmental hip abnormality. Therefore, restoration of the anatomical and biomechanical relationships of a clearly dysplastic hip may delay or prevent premature development of hip arthritis (26).

Because acetabular dysplasia is characterized by a lack of anterior and lateral coverage of the femoral head by the acetabulum, the goal of triple innominate osteotomy is to rotate the acetabulum in an anterior and lateral direction to improve coverage of the femoral head. This decreases the pressure per unit area of the weight-bearing surface of the hip by increasing the area of weight-bearing hyaline cartilage and increasing the mechanical advantage of the proximal femoral lever arm by creating a more effective fulcrum in the acetabulum (26).

The second concept is that normalization of the anatomical and biomechanical relationships of the dysplastic hip can improve or eliminate pain. Thus, triple innominate osteotomy may restore the normal physiologic equilibrium between tissue resistance and joint pressure in the hip region, resulting in a decrease in load per unit area, which may ultimately contribute to pain relief (26).

The triple innominate osteotomy in properly selected patients will postpone the need for total hip arthroplasty to a time when the patients are older and less active, thus improving the results (35). The osteotomy may also enhance the bone stock, improving support of the acetabular component. In addition, once the patients have recovered from surgery, their activity level, especially that of young adults, is closer to that of their unaffected peers compared with the activity level of patients who had total hip arthroplasties.

In a well-selected patient, triple innominate osteotomy is preferred over a salvage procedure, such as the Chiari osteotomy. The triple innominate osteotomy uses the patient's own articular surface to cover the femoral head rather than the metamorphosed raw bone and fibrous capsular tissue used in the Chiari osteotomy. The triple innominate osteotomy creates less of an anatomic alteration than the Chiari osteotomy, so it may cause less difficulty in future reconstructive surgery. Also, postoperative gait recovery after triple innominate osteotomy is faster than that following Chiari osteotomy.

Evaluation

Physical Examination

The patient's second chief complaint (the first being pain) may be gait disturbance. The patient often walks with a decreased dynamic functional range of motion to avoid the

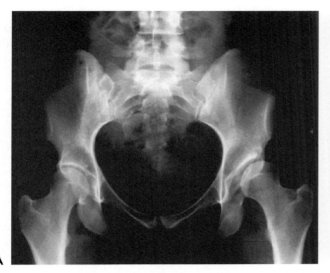 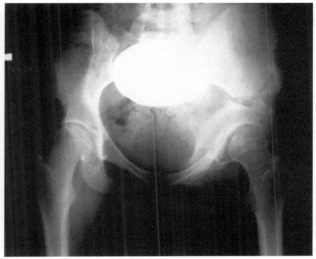

A   B

Figure 54-1 **A:** AP pelvis, standing view, showing a dysplastic left hip. **B:** AP pelvis, standing view, after surgery, showing excellent coverage of the femoral head.

"sore spot" in the joint. This abnormality can be identified easily by a gait analysis. Antalgic and Trendelenburg gaits are commonly observed abnormal gait patterns. In a patient with a significant leg-length discrepancy, a short leg limp can result. A Trendelenburg sign, either immediate or delayed, is observed in patients with abductor weakness.

A good, but not necessarily full, range of motion is important before surgery, as the osteotomy itself does not increase the range. Also, the patient needs adequate range of motion to compensate for the new acetabular position, which may redirect its arc of motions. Abduction and adduction are the most important motions needed to readjust the hip position after osteotomy so that the hip can be placed in the neutral position on standing. Usually, 30° of abduction and 90° of flexion are the minimum requirements.

Leg-length discrepancy influences pelvic tilt on standing. Depending on the length of the pathologic side, the femoral head can be either uncovered or better covered in the functional position. So, preoperative leg-length measurements, either by the usual clinical measurement from anterior superior iliac spine down to the medial malleolus and bottom of the foot or by observing the pelvic tilt in the standing position, are helpful for evaluation.

Clinical Imaging Studies

Plain radiographs should include an anteroposterior (AP) view of the pelvis in the standing position, a frog-leg lateral view, an AP view of the pelvis with both hips in abduction and internal rotation simultaneously, a shoot-through lateral view of each hip, and a *faux profil* view of each hip.

On the AP pelvis views in the standing position and the frog-leg lateral view, it is important to observe acetabular dysplasia and femoral uncovering. The center–edge angle (normally >20°) and the Sharp acetabular angle (normally <40°) are good guides for quantitating the degree of acetabular uncovering and deficiency. Congruency and relative size of the femoral head and acetabulum are important in evaluating the indication for surgery. A good clinical outcome from triple innominate osteotomy should not be expected if an incongruent

joint or an excessively large head is present. The shenton line and femoral head stations indicate the degree of proximal subluxation of the joint. Excessive lateral displacement of the femoral head produces poor mechanics for the hip. Often, this is accompanied by thickening of the medial acetabular floor and an abnormal teardrop sign. In abduction and internal rotation radiographs, it is preferred that the femoral head be medialized and that it sink into the original acetabulum.

Pelvic obliquity is another factor for consideration on the standing radiograph. The relationship of pelvic obliquity and acetabular coverage cannot be overemphasized. Asymmetry of the femoral neck–shaft angles contributes to the leg-length discrepancy and pelvic tilt, and this also needs to be addressed.

The shoot-through lateral view of both hips gives a preliminary evaluation of the posterior buttress of the acetabulum. The triple innominate osteotomy is contraindicated if there is no posterior buttress. Also, a rough evaluation of the anteversion angle of proximal femur and acetabulum can be made.

Information on anterior hip coverage is best obtained with the *faux profil* view.

A three-dimensional computed tomographic (CT) scan of both hips provides an excellent representation of the acetabulum and femoral head. The amount of joint surface uncovered can be clearly seen, as well as the relative acetabular volume and the shape and size of the femoral head. In those hips with degenerative cystic changes, the CT scan can accurately show the size and location of such areas. With subtraction images, the interior surface of the acetabulum may be viewed, but, more important, the posterior coverage (buttress) can be evaluated.

A preoperative magnetic resonance imaging scan may be valuable for evaluation of cartilage and soft tissue.

Contraindications

There are several contraindications for triple innominate osteotomy. In the physical examination, an adequate hip range of motion is essential, especially abduction and adduction, so that the patient can remain in the neutral standing position after surgery. Patients with excessive fixed external rotation should be cautioned, because the hip tends to externally rotate more after surgery.

In the radiographic evaluation, gross incongruity of the acetabulum and femoral head, either present or expected, and inability to demonstrate congruous reduction of the femoral head on the abduction radiograph are contraindications for triple innominate osteotomy. Excessive thickening of the medial acetabular floor could be an important reason that a congruous reduction may not be possible; also, it causes excessive lateralization of the femoral head. In standing radiographs, a total collapse of hip articular space is an absolute contraindication for the procedure.

Because the osteotomy rotates the acetabular fragment anteriorly and laterally, an adequate posterior buttress is important when selecting cases. Radiographs with a shoot-through lateral view of both hips and a three-dimensional CT scan will evaluate the posterior buttress. In those patients with no posterior coverage, the triple innominate osteotomy is contraindicated.

Combined Proximal Femoral Osteotomy

Concomitant proximal femoral osteotomy in selected cases may enhance the result of triple innominate osteotomy. There are two types of osteotomies that may be beneficial.

Shortening Osteotomy

A shortening osteotomy is beneficial in those patients who have leg-length discrepancy in which the longer leg is on the dysplastic hip side (Fig. 54-2A). This is evident on the standing AP radiograph of the pelvis. The triple innominate osteotomy may cause further tilt of the pelvis (i.e., by lengthening that leg), which may uncover the dysplastic side in the functional weight-bearing position. A femoral shortening osteotomy is very helpful in this situation. Actually, the slightly shorter limb

on the dysplastic side may increase coverage during functional weight bearing (Fig. 54-2B). The osteotomy is performed at the subtrochanteric region and secured using rigid fixation, without changing the neck-shaft angle.

Proximal Femoral Varus Osteotomy

In those patients who have true coxa valga on the dysplastic side (Fig. 54-3A,B), a proximal femoral varus osteotomy will improve the reducibility and coverage of the femoral head after triple innominate osteotomy. It often provides the final degree of the coverage. The proximal femoral varus osteotomy will also effectively shorten the femur. Rotational correction is not usually necessary in adults, as the rotation will not remodel and may create an unsightly external rotation gait. It is also quite important that one should not produce excess varus of the proximal femur. Usually, one should correct the neck–shaft angle to match that of the contralateral normal side or correct it to no less than 130°. Excess varus will create a permanent Trendelenburg gait, because the femur does not remodel. We prefer to perform the osteotomy at the intertrochanteric region with the proximal medial cortex cut in line with the inferior cortex of the femoral neck (Fig. 54-3C); this results in minimal distortion of the anatomy if future total hip reconstruction is needed.

Operative Technique

With the patient in a supine position, the hip and leg are draped free. Two incisions are used to perform the triple innominate osteotomy (Fig. 54-4). The first incision is made over the groin area about 0.5 cm distal to the skin crease and parallel to the crease line over the adductor longus (Fig. 54-5). After the subcutaneous tissue is incised in the line of incision, the adductor longus is exposed. Posterior to the adductor longus, using blunt dissection, the ischial tuberosity can be

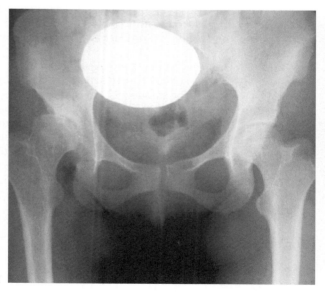

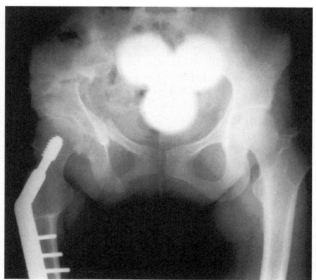

Figure 54-2 A: AP pelvis, standing view, showing a dysplastic right hip with high-riding femoral head. **B:** AP pelvis, standing view, after triple innominate osteotomy and femoral shortening osteotomy.

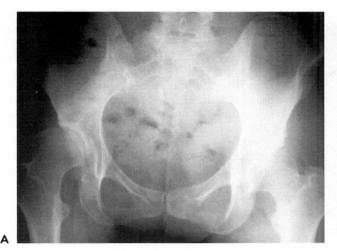

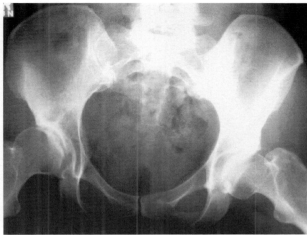

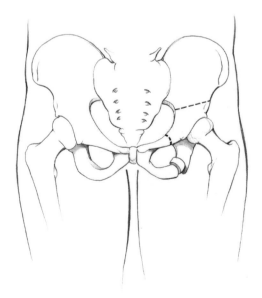

Figure 54-3   A: AP pelvis, standing view, showing dysplastic right hip with coxa valga. **B:** Abduction view showing good congruent reduction of femoral head into acetabulum. **C:** AP pelvis, standing view, after triple innominate osteotomy and proximal femoral varus osteotomy.

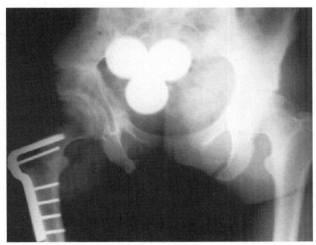

Figure 54-4   Location of osteotomies: innominate bone and superior and inferior rami.

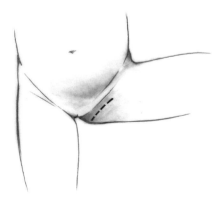

Figure 54-5   Groin incision parallel to skin crease.

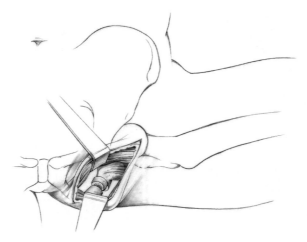

Figure 54-6 View of the inferior ramus through groin approach.

reached posteriorly and superiorly. The ischial tuberosity is then identified, and an incision is made along the inferior ramus all the way to the cortex of the bone. A subperiosteal dissection is made inferiorly and superiorly into the obturator foramen.

The muscle origins of semitendinosus, biceps, quadratus femoris, and adductor magnus are retracted to expose the inferior ramus. Using a half-inch straight osteotome, a 1-cm section of the inferior ramus at the ischial tuberosity is removed (Fig. 54-6). The site of the osteotomy should be on the lateral end of the inferior ramus. Attention is then directed to the area anterior to the adductor longus. The soft-tissue dissection goes around the anterior margin of the adductor longus and brevis, all the way to the superior ramus. The pectineus origin is then identified, and an incision is made longitudinally along the superior ramus. By using a periosteal elevator, the bone is exposed subperiosteally above and below.

After a retractor is placed, an osteotomy is made at the lateral end of the superior ramus close to the acetabulum (Fig. 54-7). There is no need to remove a segment of the bone from the superior ramus.

An anterior incision is made along the "bikini line" about 1.5 cm below the anterior superior iliac spine, parallel to the skin crease. Therefore, the direction runs obliquely from superolateral to inferomedial. The subcutaneous tissue is incised in the line of incision. The superficial fascia is exposed. The superior part of the skin flap is undermined to expose the anterior superior iliac spine. The interval between the sartorius and the tensor fascia lata is then identified and traced up to the iliac crest. An incision is made on top of the iliac crest from the anterior superior iliac spine running posteriorly. A Cobb periosteal elevator is then used to dissect the gluteal muscle and tensor fascia lata muscles from the outer table, and the iliacus muscle from the inner table of the iliac wing down distally. The sartorius muscle is retracted along with the elevated soft tissue medially, and the tensor fascia lata is retracted laterally. The dissection is taken down to the area between the anterior superior iliac spine and the anterior inferior iliac spine by sharp dissection. Again using the Cobb periosteal elevator, the dissection continues down to the acetabular area.

Using a curved periosteal elevator, the sciatic notch is then identified posteriorly. A curved retractor is inserted to protect the soft tissue behind the sciatic notch. The soft tissue over outer table is stripped all the way down until the superior edge of the capsule of the hip joint is reached. The straight head and reflected head of the rectus femoris are both visualized but not disturbed. A 90° curved Mixter clamp is inserted into the sciatic notch, and a Gigli saw is passed behind the sciatic notch. It is most important to make sure there is no soft tissue between the Gigli saw and the bone of the sciatic notch. Using a Gigli saw, an innominate osteotomy is carried out from the sciatic notch anteriorly, to exit at midpoint between the anterior superior iliac spine and the anterior inferior iliac spine (Fig. 54-8).

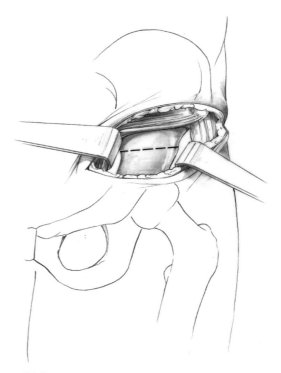

Figure 54-8 The approach to the innominate bone.

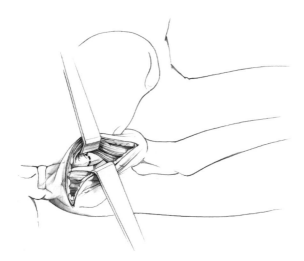

Figure 54-7 View of the superior ramus through groin approach.

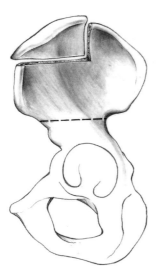

Figure 54-9 The location of the iliac bone graft.

After this is done, the acetabular fragment becomes mobile. Using a bone clamp at the anterior inferior iliac spine and with the leg in a figure-four position, the distal fragment can be displaced anteriorly and laterally. Sometimes this can be helped by using a lamina spreader at the osteotomy site. Next, the superior and inferior rami should be palpated to ensure displacement and rotation. A bone graft is taken from the iliac wing by using a power saw in a triangular shape, based posteriorly starting from the anterior superior iliac spine (Fig. 54-9). The bone graft is then placed in the osteotomy site with its base anteriorly. Fluoroscopic examination is done at this time to ensure the full coverage of the femoral head. The hip joint should not be lateralized, as this interferes with normal biomechanics. Three 3.5-mm or 4.5-mm cortical screws or threaded Steinmann pins are used to transfix the osteotomy site, starting from the bone graft donor location (Fig. 54-10). The soft tissues are closed in layers. Attention should be paid to the repair

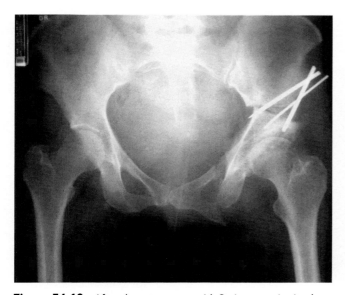

Figure 54-10 After the osteotomy, with Steinmann pins in place.

of the iliacus and gluteus muscles over the iliac crest. A subcuticular suture is used to close the skin for improved cosmesis. The patient is then placed in balanced suspension.

Postoperative Care

The patients are toe-touch weight bearing for 6 weeks, at which time partial weight-bearing is started if the AP pelvic radiograph shows adequate healing. At the same time, exercises for hip range of motion and hip muscle strengthening are started. Special emphasis is given to abductor muscle strengthening. The patient is advanced to full weight-bearing 3 to 4 months postoperatively.

Results

Steel's original publication in 1973 reported a failure rate of 23% in his series of 52 osteotomies in 45 patients with follow-up from 2 to 10 years (30). The 1977 Steel study reviewed the results of 175 hips with a follow-up period of 3 to 13 years. Average patient age was not listed, but 70% of patients ranged in age from 9 to 12 years. As with the 1973 study, results were considered satisfactory if a patient had a painless stable hip that was "reasonably mobile." Steel reported an 86% success rate and a 14% unsatisfactory rate. None of the patients with satisfactory results complained of pain, nor did any of them have radiographic evidence of degenerative joint disease (29).

Guille et al. reported on 10 children (11 hips) who underwent triple innominate osteotomy between the ages of 11 and 16 years for treatment of symptomatic acetabular dysplasia and who had greater than 10 years of follow-up. The mean length of follow-up was 12 years (range, 10 to 16). Ten of the 11 hips improved roentgenographically, and 8 improved functionally. One hip required total hip arthroplasty 16 years after the triple innominate osteotomy (13).

Dunn et al. (8) and Faciszewski et al. (10) reported on the application of pelvic osteotomy in the young adult as an alternative to total hip replacement. In the latter series (10), triple innominate osteotomy was performed on 56 hips in 44 skeletally mature patients with painful acetabular dysplasia. With an average follow-up of 7 years, there was improvement in pain and function in 53 hips. Many authors (4,13,15,16,20,23,31,32,34) reported similar results in different age groups.

Peters et al. reported on 50 patients with average age of 26 years who underwent 60 triple innominate osteotomies. At an average follow-up of 9 years, 12 hips (20%) had been converted to total hip arthroplasty, and 4 hips (7%) had incapacitating pain. Radiographically, there was significant improvement in the center–edge angle of Wiberg and the acetabular angle of Sharp. There also was a statistically significant relationship between failure of the osteotomy and severity of pre-existing hip arthrosis as measured by the Tönnis criteria. The results demonstrate that triple innominate osteotomy is effective in eliminating pain, but the fact that 27% of hips required or will require total hip arthroplasty indicates that deterioration may occur over time (26).

Conclusion

In properly selected patients, the triple innominate osteotomy can provide excellent anatomic correction of the dysplastic hip while providing excellent pain relief and improved activity tolerance. This is accomplished by covering the femoral head with the patient's own acetabular cartilage and by using sound biomechanical principles. Consequently, this construct should allow the patient's hip to function with its own biologic tissues and delay the need for total hip arthroplasty.

CHIARI OSTEOTOMY

Rationale

The Chiari osteotomy (5) is a salvage procedure that can relieve pain and increase abduction in a dysplastic hip that is too incongruous for a reconstructive procedure and too good for a hip replacement. It is a capsular arthroplasty. The newly formed roof of the acetabulum is joint capsule covered by a shelf of bone that eventually forms a fibrocartilaginous surface. An essential goal of the procedure is to increase hip abduction. This is done by abducting the limb fully while the osteotomy is free. This rotates the lower fragment medially, decreasing the head coverage by the true acetabulum and increasing total coverage achieved by medial displacement of the lower fragment. Total contact and coverage are supplemented by a bone graft that acts as a shelf and helps ensure union of the fragments (1).

Indications and Contraindications

The primary goal of Chiari's osteotomy is the relief of pain in an incongruous hip joint. It can be utilized from childhood through adolescence and into adult life, although several reports indicate that results are better in younger patients and fall off after 45 years of age (9,17,28). The antalgic component of the limp is improved, but very few patients lose the lurching Trendelenburg gait. Chiari's osteotomy is not the procedure of choice to relieve a limp (2,3,27).

Global limitation of hip joint motion is a contraindication. Although a properly done osteotomy will increase abduction, it will not increase movement in other planes. A reasonable amount of preoperative flexion and adduction is essential.

A hip that has drifted too far proximally to make the osteotomy cut with the proper slope, or a hip that is completely uncovered, is a relative contraindication. Either can only occasionally be helped by femoral shortening and open reduction in young patients.

If the head of the femur and the acetabulum can be positioned so that their surfaces are congruous, then a Chiari osteotomy is contraindicated. Proper selection of acetabular redirection, with or without an upper femoral osteotomy, can be used to reconstruct such a hip, leaving the Chiari to salvage those that are not congruous in any position (Fig. 54-11A,B).

Because the Chiari osteotomy is a salvage procedure, it has a limited life span, and it is primarily indicated in hips in which the anatomy cannot be restored to normal or near normal and in patients too young to be ideal candidates for total joint replacement.

Just how much time can be bought with the use of the Chiari osteotomy is discussed later, but the generally accepted view is that it will provide 10 to 15 years of useful service (2,3,5–7,9,17,27,28,36).

The procedure was devised by Karl Chiari in Vienna in the 1950s and first reported in English in *Clinical Orthopaedics and Related Research* in 1974 (5). Chiari described an operation in which he osteotomized the pelvis in the supraacetabular region through a small lateral incision. The operation was performed in a semiblind manner, not exposing the inner wall of the pelvis. The hip was abducted to displace the osteotomy and was medialized by pushing on the greater trochanter. No internal fixation was used. The patient was immobilized in a short hip spica in abduction for approximately 6 weeks. This immobilization in abduction was an extremely important part of the procedure, because most hips in which this osteotomy is performed have limited abduction, usually associated with lateral impingement (hinge abduction), so the achievement of increased hip abduction must be built into the technique of the procedure. Although certain improvements to Chiari's original technique have been made (e.g., better operative exposure and internal fixation to obviate casting), Chiari's key concept of increasing abduction remains.

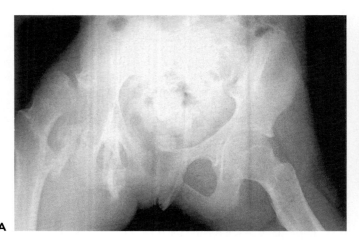
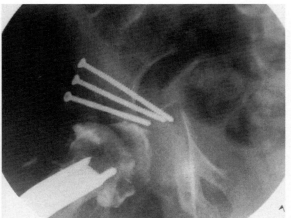

Figure 54-11 **A:** Painful dysplastic right hip. **B:** Postoperative x-ray.

Preoperative Planning

Once it has been decided that a patient is a candidate for surgery, the usual preoperative routine is followed, with general attention to past medical history, concurrent physical problems, and adequate laboratory testing of standard parameters.

Specific planning for the Chiari osteotomy will include a careful history to detect the cause of the hip dysplasia, if possible. Disorders such as congenital (developmental) hip dysplasia, Legg–Calvé–Perthes disease, slipped capital femoral epiphysis, and previous sepsis or trauma may be detected.

The type, severity, and frequency of pain will be important. Fatigue pain after prolonged usage will often indicate a hip that might respond to less severe measures or a reconstructive type of operation. Severe constant pain even at rest and restriction of activities are more usual in the candidate for the Chiari procedure.

Physical examination will include the usual survey, especially of the opposite hip and other joints, to detect generalized arthritic conditions and bilateral hip disease. The hip examination will describe the exact range of movement of both hips and the presence and severity of pain during each movement. Muscle power should be tested, especially abduction within limits of pain. The typical candidate for a Chiari osteotomy will have restricted painful active and passive motion, especially in abduction and rotation, but will have at least 90° of hip flexion and 20° to 30° of abduction. Note should be made of adductor tightness as a cause of restricted abduction, as this may necessitate a preliminary adductor tenotomy or release. This will be particularly important in patients with associated cerebral palsy or paralytic disorders. Note must be made of any leg-length discrepancy, either true or apparent.

Watching the patient walk is important for distinguishing an antalgic limp from a Trendelenburg lurch. A positive Trendelenburg test is usually present, and it should be determined whether it is caused by pain, weakness, or instability. The results of these tests will indicate whether or not gait will be improved, because usually only the antalgic component will disappear. The lurch may be even more prominent after surgery, and the patient must be made aware of this. The condition of the opposite hip will obviously affect the suitability of the patient for the procedure.

Radiologic evaluation should begin with plain radiographs taken in the AP standing position to show the pelvis and both hips. Information on anterior hip coverage is best obtained with the *faux profil* view. A true lateral film of each hip will help in assessing upper femoral shape.

These studies are often sufficient to make the decision, but in a borderline case a CT scan with three-dimensional reconstruction will be helpful.

Principles

The important principles include the following:

1. There must be adequate exposure of both lateral and medial surfaces of the ilium, the sciatic notch, and the hip joint capsule.
2. Osteotome cuts must follow the contour of the femoral head and slope upward, inward, and back.

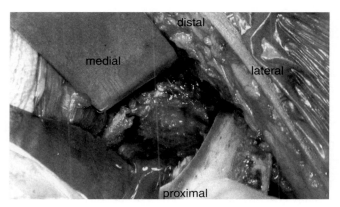

Figure 54-12   One hundred percent medial displacement.

3. Medial displacement must be sufficient to cover even 100% of the femoral head if necessary (Fig. 54-12).
4. A graft should be used to supplement the roof and to assist bony union.
5. The leg must be abducted at least 30° with respect to the pelvis, and internal fixation must be inserted in that position to maintain abduction postoperatively.

Operative Technique

The technique of the Chiari osteotomy is extremely important. If done properly, the procedure is difficult, but extra attention to detail will result in a much-improved outcome.

The patient is positioned in the lateral decubitus position. Placement of the skin incision depends on previous scars, but if there is a choice, a nearly transverse groin incision (Salter type) is preferred, extended farther laterally than for the usual innominate osteotomy. The ilium is exposed subperiosteally on both the lateral and medial surfaces until the sciatic notch is exposed posteriorly. The hip capsule must be particularly well exposed posteriorly and reflected down to the edge of the acetabulum. The capsule should not be opened. Preserving the integrity of the capsule is particularly important for the success of this procedure. If open reduction is performed as part of the procedure, the capsular incision can be made on the anterior surface and must be solidly repaired. A Gigli saw is used to cut the most posterior of the osteotomy from the anterior edge of the sciatic notch forward for about 1 cm so that it is not necessary to use osteotomes in the region of the sciatic notch. This will also prevent the propagation of spike along the sciatic notch and protect the contents of the notch.

The remainder of the osteotomy is carefully contoured, using osteotomes to follow the line of the capsule and femoral head. The direction of the individual cuts with the osteotomes or chisel is upward, inward, and posterior. This will ultimately allow a displacement of the anterolaterally subluxated femoral head with its covering capsule in an upward, inward, and posterior direction toward the thickest part of the proximal ilium.

Once the osteotomy is complete, the distal fragment is forced inward and posteriorly by medially directed pressure on the greater trochanter. The leg is then abducted as far as possible by medially directed pressure on the greater trochanter. The leg is then abducted as far as possible so that the distal osteotomy fragment and acetabulum are rotated medially. This relationship of the proximal and distal fragment, with the distal fragment relatively abducted, must be maintained until the osteotomy is internally fixed so that hip joint abduction will be maintained in the postoperative period.

If there is not perfect apposition of the proximal fragment to the capsule, this important contact must be improved by using a rongeur to remove any impinging parts of bone from the undersurface of the proximal iliac fragment. At the conclusion of the operative procedure, the undersurface of the proximal fragment must fit snugly over the joint capsule.

The anterior end of the ilium is very narrow and does not usually cover the anterior portion of the femoral head adequately. A bone graft is added to improve anterior coverage and to assist bony union (Fig. 54-13). This interposition bone graft acts as a supplemental shelf procedure, extending the coverage anteriorly (and laterally if necessary). Thus, this type of osteotomy is really a combination Chiari-shelf (1).

The amount of medial displacement is determined by the amount needed to completely cover the head and is often 100% or more. The degree of abduction is whatever can be obtained, but no less than 30°. It is vital that the osteotomy begin immediately at the capsular insertion at the acetabular edge, because a Chiari that is too high cannot function.

Internal fixation is with multiple-threaded Steinmann pins or AO screws (Fig. 54-13) that traverse the upper and lower fragments and the graft. A careful repair of the abductors is important during closure.

Postoperative Care

No external immobilization is used. Active physical therapy begins about 48 hours after surgery. A partial weight-bearing

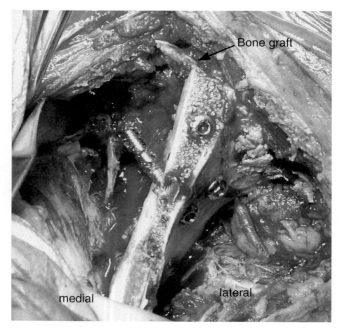

Figure 54-13 Bone graft taken from inner iliac table to supplement anterior coverage. Internal fixation with multiple screws.

gait is continued until muscle strength has returned and good osteotomy healing is seen on x-ray, usually between 6 weeks and 3 months after surgery, depending on the patient's age.

Pain relief is usually good after Chiari osteotomy. Improvement in gait is often less dramatic; it is usual for a positive Trendelenburg gait to persist (2,3,27).

Results

In 1974, Chiari (5) reported results in 200 patients, two thirds of which were excellent or good, and one third of which were improved. Subsequent reports from Vienna (17,36) on follow-up examinations of Chiari's patients have indicated durable long-term results. Colton (6) reported 68% excellent or good results. DeWaal Malefijt et al. (7) claimed 45% excellent or good results, but they had rather stringent criteria. Twenty-nine Chiari osteotomies were reported, including in 5 patients who had delivered 7 children without difficulty. Of 18 older patients with preoperative pain, 11 had good results, 2 had fair results, and 5 had poor results. The poor results were attributed to technical errors.

Fong et al. (11) reported significant radiographic improvement (center–edge angle of Wiberg, acetabular angle of Sharp, and the percentage of femoral head coverage) in their series of 14 Chiari osteotomies. They noted no significant change between postoperative measurement and the latest follow-up measurement (mean follow-up, 7.1 years). They reported that 12 patients had good results by Tönnis clinical grading and 2 had poor results.

Duquennoy et al. (9) reviewed 53 Chiari osteotomies; most were performed in patients in their thirties, but some patients were as old as 55. Most had severe pain prior to surgery, and most had no pain at follow-up. The center–edge (CE) angle was improved from an average of −5° preoperatively to +25° at follow-up. Complications included two intra-articular factures and one transient sciatic nerve palsy. Only one patient had been revised to a total hip replacement at follow-up, but one additional patient had severe limited motion. Two patients had pseudarthrosis of the osteotomy, and seven had meralgia paresthetica.

Bailey et al. (1) reported relief of preoperative pain in 17 of 18 patients after Chiari osteotomies. Wade (34) reported 33 Chiari osteotomies with 79% excellent or good results. The excellent results occurred in adolescent patients with residual hip dysplasia or subluxation following Perthes disease. Calvert et al. (3) reported 49 Chiari osteotomies after an average follow-up of 14 years, with 57% of patients having minimal or no pain, 50% a severe residual limp, and 76% a positive Trendelenburg test.

Matsuno et al. (19) reported a modified Chiari osteotomy performed using a transtrochanteric approach in which the greater trochanter is transferred distally and laterally. They reported improvement in the Trendelenburg gait. Graham et al. (12) noted an improved gait using a similar procedure in a few cases.

In 1990, Nishina et al. (24) published a series of patients who had preoperative arthrograms to detect the presence of a damaged labrum. They reported 22 out of 23 excellent results after Chiari osteotomy when the labrum was normal. Eleven out of 21 were excellent when the labrum was torn. A detached labrum resulted in only 6 excellent results in 20 cases.

Windhager et al. (36) reported on 236 Chiari osteotomies performed for hip dysplasia. Twenty-one hips (8.9%) needed revision surgery after a mean of 15.4 years. About 50% of the remaining hips had good or excellent results at a mean follow-up of 24.8 years. Lack et al. (17) reported on 100 Chiari osteotomies done for coxarthrosis secondary to dysplasia. Conversion to hip replacement was required in 20% at a mean follow-up of 15.5 years. Older age and advanced degenerative changes adversely affect the outcome of the Chiari osteotomy (18,21,22,25).

Hashemi-Nejad et al. (14) compared 28 total hip arthroplasties done in dysplastic hips after previous Chiari osteotomy (group 1) with a well-matched control group of 50 primary procedures (group 2) done during the same time period at an average follow-up of 5 years; they found that group 1 required significantly less acetabular augmentation and had significantly shorter operative times. There was no significant difference between the two groups in terms of clinical or radiographic outcome.

Conclusion

There is general agreement that the Chiari osteotomy will relieve pain in the painful incongruous unstable hip. It is not intended for those hips that can be reconstructed and adequately covered by normal hyaline cartilage. It is a difficult operation. Results will closely parallel attention to patient selection and the use of appropriate operative technique to achieve coverage of the femoral head and abduction of the hip.

REFERENCES

1. Bailey TE, Hall JE. Chiari medial displacement osteotomy. *J Pediatr Orthop.* 1985;5:635–641.
2. Betz R, Kumar SJ, Palmer CT, et al. Chiari pelvic osteotomy in children and young adults. *J Bone Joint Surg.* 1988;70A:182–191.
3. Calvert PT, Augusta AC, Albert JS, et al. The Chiari pelvis osteotomy: review of the long term result. *J Bone Joint Surg.* 1987;69B:551–555.
4. Chapchal G. Indications for the various types of pelvic osteotomy. *Clin Orthop.* 1974;98:111–115.
5. Chiari K. Medial displacement osteotomy of the pelvis. *Clin Orthop.* 1974;98:55–71.
6. Colton CL. Chiari osteotomy for acetabular dysplasia in young subjects. *J Bone Joint Surg.* 1972;59B:578–589.
7. DeWaal Malefijt MC, Hooglad T, Nielsen HK. Chiari osteotomy in the treatment of congenital dislocation and subluxation of the hip. *J Bone Joint Surg.* 1982;64A:996–1004.
8. Dunn HK, Smith JT, Coleman SS. Pelvic osteotomy: an alternative to total hip replacement in the young adult. In: *The Hip: Proceedings of the 12th Open Scientific Meeting of the Hip Society.* St. Louis: CV Mosby; 1984:3–13.
9. Duquennoy H, Miguad H, Gougeon F, et al. Osteotomie de Chiari, chez l'adulte. *Rev Chir Orthop.* 1987;73:365–376.
10. Faciszewski T, Coleman SS, Biddulph G. Triple innominate osteotomy for acetabular dysplasia. *J Pediatr Orthop.* 1993;13: 426–430.
11. Fong HC, Lu W, Li YH, et al. Chiari osteotomy and shelf augmentation in the treatment of hip dysplasia. *J Pediatr Orthop.* 2000; 20:740–744.
12. Graham S, Westin GW, Dason E, et al. The Chiari osteotomy: a review of 58 cases. *Clin Orthop.* 1986;208:249–258.
13. Guille JT, Frolin E, Kumar SJ, et al. Triple osteotomy of the innominate bone in treatment of developmental dysplasia of the hip. *J Pediatr Orthop.* 1992;12:718–721.
14. Hashemi-Nejad A, Haddad FS, Tong KM, et al. Does Chiari osteotomy compromise subsequent total hip arthroplasty? *J Arthroplasty.* 2002;17:731–739.
15. Hsin J, Saluja R, Eilert RE, et al. Evaluation of the biomechanics of the hip following a triple osteotomy of the innominate bone. *J Bone Joint Surg.* 1996;78A:855–862.
16. Kumar D, Bache CE, O'Hara JN. Interlocking triple pelvic osteotomy in severe Legg–Calvé–Perthes disease. *J Pediatr Orthop.* 2002;22:464–470.
17. Lack W, Feldner-Busztin H, Ritschl P, et al. Chiari pelvic osteotomy for osteoarthritis secondary to hip dysplasia: indications and long-term results. *J Bone Joint Surg.* 1991;73B: 229–234.
18. Macnicol MF, Lo HK, Yong KF. *J Bone Joint Surg.* 2004;86B: 648–654.
19. Matsuno T, Ichioka Y, Kaneda K. Modified Chiari pelvic osteotomy: a long-term follow-up study. *J Bone and Joint Surg.* 1992;74A:470–478.
20. McCarthy JJ, Fox JS, Gurd AR. Innominate osteotomy in adolescents and adults who have acetabular dysplasia. *J Bone Joint Surg.* 1996;78A:1455–1461.
21. Migaud H, Chantelot C, Giraud F, et al. Long-term survivorship of hip shelf arthroplasty and Chiari osteotomy in adults. *Clin Orthop.* 2004;418:81–86.
22. Millis MB, Murphy SB, Poss R. Osteotomies about the hip for the prevention and treatment of osteoarthrosis. *J Bone Joint Surg.* 1995;77A:626–647.
23. Murphy SB, Kijewski PK, Millis MB, et al. Acetabular dysplasia in the adolescent and young adult. *Clin Orthop.* 1990;261: 214–223.
24. Nishina T, Saito S, Ohzona K, et al. Chiari pelvic osteotomy for osteoarthritis, the influence of the torn and detached acetabular labrum. *J Bone and Joint.* 1990;72B:765–769.
25. Ohashi H, Hirohashi K, Yamano Y. Factors influencing the outcome of Chiari pelvic osteotomy: a long-term follow-up. *J Bone Joint Surg.* 2000;82B:517–525.
26. Peters CL, Fukushima BW, Park TK, et al. Triple innominate osteotomy in young adults for the treatment of acetabular dysplasia: a 9-year follow-up study. *Orthopedics.* 2001;24:565–569.
27. Rejholec M, Stryhal F, Rybka V, et al. Chiari osteotomy of the pelvis: a long term study. *J Pediatr Orthop.* 1990;10:21–27.
28. Reynolds DA. Chiari innominate osteotomy in adults. *J Bone Joint Surg.* 1986;68B:45–54.
29. Steel HH. Triple osteotomy of innominate bone. *Clin Orthop.* 1977;122:116–127.
30. Steel HH. Triple osteotomy of innominate bone. *J Bone Joint Surg.* 1973;55A:343.
31. Szepesi K, David T, Rigo J, et al. A new surgical approach in 8 cases of polygonal triple pelvic osteotomy. *Acta Orthop Scand.* 1993;64:519–521.
32. Tönnis D. Surgical treatment of congenital dislocation of the hip. *Clin Orthop.* 1990;258:33–44.
33. Tönnis D, Behrens K, Tscharani F. A modified technique of the triple pelvic osteotomy: early results. *J Pediatr Orthop.* 1981;1: 241–249.
34. Wade WJ. The Chiari pelvic osteotomy. *J Bone Joint Surg.* 1986; 68B:502.
35. Wedge JH. Osteotomy of the pelvis for the management of hip disease in young adults. *Can J Surg.* 1995;38[Suppl 1]:S25–32.
36. Windhager R, Prongracz N, Schonecker W, et al. Chiari osteotomy for congenital dislocation and subluxation of the hip. *J Bone Joint Surg.* 1991;79B:890–895.

Index